Clinical Anesthesia for the Newborn and the Neonate

Usha Saha
Editor

Clinical Anesthesia for the Newborn and the Neonate

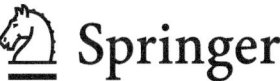 Springer

Editor
Usha Saha
Dept of Anesthesiology, Critical Care
Pain and Palliative Care
Lady Hardinge Medical College
Smt Sucheta Kriplani and Kalawati Saran
Childrens Hospitals
New Delhi, India

ISBN 978-981-19-5457-3   ISBN 978-981-19-5458-0   (eBook)
https://doi.org/10.1007/978-981-19-5458-0

This Springer imprint is published by the registered company Springer Nature Singapore Pte Ltd.
The registered company address is: 152 Beach Road, #21-01/04 Gateway East, Singapore 189721,
Singapore

Foreword

It is my proud privilege to write the Foreword for the first Neonatal Anesthesia book in India, which is the result of passionate dedication to neonatal anesthesia by my dear friend, Dr Usha Saha—an energetic, enthusiastic, straightforward, and all-for-ethics anesthesiologist. Only few books pertaining exclusively to neonatal anesthesia are available at global level. The book *Clinical Anesthesia for the Newborn and the Neonate* comprises 50 chapters, broadly divided into 5 parts so as to create a continuity of knowledge and understanding, elaborating each system and field of neonatal anesthesia, starting from basics to ethics. All 40 authors, who are experienced anesthesiologists from national and international platform, have covered the entire expanse of neonatal anesthesia, while also contributing their own experiences of this delicate and vulnerable population undergoing anesthesia. I hope this exclusive book will create its own place in the field of anesthesia.

KGMC   Anita Malik
Lucknow, Uttar Pradesh, India

Foreword

I am glad to write the foreword for *Clinical Anesthesia for the Newborn and the Neonate*.

The book is exceptional since it is one of the few that is written exclusively on the newborn and neonate anesthetic considerations. It has been very meticulously planned and organized into different parts covering all aspects of the newborn and the neonate.

It begins with the basics: magnitude of neonatal care required globally, anatomy and physiology of the newborn, and then escalates to include several topics which are relevant to those practicing neonatology. In the subsequent parts, it extensively covers all aspects of neonatal anesthesia which are very essential for the anesthesiologists interested in this specialty.

The contributors are very eminent doctors who have a vast experience in this field. The language is simple and easy to understand. Many photographs are original showcasing the contributors' expertise in the subject.

The editor, Dir. Prof. Usha Saha is a pediatric anesthesiologist of great repute. She has been practicing pediatric anesthesia for over 25 years. This book has been very well edited by her.

It is a "must read" for all the postgraduates, fellows, and those anesthesiologists who are pursuing their training in neonatal anesthesia. In addition, the first two parts are also of relevance to the physicians and students who are training in neonatology. It is highly recommended for the practicing pediatric anesthesiologists.

Institute of Anaesthesiology,   Jayashree Sood
Pain and Perioperative Medicine,
Sir Ganga Ram Hospital
New Delhi, India

Foreword

Anesthesia has changed vastly over the past 40 years, from being a routine administration of general anesthesia, to patient-tailored approach, with a goal of complete recovery after surgery.

A neonate is vastly different from a young child and adult. A special practical treatise book was required especially considering the Indian context. This book, edited by Dr Usha Saha, is a practical clinical book which will be useful for postgraduates, young, experienced consultants in anesthesia, as well as to the neonatologists.

I have known Dr Usha Saha for more than 40 years since our residency days at AIIMS Delhi and know her to be a dedicated teacher, empathetic anesthetist, who never backed off from accepting challenges in surgery. I have always felt comfortable working with her as an anesthetist at the head end, forgetting all my worries and concentrate on surgery.

She has a vast experience in pediatric anesthesia, and while working at AIIMS Delhi and PGIMER Chandigarh, she gained a lot of confidence in this field. But it was in her 30 years at Sucheta Kriplani and Kalawati Saran Children's Hospital in Delhi, that the fruits really bloomed. This is a referral hospital for children from whole of Northern India and has the maximum case load of pediatric and neonatal patients, and surgery. She is specially interested in pediatric and neonatal anesthesia. This book is her dream come true. She is an academician, a dedicated teacher, a concerted guide to her students, and a straightforward anesthesiologist, popular among surgeons and other hospital and OT staff, because of her patient-oriented attitude.

The contributing authors have used their personal experience and difficulties faced by them during their clinical practice, along with wide literature search in the writing of the chapters.

This is the first concerted effort and the first book of its kind in India. It contains developmental and physiological aspects of newborns and neonates and includes all common and rare surgical conditions and their anesthetic management. Regional anesthesia and pain management will surely be of interest to the reader in these vulnerable patients. Each chapter will captivate the reader; but a few such as anesthesia for bronchoscopy, laparoscopic, neurosurgical procedures, use of ultrasound for vascular access, and regional anesthesia in the newborn and neonates will be of great value to the budding neonatal anesthesiologists. By the way, all chapters are dedicated to the neonatal age, that is, from birth up to 28 days of life, the most critical period in the life of a human being.

I highly recommend this book to every student pursuing courses in anesthesia, to practicing anesthesiologists, especially to those interested in neonatal anesthesia. Even neonatologists and neonatal surgeons will find it highly informative.

At the end, I would like to add that incidentally I am married to her for the past 36 years, and what brought us together was our surgeon–anesthetist relationship during our residency days. I wish her all the success in her endeavors.

Sir Ganga Ram Hospital   S. S. Saha
New Delhi, India

Preface

When you are in the light, everyone will follow you
   But if you are in the dark, not even your shadow will follow you.

Neonatal age is the most vulnerable period in the life of a human being with the greatest risk of death in the pediatric age. Neonatal mortality and morbidity are is a huge burden worldwide (figures being higher in developing countries). Neonatal deaths account for 66% of infant (birth–12 months) and 40–60% of under-5 mortality rates. As per United Nations' child mortality estimates, 721,000 neonatal deaths occurred in 2018 (average 1975 deaths every day).

UNICEF, in September 2020, reported an average Global NMR (neonatal mortality rate) of 17 in 2020, 2.4 million neonatal deaths, with one-third occurring within the first 24 h, and three-fourth within the first week of life. India contributes to nearly one-fifth of global live births, to more than 25% of neonatal deaths, and to 27% of newborn deaths (figures may be higher as many deaths go unreported). Major causes of early neonatal deaths (birth–7 days) are birth asphyxia, infections, complications of premature birth (44%), and congenital anomalies. WHO and Maternal and Child Epidemiology Estimation Group (MCEE) 2018 (http://data.unicef.org) listed major causes of neonatal deaths as preterm birth complications (44%), intrapartum-related events (19%), sepsis tetanus (13%), congenital abnormalities (11%), pneumonia (5%), diarrhea (1%), and others such as low birth weight, hypothermia, and neonatal jaundice (7%). The preterm birth rate is on the increase worldwide, and so are the related complications, with mortality being inversely proportional to the gestational age. These figures are alarming, and Indian government aims to achieve the millennium goal of NMR (17 deaths/1000 live births) by 2035.

Neonatal Mortality and Bearing on Anesthesia and Surgical Risk and Outcome

Newborn and neonates are already at a high risk of mortality, and when they present for surgery under anesthesia, the risk multiplies. Despite improvement in surgical skills, better understanding of neonatal anatomy, physiology, biochemistry, and pharmacology, adverse outcomes still continue to occur in this subset of patients that includes premature (born at GA < 36 weeks), small for gestational age (SGA), and newborn (within 24 h of birth) babies. They are neither like adults nor like children in their anatomy physiology organ functions drug responses and their pharmacokinetics and pharmacodynamics, endocrine development, hemopoietic, and NM system. On top of this, there is no way they can tell their presenting complaint or give a history, and there is no past history to rely on, and limited time for evaluation and optimization.

They have all the possible ingredients for high perioperative mortality; chiefly, low birth weight, prematurity, immature and sensitive vital body systems including respiratory, cardiovascular, renal, hepatobiliary, nervous and neuromuscular system, effects of the medical and surgical condition, and unknown or undiagnosed problems (chromosomal defects, genetic syndromes, medical diseases, congenital birth defects). They thus require special care in a specialized tertiary care center with trained anesthesiologist, neonatologist, pediatric surgeons, and other supporting specialties and facilities.

Anesthesia-related morbidity and mortality are higher in newborns and neonates than in children and adults. Newborn babies must adapt to the extra uterine environment, and this continues in the neonatal period. The greatest fear of the anesthetist is the risk of reverting these changes whenever adverse conditions prevail, chiefly hypoxemia, hypercarbia, acidosis, hypovolemia, and hypothermia that may increase pulmonary vascular resistance and/or decrease systemic vascular resistance, with the return of right to left intracardiac shunting. Anesthetist must remain vigilant and proactively prevent occurrence of these events.

Postoperative outcome is better if baby is operated after post-conceptual age of 60 weeks (the safe period), earliest being at 44 weeks. Hence, a baby born at 36 weeks stands better chance of survival if operated after 8 weeks of birth, and better still after 24 weeks (6 months) of age. These figures will change with the gestational age at which baby is born (more premature the baby is, longer is the age at which it should be operated). Any surgery undertaken within these periods is considered as an emergency and life threatening.

The surgical pathology also carries its own anatomical, pathophysiological, biochemical, volume status, acid base and gas-related adverse effects, be it necrotizing enterocolitis (NEC), congenital diaphragmatic hernia, tracheoesophageal fistula (TEF), omphalocele and gastroschisis, meningomyelocele and encephalocele, or gut malrotation and volvulus. Besides, surgery itself is extremely stressful and has negative effect on the growing organs and brain, thus advisable to conduct under anesthesia, which further adds to the risk of the developing brain, of hypothermia, and of airway and ventilation related.

Recognizing the burden of perioperative mortality in neonates, it highlights the need for anesthesiologists to be better prepared for the newborn and neonates, with the caveat that they are at high risk even if no anesthesia is administered. The basic knowledge, experience, and expertise of the anesthesiologist, prevention and early recognition of complications, and prompt corrective measures will go a long way in improving outcome after general anesthesia and surgery. 88% of all postoperative complications occur within first 10 postoperative days, and if a neonate survives this period, it has a greater chance of survival as the incidence of complications reduces remarkably after that to 12%.

In 1981, when I was undergoing my PG training at AIIMS, Delhi, we were exposed to a large number of neonates coming for surgery for TEF, CDH, NEC, and intestinal obstruction. Most of them were critical, with one or more congenital problem, commonly cyanotic heart disease, with extremely high risk. All inductions and intubations were done under deep inhalation anesthesia, with or without succinyl choline, as the best available option (others available were d-tubocurarine and gallamine, long-acting NDMRs). Most surgeries were undertaken under inhalational anesthesia (Halothane) and assisted ventilation, with often good outcome. NDMRs were used conservatively, and only in less critical neonates. The reasons for minimal or no anesthesia use was mainly lack of knowledge and fear of the unknown.

Ten years later, as a teaching faculty at a children's hospital in Delhi, it came as a shock that neonates underwent surgery with minimal or no anesthesia, especially newborns, premature, and small for date babies. I started the practice of using IV and inhalational induction, intubation under paralysis with scoline, and use of NDMRs for prolonged intrathoracic or intra-abdominal surgeries. This greatly improved postoperative outcome and surgeon satisfaction. Also, pain was not managed appropriately, mainly because it was felt that neonates did not sense pain and because of the analgesics available in those days (morphine and pethidine). This has changed with the availability of newer short-acting drugs, variety of airway management equipment, use of RA and nerve blocks, and availability of pediatric mode on ventilators. But even then, it is essential that the anesthetist be fortified with full knowledge of anatomy, physiology, organ functions, complications (their prevention and management if they occur), and various modes of ventilation.

With more than 40 years of anesthesia practice as a teaching faculty in a medical college in the heart of capital of India, I have noticed the use of certain terms that pained me:

1. "Pediatric age" for all from birth to 12 years of age and today up to 18 years. Words like "neonate" and "infant" are used interchangeably, when actually neonates are uniquely different. Are these terms interchangeable?
2. Neonates also include preterms (born between 20 and 37 weeks gestation), who have a much higher global mortality, more so after anesthesia within 28 days of life. They have problems unique to this age such as respiratory distress syndrome, hyaline membrane disease, bronchopulmonary dysplasia, retinopathy, apneic spells, biliary atresia, and persistent fetal circulation.

This is the first book in the very specialized field of neonatal anesthesia published in India, and my maiden venture. The chapters in it are contributed by experts in the field of anesthesia, including pediatric and neonatal anesthesia. While didactic knowledge of neonatal anesthesia is available in anesthesiology textbooks, journals, and research publications, a compendium of information for the purpose of knowledge assessment in the subspecialty does not exist. The intent of this book is to provide a comprehensive knowledge to the anesthesiologists in both routine and complex cases based on expert opinion and referenced literature.

Hence, *Clinical anesthesia for the Newborn and the Neonate* aims to fill the gap in the knowledge of the reader and clinical reasoning regarding anesthetic management in these challenging patient categories. Each chapter has relevant additional literature citations. It covers all aspects of neonatal anesthesia concerns, anatomy, physiology, pharmacology, and all surgical conditions one is likely to encounter as a neonatal anesthesiologist, including some uncommon conditions, neonatal malignancies, palliative care, and COVID 19.

The book will guide the reader through all these aspects of neonatal anesthesia. It is divided into five parts: first being basic-general aspects of newborn diseases and care; second addresses developmental anatomical and physiological aspects; third is special aspects of neonatal anesthesia; fourth is case-based anesthesia management; and fifth includes anesthesia for newer procedures and uncommon surgeries. A chapter on ethical issues relating to treatment, use of drugs, and research in this subset of patients is also included.

The subject is vast and is expanding rapidly to keep pace with advances in medical technology, and readers will be encouraged to read more and more. No one book can cover all aspects of neonatal anesthesia. This book will be an asset to budding anesthesiologists pursuing training, certificate, or degree courses in anesthesia as well as to those practicing neonatal anesthesia. Care has been taken to explain difficult aspects for easy understanding, in simple language, and technical language at appropriate places. Each and every chapter is important, but that on transitional changes at birth is most essential to clear the concepts and will help the anesthetist and other care takers during the perioperative period.

The goal of this book *Clinical Anesthesia for the Newborn and the Neonate* is to provide ready, scientifically correct knowledge on this special subset of patients, all in one place, as a ready reference material. There is some unavoidable overlapping in some chapters, which has been kept to minimum, and reader is advised to refer back and forth in between chapters for more details on the subject.

Some rare cases, neonatal malignancies and their management, and a very upcoming branch, palliative care in neonates, have been included.

Ethics are inherent to any medical practice and ethical principles assume greater importance in neonatal anesthesia practice because the baby cannot take decisions or give consent, cannot tell if there is a problem, and must rely on parents, caretakers, and physicians. It is imperative that a neonatal anesthetist incorporate ethical principles at all times in the perioperative period.

This book has taken nearly 2.5 to 3 years from its conceptualization to its final version.

I wish to thank all the contributors to this book, whose expertise in clinical anesthesiology have made ***clinical anesthesia for the NB, NN, and premature,*** a distinctive addition to anesthesia literature. All the contributing authors are experts in the topic covered and in the field of anesthesia in children and neonates. Wide research has been involved in the writing of each chapter.

I am grateful to my husband Dr S. S. Saha, for his enduring support and encouragement, without which this book would not have come to fruition.

I dedicate this book to my parents and my extended parents, who are not here today, but their blessings are always there with me. I remember them always and wish them a peaceful life in heaven. I am grateful to my entire family for their unerring support to me. I wish to thank my son Sushank Shankar Saha, who had to bear the maximum brunt of my tough busy life as an anesthesiologist in a medical college, his wife, and my dear grandkids for their love that strengthened me to pursue with this task.

I would like to remember all the teachers in my life, chiefly Dr V. A. Punnoose, who left for his heavenly abode in 2008, Dr H. L. Kaul and Dr T. S. Jayalakshmi, who guided me during my training period and have always been a source of encouragement.

I thank all my students, who now hold senior faculty positions in the various medical colleges within and outside India, for their love and regard, for trusting me, for contributing material for the book, and also bearing with my demands during the process of writing. In the process of guiding them, I have learnt much more.

I thank Springer Nature India Pvt. Ltd. for accepting the proposal. I specially thank Gaurav Singh, Jagjeet Saini, and Christobel Gunasekaran, for patiently resolving all my queries, and guiding me in the process.

Lastly my three pet dogs, Debbie, Coco, and Mandy, and my cat Kitty, who were always there with me even into late hours, patiently waiting to go to sleep, while I worked on the book.

The years of 2020 and 2021 have been very challenging for the entire world and humanity because of the COVID-19 pandemic, where lives of some near and dear ones have been lost, others suffered, and no one has been left untouched. The book might have completed much earlier, but with God's blessings, it is finally done. This volume will be the quintessential clinical reference for perioperative care of these tiny patients.

New Delhi, India   Usha Saha

Contents

Part I

Basic: General Aspects of Newborn Diseases and Care

Neonatal Mortality and Morbidity: The Burden

Usha Saha

The greatest risk of death in the pediatric age is in the first 28 days of neonatal period life. **Neonatal Mortality Rate (NMR)** is a huge burden globally. Ninety eight percent of neonatal deaths occur in the developing countries. In 2019, 2.4 million children died in the 1st month of life (6,700/day), with 1/3rd within 1st 24 h and 3/4th within the 1st week of life. (UNICEF 2020)

Neonatal, infant, and maternal mortality rates represent the health status of a country, and can be used to compare the health of a country, state, or city, and are indicators of poor public health awareness, and inappropriate government and health department initiatives.

1.1 Causes of Neonatal Morbidity and Mortality

Global scenario: many deliveries that occur at home are unsupervised, and many newborn and neonatal deaths go unreported; hence, actual NMR is higher than that reported. Global causes of high NMR include **birth asphyxia** (21%) and **injuries** (11%), **infections** (11%) (common being pneumonia 19%, tetanus 14%, sepsis 7%, and diarrhea 2%), **congenital defects** (11%), **prematurity** (10%), and **others** (5%), such as low birth weight, hypothermia, hyperbilirubinemia, HIV, **sexually transmitted disease** (STD), and **asphyxia, infections, birth defects, and prematurity** are responsible for early neonatal deaths (in 1st week of life) [1–7].

Indian scenario: India is a huge country with many states and huge population. Neonatal deaths are not a hospital or state problem as they continue to occur across India. Most neonatal deaths occur at home, at the time of birth or later, especially in rural and remote areas, where health facilities may be inadequate or inefficient [8].

U. Saha (✉)
Department of Anesthesia, Pain and Palliative Care, Lady Hardinge Medical College,
Smt Sucheta Kriplani and Kalawati saran Childrens Hospitals, New Delhi, India

© The Author(s), under exclusive license to Springer Nature Singapore Pte Ltd. 2023
U. Saha (ed.), *Clinical Anesthesia for the Newborn and the Neonate*,
https://doi.org/10.1007/978-981-19-5458-0_1

Though most neonatal deaths occur at the time of birth, but problems start much before, preconception, and many are preventable. India contributes to 16% of global maternal deaths and 27% of global newborn deaths. Reducing the burden of maternal and newborn mortality requires active interventions at government level. In 2001, a study reported that nearly, 50% of infants developed high-risk morbidities (fatality >10%), such as **infections, birth asphyxia, birth injuries, preterm birth, and birth defects**.

As per the United Nation child mortality estimates, there were 721,000 neonatal deaths in 2018 (1975 deaths/day), with highest NMR in Bihar, Jharkhand, Uttar Pradesh, Uttarakhand, Rajasthan, Odisha, Chhattisgarh, Assam, Maharashtra, and Gujarat, common causes being **diarrhea and sepsis**. NMR was lowest in Goa, Kerala, and Tamil Nadu and mainly from **congenital or genetic causes.**

India is making an improvement in NMR, but need more focused attention to bring down NMR comparable to developed countries. A report from Rajasthan stated a decrease in NMR from 124/1000 live births in 1975–38 in 2015, over four decades [9, 10].

NMR has a wide regional variation, because variations related to:
1. **Structural issues:** lack of appropriate facility at primary centers
2. **Delayed referral to specialist care**
3. **Lack of transportation facilities**
4. **Poor quality of primary health care**, poor maternal health/antenatal/postnatal care
5. **Social problems:** malnutrition, immunization, potable water supply, and sanitation
6. **Poor living conditions:** overcrowding, indoor air pollution, and risk of pneumonia
7. **Medical causes:** prevalence of infections, diarrhea, and sepsis
8. **Congenital and genetic defects**
9. **Overcrowded tertiary care centers**

Reducing NMR Requires Stringent Simultaneous Approach at All Levels, Including:
1. Higher coverage of quality antenatal care, skilled birth care, improved postnatal care
2. Care of sick newborns
3. Institutional deliveries at hospitals with good infrastructure (rate doubled from 38.7% in 2005 to 78.9% in 2015–16) and institutions need to keep pace with this rise in numbers
4. Adoption of cost-effective neonatal care interventions, e.g., **Kangaroo care** (skin-to-skin contact with mother, thermal control, breastfeeding support, and basic care)
5. Formation of newborn care corners at every point of childbirth, of newborn stabilization units at first referral units, and of special newborn care units at district hospitals (under National Rural Health Mission 2005)

6. Sufficient qualified and experienced staff, well-equipped facilities with functioning equipment
7. Most care to be provided at district levels so as to unburden the tertiary care units, enabling them to provide care to sick and needy neonates
8. Preconceptional and antenatal care, early identification and management of risk factors
9. Preventive measures in mother—health, immunization, antenatal surveillance, timely detection, and early treatment of infections and diseases
10. Counseling on importance of healthy pregnancy, and clean, safe, assisted delivery by skilled attendant
11. Clean and safe newborn care to reduce risk of neonatal infections
12. Recognition of early signs of illness and timely medical help
13. Sensitive and empathetic attitude of officials in implementation of public health policy
14. Effective maternal and newborn health (MNH) care services and lowering the barriers to the use of such services, especially availability and accessibility
15. Saving Newborn Lives (SNL) programme, supported by Bill & Melinda Gates Foundation from 2000–2020, addresses these issues.

1.2 Causes of Neonatal Mortality (Table 1.1)

(a) **Infectious diseases** are the major cause of mortality in under 3 months of age and **major cause of death in late neonatal period (8–28 days)** [11]. Nearly, 40% of neonates die of infections. Globally, common infections are acute respiratory (30%), bacterial (40%), meningitis (40%), tetanus (70%), and diarrhea (0.6%), mortality being higher in LBW, malnourished, preterm babies, and in those not breastfed. **Maternal TB** increases the risk of fetal loss, preterm delivery, and LBW [12]. **Neonatal Diarrhea** contributes to 3% of all deaths, and early, exclusive breastfeeding, is protective. **Neonatal Tetanus is fatal within 3–10 days,** and can be contracted anytime from unimmunized mother, and unhygienic delivery and cord care [13]. **STD: syphilis** is transmitted transplacental, and is a cause of fetal death or disability [14]. **Congenital syphilis** is associated with FGR, anemia, thrombocytopenia, jaundice, hepatosplenomegaly, and neurological manifestations (mental retardation, hydrocephalus, cranial nerve palsies, and seizures) [15]. **Maternal Gonorrhea** increases the risk of conjunctivitis and blindness in the baby. **Neonatal Herpes** increases the mortality and risk of neuro-developmental sequelae [16]. **Untreated UTI** increases the risk of preterm labor and LBW babies. **Malaria** is associated with FGR and LBW. **Omphalitis** (umbilical infection) is a unique problem in developing countries, because of home deliveries in unsterile environment and poor cord hygiene, and increases the risk of neonatal sepsis and death.
(b) **Noninfectious conditions: perinatal asphyxia** defined as failure to initiate and sustain normal breathing, and includes apnea or gasping with bradycardia (<80)

Table 1.1 Causes of neonatal mortality

Factors	Effects on pregnancy/Fetus/Neonate
Infectious diseases	
Maternal infections	Fetal loss, FGR, and late neonatal deaths
Tuberculosis	High fetal loss, preterm delivery, and LBW
Untreated UTI	Preterm labor and LBW babies
Malaria	FGR and LBW
Syphilis	Fetal death/disability. Congenital syphilis associated with FGR, anemia, thrombocytopenia, jaundice, hepato-splenomegaly, and neurological manifestations
Gonorrhea	Conjunctivitis and blindness in the baby.
Neonatal infections: respiratory (30%), bacterial (40%), meningitis (40%), tetanus (70%), diarrhea (0.6%),	40% neonatal deaths. Higher in LBW, malnourished, preterm, and those not breastfed.
Neonatal diarrhea (3% of all deaths)	Early, exclusive breastfeeding, is protective.
Neonatal tetanus	Fatal within 3–10 days, can be contracted anytime from unimmunized mother, unhygienic delivery, and cord care.
Neonatal herpes	High mortality and neuro-developmental sequelae.
Omphalitis (umbilical infection)	Neonatal sepsis and death
Noninfectious conditions	
Perinatal asphyxia	Most common cause of NMR.
Birth injury	11% neonatal mortality and long-term morbidity.
Neonatal hypothermia	Risk of infection, coagulation abnormalities, acidosis, and death
Neonatal jaundice and kernicterus	Rare cause of neonatal death. Kernicterus in preterm baby and encephalopathy. Late sequel: extrapyramidal abnormalities, choreo-athetosis, involuntary muscle spasms, and sensorineural deafness.

at birth, absent or poor respiratory effort and/or gasping at 1 min, low Apgar score, and the need for assisted ventilation for more than 1 min [17–20]. The incidence is higher in developing countries because of higher prevalence of risk factors and lack of appropriate interventions [21]. Mortality is greater among preterm and LBW babies who are at risk of developing encephalopathy [7, 22–26]. Risk factors for asphyxia include: antepartum hemorrhage (APH), prolonged labor and/or prolonged rupture of membranes (PROM), drugs given to mother (magnesium sulfate, narcotics), cord accidents, vaginal breech deliveries, multiple gestation, pregnancy-induced hypertension (PIH), congenital anomalies, and IUGR/FGR with placental dysfunction.

(c) **Birth injury** contributes to 11% of neonatal deaths worldwide. It is a nonspecific term used for potentially preventable and unavoidable injuries; mechanical or hypoxic–ischemic, suffered by the neonate during labor and delivery, such as intracranial hemorrhage (ICH); blunt trauma to the liver, spleen, or other organs; injury to spinal cord or peripheral nerves, cord transaction, brachial plexus injury, and fractures (clavicles, extremities). They may result in transient or long-term morbidity and death. Predisposing factors include macrosomia, cephalopelvic disproportion, dystocia, prolonged or obstructed labor, breech presentation, and prematurity.

(d) **Neonatal hypothermia** (body temperature<36.5 °C) is frequent in newborns, especially LBW. Severe hypothermia (body temperatures <32 °C) increases the risk of infections, coagulation abnormalities, acidosis, complications of pre-term birth, and death [27, 28]. Warm environment at delivery, early breastfeed-ing and contact with mother, thermal protection, and care during transport can reduce the risk of hypothermia. Indian Kangaroo care system is specifically effective [29].

(e) **Neonatal jaundice/hyperbilirubinemia** (*s. bilirubin* >7–8 mg%) is a rare cause of neonatal death, but extreme bilirubinemia can cause devastating neu-rologic injury, long-term disability, and death from encephalopathy or kernic-terus (serum bilirubin >25 mg%). Causes include prematurity, ABO Rh incompatibility, and peripartum infection. Preterm babies are at greater risk for kernicterus. Early signs of encephalopathy are nonspecific (lethargy, poor feed-ing), bulging fontanel, opisthotonus, shrill cry, spasms, and seizures, and late sequel include extrapyramidal abnormalities, choreo-athetosis, involuntary muscle spasms, and sensorineural deafness.

1.3   Interventions

(a) **Maternal immunization against tetanus, pneumonia** (*Streptococcus pneu-moniae*, *Haemophilus influenzae* type B, and Group B streptococcal infections), and **H. influenzae**

(b) **Prevention and treatment of anemia** [30] with iron and other micronutrient supplementation, prevention of malaria and hookworm infestation, and preven-tion and treatment of maternal infections

(c) **Essential ANC:** counseling on birth preparedness and emergency readiness; provision of folic acid; tetanus immunization; prophylaxis and intermittent pre-ventive treatment for malaria and hookworm; early detection and timely man-agement of diseases/complications (anemia, hypertension, PIH, UTI, STD, and HIV), and of concurrent conditions (hepatitis, malaria, TB); and fetal malpre-sentation after 37th week [31]

(d) **Corticosteroids:** to reduce RDS, IVH, and improve survival of preterm new-borns [7]

(e) **Breastfeeding** during 1st hour of life can prevent hypoglycemia [32]. Closeness between mother and baby reduces risk of hypothermia

(f) **Vitamin A supplementation during** pregnancy and lactation is reduces neona-tal morbidity and mortality [33]

(g) **Neonatal resuscitation facilities**[21]

(h) **Require special care for improved survival:** skilled care at delivery, immedi-ate evaluation of newborn, basic resuscitation, thermal control, prevention of hypoglycemia, prevention of infections and neonatal tetanus, growth monitoring; early detection and treatment of illness, frequent home visits by trained health workers, monitoring of breastfeeding, neonatal growth, and overall well-being. Home-based Neonatal care can reduce fatality by almost 64 % [34]

(i) **Care of the newborn,** and LBW (<2500 g) and VLBW (<1500 g) [35–37]

Problems Begin Before Birth and Need to Be Addressed:

(a) **Behavior during pregnancy and postpartum**: perceived physical and supernatural threats, constellation of traditional and biomedical practices, taboos, superstitions and rituals used to mitigate them and their impact on perinatal risk
(b) **Maternal education (10 years or more):** improves outcomes
(c) **Maternal nutrition, health, and financial status:** child born to a wealthy household has three times more chance of surviving than one born to a poor family.
(d) **Time of marriage:** child marriages have higher NMR.
(e) **Less frequent ANC visits (<4):** missing out issues such as anemia, malnourishment, hypertension, diabetes. LBW (<2.5 kg) babies have high mortality (21.4%).

1.4   Conclusion

Recognition of the burden of NMR and morbidity highlights the need for health care interventions specifically targeting the newborn. The basic improvements in care that could significantly improve neonatal survival include: ANC (immunization against tetanus, preventive treatment of malaria, tuberculosis, syphilis, and urinary tract infection), clean and safe-assisted delivery by health workers skilled in neonatal resuscitation, hypothermia prevention, initiation of early breastfeeding, recognizing complications, and prompt effective referral to a tertiary care facility, and clean hygienic postnatal care of mother and baby in home care settings. **Anesthesia-related morbidity and mortality** is higher in neonates compared to infants, children and adults, more so in those with low gestational age, low birth weight, birth asphyxia, neonatal hypothermia, and hyperbilirubinemia, congenital abnormalities, compounded by the surgical condition, surgery and anesthesia. Hence, preventive initiatives can have a great impact by reducing perioperative NMR and morbidity.

References

1. WHO. Improving birth outcomes: meeting the challenge in the developing world. Washington, DC: The National Academies Press; 2003. https://doi.org/10.17226/10841).
2. Joint statement: international who recommendations on interventions to improve preterm birth outcomes. A Commitment to Action from Professional Health Organizations; 2017.

3. The Partnership for Maternal, Newborn and Child Health in Support of Every Woman Every Child (PMNCH). Strategic Plan 2016-2020. Geneva, Switzerland: PMNCH. http://www.who.int/pmnch/knowledge/publications/pmnch_strategic_plan_2016_2020.pdf.
4. WHO, UNICEF. Every newborn: an action plan to end preventable deaths: executive summary. Geneva, Switzerland: World Health Organization; 2014. https://www.everynewborn.org/Documents/Every_Newborn_Action_Plan.
5. Joint statement: health professional groups key to reducing MDGs 4 & 5. PMNCH; 2007. http://www.who.int/pmnch/events/2006/HCPjointstaterev0102207.pdf. 5.
6. Saving mothers and babies: the role of strong professional associations. FIGO; 2012. http://www.figo.org/sites/default/files/uploads/projectpublications/LOGIC/Final%20Version%20of%20LOGIC%20publication%20for%20print.pdf.
7. WHO recommendations on interventions to improve preterm birth outcomes. Geneva; 2015. http://www.who.int/reproductivehealth/publications/maternal_perinatal_health/preterm-birth-guideline/en/.
8. Bang AT, Bang RA, Baitule S, Deshmukh M, Reddy MH. Burden of morbidities and the unmet need for health care in rural neonates: a prospective observational study in Gadchiroli, India. Indian Pediatrics. 2001;38:952–67.
9. A neglected tragedy-the global burden of stillbirths. Report of the UN inter-agency group for child mortality estimation; Oct 2020. UNICEF.
10. Hug L, You D, Blencowe H, Mishra A, et al. Global, regional, and national estimates and trends in stillbirths from 2000 to 2019: a systematic assessment. Lancet. 2021(398):772–85.
11. Stoll BJ. Neonatal infections: a global perspective. In: Remington J, Klein J, editors. Infectious diseases of the fetus and newborn infant. Philadelphia: W.B. Saunders; 2000.
12. United Nations Children's Fund (UNICEF). Tuberculosis now a global threat; 2000. https://www.unicef.org/newsline/00pr24.htm.
13. WHO. Neonatal tetanus: progress towards global elimination, 1990–1997; 1999a. http://www.who.int/vaccines-diseases/diseases/Neonatal Tetanus.shtml.
14. Lumbiganon P, Piaggio G, Villar J, Pinol A, et al. WHO Antenatal Care Trial Research Group. The epidemiology of syphilis in pregnancy. Int J STD AIDS. 2002;13(7):486–94.
15. Frank D, Duke T. Congenital syphilis at Goroka Base Hospital: incidence, clinical features and risk factors for mortality. Papua New Guinea Med J. 2000;43(1–2):121–6.
16. Jacobs RF. Neonatal herpes simplex virus infections. Semin Perinatol. 1998;22(1):64–71.
17. Paul VK, Singh M, Sundaram KR, Deorari AK. Correlates of mortality among hospital-born neonates with birth asphyxia. Natl Med J India. 1997;10(2):54–7.
18. Chandra S, Ramji S, Thirupuram S. Perinatal asphyxia: multivariate analysis of risk factors in hospital births. Indian Pediatr. 1997;34(3):206–12.
19. Saugstad OD. Resuscitation with room-air or oxygen supplementation. Clin Perinatol. 1998;25(3):741–56, xi.
20. Saugstad OD, Rootwelt T, Aalen O. Resuscitation of asphyxiated newborn infants with room air or oxygen: an international controlled trial: the Resair 2 study. Pediatrics. 1998;102(1):E1.
21. Deorari AK, Paul VK, Singh M, Vidyasagar D. The national movement of neonatal resuscitation in India. J Trop Pediatr. 2000;46(5):315–7.
22. Ellis M, Manandhar DS, Manandhar N, Wyatt J, et al. Stillbirths and neonatal encephalopathy in Kathmandu, Nepal: an estimate of the contribution of birth asphyxia to perinatal mortality in a low-income urban population. Paediatr Perinatal Epidemiol. 2000;14(1):39–52.
23. Ellis M, Manandhar N, Shrestha PS, Shrestha L, et al. Outcome at 1 year of Neonatal encephalopathy in Kathmandu, Nepal. Dev Med Child Neurol. 1999;41(10):689–95.
24. Blencowe H, Lee A, Cousens S, et al. Preterm birth-associated neurodevelopmental impairment estimates at regional and global levels for 2010. Pediatr Res. 2013;74:17–34. https://doi.org/10.1038/pr.2013.204.
25. Blencowe H, Krasevec J, de Onis M, Black RB, et al. National, regional, and worldwide estimates of low birthweight in 2015, with trends from 2000: a systematic analysis. Articles. 2019;7(7):E849–60.

26. Lams JD, Romero R, Culhane J, Goldenberg RL. Primary, secondary, and tertiary interventions to reduce the morbidity and mortality of preterm birth. Preterm Birth. 2008;371(9607):164–75. https://doi.org/10.1016/S0140-6736(08)60108-7.

27. Ellis M, Manandhar N, Shakya U, Manandhar DS, et al. Postnatal hypothermia and cold stress among newborn infants in Nepal monitored by continuous ambulatory recording. Arch Dis Childhood Fetal Neonatal Ed. 1996;75(1):F42–5.

28. Manzar S. Role of hypothermia in asphyxia. Pediatrics. 1999;104(5 Pt 1):1169.

29. Choudhary SP, Bajaj RK, Gupta RK. Knowledge, attitude and practices about Neonatal hypothermia among medical and paramedical staff. Indian J Pediatr. 2000;67(7):491–6.

30. van den Broek NR, Letsky EA. Etiology of anemia in pregnancy in south Malawi. Am J Clin Nutr. 2000;72(1 suppl):247S–56S.

31. Carroli G, Rooney C, Villar J. WHO Programme to map the best reproductive health practices: how effective is antenatal care in preventing maternal mortality and serious morbidity? Paediatr Perinatal Epidemiol. 2001a;15(suppl 1):1–42.

32. Biancuzzo M. Breastfeeding the newborn clinical strategies for nurses. St. Louis, MO: Mosby; 1999.

33. Katz J, West KP Jr, Khatry SK, et al. Maternal low-dose vitamin A or β-carotene supplementation has no effect on fetal loss and early infant mortality: a randomized cluster trial in Nepal. Am Soc Clin Nutr. 2000;71(16):1570–6.

34. Bang AT, Bang RA, Baitule SB, et al. Effect of home-based Neonatal care and management of sepsis on neonatal mortality: field trial in rural India. Lancet. 1999;354(9194):1955–61.

35. World Health Organization (WHO). Essential newborn care. Geneva: WHO. 1996. http://www.who.int/reproductive-health/publications/MSM_96_13/MSM_96.

36. United Nations Children's Fund (UNICEF). The progress of nations. New York: UNICEF; 1999. www.unicef.org/pubsgen/pon99/index.html.

37. Committee on Fetus and Newborn. Levels of neonatal care. Pediatrics. 2004;114(5):1341–7. https://doi.org/10.1542/peds.2004-1697.

Impact of Maternal Health and Disease on Neonatal Outcome

Kashika Kathuria

2.1 Introduction

Low birth weight (LBW) and Preterm births make babies more vulnerable for disease and death in the neonatal period in India and Worldwide. Of 20 million LBW babies born annually, global, 97% are from low-middle income countries (nearly 40% from India), and responsible for 80% of neonatal deaths (neonatal mortality). However, incidence of preterm births is independent of income status, and is the most common cause of disability, and death. in India, premature birth rate is 14 per 1000 live births, with nearly 44% mortality rate. [1] of various factors affecting Neonatal Mortality Rate (NMR), maternal factors (undernutrition, anemia, diseases) and health have a direct and profound impact on intrauterine fetal health, the foundation of neonatal and infant health. Surgical mortality in this age group is very high, depending on a country's development and health infrastructure, nearly 6.7% in South Korea [2], 7.5% in Japan [3], 35% in India [4] and 45% in Nigeria [5]. To optimize neonatal outcome, it is extremely important to maintain good maternal health.

Health is not merely absence of disease and starts with preconceptional nutritional status of the woman, along with the absence of adverse environmental factors (smoking, alcohol, drug abuse, and stress), and encompasses supervised healthy antenatal period.

Undernutrition is an important factor, basis of most diseases in women in the reproductive age group, worldwide. Undernutrition tops the list of medical disorders, obstetric, and miscellaneous maternal factors that impact neonatal health.

Besides maternal health and disease status, other factors contributing to neonatal mortality rate (NMR) are age at delivery, educational status, nutritional status, and

K. Kathuria (✉)
Fortis Hospitals, New Delhi, India

© The Author(s), under exclusive license to Springer Nature Singapore Pte Ltd. 2023
U. Saha (ed.), *Clinical Anesthesia for the Newborn and the Neonate*,
https://doi.org/10.1007/978-981-19-5458-0_2

Table 2.1 Maternal factors that can Impact fetal health

Medical disorders	Obstetric factors	Miscellaneous factors
Undernutrition	Undernutrition	Undernutrition
Pregestational diabetes	Fetal growth restriction (FGR)/IUGR	Maternal age at delivery
Liver and renal disease	Hypertensive disorders of pregnancy—gestational hypertension, preeclampsia, eclampsia	Educational status
Anaemia in pregnancy	Gestational diabetes	Nutritional status
Cardiac and pulmonary ds	Preterm birth	Parity
Chronic hypertension	Multiple pregnancies	Addictions—alcohol, smoking, tobacco/drugs
Thyroid disease		Socioeconomic status
Under nutrition, Obesity		
Infections: TORCH, TB, HIV, COVID-19		Effect of sanitation, hygiene, environment
Neurological disorders		

parity. Risk of neonatal deaths and low birth weight (LBW) babies is 50% more in mothers under 20 years of age.

Maternal factors affecting fetal health and thereby neonatal death are listed in Table 2.1.

2.2   Undernutrition in Pregnancy

Maternal nutrition plays a key role in ensuring appropriate fetal growth and development. Nutritional requirement (macronutrient and micronutrients) is greatly augmented in pregnancy, with additional 350–450 kcal/day in the 2nd and 3rd trimesters. Adequate balanced diet is essential for good feto-maternal outcome and neonatal well-being.

Maternal undernutrition impairs the formation of placenta, uteroplacental circulation, and nutrient delivery to the fetus, resulting in FGR/IUGR, LBW, small for gestational age (SGA), preterm delivery, and birth defects.

Prematurity and congenital anomalies are two important factors of high NMR. 74.8% of all deaths due to prematurity occur in 1st week of life (30% within 1st few hours of birth). 75% of all deaths from congenital defects occur in 1st week of life (almost 50% within 24 h of birth).

Maternal weight gain and gestational weight gain are parameters of maternal nutritional status and fetal growth. Optimal maternal weight should be > 45 kg at any period of gestation, and gestational weight gain should be >300 g/week. **The Barker hypothesis** [6] postulates that undernutrition during pregnancy results in fetal programming, i.e., permanent alteration in fetal morphology and physiology. Epidemiologic studies have shown increased risk of ischemic heart disease and related disorders in later life in babies born during famine situation.

2.2.1 Micronutrients [7–10]

Deficiency of micronutrients (iron, vitamins, calcium, zinc, iodine, folic acid, and magnesium) is also associated more with feto-maternal complications.

1. **Iron** is a cofactor for synthesis of haemoglobin (Hb) and myoglobin, and various cellular functions (O2 transport, respiration, growth, gene regulation, and iron-dependent enzymes). Iron deficiency is the most common cause of anaemia in pregnancy worldwide and is associated with greater risk of preterm birth, LBW, SGA, infections, and abnormal psychomotor and cognitive function development in babies.
2. **Vitamins**
   (a) **Vitamin A** is important for growth, bone metabolism, immune and antioxidant function, gene transcription, vision, and sight. Its deficiency increases the risk of LBW and neonatal mortality. Vitamin A supplement does not reduce the incidence of complications.
   (b) **Vitamin B complex** (B_1 (Thiamine), B_2 (Riboflavin), B_3 (Niacin), B_6 (Pyridoxine), and B_{12} (Cyanocobalamin)) are required metabolism and energy production at cellular level, RBC formation, and conversion of homocysteine to methionine (role in methylation of RNA, DNA, neurotransmitters, and phospholipids). Vitamin B deficiency affects cellular growth and nerve tissue development. **B1 deficiency** impairs fetal brain development, **B2 deficiency** increases risk of CHD and LBW, and **B12 deficiency** causes macrocytic anaemia and increases the risk of abruptio placenta, still birth, LBW, and preterm delivery.
   (c) **Vitamin C and Vitamin E** promote antioxidation and reduce production of free radicals, thereby reducing oxidative stress. Vitamin C also mobilizes iron from body stores, increases GI absorption of iron, and prevents megaloblastic and iron deficiency anaemias, besides its role in collagen synthesis and connective tissue stabilization. Vitamin C by its antioxidant role, and ability to cross-placental barrier, reduces the effects of PET, IUGR, preterm birth, and premature rupture of membranes. Vitamin E cannot cross placental barrier.
   (d) **Vitamin D** has a role in calcium homeostasis and bone integrity. It also has a role in glucose metabolism, inflammatory and immune responses and angiogenesis, and gene transcription. It is important for fetal bone growth, and its deficiency is the cause of neonatal rickets, preterm, and LBW babies.
3. **Calcium** is essential for bone mineralization and maintains cell wall integrity and role in haemostasis and coagulation cascade, muscle contraction, enzyme and hormone homeostasis, neurotransmitter release, and nerve cell function. Its deficiency is a risk factor for preterm labor, LBW, preterm birth, and reduced fetal mineralization. Calcium supplement reduces the risks of these complications.

4. **Zinc** is a catalytic for various enzymes and is a part of nucleotide, proteins, and hormones. It has a role in protein nucleic acid synthesis and metabolism, cell division, gene expression, antioxidation, wound healing and immune responses, vision, and neurological function. Its deficiency is associated with LBW, IUGR, congenital defects, and pre- and post-term births and is a reason for high maternal and infant deaths in developing countries. Zinc supplement is beneficial.

5. **Iodine** is essential for growth and development and synthesis of thyroid hormones. It has a key role in fetal brain and CNS development, and myelination. Its deficiency causes fetal and neonatal hypothyroidism, goitre, and cognitive impairment. Severe deficiency leads to stunted growth (cretinism), irreversible neurological damage, and death.

6. **Folic acid** is a coenzyme for methylation process (DNA, neurotransmitters) protein metabolism, and cell multiplication, and is especially important mineral in the fetal embryonic stage. Its deficiency leads to homocysteine accumulation, fetal anomalies, and neural tube defects. Folic acid supplementation is preventive. Folic acid supplements are beneficial.

7. **Magnesium** is important for enzyme functioning, cell membrane integrity, synthesis of DNA, RNA ATP, and cAMP. Fetal effects of its deficiency are growth retardation, SGA, IUGR, and preterm birth. Magnesium supplementation can reduce these risks.

2.3 Assessment of Fetal Health

Impact on fetal growth and development and thereby neonatal outcome can be assessed by:

1. Estimated fetal weight (EFW)
2. BW

2.3.1 EFW [11–14]

Both small and large for gestational age (SGA, LGA) neonates carry high risk of morbidity and mortality. Timely detection can reduce this risk. Various methods to detect growth in antenatal period include **symphysis fundal height** (SFH in centimetres is equal to the GA in weeks), **ultrasonography** (Hadlock equation is used for GA and Shepard and Hadlock equation for fetal weight), **and biometric parameters (BPD**—biparietal diameter, **HC**—head circumference, and **FL**—femur length).

Average fetus weighs 80 g (2.8 oz) by end of 1st trimester and grows reaching weekly weight increase of 220 g (7.8 oz) up to 35 weeks, followed by a decline to weekly gain of 185 G (6.5 oz) until 40 weeks.

2.3.1.1 Fetal Growth Restriction (FGR/IUGR) [15–18]

The fetus fails to attain full growth potential, as estimated by EFW or abdominal circumference less than 10th percentile for the GA (ACOG). Moderate FGR is BW in the 3rd–10th percentile, while severe FGR is BW less than 3rd percentile.

FGR is associated with mild-to-moderate chronic O_2 and substrate deficiency and depending on the time of pathological exposure (Table 2.2), and is classified as:

1. **Symmetric** (20–30% of all FGR): exposure early in the gestation period, characterized by global impairment of cellular hyperplasia and proportional decrease in all fetal organs
2. **Asymmetric** (70–80% of all FGR): exposure late in gestation, characterized by a greater decrease in abdominal size (liver volume and subcutaneous fat tissue) than the HC. The fetus adapts by redistribution of blood flow to vital organs

Table 2.2 Causes of FGR

Fetal factors	Placental factors	Maternal factors
Chromosomal abnormalities: – Trisomy 21, 18, 13 – Turner syndrome – Chromosomal deletions – Uniparental disomy – Placental mosaicism	Abruption	Constitutional factors: Race, Height, weight
Structural malformations: Anencephaly Omphalocele/ gastroschisis CDH Renal agenesis/dysplasia Cardiac & other malformations	Placental infarction	Nutritional factors: – Low pre pregnancy weight – Poor pregnancy weight gain – Inflammatory bowel disease – Chronic pancreatitis – Gastrointestinal surgeries
Multiple pregnancies – Monochorionic gestation – Single anomalous fetus – Twin-to-twin transfusion	Preeclampsia	– Chronic hypertension – Preeclampsia – Collagen vascular disease – Antiphospholipid antibodies – Insulin-dependent diabetes
Fetal infections: – Rubella – Cytomegalovirus – Varicella-zoster	Velamentous cord insertion	Hypoxic conditions: -Congenital heart disease, Severe lung disease, Sickle cell anaemia
	Placenta previa	Environmental: high altitude, smoking, drug abuse
	Circumvallate placenta	Renal diseases: Chronic renal failure, Glomerulonephritis Renal transplantation
	Chorioangioma	Bad obstetric history: still birth, IUGR

(brain, heart, and placenta), compromising flow to nonvital organs (abdominal viscera, lungs, kidneys, and skin)

FGR causes fetal heart rate (FHR) abnormalities and fetal distress (passage of meconium, preterm births, birth asphyxia, still births, and acidosis), 10% are associated with congenital abnormalities (omphalocele, gastroschisis, diaphragmatic hernia, skeletal dysplasia, and congenital heart defects), and 20–60% of malformed neonates are SGA.

Reduced subcutaneous fat and impaired thermoregulation puts them at risk of hypothermia. Chronic intrauterine hypoxia results in polycythemia, hyperviscosity, hypoglycaemia (low hepatic glycogen reserve), and other metabolic abnormalities. They are afflicted with dual morbid states (prematurity and dysmaturity) with adverse consequences (necrotizing enterocolitis (NEC), low Apgar score, IVH—intraventricular haemorrhage, and HIE—hypoxic ischemic encephalopathy) and its sequelae, broncho pulmonary dysplasia (BPD), respiratory distress syndrome (RDS), chronic lung disease, retinopathy of prematurity (ROP), prolonged NICU stay, sepsis, and death. Long-term adverse neurodevelopmental outcomes (cognitive impairment and cerebral palsy) occur in survivors.

FGR neonates require expert care at birth and baby should be evaluated for signs of structural and chromosomal abnormalities and infections. Because of accelerated postnatal growth, they are at risk of obesity, hyperlipidaemia, metabolic dysfunction, insulin resistant type 2 diabetes, cardiovascular, and renal disease in childhood.

2.3.2   Birth Weight [19–22]

Antenatal fetal weight estimate is important because of the potential complications during labor and puerperium arising from fetal prematurity or IUGR. Common classification uses BW alone: **LBW** (1501–2500 g), **very** LBW **(VLBW)** (1001–1500 g), **extremely** LBW **(ELBW)** (500–1000 g), and **micropremies** (<400 g).

BW over 4000 g is considered as overweight (fetal macrosomia) and may be associated with birth injuries (shoulder dystocia, brachial plexus palsy, and fractures), prolonged/obstructed labor/cephalopelvic disproportion (CPD)/instrumental/Caesarean deliveries, birth asphyxia/low Apgar scores, maternal injuries, and post-partum hemorrhage (PPH).

Factors that influence BW include:

- a. **Fetal factors** (GA, gender)
- b. **Maternal factors** [race, height, weight, parity, weight gain, physical activity, Hb concentration, tobacco use, DM, pregnancy-induced hypertension (PIH), and eclampsia]
- c. **Others** (paternal factors and ambient altitude)

2.4   Maternal Diseases Affecting Neonatal Health

2.4.1   Anaemia [23–28]

Anaemia is the most common haematological disorder in women of reproductive age group. As per the World Health Statistics data 2016, almost 30% of reproductive aged and 40% pregnant women are anaemic. There is wide regional and global variation in the prevalence of anaemia in pregnancy, reflecting socioeconomic and nutritional status differences. In the South–East Asian countries, about 50% of all maternal deaths are due to anaemia or its complications. Prevalence of anaemia in pregnancy in India has decreased from 58% in NFHS-3 (National family health survey-3) to 50% in NFHS-4 survey (2015–16).

Causes of anaemia in pregnancy include:

1. Physiological (dilutional)
2. Iron deficiency
3. Other nutritional deficiencies: folate and vitamin B12
4. Hemoglobinopathies
5. Hypothyroidism
6. Chronic kidney disease (CKD)
7. Chronic infections/helminthic infections
8. Autoimmune haemolysis

There is a correlation between maternal anaemia and risk of preterm birth, low BW, SGA, low Apgar scores, and increased perinatal and maternal mortality. Iron deficiency is the most common cause of anaemia and a leading cause of anaemia-related maternal deaths [2]. Hb <10.9 g% as a cutoff to define anaemia in pregnancy. Prevalence of anaemia increases from 7% in 1st trimester to 24–39% in 2nd and 3rd trimesters. (Table 2.3)

The incidence and severity of anaemia is much higher in resource poor as compared to the developed countries, due to low socio-economic status, poor nutrition, lack of access to adequate health care facilities, prevalence of helminthic infections, malaria, inflammatory, and infectious conditions. Severity of anaemia is graded into mild (10–10.9g%), moderate (7–9.9g%), severe (4–6.9g%), and very severe (<4g%), depending on the Hb concentration.

Table 2.3 Definition of Anemia in pregnancy [23, 28]

Trimester of pregnancy	Threshold for defining anaemia
1st	Hb <11 g% (Hct <33%)
2nd	Hb <10.5 g% (Hct <31–32%)
3rd	Hb <11 g% (Hct <33%)
Postpartum	Hb <10 g% (Hct <30%)

Iron requirement in pregnancy is three times that of nonpregnant state, and the demand increases as pregnancy progresses from 4 to 6 mg/day in the 2nd trimester to 10 mg/day in the 3rd trimester. The total iron requirement is 840 mg (accounting for fetus, placenta, expansion of maternal red cell mass, and the blood loss at delivery).

Maternal iron deficiency predisposes fetus to iron deficiency. Iron is important for normal brain development, dendritic growth, synapse formation, and behaviours (grooming, timidity, poor spatial learning, and tasks requiring executive function). Long-term follow-up of infants who had iron deficiency for 3 months or more in their 1st year of life revealed that they were at high risk of cognitive impairment and autistic disorders, but since iron deficiency coexists with other nutritional deficiencies, it is difficult to attribute iron deficiency as a direct cause of cognitive impairment [29].

2.4.2 Haematological Disorders in Pregnancy

2.4.2.1 Thalassemia

Beta thalassemia minor is not associated with any higher risk of adverse outcomes in the neonates, except for higher incidence of neural tube defects due to relative folate deficiency in the mother. **β-Thalassemia major** women tend to be infertile due to chronic iron overload and associated endocrinopathies. However, pregnancies are associated with higher risk of pregnancy loss, prematurity, and FGR due to fetal hypoxia from maternal anaemia. Teratogenic effects of iron chelating agents include vertebral aplasia, abnormalities of ribs and retarded bone ossification, cephalo-pelvic disproportion, and operative deliveries.

2.4.2.2 Pregnancy in Women with Sickle Cell Disease

Pregnancy in women with **sickle cell disease** may cause worsening maternal anaemia and sickling crisis. They may also develop pyelonephritis, haematuria, PET, prematurity, IUGR, and abruption.

2.4.3 Obesity and Pregnancy

Obesity is associated with an array of maternal and perinatal complications, degree of risk amplified with increasing severity of obesity. Class II obesity or greater and high gestational weight gain are at the highest risk of complications. Obesity is defined by a body mass index (BMI) >30 kg/m^2 and can be further stratified into three severity classes, class 1 (30–34.9 kg/m^2), class 2 (35–39.9 kg/m^2), and class 3 (>40 kg/m^2). In Indian population, BMI >25 kg/m^2 is classified as obese, on account of the higher metabolic risks at lower BMI as compared to the west.

Obesity is a metabolic dysregulator. Excessive adipose tissue has a dysregulatory effect on metabolic, vascular, and inflammatory pathways, affecting placental growth and function, with risk of preeclampsia and FGR. Obesity-associated insulin resistance exposes fetus to high sugar levels, insulin, lipids, and inflammatory mediators, inducing epigenetic changes in the metabolic pathways and increasing the risk of hypertension, coronary artery disease, and diabetes in middle age (**Barker hypothesis**) [6].

Obese pregnant women are at risk of obstructive sleep apnea (OSA), early pregnancy loss, developing gestational hypertension and diabetes, occult type 2 diabetes, and PIH, and eclampsia. Multifetal pregnancy, congenital abnormalities, preterm and post-term birth, operative delivery, fetal death, still birth, birth asphyxia, and congenital defects (neural tube defects, cardiovascular anomalies, cleft palate, Anorectal atresia, and limb reduction anomalies) are also common [30].

2.4.4 Antiphospholipid Syndrome

Antiphospholipid syndrome can present with recurrent miscarriages, uteroplacental insufficiency and FGR, preterm delivery, PET, abruption, and fetal death. These occur due to impaired development of trophoblast and thrombosis of uteroplacental vasculature. Babies born are at a higher risk of vascular thrombosis (arterial, venous or small vessel).

2.4.5 Diabetes Mellitus in Pregnancy [31, 32]

Gestational diabetes mellitus (GDM) accounts for 90% cases of DM in pregnancy and 50% develop DM within 5–10 years. In 2019, there were 223 million diabetic women (20–79 years) and 20 million births. In 16% of live births, there was form of hyperglycaemia during pregnancy, and 1 in 6 births was affected by GDM. A vast majority of GDM cases were from low- and middle-income countries.

In GDM, pancreatic β-cell dysfunction prevents increase in insulin secretion, leading to maternal and fetal hyperglycaemia. In the fetus, insulin secretion increases. Insulin is an important growth factor. Hyperinsulinemia results in fetal macrosomia (BW > 4000 g), increased subcutaneous fat, and muscle mass.

2.4.5.1 Effects Maternal GDM on the Baby
The risks to the newborn are due to macrosomia, hyperglycaemia and hyperinsulinemia and increased incidence of intra uterine death (IUD) and perinatal asphyxia:

1. **Diabetic embryopathy** and congenital anomalies—heart disease, anencephaly, spina bifida, microcephaly, and caudal regression syndrome
2. **LGA**, i.e., BW at or above the 90th percentile for GA, and macrosomia (BW ≥4500 g), fetal hyperglycaemia, hyperviscosity, polyuria, hyperinsulinemia (fetal islet cell hyperplasia), and asymmetric fetal growth (broader shoulders, large thoracic, and abdomen). These increase the risk of operative or instrumental delivery, still birth and birth injuries (shoulder dystocia, brachial plexus injury, and fracture), and neonatal depression

3. Newborn **hypoglycaemia** due to islet cell hyperplasia, hyperbilirubinemia, hypocalcaemia, hypomagnesemia, polycythemia, cardiomyopathy, and birth defects
4. Risk of **RDS** from hyperinsulinemia blocking cortisol-induced lung maturation
5. **Long-term consequences**: risk of childhood obesity, diabetes, insulin resistance, cardiovascular diseases, and poor neurodevelopmental outcomes

2.4.6 Pregnancy and Infectious Diseases [33–35]

Infectious diseases are the major cause of late **neonatal death** (8–28 days). 30–40% of all neonatal deaths occur from infections, 50% occur in 1st week, 30% in 2nd week, and 20% in the 3rd–4th week of age. Common infections are acute respiratory infections (ARI) (30%), bacterial sepsis (40%), meningitis (40%), diarrhea (0.6%), and tetanus.

(a) **ARI:** commonest organism isolated is streptococci pneumonia. Mortality is high in LBW, malnourished, and preterm neonates.
(b) **Maternal tuberculosis** increases the risk of fetal loss, preterm delivery, and LBW.
(c) **Neonatal diarrhea contributes** to 3% of all deaths.
(d) **Neonatal tetanus** is contracted from an unimmunized mother, unhygienic delivery, and poor cord care. Once contracted, it is almost fatal. Newborn loses ability to suck at 3–10 days of age and develops spasms, stiffness, and convulsions, and dies.
(e) **Sexually transmitted diseases (STD):** **Syphilis** is usually transmitted from the mother via placenta and can result in fetal death or disability in 50–80% affected pregnancies. Congenital syphilis is associated with IUGR, anemia, thrombocytopenia, jaundice, hepato-splenomegaly, and neurological manifestations (mental retardation, hydrocephalus, cranial nerve palsies, and seizures) in the baby. **Gonorrhea** increases the risk of conjunctivitis in the newborn and later blindness. **Chlamydia** also exposes newborn to conjunctivitis and pneumonia. **Genital herpes** can lead to neonatal herpes with high mortality and neurodevelopmental sequelae among survivors.
(f) **UTI** and untreated bacteriuria are associated with increased risk of LBW, preterm birth, and high perinatal mortality [33].
(g) **Malaria** is associated with IUGR and LBW.
(h) **Omphalitis** (umbilical infection) is a unique problem in developing countries, attributed to unhygienic home deliveries, poor cord hygiene (nonsterile cutting and unhygienic tying), and local umbilical infection (leads to necrotizing fasciitis).
(i) **Omphalitis along with neonatal tetanus** increases the risk of neonatal sepsis and death.

2.4.6.1 Rubella (German Measles) [36–39]

Rubella is a self-limited infection, but maternal rubella can spread trans placentally to the fetus. Hematogenous spread in the fetus causes vascular cellular damage and ischemia of the affected organs. Rubella infection in pregnancy gains its significance from its teratogenic effects. Preconception or 1st trimester Rubella is associated with the risk of abortion, still birth, and birth defects. The risk of fetal infection is up to 81% in 1st trimester, 25% in 2nd, and 35% at 27–30 weeks and 100% after 36 weeks of gestation. Rubella is an important cause of severe birth defects in endemic countries. During 1996–2010 of more than one lakh infants with congenital rubella syndrome (CRS), 38% were from India.

During the global rubella pandemic of 1964–65, there were thousands of abortions, neonatal deaths, and CRS in newborns in United States. Rubella vaccine was introduced in 1969 and US has been able to eliminate CRS only in 2004. Rubella outbreaks (>2000 cases) were reported from Romania, Japan, and Poland in 2012.

Indian scenario: during a surveillance (2016–18) of 645 suspected CRS cases, 21.2% (137) were confirmed CRS. Of these 137 CRS patients, 78.8% had cardiac defects, 59.9% had eye signs (cataract, glaucoma, and retinopathy), and 38.6% had hearing impairment. 24.1% died over 2-year period.

CRS and the neonate: the classical triad of CRS includes Congenital cataract and glaucoma, congenital heart disease (CHD) patent ductus arteriosus (PDA), pulmonary stenosis (PS), and sensorineural deafness. Other effects are developmental delays, purpura, retinopathy, hepatosplenomegaly, jaundice, IUGR, myocarditis, microcephaly, and meningoencephalitis. DM, thyroid disorder, and panencephalitis can occur later in life [39].

Active rubella infection in a woman is a contraindication to conception until sero-negativity is achieved.

2.4.7 Liver Disease [40–42]

Babies of mothers with hepatitis are at risk of getting the infection from the mother:

(a) **Intrahepatic cholestasis of pregnancy (IHCP)** is associated with adverse perinatal outcomes (preterm birth, fetal distress, perinatal death, and meconium staining of liquor). Bile acids in circulation cause vasoconstriction of placental chorionic vessels, fetal asphyxia, and uterine hypertony.

(b) **Acute viral hepatitis (Hepatitis B)** may be associated with miscarriage, preterm labor, and LBW. The risk of vertical transmission to the newborn is 20–30%. If the mother is both HBsAg and HBeAg positive, the risk of transmission is 90%.

(c) In **Hepatitis C infection**, risk of vertical transmission is 5–10%.

2.4.8   Renal Disease [43–46]

Women with significant chronic kidney disease (CKD) are less likely to become pregnant. Even mild disease is associated with adverse maternal and fetal outcomes. Acute pyelonephritis can trigger preterm labor from fever-induced uterine hyperactivity but usually with no fetal loss.

CKD (with proteinuria and hypertension) is associated with higher incidence of **SGA, LBW, FGR, and preterm birth. Fetal survival** is poor when preconception blood pressure is uncontrolled (>140/90 mmHg). MAP >105 mmHg at conception carries tenfold higher risk of fetal death, higher risk of maternal events than in normotensive CKD, while during dialysis, intravascular volume and blood pressure fluctuations can be deleterious to the fetus.

Renal transplant recipients have a much lower pregnancy rate either due to infertility or from counselling (use of teratogenic drugs). There is **fetal risk of prematurity, FGR, congenital anomalies, RDS, suppressed haematopoiesis, and liver dysfunction**.

Drugs for CKD: angiotensin converting enzyme inhibitors (ACEI) and angiotensin receptor blockers (ARB) are preferred drugs because of their antihypertensive and antiproteinuric effects. However, they can cause fetal abnormalities. Diuretics also should be used sparingly and in minimal doses (to prevent volume contraction and electrolyte abnormalities). Loop diuretics (Lasix) are safe in pregnancy. Women on immunosuppressants (calcineurin inhibitors/glucocorticoids) are at higher risk of GDM, infections, and bacterial UTI and adverse fetal consequences.

2.4.9   Maternal Malignancy and the Fetus [47–49]

With advancement in perinatal care and cancer therapy, one is more likely to face a situation where pregnancy is complicated by malignancy in the mother. Malignancy is a high stress state with pathophysiological, metabolic, and biochemical effects in the body, and adverse maternal and fetal effects.

Four treatment modalities exist: surgery, chemotherapeutic (CT) drugs, radiotherapy (RT), and a combination of these:

1. Surgery can be performed during any trimester.
2. Radiotherapy can be given in the 1st and 2nd trimesters, but is associated with risk of birth defects, IUGR, miscarriage, higher risk of childhood cancer.
3. Chemotherapy is rarely used during pregnancy. The risks depend on the drug used and period of gestation. They should not be used in the 1st trimester when organogenesis is occurring because of the risk of congenital malformations and fetal loss. The effect of CT drugs on the fetus may be in the form of IUGR, LBW, SGA, bone marrow toxicity, cognitive impairment, and cardiac effects. Prematurity is most common accompanied by its own adverse effects on the baby.

4. Tamoxifen and Transtuzumab are contraindicated in pregnancy. Women with history of breast cancer are at higher risk of Preterm labor, LBW, or SGA, especially if they received CT or gave birth within 2 years of diagnosis.

However, a study in 2015 could not demonstrate a significant difference in cognitive ability, school performance or behavioral competence in children exposed to CT in utero compared to nonexposed children > 18 months of age, though prematurity was more prevalent in the CT exposed children.

2.4.10 Epilepsy in Pregnancy [50–55]

Epilepsy is a common neurological disorder with prevalence up to 1% in pregnancy. Pregnancy is usually uneventful, but they are at risk of fetal complications (poor fetal growth FGR/IUGR, congenital malformations, prematurity, preterm labor, and adverse neurodevelopmental outcomes in neonates).

Women with epilepsy suffer from anxiety and distress, for fear of harming or injuring the baby and the effect of anti-epileptic drugs (AED). Maternal AED exposure is associated with increased risk of preterm birth, FGR, and congenital malformations (4–6%). Common malformations include neural tube, congenital heart and urinary tract defects, skeletal abnormalities, and oral clefts (Table 2.4). Babies born to mothers on AED may have excessive sedation, lethargy, feeding difficulty, and withdrawal symptoms with inconsolable crying, particularly in preterms.

AEDs have anti folate reductase activity. Low serum folate level is independently associated with higher risk of congenital malformations. Folic acid supplementation diminishes this risk and improves autistic, cognitive, and behavioural outcomes. Family history of birth defects and low level of maternal education are additional risk factors.

Valproate is the major risk, while topiramate, phenytoin, and phenobarbital are of intermediate risk, and levetiracetam and Lamotrigine are least teratogenic and safer in pregnancy.

Table 2.4 Congenital Malformations associated with AED

AED exposure	Congenital malformations
Valproate	Neural tube defects: Spina bifida, lumbosacral myelocele, orofacial clefts, CVS and urogenital malformations, polydactyly, hypospadias
Phenytoin, Phenobarbitones	Orofacial clefts, cardiac malformations, genitourinary defects
Carbamazepine	Neural tube defects. Genitourinary defects, orofacial clefts, cardiac malformations
Topiramate	Oral clefts, FGR, SGA
Lamotrigine	Oral clefts in 1st trimester at high dose (200 mg/day)
Levetiracetam	Low risk of major malformations. Does not affect early development.
Pregabalin	Increased risk of major birth defects
Gabapentin	No increase in malformations. Risk of preterm, LBW, NICU admissions.

Enzyme-inducing drugs (carbamazepine, phenytoin, phenobarbital, primidone, oxcarbazepine, and topiramate) can affect the fetal microsomal enzymes and vitamin K degradation in the fetus, inhibiting clotting factor precursors, increasing the risk of haemorrhagic disease of newborn.

Maternal seizures, especially generalized tonic–clonic seizures (GTCS), are hazardous for the fetus. Hypoxia and lactic acidosis during a seizure episode leads to fetal hypoxia due to decreased placental transfer of O2 or postictal apnea in the mother, with decelerations lasting up to 30 min after the seizure. GTCS of 5 or more can cause developmental delay in the fetus and is a negative predictor of verbal intelligence quotient. Other types of seizures are associated with FGR, preterm delivery, and fetal injury. Epileptic seizures in labour are managed by benzodiazepines. There is a risk of neonatal withdrawal syndrome with use of benzodiazepines and AED.

2.5   Multiple Pregnancy

This is associated with higher miscarriage rate, preterm labour (due to overdistension of uterus, hydramnios, and premature rupture of membranes), discordant twin growth (difference of EFW of >25% between the twins), and single IUD with neurological complications in second twin. Fetal anomalies are more common in monozygotic twins including anencephaly, microcephaly, hydrocephalus, cardiac anomalies, and Down's syndrome.

2.6   COVID in Pregnancy

COVID is a new infection, and much data are not available, suggesting increased risk of miscarriage or congenital malformations, FGR, because of COVID-19. However, possibly 2/3rd pregnancies with SARS suffered FGR. Maternal COVID can lead to placental insufficiency and poor uteroplacental perfusion (chorionic intervillous inflammation, thrombosis, and focal avascularisation of the villi), fetal hypoxia, and risk of prematurity.

As per the UK obstetric surveillance system (UKOSS) cohort in 2020, of 265 newborns born to COVID positive mothers, 75% were preterm, 25% required NICU care, and 5% tested positive for COVID [56].

2.7   Conclusion

Maternal health and disease are the most important factors that can affect development and growth of the fetus. Maternal undernutrition, micronutrient deficiency, diseases commonly being anaemia, and others can have adverse effects on the fetus and the newborn baby. Common is IUGR/FGR, SGA, congenital defects, perinatal asphyxia, CHD, craniovertebral anomalies and neural tube defects, RDS, BPD, IVH, and prematurity.

Anaesthesiologist will likely face these neonates during the course of treatment in NICU or for surgery, and complete evaluation must be done for any birth defects and anomalies. Maternal details, e.g., age at delivery, educational and economic status, parity, whether ANC care provided and regarding complications during the period of pregnancy, etc., can provide a clue to the status of the neonate, and help assess risk of anesthesia and surgery, and take precautions to reduce them.

Most mishaps happen during transport of these sick premature babies from one area to another, especially if unsupervised. These neonates must be transported in preheated incubators with humidity and temperature control and facility for providing O_2 and under supervision of a medical personnel. This can go a long way in improving perioperative outcome.

References

1. Estimates generated by the WHO and Maternal and Child Epidemiology Estimation Group (MCEF) 2018: Leading Causes of Neonatal Deaths In India. http://data.unicef.org
2. Lee EJ, Choi KJ. Mortality analysis of surgical neonates: a 20-year experience by a single surgeon. J Korean Assoc Pediatr Surg. 2006. Disponível em: http://www.koreamed.org/SearchBasic.php?RID=0053JKAPS/2006.12.2.137&DT=1.
3. Taguchi T. Current progress in neonatal surgery. Surg Today. 2008;38(5):379–89.
4. Gangopadhyay AN, Upadhyaya VD, Sharma SP. Neonatal surgery: a ten year audit from a university hospital. Indian J Pediatr. 2008;75(10):1025–30.
5. Chirdan LB, Ngiloi PJ, Elhalaby EA. Neonatal surgery in Africa. Semin Pediatr Surg. 2012;21(2):151–9.
6. Barker DJ. Fetal origins of coronary disease. BMJ. 1995;311:171–4. PMC free article.
7. Blumfield ML, Hure AJ, Macdonald-Wicks L, et al. A systematic review and meta-analysis of micronutrient intakes during pregnancy in developed countries. Nutr Rev. 2013;71:118–32. https://doi.org/10.1111/nure.12003.
8. Gernand AD, Schulze KJ, Stewart CP, West KP Jr, Christian P. Micronutrient deficiencies in pregnancy worldwide: health effects and prevention. Nat Rev Endocrinol. 2016;12:274–89. https://doi.org/10.1038/nrendo.2016.37.
9. Dalton MD, Ni Fhloinn DM, Gaydadzhieva GT, et al. Magnesium in pregnancy. Nutr Rev. 2016;74(9):549–57. https://doi.org/10.1093/nutrit/nuw018. Epub 2016 Jul 21.
10. Mousa A, Nagash A, Lim S. Macronutrient and micronutrient intake during pregnancy: an overview of recent evidence. Nutrients. 2019;11(2):443. https://doi.org/10.3390/nu11020443.
11. Hadlock FP, et al. Sonographic estimation of fetal age and weight. Radiol Clin North Am. 1990;28(1):39–50.
12. Shepard MJ, Richards VA, Berkowitz RL, et al. An evaluation of two equations for predicting fetal weight by ultrasound. Am J Obstet Gynecol. 1982;142:47.
13. Hadlock FP, et al. Estimation of fetal weight with the use of head, body, and femur measurements—a prospective study. Am J Obstet Gynecol. 1985;151(3):333–7.
14. Shivkumar S, et. al., An ultrasound-based fetal weight reference for twins. Am J Obstet Gynecol 2015;213(2):224.e1-224.e9. https://doi.org/10.1016/j.ajog.2015.04.015
15. Ott WJ. The diagnosis of altered fetal growth. Obstet Gynecol Clin North Am. 1988;15(2):237–63.

16. American College of Obstetricians and Gynecologists. Fetal growth restriction. Practice Bulletin No. 134. Obstet Gynecol. 2013;121:1122–33.5.
17. Society of Obstetricians and Gynaecologists of Canada. Intrauterine growth restriction: screening, diagnosis, and management. SOGC Clinical Practice Guideline No. 295, August 2013. J Obstet Gynaecol Can. 2013;35(8):741–8.
18. http://sogc.org/wp-content/uploads/2013/08/August2013-CPG295-ENG-Revised.pdf
19. Unterscheider J, Daly S, Geary MP, Kennelly MM, et al. Optimizing the definition of intrauterine growth restriction: the multicenter prospective PORTO Study. Am J Obstet Gynecol. 2013;208(4):290.e1–6. https://doi.org/10.1016/j.ajog.2013.02.007.
20. American College of Obstetricians and Gynecologists. Fetal macrosomia number 22, November 2000 (Reaffirmed 2015). http://www.acog.org/Resources_And_Publications/Practice_Bulletins/Committee_on_Practice_Bulletins_Obstetrics/Fetal_Macrosomia
21. Boulet SL, Alwxander GR, Salihu HM, Pass MA. Macrosomic births in the united states: determinants, outcomes, and proposed grades of risk. Am J Obstet Gynecol. 2003;188(5):1372–8. https://pubmed.ncbi.nlm.nih.gov/12748514
22. Faschingbauer F, Dammer E, Raabe E, Schneider M, et al. Sonographic weight estimation in fetal macrosomia: influence of the time interval between estimation and delivery. Arch Gynecol Obstet. 2015;292(1):59–67. https://doi.org/10.1007/s00404-014-3604-y.
23. Kriplani A, Sharma A, Radhika AG, Rizvi ZA, et al. Management of iron deficiency anaemia in pregnancy. FOGSI General Clinical Practice Recommendations. https://www.fogsi.org/wp-content/uploads/2017/07/gcpr-recommend
24. American College of Obstetricians and Gynecologists. ACOG Practice Bulletin No. 95: anemia in pregnancy. Obstet Gynecol. 2008;112(1):201–7. https://doi.org/10.1097/AOG.0b013e3181809c0d. Erratum in: Obstet Gynecol. 2020 Jan;135(1):222.
25. Auerbach M, Abernathy J, Juul S, Short V, Derman R. Prevalence of iron deficiency in first trimester, nonanemic pregnant women. J Matern Fetal Neonatal Med. 2021;34(6):1002–5. https://doi.org/10.1080/14767058.2019.1619690. Epub 2019 Jun 3.
26. Juul SE, Derman RJ, Auerbach M. Perinatal Iron deficiency: implications for mother and infants. Neonatology. 2019;115(3):269–74.
27. Ren A, Wang J, Ye RW, et al. Low first trimester haemoglobin and low birth weight, preterm birth and small for gestational age newborns. Int J Gynaecol Obstet. 2007;98:124.
28. Rohilla M, Raveendran A, Dhaliwal LK, Chopra S. Severe anaemia: a tertiary hospital experience from northern India. J Obstet Gynaecol. 2010;30:694.
29. Hemoglobin concentrations for diagnosis of anaemia and assessment of severity. Vitamin and mineral nutrition information system. Geneva, World Health Organization; 2011.
30. Robinson HE, O'Connell CM, Joseph KS, McLeod NL. Maternal outcomes in pregnancies complicated by obesity. Obstet Gynecol. 2005;106:1357.
31. Stewart A, Malhotra A. Gestational diabetes and the neonate: challenges and solutions. Res Reports Neonatol. 2015;5:31–9. https://doi.org/10.2147/RRN.S30971.
32. International Diabetes Federation. IDF Atlas. 9th ed. Brussels, Belgium: International Diabetes Federation; 2019.
33. Sobel JD, Kaye D. Urinary tract infections. In: Mandell GL, Bennett JE, Dolin R, editors. Mandell, Douglas, and Bennett's principles and practice of infectious diseases, 7, vol. 1. Philadelphia: Elsevier; 2010. p. 957.
34. Nicolle LE, Gupta K, Bradley SF, et al. Clinical practice guideline for the management of asymptomatic bacteriuria: 2019 update by the infectious diseases Society of America. Clin Infect Dis. 2019;68:e83.
35. Smaill FM, Vazquez JC. Antibiotics for asymptomatic bacteriuria in pregnancy. Cochrane Database Syst Rev. 2019;2019
36. Documentation and verification of measles, rubella and congenital rubella syndrome elimination in the region of the Americas United States National Report, March 28, 2012. pdf icon. [1.4 MB, 62 pages].
37. Rubella and congenital rubella syndrome control and elimination—global progress, 2000–2012. Morbid Mortal Wkly Report. 2013;62(48):983–6.

38. Papania M, Wallace GS, Rota PA, Icenogle JP, et al. Elimination of endemic measles, rubella, and congenital rubella syndrome from the western hemisphere—the US Experience. 2014 external icon. JAMA Pediatr. 2014;168(2):148–55.
39. Murhekar M, Verma S, Singh K, Bavdekar A, Benakappa N, et al. Epidemiology of congenital rubella syndrome (CRS) in India, 2016-18, based on data from sentinel surveillance. PLoS Negl Trop Dis. 2020;14(2):e0007982. https://doi.org/10.1371/journal.pntd.0007982.
40. Tran TT, Joseph A, Reau N. ACG clinical guideline: liver disease and pregnancy. Am J Gastroenterol. 2016;111(2):176–94. https://doi.org/10.1038/ajg.2015.430.
41. Westbrook RH, Dusheiko G, Williamson C. Pregnancy and liver disease. J Hepatol. 2016;64j:933–45.
42. Mikolasevic I, Filipec-Kanizaj T, Jakopcic I, Majurec I, et al. Liver disease during pregnancy: a challenging clinical issue. Med Sci Monit. 2018;15(24):4080–90. https://doi.org/10.12659/MSM.907723.
43. Millar LK, DeBuque L, Wing DA. Uterine contraction frequency during treatment of pyelonephritis in pregnancy and subsequent risk of preterm birth. J Perinat Med. 2003;31:41.
44. Tangren J, Nadel M, Hladunewich MA. Pregnancy and end-stage renal disease. Blood Purif. 2018;45:194–200. https://doi.org/10.1159/000485157.
45. Gonzalez Suarez ML, Kattah A, Grande JP, Garovic V. Renal disorders in pregnancy: core curriculum. 2019;73(1):119–30. https://doi.org/10.1053/j.ajkd.2018.06.006.
46. Hui D, Hladunewich MA. Chronic Kidney Disease and Pregnancy. Obstetrics & Gynecology. 2019;133(6):1182–94. https://doi.org/10.1097/AOG.0000000000003256.
47. Brewer M, Kueck A, Runowicz CD. Chemotherapy in pregnancy. Clin Obstet Gynecol. 2011;54(4):602–18. https://doi.org/10.1097/GRF.0b013e318236e9f9.
48. Dekrem J, Van Calsteren K, Amant F. Effects of fetal exposure to maternal chemotherapy. Paediatr Drugs. 2013;15(5):329–34. https://doi.org/10.1007/s40272-013-0040-6.
49. Cardonick EH, Gringlas MB, Hunter K, Greenspan J. Development of children born to mothers with cancer during pregnancy: comparing in utero chemotherapy-exposed children with nonexposed controls. Am J Obstet Gynecol. 2015;212(5):658.e1–8. https://doi.org/10.1016/j.ajog.2014.11.032. Epub 2014 Nov 27.
50. MacDonald SC, Bateman BT, McElrath TF, et al. Mortality and morbidity during delivery hospitalization among pregnant women with epilepsy in the United States. JAMA Neurol. 2015;72:981.
51. Kapoor D, Wallace S. Trends in maternal deaths from epilepsy in the United Kingdom: a 30-year retrospective review. Obstet Med. 2014;7:160.
52. Tomson T, Battino D, Bromley R, et al. Management of epilepsy in pregnancy: a report from the International League Against Epilepsy Task Force on Women and Pregnancy. Epileptic Disord. 2019;21:497.
53. Meador KJ, Pennell PB, May RC, et al. Fetal loss and malformations in the MONEAD study of pregnant women with epilepsy. Neurology. 2020;94:e1502.
54. Hernández-Díaz S, Werler MM, Walker AM, Mitchell AA. Folic acid antagonists during pregnancy and the risk of birth defects. N Engl J Med. 2000;343:1608.
55. Tomson T, Battino D, Bonizzoni E, et al. Dose-dependent risk of malformations with antiepileptic drugs: an analysis of data from the EURAP epilepsy and pregnancy registry. Lancet Neurol. 2011;10:609.
56. Characteristics and outcomes of pregnant women admitted to hospital with confirmed SARS-CoV-2 infection in UK: national population based cohort study. BMJ. 2020;369:m2107. https://doi.org/10.1136/bmj.m2107.

Changes in the Newborn at Birth: Fetal-to-Newborn Transition

3

Usha Saha

3.1   Introduction

In the intrauterine life, fetus is totally reliant on the mother for nutrition for growth and development, for gas exchange (oxygenation and carbon dioxide removal), and for clearing of metabolic waste products.

Placenta is the link between the mother and the fetus. Maintenance of normal maternal–placental–fetal physiology and metabolism, and regulation of placental circulation is extremely important.

At birth, this equation changes and the newborn baby must adapt to the extrauterine life when it needs to fend for itself. Transition is a complex process, and several factors interplay to make it a success. Of significance is the short time over which these changes must take place. All body systems undergo changes, cardiovascular and respiratory being prime, others being endocrine, metabolism, hepatic, hemopoietic, and thermoregulatory [1–3].

Abnormal adaptation increases the morbidity and mortality in the newborn baby and is more common in in-hospital and operative deliveries, and in premature and syndromic babies [4].

Neonatal anesthesiologists must understand and have complete knowledge of the intricacies of the transition process, **normal and abnormal adaptation,** factors in the perioperative period that can revert these changes (fetal asphyxia, respiratory distress in the newborn, neonatal hypoxia), and role of Surfactant.

U. Saha (✉)
Department of Anesthesia, Critical Care, Pain and Palliative Care, Lady Hardinge Medical College, Smt Sucheta Kriplani and Kalawati Saran Childrens Hospitals, New Delhi, India

© The Author(s), under exclusive license to Springer Nature Singapore Pte Ltd. 2023
U. Saha (ed.), *Clinical Anesthesia for the Newborn and the Neonate*,
https://doi.org/10.1007/978-981-19-5458-0_3

3.2   Placenta

Placenta is a temporary fetal organ, formed soon after implantation of the embryo. Its role is to provide nutrition and oxygen to the fetus and remove waste products. It is a barrier between fetal and maternal circulation, preventing direct mixing of maternal and fetal blood. Umbilical cord, the link between placenta and the fetus, contains two arteries and one vein. Umbilical arteries carry waste material and deoxygenated blood from the fetus to the placenta, while the umbilical vein carries nutrients and oxygen from the mother to the fetus. Placenta assumes its full function by the end of 1st trimester and continues to grow with the fetus.

Placenta also has an important role in the transitional process after birth and baby's adaptation to the external environment.

3.2.1   Feto-placental Maternal Circulation

This consists of two circulations: **1. utero-placental circulation and 2. feto-placental circulation.**

There is no mixing of maternal and fetal blood and exchange occurs by diffusion. Placenta is highly vascular. At term, it weighs about 500 g and has blood flow of 600–700 mL/min (80% of uterine perfusion).

Uterine arterial pressure is 80–100 mmHg and it drops to 10 mmHg in the inter-villous spaces on the maternal side. Pressure in the umbilical arteries is 50 mmHg which falls to 30 mmHg on the fetal side. Umbilical venous pressure is 20 mmHg. Higher uterine arterial pressure allows forward flow through the placenta. Maintenance of maternal systolic blood pressure (SBP) and uterine blood flow is essential for normal utero-placental fetal circulation. Maternal hypotension, hypo-volemia, anemia, and poor oxygenation (lung disease and high altitude) may adversely affect placental circulation and fetal growth. Placental circulation has poor neurovascular regulation and is not affected by catecholamines. Feto-placental circulation is vulnerable to hypoxia. Reoxygenation is associated with release of excessive free radicals, contributing to pre-eclampsia and other pregnancy-related complications. Endothelins and prostanoids cause vasoconstriction, while nitric oxide (NO) has a vasodilatory effect. Melatonin has an anti-oxidant role.

3.2.2   Functions of Placenta

1. **Nutrition** and **gas exchange** between fetus and mother
2. **Removal of waste** products (urea, uric acid, creatinine, and CO_2)
3. Placental nutrient metabolism plays a key role in limiting transfer of some nutrients. Conditions such as diabetes and obesity affect nutrient transport, resulting in over or restricted growth (IUGR)
4. **Physical barrier** to microbe transmission from the mother
5. **Immune role:**
   (a) **IgG** antibodies can pass through placenta by 20th week, providing immunity to the fetus and newborn up to first few months of life.

(b) **IgM** antibodies cannot pass through the placental barrier. They are the first immunoglobulins expressed in the fetus, at 20 weeks, and are the first responders to an infection. Intravenous immune globulin (IVIG) can prevent neonatal infections, and sepsis in premature and low birth weight (LBW) neonates.

(c) **Immunological barrier**: small lymphocytic suppressor cells in the fetus inhibit maternal cytotoxic cells and prevent maternal rejection of the fetus as foreign body.

6. **Endocrine function**: placenta produces hormones that regulate maternal fetal physiology during pregnancy

(a) Chorionic gonadotrophic hormone (CGH):
   - Is responsible for fetal survival
   - Stimulates release of progesterone and estrogen
   - Protects fetus from being rejected by the maternal body
   - Its deficiency is associated with risk of spontaneous abortions
   - Stimulates testis to produce testosterone and sex organ development in male fetus

(b) Progesterone:
   - Helps in implantation of the embryo
   - Its uterine relaxant effect decreases the risk of spontaneous abortions

(c) Estrogen:
   - Crucial for proliferation process (breasts, milk production, uterus, and fetus)
   - Increases blood supply (vasodilator effect) near end of pregnancy
   - Level is 30 times more than nonpregnant female

(d) Human placental lactogen (hPL):
   - Necessary for fetal growth, development, and metabolism
   - Stimulates production of insulin-like growth factor that regulates intermediary metabolism
   - Necessary for production of IgF, insulin, surfactant, and adrenocortical hormone
   - Higher levels in multiple pregnancies, diabetes, molar pregnancy, and in RH incompatibility
   - Low levels in toxemia, choriocarcinoma, and placental insufficiency

(e) It is a reservoir of blood for the fetus (500 mL), delivering to it in case of hypotension and viceversa.

3.3 Lung Development

Primordial lung appears as a lung bud off the esophagus, caudal-to-laryngotracheal sulcus by about 3–4 weeks of gestation. It elongates, divides, and stems into future lung.

i. 16–26 weeks: canalicular stage—peripheral lung development and differentiation of epithelium takes place.

ii. 20 weeks: surfactant production starts.

iii. 32 weeks: 17 generations of airways have developed.

iv. 36 weeks: 4 million distal saccules (respiratory bronchioles and alveolar ducts) are present.

v. Alveolarization (increase in number of alveoli) begins 36 week preterm (3–4 weeks of gestation) and continues until 36 months postnatal (3 years of age).

vi. Alveoli are lined by two types of epithelial cells (pneumocytes)—type 1 and type 2.

vii. Type 2 Pneumocytes produce and secrete surfactant.

viii. Alveoli have a property to collapse because of their spherical shape, but are prevented by surfactant (natural surfactant reduces ST to < 6 dynes/cm).

3.4   Surfactant [5]

Surfactant is a phospholipid, a surface-active lipoprotein, produced by the type 2 pneumocytes. The main active component is dia-palmitoyl-phosphatidyl-choline (DPPC). Surfactant forms a layer inside the alveolus to stabilize it and reduce the surface tension (ST). It has a hydrophobic area (facing air) and a hydrophilic area (facing water). ST acts as air–water interface of a bubble and makes it smaller by decreasing the surface area at the interface. Lowering of ST prevents the collapse of the alveolus. With decrease in ST, surface pressure increases, according to Laplace Law, i.e., gas pressure (P) needed to keep equilibrium between collapsing forces (ST = y) and expanding forces of gas in an alveolus of a radius (r) is represented by the formula:

$$P = 2y/r$$

3.4.1   Surfactant Production

Surfactant production begins by the 20th week and gradually increases. It appears in the amniotic fluid by 28 weeks, and by 35 weeks, fetus has adequate quantity of surfactant. A term newborn has alveolar surfactant pool of about 100 mg/kg, which is much lower in preterm newborns (4–5 mg/kg), as in an adult. Once secreted, it has a half-life of 5–10 h. Its unique property is that it is recycled. Up to 90% is reabsorbed by the pneumocytes themselves and remaining 10% is digested by the macrophages. Metabolism of surfactant is slower in newborns as compared to in adults.

3.4.2 Role of Surfactant

ST of water is 70 dynes/cm, and in lungs, it is 25 dynes/cm. At the end of expiration, as alveoli reduce in size, ST will reduce to zero (in the absence of surfactant). Surfactant reduces ST to 5–6 dynes/cm (preventing it to reach zero), and thereby prevents complete collapse at end of expiration, allowing alveoli to inflate more easily, with less work of breathing and less energy expenditure. Clinical surfactants reduce the ST to 5–10 dynes/cm. Role of surfactant:

- ↑**Pulmonary compliance**: by reducing ST, allowing alveoli to inflate more easily, with less work of breathing and less energy expenditure
- **Facilitate recruitment of collapsed alveoli**: by decreasing the required inflation pressure
- **Prevention of atelectasis**: smaller the alveolar size, greater the effect of surfactant
- **Reduces fluid accumulation** and keeps airways dry
- **Immune role**—by regulating inflammatory responses and interacting with adaptive responses. Two constituent proteins (SP-A and SP-D) bind to sugars on the surface of the pathogens and opsonize them, facilitating their phagocytosis
- **Surfactant deficiency** has two consequences: (**a**) Shrunken and fibrotic alveoli [as in respiratory distress syndrome (RDS)] and (**b**) enhanced pulmonary inflammation and infections.

3.4.3 Clinical Effects of Surfactant

1. Increase in pulmonary compliance
2. Prevention of atelectasis at the end of expiration
3. Facilitate recruitment of collapsed airways and alveoli

Adaptations at Birth - At birth, fetus must make several changes to adapt to the extrauterine life. Timing and appropriateness of these changes are essential for successful transition and survival of the newborn baby. Two systems undergo major changes—a respiratory and b cardiovascular system. In most newborns, complete changes occur at birth itself, but in some, it may take a few hours, latest 24 h of birth. Various factors can interfere with normal transition (Fig. 3.1).

Neonatal anesthesiologists need to be aware of these changes and factors affecting. Functional changes occur at birth, but permanent changes take place over a period of weeks to months. If care is not taken during the peri-operative period of the surgical neonate, these changes revert, with adverse postoperative outcome and high morbidity (delayed recovery, failure to extubate, need for prolonged, and more intense care), and mortality.

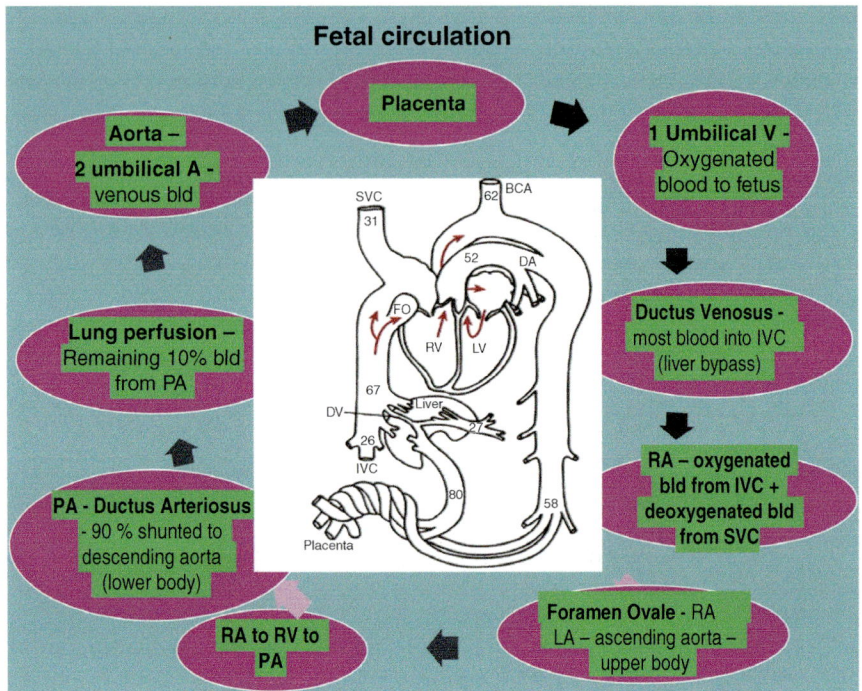

Fig. 3.1 Fetal circulation, *DA* Ductus Arteriosus, *DV* Ductus Venosus, *FO* Foramen Ovale

3.5   Fetal Circulation

In utero, blood, rich in nutrition and oxygen, is delivered to the fetus via the umbilical vein. Umbilical arteries carry venous blood back to the placenta. Heart acts as a conduit to blood flow and fetal lungs are non-functional. Pulmonary vascular resistance (PVR) is high due to hypoxic pulmonary environment ($PaO_2 = 17$–19 mmHg). Systemic vascular resistance (SVR) is low. Left atrial saturation is about 65%, which falls to 30% during labor, and within 5 min of birth, it increases to 90% (preductal SpO_2).

In a term fetus, cardiac output from both the ventricles is about 450 mL/kg/min, that of right ventricle (RV) being double of left ventricle (LV). At birth, circulation changes from "parallel" to "series", and total cardiac output increases to 800 mL/Kg/min. LV output increases and that of RV decreases, to become equal (LV output = RV output = 400 mL/kg/min), keeping pace with the increased O_2 consumption. Blood flow to lungs, heart, kidneys, liver, and the gastrointestinal tract increases. Cortisol, catecholamines, rennin–angiotensin system, vasopressin, and thyroid hormones, all play an important role.

Characteristic feature of Fetal circulation is the presence of three shunts: **ductus venosus (DV), ductus arteriosus (DA), and foramen ovale (FO).**

Umbilical vein carries blood from the placenta, toward the liver, where >80% blood bypasses the liver via the 1st shunt, DV (between portal vein and inferior vena cava (IVC)) toward the right atrium (RA). With increasing gestational age, blood flow to the liver increases. By 32 weeks, it is almost 80% of umbilical blood flow. Blood from the IVC (venous, from the lower body) mixes with the arterial blood from the DV. In the RA, blood from the IVC (O_2 rich) and superior vena cava (SVC) (venous, from head and upper extremities) mix. RA contains mixed venous blood (O_2 content < than in IVC but > than of SVC). 50–60% of blood in the RA is directed through the 2nd shunt, FO into the left atrium (LA), LV, and ascending aorta, to be supplied to the upper part of the body. This is facilitated because of low SVR and the flaplike aperture of FO, which acts as a one way valve, allowing blood flow from right to left only. Remaining 50–40% blood enters the RV and pulmonary artery (PA).

Fetal lungs are fluid filled, not fully developed, have high airway and PVRs. They have no role in fetal gas exchange. In the PA, 90% blood is shunted off into the descending aorta through the 3rd shunt, DA, to perfuse the lower part of the body, and eventually drains back to the placenta through the umbilical arteries. Remaining 10% blood in the PA (8% of cardiac output) perfuses the lungs to meet its metabolic demands. After 30 weeks of gestation, lung perfusion gradually increases.

3.6   Transition from Fetus to Newborn (Fig. 3.1)

This is a complex physiological process that takes place rapidly, over a short period, at the time of delivery [6]. **Two events initiate these changes:**
1. **Newborn baby's 1st cry or breath**
2. **Clamping of the umbilical cord**

1. **Newborn baby's cry or 1st breath** (Box 3.1): at birth, exposure of the head to cold, stimulates the baby to gasp (1st breath). Air rushes into the airways and alveoli, opening them up, and airway pressure falls. As air enters the lungs, pul-

---

Box 3.1 1st Breath: What Happens?
- **Delivery of Head**: Gasp—1st breath
- Generates -ve intrathoracic pressure: air flows into the lungs—lung expansion
- Opening of airways and alveoli: ↑FRC (functional residual capacity)
- Blood flows from PA to pulmonary capillaries: ↓ PVR (pulmonary vascular resistance)
- ↓ Blood flow through DA and FO—functional closure
- During vaginal delivery: chest gets compressed—**1/3rd lung fluid expelled** thru nose/mouth
- **After delivery:** chest wall relaxes—-ve intrathoracic pressure—air flows into the lungs
- **Crying:** generates +ve Intrathoracic P—keeps alveoli open and remaining fluid forced out

---

Box 3.2 Cord Clamping: Cutoff from Maternal Circulation

(a) Stimulation of aortic and carotid chemoreceptors, respiratory center from hypoxia, hypercarbia and acidosis
(b) ↑ SVR, SBP and LV pressure; ↓ flow through FO and DA
(c) Functional closure of foramen ovale: at birth (anatomic closure 3 months–1 year age)
(d) PA to DA flow ↓: functional closure—within 10–15 h of birth (anatomical closure—4–6 weeks)
(e) ↓ Prostaglandins from the placenta: DA closure
(f) Umbilical vessels and ductus venosus: become nonfunctional—anatomic closure by the end of 1st week

---

Box 3.3 Facilitation of Transitional Changes at Birth

1. Hormone surges at labor: cortisol, catecholamines, and thyroid hormones
2. Negative intrathoracic pressure by chest compression during vaginal delivery
3. Exposure to cold: gasping—1st breath—alveolar expansion, increase in FRC
4. ↑ PaO_2 and ↓ PGE2 stimulate DA spasm and closure
5. Clamping of umbilical cord: ↑ SVR–↑ Resistance to flow through Ductus Arteriosus
6. Alveolar expansion, loss of HPV: decrease in PVR, ↑ pulmonary blood flow
7. Activation of sodium pump and clearance of lung water
8. ↑ SVR–↑ LAP: closure of FO
9. Cord ligation: cessation of blood flow to umbilical vein–passive closure of DV
10. Lungs take over its function: gas exchange

---

monary vascular bed dilates [elimination of hypoxic pulmonary vasoconstriction (HPV)], PVR decreases, allowing forward blood flow from PA into pulmonary capillaries. RA, RV, and PA pressures decrease, with cessation of flow through the FO and DA. Further cries of the newborn generate +ve intrathoracic pressure that keeps airways and alveoli open and forces out remaining lung fluid.

2. **Clamping of the Umbilical cord** (Box 3.2)

   With the clamping of the umbilical cord two things take place:

   (a) Pulmonary arteries face resistance and can no longer drain into the placenta, with resultant increase in SVR, SBP, LV, and LA pressures.
   (b) Pulmonary vein is no longer fed by the placenta, with cessation of flow through DV. Systemic venous pressure falls, umbilical vessels constrict, with immediate closure of DV (Fig. 3.1).

Factors that facilitate transition at birth are summarized in Box 3.3

Prostaglandins are secreted by the Placenta and metabolized in the lungs. Fetal Prostaglandin levels are high because lung is unable to metabolize them. Prostaglandins maintain the patency of the DA, important for fetal circulation. With clamping of the cord and removal of placenta, airways open, alveoli expand, and pulmonary perfusion increases. Lungs start the process of gas exchange and can metabolize prostaglandins. As levels of prostaglandins fall, DA goes into spasm and closes.

3.7 Other Adaptations

3.7.1 Respiratory Adaptaions

Fetal lungs are filled with fluid secreted by the lung epithelium, and alveoli are collapsed. Lungs are in a hypoxic environment, initiating pulmonary vasospasm (HPV). Lung fluid is rich in chloride and low in protein. Toward the end of gestation, production of lung fluid gradually diminishes. Endocrinal adaptations (cortisol, catecholamines, and thyroid) are critical to lung fluid clearance.

3.7.2 Pulmonary Changes at Birth:

- **Exposure** of the newborn to external cold environment stimulates a gasping breath.
- Lungs are **HEAVY–HIGH inspiratory pressures are** required to open the Alveoli.
- **One (1st) breath may not be enough, and MORE BREATHS** are required.
- **Initiation of 1st breath** is a complex process, involving several biochemical, neural, and mechanical factors. Hypoxia, hypercarbia, and acidosis stimulate aortic and carotid chemoreceptors, and trigger medullary respiratory center at birth.
- **Vaginal delivery**—1/3rd fluid expelled thru nose/mouth, and remaining gradually drains via the lymphatics.
- **How quickly fluid leaves the lungs depend on the effectiveness of the 1st few breaths in expanding the alveoli.**
- **Crying** creates a positive intrathoracic pressure, keeps alveoli open and forces fluid out.
- **Simultaneous** ↓ PVR **and** ↑ pulmonary blood flow occurs.
- As the baby's breathing becomes regular, lungs resume their function.
  In 90% newborns, lungs assume their normal function, but 10% require assistance, while 1% newborns need extensive resuscitative measures.

Pulmonary Response:
- Pulmonary vasoconstriction occurs in response to hypoxia, acidosis, and hypercarbia
- Arteriolar constriction in the gastrointestinal tract, kidneys, muscles, skin occurs allowing redistribution of blood flow to vital organs (heart and brain)
- In prolonged asphyxia, myocardial function gets adversely affected, with decrease in Cardiac output and cerebral and myocardial ischemia.

Table 3.1 Cortisol levels

Gestational age	Fetal cortisol levels
30 weeks	5–10 µg/mL
36 weeks	20 µg/mL
Pre labor	45 µg/mL
Few hours post delivery	200 µg/mL

3.7.3 Endocrine Adaptations

Cortisol, vasoactive mediators, and thyroid hormones play an important role in transition at birth.

1. **Cortisol**: fetal cortisol synthesis and release is under fetal hypothalamic control. Fetal levels are low and increase with the period of gestation. (Table 3.1)

   Role of cortisol in adaptation process:
   (a) **Pulmonary effects**: in lung maturation, surfactant production, and clearance of lung fluid
   (b) **Increased β receptor density** in heart and lungs
   (c) **In catecholamine release**
   (d) **In conversion of T_4 to T_3**
   (e) **Maturation of thyroid axis**
   (f) **Metabolic and energy substrate** metabolism in the liver
   (g) **Gut maturation** and increase in digestive capacity

2. **Vasoactive substances:** catecholamines (norepinephrine, epinephrine, and dopamine), Angiotensin II and renin increase at birth, indicating presence of stress response in fetus and neonates. Levels are higher in preterms, probably because organs immature and less responsive, and lower in Cesarean delivery, when there is no stress of labor.

   Role of catecholamines in adaptation process:
   (a) Increase in blood pressure
   (b) Metabolic (glucose and fatty acids)
   (c) Brown fat thermogenesis

3. **Thyroid Hormones:** at birth, there is an increase in levels of T_3 and T_4 in response to cortisol surge, cord clamping and cold stimulus of birth.

   Role of thyroid hormones in adaptation process:
   (a) **In fetal lung fluid clearance** (activating the Na^+, K^+, ATPase)
   (b) **Congenital hypothyroidism:** no adaptation abnormality
   (c) **Very preterm babies**: blunted thyroid functional transition from fetal to newborn life (depressed adaptive behavior)

3.7.4 Metabolic Adaptations

Fetal energy needs are met with transplacental transfer of glucose. Fetal liver stores glycogen fat and other substrates. In early hours of birth plasma, glucose levels fall.

Catecholamine and cortisol surge and fall in insulin levels at birth help maintain plasma glucose and free fatty acid levels at birth.

Preterm babies have abnormal responses to cortisol and catecholamines, with increase in catecholamine release. They have minimal glycogen and fat stores and low substrate pool, which make birth adaptation difficult. They need glucose infusion to prevent hypoglycemia and as substrate for energy production.

Fetal heart is a mere conduit, and not much energy is consumed by the myocardial activity. At birth, it assumes its role in maintaining cardiac output, peripheral circulation, and vascular resistance. This is high energy consuming. Availability of substrates to the newborn depends on:

(a) Adequate gas exchange in the lungs
(b) Coronary blood flow
(c) Nutritional intake
(d) Efficiency in shifting from carbohydrate to fatty acid utilization

Neonatal myocardium is capable of anaerobic energy production and can maintaining cardiac function even at low PaO_2, providing some protection from ischemic injury to the myocardium in conditions of hypoxemia. However, persistent hypoxia or asphyxia adversely affects transitional changes much before the direct myocardial effects become apparent.

3.7.5 Thermal Adaptation and Thermogenesis

Core temperature of the fetus is 0.5 °C above the maternal temperature. Fetus does not expend energy to maintain body temperature and glucose is converted to glycogen in the liver and stored. After birth, the newborn utilizes these stores to maintain body temperature and other organ functions. Heat production is twice as much in a growing baby than adult.

Hormone surge (cortisol, catecholamines, and thyroid) at birth activates brown fat thermogenesis. Brown fat is 1% of body weight and is abundant around the kidneys and in the intrascapular areas. It generates heat by uncoupling of mitochondrial oxidative metabolism from ATP synthesis. **Neonates are extremely prone to hypothermia,** due to:

1. Large body surface area in relation to body weight, and greater heat loss
2. Limited fat reserves
3. Inability to shiver
4. Higher energy utilization for maintaining body functions.

Methods by Which Term Neonate Maintains Core Body Temperature:
1. **Brown fat metabolism** (non-shivering thermogenesis), that produce twice the amount of heat as compared to white fat metabolism
2. **Shivering thermogenesis** (from physical activity of kicking and crying)—minor role in heat production
3. **Peripheral vasoconstriction** secondary to exposure to cold, and decreased heat loss from skin surface

Key Points
1. Heat production is an active process needing O_2 and glucose—newborn should be allowed to breathe O_2 rich air for a few hours after birth.
2. Persistent hypothermia will result in metabolic acidosis, hypoglycemia, and decreased surfactant production, growth retardation and long-term effects—newborn should be kept in a warm environment.
3. Catecholamine surge at birth mobilizes glycogen, still glucose levels decline to a lowest point at 1 hour of age. Newborns should be given dextrose water orally or IV until initiation of regular feeds.

3.7.6   Hepatic Adaptation

Fetal liver is the main erythropoietic tissue at midterm. Besides storing glycogen, it is also the major store for Iron. Fetal liver is involved in all the three mechanisms of RBC formation:
1. **Initiation of erythropoiesis** in the embryonic liver
2. **Conservation of a high erythropoietic activity** for several weeks until bone marrow can take over
3. The **switch mechanism** from fetal to adult hemoglobin
   This process is regulated by two hormones:
   (a) **Testosterone** which stimulates heme and hemoglobin synthesis in liver at about 10–13 weeks of gestation
   (b) **Erythropoietin** in 2nd trimester (>12 week gestation)
       After birth, liver gradually takes on all the functions, chiefly:
       i. Production of clotting factors
       ii. Breakdown of glycogen to glucose
       iii. Anabolic and catabolic processes
       iv. Bilirubin metabolism: defects in bilirubin metabolism can lead to newborn jaundice

3.8   Normal Transitional Findings

Most of transitional changes occur within a few hours of birth, but permanent changes occur earliest by 6 weeks. This period is critical in the life of a newborn because of the risk of reversal to fetal status and reopening of the functionally closed shunts in event of hypoxia, acidosis, hypothermia, or respiratory infections. Some tachypnea, lung crackles from remaining fluid, tachycardia, flow or systolic murmur, and acrocyanosis for a few hours, but usually settles by 24 h of age [transient

Table 3.2 PVR and factors affecting PVR

↓ **PVR**: promote closure of DA and FO	↑ **PVR**: Encourages PFC/PPHT
i. High FiO_2	i. Airway resistance/pressure
ii. Alkalosis	ii. Poor RV function
iii. Nitric oxide	iii. Hypoxia
iv. Magnesium	iv. Asphyxia
v. Histamine	v. Acidosis
vi. Acetyl choline	vi. Hypercarbia
vii. ß-Sympathetic stimulation	vii. α-Sympathetic hyperactivity
viii. K+ channel activation	viii. Ca++ activation

tachypnea of the newborn (TTN)]. Several factors can interfere with the normal transition process at birth, by affecting **normal breathing or respiratory responses to hypoxia.** In an attempt to establish normal respirations, newborn can develop two problems:

1. Fluid may remain in the alveoli
2. Pulmonary blood flow may not increase as desired.

This can have several adverse consequences. Basic pathophysiology is continued high PVR, and all consequences are severe or minor forms of raised PVR. Decrease in **PVR** promotes functional closure of the DA and FO. High **PVR** encourages persistence of fetal circulation (PFC)/persistent pulmonary hypertension of the newborn(PPHN), patent DA (PDA)/patent FO (PFO), and shunt reversal. Factors that affect PVR are listed in Table 3.2.

3.9   Abnormalities of Transitional Changes at Birth

Incomplete removal of alveolar fluid has several adverse consequences, with immediate- and long-term impacts (Box 3.4). Several factors can interfere with complete removal of fluid from the lungs:

1. **APNEA at birth/birth asphyxia:** alveoli do not expand and remain small, collapsed, HEAVY, and fluid filled—more number of breaths with additional inflatory pressure are required to inflate them.
2. **Gasping irregular respiration following primary apnea**: poor alveolar expansion.
3. **Poor muscle tone and weak respiratory efforts.**
4. **Absent or weak crying.**
5. **High PVR.**
6. **Surfactant deficiency,** as in premature birth.

Box 3.4 Clinical Implications of Incomplete Lung Clearance
1. Inadequate lung expansion
2. Pulmonary crackles, noisy breathing, and wheeze
3. Transient tachypnea of the newborn (TTN)
4. Recurrent chest infections
5. Failure to thrive
6. Persistence of fetal circulation (PFC)
7. Risk of respiratory distress syndrome (RDS)

Table 3.3 High-risk pregnancies

Maternal Factors	Prepartum Factors	Intrapartum Factors	Intrinsic Factors
age >35, alcohol/substance abuse, Diabetes Mellitus, Hypertension, Cardiac disease Respiratory disease Severe anemia Infections	APH, PET, multiple births, no ANC IUGR, Placenta previa/ Abruptio Fetal–maternal hemorrhage PIH Illicit or drug exposure	Preterm/post term delivery Amnionitis Fetal distress/meconium- stained liquor/Prolapsed cord Premature rupture of membranes (PROM) Narcotic, MgSO₄ administration Malpresentations Prolonged labor Instrumental/Operative delivery	Prematurity, Congenital defects RDS Birth trauma

3.9.1 Apnea at Birth

Apnea at birth: babies of all high-risk pregnancies are at a risk of developing Apnea, primary and secondary (Table 3.3).

  Primary apnea: in response to O_2 deprivation, there is initial rapid breathing, and if asphyxia/hypoxia continues, there is a decrease in respiratory movements (apnea) and bradycardia. Initial management consists of high FiO_2 and tactile stimulation. Usually, these suffice, but if apnea persists, management is as for secondary apnea.

  Secondary apnea: if primary apnea remains unresolved, *secondary apnea occurs, during which HR, BP, and* PaO2 fall further. Management includes

(a) **High FiO₂** (50–60%)
(b) Check for any **obstruction** to respiration: use oropharyngeal (preferred)/nasopharyngeal airway
(c) **Respiratory support:** in a baby who has spontaneous efforts, continuous positive airway pressure (CPAP) should be tried through oropharyngeal or nasopharyngeal route

Table 3.4 Factors that affect respiration at birth

Stimulate respiration	Depress respiration
Mild acidosis	Severe acidosis
Hypercarbia	CNS damage
Hypoxia	Hypoxia
Sensations—pain, cold, touch, noise	**Drugs**—magnesium, alcohol, opioid, barbiturates

(d) **Mechanical ventilatory support (IPPV)**: babies with no respiratory effort or who do not respond to above measures, will need to be intubated and provided positive pressure ventilation

(e) **Early O$_2$ and IPPV** to prevent hypoxic ischemic injury to the brain

(f) Provide care in a **thermoneutral** environment

(g) Once stabilized, look for additional **avoidable causes of apnea** and accordingly manage

Important to Note:
- **Avoid nasal instrumentation** as far as possible because of narrow nares and they are obligate nasal breathers
- **Avoid 100% O$_2$**, and if required, use for the shortest duration (risk of developing ROP and BPD).
- Eliminate **other causes of apnea** that depress respiration (Table 3.4)

3.9.2 Vaginal vs Cesaritan Delivery

There is some difference in clearing of alveolar fluid in a baby born by normal labor and vaginal route compared to one born by cesarian section. The catecholamine surge during labor and the process of baby squeezing out through the cervix and vagina, helps in two ways:

1. **Compression of the chest** of the fetus during its passage down the birth canal and the elastic recoil of the thorax after birth creates a negative intrathoracic pressure, allowing air to gush in and expand the lungs.
2. **Expulsion of lung fluid**: 1/3rd fluid is expelled through nose/mouth during vaginal delivery, while remaining gradually passes into the interstitial spaces, to be carried away by the Lymphatics over a few hours after delivery.
3. **Crying** of the baby generates a positive intrathoracic pressure, further aiding in alveolar expansion, distribution of air throughout the lung, and exudation of lung fluid.

This benefit is lost during operative delivery, with cesarian babies more likely to have residual lung fluid, noisy breathing, wheeze, and pulmonary crackles. They are at a greater risk of developing TTN, recurrent chest infections, and failure to thrive.

3.9.3 Persistence of Fetal Circulation (PFC)/Persistent Pulmonary Hypertension of Newborn (PPHN)

PFC/PPHN [7, 8]: this is an extremely rare condition associated with poor survival, high morbidity and mortality in the newborn baby. Fetal circulation persists even after birth, i.e., right-to-left shunts at atrial and pulmonary arterial levels, high PVR, with PPHN, hypoxemia, and cyanosis. **Newborns at risk of PFC** include all high-risk pregnancies (Table 3.3) fetal or birth asphyxia, meconium aspiration syndrome (MAS), RDS, and sepsis. **Prevention is the only cure** (avoidance of factors that increase PVR, antenatal and neonatal care, and use of antenatal steroids in high-risk cases). **Management** includes early diagnosis and prompt intervention. **Baby presents with features of** severe hypoxemia, low Hb SpO_2, need for high FiO_2 and respiratory support, initial tachycardia followed by bradycardia, cyanosis and cardiac arrest. **Investigations include** hematocrit, platelet counts, serum glucose and calcium levels, X-ray chest (pulmonary haze or ground glass appearance), and ECG pattern of right axis deviation, RV strain and arrhythmias. **Hyperoxia (100% oxygen) challenge test**: if the shunt is >30% of the cardiac output, even 100% O_2 will not relieve cyanosis. Preductal PaO_2 >postductal PaO_2 is diagnostic. Echocardiography is indicated to rule out cyanotic congenital heart disease. Monitoring includes SpO_2, NIBP, ECG, and PaO_2. **Treatment** is by surfactant replacement, NO inhalation, beta-adrenergic drugs, and respiratory support.

3.9.4 Patent Foramen Ovale PFO/Patent Ductus Arteriosus PDA

PFO/PDA: in few newborns, there is minor maladaptation at birth that can lead to incomplete closure of FO or DA. Pressure changes occur as in normal transition with increase in SVR and decrease in PVR. The shunt is usually left to right, because of high left-sided pressures, or through the PFO/PDA. There is no cyanosis, and symptoms are due to pulmonary congestion. In PFO, left-to-right shunting leads to high pulmonary blood flow, and pulmonary congestion. In PDA, shunt is from the descending Aorta to the PA, and outflow of aortic blood leads to low diastolic blood pressure with wide pulse pressure. These babies are at **risk of complications,** such as necrotizing enterocolitis (NEC), intraventricular hemorrhage (IVH), bronchopulmonary dysplasia (BPD), and sudden death. **Management** is **medical** (O_2 supplement, fluid restriction, diuretics, NSAIDS), and **surgical** (usually undertaken by 3–6 months of age).

3.9.5 Reversal of Shunt

Reversal of shunt: these are situations of PFO/PDA, with left-to-right shunts. As already stated, at birth closure of all shunts is functional. Permanent closure of DV takes place by 1 week, DA by 3–4 weeks and FO by 3–12 months of life. Any insult or exposure to factors that can increase PVR, in the neonatal period can lead to reversal of shunt, which now becomes right to left through the PFO or PDA. Acyanotic congenital cardiac defect converts to cyanotic cardiac disease. **Resultant shunt is an interplay of SVR and PVR. Caution must be exercised by the anesthesiologist in such all neonates to avoid causative or precipitating factors** (Table 3.2). **Broadly speaking, increases in right-sided pressures and decrease in left-sided pressure must be always avoided. The goal is to maintain high SVR and low PVR.**

Reversal of shunt results in increased venous admixture, decreased O2 carrying capacity, desaturation and low SpO_2, hypoxemia, cyanosis, pulmonary edema, and sudden death.

3.9.6 Pulmonary Consequences of Lung Fluid Retention

Pulmonary consequences of lung fluid retention include TTN and RDS.

TTN is the mildest and transient complication of incomplete clearance of fetal lung fluid. It is more frequent in preterm babies. They are tachypneic, have lung crackles, crepitations on auscultation, tachycardia, flow (systolic) murmur, and acrocyanosis for a few hours, but usually settle by 24–48 h of age. Factors contributing are decreased Na^+ transport, and low surfactant. If surfactant deficiency is severe, features of become evident.

Note **L → R shunt is Preferable over R → L shunt**

Key Points for an Anesthesiologist
1. DA is thick and muscular, and its constriction is a gradual process. With increase in PaO_2, ductus goes into spasm and its functional closure occurs at birth. Spontaneous closure occurs over a period of 96 h (4 days) of life in almost all babies. Most newborns have a PDA in the first 8 h of life, in 505 newborns at 24 h, and in 10% by 48 h of age. Permanent anatomic closure occurs by fibrosis by 4–6 weeks. It can reopen any time there are factors similar to intrauterine life, hypoxemia, acidosis, increase in PVR, and decrease in SVR, with reversal to fetal circulation (R–L shunt). It is crucial that neonatal anesthesiologist takes special care and precautions in the perioperative period, especially in the first 4 days of life, but through the entire neonatal period, to prevent this from happening.
2. Fetal pulmonary vessels have a thick layer of smooth muscle, thereby prone to vasoconstriction. It takes about 6–8 weeks for the muscle layer to thin out and less prone to vasospasm. Hypoxia is a very potent stimulus to pulmonary vasospasm and should be avoided.
3. Functional closure of FO occurs at birth or within 24 h. Permanent closure occurs by 3 months to 1 year of age. This also can reopen any time.
4. Cyanosis is a late sign of distress in neonates. It becomes visible in the presence of at least 5 g% of deoxygenated hemoglobin. A polycythemic baby, with high Hb concentration, may have cyanosis even at higher or normal O_2 saturation

levels, while an anemic baby with low total Hb concentration may be quite hypoxic before becoming visibly cyanotic.

In all newborns, neonates, especially premature, present for surgery, anesthesiologist must carry out a thorough detailed evaluation in the form of detailed antenatal and birth history, APGAR scores, examination and evaluation of investigations, to establish or rule out any other medical disease or metabolic derangement or congenital abnormality, besides the surgical condition, that may impact anesthetic management, and appropriate perioperative anesthetic care can be provided, to reduce morbidity and mortality, in the already high risk baby.

Make Special Note of

- **Medications received by the newborn:** in general, all newborns receive intramuscular Vit K to facilitate normal clotting and preventing Hemorrhagic disease of the Newborn, until intestinal bacteria can start synthesizing Vit K.
- **APGAR Score** as it provides an estimate of how well the newborn is adapting. It takes into consideration Color, HR, Resp, Reflex Response, Muscle tone and each is scored as 0, 1, 2. Max score is 10. A 10 min Apgar is significant and is graded as 7–10 normal, 4–6 is low, and 3 is critically low.

Special Care and Precautions:

(a) Supplemental O_2
(b) Maintenance of airway and ventilation
(c) Temperature controlled environment: incubator
(d) Strict maintenance of IV fluid transfusion, acid base, serum electrolytes and glycemic balance
(e) Maintenance of systolic perfusion pressures and need for vasoactive drug support
(f) Avoidance of triggering factors: hypoxia, hypercarbia, acidosis, hypotension and peripheral vasodilatation, increase in PVR

Anesthetist has a great responsibility during the perioperative management of neonates because of the potential to reopen these shunts and revert to fetal circulation with postoperative adverse outcome (delayed recovery, failure to extubate, need for prolonged and more intense care), high morbidity with long-term consequences, and mortality. Premature babies are at a greater risk.

3.10　Key Points

i. The transition from fetal to extrauterine life involves rapid adaptations of several organs in a very short time.
ii. Hormones play an important role in normal transition process, namely, cortisol, catecholamines and thyroid hormones.
iii. Pulmonary adaptation requires clearance of lung fluid, surfactant secretion, and onset of breathing.
iv. Cardiovascular adaptation requires changes in pulmonary and SVRs, pressures blood flow, and closure of shunts.
v. Abnormalities in adaptation are more frequent preterm birth or operative delivery.

References

1. Marcdante KJ, Kliegman RM. Assessment of the mother, fetus, and newborn. In: Marcdante KJ, Kliegman RM, editors. Nelson essentials of pediatrics. 8th ed. Elsevier; 2019: chap 58.
2. Olsson JM. The newborn. In: Kliegman RM, St. Geme JW, Blum NJ, Shah SS, Tasker RC, Wilson KM, editors. Nelson textbook of pediatrics. 21st ed. Philadelphia, PA: Elsevier; 2020 chap 21.
3. Goyal NK. The newborn infant. In: Kliegman RM, St. Geme JW, Blum NJ, Shah SS, Tasker RC, Wilson KM, editors. Nelson textbook of pediatrics. 21st ed. Philadelphia, PA: Elsevier; 2020: chap 113.
4. Rozance PJ, Wright CJ. The neonate. In: Landon MB, Galan HL, Jauniaux ERM, et al, editors. Gabbe's obstetrics: normal and problem pregnancies. 8th ed. Philadelphia, PA: Elsevier; 2021: chap 23.
5. Nkadi PO, Merritt TA, Pillers DM. An overview of pulmonary surfactant in the neonate: genetics, metabolism and the role of surfactant in health and disease. Mol Genet Metab. 2009; 97(2):95–101. https://doi.org/10.1016/j.ymgme.2009.01.015.
6. Hillman N, Kallapur SG, Jobe A. Physiology of transition from intrauterine to extrauterine life. Clin Perinatol. 2012;39(4):769–83. https://doi.org/10.1016/j.clp.2012.09.009. PMCID: PMC3504352. PMID:23164177.
7. Perkins RM, Anas NG. Pulmonary hypertension in pediatric patients. J Pediatr. 1984;105:511–22.
8. Dworetz AR, Moya FR, Sabo B, Gladstone I, Gross I. Survival of infants with persistent pulmonary hypertension without extracorporeal membrane oxygenation. Pediatrics. 1989;84(1):1–6. PMID: 2740158.

Common Medical Conditions in the Neonates

4

Sadiya Zinjani

4.1 Introduction

The **neonate** is the smallest of all human beings, whose arrival in this world is perhaps one of the most eagerly awaited event in the lives of the 'to be parents' and their extended families. This little bundle of joy brings not only immense happiness but sometimes also brings much anxiety and worry. This small human offspring may carry with it certain genetic disorders or may develop medical or surgical issues demanding rapid intervention. With regard to surgical issues and other invasive procedures, the necessity to administer anesthesia to these babies arises. Safe methods of anesthesia are now available for even the most premature and sickest of neonates. However, it must be remembered that neonates are not small adults, their physiology is at a complete variance with adult humans, their anatomy is still developing and their physiology is still immature.

Therefore, in the highly specialized field of neonatal anesthesia, there is a definite need to highlight various medical aspects which must be dealt with before proceeding to administer anesthetic agents and analgesic drugs to them.

In addition, before delving into the vast realm of medical problems which a newborn is either born with or may develop, it is probably appropriate to define various terminologies used for a neonate and simultaneously give a meaning to important time spans in the life of these little babies.

S. Zinjani (✉)
Department of Paediatrics, Max Smart Super Speciality Hospital, Saket, New Delhi, India

© The Author(s), under exclusive license to Springer Nature Singapore Pte Ltd. 2023
U. Saha (ed.), *Clinical Anesthesia for the Newborn and the Neonate*,
https://doi.org/10.1007/978-981-19-5458-0_4

49

4.2   Definitions Terminologies

A newborn may be born after completion of the normal gestational period or may be delivered earlier or later than the expected date, and the body weight (BW) may be appropriate, less or more than that expected for the gestational age (GA). Both the BW and GA have an important bearing on the survival as well as the development of the newborn. In addition, the outcome of several medical and surgical issues are weight and gestational age related, hence the significance of knowing these terminologies [1, 2].

4.2.1   As Per Gestational Age (GA)

Term babies are babies born between 37 and 42 weeks of pregnancy. They are subdivided into three categories: **early term** (37–38 weeks), **full term** (39–40 weeks), and **late term** (40–42 weeks).

Babies born before completion of 37 weeks of pregnancy are considered **preterm.** They are categorized as **extreme preterm** (GA <28 weeks), **very preterm** (GA 28–32 weeks), and **moderate-to-late preterm** (GA 32–37 weeks).

Babies born at and beyond 42 weeks of gestation or expected date of delivery (EDD) + 14 days, are considered as **post-term**.

4.2.2   As Per Birth Weight (BW)

Low birth weight (LBW) babies are those with BW less than 2500 g irrespective of GA. This may be due to prematurity or fetal growth retardation (FGR), which account for 1/3rd LBW babies, or small for gestational age (SGA) babies, which accounts for 2/3rd of LBW babies. They are further categorized as **very** LBW (VLBW) with BW less than 1500 g and **extremely** LBW (ELBW) with BW less than 1000 g.

Appropriate for gestation age (AGA) babies are those with BW appropriate for the GA, i.e., >2500 g or between the 10th and 90th percentile on the intrauterine growth curves. SGA babies are smaller than usual for the GA and their BW is below the 10th percentile (they are smaller than other babies of the same GA), and **large for gestational age (LGA)** babies have BW greater than 97th percentile for that GA and refers to babies with BW more than 4000 g. (Stanford Children's Health)

Note: LBW is a valuable public health indicator of a country's healthcare system in terms of maternal health and nutrition and in socio economic stratification. Mortality and risk of developing neurologic sequelae with impairment in cognitive skills and chronic diseases is significantly higher in LBW babies. Due to immaturity of multiple organ systems, preterm babies carry higher morbidity and mortality risks, and are the leading cause of all under-5 mortality, globally.

Intrauterine growth retardation (IUGR) is defined as fetal growth rate less than normal for the growth potential of the baby (AAP) at that gestational age. It is not defined by the subsequent BW, whereas BW is used to define SGA. It is therefore possible for a newborn to be SGA without being FGR.

Certain vital periods in the life of a baby are major determinants in the outcome of pregnancy, neonatal wellbeing, morbidity, and mortality. **Perinatal period** extends from 20 weeks (140 days) of gestation to 28 completed days (4 weeks) after birth. This is an extremely vulnerable period for the developing organs. Any misstep in this period carries with it the possibility of disastrous and serious ill effects, which may result in profound and long-lasting deficits. The **neonatal period** is the most crucial phase of life and survival during this period is of paramount importance for a baby to reach adulthood. Nearly 41% of all under-5 deaths involve neonates. Neonatal period is divided into two, **early neonatal period** (birth to 7 days of age this period accounts for 75% of neonatal deaths) and **late neonatal period** (8th day to 28 days of life). **Infancy** period includes the period from birth to 12th months (1 year) of life. The 'Golden 1000 days' time span is a unique period during which there is the laying down of the foundation of optimum health, growth and neurodevelopment, and stretches right from the time of conception to 2 years of age.

4.3   Special Considerations [3]

4.3.1   Prematurity

Despite advances in neonatal care, preterm birth remains the leading cause of infant mortality, globally. Due to their LBW and organ immaturity, preterm babies may have various problems:

(a) Their **caloric needs** are high but due to the lack of sucking and swallowing reflexes, difficulties with oral feeding are often encountered.
(b) **Gastrointestinal** immaturity impairs digestion, absorption of carbohydrates and lipids, and increases the risk for necrotizing enterocolitis (NEC).
(c) **Pulmonary** immaturity makes them more prone to apnea and respiratory distress both of which call for very specialized care.
(d) **Neurological** immaturity contributes to the increased risk of CNS insults, which may later manifest as a poor cognitive ability, developmental delays, and other neurological sequelae.
(e) **Visual** issues such as retinopathy of prematurity (ROP) have to be guarded against.
(f) They are at increased risk for sudden infant death syndrome (SIDS).
(g) **Metabolic** immaturity, poor fat insulation, decreased glycogen stores, immature skin with increased water loss, poor vascular control, and lower maximal metabolism, narrows the range of thermal control, and makes them prone to hypothermia.

(h) Immaturity of the **immune** system places them at high risk for contracting life-threatening infections.
(i) Congenital **cardiac anomalies** such as patent ductus arteriosus (PDA) and blood pressure variations need regular monitoring and specialist referrals.

Premature newborns need continuous and prolonged specialized care and must be observed for onset of anemia and jaundice which call for prompt attention and remedial measures. Round the clock monitoring of blood sugar is essential since hypoglycemia is a potential danger that needs urgent attention.

4.3.2 Fetal Growth Restriction (FGR)

This refers to a fetus smaller than it should be. FGR may be symmetrical or asymmetrical depending on the time of development of restriction in fetal growth. FGR with associated inability to handle stress puts these babies at a health risk during pregnancy, delivery and even after birth, thus increasing the probability of adverse short- and long-term outcomes. The acute neonatal consequences of FGR/IUGR are perinatal asphyxia and neonatal adaptive problems. Respiratory distress due to meconium aspiration is an adaptive issue in these neonates which may sometimes necessitate the use of mechanical ventilation. Hypoglycemia and hypocalcemia are commonly encountered metabolic imbalances. Due to a compromise in their resistance to infection, there is an increase in the incidence of sepsis. Polycythemia is another cause of high morbidity.

4.3.3 Large for Gestational Age (LGA)

As already defined includes babies with BW larger than expected for their GA or BW greater than the 90th percentile. Causes attributed are genetic, maternal, or due to a medical condition in the baby. Due to their large size, these neonates have specific problems which necessitate their inclusion in a separate group. Their delivery poses a risk for the mother with increase in operative/instrumental deliveries, more frequent genital tract lacerations, and PPH. The incidence of birth injuries (BI) (shoulder dystocia, clavicle or limb fractures, and nerve injuries) is high during normal vaginal delivery. Other common problems are perinatal asphyxia, respiratory distress, meconium aspiration, hypoglycemia, and polycythemia.

4.3.4 Hypothermia/Hyperthermia

Medical issues in neonates may be initially mild and delay in addressing them may assume serious proportions due to the inability of the 'little one' to compartmentalize the problem. Thus, all health issues in the neonates underscore the need for a quick assessment and rapid initiation of remedial measures. The resuscitation of the newborn may sometimes produce temperature fluctuations which may be detrimental to life, rendering it of utmost importance to ensure that the newborn is resuscitated in a thermoneutral environment, i.e., the temperature of the resuscitation area should be maintained around 25 °C (WHO). Overexposure in a cold room will quickly result in hypothermia, which may be mild (36–36.4 °C), moderate (32–35.9 °C), and severe (<32 °C). Signs of hypothermia may be nonspecific or absent, and include pallor with bluish extremities, lethargy, and refusal of feeds. Gentle warming and adequate wrapping may ameliorate the problem. However, adoption of the preventive measures is the best policy.

Hyperthermia refers to a temperature record >37.5 °C and may be due to over-wrapping or keeping the baby directly in front of a warmer or heater. This can be easily corrected by reducing the layers of clothing and removing the source of external heat.

Fever may be due to high environmental temperature or dehydration (poor oral intake). Ensuring adequate feeds at frequent intervals may help in relieving fever. Sometimes, sepsis may be the cause, and appropriate measures such as sepsis workup should be done and relevant antibiotics started.

4.3.5 Birth Injuries (BI) [4–8]

These injuries are sustained by the newborn during delivery from compression or trauma. The incidence is 3.7 per 100,000 live births. Risk factors include abnormal presentations, instrumental delivery, intra uterine versions, prolonged/precipitous labor, short maternal stature, extreme prematurity, LGA, large fetal head, and fetal anomalies, etc. BI's may be grouped as cranial, head and neck, facial (nasal, ocular, and ear), muscular, nerve, bony, soft tissue, and abdominal injuries. They may manifest as mild bruising, superficial cuts, bony fractures or bleeding into the body cavities. The most frequently encountered injuries are swelling or bruising of the head (caput succedaneum or chignon), bleeding underneath a cranial bone (cephal hematoma, subgaleal hemorrhage), subconjunctival hemorrhage, facial nerve injury, and clavicle fracture. Treatment varies from no intervention to appropriate therapy. For nerve injuries, physiotherapy is advised, and fracture clavicle requires no treatment except to pin the affected arm of the baby to the front of the clothing and reducing movement of that arm.

Note: Caput succedaneum is an extra periosteal fluid collection due to molding of the baby's head and needs no treatment. Cephal hematoma is a sub periosteal accumulation of blood following the rupture of blood vessel because of trauma during the birth. Chignon is the swelling left on an infant's head after delivery with a ventouse suction cap and usually resolves without any intervention.

4.3.6 Neonatal Asphyxia (Includes Birth Asphyxia and Perinatal Asphyxia) [9–13]

This is one of the most feared outcomes of fetal life, labor or a complicated delivery. There is lack of oxygen to the newborn during birthing leading to the inability to establish or sustain spontaneous or adequate respiration on delivery. This produces perfusion deficit to various organs causing a hypoxic damage and can thus result in significant morbidity and mortality. If ventilation and adequate pulmonary perfusion are not established soon after birth a worsening cycle of hypoxia, hypercapnia, and metabolic acidosis sets in. The damage to the brain is of tremendous concern, since it is least likely to completely heal and may manifest in a surviving infant with either or both mental and physical deficits. **Perinatal asphyxia** is oxygen deficit from 28th week of gestation to the 7th day of life. **Neonatal asphyxia** is oxygen deficit occuring after birth. It can result in hypoxic ischemic encephalopathy (HIE) or intraventricular hemorrhage (IVH) especially in preterm newborns. A baby with severe neonatal asphyxia is cyanosed, hypotonic, has absent or poor respiratory effort and poor responses, all adding up to a low 5 min Apgar Score. Extreme asphyxia can cause cardiac arrest and death. The incidence of neonatal asphyxia has a multifactorial dependence with GA and BW being important determinants, others being maternal, fetal, placental, labor related, and cord related. Some of the maternal risk factors are age (elderly or very young mothers), lack of antenatal care, anemia, diabetes, heart disease, hypertension, and toxemia. Placental and labor related causes are placental insufficiency, placenta previa, prolonged membrane rupture, and difficult/prolonged labor. A short or a nuchal cord, a true knot, cord prolapse, and cord compression are important cord relevant risk factors. Fetal causes include both pre- and postmaturity, FGR, malpresentations, multiple pregnancies, fetal distress, and meconium aspiration.

Long-term adverse effects of birth asphyxia are cerebral palsy, motor disorders, seizure disorders and epilepsy, developmental delays, speech disorders, learning disabilities, visual and auditory impairment, respiratory problems, behavioral and emotional disorders, and feeding problems.

Prognosis: GA is an important mortality predictor in babies asphyxiated at birth. When compared to respiratory acidosis, metabolic acidosis scores far worse. A very low Apgar Score at 20 min is a reliable predictor of neurological morbidity, and a prolonged delay in the establishment of spontaneous respiration points to the development of irreversible brain damage. Babies with severe HIE have mortality rates ranging from 50–100%, and survivors may have up to 75% of residual disability rates.

4.3.7   Hypoxic Ischemic Encephalopathy (HIE) [4]

Severe birth asphyxia causing injury to the brain leads to the development of HIE, which may progress to permanent brain damage, manifesting as cerebral palsy. Treatment includes (a) airway management (suction, positioning to maintain airway patency, and tracheal intubation), (b) breathing stabilization [tactile stimulation, O_2, bag mask ventilation, and positive pressure ventilation (PPV)], (c) circulation improvement (chest compressions, IV fluids, and medications), (d) drug administration (to regulate heart rate, blood pressure, renal function, and control seizures), and (e) **hypothermia induction** (to help brain cells recover, thus preventing spread and severity and permanent brain damage).

4.3.8 Birth Defects

These may be structural or metabolic defects.

(a) **Structural birth defects** [14–16], as defined by the center for disease control (CDC), are problems present in the newborn structure that can affect almost any part or parts of the body, involving either the appearance or the function of the body, or both. The incidence is 3–4%. The well-being of the baby affected with a birth defect depends on which organ or body part is involved and extent of affectation. The severity of the defect as well as the body part affected may or may not influence the expected lifespan of the afflicted baby. The most common causes of birth defects are genetic disorders, chromosomal abnormalities, and pregnancy-related issues (infections, smoking, drugs, alcohol, or substance abuse). All birth defects may not be preventable, since the cause of many may be unknown. However, adoption of a healthy lifestyle, prior and during pregnancy, will increase the chances of having a healthy baby. When planning a pregnancy, a woman should consult a health care professional, and any existing problems such as diabetes, obesity, hypertension, asthma should be addressed. Once pregnancy is confirmed, women should enroll in a prenatal care program. Major brain and spine birth defects may be prevented by ensuring an adequate intake of folic acid. Avoidance of all harmful substances in the form of drugs, cigarettes, and alcohol should be mandatory throughout pregnancy. Equally important is avoidance of all infections. All medications and vaccinations as advised by the health care provider should be taken. The most common birth defects are Cardiac, Cleft lip/palate, Down syndrome, and Spina Bifida.

The common **cardiac defects** include atrial septal defect (ASD), AV septal defect, coarctation of the aorta, transposition of the great arteries (TGA), hypoplastic left heart syndrome, Pulmonary Atresia, tetralogy of fallot (TOF), and total anomalous pulmonary venous drainage (TAPVD).

Cleft lip/palate are common birth defects and may be isolated or a part of a syndrome. Symptoms arise from the opening in the mouth as feeding difficulties during the neonatal period and infancy, and later as problems with speech. Lip repair is done at 4–6 weeks and palate repair at about 9 months to one year of age. Corrective surgery followed by speech therapy can restore normal function.

Down syndrome or Trisomy 21 is by far the most common and best-known chromosomal disorder in human with a global incidence of 1:1000–1:1100 live births (WHO). It is one of the most common cause of moderate-to-severe intellectual disability. Down syndrome is strongly associated with increasing maternal age resulting in maternal meiotic nondisjunction. Unbalanced translocation accounts for up to 4% of cases.

Spina bifida is thought to result from a combination of genetic, nutritional, and environmental factors, in which folic acid deficiency and family history of neural tube defects (NTDs) play an important role. Incidence is 1:1000 births globally, with marked geographical variations. It is a spinal disorder involving improper closure of the neural tube. The three common types often encountered are Meningomyelocele, Meningocele, and Spina Bifida Occulta. The plethora of presentations, treatment, and time of treatment of babies with Spina Bifida is extremely variable.

Often babies with birth defects require to undergo corrective surgery during the neonatal period, which increases the risk of morbidity.

Note: Birth defects are commonly called congenital anomalies or abnormalities. A genetic disorder is a disease caused by a change in the DNA sequence, either wholly or partly. A Chromosomal disorder is a syndrome characterized by malformations or malfunctions in any of the body systems and caused by abnormalities in either the number or constitution of the chromosomes.

(b) **Metabolic birth defects: inborn errors of metabolism (IEsM)** [17–19] are disorders present from birth, affecting either the process of food breakdown or food absorption, or affecting various enzymes involved in these processes. Left untreated, some of these disorders affect the baby's development or cause organ damage and death. Neonates with IEsM may remain normal for the first few hours or days of life, and then become symptomatic with signs mimicking neonatal sepsis. Diagnosis is based on a high level of suspicion and is essential both for treatment as well as genetic counseling. The common IEsM are congenital hypothyroidism (CH), congenital adrenal hyperplasia (CAH), glucose 6 phosphate dehydrogenase (G6PD) deficiency, biotindase deficiency, galactosemia (galactose-1-phosphate uridyl transferase) (GALT), phenylketonuria (PKU), and maple syrup urine disease (MSUD). Pregnancy and delivery are generally uneventful. Accompanying sepsis may mask the disorder. Babies with IEsM may present with extreme hypotonia, sluggishness, dysmorphic features, poor feeding, jaundice, hypoglycemic, altered sensorium, or seizures. Parental consanguinity with history of a similar presentation in an earlier issue is a valuable pointer towards the suspicion of IEsM. Prognosis depends on several factors such as time of diagnosis, type and severity of the disorder, availability of specific treatment options, and definitive therapeutic interventions. Some IEsM have a relatively better prognosis than others. Some children may live longer but be at risk of developing progressive neurologic deficits, learning disabilities, and mental retardation. It is, therefore, important for primary care providers to know how to recognize IEsM, manage them in the interim while awaiting definitive diagnosis, and refer them to the appropriate metabolic specialist for the collaborative management.

Note: Prompt detection requires a high index of suspicion and the early measurement of biochemical markers such as blood ammonia.

Routine antenatal and neonatal screening tests cover a wide range of IEsM [20]. A special mention is to be made of 2 IEsM: **CH** and **CAH**, where the defect lies in either the paucity of hormone produced or in the buildup of certain intermediate hormones.

(i) **Congenital Hypothyroidism (CH)** [21, 22] is a birth defect due to the absence or under development of the thyroid gland or a problem in the production of the thyroid hormone. It is one of the most common treatable causes of intellectual disability which makes it empirical to diagnose it early and simultaneously initiate the thyroid replacement therapy. With early diagnosis and treatment, the baby is likely to have a normal, healthy life. CH is mostly sporadic, with incidence of 1: 3500 live births. Babies may be asymptomatic or present with hypotonia, hypothermia, jaundice, delayed stooling, and poor feeding. Thyroid screening is a part of routine newborn screening tests. Treatment is lifelong thyroid replacement therapy. Neonatal Hyperthyroidism is transient due to the transplacental passage of thyroid stimulating antibodies by a mother with Grave's disease.

(ii) **Congenital Adrenal Hyperplasia (CAH)** [23–26] is a group of autosomal recessive disorders that occur in 1:1600 live births. The most common cause is the absence of enzyme 21-hydroxylase, due to gene mutations, resulting in varying levels of the enzyme, producing a spectrum of effects. There are other rarer enzyme deficiencies which may also cause CAH. The two main forms of CAH are "**classic**" and "**non-classic.**" The classic CAH is more severe, and is usually detected at birth or in infancy, and may be of the "**salt losing form**" which forms 2/3rd of this group while the remaining 1/3rd is constituted by the "**simple-virilizing form.**" The nonclassic CAH is milder, more common and may not become evident until childhood or early adulthood. The sign and symptoms of classic CH include those due to cortisol deficiency (high blood sugar), life threatening adrenal crisis, atypical genetalia, high androgens (short height, early puberty, acne), altered growth, and fertility issues. Prenatal amniocentesis and Neonatal Screening tests should also include screening for CAH. An out of range result for CAH in the neonatal screening tests will necessitate further confirmation by urine and blood sampling. Treatment depends on the presenting form and includes medications (corticosteroids, mineralocorticoids, and supplements) reconstructive surgery, and psychological support [8].

(c) **Hypoglycemia:** [27, 28] Glucose is crucial for brain development as it is the main source of energy for the brain. A low blood sugar in a newborn may lead to injury and then death of the brain cells resulting in permanent damage. Neonatal hypoglycemia (NH) is one of the most common metabolic problems, and severe NH is one of the leading causes of neonatal brain injury. It is easy to recognize and treat. In the fetus, glucose diffuses across the placenta, so the fetal glucose levels are 2/3rd the maternal level. Once the umbilical cord is severed after the birth, blood glucose level may fall to dangerously low levels for the next 1–2 hrs before stabilizing by 3–4 hrs to a mean of 70 mg/dL. Monitoring of hypoglycemia in high risk neonates is of utmost importance. Babies at risk of NH are SGA, LGA, IUGR and preterm babies, those born to diabetic mothers, babies with birth asphyxia (HIE), and pregnancy with intrauterine stress and sepsis. Babies with some genetic disorders may also present with NH. Signs and symptoms include cyanosis or pallor, breathing problems (tachypnea, apnea, or grunting sounds), lethargy or irritability, muscular weakness (hypotonia), vomiting, poor feeding, weak or high pitched cry and tremors, shakiness, sweating, or seizures. Blood sugar should be tested within seconds of appearance of symptoms. A low initial blood glucose is rechecked every 2–3 hrs for the first 24–48 hrs and close monitoring is continued until the blood sugar stabilizes. If conditions permit, then the initiation of feeding in high risk and babies with symptoms of NH should be early and repeated every 2 hrs. Babies who cannot be put on oral feeds should be treated aggressively with IV dextrose while monitoring is continued. In babies with severe hypoglycemia, glucagon may be used subcutaneously or intramuscularly.

Neonatal hyperglycemia: [9] This refers to blood sugar levels over 150 mg/dL and is very frequently iatrogenic or due to insulin resistance, glucose intolerance or inability of the neonate to control hepatic glycogenolysis. It is frequently encountered in preterm babies during parenteral glucose infusion. Other precipitating factors include infection and stress. Treatment is reduction of the dextrose infusion rate or IV Insulin infusion.

(d) **Hypocalcemia** [27, 29] is also frequently encountered metabolic disorder in the newborns. Following the transition from intrauterine to a life outside the womb, after cord clamping, there is cessation of placental transfer of calcium (Ca). Consequently, neonatal Ca levels drop to about 8–9 mg/dL (2–2.25 mmol/L), and ionized Ca falls to 4.4–5.4 mg/dL (1.1–1.35 mmol/L) by 24 hrs of birth. Serum Ca concentration subsequently rises, reaching normal levels by 2 weeks of age. Neonatal hypocalcemia may be early onset when it manifests within the first 2 days of life or late onset when symptoms appear after the 3rd postnatal day, usually by the end of the first week of life. Risk factors include prematurity, SFD, IUGR, birth asphyxia, due to immaturity of the parathyroid gland or decreased transplacental passage of calcium. Babies of diabetic mothers are also likely to manifest with signs and symptoms of hypocalcemia. The most common causes of late-onset hypocalcemia are excessive phosphate intake, hypomagnesemia, hypoparathyroidism, and vitamin D deficiency. Hypocalcemia may be asymptomatic or the baby maybe irritable, have muscle twitches, tremors, or jitteriness, lethargic with refusal of feeds, or may present with frank seizures. Treatment of early onset hypocalcemia is 10% calcium gluconate given IV slowly under heart rate monitoring. After initial acute correction of hypocalcemia, calcium gluconate is added to the IV infusion. When oral feeds are started the formula is supplemented with oral calcium gluconate. This supplementation is required usually for a few days only. Late onset hypocalcemia is treated by addition of calcitriol or calcium to infant formula until normal calcium levels are maintained. A low mineral and low phosphate formula is advised for neonates with renal impairment.

Hypercalcemia (10): neonatal hypercalcemia is said to occur when total serum calcium level is >12 mg/dL or ionized calcium level >6 mg/dL. Most common cause is iatrogenic, though hyperplasia of the parathyroid and subcutaneous fat necrosis may be sometimes implicated as causative factors. When no cause is found, it is labeled as idiopathic. Maternal hypoparathyroidism and hypocalcemia, by its stimulatory action on fetal parathyroid gland, produce hypercalcemia in the baby. It may manifest as generalized irritability, lethargy, refusal of feeds or frank seizures. Treatment is IV saline and diuretics.

4.3.9 Hematological Disorders and Bleeding

(i) **Anemia** [30–33] is defined as hematocrit (Hct) or hemoglobin (Hb) concentration >2 SD below mean for the age. Normal Hct for a term baby is around 53%, while in a 32-week baby, it is 47%. Causes of neonatal anemia are:

   (a) **Blood loss** is the most common cause. This loss may be due to obstetric causes, or feto-maternal/feto-placental transfusion. In a twin pregnancy, there may be a twin to twin transfusion in which case one twin may be anemic while other may be polycythemic. Any cause leading to internal hemorrhage in the neonate may manifest as anemia. Repeated and frequent blood sampling is another reason of anemia in the neonate.

   (b) **Hemolysis -** Increased RBC breakdown may be due to intrinsic causes (hereditary RBC disorders, RBC enzyme defects (G6PD deficiency), RBC membrane defects (hereditary spherocytosis), and hemoglobinopathies (alpha thalassemia)), or extrinsic causes (immune hemolysis Rh or ABO incompatibility acquired e.g., infection, sepsis, or drug-induced hemolysis).

   (c) **Decreased RBC production** includes anemia of prematurity seen in preterm babies due to the transient deficiency of erythropoietin, congenital hypoplastic anemia (Diamond Blackfan syndrome), and anemia due to bone marrow suppression (congenital leukemia/infections/drug induced).

   The clinical signs and symptoms depend on the severity and the cause of anemia. The neonate besides looking pale may have both tachypnea and tachycardia, may be lethargic and feed poorly. Diagnosis is based on a detailed history (family, antenatal, obstetric, and postnatal history), and blood investigations. Radiological and imaging studies may also be required to establish a cause. Management depends on the cause and severity of the anemia. Prenatal fetal transfusion (intra uterine) may be needed in severe anemia resulting from hemolytic disease of the newborn (HDN). Postnatal anemia of prematurity may require treatment with human recombinant erythropoietin. Severe anemia may require packed RBC (PRBC) transfusion. Other causes of the anemia should be simultaneously treated.

(ii) **Neonatal polycythemia** [34] is defined as abnormally high RBC concentration with venous Hct >65%. It refers to a venous Hct greatly exceeding normal values for GA and postnatal age, and affects 0.4–5% of newborns. The effects of polycythemia are increase in the blood viscosity and reduced blood flow. With increase in blood viscosity, tissue oxygenation and perfusion are hampered and the tendency to form microthrombi sets in. The occurrence of these events in the cerebral cortex, kidneys, or adrenal glands can be disastrous, necessitating urgent management. The causes include increased erythropoiesis, as in utero hypoxia (SGA babies, postmature neonates, toxemia of pregnancy, severe maternal heart disease, maternal smoking, and other causes of placental insufficiency), maternal diabetes, neonatal hypothyroidism/hyperthyroidism, CAH, chromosomal abnormalities (trisomy 21), and transfusion related (which may occur due to delay in clamping of the cord or maternal to fetal or twin to twin transfusion). Clinical features—most polycythemic babies are asymptomatic and nonspecific symptoms seen in many neonatal disorders, may be present, such as lethargy, hypotonia, cyanosis, and poor feeding. They may sometimes manifest with tachypnea, tachycardia, and other signs of congestive heart failure. They tend to have increased jaundice. Renal involvement may result in renal vein thrombosis, hematuria, and proteinuria. Diagnosis is established by the measurement of capillary or peripheral venous hematocrit. Management—if the venous Hct of a plethoric neonate or neonate with features suggestive of polycythemia is above 65%, a partial exchange transfusion (PET) is the treatment of choice, which involves removing some volume of blood and replacing it with saline.

(iii) **Bleeding neonate:** [35] In comparison with older children and adults the physiological immaturity in neonates results in both qualitative and quantitative differences in the various components of the hemostatic system. Most of the coagulation factors other than factors I, V, VII and platelets are reduced in term neonates. Preterms have the added disadvantage of increased vascular permeability as well as an inability to effectively utilize Vitamin K for the synthesis of coagulation factors, thus enhancing the vulnerability of these babies to bleeding, in utero or after birth. Fetal hemorrhage may be associated with twin-to-twin transfusion, APH secondary to bleeding from the fetal side of the placenta, feto-maternal transfusion, maternal anticoagulation therapy (Coumarin), and accidental injury of the placenta during caesarean section. Neonatal hemorrhage may occur due to defects in any of the steps of the hemostatic pathway, such as defects in the platelets or in the coagulatory mechanism. These defects may present in isolation or in combination. Bleeding may also result from defects in the vessel wall.

(iv) **Coagulation defects** include hemorrhagic disease of the newborn (HDN) and inherited coagulation disorders. HDN may be early, classic, or late depending on the time of presentation. Early HDN is seen in neonates born to mothers who have been on certain medications antenatally (anticonvulsants/antibiotics/antitubercular) and may manifest within the first 24 h with a large cephal hematoma, umbilical bleeding, or even with intracranial hemorrhage. Treatment is administration of Inj. Vitamin K and FFP if bleeding persists. Classic HDN manifests within 48–72 h due to lack of administration of prophylactic Vitamin K. The neonate may present with bleeding from the GIT, umbilical cord, nose, or from the circumcision site. The response to Vitamin K is dramatic. Late HDN presents after the first week of life, sometimes at 8–12 weeks, in infants on prolonged antibiotic therapy or with malabsorption (liver disease/cystic fibrosis). They may bleed from the GIT or present with mucocutaneous or intracranial bleeding. Parenteral Vitamin K therapy is the treatment of choice.

Inherited deficiency of coagulation factors rarely manifest in the neonatal period except when the deficiency is very severe. These include Hemophilia, Von Willebrand disease, and Dysfibrinogenemia. Treatment includes the administration of FFP or specific factor concentrates.

Platelet defects may be quantitative or qualitative. Neonatal thrombocytopenia has platelet count <150,000/cu mm. Most neonates with thrombocytopenia have a modest reduction in platelet count which is frequently self-resolving. However, in the NICU, incidence of thrombocytopenia is quite significant. Quantitative platelet disorders are seen secondary to placental insufficiency, perinatal asphyxia, immune disorders, disseminated intravascular coagulation (DIC), intrauterine infections, neonatal sepsis, and NEC. Qualitative platelet disorders are uncommon and may be induced by drugs (indomethacin/antihistaminic) or may be part of a syndrome (Bernard Soulier syndrome).

Combined defects include coagulation defects as well as defects in the platelets and is classically seen in DIC. Various factors predispose to development of DIC, such as septicemia, hypothermia, asphyxia, prematurity, HMD, NEC, and severe Rh isoimmunization.

Vascular defects neonates with vascular malformations, hemangiomas, and trauma may also present with bleeding. Cavernous hemangiomas are large and deep set, and though they usually regress, they may be associated with complications which necessitate surgical removal. Clinical features are determined by the site, severity, and cause of bleeding. A baby presenting with pallor, tachycardia, fast breathing, and falling blood pressure indicates a significant blood loss. Diagnosis in a bleeding neonate involves a battery of blood investigations. Management is by Vitamin K administration once blood has been collected for investigations. When the signs point to a significant blood loss, fresh blood transfusion will be required. In DIC and specific clotting factor deficiencies, FFP and platelets are indicated.

4.3.10 Perinatal Infections [36–41]

These include intrauterine (congenital) infections and neonatal sepsis. The fetus may get infected in utero, during the passage through the birth canal or after birth. Neonatal bacterial sepsis is one of the most common causes of neonatal mortality.

(i) **Congenital infections** occur due to transplacental passage of the infecting agent or secondary to the infection of the placenta. Ascending infection causing amnionitis may result in in-utero bacterial infection of the fetus. The acronym TORCH is used to list infections caused by toxoplasma, other (syphilis, varicella zoster, and parvovirus) rubella, cytomegalovirus, and herpes simplex. Infections acquired in utero may cause fetal loss, FGR, premature birth and postnatal effects in the form of hepatosplenomegaly, CNS abnormalities, bleeding disorders, and features specific to the infection. Toxoplasmosis may manifest with hydrocephaly, intracranial calcifications, chorioretinitis, and convulsions. Congenital syphilis may present with interstitial keratitis, meningoencephalitis, rashes, snuffles, periostitis, and chondritis. Parvovirus B 19 infection may result in hydrops fetalis due to severe anemia. Varicella Zoster infection may result in skin lesions, microcephaly, mental retardation, cataracts, and limb hypoplasia. Congenital rubella may result in cardiac defects (PDA, PS, VSD), meningoencephalitis, and multiple ophthalmic defects (cataract, micro-ophthalmia, corneal opacities, retinitis). Cytomegalovirus may produce diffuse peripheral chorioretinitis, micro-ophthalmia, microcephaly, periventricular calcifications, and psychomotor retardation. Herpes simplex infections are acquired by direct contact with an infected mother, and signs usually appear 8–10 days after exposure as cutaneous lesions or features suggestive of sepsis. HIV infection may be acquired trans placentally, during delivery due to blood exposure or post natally from breast milk. Careful perinatal management reduces the risk of transmission. In congenital intrauterine infections, much of the damage has already occurred when the baby is born, so emphasis is more on prevention rather than treatment.

(ii) **Neonatal sepsis** includes various systemic infections such as septicemia, pneumonia, meningitis, osteomyelitis, arthritis, and urinary tract infection. The incidence varies between 1 and 8 cases per 1000 live births. Approximately 1/3rd of septic newborns develop meningitis. Several maternal and neonatal predisposing factors have been identified. Depending on the onset of symptoms, it may be **early onset** (within 72 hrs) or **late onset** (after 72 hrs). Clinical features—initial signs may be nonspecific, or may manifest as hyperthermia, refusal of feeds, poor cry and decreased activity. Involvement of the various systems may produce specific features. A high index of suspicion is necessary for early diagnosis which is then confirmed by a sepsis work up. Management is supportive including care in a thermoneutral environment. Appropriate antimicrobial therapy is the mainstay of the treatment.

4.3.11 Cutaneous Manifestations [42, 43]

An important part of neonatal management is skin care. The skin is a protective organ and any break in the skin may create an opportunity for infection to set in. Common skin problems in the neonate are—traumatic injuries—these may occur during instrumental delivery or following indiscriminate chemical use. Thermal injuries may occur from the use of warming devices. Necrosis -Due to extravasation of IV solutions may cause tissue necrosis and sloughing, while prolonged use of O_2 mask or nasal tubes may result in pressure necrosis, other skin conditions - Milia are pearly white or yellow papules (sebaceous follicles) seen mainly on the nose, forehead or chin and usually disappear within few weeks of life. Neonatal acne appears as raised red or white spots on the cheeks, nose and forehead, often develop within 2–4 weeks of birth, secondary to maternal androgen stimulation. It clears up on its own. Erythema toxicum is a macular, papular or occasionally vesicular rash over the face, trunk or extremities within first 48 hrs of life and is presumed to be allergenic in nature. It is self-limiting. Abnormalities of pigmentation may present as Mongolian spots, café-au-lait spots or Naevi. The baby may have diffuse hyperpigmentation or extensive or scattered hypopigmented areas on the skin. Since some of these conditions may be syndromic, diagnosis is essential. Vascular abnormalities include various hemangiomas (port wine stain, strawberry hemangiomas) which necessitate early diagnosis as they may be suggestive of a syndrome with more generalized effects. The presence of purpuric lesions on the skin may be a pointer to the presence of intrauterine or perinatal infections. Transient neonatal pustular melanosis is a benign idiopathic skin condition characterized by pustules, vesicles, and pigmented macules. Lesions are usually transient and resolve spontaneously. Infections may be bacterial or viral. Bacterial may manifest as impetigo which appear as pustular lesions, commonly on the face or at the skin folds, and are caused primarily by Streptococcus pyogenes or Staphylococcus aureus. These are highly contagious, and treatment should be prompt and aggressive with the use of topical antibiotic for local skin care, and systemic antibiotics for more fulminant lesions.

4.3.12 Central Nervous System

(i) **Congenital CNS malformations** are caused by either isolated or a combined array of genetic and environmental factors. Common amongst these are NTD. This is described in a separate chapter.

(ii) **Intra Ventricular Hemorrhage (IVH)** is a highly fatal condition from bleeding in the subependymal germinal matrix which may be induced by fluctuations in the cerebral blood flow, increase in cerebral venous pressure, defects in coagulation, qualitative, or quantitative defects in platelet function or due to certain vascular defects. This causes cerebral parenchymal destruction which is in turn is responsible for the associated increased mortality and in case of survivors to seizures, cerebral palsy, mental retardation, and hydrocephalus. This is more common in preterm babies (<32 weeks), but may occur in term neonates with trauma or perinatal asphyxia. Treatment is symptomatic and supportive.

(iii) **Seizures** [44, 45] is the most distinctive manifestation of an underlying cerebral or biochemical abnormality. The incidence is inversely proportional to GA and BW, being twice as common in preterms. Neonatal seizures describe the occurrence of stereotyped muscular activity or autonomic changes secondary to abnormal electric discharges in the neonatal CNS. They are classified according to their clinical presentation and may be **Subtle seizures** (commonest, mild twitching of limbs, fixation of the eyes, repeated lip movements, tachycardia or bradycardia or occasionally with apnea, which may be missed sometimes), **Clonic seizures** (may be limited to one side of the body and may present as rhythmic movements of certain muscle groups), **Tonic seizures** (generalized or focal, may involve more sustained contraction of the muscles of the limbs and autonomic changes), and **Myoclonic seizures** (worst prognosis with regard to development of neurological sequelae and seizure recurrence) manifest as quick jerky movements produced by episodic contractions of limb muscles. The causes include perinatal complications (HIE), metabolic causes (hypoglycemia, hypocalcemia, hypomagnesemia, and IEsM), infections (meningitis, TORCH), ICH, developmental defects (hydrocephalus, microcephaly, microgyria, and porencephaly), maternal drug withdrawal, accidental injection of LA into fetal scalp, drug toxicity (phenothiazine), and dyselectrolytemia). Diagnosis is by a detailed antenatal, natal, and postnatal and family history, various laboratory investigations, imaging studies, and EEG. Treatment must be prompt. The neonate is nursed in a thermoneutral environment, airway is kept patent and necessary circulatory, and respiratory support provided. After collection of all relevant samples, the metabolic parameters are attended to, and correction of hypoglycemia, hypocalcemia and hypomagnesemia addressed. The occurrence of seizure activity makes use of antiepileptic drugs (AED) mandatory, first choice being phenobarbitone. If, however, seizures persist then midazolam or lidocaine, and second line AEDs are brought into play. In case of pyridoxine dependency, injectable pyridoxine is administered. Exchange transfusion may be resorted to in overwhelming metabolic disorders, bilirubin encephalopathy, or accidental injection of LA. Phenobarbitone and other AEDs are continued till seizures are controlled and baby appears neurologically normal. However, if abnormal neurological signs persist, AEDs are continued and the baby reassessed at monthly intervals.

4.3.13 Cardiovascular System

Many neonatal CVS issues have been dealt with in other chapters in this book, so we shall focus on those CVS problems which have remained untouched so far (**shock**, **hypertension**).

(i) **Shock** [46–48] is an acute state of pathophysiological dysfunction due to inadequate and ineffective tissue perfusion. Though initially reversible, persistent tissue hypoperfusion may progress to a state of decompensation which is ultimately fatal. Shock may manifest with signs of tissue hypoperfusion (cold extremities, cyanosis, and prolonged CRT), hypotension, initial tachycardia progressing to end stage bradycardia, tachypnea, apnea, oliguria, hypotonia, and gradually increasing poor responsiveness.

Note: The recognition of hypotension in the neonate is important to prevent the secondary effects of cerebral ischemia or IVH. Treatment besides being prompt must be aggressive. In neonates, the BP varies according to the BW, GA and postnatal age. An arbitrary range of the normal systolic BP in preterm ranges between 50 and 62 mmHg and diastolic between 26–36 mmHg. In term babies, a systolic BP of 70 mmHg with a diastolic of 44 mmHg is considered normal. Shocks are classified into five types—(a) hypovolemic, (b) cardiogenic, (c) obstructive, (d) septic, and (e) distributive (*secondary to impairment of the vascular tone as is seen in sepsis and anaphylaxis*). Various causes attributed are blood loss (IVH, abruptio placenta), congenital cardiac defects, birth asphyxia, pneumothorax, severe anemia, hypoxic ischemic cardiac/pulmonary injury, fulminant sepsis, and DIC. Treatment is preventive. Once the signs of shock appear, management should be aggressive since reversal of secondary complications is extremely difficult. Establishment of adequate tissue perfusion and oxygenation is the goal of therapy with administration of fluids, appropriate blood products, and vasopressor infusion.

(ii) **Hypertension** [49–51] is seen in 3% of NICU admissions, and is usually secondary to cardiac or renal cause. In a term neonate a systolic of >90 mmHg with diastolic >60 mmHg, while in a preterm, a systolic >80 mmHg with diastolic >50 mmHg, is labeled as hypertension. Clinical features may be nonspecific, such as feeding difficulties, tachycardia, tachypnea, apnea, hematuria, lethargy, skin mottling, and rarely seizures. Causes of neonatal hypertension are listed as renal (renal artery stenosis, acute tubular necrosis, polycystic kidney disease, hydronephrosis, renal artery thromboembolism secondary to umbilical catheterization, renal cortical necrosis secondary to asphyxia or polycythemia, obstructive uropathy and renal tumors), CVS (coarctation of aorta, abdominal aortic atresia), endocrinal (CAH, hyperaldosteronism, hyperthyroidism, hypercalcemia and SIADH (syndrome of inappropriate secretion of ADH), and drug induced (aminophylline). Investigations include assessment of renal functions, TFT (thyroid function test), plasma rennin activity, cortisol, 17-OHP (hydroxy progesterone), aldosterone levels, Xray chest, renal USG and Echocardiography.

  Treatment depends on the severity and cause of hypertension. Medications include Beta blockers, ACE inhibitors, diuretics, and calcium channel blockers.

  Note: Coarctation of aorta is suspected when femoral pulses cannot be palpated, and arm BP is higher than in the legs. While treating hypertension it is important to avoid drastic falls in the BP during drug therapy.

4.3.14 Respiratory System

(i) **RDS** [52, 53] is one of the more common causes of NICU admission, with an incidence as high as 30% in preterm, 21% in post-term and 4% in term neonates. The National Neonatal Perinatal Database of India (NNPD) defines respiratory distress as the presence of any two of the three features—RR >60/min, subcostal/intercostals recession, and expiratory grunt/groaning. Additional features are nasal flaring and suprasternal retraction. RDS occurrence is largely dependent on the gestational age, surfactant deficiency (in preterm), and Transient Tachypnea of Newborn (TTN) (in post-term and term neonates). *RDS is discussed in another chapter of this book.*

(ii) **Apnea** is defined as cessation of breathing associated with bradycardia (HR<80 bpm) and changes in skin color (pallor/cyanosis). This pause in breathing may extend to 20 sec or more. Apnea may be a manifestation of immaturity of the respiratory system as seen in preterms or it may be a feature of other neonatal problems. Occurrence of apnea prompts immediate intervention in the form of ensuring airway patency, O_2 administration, treatment of the underlying cause, and other supportive measures.

(iii) **Bronchopulmonary dysplasia (BPD)** [54, 55] is a chronic lung disease of neonates predominantly preterms who require assisted ventilation and or O_2

therapy. BPD may develop due to several causes, prematurity being most important, others being mechanical ventilation, O_2 therapy, infections, cardiac defects (PDA), and genetic factors. Positive pressure ventilation (PPV) with high FiO_2 predisposes the immature lung to oxidative stress and barotrauma followed by defective lung repair. The presence of inflammation due to underlying infections worsens lung injury. Neonate may present with rapid shallow respiration, which may be paradoxical, and coarse crepitations and rhonchi on auscultation. Diagnosis is confirmed by radiological evidence of generalized haziness with occasional areas of pneumonic infiltrates or segmental atelectasis. Prevention forms an important part of **management**, with antenatal steroids to mothers at risk for premature labor. In the labor room, delayed cord clamping, early use of CPAP and selective use of surfactant, plays an important role in the reducing the severity and incidence of BPD. Time targeted O_2 use for resuscitation is also beneficial. Early initiation of parenteral feeding with rapid switch to enteral feeds also has a protective effect. Newer ventilation strategies are being adopted in the management of BPD. Surfactant, Vitamin A, methylxanthine, and steroids are the mainstay of preventional pharmacological strategies. Treatment is aimed at maintaining sufficient ventilation with minimal support, in which early CPAP plays an important role. When mechanical ventilation becomes imminent, regular titrating of the settings to minimize lung trauma is important. Pharmacological therapy forms a part of the treatment of established BPD. Significant morbidity with the development of asthma like symptoms and other compromised lung functions are the long-term sequelae in babies who recover from BPD.

4.3.15 Liver and GIT

(i) **Neonatal jaundice or hyperbilirubinemia** [56, 57] is the most common morbidity in the neonates in the 1st week of life, occurring in 60% of term and 80% of preterm babies. It is visible as a yellow staining of the skin and eyes resulting from an increase in the total bilirubin beyond 5 mg/dL. Detection and monitoring of jaundice are important since hyperbilirubinemia can have adverse effects and induce bilirubin encephalopathy. Pathogenesis of neonatal jaundice is explained by three main factors—increased bilirubin production due to larger volume and shorter life span of fetal RBCs, immature hepatic functions which is responsible for reduced hepatic uptake, conjugation and bilirubin clearance, and bilirubin reabsorption by the enterohepatic circulation.

Physiological jaundice is a normal occurrence in the nearly 60% term and 70% preterm neonates and is due to the physiological immaturity of the newborn to handle high bilirubin load. Detectable jaundice appears by 30–72 hrs, peaks by days 3–4 to a maximum of 12 mg/dL and then starts declining. In preterm babies the onset is similar, the peak is higher (15 mg/dL), appears slightly later (days 5–7), and decline is more gradual. Diagnosis is based on the time of appearance of jaundice, peak level, time of decline, and absence of pathological factors. **Pathological Jaundice** is defined as total bilirubin level more than 5 mg/dL in 24 hrs (beyond physiological limits). The distinction between physiological and pathological jaundice is arbitrary and the two conditions frequently overlap. Causes attributed are—blood-related (Feto maternal blood incompatibility, hereditary spherocytosis/ elliptosis, non-spherocytic hemolytic anemias, G6PD/pyruvate kinase deficiency, alpha thalassemia, drug-induced hemolysis, hematomas, cerebral or pulmonary hemorrhage, and polycythemia, metabolic and endocrine (galactosemia, familial nonhemolytic jaundice types 1and 2, Gilbert's disease, hypothyroidism, tyrosinosis, infants of diabetic mothers, hypermethioninemia, and hypopituitarism), Obstructive (biliary atresia, dubin johnson/rotor's syndrome, choledochal cyst, pyloric stenosis, intestinal atresia/stenosis, meconium plug syndrome, and Hirschsprung's disease), and Others (sepsis, intrauterine infections, RDS, HIE, and breast milk jaundice). Clinical assessment should be done 12 hrly intervals in hospital admitted babies and reassessed within 48 h postdischarge. Any doubt in the clinical assessment should be confirmed by a laboratory measurement of the total serum bilirubin. At risk neonates, should be kept under enhanced surveillance, such as preterm/SGA/IDM neonates, babies with a large cephalhematoma or significant bruising, newborn's with ABO/Rh incompatibility or G6PD deficiency, babies with siblings with history of significant jaundice, and a rate of rise of total bilirubin >5 mg/dL per day. Clinical tests are done in both the mother and the baby and depending on the level of the unconjugated bilirubin fraction further treatment suggested. Hospitalization and double surface phototherapy are offered to babies with the bilirubin level above the age specific cutoff. If however, the unconjugated bilirubin fraction is in the critical range or the neonate shows signs of bilirubin encephalopathy then a double volume exchange transfusion is done. In all cases, other supportive and specific treatment is continued.

Note: AAP (American Academy of Pediatrics) has laid down age specific nomograms for phototherapy and exchange transfusion which are referred to for deciding the treatment to be followed in jaundiced neonates.

Direct or unconjugated hyperbilirubinemia occurs due to ineffective or failed excretion of conjugated bilirubin into the duodenum. The level of conjugated bilirubin is >2 mg/dL. It may develop due to damage to the liver cells by infective/toxic or metabolic factors or due to obstruction in the bile flow, due to **extra or intrahepatic biliary atresia (EHBA).** EHBA results from obstruction or stenosis of the extrahepatic biliary tree and accounts for 25–30% cases of neonatal cholestasis. In the absence of medical or surgical intervention, the disease progresses rapidly to liver failure and death within 2–3 years. Primary treatment of EHBA is surgical and if applied early may effectively restore bile flow from the liver to the intestines. Liver transplant may be lifesaving in infants in whom this surgery fails.

Kernicterus or bilirubin encephalopathy occurs when unconjugated bilirubin crosses the blood brain barrier and gains access into the neonates' brain leading to varying degrees of neuronal injury. The unconjugated bilirubin level at which kernicterus occurs varies. However, the presence of Rh/ABO incompatibility along with family history of RBC abnormalities add to the increased risk of development of pathological hyperbilirubinemia. Clinical features include lethargy, refusal of feeds, a shrill cry, opisthotonus, rigidity, sensory–neural deafness, visual abnormalities, and convulsions.

Prevention of neurotoxicity is the bottom line in the management of hyperbilirubinemia. Exchange transfusion remains the undisputed definitive mode of clearing blood of bilirubin.

(ii) **Necrotizing Enteroclitis (NEC)** [58–60] is one of the common GIT emergencies seen in the NICU. It generally occurs in premature formula fed neonates, by about 2–3 weeks age. It has also been seen in term and border line term babies. It results from damage to the intestinal tract, ranging from mucosal injury to full thickness necrosis and perforation. Depending on the severity of the intestinal damage, mortality rate may even go up to 50%. Clinical features include abdominal distension, erythema of abdominal wall, increased gastric aspirate, signs of peritonitis, and bloody diarrhea. There may be respiratory distress with frequent episodes of apnea/bradycardia, temperature fluctuations, pallor, hypo/hyperglycemia, and bleeding from various sites. Along with biochemical investigations, abdominal radiography helps in confirming the diagnosis with demonstration of Pneumatosis Intestinalis. Treatment is initially medical with the stoppage of oral feeds, gastric decompression, aggressive antibiotic therapy, and CVS and respiratory support. Development of pneumoperitoneum (indicative of intestinal perforation) makes surgical treatment mandatory.

(iii) **Intestinal obstruction** is one of the most frequent neonatal emergencies with an incidence of 1:2000 live births, and includes gastric outlet obstruction, duodenal obstruction, intestinal malrotation and atresia, Hirschsprung's disease, and anorectal malformations.

These are dealt with in detail in a separate chapter.

4.4 Conclusion

The immaturity of many organ systems and metabolic processes together with the "circulation in transition" in the neonate, more particularly the preterm neonate make the administering of anesthesia in these small human beings a more than usual risky proposition. The commonly encountered medical issues which need to be carefully looked into while planning any invasive/surgical procedure have been enumerated in the earlier pages. This discussion on anesthesia relevant medical issues in the neonate will help in guiding upcoming neonatal anesthetists in ensuring the administration of "safe" and effective anesthesia to these precious little souls.

References

1. Definition of term pregnancy. ACOG Committee Opinion No.579. Obstet Gynecol. 2013;122:1139–40. https://www.acog.org › clinical › articles › 2013/11 › d.
2. Diagnosis and Management of Fetal Growth Restriction. SMFM recommendations 2012. https://www.smfm.org › publications › 289-smfm-cons… https://www.smfm.org › publications › 289-smfm-cons…

3. Preterm or early term delivery. WIC-Minnesota Department of Health. 142(pdf); 2019. https://www.health.state.mn.us > nutrition > riskcodes > antrhro (pdf)

4. Rosenberg AA. Traumatic birth injury. NeoReviews. 2003;4(10):e270–6.

5. Uhing MR, Management of birth injuries. Clin Perinatol. 2005;32:19–38.

6. Moczygemba CK, Paramsothy P, Meikle S, etal. Route of delivery and Neonatal birth trauma. Am J Obstet Gynacol 2010; 202:361.e1-361.e6

7. Abdulhayoglu E, Birth trauma Chapter 6. In Cloherty, Eichenwald, Hansen, Stark manual of neonatal care, 7th ed., pp. 63–73, SAE, LWW; 2012.

8. Hansen AR, Eichenwald EC, Stark AR, Martin CR. Birth injuries. In Cloherty and Stark's manual of neonatal care, 8th ed.; 2016.

9. Hansen AR, Soul JS. Perinatal asphyxia and HIE. Chapter 55, Cloherty, Eichenwald, Hansen, Stark, manual of neonatal care, 7th ed. pp. 711–789. SAE, LWW; 2012.

10. Levene MI. The asphyxiated newborn infant. Fetal and neonatal neurology and neurosurgery. Edinburgh: Churchill Livingstone; 1995. p. 405–26.

11. Thompson CM, et al. The value of a scoring system for hypoxic encephalopathy in predicting neurodevelopmental outcome. Acta Paediatr. 1997;86:757.

12. Robert C, Finer N. Term infants with HIE: outcome at 3.5 years. Dev Med Child Neurol. 1985;27:473–84.

13. Agarwal R, Deorari A. Neonatal Asphyxia/HIE. AIIMS protocols in neonatology.pdf. online 26 sept 2021.

14. WHO fact sheet on congenital anomalies 1 December 2020. https://www.who.int/news-room/fact-sheets/detail/congenital-anomalies.

15. Congenital Anomalies- Definitions| CDC https://www.cdc.gov.>chapters>chapter-1>chapter1-44

16. Jones KL. Smith's Recognizable patterns of Human Malformations. 6th ed. Philadelphia: Elsivier Saunders; 2006.

17. Jeanmonod R, Asuka E, Jeanmonod D. Inborn errors of metabolism. In: StatPearls [Internet]. Treasure Island (FL): StatPearls Publishing; 2021 Jan.2021 Jul 20.

18. Ayman W. El Hattab, V. Reid Sutton. Inborn errors of metabolism, Chapter 6, Cloherty, Eichenwald, Hansen, Stark, manual of neonatal care, 7th ed, pp. 767–789, SAE, LWW.

19. Behrman ER, Kliegman R, Jensen H, etal. Metabolic diseases. In Nelson textbook of pediatrics.16th ed. Philidelphia: WB Saunders; 2000.

20. National Newborn Screening and Genetic Resource Centre. http://genes-r-us.uthscsa.edu/resources/newborn/00/ch4_complete.pdf

21. Congenital Hypothyroidism. British Thyroid Foundation. https://www.btf-thyroid.org > congenital hypothyroidism

22. Rose SR, Section on Endocrinology and Committee on Genetics, American Thyroid Association, et al. Update of newborn screening and therapy for congenital hypothyroidism. Pediatrics. 2006;117(6):2290–303.

23. Congenital adrenal hyperplasia. https://www.mayoclinic.org › syc-20355205

24. Congenital adrenal hyperplasia. https://www.mayoclinic.org › drc-20355211

25. White PC, Spenser PW. Congenital adrenal hyperplasia due to 21 –hydroxylase deficiency. Endocr Rev. 2000;21(3):25–291.

26. Congenital adrenal hyperplasia -Symptoms and causes. Mayo Clinic; 2020. https://www.mayoclinic.org/diseases-conditions/congenital-adrenal...

27. Dysart KC. Neonatal Hypoglycemia—Pediatrics—MSD Manuals 2021. https://www.msdmanuals.com › professional › pediatrics.

28. Wilker RE. Hypoglycemia and hyperglycemia. Chapter 24, Cloherty, Eichenwald, Hansen, Stark manual of neonatal care, 7th ed, pp. 284–296. SAE, LWW.

29. Abrams SA. Abnormalities of serum calcium and Magnesium, Chapter 25, Cloherty, Eichenwald, Hansen, Stark manual of neonatal care, 7th ed, pp. 297–303, SAE, LWW.

30. Neonatal Anemia. https://www.ucsfbenioffchildrens.org › 37_anemia PDF.

31. Christou HA, Anemia, Chapter 45, Cloherty, Eichenwald, Hansen, Stark manual of neonatal care, 7th ed., pp. 563–570, SAE, LWW.

32. Bifano EM, Ehrenkranz Z, editors. Perinatal hematology. Clin Perinatal, 1995;23(3).

33. Iron deficiency anemia. https://www.ucsfbenioffchildrens.org/conditions/iron-deficiency-anemia

34. Agarwal R, Deorari A, Paul V, Sankar MJ, Sachdeva A, Polycythemia. chapter 33, AIIMS protocols in neonatology, Vol. 1, 2nd ed., pp. 407–414; 2019.

35. Agarwal R, Deorari A, Paul V, Sankar MJ, Sachdeva A. Approach to bleeding neonate. Chapter 32, AIIMS protocols in neonatology, Vol. 1, 2nd ed., pp. 396–406; 2019.

36. Murray M, Richardson J. Intrauterine congenital infections. In Neonatology. Core concepts of pediatrics. 2nd Ed. 1991 UTMB Health Pediatrics. Niebuhr V, Urbani MJ, editors.

37. Intrauterine (congenital) infections. https://www.utmb.edu › Neonatology › Neonatology31

38. Burchett SK. Viral infections. Chapter 48. Cloherty, Eichenwald, Hansen, Stark, manual of neonatal care, 7th ed., pp. 588–622, SAE, LWW.

39. Committee on Infectious Diseases. 2009 Red book: report of the Committee on Infectious Diseases. 28th ed. Elk Grove Village, IL: American Academy of Pediatrics; 2009.

40. Agarwal R, Deorari A, Paul V, Sankar MJ, Sachdeva A, Sepsis in the newborn. Chapter 24, AIIMS protocols in neonatology. Vol. 1, 2nd ed, pp. 303–314; 2019.

41. Wolach B. Neonatal sepsis: pathogenesis and supportive therapy. Semin Perinatol. 1997;21:28–38.

42. Izatt SD. Skin care. Chapter 34. Cloherty, Stark manual of neonatal care, 4th ed., pp. 633–642, Lippincott-Raven

43. AAP Committee on the Fetus and New Born. Guidelines for perinatal care. 3rd ed. Elk Grove, IL: ACOG Committee on Obstetrics: Maternal and Fetal Medicine; 1992.

44. Agarwal R, Deorari A, Paul V, Sankar MJ, Sachdeva A, Neonatal seizures. Chapter 8. AIIMS protocols in neonatology, Vol. 1, 2nd ed., pp. 71–86, 2019.

45. Rennie JM. Neonatal seizures. Eur J Pediatr. 1997;156:83–7.

46. Kourembanas S. Shock. In: Cloherty JP, Eichenwald EC, Stark AR, editors. Manual of Neonatal Care. 6th ed. Lippincott; 2008. p.176.

47. Neonatal shock: etiology, clinical manifestations, and evaluation. https://www.uptodate.com › contents › neonatal-shock-eti…

48. UpToDate Neonatal Shock 2018 | PDF | Shock (Circulatory) | Sepsis. https://www.scribd.com › document › UpToDate-Neonata…

49. Blood pressure disorders | Better Safer Care. https://www.bettersafercare.vic.gov.au › neonatal › blo...

50. Flynn JT. Neonatal Hypertension: diagnosis and management. Pediatr Nephrol. 2000;14:332–41.

51. Fanaroff JM. Blood pressure disorders in the neonate; 2006. https://pubmed.ncbi.nlm.nih.gov

52. Agarwal R, Deorari A, Paul V, Sankar MJ, Sachdeva A, Respiratory distress. Chapter 15, AIIMS protocols in neonatology. Vol. 1, 2nd ed., pp. 167–182; 2019.

53. Bhakta KY. Respiratory distress syndrome. Chapter 33. Cloherty, Eichenwald, Hansen, Stark, manual of neonatal care, 7th ed., pp. 406–416 SAE, LWW.

54. Agarwal R, Deorari A, Paul V, Sankar MJ, Sachdeva A, Bronchopulmonary dysplasia. Chapter 17. AIIMS protocols in neonatology. Vol. 1, 2nd ed., pp. 195–210; 2019.

55. Parad RB. Bronchopulmonary dysplasia/chronic lung disease. Chapter34. Cloherty, Eichenwald, Hansen, Stark manual of neonatal care. 7th ed., pp. 417–428. SAE, LWW.

56. Lucia M, P Gregory, Martin CR, Cloherty JP. Neonatal hyperbilirubinemia. Chapter 26. Cloherty, Eichenwald, Hansen, Stark, manual of neonatal care, 7th ed., pp. 304–339. SAE, LWW; 2012.

57. American Academy of Pediatrics Subcommittee on Hyperbilirubinemia. Management of hyperbilirubinemia in the newborn infant 35 or more weeks of gestation. Pediatrics. 2004;114:297–316.

58. Springer SC. What is necrotizing enterocolitis (NEC)? Updated: Dec 27, 2017. Ed: Muhammad Aslam.

59. Premkumar MH. Necrotizing enterocolitis. Chapter 27. Cloherty, Eichenwald, Hansen, Stark manual of neonatal care, 7th ed., pp. 340–349. SAE, LWW.

60. Necrotizing enterocolitis | Genetic and Rare Diseases Information. https://rarediseases.info.nih.gov/diseases/9767/necrotizing-enterocolitis.

Neonatal Screening for Metabolic Diseases

5

Anju Gupta and Swathi Pandurangi

5.1   Introduction

The screening of neonates for various disorders has increased over the last few decades worldwide, including in the developing countries. Metabolic disorders, such as congenital hypothyroidism (CH), congenital galactosemia, and phenylketonuria (PKU), have been immensely benefitted by mass screening. Their early detection implies that neonates will be better evaluated and controlled before they come for surgeries, emergent or elective, under general anesthesia. Knowledge of the presence of such disorders, especially in asymptomatic neonates, will embolden the anaesthesiologist with the knowledge, who will be better prepared to provide high degree of care in the perioperative period for a good postoperative outcome.

In 1960s, Guthrie introduced Guthrie's test for detection of high levels of phenylalanine, making PKU the first disorder to benefit from mass screening of newborns and neonates. Heel-prick test, cord blood sampling, and tandem mass spectrometry of dried blood spots are some of the commonly used methods of screening neonates. However, in many parts of the world, especially Asian countries, universal screening facilities are not available or are not incorporated into the regular health care system. This is attributable to large population densities, limited health care resources, and the relatively uncommon nature of these diseases. This is of particular significance, as more than 50% of neonates globally, are born into these populations [1]. More widespread screening, training health care personnel in interpreting test results, their subsequent follow-up, and allocating a fair share of health care resources to the screening of neonates will lead to a substantial increase in their

A. Gupta (✉)
Anaesthesia, Pain medicine and Critical Care, All India Institute of Medical Sciences, New Delhi, India

S. Pandurangi
Vardhman Mahavir Medical College and Safdarjung Hospital, New Delhi, India

© The Author(s), under exclusive license to Springer Nature Singapore Pte Ltd. 2023
U. Saha (ed.), *Clinical Anesthesia for the Newborn and the Neonate*,
https://doi.org/10.1007/978-981-19-5458-0_5

Table 5.1 Screening tests for various metabolic diseases of newborn

	Disease	Incidence	Screening entity	Mass screening method
1	**Congenital Hypothyroidism**	1:1000–3500	TSH and T4	ELISA kits using dried blood spots
2	**Congenital Galactosemia**	1: 60000	GALT, Galactose-1-Phosphate	Fluorometric based methods
3	**Phenylketonuria**	1:10000–20000	Phenylalanine	Tandem mass spectrometry
4	**Maple Syrup Urine Disease**	1:120000	Leucine + Isoleucine + allo-isoleucine + hydroxyproline	Tandem mass spectrometry (TMS)
5	**Congenital Adrenal Hyperplasia**	1:15000	17-hydroxyprogesterone	Fluoro immunoassay

diagnosis, thus preventing or at least reducing their long-term implications and consequences, and the quality of life of affected individuals.

Over the years, newborn screening systems have been revised by the paediatric committees and associations and updated with evolving technologies. In 1996, AAP revised neonatal screening strategies and came up with a five-part system of newborn testing (Table 5.1); follow-up of abnormal screening results to facilitate timely diagnostic testing and management; diagnostic testing; disease management, which requires coordination with the medical home and genetic counselling; and continuous evaluation and improvement of the newborn screening systems [2].

Many a times, neonates presenting to the anaesthetist, especially in an emergency, will not have a diagnosis for these diseases, and thus a sound understanding of the etiology, pathophysiology, clinical presentation, and treatment strategies, along with a high degree of suspicion, is a must for every neonatal anaesthesiologist.

5.2 Congenital Hypothyroidism (CH) and Its Anaesthetic Implications

CH, inadequate production of thyroid hormone, is the most common neonatal endocrine disorder. The most appropriate time for screening is after the 3rd day of life because of the transient high levels of TSH in the initial 48 h of birth. This can be due to either an absent, ectopic, or nonfunctioning thyroid gland. The initial elevation of TSH should not be inadvertently classified as CH and treated [3].

Neonates with CH may have associated cardiac, neurological, and ocular anomalies, making perioperative workup and management challenging for the anaesthetist. Some common syndromes associated with CH include Pendred syndrome (deafness, goitre, and hypothyroidism), Bamforth–Lazarus syndrome (hypothyroidism, cleft palate, and spiky hair), Benign chorea–hypothyroidism (brain–lung–thyroid syndrome), Kocher–Deber Semilange syndrome (muscular pseudohypertrophy and hypothyroidism) [4], and Downs syndrome [5]. As many as 11% of Downs syndrome babies have associated CH [6].

The incidence is 1 in 1000 to 1 in 3500 with regional variations [5]. Countries such as Chad, Nepal, Bangladesh, Peru, and Zaire have a higher incidence. In recent times, the incidence has increased because of improved and more widespread screening of neonates. It is twice as common in female than male neonates [3].

The various surgeries that a neonate with CH may require, include cardiac (ASD, VSD), ocular (congenital cataract and glaucoma), and for cleft lip repair [5].

5.2.1 Preanaesthetic Evaluation of a Neonate Presenting with CH

The classic features of CH are large anterior fontanelle and wide sutures, large tongue, decreased deep tendon reflexes, and umbilical hernia. Apart from these, features of associated syndromes, such as cardiac defects, congenital cataract, cleft of the lip, and palate, may be present. CH with Down's syndrome in the neonate (small head (brachycepahaly), flat face (missing nasal bone or small flat nose), large tongue, epicanthus folds, nuchal translucency, short stature, and short femur, single palmar crease (clinodactyly), hypotonia or floppy baby, developmental delays, and birth defects), pose additional anaesthetic challenges, and should not be missed during evaluation. Presence of laryngomalacia, and or subglottic stenosis require special readiness for airway-related problems [7]. Large floppy tongue makes babies susceptible to airway obstruction during sleep, apnea, and hypoxemia. This should be especially made a note of. Although rare, severe hypothyroidism may be associated with hyponatremia, cardiovascular collapse, and hypothermia [8].

Laboratory investigations include routine (CBC, LFT, KFT, and serum electrolytes) (Table 5.2), and tests specific for CH (TSH. T4, TBG, USG, thyroid antibodies, radiography, and scintigraphy, where indicated (Table 5.3). Genetic evaluation for establishment of associated syndromes is essential. The etiopathogenesis of the disease should be established, whether it is thyroid gland dysgenesis, or an inborn error of metabolism, though the treatment in both is thyroid hormone substitution. Earlier the diagnosis and initiation of treatment, better is the outcome with fewer

Table 5.2 Routine laboratory investigations

Investigation	Significance	Remarks
Complete Blood Count	Baseline haemoglobin	Anaemia is common
Kidney Function Test	Baseline values	Decreased renal clearance of drugs
Liver Function Test	Hyperbilirubinemia	Can be due to decreased excretory function [7].
Serum Electrolytes	Hyponatremia	A feature of severe hypothyroidism due to decreased Atrial Natriuretic Peptide [9].

Table 5.3 Tests specific for congenital hypothyroidism (CH)

Test	Significance	Remarks
TSH	Raised	Along with Low T4 suggestive of CH[a]
T4 (Total and Free)	Low	If TSH normal—suggests TBG deficiency
TBG	Low	TBG deficiency, has no pathological consequences, and should not be treated
THYROID USG	Absent in agenesis of thyroid gland.	Lingual/sublingual thyroid not detected. USG is good to measure thyroid dimensions
SCINTIGRAPHY (Tc[99], I[123])	Uptake of the dye if thyroid gland is present	Can detect ectopic gland tissue
ANTITHYROID ANTIBODY	Can be seen in maternal antibody mediated CH	A very rare cause
RADIOGRAPHY	Lateral X-ray of knee in term/post term infants. Absence of distal femoral epiphysis suggests prenatal hypothyroidism.	Cannot be used in preterm infants as the epiphysis occurs at 36 weeks of age

[a]TSH >40 mIU/L and T4 <85 nmol/L is suggestive of Congenital Hypothyroidism [3]

neurological complications. Thyroid dysgenesis accounts for around 80 % of the cases [3], and can be easily detected by thyroid ultrasonography, although ectopic gland may be missed. For detection of ectopic thyroid tissue, thyroid scintigraphy with Tc[99] and I[123] can be done. A bilobed thyroid gland on ultrasound, no ectopic gland, and deranged thyroid function tests, is suggestive of inborn errors in the synthesis of thyroid hormone [3].

There is increased stress on gradual correction Thyroid hormone levels, over a period of 2 weeks, prior to elective surgery, starting with 6–8 µg/kg/day, with gradual increment over 2–4 weeks, until maintenance dose is reached [8]. Emergency surgeries, however, do not give us the luxury of preoperative optimization. Invasive monitoring, and postoperative NICU bed may be required in the event of occurrence of complications such as cardiovascular instability, hypothermia, and myxoedema coma.

5.2.2 Perioperative Care of a Neonate with CH

Neonates with CH are considered as full stomach babies because of the delayed gastric emptying time. Initiating anti-aspiration prophylaxis, and anti-sialagogue medication may be considered prior to the procedure. Some cases may be associated with adrenaline insufficiency, so adequate steroid coverage is required. Securing the airway in such a patient poses unique challenges. Presence of large tongue makes laryngoscopy difficult. In addition, if cleft palate is present as seen in Lazarus syndrome, the tongue may flop over the laryngoscope and obstruct vision of the glottis. Babies with Down's syndrome, with short neck and subglottic stenosis, will need a smaller endotracheal tube [7]. Large goitre can make laryngoscopy and glottis visualisation challenging. All infusion sets and syringes must be air free due to the possible presence of an intracardiac shunt and risk of paradoxical air embolism.

Appropriate reduction of dose in anaesthetic agents should be done in CH. They generally require lower MAC, and lower doses of muscle relaxants and lower opioid doses [8], as they have lower rates of drug metabolism and excretion. Invasive monitoring may be indicated in nonoptimised neonates, as large volume shifts can lead to severe hemodynamic instability. Neuromuscular and TOF monitoring is useful for accurate dosing of neuromuscular blocking agents and is beneficial at the time of reversal. All throughout, normothermia should be maintained as they are susceptible to hypothermia, using additional warmers, infusion of warm fluids and use of warm humidified gases. All these babies must be cared for in NICU postoperatively, especially in the events of delayed awakening, hemodynamic instability requiring inotropic support [8], and stridor [10]. Non opioid analgesics are preferred [11].

With all these anaesthetic considerations, it is possible for conduct of safe anaesthesia in neonates with CH. It is imperative to further increase screening and management of CH as it is one of the most common preventable causes of mental retardation later in life [12].

5.3 Congenital Galactosemia (CG) and Its Anesthetic Implications

Congenital galactosemia is a rare metabolic disorder, genetically inherited through autosomal recessive pattern, i.e., both the parents are carriers. The culprit gene is galactose-1-phosphate uridyl transferase (GALT), and more than 230 mutations are noted. It is located on chromosome 9p13. It manifests equally in male and female babies, with incidence ranging from 1 in 60,000 in United States to 1 in 10,00,000 in Japan and is more prevalent in Europe and North America compared to Asian countries [13].

Basic defect is inability of the neonate to effectively metabolise galactose into glucose due to absence of GALT enzyme, leading to accumulation of galactose-1-phosphate (Leiloir Pathway) [14]. When partial activity of the GALT enzyme is present, it results in milder clinical symptoms, often not requiring treatment. The most common variant goes by the name of Duarte variant. Other variants, relatively uncommon and present with milder clinical picture, include Galactokinase and galactose-4-epimerase (GALE) enzyme deficiencies.

Foods that contain lactose (breaks down into galactose) and galactose include milk and milk products, breast milk, formula feeds, some fruits and vegetables, various of nuts and other food items [13]. The significance of the diagnosis of CG is that all galactose containing food items, including breast milk, must be stopped (Box 5.1). Most formula preparations contain galactose, but galactose free preparations are also available [15].

Box 5.1 Galactose and lactose containing foods
Breast milk
Bovine milk
Milk formula
Milk products: cheese, curd, butter, whey
Vegetables: artichoke, mushroom, olives, tomato, cucumber
Fruits: plum, pear, blackberry
Peanut

5.3.1 Clinical Features of CG

Neonatal galactosemia is easily picked up on screening. In many parts of the world, particularly, Asian countries, where CG is relatively rare, screening not done routinely. Symptoms usually appear after initiation of breast feeding (48–72 h of life) in the form of poor feeding, low weight gain, jaundice, vomiting, diarrhoea, lethargy, hypotonia, and easy bruisability. Other features include neonatal cataract, liver dysfunction, raised clotting time, albuminuria, haemolysis, hypoglycaemia, and sepsis, largely due to accumulation of galactose-1-phosphate in hepatic, nervous and ocular tissues. These patients have low plasma glucose levels, high plasma galactose and galactose-1-phosphate levels and increased urinary excretion of galactose, albumin, and amino acids in some patients with high levels of certain amino acids [14]. Even the slightest of doubts of CG should alert one to promptly stop breast feeding and eliminate galactose from baby's diet. The earlier it is detected, and dietary changes initiated, better is the long-term outcome. Despite utmost care with reference to diet, long-term impact of CG (impaired speech, cataract, neurological sequel, mental retardation, and seizure disorder) cannot be eliminated completely because of endogenous galactose production. Low oocyte production, delayed onset of puberty and early menopause is noted in adult females [16].

There is not much evidence of primary galactosemia having any syndromic associations. Neonatal management of CG includes mostly dietary changes, management of metabolic emergency, such as metabolic acidosis, sepsis, hypoglycaemia, hyperbilirubinemia, and dehydration due to vomiting and diarrhoea. These neonates respond well to intravenous (IV) fluids, antibiotics, and phototherapy [14]. Choosing an appropriate nonhepatotoxic antibiotic is importance [17].

There is little literature available on surgeries performed in the neonatal period in primary galactosemia patients. Often, if a cardiac or other major surgery is required, then preoperative optimization and postponement of surgery for a later date (post neonatal period) is a preferred approach [17, 18].

The chief perioperative anaesthetic concern is avoiding catabolic states. This can be achieved by keeping the fasting period to minimum and providing glucose containing IV fluids during this period [19].

Preoperative workup includes routine investigations (CBC, LFT, KFT, serum electrolytes), plasma glucose level, and coagulation profile (bleeding and clotting time) (Table 5.4).

Babies with classic galactosemia need to undergo further investigations (Table 5.5), especially where routine screening not done, there is suspicion of CG, and if serum galactose and galactose-1-phosphate levels are evaluated. A genetic evaluation to rule out cardiac and other systemic involvement is advisable. Invasive monitoring may be required for unstable patients, or those in severe sepsis. Non-invasive pulse pressure variation can also guide fluid therapy. Arterial cannulation may be considered for blood gas analysis and lactate levels in case metabolic acidosis is suspected. In such cases, avoid infusion of Ringer's lactate, as lactate does not metabolise to bicarbonate in the compromised liver. All procedures should be done under utmost aseptic precautions as these patients are particularly susceptible to infection, possibly because of high levels of galactose that may prevent neutrophil chemotaxis and chemiluminescence, essential for killing bacteria [13]. The choice of antibiotics and anaesthetic agents should be made carefully, avoiding hepatotoxic drugs to an already compromised liver [17]. Adequate blood and blood products should be reserved, even for minor surgeries because of elevated clotting

Table 5.4 Workup for a patient with primary galactosemia

Investigations	Significance	Remarks
CBC	Baseline values	Anaemia due to poor nutrition, Elevated TLC may indicate infection and sepsis
KFT	Baseline values	Drug excretion
LFT	Hyperbilirubinemia	Due to accumulation of galactase-1-phosphate in liver
CLOTTING TIME	Elevated	Risk of intraoperative bleeding, increased bruisability.
PLASMA GLUCOSE	Hypoglycemia	Galactose does not metabolise to glucose
S. ELECTROLYTES	Deranged	Fluid and electrolyte loss due to vomiting and diarrhoea, Sepsis and metabolic acidosis induced dyselectrolytemia

Table 5.5 Investigations specific to classic galactosemia

Investigation	Significance	Remarks
S. GALACTOSE	Elevated	Values >5mg/dl should prompt further evaluation [13].
GALT Assay	Insignificant level of GALT	Can be done in the prenatal period as well, by testing fibroblasts from amniotic fluid, chorionic villous biopsy. Done if sibling has primary galactosemia or any of its variants [13]
Galactose-1-phosphate	Elevated Red cell levels	>150 µmol/L indicative of primary galactosemia [16]
URINE GALACTICOL	Elevated	Is of particular importance when cataract does not resolve

time and increased chances of blood loss. Albuminuria may be present [16], so albumin binding drugs, such as barbiturates, benzodiazepines, and penicillin, should be avoided. In all cases, a postoperative NICU bed should be reserved in view of hemodynamic instability, delayed awakening due to decreased hepatic metabolism, and sepsis.

Anaesthetist encountering such a patient should bear these considerations in the perioperative period. Such diseases are rare and are often missed in the initial days of life. As screening is not universal, diagnosis may be delayed. More widespread screening can potentially detect galactosemia and its variants at an earlier stage and reduce its long-term effects.

5.4   Congenital Phenylketonuria (PKU) and Its Anesthetic Implications

The concept of testing new-born babies in large numbers was introduced by Guthrie in the 1960s for detecting high levels of phenylalanine, thus making it the first disease to benefit from neonatal screening [20]. PKU is an inborn error of metabolism. Accumulation of high levels of phenylalanine in the blood occurs due to genetic mutation encoding phenylalanine hydroxylase (PAH) enzyme that metabolises phenylalanine into tyrosine with tetrahydrobiopterase (BH4) as a cofactor. Mutation in the gene encoding BH4 can also lead to variants of PKU [21]. Phenylalanine is an essential amino acid, and is present in large number of protein rich foods.

PKU is autosomal recessive, both males and females equally affected, and with the incidence of 1 in 10,000–20,000. It is most prevalent in Caucasians [21].

Another condition worth mentioning is maternal PKU. If a pregnant woman has untreated or poorly controlled levels of phenylalanine, it crosses the placenta and has teratogenic effects on the fetus. High preconceptual levels of phenylalanine hamper normal fetal growth and development, resulting in microcephaly, facial dysmorphism, growth defects, developmental delay, and congenital heart disease. Babies born to mothers on strict diet control right from the preconceptual stage and tend to fare better than those born to mothers with poor or no diet control during pregnancy [20].

There is no treatment for PKU except for early recognition and dietary changes, with relatively good outcome, in the form of phenylalanine free diet, and addition of tyrosine and BH4 rich foods. The exact age to discontinue treatment is not standardised. Patients who are 12 years or older, do not require dietary restrictions, if blood phenylalanine levels are <600 μmols/L. [22] According to Medical Research Council, there is merit in continuing dietary restrictions well into adulthood [23].

5.4.1 Clinical Features

PKU in a newborn is detected mostly through the screening process, as it is asymptomatic in the neonatal period. However, early detection and prompt change in diet have a significant impact in the growth and development of the infant and the long-term consequences. These include various cognitive, neuropathological, and neuropsychological dysfunctions [22].

5.4.2 Perioperative Management of PKU

As screening is not prevalent in many parts of the world, the patient often presents during early childhood or adolescence, most commonly with neurodevelopmental delays, seizure disorders, and mental retardation. Teratogenic effects of maternal PKU may lead to early symptoms. The various laboratory investigations include complete blood count, Renal function tests, liver function tests, ECG. Echocardiography is done if cardiac defects are suspected. MRI brain can be considered in patients with neurological involvement. Phenylalanine levels should be evaluated in the perioperative period. (Table 5.6) The perioperative fasting should be kept to the minimum in a bid to avoid catabolic states, and continuation of the protein-restricted diet is essential [21]. Apart from fasting status, surgical stress can also increase enzymatic activity and increase in protein catabolism [24]. Check for supplementary BH4 and tyrosine in the diet. Facial dysmorphism and microcephaly can lead to difficulty in securing the airway. Perioperative genetic evaluation can rule out other syndromic involvement. Short acting drugs such as propofol and remifentanyl are preferred for providing high controllability and early recovery. Adequate depth and analgesia also reduce surgical stress and thus prevent increase in phenylalanine levels by decreasing protein catabolism [24].

Table 5.6 Investigations in a case of phenylketonuria (PKU)

Investigation	Remarks	
Complete Blood Count	Baseline values	
Renal Function Tests	Baseline values	
Liver Function Tests	Baseline values	
ECG/Echocardiography	To rule out Congenital cardiac disease	
MRI Brain	To rule out structural brain involvement	
Phenylalanine Levels	<600 µmol/L	Hyperphenylalanemia
	600–1200 µmol/L	Mild PKU
	>1200 µmol/L	Classic PAH deficiency [20]

The Medical Research Council recommends that neonates should be screened by 20 days of life or earlier, if possible. The outcome of adhering to dietary restrictions is relatively good, and in some cases may even lead to a normal adulthood. Thus, the more widespread screening of this disease becomes important. The challenges for the anaesthetist remain manyfold, but a sound understanding of the disease, its pathogenesis, and associated conditions, can lead to a safe perioperative experience for these patients.

5.5   Maple Syrup Urine Disease (MSUD) and Anesthetic Implications

MSUD is an autosomal recessive inborn error of metabolism, where there is deficiency of the enzyme branched chain alpha ketoacid dehydrogenase kinase (BCKDK) [25]. In its classic form, there is complete absence, and in the variants, there is varying deficiency of BCKDK. The incidence is 1 in 1,20,000. Neonates are not universally screened [26].

The absence of BCKDK leads to accumulation of branched chain amino acids leucine, isoleucine, and valine, and their toxic metabolites. Symptoms usually present within 48 h to 1 week of life [25]. The disease gets its name because of the maple syrup, such as odour of the urine. Early detection and initiation of protein restricted diet reduce the neurological and metabolic sequel. If untreated, dangerous levels of Leucine accumulate, leading to severe metabolic acidosis, hypoglycaemia, cerebral edema, seizures, dystonia, and neurodevelopmental delays. Due to protein restricted diet, patients are often malnourished [26].

Perioperative evaluation includes thorough assessment of metabolic status of the patient, and it is important to minimise stress of surgery and catabolic states. Fasting times are to be kept to the minimum and careful selection of the choice of fluids. Use of specialised dextrose containing TPN should be used in the perioperative period [25]. Glucose containing fluids are preferred to prevent hypoglycemia. While using hypertonic dextrose to maintain hydration and prevent hypoglycemia, conservative fluid management can reduce the risk of overhydration and cerebral edema [27]. Hypotonic solutions should be avoided to prevent cerebral edema [25]. Arterial cannulation may be justified as repeated blood gas sampling is required for monitoring perioperative metabolic acidosis. Intraoperative monitoring includes ECG, NIBP, and SpO2. There is no evidence that any particular anaesthetic agent is contraindicated, so agents should be selected on case-to-case basis [26]. Short acting drugs are preferred to minimise the total anaesthetic period. Drugs that may increase intracranial pressure and precipitate seizures should be avoided [27]. Postoperatively, babies must be kept in NICU.

There is little literature available on surgeries performed in the neonatal period. In a case report, a 2-month infant diagnosed with MSUD at 14 days of life underwent peritoneal dialysis to wash out excess branched chain amino acids [27]. Domino liver transplantation, i.e., donor liver from MSUD patient, is transplanted into a patient with end-stage liver disease, expecting it to function normally in the recipient, as they do not have the genetic defect [25].

5.6   Congenital Adrenal Hyperplasia (CAH) and Anesthetic Implications

CAH is an autosomal recessive condition with deficiency of one of the five enzymes responsible for synthesis of cortisol and aldosterone from cholesterol. In 90% cases, 21 hydroxylase deficiency is present. Its incidence is 1 in 15,000 [28], and is seen equally in males and females.

Female babies are usually born with ambiguous genitalia, whereas male babies appear to be normal. By the first to fourth week of life an undetected case of CAH can present with severe salt wasting, hyponatremia, hyperkalaemia, vomiting, diarrhoea, and shock [29].

Perioperative management is challenging. As there is no universal screening for CAH, there is no standard steroid replacement protocol. The challenge lies in minimising stress of surgery and sickness and identifying signs of adrenal insufficiency. Usual procedures in the neonate are cystoscopy, vaginal reconstruction, and hypospadias [28]. Undetected CAH can also present with acute abdomen requiring exploratory laparotomy [8]. It is essential to get a complete blood count, baseline renal and liver function tests, serum electrolytes, and preoperative cortisol levels. Fasting should be kept to the minimum, and catabolic states need to be avoided. Steroid coverage the night before surgery, and post induction is essential. The recommended dose varies among practitioners and institutes. One study recommends methyl prednisolone 10 mg/m^2/dose [28]. The goal is to minimise surgical stress. Standard monitoring includes ECG, SpO$_2$, and EtCO$_2$. Invasive arterial BP monitoring may be justified, to identify hypotension as a sign of adrenal crisis intraoperatively. A close lookout for bradycardia and hypotension as a sign of adrenal crisis may warranty an additional dose of steroid intraoperatively. Short acting anaesthetic agents should be used. Etomidate is known to cause adrenal suppression and should be avoided [28]. It is advisable to reserve a bed in NICU for such patients, as close postoperative monitoring is required, to detect signs of adrenal crisis.

5.7   Conclusion

Inborn errors are relatively rare diseases. More widespread screening, training health care personnel in interpreting test results, and their subsequent follow-up, and allocating a fair share of health care resources to the screening of neonates will lead to a substantial increase in diagnosing these diseases, and thus reducing their long-term implications and improving the quality of life of affected neonates. These neonates may present to the anaesthetist, either for emergency or for routine procedures. Hence, a sound understanding of the etiology, pathophysiology, clinical presentation, and treatment initiation strategies, along with a high degree of suspicion, is a must for every anaesthetist.

References

1. Padilla CD, Therrell BL Jr. Consolidating newborn screening efforts in the Asia Pacific region: networking and shared education. J Community Genet. 2012;3(1):35–45.
2. Kaye CI, Committee on Genetics, Accurso F, La Franchi S, Lane PA, Hope N, Sonya P, et al. Newborn screening fact sheets. Pediatrics. 2006;118(3):e934–63.
3. Daniel MS, Bowden SA. Congenital hypothyroidism workup. Medscape. Oct 14, 2017.
4. Rastogi MV, LaFranchi SH. Congenital hypothyroidism. Orphanet J Rare Dis. 2010;5:17.
5. Prakash KS, James JN, Kumar K, Chandy TT. Anaesthetic considerations in a prematurely born infant with congenital hypothyroidism presenting for cataract surgery. South Afr J Anaesth Analg. 2013;19(2):127–9.
6. Razavi Z, Yavarikia A, Torabian S. Congenital anomalies in infant with congenital hypothyroidism. Oman Med J. 2012;27(5):364–7.
7. Gregory GA, Claire B. Neonatology for anesthesiologists. In: Davis PJ, Cladis FP, Motoyama EK, editors. Smith's anesthesia for infants and children. 8th ed. Elsevier; 2011.
8. Maxwell GL, Goodwin SR, Mancuso TJ, Baum VC, et al. Systemic disorders. In: Davis PJ, Cladis FP, Motoyama EK, editors. Smith's anesthesia for infants and children. 8th ed. Elsevier; 2011.
9. Ellis D. Regulation of fluids and electrolytes. In: Davis PJ, Cladis FP, Motoyama EK, editors. Smith's anesthesia for infants and children. 8th ed. Elsevier; 2011.
10. Vavilala MS, Soriano SG. Anesthesia for neurosurgery. In: Davis PJ, Cladis FP, Motoyama EK, editors. Smith's anesthesia for infants and children. 8th ed. Elsevier; 2011.
11. Landsman IS, Werkhaven JA, Motoyama EK. Anesthesia for pediatric otorhinolaryngologic surgery. In: Davis PJ, Cladis FP, Motoyama EK, editors. Smith's anesthesia for infants and children. 8th ed. Elsevier; 2011.
12. Agrawal P, Philip R, Saran S, Gutch M, Razi MS, etal. Congenital hypothyroidism. Indian J Endocrinol Metab 2015;19(2):221-227.
13. Grady NEG, Millard D. Congenital galactosemia. NeoReviews. 2017;18(4):e228–33.
14. Berry GT. Chapter 55. Disorders of galactose metabolism. In: Rosenberg RN, Pascual JM, editors. Rosenberg's molecular and genetic basis of neurological and psychiatric disease. 5th ed. Academic Press; 2015. p. 615–26.
15. Gross KC, Acosta PB. Fruits and vegetables are a source of galactose: Implications in planning the diets of patients with galactosaemia. J Inherit Metab Dis. 1991;14:253–8. https://doi.org/10.1007/BF01800599.
16. Walter JH, Collins JE, Leonard JV. Recommendations for the management of galactosaemia. Arch Dis Childhood. 1999;80:93–6.
17. Choudhury A, Das S, Kiran U. Anaesthetic management of a newborn with galactosaemia for congenital heart surgery. Indian J Anaesth. 2009;53(2):219–22.
18. Banerjee A, Yee J, Sood V. A case report of a newborn with hypergalactosemia and congenital intrahepatic portosystemic shunt. Pediatrics. 2018;142. (1 Meeting Abstract 477).
19. Trapani L. Anesthesia for children with inborn errors of metabolism: opening up the black box. International Anesthesia Research Society; 2018.
20. Lee PJ, Ridout D, Walter JH, Cockburn F. Maternal phenylketonuria: report from the United Kingdom Registry 1978-97. Arch Dis Child. 2005;90(2):143–6.
21. Kumari JP, Nalin C, Abhinav P. A case report: phenylketonuria in a one-year-old child from India. Int Arch Integr Med. 2017;4(9):195–206.

22. van Wegberg AMJ, MacDonald A, Ahring K, et al. The complete European guidelines on phenylketonuria: diagnosis and treatment. Orphanet J Rare Dis. 2017;12(1):162.
23. Narayanan D, Barski R, Henderson MJ, Luvai A, etal. Delayed diagnosis of phenylketonuria: a case report of two siblings. Ann Clin Biochem 2014; 51(Pt 3):406-408.
24. Matsushita Y, Momota Y, Kishimoto N, Junichiro K. Dental management under general anesthesia in an intellectually disabled adult patient with phenylketonuria. J Dental Sci. 2013;8:96–7.
25. Scott VL II, Wahl KM, Soltys K, Belani KG, et al. Anesthesia for organ transplant. In: Davis PJ, Cladis FP, Motoyama EK, editors. Smith's anesthesia for infants and children. 8th ed. Elsevier; 2011.
26. Karahan MA, Sert H, Havlioğlu İ, Yüce HH. The anaesthetic management of a patient with maple syrup urine disease. Turk J Anaesthesiol Reanim. 2014;42(6):355–7.
27. Fuentes-Garcia D, Falcon-Arana L. Perioperative assessment of supracondylar fracture in a patient affected with maple syrup urine disease. Br J Anaesth. 2008;101, Issue eLetters Supplement.
28. Baş SŞ. General anesthesia for congenital adrenal hyperplasia: a single institution's experience. Pediatric Anesth Crit Care J. 2019;7(2):47–52.
29. Wilson TA, Bowden SA. Congenital adrenal hyperplasia. Medscape. 2020; Oct 06.

Ophthalmological Surgical Conditions in the Newborn and Neonate

6

Siddharth Madan and Sarita Beri

6.1 Introduction

Eye is aptly labeled as a window to the body. It is among the most important of the basic senses that an individual possesses [1]. Loss of vision can have huge effects on the quality of life of a person. Therefore, tackling these diseases in the neonatal period is of utmost importance [2, 3]. The eye of a newborn baby differs from that in infants and adults in various aspects (Table 6.1).

Any intervention in a neonate and newborn raises a call for general anesthesia and vigilant monitoring. A preanesthetic evaluation (PAE) for medical and surgical fitness and clearance for administration of anesthesia is indispensible. Some ophthalmic conditions may have accompanying systemic comorbidities that make administration of anesthesia more challenging and difficult. This involves a battery of investigations as advised by the attending anesthesiologist, which may be time consuming. Moreover, various drugs used for anesthesia may have potential effects on the IOP and other toxicities that should be kept in mind.

6.1.1 Ophthalmic Conditions of Importance in the Neonatal Period that Require Anesthetic Attention, Include

1. Congenital cataract
2. Congenital glaucoma
3. Retinopathy of prematurity (ROP)

S. Madan
Department of Ophthalmology, UCMS and GTB Hospital, New Delhi, India

S. Beri (✉)
Department of Ophthalmology, Lady Hardinge Medical College, SSK and Kalawati Saran Children's Hospitals, New Delhi, India

85

Table 6.1 Comparison of the Eye of a Newborn, Infant and Adult

	At Birth	Infancy	Adult
Orbital Volume	7 cc	16 cc	30 cc
Ocular Volume	2.8 cc	3.9 cc	6.8 cc
Palpebral fissure (Horizontal)	17 mm	23.5 mm	27 mm
Corneal thickness	581 microns	530 microns	510 microns
(Mean Keratometry)	55 D	47.5 D	43 D
Lens Thickness	3.2 mm	3.4 mm	4 mm
Optic nerve length	24 mm		30 mm
Refraction	−4 to +6 D	−3 to +5 D	Emmetropization
Axial Length	16.8 mm	20.19 mm	23 mm
IOP	7.8–11.4 mmHg	10–15 mmHg	12–21 mmHg

4. Retinoblastoma
5. Child abuse and shaken baby syndrome and vitreous hemorrhage
6. Coloboma of the eyelid
7. Congenital dacryocystitis
8. Cryptophthalmos and Ankyloblehpheron
9. Congenital entropion
10. Keratomalacia, corneal ulceration, and
11. Trauma

6.2 Congenital Cataract

Congenital cataract may occur in isolation or associated with other congenital conditions. Childhood cataract accounts for 7.4–15.3% of childhood blindness and a significant amount of preventable disability-adjusted life years, with a prevalence of 1.03/10,000 children (0.32–22.9/10,000) and annual incidence of 1.8–3.6/10,000 [4]. In high-income economies' prevalence rate is 0.42–2.05 compared to 0.63–13.6 in low-income economies per 10,000 children. There is no difference in prevalence of cataract based on laterality or gender [5]. India has around 280,000–320,000 visually impaired children [6, 7]. It is associated with ocular abnormalities in 27% of cases and with systemic abnormalities in 22% of cases. The diagnosis is incidental, made on routine screening in 41% of cases, whereas leukocoria and strabismus are pointers in 24% and 19% cases, respectively. Management of pediatric cataract has changed in the past decade and there is an increasing trend toward surgical removal and implantation of an intraocular lens (IOL) in the neonatal period.

The most common cause of congenital cataract is genetic mutation with autosomal dominant pattern of inheritance in nearly 25% of cases. Other causes include chromosomal abnormalities [Down's syndrome (trisomy 21) and Edwards Syndrome (trisomy 18), Lowe syndrome], metabolic disorders [Galactosaemia (central oil-droplet like morphology of cataract), Wilson's disease, hypocalcemia, hypo/

hyperglycemia] and as part of syndromes associated with congenital infections (rubella, toxoplasmosis, cytomegalovirus, syphilis, and varicella zoster virus) [8, 9].

Clinical features include the absence of red fundal glow, nystagmus, and inability to fix and follow light. Evaluation of an underlying cardiac disease is important in newborns suffering from congenital rubella syndrome (CRS). Other manifestations of CRS include microphthalmia, glaucoma, retinopathy, iris atrophy, keratitis, and uveitis [10]. With the introduction of the measles, mumps and rubella (MMR) vaccine in 1988, the incidence of CRS has decreased significantly.

Congenital varicella syndrome due to maternal infection with varicella zoster virus in the 1st or 2nd trimester can cause cataract in about 2% babies [11]. Other features include skin lesions, neurological defects, skeletal limb deformities, microphthalmia, chorioretinitis, and optic atrophy [12]. Newborn is kept isolated from the mother until all her lesions have crusted and dried. When infection occurs near the time of delivery (5 days prior–2 days after delivery), risk of development of varicella in the newborn is considerable. Immediate treatment involves Varicella Zoster immunoglobulin and antiviral therapy (acyclovir). Cataract surgery can be undertaken once the disease becomes quiet.

Cataract may be associated with **microphthalmos**, where total axial length is 2 SD below similar age controls. In Nanophthalmos, a subtype of microphthalmos, both anterior and posterior segments are shortened, lens is enlarged and sclera is thickened. These have implications during cataract surgery as babies may have to be left aphakic with IOL implantation planned later.

Aniridia (hypoplasia or absence of iris) usually involves both eyes and is often associated with other ocular abnormalities including macular/optic nerve hypoplasia, cataract, glaucoma, and corneal opacification [13]. Sporadic aniridia exposes babies to increased risk of developing Wilm's tumor and, therefore, must be screened using serial ultrasounds of the abdomen. Treatment is in the form of lubricants, opaque contact lenses (to create an artificial pupil), and cataract surgery.

Cataract in microphthalmia is usually associated with persistent hyperplastic primary vitreous (PHPV) and requires intraoperative diathermy, need for pars plana vitrectomy along with lens extraction. In continentia pigmenti, underlying toxocariasis needs to be ruled out before proceeding with surgery as both conditions present with leukocoria (white pupillary reflex). Fundal screening is imperative under sedation or anesthesia. Other causes of leukocoria are retinoblastoma, ROP, vitreous hemorrhage, retinal detachment (RD), and persistent fetal vasculature.

Dislocation of the crystalline lens is associated with Marfan's syndrome. These babies usually have underlying cardiac disease, requiring 2-D Echo.

6.2.1 Management

Surgery is not necessary if the cataract does not obscure the visual axis. Unilateral cataracts need surgery at an earlier date as it has significant risk of development of recalcitrant amblyopia compared to bilateral cataract. Prognosis is better if cataract is diagnosed and treated before the age of 2 months. Intraoperatively in cataract surgery because of the low scleral rigidity in Paediatric age group, the anterior chamber shallows and Vitreous pressure increases, making surgery difficult. Hyperventilation during General Anesthesia helps reduce the Vitreous pressure and allows easier anterior chamber manipulation.

Staphylomas may be congenital or comorbid in high myopia, although their actual incidence in pediatric population is unknown [14]. Intraconal eye blocks in congenital cataracts or when a staphyloma defect is suspected requires extreme caution. Posterior staphyloma (defect in the scleral wall) causes outward pouching of the pigmented retina, and this increases the risk of scleral perforation during needle blocks [15]. Extraconal or sub-Tenon block are safer options.

6.3   Congenital Glaucoma

Isolated trabeculo-dysgenesis (obstruction to the pathway for aqueous outflow) is the underlying cause for primary congenital glaucoma (PCG). This rare disorder contributes to 0.01–0.04% of total blindness. Incidence of PCG is 1:10 000 to 1:20 000 in western countries. The disease usually manifests at birth or early under the age of 3 years [16]. Gene mutation in PCG shows a recessive pattern of inheritance, with CYP1B1, MYOC, and FOXC1 genes being the commonest. The risk of developing PCG is more in consanguineous marriages. A classical triad of epiphora, photophobia, and blepharospasm is observed but seldom evident in neonates. Other features are buphthalmos (large eyeball) and corneal haze or red eye. A comprehensive ophthalmic EUA is done to confirm the diagnosis and IOP measurement. Most anaesthetics reduce IOP, and injudicious anaesthesia will reduce the IOP to an extent to mask raised IOP, affecting management. Ketamine is frequently used. A slight increase in IOP may occur, but this does not much interfere with management. Sevoflurane-based anesthesia is a good alternative, but IOP reading should be taken at the beginning of the induction of anesthesia as higher concentrations (>5%) and prolonged exposure may result in underestimation of IOP.

The congenital phacomatosis, a group of neuro-oculo-cutaneous disorders that include the Sturge–Weber syndrome, neurofibromatosis, tuberous sclerosis, and von Hippel–Lindau disease are all associated with ocular lesions and need surgery at some point in the course of their disease. Seizures, intracranial, and cardiac lesions necessitate appropriate PAE. Pheochromocytoma may rarely be associated.

Regional eye blocks have shown to provide better perioperative hemodynamics and less incidence of OCR and hence beneficial in syndromic babies with comorbid cardiovascular conditions [17, 18].

6.3.1   Management

Medical treatment with topical anti-glaucoma is usually supportive. The definitive treatment is surgery in the form of goniotomy, trabeculotomy, or trabeculectomy with/without anti-fibrotic agents, such as mitomycin C. Deep sclerectomy and visco-canal-ostomy are alternative methods with satisfactory results. Glaucoma drainage implants and cyclo-destructive procedures have also been tried. The earlier detection and management of glaucoma has a good prognosis. However, the prognosis is worse when the disease presents at birth.

6.4   Retinopathy of Prematurity (ROP)

ROP is one of the most important causes of childhood blindness, worldwide, accounting for 3% of all childhood vision losses. ROP needs to be identified in the neonatal period before development of sight threatening sequel. Prematurity results in a failure of the vessels to reach the temporal periphery and increases the susceptibility of the retina to O_2 damage and halt in retinal vascularization. Newborns with a low birth weight are also susceptible to O_2-related damage as they may have increased periods of stay in the incubator. Increased metabolic demand of the eye stimulates excessive production of vascular endothelial growth factor (VEGF) that causes neovascular complications and blood vessels grow into the vitreous cavity with accompanying fibrovascular proliferation causes contraction of the latter and may cause partial or complete retinal detachment. Birth weight and gestational age are most important risk factors for ROP [19]. Other risk factors are early exposure to high levels of O_2, anaemia, sepsis, intraventricular hemorrhage (IVH), NEC, and mechanical ventilation. Differential diagnosis includes Norrie disease (inherited eye disorder leading to blindness in male babies at birth) and familial exudative vitreo-retinopathy.

6.4.1   Indications for Screening

With increasing number of NICUs and poor neonatal care, the incidence of ROP is on the rise. Early screening (2–3 week age) is recommended to enable early identification of aggressive posterior (AP-ROP), in India as per the national neonatology forum (NNF) [19]:

- Newborns ≤1750 g and/or <34 weeks
- Newborns <2000 g and 36 weeks with a bad postnatal period
- All newborns with birth weight (BW) <2000 g
- All newborns with gestational age <28 weeks or BW <1200 g

   Western screening criteria is BW <1500 g or <32 week gestation.

6.4.2   Management

Goal of management is to convert the hypoxic retina into ischemic retina and thereby reduce the aberrant neovascularization from continuing and progressing into RD.

Screening is usually under topical anesthesia, in presence of a pediatrician and anesthesiologist, as babies can go into apnea.

Topical medications used to dilate the pupils vary from place to place. Commonly used combination is of tropicamide (0.4%) and phenylephrine (2.5%), in half dose as in adults. Higher dose can result in a hypertensive episode [19]. The initial dose is given 30–60 min prior to the examination. Atropine, a potent mydriatic, can result in severe gastrointestinal effects, tachycardia, flushing, and fever.

Topical local anesthetic application, just before the examination, helps reduce pain and discomfort of the corneal and conjunctiva from the bright light of the ophthalmoscope. Proparacaine is commonly used but excessive instillation can weaken the intercellular attachments of the corneal epithelium resulting in corneal haze. Administration of paracetamol or oral sucrose provides additional analgesia, but repetitive sucking by the infant can make the procedure difficult.

Treatment depends upon the progression and stage of ROP and zones involved:

i. **Cryosurgery** or cryotherapy was the initial treatment modality, but it was painful and was associated with significant postoperative pain and discomfort from conjunctival swelling. Hence, it was done under general anesthesia. Cryotherapy is not used anymore due to its complications.

ii. **Laser photocoagulation** is the gold standard of treatment today. It is performed under topical anesthesia, sedation or general anesthesia depending on the ophthalmologist, the stability, and cooperativeness of the baby. It is less painful and lasts approximately 30–40 min per eye. Babies are sensitive to the burns themselves, but the procedure also is stressful as it involves manipulation of the globe and discomfort with the bright light of the indirect ophthalmoscope, which predisposes them to development of apnea and bradycardia. Hence, it is important to monitor SpO_2 throughout the procedure [20–22]. General anesthesia reduces the procedure time, but comes with the usual complications. Sedation (e.g., chloral hydrate) and morphine (0.5 mg/kg) may be used.

iii. **Anti-VEGF treatment** promotes rapid regression of acute-phase of ROP, allows potential for retinal vascularization, approaches eyes with a rigid pupil, and minimizes stress of laser to the baby [19, 23, 24]. These potential benefits are a reason for their growing popularity in the management of ROP.

iv. Other treatment options include **vitreoretinal surgery** for severe ROP, under general anesthesia.

6.5   Retinoblastoma

Retinoblastoma, though rare, is the most common intraocular malignancy of childhood, contributing to 3% of all childhood cancers [25]. The peak incidence is in under 1 year age and most cases are seen in under 5 year age. Somatic type of retinoblastomas contributes to 60% of cases and presents at a later age. Remaining 40% are due to autosomal dominant mode of inheritance and retinoblastoma (Rb1) gene mutation. Most common presentation is a white pupillary reflex, others being strabismus, change in color of the iris, and painful/red eye or orbital cellulitis [26].

6.5.1 Management

The tumor has a very low mortality rate if identified early and if timely treatment is initiated. The available treatment modalities are laser trans-pupillary thermotherapy, trans-scleral cryotherapy, laser photocoagulation, enucleation, external beam radiotherapy, and chemotherapy. General anesthesia is required for treatment in newborns and neonates and thus calls for an anesthesia backup. Eye blockade in the presence of retinoblastoma is relative contraindication. Inadvertent globe penetration during needle block may lead to extraocular seeding, and orbital retinoblastoma with distant metastasis, that necessitates adjuvant orbital radiotherapy after enucleation [27, 28].

6.6 Child Abuse and Shaken Baby Syndrome

Shaken baby syndrome (SBS) is a form of abuse in children under 6 months of age using physical force resulting in damage to the nervous system of the baby. In 78% cases it is associated with retinal hemorrhages, usually bilateral, severity correlating with the intensity of the abusive trauma [29, 30]. The underlying mechanism is acceleration and deceleration forces that cause rigorous movements and displacement of the vitreous, with resultant traction on the retina and its vessels, which eventually rupture and bleed. A classical triad of cerebral damage, subdural/subarachnoid hemorrhage and retinal hemorrhage is observed. The diagnosis requires retinal examination under sedation or general anesthesia.

6.6.1 Management

Pars plana vitrectomy might be required in cases with a non-resolving vitreous hemorrhage, macular hole, or underlying RD. Babies with an underlying intracranial bleed have poor prognosis. Ophthalmic and/or neurosurgical interventions require general anesthesia.

6.7 Coloboma of the Eyelid

Colobomas of the eyelid are rare malformations because of failure of the mesodermal folds of the eyelid to fuse during embryogenesis. This results in a triangular shaped defect usually located at the junction of the medial and middle 1/3 of the upper eyelid [31, 32]. They may be solitary or as a part of Goldenhar or Fraser syndrome. Large eyelid defects can cause exposure keratopathy and development of corneal ulcers, potentially blinding.

6.7.1 Management

Correction of large upper eyelid defects in the neonatal period present unique challenges, because unilateral procedures on the eyelid may result in development of amblyopia. If possible surgery should be delayed till the age of 3 or 4 years, but in case of larger defects, a prompt, immediate surgery is advocated to prevent exposure keratopathy [33–35].

6.8 Congenital Dacryocystocele

Congenital dacryocystocele presents with a cystic distension of the lacrimal sac, of bluish appearance. The swelling is usually located just inferior to the medial canthus at birth. It can get infected and drainage with a reverse lacrimal sac massage is advocated. If contents of the sac get infected, surgical probing, drainage, and decompression are performed under general anesthesia, along with systemic antibiotics [36].

6.9 Cryptophthalmos and Ankyloblehpheron

Cryptophthalmos that is complete is characterized by complete covering of the eye with the eyelid skin. In incomplete/partial cryptophthalmos, the skin of the eyelid fuses with the conjunctiva or cornea. Bilateral cryptophthalmos is associated with Fraser syndrome [37]. There may be malformation of the underlying ocular structures.

Ankyloblehpheron presents with an adhesion of the edges of the upper and lower eyelids.

6.9.1 Management

Prognosis following a surgical repair has a good prognosis if underlying structures are normal [38].

6.10 Congenital Entropion

Entropion is defined as inversion of the eyelid margin and in-turning of the eyelashes. This requires surgical correction as the in-turned eyelashes can damage the cornea and cause corneal ulcers.

6.11 Keratomalacia, Corneal Ulceration

Vitamin A deficiency (VAD) due to malnutrition is endemic in developing countries in Southeast Asia and sub-Saharan Africa, where it is a leading cause of childhood blindness and accounts for 19–26% of cases of corneal blindness [39–41]. Over 5 million children develop xerophthalmia annually and one-fourth of these become blind. Keratomalacia following severe VAD, seen at 3–4 years is mostly associated with underlying malnutrition. However, VAD in neonates may occur from maternal deficiency of Vitamin A, thus stores are not built-up in the baby. VAD can be precipitated if the neonate develops severe diarrhea [42, 43]. Infection with virulent microorganism such as *Neisseria gonorrhea*, *Pneumococcus*, *H. influenza*, and *listeria* are responsible for penetration of the intact cornea and corneal perforation.

6.11.1 Management

A therapeutic graft may be required as a sight saving measure apart from retrieval of corneal scrapings for isolation of the infecting organism and initiation of appropriate antimicrobial therapy. Cornea transplantation is difficult in pediatric eyes as there are increased chances of graft failure. Optic iridectomy is an option apart from penetrating keratoplasty requiring a donor cornea. These procedures require general anesthesia in the neonate.

6.12 Trauma

Surgery in cases of trauma in children is indicated when the integrity of the globe is compromised with loss of intraocular contents. Excessive crying, coughing, Valsalva, or any maneuver that causes an increase in IOP will further complicate the integrity of the globe, exacerbating risk of extrusion of intraocular contents, and must be avoided. Regional anesthesia may be beneficial by avoiding the need of laryngoscopy, which itself may raise the IOP. Literature supports the fact that no difference in long-term visual outcomes is observed in patients with open globe injuries when comparing regional blockade versus general anesthesia [44, 45]. However, in neonates, general anesthesia remains the technique as it helps to lower IOP for comfortable intraoperative manipulations.

6.13 Conclusion

A multitude of eye disorders affect the newborns, and if not attended to timely, these may lead to vision disturbances, including blindness. Early identification of these conditions is based on a comprehensive history, clinical examination, and necessary ancillary investigations. Screening in newborns and neonates under general anesthesia might be indicated for establishment of appropriate diagnosis. In neonates, adjunctive regional eye blocks, improve postoperative pain scores [46, 47]. They can reduce many risks of general anesthesia, opioid use, postoperative apnea, desaturation, and bradycardia [48, 49].

Intraconal block is relatively contraindication in neonates, because their extra ocular orbital volume is significantly low. In strabismus surgery or where muscles are being stretched, oculocardiac reflex can cause bradycardia, hypotension, arrhythmias, and asystole. Intraconal or regional blocks can be given to prevent the oculocardiac reflex by blocking the ciliary ganglion.

Extraconal nerve blockade is preferred in neonates. Its safety profile, with regard to adverse events (postoperative apnea and NICU admissions), has been demonstrated in ex-premature neonates undergoing vitreoretinal surgery [50]. Timely management can help preserve the vision of the baby in childhood.

References

1. Mansoor N, Mansoor T, Ahmed M. Eye pathologies in neonates. Int J Ophthalmol. 2016;9(12):1832–8.
2. Litmanovitz I, Dolfin T. Red reflex examination in neonates: the need for early screening. Isr Med Assoc J. 2010;12(5):301–2.
3. Davidson S, Quinn GE. The impact of pediatric vision disorders in adulthood. Pediatrics. 2011;127(2):334–9.
4. Rahi JS, Sripathi S, Gilbert CE, Foster A. Childhood blindness in India: causes in 1318 blind school students in nine states. Eye (Lond). 1995;9(5):545–50.
5. Sheeladevi S, Lawrenson JG, Fielder AR, Suttle CM. Global prevalence of childhood cataract: a systematic review. Eye (Lond). 2016;30:1160–9.
6. Titiyal JS, Pal N, Murthy GV, Gupta SK, Tandon R, et al. Causes and temporal trends of blindness and severe visual impairment in children in schools for the blind in North India. Br J Ophthalmol. 2003;87(8):941–5.
7. Shamanna BR, Dandona L, Rao GN. Economic burden of blindness in India. Indian J Ophthalmol. 1998;46(3):169–72.
8. Chan WH, Biswas S, Ashworth JL, Lloyd IC. Congenital and infantile cataract: aetiology and management. Eur J Pediatr. 2012;171(4):625–30.
9. Mets MB. Eye manifestations of intrauterine infections. Ophthalmol Clin North Am. 2001;14(3):521–31.
10. Givens KT, Lee DA, Jones T, Ilstrup DM. Congenital rubella syndrome: ophthalmic manifestations and associated systemic disorders. Br J Ophthalmol. 1993;77(6):358–63.
11. Sauerbrei A, Wutzler P. Herpes simplex and varicella-zoster virus infections during pregnancy: current concepts of prevention, diagnosis and therapy. Part 2: Varicella-zoster virus infections. Med Microbiol Immunol. 2007;196(2):95–102.
12. Kohli U, Rana N. Congenital varicella syndrome: presenting with eye complications. Indian Pediatr. 2006;43(7):653–4.
13. Wan MJ, VanderVeen DK. Eye disorders in newborn infants (excluding retinopathy of prematurity). Arch Dis Child Fetal Neonatal Ed. 2015;100(3):F264–9.
14. Guise PA. Sub-Tenon anesthesia: a prospective study of 6,000 blocks. Anesthesiology. 2003;98(4):964–8.
15. Edge R, Navon S. Scleral perforation during retrobulbar and peribulbar anesthesia: risk factors and outcome in 50,000 consecutive injections. J Cataract Refract Surg. 1999;25(9):1237–44.
16. François J. Congenital glaucoma and its inheritance. Ophthalmologica. 1980;181(2):61–73.

17. Gupta N, Kumar R, Kumar S, Sehgal R, Sharma KR. A prospective randomised double-blind study to evaluate the effect of peribulbar block or topical application of local anaesthesia combined with general anaesthesia on intra-operative and postoperative complications during paediatric strabismus surgery. Anaesthesia. 2007;62(11):1110–3.
18. Subramaniam R, Subbarayudu S, Rewari V, etal. Usefulness of pre-emptive peribulbar block in pediatric vitreoretinal surgery: a prospective study. RegAnesth Pain Med 2003;28(1):43-47.
19. Beri S, Madan S, Shandil A, Nangia S, etal. Management of retinopathy of prematurity: quest for the best Official Sci J Delhi Ophthalmol Soc 2020;30(3):27–31.
20. Jacqz-Aigrain E, BartinP . Clinical pharmacokinetics of sedatives in neonates. Clin Pharmacokine 1996; 31(6): 423–443.
21. Carbajal R, Lenclen R, Jugie M, Paupe A, et al. Morphine does not provide adequate analgesia for acute procedural pain among preterm neonates. Pediatrics. 2005;115(6):1494–500.
22. Pokela ML, Olkkola KT, Seppala T, Koivisto M. Age-related morphine kinetics in infants. Dev Pharmacol Ther. 1993;20(1–2):26–34.
23. Mintz-Hittner HA, Kennedy KA, Chuang AZ. BEAT-ROP Cooperative Group. Efficacy of intravitrealbevacizumab for stage 3+ retinopathy of prematurity. N Engl J Med. 2011;364(7):603–15.
24. Fleck BW. Management of retinopathy of prematurity. Arch Dis Child Fetal Neonatal Ed. 2013;98(5):F454–6.
25. Jenkinson H. Retinoblastoma: diagnosis and management—the UK perspective. Arch Dis Child. 2015;100(11):1070–5.
26. Goddard AG, Kingston JE, Hungerford JL. Delay in diagnosis of retinoblastoma: risk factors and treatment outcome. Br J Ophthalmol. 1999;83(12):1320–3.
27. Honavar SG, Manjandavida FP, Reddy VAP. Orbital retinoblastoma: an update. Indian J Ophthalmol. 2017;65(6):435–42.
28. Pandey AN. Retinoblastoma: an overview. Saudi J Ophthalmol. 2014;28(4):310–5. https://doi.org/10.1016/j.sjopt.2013.11.001. Epub 2013 Nov 21.
29. Maguire SA, Watts PO, Shaw AD, Holden S, et al. Retinal hemorrhages and related findings in abusive and non-abusive head trauma: a systematic review. Eye (Lond). 2013;27(1):28–36.
30. Binenbaum G, Mirza-George N, Christian CW, Forbes BJ. Odds of abuse associated with retinal hemorrhages in children suspected of child abuse. J AAPOS. 2009;13(3):268–72.
31. Lodhi AA, Junejo SA, Khanzada MA, et al. Surgical outcome of 21 patients with congenital upper eyelid coloboma. Int J Ophthalmol. 2010;3(1):69–72.
32. Zhang DV, Chundury RV, Blandford AD, Perry JD. A 5-day-old-newborn with a large right upper eyelid coloboma. Digit J Ophthalmol. 2017;23(3):88–91.
33. Ortega Molina JM, Mora Horna ER, Salgado Miranda AD, Rubio R, Pérez S, de Larraya A, SalcedoCasillas G. Congenital upper eyelid coloboma: clinical and surgical management. Case Rep Ophthalmol Med. 2015;2015:286782.
34. Sinkin JC, Yi S, Wood BC, Kwon S, Gavaris LZ, etal. Upper eyelid coloboma repair using accessory preauricular cartilage in a patient with goldenhar syndrome: technique revisited. Ophthalmic Plast Reconstr Surg 2017;33(1):e4-e7.
35. Hashish A, Awara AM. One-stage reconstruction technique for large congenital eyelid coloboma. Orbit. 2011;30(4):177–9.
36. Cavazza S, Laffi GL, Lodi L, Tassinari G, Dall'Olio D. Congenital dacryocystocele: diagnosis and treatment. Acta Otorhinolaryngol Ital. 2008;28(6):298–301.
37. Slavotinek AM, Tifft CJ. Fraser syndrome and cryptophthalmos: review of the diagnostic criteria and evidence for phenotypic modules in complex malformation syndromes. J Med Genet. 2002;39(9):623–33.
38. Alami B, Maadane A, Sekhsoukh R. Ankyloblepharon filiforme adnatum: a case report. Pan Afr Med J. 2013;8(15):15.
39. Thylefors B, Négrel AD, Pararajasegaram R, Dadzie KY. Global data on blindness. Bull World Health Organ. 1995;73(1):115–21.

40. Maharana PK, Nawaz S, Singhal D, Jhanji V, Agarwal T, Sharma N, et al. Causes and management outcomes of acquired corneal opacity in a preschool age (0-5 years) group: a hospital-based study. Cornea. 2019;38(7):868–72.
41. Vajpayee RB, Vanathi M, Tandon R, Sharma N, Titiyal JS. Keratoplasty for keratomalacia in preschool children. Br J Ophthalmol. 2003;87(5):538–42.
42. Rahmathullah L, Raj MS, Chandravathi TS. Aetiology of severe vitamin A deficiency in children. Natl Med J India. 1997;10(2):62–5.
43. Varughese S. Vitamin A deficiency in children under 6 months. Trop Doct. 2007;37(1):59–60.
44. Scott IU, Mccabe CM, Flynn HW, Lemus DR, Schiffman JC, Reynolds DS, Pereira MB, Belfort A, Gayer S. Local anesthesia with intravenous sedation for surgical repair of selected open globe injuries. Am J Ophthalmol. 2002;134(5):707–11.
45. Scott IU, Gayer S, Voo I, Flynn HW Jr, Diniz JR, Venkatraman A. Regional anesthesia with monitored anesthesia care for surgical repair of selected open globe injuries. Ophthalmic Surg Lasers Imaging. 2005;36(2):122–8.
46. Sinha R, Maitra S. The effect of peribulbar block with general anesthesia for vitreoretinal surgery in premature and ex-premature infants with retinopathy of prematurity. A A Case Rep. 2016;6(2):25–7.
47. Chhabra A, Sinha R, Subramaniam R, etal. Comparison of sub-Tenon's block with i.v. fentanyl for paediatric vitreoretinal surgery. Br J Anaesth 2009;103(5):739-743.
48. Pinho DFR, Real C, Ferreira L, Pina P. Peribulbar block combined with general anesthesia in babies undergoing laser treatment for retinopathy of prematurity: a retrospective analysis. Rev Bras Anestesiol. 2018;68(5):431–6.
49. Waldschmidt B, Gordon N. Anesthesia for pediatric ophthalmologic surgery. J AAPOS. 2019;23(3):127–31.
50. Khokhar S, Nayak B, Patil B, Changole MD, etal. Subperiosteal hematoma from peribulbar block during cataract surgery leading to optic nerve compression in a patient with parahemophilia. Int Med Case Rep J 2015; 3;8:313-316.

Neonatal Transfusion

7

Anita Nangia

7.1 Introduction

The guidelines for adult transfusions are well-documented and known to most practicing clinicians; however, special care needs to be taken regards donor selection, selection of appropriate blood product, dosages, and storage conditions for neonatal transfusion. Neonates are a vulnerable clinical group with unique requirements for blood products. Moreover, the WHO bleeding scale which assigns grades between 1 and 4 for clinically significant bleeding is applicable primarily to adults [1]. The process of transfusion requires a control of large number of factors in the pretransfusion, transfusion, and post-transfusion stages.

7.2 Pretransfusion Factors

The guidelines for pretransfusion testing in neonates and infants are provided by BCSH in 2013 (British Committee for Standards in Hematology) [2]. Certain blood safety procedures are to be strictly endured in setting of neonatal transfusions. Points to remember are:

1. **Donor selection**: the components for neonatal transfusion are best prepared from repeat blood donors/donors who have given at least one donation within previous 2 years. The donors should be negative for all mandatory microbiological markers.
2. **Choice of correct component:** based on clinical condition and indication.
3. **Leucodepletion**: Components with WBC $<1 \times 10^6$/unit help to:
   (a) Prevent nonhemolytic febrile reactions
   (b) Reduce the risk of alloimmunization

A. Nangia (✉)
Department of Pathology, Lady Hardinge Medical College, SSK and Kalawati Saran Childrens Hospitals, New Delhi, India

U. Saha (ed.), *Clinical Anesthesia for the Newborn and the Neonate*,
https://doi.org/10.1007/978-981-19-5458-0_7

4. **Cytomegalovirus (CMV) safe blood**: Recommended for most components in babies less than 4 weeks of age, especially for:
   (a) Intrauterine transfusion of red blood cells (RBC) and platelets
   (b) VLBW ($\leq$1500 g) and/or with a gestational age $\leq$30 weeks
   (c) Neonates with congenital or acquired immunodeficiency
5. **Irradiation**: RBC and platelets are irradiated with 25–50 Gray (2500–5000 rad) to prevent graft-versus-host disease for:
   (a) Intrauterine transfusion of RBC and platelets
   (b) Exchange transfusion of RBC
   (c) Transfusion in VLBW neonates ($\leq$1500 g) and/or with a age $\leq$30 weeks
   (d) Neonates with congenital or acquired immunodeficiency
6. **Pretransfusion tests**: ABO typing in neonates is based on the identifying RBC antigens as anti-A/-B iso-agglutinins, are absent in first 4 months of age. In addition, there is weak expression of erythrocyte antigens on the neonatal RBC. Circulating maternal IgG ABO antibodies may be detected in neonatal plasma due to placental transfer. So always test dual sample: maternal and neonate:
   (a) Tests on the mother sample:
       • Determination of ABO/Rh phenotype
       • An indirect antiglobulin test (IAT) to screen for unusual antibodies against RBCs
   (b) Tests on the neonate:
       • Determination of ABO/Rh phenotype (2 samples always—cord blood and second capillary sample)
       • Direct antiglobulin test (DAT)
7. **Pretransfusion compatibility tests:**

When maternal IAT and neonatal DAT are negative, top-up transfusions are given with ABO Rh compatible blood in the first 4 months of life.

Note: *If maternal IAT is positive, transfuse with RBCs lacking the antigen to which the antibody is directed. Following first transfusion, neonate's serum/plasma must be used.

*In case of major incompatibility issues, O Negative fresh RBC are the best option.

*A contact list of rare blood group donors is always available in blood bank, which can be requested for planned surgeries and transfusions.

7.3   Red Cell Transfusion in Neonates

Neonatal transfusions can be small volume (TopUp), large volume and/or exchange transfusions. The most common indications are:

• **Severe anemia**
• **Severe hyperbilirubinemia**
• **Prematurity (<32 weeks)**
• **Low birth weight (<1500 g)**
• **Neonatal surgery**

Neonates with severe anemia are at risk of associated high mortality. Additional illnesses (acute infections, diarrhea, pneumonia etc.) make them even more vulnerable. Low Hb affects tissue oxygenation, growth, neurodevelopment, and immunity. Determining the level of Hb and Hematocrit (Hct) at which tissue oxygenation is inadequate, and to cause critical hypoxemia in term or preterm neonates is difficult, making the timing of transfusion challenging [3–5].

7.3.1 Small Volume (TOP UP) Transfusions in Neonatal Anemia

Most of the RBC transfusions in neonates are **small volume transfusions (TOP UP)** involving 10–20 mL/kg body weight given at 5 mL/kg/h over 2–4 hours, usually to treat anemia of prematurity. Top-up transfusions more than 20 mL/kg are not recommended because of the risk of transfusion-associated circulatory overload (TACO) [6, 7]. Neonatal anemia is defined as decrease in Hb (g/dL)/RBC volume below the normal for healthy babies (Box 7.1).

Experts vary in their views regarding a cautious/restrictive transfusion policy [8, 9] versus a liberal one [10, 11] (Table 7.1).

Repeated transfusions may be required to make up for decreased RBC production, as also for losses from repeated blood testing. Most preterm LBW neonates (<1500 g) will require at least 1 or 2 transfusions. The new BCSH Transfusion Guidelines for Neonates and Older Children (https://b-s-h.org.uk/) [6] suggest the following thresholds based on Hb concentration and cardiorespiratory status of the baby [10–12] (Table 7.2).

7.3.2 Goal of Blood Transfusion

The goal of BT is to achieve Hct of approximately 45%, maximum volume of transfusion being 15 mL/kg [14] (UI NICU G). PRBC has a hematocrit of 80–90%. 1 mL/kg of PRBC transfused should increase hematocrit by 1%, (15 mL/kg should increase hematocrit by 15%). The RBC units are selected carefully for neonatal transfusion (Box 7.2).

Box 7.1 Normal Hb Concentrations

Cord blood (term)	±16.5 g/dL
Newborn: day 1	±18.0 g/dL
Neonate (4 weeks)	±14.0 g/dL

Table 7.1 Hb Transfusion Thresholds for Restrictive Transfusion Policies

Postnatal age	Respiratory support	No respiratory support
Week 1	11.5 G%	10 G%
Week 2	10 G%	8.5 G%
Week 3	8.5 G%	7.5 G%

Table 7.2 Summary of BCSH Recommendations for Neonatal Top-Up Transfusions—Hb in g/L

Postnatal age	Ventilated	On O$_2$/CPAP	Off O$_2$
First 24 h	<120	<120	<100
<1 week (1–7 days)	<120	<100	<100
Week 2 (8–14 days)	<100	<95	<75–85 depending on clinical situation
3 weeks (day 15 onwards)		<85	

Note: *Neonates clinical condition and low hematocrit besides blood loss are important factors before deciding on transfusion. *Micro sampling technique to reduce the risk of iatrogenic anemia. *Use of **peadipacks** [12, 13] single donor, 50 mL, leuco-depleted, CMV negative, group O Positive or O Negative RBC units, to neonates who are likely to need one or more transfusions, increase safety in transfusion.

Box 7.2 Selection of RBCs for Small-Volume Transfusion of Neonates and Infants (Top Up)

1. Hematocrit 0.5–0.7

2. Unit should be less than 35 days old (from date of collection)

3. In SAG-M anticoagulant/additive solution (approximately 20 mL residual plasma) (SAG-M - saline, adenine, sugar, mannitol)

4. Irradiated at time of issue[a]

5. Group O ABO-compatible with baby and mother, and RhD −ve/ RhD compatible with baby[b]

6. CMV seronegative for neonates

7. Commence transfusion within 30 min of product receipt and complete within 4 h

8. HIV, hepatitis B and C, and HTLV I/II negative

Note: Always do dual testing (maternal and neonatal) before transfusion.
[a]In the case of multiple transfusion of small volumes irradiate only the fraction needed for transfusion
[b]Check ABO group on both mother and neonate. Perform IAT on maternal and DAT on neonatal sample. SAG-M saline–adenine–glucose–mannitol.

Always check neonatal blood group on two separate samples (cord blood and capillary). Following the transfusion, improvement in Hb level can be assessed and monitored [13] (Table 7.3).

7.3.3 Neonatal Red Cell Exchange Transfusion (EBT)

The **main indication** for neonatal RBC exchange blood transfusion (EBT) is to **treat severe hyperbilirubinemia or severe anemia** usually due to hemolytic disease of fetus and newborn (HDFN). This helps in removing antibody coated RBC and reduce the level of unconjugated bilirubin in the plasma, to prevent or reduce the risk of encephalopathy. Neonatal hyperbilirubinemia due to glucose-6-phosphate dehydrogenase (G6PD) deficiency is also treated with EBT. A single blood volume (80–100 mL/kg) EBT is capable of extracting 75% of the RBCs whereas a 'double volume exchange' (160–200 mL/kg) can remove almost 90% of neonatal

Table 7.3 Assessment of Improvement in Hb Status After Transfusion Volume [13]

Pretransfusion Hb(g/L)	Expected Hb in g/L Post transfusion		
	@ 10 mL/kg	@ 15 mL/kg	@ 20 mL/kg
1. Very preterm neonate with estimated blood volume 100 mL/kg			
70	91	102	112
80	101	112	122
90	111	122	132
2. Term neonate with estimated blood volume 80 mL/kg			
70	96	109	123
80	106	119	133
90	116	129	143

Box 7.3 Red Cells for Neonatal Exchange Transfusion

1. Plasma reduced, Hct 0.5–0.6 (NHSBT) to reduce risk of post exchange polycythemia (National Health Service Blood and Transplant)
2. CPD anticoagulant
3. <5 days old to prevent hyperkalemia
4. Irradiated, essential if baby has received IUT
5. CMV negative
6. Sickle screen negative
7. Usually group O (with low titer hemolysins Anti A and Anti B)
8. Rh D −ve (or Rh D identical with neonate) and Kell −ve
9. Red cell antigen −ve for maternal alloantibodies
10. IAT (indirect antiglobulin test) crossmatch compatible with maternal plasma

---

RBCs and approximately 50% of bilirubin [15–17]. The red cell units for exchange transfusion are selected first (Box 7.3).

The volume to transfuse is calculated using the following formula:

$$\text{Volume to transfuse} (\text{mL}) = \text{Desired Hb} - \text{actual Hb} (g/dL) \times \text{weight} (\text{kg}) \times \text{factor}/10$$

Factor between 3 and 5 are recommended [18]. (Factor is a correlation gradient between mL/kg blood transfused and increase in Hb). **Now the new modified formula has replaced factor/10 with factor/hematocrit (Hct)** [18]. The rate of transfusion is 5 mL/min and 2–3 mL/min in a severe hydrops. The unit should be warmed to 37 °C before transfusion using a blood warmer. Use of radiant heater on exposed infusion line is not recommended (red cell hemolysis) [19].

7.4 Surgery and Large Volume Neonatal Red Cell Transfusion

The total circulating blood volume is approximately 80 mL/kg [4, 5]. Large-volume transfusion is defined as transfusing either a single circulating blood volume (approximately 80 mL/kg) over 24 h or almost 50% of the circulating volume (40 mL/kg) within 3 h or at a rate of 2–3 mL/kg/min. The **main use is in neonatal**

cardiac, hepatic, scoliosis or craniofacial surgery. The thresholds given in Table 7.2 can be used for preoperative surgical assessment in neonates. The RBC unit supplied has a mean volume of 294 mL, in SAG-M anticoagulant but preferably less than 5 days to prevent hyperkalemia [20]. The other specifications are similar to that used for neonatal 'top-up' transfusions (Box 7.2). Dosage is 10–20 mL/kg.

Note: All large volume transfusions should be given via a blood warmer to maintain temperatures close to 37 °C to avoid development of hypothermia. The core temperature of the neonate should be carefully monitored [21, 22].

Irradiated blood is an essential requirement for known or suspected T-cell immunodeficiency, e.g., DiGeorge syndrome. The transfusion time of the unit should be within 24 h of irradiation. Electrolyte monitoring is essential especially for potassium and calcium (hypocalcemia due to citrate overload) [6].

7.5   Bleeding in Neonates

The causes of bleeding in neonates can be due to platelet deficiency or due to coagulation defects.

7.5.1   Neonatal Platelet Transfusions

Normal platelet counts in neonates is $150–450 \times 10^9$/L. The counts fall after birth up to 1 week but then rise. Neonates have a risk of bleeding due to birth trauma, sepsis, intrauterine hypoxia, TORCH infections, disseminated intravascular coagulation (DIC), inborn errors of metabolism, drugs, and pre-eclampsia in mother. Neonatal autoimmune thrombocytopenia (NAIT) causes pronounced thrombocytopenia and is most commonly due to maternally derived anti-HPA-1a or 5b platelet antibodies which cross placenta in utero [23].

Severe thrombocytopenia ($<50 \times 10^9$/L) is a common finding in patients in NICU, especially sick preterm neonates. Risk for bleeding is minimal at 20×10^9 to 100×10^9/L, moderate between 5×10^9 to 20×10^9/L and severe below 5×10^9/L. Intraventricular hemorrhage (IVH) depends not only platelet count but other clinical factors as well (Table 7.4) [24].

Single donor apheresis platelets are used. The unit should be CMV negative, ABO Rh D identical or compatible, dose 10–20 mL/kg body weight, preferably irradiated, and used within 5 days of collection. One 1 unit (50 mL)/10 kg raises count by 50,000/cu mm. A post-transfusion platelet count is done to check

Table 7.4 Transfusion Thresholds for Neonatal Transfusion (Excluding NAIT)

Platelets <20 or 30 × 10⁹/L	Stable term or preterm baby, asymptomatic thrombocytopenia, no bleeding
Platelets 30–50 × 10⁹/L	Sick preterm neonate with thrombocytopenia
Platelets <50 × 10⁹/L	Term/preterm neonate, symptomatic thrombocytopenia, minor bleeding, current coagulopathy, planned surgery or exchange transfusion
Platelets <100 × 10⁹/L	Term/preterm baby, symptomatic thrombocytopenia, major bleeding, major surgery (neuro, cardiac, abdominal)

increment. If cranial ultrasound reveals ICH, platelets should be transfused to maintain count of 50–100×10^9/L. **Intraoperative indications** of platelet transfusion are persistent surgical ooze, massive blood transfusion, and thrombocytopenia.

7.5.2 Neonatal FFP and Cryoprecipitate Transfusion

Vitamin-K-dependent clotting factor levels are approximately half that of adults at birth and even lower in preterm babies. The hemostatic tests [prothrombin time (PT), thrombin time (TT), and activated partial thromboplastin time (APTT)] may be prolonged even if overall coagulation is normal. BCSH guidelines recommends PT/APTT values of greater than 1.5 times midpoint of normal range as a guide for use of FFP in [6]:

i. Congenital factor V deficiency
ii. Vitamin K deficiency
iii. Disseminated Intravascular Coagulation (DIC)
iv. Congenital thrombotic thrombocytopenic Purpura (ADAMTS 13 deficiency*)—rare
v. Cardiopulmonary bypass surgery—hemodilution induced low platelets and coagulation factors.

Intraoperative indications include massive blood transfusion, abnormal surgical ooze, clotting factor deficiency, DIC, PT >15 s (INR >1.4), PTT >60 s (INR >1.5).

NOTE: ADAMTS = A Disintegrin and Metalloproteinase with Thrombospondin motifs. The ADAMTS 13 gene provides instructions for making an enzyme that is involved in regulating blood clotting. After an injury, clots normally protect the body by sealing off damaged blood vessels and preventing further blood loss. The ADAMTS13 enzyme processes the large protein called von Willebrand factor [25].

Routine and repeated tests for coagulation are not recommended as it leads to unnecessary blood loss due to sampling. Coagulation screening is however recommended in neonates with active bleeding or those at high risk of DIC, e.g., NEC, severe sepsis, and TORCH infection.

For FFP transfusion in neonate, the guidelines and prerequisites must be followed (Box 7.4).

Box 7.4 Guidelines for FFP transfusion in neonates
1. Blood group identical or Group AB
2. Volume 60 mL
3. Dose 10–20 mL/kg
4. Thawed to 37 °C over 30 min
5. No leucocyte depletion or irradiation needed

Note: The amount of correction in clotting tests is unpredictable and should be repeat tested. BCSH recommends FFP transfusion for PT >1.5 times normal while treating the underlying cause (including adequate reversal of heparin). **Do not use FFP for routine prophylaxis against ICH in preterm neonates, or as substitute for volume replacement or as blanket therapy to correct coagulation screen abnormalities**.

Cryoprecipitate is an extremely concentrated source for fibrinogen and is used in bleeding due to h-ypofibrinogenemia (<150 mg/dL), when fibrinogen concentrate is not available. It also has the additional advantage of lower transfusion volumes as compared to FFP for correction of hypofibrinogenemia especially in preterm neonates. Guidelines are similar to FFP (Box 7.4) but less volume. 1 unit (10–15 mL with 150 mg of fibrinogen)/10 kg, (dose 1.0 mL/kg). It contains factor VIII, Von Willebrand factor, XIII, fibrinogen, and fibronectin. Prophylactic use is not recommended in non bleeding stable neonates [5]. However it is used for hypofibrogenemia persisting after FFP use.

Combined factor deficiencies (except Factor V) are best managed using cryoprecipitate [22, 26]. It is also used to treat congenital TTP (thrombotic thrombocytopenic purpura). Factor VIII concentrate has ADAMTS13.

Note: In case of individual factor deficiency, especially hypofibrinogenemia, use single factor recombinant factor for therapy.

7.6 Neonatal Granulocyte Transfusion

Granulocyte for transfusion can be prepared by apheresis or from buffy coat of whole blood [27]. They are requested in older children with hematology/oncology/immunology neutropenia patients at high risk for developing severe infections [28]. **Current BCSH guidelines do not recommend their routine use or even in neutropenic septic neonates,** and only in selected cases of neutropenia in older children [22, 26, 28].

7.7 Erythropoietin (EPO)

There are no clear guidelines for the use of erythropoietin in neonates. It provides a marginal benefit in VLBW neonates (Multicenter U.S. and European VLBW clinical trial). EPO is believed to reduce the need for multiple blood transfusions thus repeated donor exposure but increases the risk for development of retinopathy of prematurity (ROP) in the neonates [5]. If EPO therapy is considered, the dose is 200–300 U sq./kg/ad. + Fe intake of 6 mg/kg/d. Delayed cord clamping, by a minute, in both term and preterm neonates not requiring resuscitation is a great way to improve blood hemoglobin and hematocrit post delivery. It is also shown to reduce the red cell transfusion requirements as well as decrease the risk for iron deficiency between 2–6 months of age [5].

7.8 Hb Triggers as Per Ventilation Status [14]

(a) **On IPPV:** (a) FiO_2 >70% /ECMO = Hb <15 g%, (b) FiO_2 40–70% = <13 g%, (c) FiO_2 <40% = <11.5 g%.
(b) **On CPAP:** FiO_2 <40%/nasal cannula/preoperatively (on or off O2)—<10 g%.

(c) **Not on O₂ therapy**, but signs of anemia, apnea, tachycardia (>180/min), tachypnea (>80/min), poor growth = <8 g%.
(d) **No O₂ therapy**, clinically well = <7 g%.

7.9   Intrauterine Transfusion (IUT)

Intrauterine transfusions are invasive procedures carried out between 16 to 35 weeks of gestation and carry a risk of fetal death of 1–3%, which is higher for hydrops foetus (20%). IUT with RBC is needed most commonly for HDN usually caused by anti-D or anti-K [29], severe anemia, and fetal parvovirus infection. The procedure is required every 15–20 days and aims at raising/maintaining Hct of 0.45. Babies who received IUT for HDN, generally are anemic post delivery too. This may persist for a few weeks due to passively acquired maternal antibodies and transient suppression of erythropoiesis in neonate due to transfusion.

RBCs used should be of high Hct, irradiated to prevent graft versus host disease (GVHD), transfused as early as possible (shell life 24 h), warmed, and free of the offending antigen. The amount to be transfused can be calculated based on donor and fetal Hct and fetoplacental volume. In case of emergency non-irradiated but leuco-depleted fresh (<5 days) RBCs are used. IUT with platelets are needed in case of foetal thrombocytopenia commonly occuring as a result of NAIT. It can be best avoided by treating mother with intravenous Immunoglobulis or corticosteroids. However, when the thrombocytopenia, is severe, especially <50 × 10/L, IUT is performed. The Platelet unit is irradiated and HPA compatible to maternal antibody. The transfusion is given slowly to prevent foetal blood stasis and stroke [5].

7.10   Post-transfusion Complications

Severe hemolytic transfusion reactions may occur in neonates who receive red blood cell or FFP transfusions containing anti-T antibodies. (Box 7.5) All adult plasma contains anti-T. The T-antigen gets exposed on the RBC surface in neonates suffering from NEC due to neuraminidase-producing bacteria of Clostridium species which could exacerbate hemolysis. It is best to request for washed red cell products in neonates with significant hemolysis, to avoid exposure to plasma and by avoiding all nonessential transfusions of FFP and platelet. Judicious and restrictive use policy are associated with better outcomes especially in preterm neonates [29, 30]. Large volume blood transfusions given for blood loss greater than 10% of blood volume, multiple transfusions and low platelet counts are associated with increased odds for 30 day mortality rates in surgical neonates [31, 32]. Risk for complications following surgery can be calculated and prognosis assesed [32, 33].

> **Box 7.5 Complications of Blood Transfusion**
> - Infectious disease transmission.
> - Transfusion reactions: TRALI/TLI.
> - Haemolysis, especially in NEC
> - Metabolic: Acidosis, Hypothermia, Hyperkalaemia (>10 days old blood), Hypocalcaemia.
>
> **Note**: At high transfusion rates: severe hypocalcemia, cardiac depression, hypotension—aggravated under anesthesia. **Management under anesthesia**—calcium replacement (Ca gluconate—7.5–15 mg/kg or Ca chloride 2.5–5 mg/kg).

7.11   Special Care During Surgery

1. **Minimize use of blood products**: decrease surgical loss, reduce blood sampling losses, preoperative nutrition and TPN, manage 10–20% losses by crystalloids, prefer to use lower Hct (30%) and Hb (10 g%) targets as possible.
2. **Transfusion specifics**: PRBC (mL) = (Desired Hct − Present Hct) × EBV transfused/Hct of PRBC, at slow rate (<5 mL/kg/h), Fresh blood (<7 days), Wider bore cannula (22G), Infusion pump if smaller cannula (24G), or with a syringe.
3. **Calculate allowable blood loss meticulously:** maximum allowable blood loss (MABL) − EBV × (Starting Hct − Target Hct)/Starting Hct (EBV in term neonate 80 mL/kg and in preterm 90–100 mL/kg).
4. Use restrictive transfusion than liberal transfusion

7.12   Conclusion

Blood transfusion is very common in premature and low birth weight newborns in the NICU setting. Neonates undergoing major surgeries under general anesthesia almost always require blood transfusion. Clinicians and anesthesiologists need to be conversant with the various indications, recommendations, safe transfusion volumes or dosages, and complications, thereof. During surgery, it is the responsibility of the anesthesiologist to cross check the blood before transfusion, a precaution to prevent transfusion related iatrogenic problems in the neonate, under anesthesia.

Anti A/B iso agglutinins are absent in a neonate. They usually develop by the age of 4 months. Maternal antibodies may be present in the neonate, due to passive placental transfer, creating compatibility issues. Hence, dual testing must be done [IAT on the mother and DAT on the baby]. When both are −ve, ABO Rh compatible blood should be used, and if IAT is +ve, RBCs lacking that antigen should be given to the baby. Ideally, all transfusions should be ABO RH compatible. In case of major compatibility issues, fresh O −ve blood is best.

Change in trends from whole BT to component therapy, requires a detailed insight into the pre requites for these components in the neonate, e.g., indication and choice of component, need for leucodepletion and gamma irradiation, and prevention of alloimmunization, hemolytic reactions, and infections. Common products used in the neonates are PRBC, FFP, Cryoprecipitate and Platelet concentrates. Follow the guidelines as mentioned in the chapter.

In neonates, it is advocated to use small volume transfusions (top ups) 10–20 mL/kg given at 5 mL/kg/h over 2–4 h, as there is risk of TACO in higher doses. Usually, preheating is not required. Blood is transfused slowly using infusion pump or a syringe at room temperature. For large volume transfusions, blood should be warmed up to 37°C, immediately before transfusing.

Research and experience suggest that the Hb trigger for transfusion is higher in anemic, premature, low birth weight babies, and those on ventilatory support, and FiO_2. The goal of transfusion is to maintain Hct of 45%. The maximum volume should not exceed 15 ml/kg, transfused (@5 mL/kg/h, less than 35 days (preferably within 5 days), leukodepleted and gamma irradiated ABO RH compatible, CMV, HIV, Hep B and C, and HTLV I/II negative. Volume for transfusion should be calculated meticulously using the initial and target Hct. With PRBC (Hct >80%) expect an increase in Hct of 1%/1 mL/kg of PRBC.

References

1. National Institute for Health and Clinical Excellence (NICE). NG 24 Blood Transfusion. London: NICE; 2015. https://www.nice.org.uk/guidance/ng24
2. British Committee for Standards in Haematology. Guidelines for pre-transfusion compatibility procedures in blood transfusion laboratories. Transfusion Med. 2013b;23:3–35.
3. Transfusion Handbook: Neonatal transfusion, Joint United Kingdom Blood Transfusion and Tissue Transplantation Services Professional Advisory Committee (JPAC); 2021. https://www.transfusionguidelines.org
4. Neonatal Red Blood Cell Transfusion Indian Society of Blood Transfusion. https://www.isbtweb.org
5. Guidelines on transfusion for foetus, neonates and older children. British Committee for Standards n Hematology, (BCSH 2016). https://b-s-h.org.uk
6. British Committee for Standards in Haematology. Guideline on the administration of blood components. addendum: avoidance of transfusion associated circulatory overload (TACO) and problems associated with over transfusion; 2012a. https://www.bcshguidelines.com/documents/BCSH_Blood_Admin_-_addendum_August_2012.pdf
7. Aher S, Malwatkar K, Kadam S. Neonatal anemia. Semin Fetal Neonatal Med. 2008;13:239–47.
8. Venkatesh V, Khan R, Curley A, et al. The safety and efficacy of red cell transfusions in neonates: a systematic review of randomized controlled trials. Br J Haematol. 2012;158:370–85.
9. Venkatesh V, Khan R, Curley A, New H, Stanworth S. How we decide when a neonate needs a transfusion. Br J Haematol. 2013;160:421–33.
10. Whyte RK, Kirpalani H, Asztalos EV, et al. Neurodevelopmental outcome of extremely low birth weight infants randomly assigned to restrictive or liberal hemoglobin thresholds for blood transfusion. Pediatrics. 2009;123:207–13.
11. Whyte R, Kirpalani H. Low versus high haemoglobin concentration threshold for blood transfusion for preventing morbidity and mortality in very low birth weight infants. Cochrane Database Syst Rev. 2011:CD000512. https://doi.org/10.1002/14651858.CD000512.pub2.
12. National Comparative Audit of Blood Transfusion. National comparative audit of the use of red cells in neonates and children; 2010. http://hospital.blood.co.uk/media/26872/ncared_cells_neonates_children.pdf

13. The Royal Children's Hospital Melbourne guidelines for transfusion in neonates. https://www.rch.org.au/home
14. Bell EF. When to transfuse preterm babies. Arch Dis Child Fetal Neonatal Ed. 2008;93:F469–73.
15. Lathe GH. Exchange transfusion as a means of removing bilirubin in haemolytic disease of newborn. Br Med J. 1955;22:192–6.
16. Sproul A, Smith L. Bilirubin equilibration during exchange transfusion in hemolytic disease of newborn. J Pediatr. 1964;65:12–26.
17. Thayyil S, Milligan DW. Single versus double volume exchange transfusion in jaundiced newborn infants. Cochrane Database Syst Rev. 2006:CD004592. https://doi.org/10.1002/14651858. CD004592.pub2.
18. New HV, Grant-Casey J, Lowe D, et al. Red blood cell transfusion practice in children: current status and areas for improvement? A study of the use of red blood cell transfusions in children and infants. Transfusion. 2014;54:119–27.
19. Neonatal Transfusion Guidance; 2012. AABB, Bethesda, MD. ISBN: 978-1-56395-848-9.
20. Lee AC, Reduque LL, Luban NL, Ness PM, et al. Transfusion associated hyperkalaemic cardiac arrest in paediatric patients receiving massive transfusion. Transfusion. 2014;54:244–54.
21. National Institute for Healthcare and Excellence (NICE). CG 65. Hypothermia: prevention and management in adults having surgery. London: NICE; 2008. https://www.nice.org.uk/guidance/cg65
22. Neonatal Pediatric Transfusions. National Blood Authority Australia; 2016. https://www.blood.gov.au/pbm-guidelines
23. Sillers L, Slambrock VC, Lapping-Carr G. Neonatal thrombocytopenia: etiology and diagnosis. Pediatr Ann. 2015;44(7):e175–80. https://doi.org/10.3928/00904481-20150710-11.
24. Lieberman L, Liu Y, Portwine C, et al. An epidemiologic cohort study reviewing the practice of blood product transfusions among a population of pediatric oncology patients. Transfusion. 2014;54:2736–44.
25. Kelwick R, Desanlis I, Wheeler GN, Edwards DR. The ADAMTS (A Disintegrin and Metalloproteinase with Thrombospondin motifs) family. Genome Biol. 2015;16(1):113. Published online 2015 May 30. https://doi.org/10.1186/s13059-015-0676-3.
26. Girelli G, Antoncecchi S, Casadei AM, et al. Recommendations for transfusion therapy in neonatology. Blood Transfus. 2015;13(3):484–97.
27. Bashir S, Stanworth S, Massey E, et al. Neutrophil function is preserved in a pooled granulocyte component prepared from whole blood donations. Br J Haematol. 2008;140:701–11.
28. Strauss RG. Role of granulocyte/neutrophil transfusions for hematology/oncology patients in the modern era. Br J Haematol. 2012;158:299–306.
29. Kirpalani H, Whyte RK, Andersen C, Asztalos EV, et al. The Premature Infants in Need of Transfusion (PINT) Study: a randomized, controlled trial of a restrictive (low) versus liberal (high) transfusion threshold for extremely low birth weight infants. J Pediatr. 2006;149:301–7.
30. Bell EF, Strauss RG, Widness JA, Mahoney LT, et al. Randomized trial of liberal versus restrictive guidelines for red blood cell transfusion in preterm infants. Pediatrics. 2005;115:1685–91.
31. Puri A, Yadav PS, Saha U, et al. A case series study of therapeutic implications of type IIIb4: a rare variant of esophageal atresia and distal tracheoesophageal fistula. J Pediatr Surg. 2013 Jul;48(7):1463–9.
32. Stey AM, Kenney BD, Moss RL, Hall BL, Berman L, et al. A risk calculator predicting postoperative adverse events in neonates undergoing major abdominal or thoracic surgery. J Pediatr Surg. 2015;50(6):987–91.
33. Manchanda V, Sarin YK, Ramji S. Prognostic factors determining mortality in surgical neonates. J Neonatal Surg. 2012;1(1):3.

Effect of Anaesthesia on Developing Brain

8

Pratishtha Yadav and Nishkarsh Gupta

8.1 Introduction

Brain is one of the most vital organs that influence an organism throughout the life. In the last two decades, animal studies have highlighted the neuroapoptotic and neurodegenerative effects of the anaesthetic drugs. This paved way for the numerous studies in humans, albeit retrospective. Most of them have clearly demonstrated an association between exposure to anaesthesia in infancy and development of behavioral problems later in life. So far, maximum evidence suggests that anesthetic drugs can influence the neurodevelopmental outcome of pediatric patients.

Recently, US Food and Drug Administration (FDA) has updated their statement that repeated or lengthy use of general anesthesia and sedative drugs during surgeries or procedures in children younger than 3 years or pregnant women during their 3rd trimester may affect the development of child's brain [1]. Thus, it is important to understand the role of anesthetic drugs in neurodevelopment so as to avoid long-term deleterious effects.

8.2 Brain Growth and Development

Differentiation of progenitor cells in the 3rd week of gestation marks the beginning of development of brain. It is an extensive process that progresses through multiple stages (Fig. 8.1). First is the formation of a neural tube. The ectodermal plate folds around a liquid-filled cavity creating the neural tube. This later gives rise to spinal cord enclosed in the spinal canal. Rest of the primary brain structure and ventricles arise from the vesicle-filled bulges at the anterior end of ectodermal plate. This whole process is the first step of brain development called **neurulation.** This is

The original version of this chapter has been revised by correcting an incorrect spelling of one of the author's names. A correction to this chapter can be found at https://doi.org/10.1007/978-981-19-5458-0_51

P. Yadav · N. Gupta (✉)
Onco-Anaesthesiology and Palliative Care, DR BRAIRCH, AIIMS, New Delhi, India

U. Saha (ed.), *Clinical Anesthesia for the Newborn and the Neonate*, https://doi.org/10.1007/978-981-19-5458-0_8

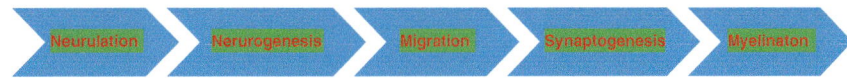

Fig. 8.1 Stages in the Development of Brain

followed by the process of **neurogenesis,** which takes place in the early weeks of gestation, in the germinal matrix and subventricular zone. Epithelial progenitor cells lining the early ventricles differentiate into neurons and glial cells. At 12–20 weeks of gestation, neurons migrate to their final destination, the brain. At 20th weeks, the process synaptogenesis starts. The proliferation of neuronal synapses reaches its peak at 1–2 years of age. Synapse formation is the basis of learning throughout our life. Neuro-apoptosis or programmed cell death begins at 24th week of gestation and continues till 4th week after birth, i.e., in the neonatal period. Natural neuro-apoptosis takes place at a rate of 1% neurons per day, which reaches a peak in late gestation or early infancy. Final is the myelination of the axons which begins in the 2nd trimester and continues throughout childhood.

Neurotransmitters such as γ-aminobutyric acid (GABA), glutamate, and receptor system play a crucial role in neurodevelopment and are essential for maintenance of neuronal connections and in transmission of impulses. On the other hand, the absence of neuronal transmission and binding of GABA and glutamate stimulates neuro-apoptosis or cell death [2]. In the next section, we will discuss the impact of anaesthetic drugs on neuronal transmission and how they influence the complex process of neurodevelopment.

8.3   Suspected Pathways of Neurotoxicity

Anaesthetic drugs and sedatives are suspected to interfere with development of the brain by inducing neuro-apoptosis and disturbing the cerebral cytoarchitecture.

Role of GABA and NMDA receptors: Commonly used anaesthetic drugs and sedatives act via GABA receptor, or N-methyl-D-aspartate receptor (NMDA—a subtype of glutamate receptor). GABA-binding agents include volatile anaesthetic agents, propofol, benzodiazepines, barbiturates, etomidate, and chloral hydrate (Table 8.1). Nitrous oxide, and ketamine bind to NMDA receptors [3].

GABA receptors are inhibitory in nature, but due to an unknown mechanism, they act as excitatory during the developmental phase [4]. It is seen that refinement of the neuronal circuits takes place by activation of GABA receptors. Activation of the receptors induces cell migration, synaptogenesis, DNA synthesis, and cell proliferation. Antagonistic action of anaesthetic agents on these receptors can disturb this physiological neurodevelopment. Animal studies have confirmed the neurotoxic profile of NMDA antagonists and GABA agonists [5].

Synapse formation is an important component of brain development. Anaesthetic exposure in rodents leads to decrease (postnatal days 5–10) as well as increase (postnatal days 15–20) in the synapse density [6]. This brings forth the fact that exposure to clinically relevant doses of anaesthetics, whether short, prolonged, or multiple, can modify neuronal cytoarchitecture.

Table 8.1 Anesthetic drugs and their effect on various receptors

Agent	GABA	NMDA	Opioid receptor	Alpha2 adrenergic
Halogenated agents (sevoflurane, isoflurane, desflurane)	+			
Nitrous oxide		−		
Benzodiazepines	+			
Propofol	+			
Barbiturates	+			
Etomidate	+			
Chloral hydrate	+			
Ketamine		−		
Opioids			+	
Dexmedetomidine				+

GABA γ-Aminobutyric acid, *NMDA* N-methyl-D-aspartate; + Agonist; − Antagonist

Apart from neurogenesis, DNA-programmed neuronal death is equally important. During early developmental phase, excess of neurons and synapses are generated, which are reduced to less than 50% in adult life. Any interference with the normal apoptotic process can be detrimental to the neural architecture. Interference with the normal functioning of the GABA and NMDA receptors can lead to synaptic deprivation which in turn activates intrinsic neuro-apoptotic cascade.

Another mechanism is the anaesthesia-mediated mitochondrial disruption with release of caspase 9, the final executioner of cell death [2].

Role of calcium: calcium is for neuronal transmission. Endoplasmic reticulum (ER) is the primary regulator and source of calcium. Elevation of intracellular calcium is necessary for signalling, but excessive and prolonged exposure can be lethal. ER is considered an important initial target for anaesthetic agents. Exposure of anaesthetic agents in young animals is associated with prolonged elevation of intracellular calcium triggering neurotoxicity. Other suggested mechanisms include mitochondrial inhibition and energy depletion.

Neurotrophins: brain-derived neurotrophic factor (BDNF) is a type of neurotrophin. It plays a crucial role in neuronal survival and differentiation by activation of Trk receptors. It has been observed that if BDNF acts via p75NTR, it inhibits neurogenesis. Volatile anaesthetics and propofol increase the affinity of pro-BDNF toward p75NTR than Trk receptors, decreasing the neuronal survival [7]. Gross morphological changes can be easily detected by histological assessment, but sometimes even in the presence of normal looking neurons, abnormality may lie in the neuronal communications. Significant impairment in synaptic transmission in hippocampus of adolescent rats has been reported when exposed to anaesthesia on PD 7. Normal functioning of these circuits plays a crucial role in memory and learning later in life. Connections carrying inhibitory transmission are affected more.

Epigenetic Modification: Epigenetics is the study of heritable changes in the gene expression without changes in DNA. Recent reports have suggested that intrauterine exposure to anaesthetic drugs can induce cognitive impairment in 2nd generation off springs [8]. The mechanism is still unknown, but there is a risk of intellectual disability and autism due to epigenetic changes in the progeny as well.

8.4   Human Studies vs Preclinical Studies

Attention was drawn toward the effect of anaesthesia exposure on neurodevelopment only after findings in the laboratory. Prior to this, anaesthesia-related toxicity was not considered. With growing evidence from preclinical studies, it has become even more important to determine if anaesthesia exposure can lead to clinically relevant neurode-velopmental side effects. The question is not straight forward. There are multiple domains associated with it, like time/duration of anaesthesia exposure, subpopulation affected, and type of neurodevelopmental function affected. However, direct recipro-cation of preclinical data onto the human population may be imprecise.

Research has been conducted to study impact of anesthetic exposure in utero in rodent and non-human primate fetuses. Anesthetic drugs (isoflurane, propofol) administered for the duration of 4–5 h at the gestational age, equivalent to the 2nd and late 3rd trimester in humans, led to anaesthesia-induced neuro-apoptosis [9]. Another ovine study with isoflurane exposure in the mid-gestation failed to demon-strate any adverse effect with single exposure but, repeated exposures led to signifi-cant neuronal cell damage. However, these studies involved only anaesthesia and no surgery, which can confound the results. Another rodent study, with both anaesthe-sia and surgical exposure, has demonstrated conflicting results.

So far, majority of the studies have been done in the animal fetal and neonatal models, but they have several shortcomings. First, the interspecies differences in the brain development cannot be ignored. Second, most studies lack surgical stimulation. The negative impact of surgical stress, pain, tissue trauma on neurodevelopment is still unknown, but cannot be ignored. Third, the standard multiparameter monitoring done in humans is usually not practiced in majority of animal studies. This may be due to small size of neonatal animals and small circulating blood volumes precluding repeated blood gas analysis and glucose measurements. Fourth, most preclinical stud-ies lack precision with regard to duration of exposure, specific age group, and specific functional defect. However, the consistent and reproducible adverse neurodegenera-tive and neurobehavioral effects seen in the animal models encourage scientists to explore the same on human fetus, infants, and young children exposed to anaes-thetic agents.

8.5   Effect of Drugs in Utero and Maternal Exposure

8.5.1   Anaesthesia and Pregnant Mother

A large number of pregnant women require anaesthesia for obstetric and nonobstet-ric surgeries each year. Most commonly neuraxial anaesthesia is administered for caesarian surgeries. Majority of the surgeries take place at or near term, but emergent surgeries can take place any time during the gestation. In case of an emergent surgeries or maternal contraindication for neuraxial anaesthesia, inhalation-based general anaesthesia is the preferred mode. Considering the duration of cesarian delivery, the anaesthesia exposure time is usually short. So far, the results are rather conflicting. A retrospective study in patients undergoing caesarian delivery found no differences between the two modes of anaesthesia (general anaesthesia and neuraxial anaesthesia) as well as vaginal delivery without any anaesthetic. However, a population-based study of neonates following cesarian delivery under general anaesthesia demonstrated higher incidence of autism as compared to neonates delivered under neuraxial anaesthesia or vaginal delivery without any anaesthetic [10].

8.5.2 Anaesthesia and Fetus

With advancement in fetal surgery, there is a surge in the incidence of in-utero surgeries. The commonly known indications are fetal surgeries for myelomeningocele, sacrococcygeal teratoma, and other congenital anomalies, also ex-utero intrapartum therapy (EXIT). These procedures demand general anaesthesia with adequate uterine relaxation, maternal and fetal analgesia, and appropriate surgical access. With inhalational agents, one is able to achieve adequate, precise, and predictable uterine relaxation, most suitable for in-utero surgeries. Other surgeries such as fetoscopy-guided selective laser photocoagulation for twin–twin transfusion syndrome (TTTS) and tracheal occlusion for congenital diaphragmatic hernia (CDH) can be performed with maternal local anaesthesia and sedation (fentanyl or remifentanil) along with fetal medications. With the growing concern associated with the negative impact of anaesthesia on fetal neurodevelopment, we face few important questions. First, utility or need of fetal procedure requiring anaesthesia exposure. Some of the surgeries such as myelomeningocele and TTTS have proven beneficial to the fetus, unlike others like tracheal occlusion for CDH, benefits of which are still under review. Second, significant number of paediatric patients with congenital cardiac anomalies suffers from neurological impairment independent of treatment.

Information regarding in-utero studies is very limited. Duration may vary from standard to lengthy surgeries depending upon the urgency and type of procedure. Information regarding pharmacokinetics and pharmacodynamics of anaesthetic drugs in fetus is also very limited. Moreover, there is always an ethical dilemma associated while conducting any such study specifically in humans. Like, randomization of patients to regional anaesthesia group may pose a challenge as general anaesthesia is usually considered appropriate as per maternal and fetal safety is concerned. Suitable alternative is prospective follow-up of children undergoing in-utero surgery with respect to neurological development. Plasticity or ability of the fetal brain to recover from neuronal/axonal injury during the early phase of brain development is still unclear. More research is urgently required in this field.

Neuraxial anaesthesia can be considered as the primary mode of anaesthesia whenever feasible. General anesthesia via inhalational agents can be kept as a reserve for emergent nonobstetric surgeries or procedures/patients with contraindication for neuraxial anaesthesia. Only sedation requiring fetal procedures can be performed with the help of intravenous opioids such as fentanyl, remifentanil as monotherapy or with neuraxial anaesthesia with local anesthetics such as lidocaine, and bupivacaine, instead of agents implicated by FDA (midazolam, propofol). Communication and allaying maternal anxiety is equally important. For uterine relaxation, specially of prolonged duration (>3 h), other tocolytic agents, such as intravenous nitroglycerine (NTG) or magnesium sulfate ($MgSO_4$) or Atosiban, may be considered. There are limitations with these drugs, e.g., titrating the dose of NTG, while Atosiban and $MgSO_4$ have limited efficacy, making them unsuitable as sole tocolytics, but can be used as adjuncts to enhance uterine relaxation and reduce the requirement of inhalational agents. Another alternative is opioid supplementation with sparing effect on inhalational agents at the critical period when maximum relaxation is required during fetal manipulation.

Most preclinical studies suggest detrimental effect of high concentration and prolonged exposure of inhalational agents (Table 8.2). However, the exact concentration and duration have not been elucidated. FDA warning also lacks recommendations for exact dose or concentration of the anaesthetic agents to avoid.

Table 8.2 Type of surgery and choice of anesthesia technique

Type of surgery	Anaesthetic technique	Suggested modifications
Obstetric	Neuraxial block—LA ± opioids	None
Nonobstetric, Nonemergent	Neuraxial block—LA ± opioids	None
	Inhalation-based GA	<3 h duration—no change >3 h durations—consider deferring until postpartum
Nonobstetric (emergent)	Inhalation-based GA	Limit times: (a) Between induction and start of surgery (b) Between end of surgery and end of anesthesia.
Fetal procedures	LA/neuraxial anaesthesia	None
	IV sedative-hypnotic—propofol/ Midazolam	<3 h duration—no change >3 h duration—discuss risk/benefit Consider IV opioids (fentanyl or remifentanil) or dexmedetomidine
	GA with inhalational agents	<3 h duration—no change >3 h duration—discuss risk/benefit
	GA with increased concentration of inhalational agents for uterine relaxation	Consider supplementing with $MgSO_4$, Atosiban or NTG for tocolysis

LA Local anesthesia, *GA* General anaesthesia

8.6   Factors Affecting Neurotoxicity

8.6.1   Drug Type

Effect of inhalational agents on neurodegeneration and behavioral deficits is now accepted.

Isoflurane activates inositol 1,4,5-triphosphate receptors and induces excessive release of calcium from ER, modulating mitochondrial Bcl-xl protein ultimately initiating neural cell apoptosis. Similar mechanism is also reported with propofol, desflurane, and sevoflurane leading to uncontrolled release of pro-apoptotic factors [11].

Histopathological examination of brain of PD6 rhesus monkey after 5 h exposure to surgical plane of isoflurane anaesthesia revealed significant neuro-apoptotic changes as compared to age-matched controls. It was interesting to note that apoptosis was not confined to neurons, but large proportion of glial cells were also affected. Oligodendroglia plays a crucial role in the myelination of the neuronal axons. The study was repeated at the timepoint corresponding to the early stage of myelogenesis (gestational age of 120 days in monkeys). On examination, widespread neuronal apoptosis was noted in several cerebral cortical regions along with dispersed apoptosis of oligodendrocytes in the white matter region. Similar observations were made with propofol. Very recent reports have reported similar damage even with shorter exposure times (<3 h) also.

Prolonged exposure of sevoflurane (2.5% for 9 h) in nonhuman primates is associated with modulation of gene expression and impairment of lipid metabolism. Ketamine, widely used in children, is also associated with developmental abnormalities. A study reported that early developmental stages (122 days of gestation and 5 PD) are more susceptible to ketamine-induced neuronal death as compared to late that is 35 PD in resus monkeys. Long-term cognitive impairments such as learning, psychomotor skills, concept formation, and motivation were also affected, in the coming years. However, in this study, ketamine was administered for 24 h, which is quite unusual in clinical scenario. Later, shorter exposure times (5 h),, also demonstrated significant neuro-apoptosis.

8.6.2   Exposure Time

When it comes to exposure time, whether short or long, the results are unclear, both in animal and human studies. The positive vs negative studies ranged between 40 and 50% for exposure time of less than 1 h. However, the same ratio increases to 80% when exposure time is increased to more than 3 h. Most recent randomized control trials have also failed to demonstrate any effect with single and brief exposure in early infancy [12]. PANDA study also failed to detect any significant difference in IQ in between siblings with and without anaesthesia exposure (median exposure time of 80 min). On the contrary, in a cohort study from Western Australia, extensive neurobehavioral testing was done in children who underwent anaesthesia and surgery prior to the age of 3 years. They reported that with exposure as low as 15 min was associated with defective language and abstract reasoning later in life as compared to unexposed children.

8.6.3   Number of Exposures

Multiple anaesthesia exposures lead to cumulative effect and may be cause functional and structural alterations in the brain. On the other hand, single exposure is not completely devoid of any adverse neurodevelopmental effects. Wilder et al. studied the impact of single vs multiple exposures in more than 500 children and found that those with more than one exposure developed learning disabilities later in life [13].

8.7   Age of Exposure

8.7.1   Window of Vulnerability

Exposure to anaesthetic agents leads to neuronal cell death in the developing brain, which ultimately leads to neurodevelopmental defects as the child grows [14]. It is postulated that there is a specific time-period, the **window of vulnerability,** when the anaesthetic exposure may be particularly deleterious. In rodents, peak sensitivity is expected between postnatal days 7 and 10, followed by reduced sensitivity after day 10, and no effect beyond 60 days. However, this may be different in humans considering the developmental differences between the two species. As per current scientific evidence suspected period of vulnerability is expected to be during synaptogenesis, which ranges from birth to 2–4 years of age. However, high level of heterogenicity in the current evidence adds uncertainty to the acceptance of this hypothesis especially as to the period of vulnerability.

A recent large-scale observational cohort study concluded that children undergoing minor surgery and anaesthesia exposure before the age of 5 years are at a statistically significant increased risk of mental disorders, developmental delays, and attention deficit hyperactivity disorders (ADHD). The most significant observation was that the risk was found to be uniform regardless of age of exposure in the 5 year age period [15].

Based on the results of animal studies, it can be understood that the immature stages of human brain development in the antenatal period are most vulnerable to anaesthetic agents. On the other side, studies beyond the prenatal period also have failed to ensure safety of anaesthetic agents. Thus, there is still no specific age beyond which anaesthetic agents can be considered safe.

With all these considerations and limitations, FDA warns against use of anesthetics in children under the age of 3 years.

However, as a clinician and anesthetist, one must balance delaying the anaesthesia exposure with the unintended harmful consequences of delaying the surgery (Fig. 8.2) [1].

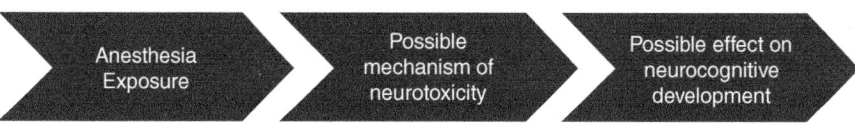

- Drugs (? Inhalation agents)
- Exposure time
- Number of exposures
- Age during exposure

- Neuroapoptosis
- Nerve function
- Structural changes
  - synaptogenesis
  - demyelination

- Decreased IQ
- Attention deficit
- Mental retardation
- Psychomotor changes
- Memory impairment

Fig. 8.2 Anesthetic Agent Induced Neurotoxicity

8.8 Clinical Implications of Potential Anesthesia-Related Neurotoxicity

The greatest dilemma for the anaesthesiologist will arise at the time of informed consent taking from the parents and ensuring safety of their child. All anesthetic agents, including nitrous oxide, have been implicated in causing cerebral neurotoxicity, affecting brain development and growth, with potential long-term deficits. Question arises then should we give anesthesia to these babies?? Unlike animal studies, whose data are being extrapolated to humans, and where anaesthetics are given without surgical indications, in human babies, anesthesia is provided for a surgical procedure. Because of the surgical condition, there may already be effects on various organ systems (pulmonary and gas exchange, hepatic renal and cardiac effects, metabolic, and acid base changes neurological changes (lethargy, somnolence, seizures, etc.).

On top of that blaming anesthesia for potential adverse neurotoxicity and long-term effects, seems unfair, as is depriving a surgical neonate of anesthesia.

Still, considering the scientific data in this field, however, limited and mostly from animals, it is imperative that proper precautions are taken while dealing with procedures requiring anesthetic exposure to prevent add-on effects on the growing brain of the fetus, or newborn, or neonate, depending on the situation.

Hence, safest course to be adopted by the concerned clinicians includes:

1. Undertake only that surgery which is urgent, life or organ saving
2. Use of adjuvant techniques (regional, local, or neuraxial anesthesia) so as to reduce the requirement of general anesthetic drugs
3. Precautions during regional anesthesia to use diluted concentrations of the LA drugs and never exceed toxic dose
4. Use the lowest possible anesthetic doses for shortest possible times, minimizing any potential brain effects
5. Use of safer drugs, e.g., fentanyl, remifentanil instead of morphine and pethidine, and avoiding propofol, and inhalational agents, as far as possible
6. Limited duration of surgery and hence anesthesia—total duration of anesthesia should not exceed 3 h

7. Minimising the duration of anaesthetic exposure for fetal, obstetric and nonobstetric procedures, by reducing the time interval between anaesthesia induction and start of surgery
8. Using of drugs and in doses, so that it does not prolong recovery time after anesthesia (i.e., end of surgery to extubation or recovery), for example, following a short surgery of 30 min should not be accompanied by prolonged or delayed recovery from anesthesia
9. Intrauterine surgeries and EXIT procedures require good uterine relaxation, so that surgical manipulations do not stimulate uterine contractions, and fetal morbidity and mortality. This is usually achieved by high doses of volatile anesthetic agents. Hence, to reduce their requirement, adjuvant tocolytic agents should be used instead, e.g., Corticosteroids, $MgSO_4$, Terbutaline, and Ritodrine
10. Use of alternative analgesic drugs and techniques Remifentanyl, Fentanyl, local infiltration, and reginal blocks including caudal block
11. BP, blood flow to brain and levels of CO_2 and O_2, may also play a role in protecting the brain. Using drugs and techniques that will create minimal hemodynamic and gas exchange disturbances and careful intraoperative monitoring

8.9   Future Direction

1. There is an urgent need to conduct research in the future keeping in mind the lacunae in the current evidence, with a multifaceted approach involving preclinical scientists, neuropsychologists, neonatologists, developmental paediatricians, neurologists, toxicologists, epidemiologists, and the anaesthesia community
2. Basic and translational high-quality preclinical studies to evaluate mechanism of toxicity with proper documentation of the anaesthesia technique and duration of exposure
3. Cohort studies with large sample size to detect small outcome differences in the neurodevelopmental domains, sufficient enough to establish clinical risk modifiers
4. Planning of high-quality clinical trials with adequate power in specific age groups focusing on specific interventions to achieve clinically relevant results

8.10   Conclusion

Exposure to general anaesthesia in fetus and early childhood is associated with neurodevelopmental anomalies later in life. Several preclinical studies have pointed toward possible mechanisms for neurotoxicity, but their implications on humans are still unclear. Genetic, physiological, and developmental interspecies differences limit the translation of animal and preclinical results to humans. Recent FDA warning cautioning against frequent prolonged anesthesia in small children **"repeated or lengthy use of general anesthesia and sedation drugs during surgeries or**

procedures in children younger than 3 years or pregnant women during their third trimester may affect the development of children's brains" must be paid heed to.

References

1. FDA Drug Safety Communication: FDA approves label changes for use of general anesthetic and sedation drugs in young children. Nov, 2017; https://www.fda.gov/drugs/drug-safety-and-availability/fda-drug-safety-communication-fda-approves-label-changes-use-general-anesthetic-and-sedation-drugs
2. Sanders RD, Hassell J, Davidson AJ, Robertson NJ, Ma D. Impact of anaesthetics and surgery on neurodevelopment: an update. Br J Anaesth. 2013;110(suppl 1):i53–72.
3. Istaphanous GK, Ward CG, Loepke AW. The impact of the perioperative period on neurocognitive development, with a focus on pharmacological concerns. Best Pract Res Clin Anaesthesiol. 2010;24:433–49.
4. Tashiro A, Sandler VM, Toni N, et al. NMDA receptor mediated, cell-specific integration of new neurons in adult dentate gyrus. Nature. 2006;442(7105):929–33.
5. Gentry KR, Steele LM, Sedensky MM, et al. Early developmental exposure to volatile anesthetics causes behavioral defects in Caenorhabditis elegans. Anesth Analg. 2013;116(1):185–9.
6. Head BP, Patel HH, Niesman IR, et al. Inhibition of p75 neurotrophin receptor attenuates isoflurane mediated neuronal apoptosis in the neonatal central nervous system. Anesthesiology. 2009;110(4):813–25.
7. Suehara T, Morishita J, Ueki M, et al. Effects of sevoflurane exposure during late pregnancy on brain development of offspring mice. Paediatr Anaesth. 2016;26(1):52–9.
8. Chalon J, Tang CK, Ramanathan S, et al. Exposure to halothane and enflurane affects learning function of murine progeny. Anesth Analg. 1981;60(11):794–7.
9. Creeley C, Dikranian K, Dissen G, Martin L, et al. Propofol induced apoptosis of neurones and oligodendrocytes in fetal and neonatal rhesus macaque brain. Br J Anaesth. 2013;110(Suppl 1):i29–38. https://doi.org/10.1093/bja/aet173.
10. Chien LN, Lin HC, Shao YH, et al. Risk of autism associated with general anesthesia during cesarean delivery: a population-based birth-cohort analysis. J Autism Dev Disord. 2015;45(4):932–42. https://doi.org/10.1007/s10803-014-2247-y.
11. Inan S, Wei H. The cytoprotective effects of dantrolene: a ryanodine receptor antagonist. Anesth Analg. 2010;111:1400–10.
12. Davidson AJ, Disma N, de Graaff JC, Withington DE, et al. Neurodevelopmental outcome at 2 years of age after general anaesthesia and awake regional anaesthesia in infancy (GAS): an international multicentre, randomised controlled trial. Lancet. 2016;387:239–50.
13. Wilder RT, Flick RP, Sprung J, Katusic SK, et al. Early exposure to anesthesia and learning disabilities in a population based birth cohort. Anesthesiology. 2009;110:796–804.
14. Jevtovic-Todorovic V, Hartman RE, Izumi Y, et al. Early exposure to common anesthetic agents causes widespread neurodegeneration in the developing rat brain and persistent learning deficits. J Neurosci. 2003;23:876–82.
15. Ing C, Sun M, Olfson M, DiMaggio CJ, et al. Age at exposure to surgery and anesthesia in children and association with mental disorder diagnosis. Anesth Analg. 2017;125(6):1988–98. https://doi.org/10.1213/ANE.0000000000002423.

Neonatal Rehabilitation and Outcome

9

Ritu Majumdar

9.1 Introduction

Neonatal rehabilitation includes strategies to restore the developmental milestones and improve the neurodevelopmental outcome in neonates who have suffered injury to the brain before, during or after birth.

Common causes of neonatal morbidity include preterm birth complications, intrapartum-related factors: hypoxic–ischemic encephalopathy (HIE), infections (sepsis, meningitis and neonatal tetanus) and other conditions: jaundice and congenital infections (cytomegalovirus, toxoplasma, syphilis, and rubella).

Neonatal encephalopathy is diagnosed in neonates with significant neurologic dysfunction, including respiratory difficulties, altered tone, low consciousness, or seizure activity. It is the best predictor of Cerebral palsy in term infants, regardless of the cause of encephalopathy [1].

Before planning rehabilitation, it is important to learn about the following terms which will affect the overall neonate outcome:

9.2 Growing Brain and Neural Plasticity

In infancy, the sensory and motor systems interact with the environment and construct more complex systems, and thus learning is achieved. Neural processes such as the formation of multisensory connections and higher order networks are all built upon the more basic functions (e.g., hearing, vision). Preterm birth and its complications or injuries resulting from insults such as prolonged hypoxia or illness change the order of normal neurodevelopment. Growth and environment are critical for

R. Majumdar (✉)
Department of Physical Medicine & Rehabilitation, Lady Harding Medical College & Associated Hospitals, New Delhi, India

© The Author(s), under exclusive license to Springer Nature Singapore Pte Ltd. 2023
U. Saha (ed.), *Clinical Anesthesia for the Newborn and the Neonate*, https://doi.org/10.1007/978-981-19-5458-0_9

early neurodevelopment making nutritional, social–emotional and physical environmental factors as essential components of evaluation and treatment in infancy [2]:

- Neural plasticity is the capacity of the nervous system to modify itself, functionally and structurally, in response to experience and injury.
- It is a key component of neural development and normal functioning of the nervous system as well as a response to the changing environment, aging or pathological insult.
- Plasticity is necessary not only for neural networks to acquire new functional properties but also for them to remain robust and stable [3].
- It is the process of reorganization of neural connections after injury or experiences and can be harmful also. Compensation for a brain lesion or a poorly functioning pathway can be re-established at the expense of another pathway, even of a higher order process.
- Hence, a rehabilitation expert should have an in depth knowledge about the good and ill effects of neural plasticity before applying its fundamentals for neurorehabilitation [2]

9.3   Development Process of a Child

Development is a continuous process; it proceeds stage by stage in an orderly sequence, despite individual variations. As the nervous system matures, increasingly complex behaviors unwind. Each stage of development represents a higher level of maturity where features are qualitatively different, yet dependent and derived from earlier stages [4].

There are four components or domains of developmental growth: physiological, sensorimotor, Cognitive and psychological.

1. **Physiologic domain**: at birth, a full-term neonate adapts to the new environment and is independent in respiration, circulation, digestion and temperature regulation.
2. **Sensorimotor domain**: newborns and neonates exhibit specific behavioral states of arousal: deep sleep, light sleep, drowsy, quiet, alert, active, awake and crying. There is a gradual transition from one state to another, and the response to stimulation is influenced by the neonate's behavioral state.
   (a) **Gross motor skills**: neonate's gross motor activity is developed from movement patterns that begin in the intrauterine environment and from the maturation of reflex behavior which is under control at two levels—spinal and brainstem. Apart from reflex behavior, a neonate demonstrates orientation, attention, and habituation to visual, auditory, and tactile stimuli. Motor responses in head control, sitting, rolling, and locomotion continue to develop from simple to complex skills. At 4 weeks, the neonate can move its head side to side. Head lag is noted from pull to sit position.
   (b) **Fine motor skills**: grasping reflex is present at birth. This allows the infant to have automatic contact with anything placed in the palm, though the hands are predominantly closed and the contact with the object is more with

the eyes than with hands. They look, stare and track objects within their visual fields.

3. **Cognitive domain**: According to Jean Piaget's theory, a child from birth to 2 years of age responds to and learns about the environment directly through sensations and motor responses. The emphasis is on sensory, movement and manipulative experiences with objects.
   (a) This is the shortest period of mental development but is the most active.
   (b) This accounts for the reflexive stage with simple biologic reflexes that are primitive, general, and related to survival.
   (c) Sucking and palmar reflexes which help to promote oral and manipulative exploration are most critical to early mental development.
   (d) The taste of food later in life depends on kinesthetic sensations derived from reflexive movements of sucking.
   (e) The development of communication is also related to the infant's cognitive abilities. The ability to produce different sounds is evidenced in crying. Lack of crying ability indicates neurologic impairment.

4. **Psychological domain**: after birth, there is emotional transition as the baby moves out of the protected environment of the womb. A sense of trust and mistrust starts developing. The ease of feeding, depth of sleep, and relaxation of bowels are signs of neonate's development of trust which is highly dependent on its relationship with primary caregivers. Position of face and early eye-to-eye contact between parents and neonate, help in the attachment process.

9.4 History Taking

- A detailed neonatal history is essential, including birth age and weight, Apgar scores, onset and success of breastfeeding, medications, and supportive measures given while hospitalized.
- Age, weight, and condition on discharge, means of feeding, need for ventilatory or other support at home, help predict subsequent, continuous, or recurrent problems.
- Weak lip closure, weak sucking force, and inadequate feeding may be preliminary signs of oral-motor dysfunction.
- Neonatal seizures may signal perinatal brain damage.
- Prematurity, particularly with low birth weight, is a frequent cause of cerebral palsy [2].
- Large birth weight may lead to intrapartum trauma, brachial plexus injury, and palsy, particularly with breech or other fetal malposition.

9.5 Examination

In newborns and young infants, state of alertness, activity, and comfort influence muscle tone. If the baby is restless and crying (anxious, upset), examination for muscle tone should be postponed.

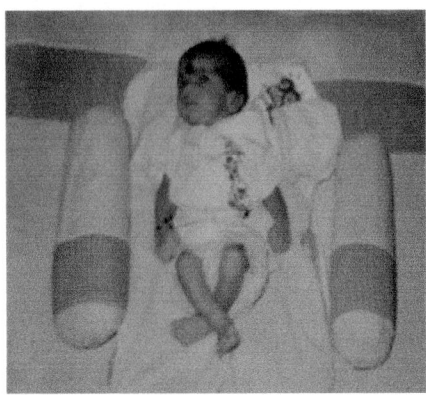

Fig. 9.1 High-risk neonate with increased tone of all four limbs

- Increased tone is the symptom of corticospinal or basal ganglion damage (Fig. 9.1).

Intrauterine and neonatal insults carry a high risk of substantial long-term neurological morbidity.

- Neurological abnormalities should always be routinely sought as part of neonatal care in babies who survive significant Hypoxic Ischemic Encephalopathy.
- Persistent generalized disturbances of tone, seizures, continued irritability or decreased alertness, persistent asymmetry of posture, movement and delay in establishing efficient feeding, are all indicative of neurological abnormalities of the infant beyond the neonatal period [5].

9.6   Posture and Movement Patterns

A fetus in the womb is flexed with midline orientation of the head and extremities.

- Due to effects of gravity, prematurity, illness, low tone, primitive reflexes and immature neuromotor control, the resting posture of a neonate without therapeutic positioning will be flat, extended, asymmetrical with the head to one side and with the extremities abducted and externally rotated.
- Lack of appropriate positioning can create short-term and long-term functional problems even in the absence of overt brain pathology [6].

The best known neuromotor assessment is the general movement assessment (GMA).

- General movements are the most frequently used movements from early fetal age until 3–4 month post-term.
- Quality of these movements provides information about the integrity of the brain, especially about the connectivity in the periventricular white matter [7].
- Movements are assessed when the neonate is awake, calm, alert, and lying on the back.
- Baby should not have any toys or pacifiers and parents should not be interacting with the baby.
- The baby is videoed for 3–5 min and used for assessment and scoring.
- Babies with absent or abnormal general movements are at higher risk of neurological conditions, particularly, cerebral palsy.

9.7 Muscle Tone

- Muscle tone gradually increases with age, in caudal-to-cephalic (feet-to-head) and distal-to-proximal (extremities-to-trunk) directions.
- Active muscle tone, observed during spontaneous movement or elicited by righting reactions when the infant is handled, develops before passive flexor tone seen at rest [8].
- Hypotonia is normal for extremely preterm neonates, and at term demonstrates greater extension and less physiologic flexion than a full-term newborn.
- Twitches, tremors, and startles are common in preterm infants, but movements typically become even and tremors less prevalent as term equivalency nears.
- Assessment of muscle tone also depends on state of arousal and medical status. A preterm neonate may be active when awake but hypotonic if assessed while drowsy or asleep.
- Evaluation of muscle tone is not accurate when the baby is ill. It changes as the baby recovers.
- Many medications have neuromotor side effects [9].
- Atypical findings and unusual movement patterns improve with maturation and physical recovery.

Bone layout and joint mobility change during the growing years:

- Full-term infants have predominant flexor tone and lack around 25° of elbow extension.
- Joint hyperextensibility and hypotonia allow increased passive motion in preterm infants.
- **Scarf sign** is a good example of excessive joint mobility in premature babies. Holding the baby's hand, the examiner draws one arm across the chest, like a scarf, toward the contralateral shoulder, round the neck. In premature infants, the

elbow crosses the midline, indicating hypotonic laxity of the shoulder and elbow joints.

- In full-term neonates, due to early flexor tone predominance, there is incomplete hip extension with a mean constraint of 30°, which decreases to less than 10° by 3–6 months [10]. At birth and during early infancy, hip external rotation surpasses internal rotation due to early hip flexion attitude. Differences between bilateral hip abduction, apparent shortening of one leg and asymmetric gluteal and upper thigh skin folds are highly suggestive of congenital or acquired hip dysplasia or dislocation [11]. Alignment of the femoral neck in neonates is consistent with prenatal coxa valga and increased anteversion. Femoral inclination is 160° and the angle of anteversion is 60°. Respective adult measurements of 125° and 10–20° develop postnatally and are accelerated by weight bearing.

Screening of eyes and ear are part of routine examination at birth to rule out congenital visual impairment and hearing loss, respectively [12].

Early onset brain damage, especially of the prefrontal cortex, can result in behavioral problems, making assessment exceedingly difficult during the early years, especially when other impairments (motor and cognition) are also present.

9.8   Neonatal Rehabilitation - Early Interventions

The aim of neonatal rehabilitation is early intervention in the high-risk neonate in all areas of development to achieve functional independence as an individual. This should be an integral part of the management for early and effective planning from day one for on-going care.

Early intervention is defined as child-oriented training activities and parent-oriented guidance activities which are implemented after identification of the developmental condition. Early age period from 0 to 3 years is the most appropriate period to lay the basic foundation for further development and learning as brain is characterized by high plasticity during this period. Early intervention involves interaction of the child, parents, family, society, and environment. These services are designed to identify and meet child's needs in five developmental areas:

(a) Physical
(b) Cognitive
(c) Communication
(d) Social or emotional development
(e) Sensory and adaptive development

Early intervention includes provision of services to children with developmental delays or disability and their families for the purpose of lessening the effects or burden of the condition. Early intervention can be **remedial** or **preventive** in nature—remediating the existing developmental problems or preventing their occurrence [13]. All children who are subjected to developmental risk or developmental disability should have access to these services.

1. **Caregiving:** the sense of touch is highly developed in utero, and gentle human touch after birth, provides consistent positive tactile inputs. Caregiving procedures may contribute to the neonate's physiologic instability (increased heart rate, fluctuations in blood pressure, alterations in cerebral blood flow, and hypoxemia), motor stress, energy depletion, and agitation. Caregiving based primarily on fixed schedules for vital signs and feeding often delays the caregiver's response to baby cues and thus baby's efforts to communicate are wasted.

   Synaptogenesis (formation of billions of connections between neurons) is a primary ongoing event in the development of brain and sensory system during the last trimester. After 28 weeks of gestation, endogenous synaptogenesis generates brain complexity and plasticity, and occurs only during REM sleep. Undisturbed sleep is **absolutely essential** for normal development of the fetal brain and sensory systems during the last trimester.

   Caregivers should focus for an optimum sleep of their child.

   (a) Unnecessary handling and movement should be avoided.
   (b) Caregivers should prepare the baby for touch or movement by speaking softly and containing extremities during movement and lifting.
   (c) Social touch and noninvasive care giving procedures can disturb and stress neonates, requiring caregiver efforts to comfort and promote recovery.
   (d) Comfortable bedding, containment, parental skin-to-skin holding (kangaroo care) and reduction of environmental light and sound are supportive measures [14].

   Maternal depression after birth of a high-risk child increases stress and delays parental responsibilities:

   (a) Parents have multiple roles as caregivers, educators, and facilitators of their child's development.
   (b) They should be encouraged to ask questions about what they understand and want to know.
   (c) The response of the treating physician and other staff involved in care of the child should be honest and understandable.
   (d) Parents are often frustrated and anxious when information is incomplete and conflicting.
   (e) Printed material such as pamphlets/booklets with information about early intervention in simple language along with pictures can be provided for parent education.
   (f) Parent support groups/peer group counselling can also be helpful in providing information and support.
   (g) Inclusion of siblings, extended family members, and volunteers should be encouraged.

   Parents should be helped with the following for a long-term positive outcome:

   (a) To gain competence and confidence in recognizing and responding to their infant's cues of stress
   (b) Providing therapeutic positioning and developmentally supportive handling
   (c) Regulating sensory input to avoid overstimulation

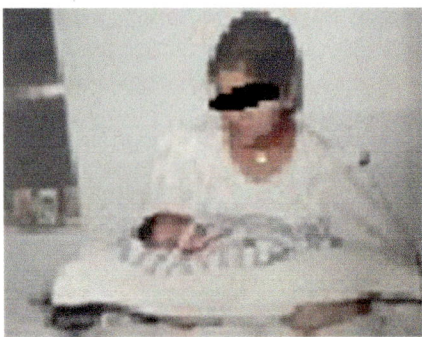

Fig. 9.2 Mother–infant bonding

(d) Facilitating functional oral feeding
(e) Meeting the neonate's long-term developmental needs
(f) Promoting parent–infant attachment (Fig. 9.2).

2. **Developmental stimulation** is not appropriate until the neonate is near term and sufficiently stable medically, for seeking attention and interaction. Each child is different. Stable term infants may demand more attention. Prolonged crying must not be ignored. Lullabies and musical toys can be used for stimulation [9].

3. **Touch, Smell and movement sensations:** These sensations help the newborn to maintain contact with the caregiver. Touch or Tactile sensations are critical in establishing a mother infant bond and help in forming feelings of security in the infant. Tactile system plays an important role regarding emotions as it is directly involved in making physical contact with others. Proprioception also plays an important role in mother infant relationship. The phasic movements of the infant's limbs generate additional proprioceptive inputs which help in development of body awareness [4]. Of all the sensory systems, Vestibular is first to mature. It is fully functional at birth, although its integration with visual and proprioceptive systems continues through childhood. This is seen when rocking and carrying to calm the baby. Lifting into an upright posture against the caregiver's shoulder increases alertness and visual tracking.

4. **Oromotor impairments** can cause feeding difficulties in preterms, who may have encephalopathy. Rehabilitation aims at re-establishing patterns of suck–swallow–breathe coordination and increased endurance and efficiency during oral feeding.

5. **The visual and auditory systems are immature at birth**—the neonate orients to some visual and auditory inputs, particularly human face, and voice. For a proper developmental care, there should be interaction among the neonate, family, and surroundings wherever the neonate is cared for. The surroundings should be lively and positive and promote involvement of family members as primary caregiver hospital environment (Fig. 9.3).

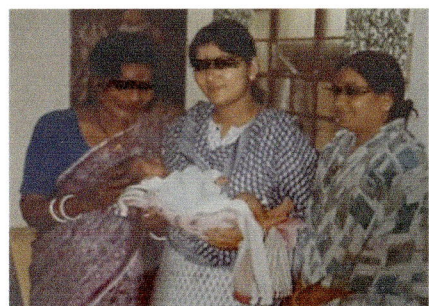

Fig. 9.3 Interaction by paternal and maternal grandmothers in an Indian setting

A preterm infant's immature CNS is generally competent for protected intrauterine life, but is not sufficiently developed to adjust to the demands of extrauterine life, which may stress the already vulnerable and disorganized CNS. Excessive sensory stimulation can cause insults to the developing brain (from repeated hypoxic episodes related to stress) and create maladaptive behaviors that contribute to later poor developmental outcome [15]. It becomes a priority to reduce avoidable stressors and help the preterm baby remain calm, without sleep deprivation.

Auditory stimuli: sufficient opportunities should be provided to hear interactive parent voices by the high-risk neonate [15]. Audio recordings should be played only for brief periods, be less than 55 dB and at a reasonable distance from ear, and should not affect sleep.

Visual stimulation: protection of eyes from direct light exposure and avoid abrupt light fluctuations [16]. Black & white patterns drawn on a cardboard placed near the child can be used for visual stimulation.

Developmental interventions that support neonate's physiologic stability and brain development include:

(a) Proper lighting (bright lights can disrupt sleep)
(b) Sound modifications (loud noise can contribute to apnea, bradycardia, sleep disruption)
(c) Therapeutic positioning, nurturing touch, non-nutritive sucking
(d) Alteration of caregiver timing and handling techniques
(e) Preservation of sleep and
(f) Increased family involvement

6. **Therapeutic positioning:** positioning replicates the in utero posture. External support and positioners can provide a temporary substitute for the premature neonate's poor motor control. Proper positioning is an important neuromotor developmental intervention to minimize positional deformities and to improve muscle tone, postural alignment, movement patterns, and developmental milestones [9]. Active infant movement is potentially important for normal muscle tension on bone and necessary for mineralization and bone density. Mother should be given training regarding holding techniques specially in neonates with increased tone.

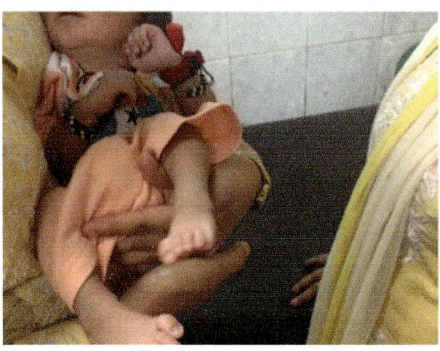
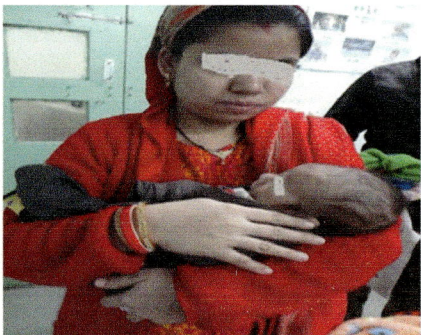

Fig. 9.4 Proper posture and positioning

7. **Range of motion:** passive range of motion (PROM) (Fig. 9.4) may be appropriate for neonates who demonstrate structural or neuromuscular limitation of movement and are stable enough to tolerate a rehabilitation approach. It is less beneficial in hypertonicity neonate, where sustained stretch is advocated. Gentle PROM can be useful in sedated neonates to avoid development of contractures.

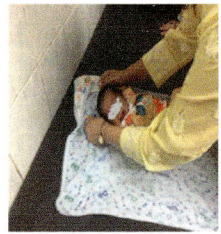
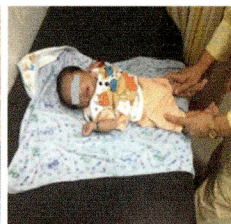
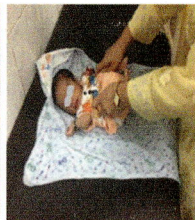
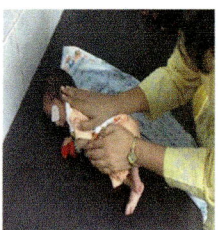

Gentle PROM exercises

8. **Massage:** massage is an art and a science that the caregiver should be taught in terms of techniques, precautions, and warning signs. This allows an active engagement and bonding between the neonate and the caregiver.
9. **Splinting:** splinting is rarely needed in neonates as rigid contractures are uncommon and neonates are notably flexible. Over time improvement is achieved with gentle stretches, and therapeutic positioning. Rigid splints inhibit spontaneous movements and should be avoided for long periods of time. Protecting skin integrity and encouraging active movements are priorities in designing a neonatal splint. Simple splints made of light material-like foam is well-tolerated.
10. **Feeding:** breast milk is the optimal nutrition for neonates. Any breast milk the child receives is valuable. Mothers of preterm or ill infants who are educated about the benefits of breast milk often choose to pump milk for

their infants; many are unable to maintain sufficient lactation for successful or exclusive breastfeeding at discharge. Early initiation of frequent breast pumping, skin-to-skin holding as soon and as often as possible, non-nutritive sucking at breast (breast pumped first, although the breast is never truly empty and milk may "letdown") and establishing the basics of breastfeeding [17]. Milk banks are now associated with Neonatology units in tertiary care Hospitals.

9.9 Outcome

- Prediction of future developmental outcome is difficult, as change is one of the main characteristics of the developing brain.
- Many neonates survive major insults without any evidence of impairment because of the plasticity of the developing brain and improvements in medical care.
- In some newborns, insults can cause varying degrees of long-term neuro developmental impairment, with huge socioeconomic burden, especially in resource-poor countries, and affect the global burden of disease as it contributes to both premature mortality and long-term disability.
- There is less information about the severity and distribution of long-term impairments after intrauterine or neonatal insults. Few studies provide supportive evidence that intrauterine and neonatal insults result in significant long-term neurological morbidity and that these insults have a high risk of affecting more than one domain [e.g., cognitive impairment, motor impairment, hearing and vision loss [18]].
- Presence of widespread neural impairment reduces the probability for neuro plasticity of the nervous system and chances of beneficial effects of intervention decrease with the extent of brain pathology.
- High-risk neonates are at increased risk of developing behavioral problems throughout childhood, such as autism spectrum disorder, potential precursors of anxiety and depression in childhood and adolescence [2].
- Stress during early life is known to have lifelong consequences, as it induces permanent changes in the brain, especially the mono-aminergic and dopaminergic systems. Alterations in the dopaminergic system are associated with impaired motor learning [19].

Rehabilitation, by early intervention, helps in attainment of developmental milestones and prevention of development of complications, such as contracture in limbs and pressure sores.

Along with motor outcome, improving cognition, socio-emotional skills and mental health is the focus of early intervention programs.

Family counseling and timely guidance improve outcome of high-risk babies.

These include providing:

1. Family education concerning the issues being faced by the child and its management
2. Peer counseling by caregivers of other high-risk babies
3. Education to caregivers regarding importance of sensory and environmental stimulation
4. Basic rehabilitation in home settings, such as proper handling, positioning, therapeutic exercises, daily care (bathing, dressing, feeding), and use of simple aids
5. Family support essential for positive outcome

9.10   Pearls of Wisdom

1. Proper Antenatal care with identification of high-risk pregnancies and parental counseling regarding care of the neonate is a must.
2. Timely referral to rehabilitation specialist is the need of hour.
3. Awareness regarding rehabilitation and timely utilization of these services to prevent secondary complications of motor impairments (contractures, feeding difficulties, later psychological, and cognitive impairments).
4. District health care workers should be trained in basic rehabilitation techniques and motion exercises.
5. The plastic changes may fade away the affliction present at early age—infants grow out of their deficit. The reverse is also possible: children may be effectively free from signs of dysfunction at early age, but grow with functional deficit due to age-related increase in complexity of neural functions [20].
6. In view of the poor outcome, prevention, and improved treatment of complications during birth and neonatal period, along with research into adjunct treatment approaches cannot be overemphasized [21].
7. Involvement of caregivers is the key to successful rehabilitation program.

References

1. Alexander MA, Mathews DJ. Pediatric rehabilitation. Principles and practice. 4th ed. Demos Medical; 2009.
2. Maitre NL. Neurorehabilitation after neonatal intensive care: evidence and challenges. Arch Dis Child Fetal Neonatal Ed. 2015;100(6):F534–40. https://doi.org/10.1136/archdischild-2013-305920. Epub 2015 Feb 20.
3. von Bernhardi R, Eugenín J, Muller KJ. The plastic brain. Springer; 2017. https://link.springer.com/book/10.1007/978-3-319-62817-2
4. Nuse Clark P, Allen S. Occupational therapy for children. Am J Occup Ther. 1988;42(6):359–63.
5. Sabrine N, Singh J, Sinha SK. Medical management of birth asphyxia. Indian Pediatrics. 1999;36:369–76.
6. Spear ML, Leef K, Epps S, etal. Family reactions during infant hospitalization in the neonatal intensive care unit. Am J Perinatol 2002;19: 205–213.

7. Prechtl HRF. Qualitative changes of spontaneous movements in fetus and preterm infant are a marker of neurological dysfunction. Early Hum Dev. 1990;23:151–8. https://doi.org/10.1016/0378-378290)90011-7.

8. Blackburn ST. Neuromuscular and sensory systems. In: Blackburn S, editor. Maternal, fetal, and neonatal physiology: a clinical perspective. 2nd ed. St. Louis: Saunders; 2003. p. 546–98.

9. O'Brien S. 'Neonatal intensive care unit': occupational therapy for children. 6th ed. Mosby; 2010.

10. Steindler A. Kinesiology of the human body. Springfield, IL: Charles C Thomas; 1955.

11. Tachdjian MO. Pediatric orthopedics. 2nd ed. Philadelphia: WE Saunders; 1990.

12. Rashtriya bal swasthya karyakram: Ministry of Health & Family Welfare, Government of India; 2017. http://nhm.gov.in/nrhm-components/rmnch-a/child-health-immunization/rashtriya-bal-swasthya-karyakram-rbsk/background-html.

13. Organization of Early Intervention Services. National Institute for the Mentally Handicapped Secunderabad; 2008

14. Gardner SL, Goldson E. The neonate and the environment: impact on development. In: Merenstein SL, Gardner GB, editors. Handbook of neonatal intensive care. 6th ed. St. Louis: Mosby; 2006. p. 273–349.

15. Graven SN. Sound and the developing infant in the NICU: conclusions and recommendations for care. J Perinatol. 2000;20:S88–93.

16. Graven SN. Early neurosensory visual development of the fetus and newborn. Clin Perinatol. 2004;31:199–216.

17. Howe TH, Wang TN. Systematic review of interventions used in or relevant to occupational therapy for children with feeding difficulties ages birth–5 years. Am J Occup Ther. 2013;67:405–12.

18. Kolb B, Mychasiuk R, Williams P etal. Brain plasticity and recovery from early cortical injury. Dev Med Child Neurol 2011; 53(Suppl 4):4–8. https://doi.org/10.1111/j.1469-8749.2011.04054.x

19. Weinstock M. The long-term behavioral consequences of prenatal stress. Neurosci Biobehav Rev. 2008;32:1073–86. https://doi.org/10.1016/j.neubiorev.2008.03.002.

20. Hadders-Algra M. Two distinct forms of minor neurological dysfunction: perspectives emerging from a review of data of the Groningen Perinatal Project. Dev Med Child Neurol. 2002;44:561–71. https://doi.org/10.1111/j.1469-8749.2002.tb00330.x.

21. Mwaniki MK, Atieno M, Lawn JE, et al. Long-term neurodevelopmental outcomes after intrauterine and neonatal insults: a systematic review; 2012, p. 379. www.thelancet.com.

Part II

Developmental Anatomical and Physiological Aspects

General Anatomical and Physiological Considerations in the Newborn and Neonates

10

Usha Saha

10.1 Introduction

Neonatal period is a very high-risk period, especially the first 24 h of life, because of the ongoing transitional changes. The anesthesiologist faces several challenges when faced with delivery of anesthesia for various surgical procedures in newborns, and term and premature neonates. The dilemmas are several, all culminating into the two goals of anesthesia: adequacy of anesthesia appropriate for the surgery and its duration, and adequacy of recovery at the end. Though they may appear simple and easy to attain, in reality, anesthesiologist is often confronted with either too less or too much of ANESTHESIA, and delayed recovery, with need for ventilatory support, prolonged duration of hospital stay, increased cost of perioperative care, and not always an optimum outcome. Their anatomical, physiological, biochemical, and organ functions are different from those in an adult or child, knowledge of which is essential for the anesthesiologist to fulfill the goals and have a good outcome [1–9].

Various parameters and methods have been used to assess this risk, gestational age (GA) at birth, and birthweight (BW) being commonly used. Worldwide, more than 1 million neonates need surgery, and nearly 6% of total live births are premature. At birth, there are incomplete organogenesis, immature physiology, and poor organ functioning. They may require surgery on day of birth itself or during the neonatal period. This number is on the rise with improvement in perinatal and neonatal care.

They are extremely prone to deleterious effects of stress and pain itself, and anesthetic and analgesic drugs further add on to these adverse effects, with very high postoperative morbidity, poor survival, apnea, proneness to RDS, IVH, ROP, hypothermia, hypoglycemia, infections, seizures, PFC, reopening of shunts, and death. Because of this, many elective operations are deferred during the neonatal

U. Saha (✉)
Department of Anesthesia, Critical Care, Pain and Palliative Care, Lady Hardinge Medical College, Smt Sucheta Kriplani and Kalawati Saran Childrens Hospitals, New Delhi, India

© The Author(s), under exclusive license to Springer Nature Singapore Pte Ltd. 2023
U. Saha (ed.), *Clinical Anesthesia for the Newborn and the Neonate*, https://doi.org/10.1007/978-981-19-5458-0_10

period. Anesthesiologists can also apply these criteria to assess perioperative risk of anesthesia and surgery and take special precautions during administration of anesthesia. Perioperative morbidity and mortality are inversely proportional to GA and BW. The goal of anesthetic management is early recovery after anesthesia and surgery and some guidelines have been proposed for neonates undergoing intestinal surgeries [10, 11].

This chapter will discuss all these aspects and their implications in the anesthetic management.

Before advancing into the details of this topic, several queries that arise in the mind are:

1. How are newborns and neonates different? And its significance to the anesthetist.
2. What is anesthetically safe period?
3. Fetal circulation, transitional changes or adaptations at birth, and consequences of abnormal adaptation,
4. Anatomy and physiology of a newborn, neonate, and premature—growth and maturation of the body organs.
5. What are the common medical diseases likely to be encountered, and their impact on anesthesia delivery and outcome?
6. What are the conditions likely to require surgical intervention in the neonatal period, and their impact on body anatomy, physiology, biochemical and metabolic functions, and anesthetic management?
7. Perianesthetic or perioperative concerns.

10.2 Categorization (Table 10.1)

In the fetus, organogenesis occurs in the first trimester, growth and development in the second, and anatomical and functional maturation, including surfactant production in the 3rd. Mortality is inversely proportional to GA at birth. Accordingly, newborns are categorized into two: **"TERM" and "PRETERM".**

Table 10.1 Categorization and terms used for neonates

		GA (week)/age	Birth Weight (grams)
A. Categorization according to GA			
1.	**Term**	≥37 weeks (37–42) weeks	
	Early term	37 weeks 0 days to 38 weeks 6 days	
	Full term	39 weeks 0 days to 40 weeks 6 days	
	Late term	41 week 0 day to 41 week 6 day	
2.	**Newborn**	C	
	Neonate	0 h–28 day age	
	Infant	29 day–1 year age	
3.	**Perinatal period**	28-week GA (1 kg)—seventh day of life	
	Extended perinatal period	20-week GA (>0.5 kg) - seventh day of life	
	Prematurity	<37 weeks GA	And <2500

Table 10.1 continued

		GA (week)/age	Birth Weight (grams)
4.	**Micropremies**	ELBW	And 400–1000
	Dysmaturity (postmaturity syndrome)	>42-week GA	And cessation of weight gain (placental insufficiency)
	Post-term	>42-week GA	And no signs of dysmaturity
	Fetal macrosomia	>4000 g (8 lb 13 oz)	
	Ex premature	Premature + >38 weeks PCA	
B. Categorization according to BW			
1.	**Low birthweight (LBW)**		<2500
2.	**Very low birthweight (VLBW)**		<1500
3.	**Extremely low birthweight (ELBW)**		<1000 (2 lb 3 oz)
4.	**AGA**	37–42	And >2500
5.	**SGA**	>37	And <2500
6.	**LGA**	Any GA	>Appropriate weight

Note—(a) Neonate is from birth up to 28 days past due date. If born at 40 weeks, he is a neonate for 4 weeks, and if born at 30 weeks, it will be a neonate for 14 weeks. (10 weeks to correct to term age + subsequent 28 days). (b) Dysmaturity or postmaturity syndrome refers to the fetus whose weight gain after the due date has stopped, usually due to placental insufficiency leading to malnourishment, Marasmic appearance, desquamation of skin, loss of subcutaneous tissues, and yellow meconium staining of skin, nails, and umbilical cord. (c) Post-term includes those born after 42 weeks but with no signs of dysmaturity. They have dry, loose, peeling skin, overgrown nails, abundant scalp hair, visible palm and sole creases, minimal fat deposits, and green or brown staining of skin from passage of stools into amniotic fluid. (d) Fetal macrosomia describes a newborn who is much larger than average, with BW more than 4000 gm (8 lb 13 oz). Worldwide, incidence of fetal macrosomia is about 9% of all births

10.2.1   As Per Gestational Age (GA)

1. **TERM** babies are born at ≥37 weeks GA (37–42 weeks) and BW >2.5 kg. This is further subcategorized into **early term** (37 weeks 0 days to 38 weeks 6 days), **full term** (39 weeks 0 days to 40 weeks 6 days), and **late term** (41 weeks 0 days to 41 weeks 6 days).
2. **PREMATURE** babies are those born at <37 weeks GA and <2.5 kg BW. They are further subcategorized into

Borderline premature (near term)	36–37 GA	0% mortality
Moderately premature	31–36 GA	50% mortality
Severely premature	28–24 GA	>70% mortality
Extreme prematurity	24–28 GA	> >>>% mortality

Surgical and medical diseases and anesthesia further increase mortality.

10.2.2 As Per Birthweight (BW)

BW is an important indicator of newborn's health and well-being, and several peri-natal complications are associated with it. Incidence of perioperative complications is inversely proportional to BW.

1. **Normal BW** ranges between 2500 and 3500 g. These babies are born full term, pulmonary development and surfactant amounts are adequate, and organs are mature and take over their individual functions in the extrauterine life. They have less incidence of congenital abnormalities or severe form of surgical diseases. When these newborns present for surgery, they have the best perianesthetic outcome, with nil or minimal morbidity [12].
2. **Low BW (LBW)** newborns have BW <2500 g. (India <2000 g).
3. **Very low BW (VLBW)** newborns have BW <1500 g.
4. **Extremely low BW (ELBW)** newborns have BW of 1000 g (2 lbs 3 oz) or less. These are usually born prematurely (GA <28 weeks). Though fetus is viable, organs are not fully mature and are deficient in surfactant too.
5. **AGA** (appropriate for GA) includes newborns with BW appropriate for GA.
6. **SFD** (small for date)/**SGA** (small for GA)—newborns with BW less than expected for GA, and includes those born >37 weeks but BW <2500 g, and usually have IUGR.
7. **LFD** (large for date)/**LGA** (large for GA)—are newborns with BW more than expected for GA.
8. **IUGR** (intrauterine growth retardation) or **FGR** (fetal growth restriction) is often due to placental insufficiency, and viral infection (TORCH complex—toxoplasmosis, rubella, cytomegalovirus, herpes) (Fig. 10.1).

As per the reported data of 3,952,841 births in USA in 2012, approximately 8% were LBW (<2500 g) and 1.4% VLBW (<1500 g). The incidence of low BW and related problems is more in developing countries like India. With improvement in antenatal and perinatal care (maternal steroids, surfactant replacement, and advanced neonatal care), survival of LBW, VLBW, and ELBW newborns has improved remarkably. Currently, accepted minimal age of viability is 23 weeks, a decline

Fig. 10.1 LBW newborn (BW 1500 g)

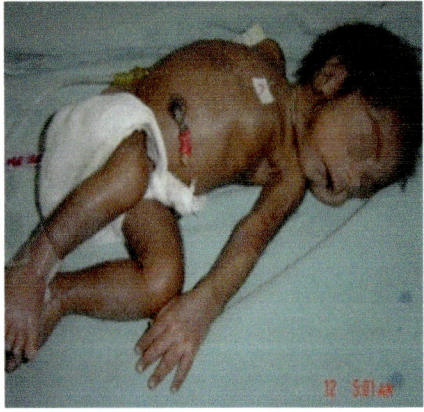

from old figure of 28 weeks. Neonatal anesthesiologists are likely to face challenges when managing these babies presenting for surgery, especially during their neonatal period. ELBW survival has improved with the widespread use of exogenous surfactant agents, maternal steroids, and advancements in neonatal technologies. Current minimum age of viability is 23 weeks' gestation, with scattered reports of survivors at 21–22 weeks too.

10.2.3 The Ballard Maturational Assessment

The Ballard Maturational Assessment (**Ballard Score**) introduced in 1979 is a reliable tool for assessing fetal maturation and gestational age. A score is assigned to various physical and neurological criteria, and sum total is extrapolated to estimate the GA in the range of 26–44 weeks [13]. The New Ballard Score includes extremely preterm babies (20 weeks) [14].

10.2.4 APGAR Score

APGAR Score [15] was developed by an anesthesiologist Virginia Apgar in 1952 to assess the status of the newborn after birth. It gives an estimate of how well the newborn is adapting to extrauterine environment. It gives numerical scores (0–2) to 5 parameters (Appearance, Pulse, Grimace, Activity and Respiration APGAR), assessed at 1, 5, and 10 min. 1-min score reflects the status at delivery and is low in almost all newborns. 5- and 10-min score is an estimate of how well a newborn has adapted. Low score at 10 min is associated with poor survival or survival with severe disability. Maximum score is 10, but score of 7–10 is accepted normal at both 5 and 10 min, 3 as critically low, and 4–6 as fairly low. (Table 10.2) Normal values of vital parameters at birth are RR 60–80/min, HR 120–160/min, and Temp 36.3–37.2 °C

Factors that influence Apgar score include maternal conditions (drugs, infections, high-risk pregnancy), labor and delivery (complicated labor and delivery, trauma, resuscitative measures, operative delivery), and fetal factors (GA, BW, congenital anomalies, hypoxia, hypovolemia, and cardiopulmonary and neurologic dysfunction) (Table 10.3).

Table 10.2 Apgar score

Criteria	0	1	2
Appearance	Entire body pale or blue	Good color with bluish hands or feet	Good color all over
Pulse (HR)	Absent	<100	>100
Respiration (breathing)	Absent	Slow irregular	Good rate and effort with strong crying
Grimace (reflexes)	No response to stimulation	Facial grimace during stimulation	Pulls away, cries vigorously, or sneezes on stimulation
Activity (muscle tone)	Absent, limp, floppy loose muscles	Some muscle tone, some flexing of arms and legs	Active spontaneous motion, flexed arms and legs that resist extension

Table 10.3 Major problems in ELBW neonates

System	Pathology
Respiratory	Apnea, Resp failure, RDS, CLD (chronic lung disease)
CVS	PDA (patent ductus arteriosus)
CNS	IVH, PVL (periventricular leak), seizures
Renal	Electrolyte imbalance, acid-base disturbances, renal failure
Ophthalmologic	ROP, strabismus, myopia
GI & Nutritional	Feeding intolerance, NEC, inguinal hernia, cholestatic jaundice
Immunologic	Poor defense mechanism, infections (perinatal, nosocomial)

Table 10.4 Anesthesia Risk

GA at birth	Critical period—44-week postconception	Safe period—60-week postconception
28 (severe premature)	16 (4 months age)	32 (8 months age)
32 (mod premature)	12 (3 months age)	28 (7 months age)
36 (borderline, near term)	8 (2 months age)	24 (6 months age)
40 (full term)	4 (1 months age)	20 weeks (5 months age)
44 (post-term)	0 (0 months age)	16 weeks (4 months age)

10.2.5 Anesthesia Risk

Anesthetists can use 10-min score to estimate the risk to the neonate and take appropriate care during anesthetic management. Newborns with low score are at a greater risk of anesthesia and related complications because of their immaturity. (Table 10.4).

10.3 Anatomical and Physiological Considerations

All body systems each and every system is different. We will consider each system separately along with its anesthetic implications—respiratory system, airway and apnea, cardiovascular system, central nervous system, thermoregulation endocrinology, metabolic, hepatic and metabolic, renal, body H2O distribution, hemopoiesis and coagulation, NM transmission, pharmacokinetic, pain, feeding and intestine physiology, immune system, ophthalmic considerations, and skin physiology.

Box 10.1 General Features at Birth

(a)   Head is large, nearly one-third of body length—Great heat loss. Molding of skull bones for delivery causes a prominent crown and neck flexion and airway obstruction.
(b)   Copious secretions may be present for hours after delivery.
(c)   Term newborns have brown fat stores as internal heat source; they do not have the ability to shiver.
(d)   Respiration may be irregular and erratic, and heart rate is high 120–160 min.
(e)   Mild jitteriness, uncoordinated, and acrocyanosis are normal.
(f)   Reflexes present—Grasp, sucking, rooting, and startle reflex.

10.3.1 General Features at Birth

General features at birth are listed in Box 10.1.

10.3.2 Common Medical and Conditions

The medical and surgical derangements seen in the neonatal age are different from those in children and adults. (Boxes 10.2 and 10.3) They are only seen in this age and, if not treated or managed, can have adverse outcomes or long-term sequelae.

Not all of these conditions are necessarily life-threatening. Incidence of congenital anomalies is 3% of all live births, and its presence may convert a simple condition to that with higher perioperative risk:

(a) **Life threatening**—related to the airway, cardiac anomalies, facial anomalies, open lesions of the spinal cord, abdominal wall defects, and from birth trauma, while.
(b) **Non-life threatening** includes birth marks, extra fingers or toes, and club foot.

Box 10.2 List of Common Medical Conditions in the Neonatal Period

1. Prematurity
2. Problems of transition—PFC, PPHN, RDS
3. Resp system—Apneic spells, RDS, BPD, MAS, HMD, air lock (emphysema, pneumothorax, pneumomediastinum), pulmonary hemorrhage, lung cysts, pneumatoceles, congenital lobar emphysema, lung hypoplasia, vascular rings, TEF, micrognathia, glossoptosis.
4. Nonpulmonary causes of respiratory disease—ICH/IVH, CHD, hemolytic, and NM ds.
5. Anemia, polycythemia, hematological disorders, hemolytic ds of newborn
6. Inborn errors of metabolism
7. CVS—Congenital birth defects
8. CNS—ICH/IVH, seizures
9. Hepatic—Jaundice, hyperbilirubinemia, kernicterus
10. Metabolic—Hypoglycemia, hypocalcemia, hyponatremia
11. Immune system—Infections, sepsis
12. Eye—ROP, RLF
13. GI related—Feeding problems, diarrhea, acute abdomen, vomiting, dehydration
14. Congenital anomalies, genetic syndromes
15. Endocrine—Thyroid disorders, insulinoma (nesidioblastoma)
16. NM diseases, muscular dystrophy
17. Vertebral defects—Spina bifida

10.3.3 Common Surgical Conditions

Box 10.3 List of Common Surgical Conditions in the Neonatal Period

1. CDH, eventration of the diaphragm
2. Tef
3. Abdominal wall defects—Omphalocele/gastroschisis
4. Thoracic/pulmonary—Lobar emphysema/BPD, lung cyst, abscess, lobar/pulmonary agenesis, congenital pneumothorax
5. Airway related—Tracheal webs, narrowing, stenosis, tracheomalacia, laryngomalacia, choanal atresia
6. Congenital cardiac defects—PFO/VSD/PDA, TAPVD, TOF, ASVR (anomalous systemic venous drainage), persistent LSVC (left superior vena cava), cardiac failure
7. GIT—NEC/bowel perforation and peritonitis, PVID (patent vitello intestinal duct), obstruction, malrotation, intussusception, Hirschsprung's disease, IHPS (idiopathic hypertrophic pyloric stenosis), umbilical hernia, inguinal hernia. GI atresia (duodenal, jejunal, ileal), ARM (anorectal formation), imperforate anus, cloacal anomalies
8. Genitourinary—PUV, ectopia vesicae, Wilm's tumor, nephrectomy, congenital hydronephrosis, obstructive uropathy, exstrophy bladder, undescended/torsion testis, hypo-epispadias, hydrocele
9. Vertebral defects and neural tube defects—Meningomyelocele, meningocele, encephalocele
10. CNS—Congenital hydrocephalus, craniosynostosis, craniopharyngiomas
11. Cystic hygroma, teratomas—Cervical, sacrococcygeal
12. Hepatic—Biliary atresia,
13. Eye—RD (laser, cryosurgery), vitrectomy
14. Birth and neonatal care injuries [16],
15. Orthopedic—CTEV, hip dislocation, shoulder dislocation.

10.4   The Airway Anatomy and Respiratory Physiology in Newborns

Respiratory system in the newborn baby is still in a developing phase and respiratory mechanics are immature (Box 10.4). The central control and responses to hypoxemia and hypercarbia are also not fully functional. The alveoli are small, have little elastin, are stiff, and are poorly compliant. Vasomotor tone is not developed and pulmonary capillaries have high resistance [17–19]. Of the autonomic nervous system components, parasympathetic is most predominant.

Box 10.4 Respiratory System—Development

- 17–28 weeks GA—Alveolar formation
- 8–36 weeks GA—Pulmonary capillary formation
- 24 weeks GA—Surfactant production starts
- 36 weeks GA—Marked surge in synthesis of surfactant
- 20 million alveoli at birth and 300 million 8 months age
- Full maturation only by 36 weeks GA.

10.4.1 Airway Anatomy

Airway anatomy is different not only in dimensions, but also in its functionality. Clinical assessment is nearly impossible unless the anesthesiologist is familiar with the anatomy and physiology of the pulmonary system and airways. **Neonatal airway is described as a difficult airway.** All aspects of airway difficulty are present due to the unique anatomy of the head and trachea (Box 10.5, Fig. 10.2): mask holding, laryngoscopy, intubation, and ventilation.

The differences in anatomy are related to the **large head size** and prominent occipital bone. Laryngoscopy and intubation require the head in sniffing position. In older children and adults, a small pillow placed under the head extends the neck and provides correct position, but placing a small pillow under the occiput in a neonate will flex the head on the neck instead of extending it, with potential airway obstruction, difficult laryngoscopy and its view, and difficult intubation. Hence, it is preferable to place a small pad under the neck and shoulders, with a large ring under the head to accommodate the occiput (and stabilize the head) for induction, laryngoscopy, and intubation. **Improper mask size** and forceful grip on the jaw and surrounding soft tissue will also obstruct the upper airway. Hence, mask holding should be gentle, using a C or E technique. **Nares are narrow** and any nasal instrumentation must be avoided to prevent trauma to nasal mucosa and postoperative problems in breathing after tracheal extubation. **Larynx is high** (C3–4) and more **anteriorly placed**, cricoid cartilage (subglottic) is the narrowest part of the airway (debatable), and even small edema will have a greater narrowing effect, and **short tracheal length** puts them at risk of endobronchial intubation and accidental extubation even with minimal head manipulations. They are **obligate nose breathers** and relatively large tongue and more complaint pharyngeal tissue, makes them liable to obstruction during sleep and periods of relaxation (as at anesthetic induction).

Box 10.5 Neonatal Airway—Difficult Mask Holding, Laryngoscopy, Intubation, Ventilation

1. Large unstable head
2. Small jaw, short neck—No chin lift, avoid pressure over soft tissues of neck and jaw
3. Macroglossia—Use oropharyngeal airway to keep oropharyngeal airway patent
4. Obligate nasal breathers, small nares—Prone to obstruction
5. Narrow nares—No nasal instrumentation
6. Larynx—High C 2–3 and anterior—(external manipulation, BURP)
7. Epiglottis—Long floppy, omega shaped, 45° to the tongue
8. Straight blade laryngoscope preferred and epiglottis lifted at laryngoscopy
9. Cricoid—Narrowest, conical/cylindrical—Selection of ET tube
10. Face mask or supraglottic device or definitive airway
11. Angle of tracheal bifurcation (45°)—Equal chance of right or left endobronchial intubation

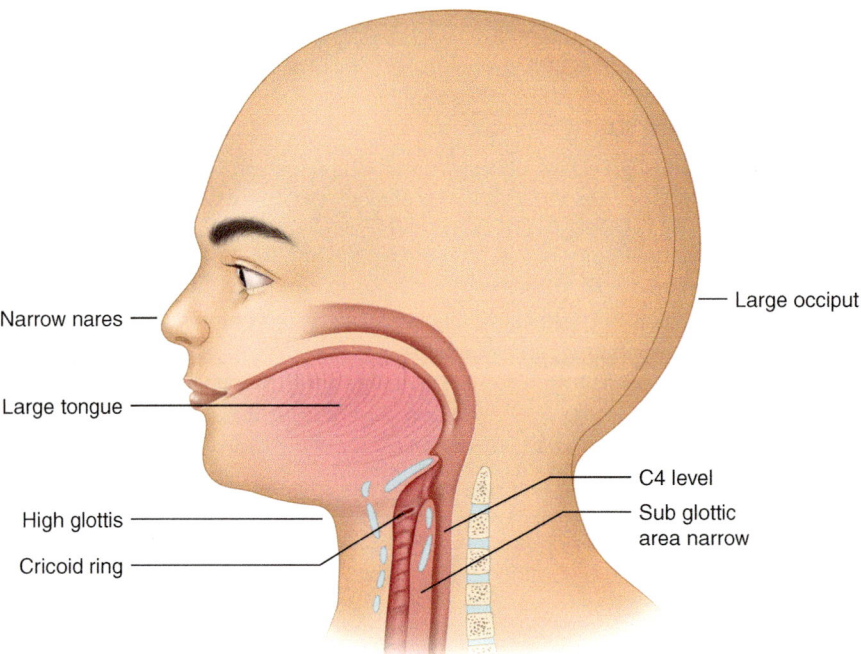

Fig. 10.2 Airway anatomy—unique features

10.4.2 Respiratory Physiology

Unique features of the neonatal **respiratory physiology** arise from the fact that their metabolic demand of O_2 is high to cater to the ongoing growth and maturation after birth. Important aspects of significance to the anesthesiologist are as follows:

(i) **Airways are narrower**, are **poorly supported by the surrounding structures** and can easily give in and collapse, causing further narrowing, and obstruction to flow of air or O_2, and **increased work of breathing and O_2 demand**.

(ii) **Chest wall is highly compliant** and ribs provide little or no support to the lungs. The negative intra thoracic pressure is poorly maintained, which essential for generation of inspiration, hence decreased lung volumes and capacities.

(iii) The **lung volumes and capacities** are small but appropriate for weight and age. (Note—Vt in a 3 kg baby is just 15–20 mL) (Table 10.5) **FRC** is low and CV and CC are high. They have poor O_2 reserves.

(iv) Basal **respiratory rate** is high (60–70/min at birth) which decreases over the period of 4 weeks to 30–50/min. This increases the demand of O_2 by the respiratory muscles. Work of breathing is three times and O_2 consumption is twice that in adults (5–6 mL/kg/min vs 2–3 mL/kg/min).

(v) The **respiratory muscles** are immature. The fatigue-resistant type I muscle fibers are deficient in neonates. Adult fiber configuration is reached only by 2 years of age [20].

(vi) The **ribs are more horizontally** placed. **Chest wall** lacks the **bucket handle movement** that allows increase in Tv by increasing the transverse diameter of the chest in adults.

(vii) **Diaphragm**, the chief muscle of respiration, is deficient in the proportion of high oxidative contractile fibers type 1. Adults have 55%, term newborns have 25%, and premature (at 30 weeks gestation) have 10%. Diaphragm easily tires, **with high risk of apnea.**

(viii) **Early fatigue and tachypnea cause further reduction in Vt and increase in O_2 demand.**

(ix) The **respiratory pattern** is also different. There is no pause between inspiration and expiration; i.e., no expiratory or inspiratory pauses and the respiratory movements are **see-saw like**. During the **inspiratory pause,** air gets redistributed from the fast to the slow alveoli, allowing their expansion through alveolar recruitment. Extruded alveolar fluid drains via the venous and lymphatic systems, thereby further improving gas exchange. During the **expiratory pause**, intrathoracic pressure is low, which allows better venous return to the heart, improved cardiac filling, and improved CO and better peripheral perfusion. **With the see-saw like pattern, the advantage of the inspiratory and expiratory pauses is LOST.**

(x) There are **two types of alveoli—fast and slow**. Fast alveoli have low resistance and are very compliant and fill and expand quickly, and slow alveoli have high resistance and slow compliance and fill slowly and are unable to expand fully. In the newborns, especially the premature, **alveoli are slow** (stiff or collapsed and have residual fluid).

(xi) During periods of complete relaxation, as at induction and during anesthesia, use of muscle relaxants, FRC decreases further (to 10–15% of TLC), nearing CC, leading to Atelectasis, V: Q mismatch, and Hb desaturation.

(xii) Increase in O_2 supply can only be met with by increasing the RR (as they cannot increase their Vt). Minute ventilation is high (>200 mL/kg/min) compared to 100 mL/kg/min in adults.

(xiii) **Poor cough reflex**

(xiv) **Response to hypoxia** is different, and an initial brief increase in ventilation is followed by sustained depression. Immature central respiratory center is prone to greater depression after anesthetic drugs.

(xv) **Oxygen dissociation curve** in neonates is placed more leftward, an indication of high affinity of Hb F to O_2 and reduced release at tissue level. Both presence of Hb F and poor medullary response make neonates prone to hypoxia and apnea.

(xvi) **CO2 response curve** is shifted to left.

(xvii) **Pulmonary circulation** is high resistance system in neonates. Asphyxia, acidosis, and hypercarbia cause pulmonary vasoconstriction and increased pulmonary arterial pressure. Splanchnic, renal, skeletal muscular, and cutaneous arterioles are vasoconstricted allowing redistribution of flow to the vital organs.

(xviii) **Prolonged asphyxia** causes further myocardial depression and decrease in cardiac output and poor peripheral perfusion.

All these factors contribute to early respiratory fatigue, O_2 deficiency, CO_2 retention, respiratory failure, and APNEA in neonates.

Table 10.5 Pulmonary Parameters

Pulmonary Indices	Term	Premature	Adult
O2 consumption mL/kg/min	6.4	7	3.5
Alveolar ventilation mL/kg/min	130	120–130	60
CO2 production mL/kg/min	6	5–6	3
VT mL/kg	6	4–5	6
RR/min	35	50–60	12–16
VC mL/kg	35	<35	70
FRC mL/kg	30	<30	35
Closing capacity mL/kg	35	>35	23
Tracheal length cm	5.5	Less	12
PaO_2 on air mmHg	65–85	60–70	95–97
$PaCO_2$ mm hg	30–36	30–36	36–44
pH	7.34–7.4	7.3–7.35	7.36–7.44
SpO_2%	85–95	80–90	95–100

Table 10.6 ETT size and length

Body Weight kg	ID mm	Length cm (at angle of mouth)
1	2–2.5	7
1.5	2.5–3	7.5
2	2.5–3	8
3 preterm	3	8–9
3 term	3.5	10

Guide—1, 2, 3, 4 kg = 7, 8, 9, 10 cm length

10.4.3 Airway Management

With the airway anatomy and respiratory physiology in the newborn and neonate, it is preferred to secure and maintain the airway by endotracheal intubation, and assisted or controlled respiration, during surgery under anesthesia, size appropriate (Table 10.6). Uncuffed ETT is preferred; however, special microcuff ETT are now available for use in neonates.

10.5   Respiratory Abnormalities at Birth

Most of transitional changes occur within a few hours of birth. They are functional changes and permanent changes occur earliest by 4 weeks. Several factors can interfere with normal transition at birth and cause pulmonary-related problems [21], chiefly;
1. Apnea of the newborn.
2. TTN—transient tachypnea of the newborn.
3. Respiratory distress syndrome (RDS)—BPD, MAS, HMD.

10.5.1 Apnea of the Newborn

Apnea is one of the very common causes of neonatal death. The compensatory responses to hypoxemia and hypercarbia are weak in the newborn because of immature medullary respiratory centers, contributing to the high mortality following apnea in these babies [22–24].

Periodic breathing, short episodes (about 3 s) of shallow breathing or apnea, followed by periods of regular breathing lasting 10–15 s, is normal in neonates. Irregular breathing is of common occurrence in late premature or near-term newborns. The incidence of apnea varies from 25 to 85%, more in LBW and premature babies.

Apnea in neonate is defined as cessation of breathing for 20 s or more, or cessation of breathing of less than 20 s accompanied with bradycardia (decrease of 30 beats/min or of more than 20% from baseline), or cessation of breathing (of any duration) accompanied with cyanosis, pallor, or hypotonia. Heart rate may remain normal. Apnea may be primary or secondary.

Primary Apnea—Failure of newborn to breathe at birth (no alveolar expansion, alveoli remain fluid filled), or initial breathing followed by apnea, leading to hypoxia. Normal response to hypoxia is respiratory stimulation. If the newborn fails to respond, hypoxia will lead to further inhibition of breathing (apnea) and bradycardia. This must be managed as soon as it is identified, by tactile stimulation and high FiO_2 (40–50%) via face mask. If apnea persists, management is as for secondary apnea.

Secondary Apnea—Unresolved primary apnea or neonatal apnea, and there is further fall in heart rate, blood pressure, and PaO_2 (bradycardia, hypotension, hypoxemia). Management includes -

(a) High FiO_2 (50–60%),
(b) Check for any obstruction to respiration—use oropharyngeal/nasopharyngeal airway,
(c) Respiratory support—in a baby who has spontaneous efforts, CPAP should be tried through oropharyngeal or nasopharyngeal route. Tracheal intubation and mechanical ventilatory support are reserved for newborns with no respiratory effort or who do not respond to initial measures.
(d) Provide care in a thermoneutral environment.

Once stabilized, additional avoidable causes of apnea must be looked for and managed.

The consequences of apnea are grave because of hypotension, bradycardia, hypoxemia followed by death, and needs urgent intervention. Early O_2 therapy and IPPV are advised to prevent hypoxic ischemic injury to the brain.

10.5.1.1 Risk Factors for Apnea in Neonates

- **Maternal related**—elderly age >35 years, diabetes mellitus, hypertension, cardiac disease, respiratory disease, severe anemia, infections, alcohol, and/ or drug abuse,
- **Pregnancy related**—APH, toxemia of pregnancy, multiple births,
- **Delivery related**—Abnormal presentations, prolonged or difficult labor, cord prolapse, fetal distress, narcotic or MgSO4 administration, malpresentation, instrumental/operative delivery.
- **Fetal factors**—prematurity, congenital malformations, birth trauma, fetal distress.

Diagnosis is made by exclusion of treatable causes.

Etiologically, apnea is of three types—central—due to immature medullary centers, **obstructive**—nasal, pharyngeal, laryngeal pathology, and **mixed**—is the most common, combination of both central and obstructive types.

Monitoring includes vitals (HR, RR), SpO_2, temperature, and ECG.

Management depends on the cause, frequency, and severity of apneic episodes. All premature babies should be monitored for apnea in the NICU settings in O_2 tent in a thermal controlled environment.

1. Nonpharmacological measures include elimination of treatable **causes of apnea** (Table 10.7), monitoring, tactile stimulation, repositioning to lateral or semi lateral position, and clearing of nasal and oral cavities.

Table 10.7 Factors that affect respiration

Stimulate respiration/tachypnea	Depress respiration/apnea
Mild acidosis	Severe acidosis
Hypercarbia	CNS damage
Hypoxia	Hypoxia
Sensations—Pain, cold, touch, noise	Drugs—Magnesium, alcohol, opioid, barbiturates

2. Maintenance of Hb saturation by O_2 therapy, high FiO_2 (50–60%), bag mask ventilation, noninvasive CPAP, or tracheal intubation and assisted ventilation, and extracorporeal membrane oxygenator (ECMO).
3. Drug therapy—Three drugs used with varying success rates, either alone or in combination, are caffeine, theophylline, and doxapram.
   (a) **Caffeine citrate** is a central medullary stimulant and improves the response to hypoxia and hypercarbia by diaphragmatic contractility, and increase in minute ventilation and metabolic rate. It can be given IV in a dose of 5–10 mg/kg, and if administered preoperatively, it can reduce the incidence of postoperative apnea in risky neonates.
   (b) **Theophylline** is administered IV in a dose of 5 mg/kg, followed by a maintenance dose of 2 mg/kg two to three times a day. Risks associated are tachycardia, arrhythmias, and seizures.
   (c) **Doxapram** can be administered IV in a dose of 1–2 mg/kg. Its side effects are hypertension and seizures (because of additive benzyl alcohol).

10.5.1.2 Neonatal Apnea and the Anesthesiologist

Postoperative apnea is of grave concern to the anesthesiologist, critical period being the first 12 h, but the risk persists up to 72 h, especially after general anesthesia. Hence, all neonates should be kept admitted in the hospital for observation for minimum of 24 h postoperatively. Risk factors for postoperative apnea include **patient factors** (prematurity (<35 weeks GA), anemia, H/o birth apnea, CNS/lung disease), and **iatrogenic factors** (hypoxia, hypercapnia, hypoglycemia, anemia, hypothermia, ICH, sepsis, heart failure, drugs).

10.5.1.3 Premature Neonates are at Extreme Risk of Perioperative Hypoxemia, Due to

- Greater central immaturity and lack of compensatory responses
- Weak muscles of respiration and diaphragm
- High incidence of birth apnea
- High metabolic rate and O_2 requirement
- Low FRC (less than CC) and poor respiratory reserve

10.5.1.4 Care During Anesthesia Management to Prevent Hypoxemia

- Avoid nasal instrumentation as far as possible.
- Avoid 100% O_2, and if required, use for the shortest duration (risk of developing ROP, BPD).
- Use of minimal FiO_2 to maintain target SpO_2 (88–92%).

- Use low PEEP to prevent basal collapse.
- NO crash induction/RSI, as they cannot tolerate even short periods of apnea.
- General care—prevention of hypothermia, maintaining heart rate, rhythm, and volume status.
- Avoidance of anemia and maintaining Hct.
- Thorough asepsis in handling them and during procedures and drug administration.
- Always assist ventilation. No spontaneous ventilation during aesthesia.
- Adequate analgesia and muscle relaxation
- Provision for postoperative ventilatory support.

10.5.2 Transient Tachypnea of the Newborn (TTN)

TTN is the mildest and transient complication of incomplete clearance of fetal lung fluid. It is more frequent in preterm and male babies and presents as tachypnea (RR >60/min), lung crackles, crepitations on auscultation, tachycardia, flow murmur, and acrocyanosis.

Contributing factors are decreased Na^+ transport and low surfactant. If surfactant deficiency is severe, features of RDS become evident. Babies at risk are those who have problem with clearing of lung fluid at birth (operative deliveries, diabetic or asthmatic mothers, and multiple pregnancies).

Management includes O_2 by mask to maintain SpO_2. Other care includes care of nutrition and antibiotic cover. Outcome—as the name implies, it is transient and usually resolves within 48 h. If it persists, it is known as malignant TTN, which is a precursor of RDS.

10.5.3 Respiratory Distress Syndrome (RDS)

RDS is the most common cause of morbidity and mortality worldwide, with preponderance in male and preterm neonates, and can be because of BPD (bronchopulmonary dysplasia, arrest of lung development, evolving chronic lung disease, neonatal chronic lung disease, respiratory insufficiency), MAS (meconium aspiration syndrome), HMD (hyaline membrane disease).

10.5.3.1 Pathophysiology

Surfactant production starts in the second trimester (24 weeks) and continues up to 32 weeks, with a surge at 36 weeks, in preparation for the birth of the baby. Babies born prematurely have deficiency of surfactant and may develop BPD, HMD, and RDS. Prematurity (<30 weeks GA) and LBW (<2 lbs) are risk factors for BPD, and risk factors for HMD include (high risk—prematurity, asphyxia, maternal diabetes and hemorrhage, operative delivery, and multiple births, and low risk—IUGR, maternal hypertension, steroid therapy, placental insufficiency, and heroin addiction). MAS, hypoxia, acidosis, hypotension and shock, and pulmonary hemorrhage all cause endothelial damage and affect surfactant production (refer to the chapter on transitional changes at birth).

Pathological changes in the lung are alveolar collapse, alveolar and interstitial edema, diffuse hyaline membrane in the distorted small airways, reduced pulmonary and alveolar compliance and lung distensibility, stiff alveoli, poor alveolar stability, increased airway resistance (rigid bronchioles), reduced FRC, right-to-left shunt, reduced effective pulmonary blood flow, inefficient gas exchange, hypoxemia, and pulmonary hypertension.

10.5.3.2 Presentation—Clinical Features Appear Soon After Birth
- At birth—apnea, cyanosis, grunting, stridor, tachypnea, intercostal and sub-costal retraction, hypotension.
- Chest radiology—ground glass appearance because of alveolar collapse, and signs of inflammation.
- ABG—low PaO_2, elevated $PaCO_2$, acidosis.
- ECHO—to rule out cardiac defects as cause of pulmonary hypertension.
- Autopsy finding—alveolar collapse, alveolar and interstitial edema, and diffuse hyaline membrane in the distorted small airways.

10.5.3.3 Management—Aims at Improving Oxygenation and Correcting Hypoxemia. Preventive/Prophylactic
Goal—PaO_2 of >55 mmHg, with normal $PaCO_2$ (40–60 mmHg).
- (a) High FiO_2 and airway pressures.
- (b) Noninvasive CPAP of 4–6 cm H_2O using face mask, in a spontaneously breathing neonate.
- (c) If the baby is apneic with severe hypoxemia, or acidosis (pH <7.20)—immediate tracheal intubation and ventilation must be instituted.
- (d) Premature and VLBW newborns—O_2 supplementation, ventilatory support—CPAP, IPPV with PEEP may be necessary for prolonged period.
- (e) Drug therapy—bronchodilators, steroids, diuretics, antibiotics.

Special Care
- These babies are at risk of barotrauma and BPD during IPPV and high FiO_2.
- Use lowest peak inspiratory pressures and lowest FiO_2 to maintain PaO_2 and pH.
- Increase in minute ventilation can be achieved by increase in RR.
- O_2 requirement is increased, but even with 100% FiO_2, gas exchange and tissue oxygenation may not improve.
- Avoid use of 100% O_2 (high FiO_2 may inflame the lining of the lungs, injure the airways, and slow lung development in premature newborns).

Supportive care includes maintenance of body temperature, intravascular volume and electrolyte status, nutritional support (100–120 calories/kg/day), higher in LBW, correction of metabolic acidosis (base deficit (mEq) = base excess × 0.6 × body weight (kg)), oral feeds started once the baby is stable to provide 100–120 calories/kg/day, and vigorous monitoring of intake/output, body weight, electrolytes, acidbase, blood gases, serum and urine osmolality, and X-ray chest. **Advanced measures** include surfactant replacement therapy, ECMO, whole lung lavage, and lung transplantation [25–30].

10.6 Cardiovascular System (CVS)

The heart undergoes marked adaptation at birth. In utero it behaves as a conduit between right and left side of the heart. After birth, there is a change in the available energy substrate, its utilization, and in the cardiac metabolic activity, with shift from CHO to fatty acid utilization. In O_2 lack situations, neonatal heart can undergo anaerobic energy production and still maintain cardiac function. The load on the newborn heart is huge as it must take over the complete function. How efficiently it works depends on adequacy of pulmonary gas exchange, coronary blood flow, and nutrient intake [31].

Neonatal cardiac myocytes are poorly contractile. Both, the intracellular contractile protein- and calcium-dependent sarcoplasmic reticulum, are immature and cellular mass is less. Myocardium has more connective or non-contractile tissue. Both ventricles are equal unlike in adults where LV is predominant. Starling law is not applicable. Poor myocardial contractility and poor ventricular compliance prevent both early and late diastolic filling, with decrease in stroke volume and cardiac output.

Cardiac output (SV x HR) in the neonate is high, almost 200 mL/kg/min. Myocardial force of contraction and hence, stroke volume, cannot increase, so CO is HR dependent; such that if HR decreases, CO also decreases. Starling's law does not apply. With increase in HR, CO increases, but excessive tachycardia is also detrimental by limiting diastolic filling and SV, and while there is no increase in CO, but myocardial O_2 demand becomes excessive, with risk of myocardial damage. Net result is that both bradycardia and excessive tachycardia reduce CO and blood pressure markedly.

Heart rate in a newborn is 120–180/min, and by 1 month of age, it should not exceed 160/min in term neonate. **It is utmost important to maintain HR in within a range of 120–180/min.**

Vasomotor tone—Parasympathetic innervation of the neonatal heart is more developed compared to sympathetic innervation. Baroreflex mechanism is also weak. Catecholamine stores are small and inadequate, and all stress responses are blunted. Thus, the initial response to any stimulation or stress is bradycardia (parasympathetic), unlike tachycardia in older children and adults. Premature heart is extremely susceptible to bradycardia and hypotension. Vasoconstrictive responses to volume change are weak and hypotension is poorly compensated. Besides, volume changes as in hypovolemia, hypotension, and hemorrhage, are not accompanied by increase in HR. They cannot tolerate fluid and blood loss.

Systemic blood pressure (SBP) varies with GA and normalizes by 36 h of life. In a term neonate, it is >90/65 mmHg and >80/45 mmHg in a preterm neonate. MAP ranges between 45 and 50 mmHg and DBP between 30 and 35 mm Hg. Table 10.8 shows mean circulatory values with BW.

MAP should not be allowed to drop below 20% of baseline or below an absolute value of 30 mm Hg. A rough guide for the lowest acceptable MAP is a value equal to the GA of the neonate in weeks. **ECG**—unlike a mature heart, newborn heart has right predominance. ECG shows right axis deviation (tall R, (right lead), deep S (left lead).

Patent ductus arteriosus (PDA) more common in premature infants; normally closes 10 days to 2 weeks after birth. It is associated with increased pulmonary flow and pulmonary congestion, and low DBP. These neonates are prone to NEC, IVH, BPD. May reopen whenever pulmonary arterial pressure rises (hypoxemia, hypercarbia, acidosis, or respiratory distress syndrome), causing **shunt reversal**. Therapeutic strategies include administration of O_2, prostacyclin and/or indomethacin, nitric oxide, or surgical ablation. **PFC** occurs due hypoxia, hypercarbia, and acidosis, all that cause pulmonary vasoconstriction and high PVR (Table 10.9).

- Find this author on Google search
- Find this author on PubMed
- Search for this author on this site
- Find this author on Google Scholar
- Find this author on PubMed
- Search for this author on this site

Care during anesthetic management must be taken to prevent increase in PVR and decrease in SVR, so as to prevent reversal of shunt, meticulous fluid management (Table 10.2), avoidance of bradycardia, arrhythmias, undue tachycardia.

Table 10.8 Mean circulatory values and birthweight

BW kg	0.75	1	2	3	>3
SBP	44	49	54	62	66
MAP	33	34	41	46	50
HR	160–180	160–180	120	120	

Table 10.9 Ductus arteriosus and foramen ovale closure

	Functional closure	Anatomical closure	Initiation of closure	Reopening risks/shunt reversal
Ductus arteriosus	10–15 h	2–3 weeks	↑ PaO_2	Hypoxia, acidosis (CDH, MAS, RDS),
Foramen Ovale	At birth (within 24 h)	3 mth-1 yr.	↑ LAP	Hypothermia, Excessive airway pressure—Crying

10.7 Central Nervous System

The central nervous system is immature and incompletely developed at birth, cerebral cortex is poorly developed, and myelination is incomplete. Newborn brain has high water content. As cerebral maturation occurs, water content decreases steadily, and myelin and protein concentration increase.

10.7.1 Anatomy

A newborn brain weighs 350–400 g (nearly 1/fourth the size of adult brain). Rapid growth and maturation occur after birth, and its weight doubles by the end of first year. By 5 years of age, brain weighs 90% of the adult size, which is reached by teenage.

Major bones that compose the skull of a newborn include 2 frontal bones, 2 parietal bones, and 1 occipital bone, held together by fibrous sutures. Sutures allow the bones to move during the vaginal birth process. They are like expansion joints that allow the bone to enlarge evenly as brain grows and the skull expands into a symmetrical shaped head. (Fig. 10.3) **Important sutures are**

- **Metopic or frontal suture**, from the top of the head down the middle of the forehead, toward the nose, between 2 frontal bone plates.
- **Coronal suture** extends from ear to ear, between each frontal and parietal bone plates.
- **Sagittal suture** extends from the front of the head to the back, down the middle of the top of the head, between the 2 parietal bone plates.
- **Lambdoid suture**, across the back of the head, between each parietal and occipital bone plates.

Fontanelles are spaces where the sutures intersect and are present in the newborns and infants. There are 2 fontanelles which are covered by tough membrane that protects the underlying brain tissue:

- **Anterior fontanelle or the soft spot** is diamond shaped membrane, at the junction of the 2 frontal and 2 parietal bones. It remains soft until about 18 months to 2 years of age and is normally flush with the outer skull. Any fullness is indicative of raised ICP.

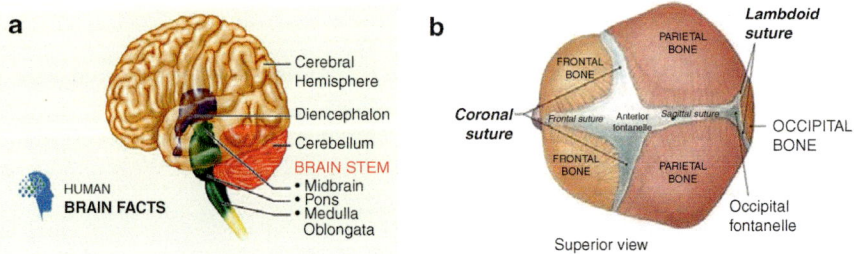

Fig. 10.3 (a) Newborn brain and (b) Newborn skull

- **Posterior fontanelle** is at the junction of the 2 parietal and the occipital bone. It usually closes earlier, during the first few months of life.

10.7.2 Blood–Brain Barrier (BBB)

Blood–brain barrier (BBB) is immature at birth, but matures soon after. It is permeable to many large lipid soluble molecules, such as volatile anesthetic agents and bilirubin. The partition coefficient of inhalational anesthetic agents is high, with a rapid wash in and wash out, and the clinical effect is achieved at lower concentrations and more rapidly. This also increases the susceptibility of the developing brain to anesthesia neurotoxicity. Permeability to bilirubin makes the newborn, especially the premature, at high risk of developing kernicterus.

10.7.3 Cerebral Blood Flow (CBF)

Brain receives almost 15% of cardiac output, 30–40 mL/100 g brain tissue. Newborn brain has a high metabolic activity. Higher CBF takes care of the O_2 and nutritional demand and for removal of CO2 and metabolic waste. CBF or cerebral perfusion pressure (CPP) is a factor of mean arterial pressure (MAP) and intracranial pressure (ICP). Any decrease in MAP of more than 20% from the baseline or increase in ICP above 15 mmHg reduces CPP. Cerebral venous drainage occurs through the 3 sinuses, which drain into the jugular veins—superior sagittal sinus, 2 transverse sinuses, and sigmoid sinus. In infants with open fontanelles, CPP varies in accordance with arterial blood pressure. Immaturity of the central nervous system also contributes to the development of ROP, where retinal vascular narrowing and obliteration are followed by neovascularization, hemorrhage, and in retinal detachment in severe cases [32].

10.7.4 Neonatal Brain Is Protected from Hypoxic Insults by Four Mechanisms

1. **Dual blood supply**—The anterior part is supplied by the two internal carotid arteries, branches of the arch of aorta, and posterior part by the two vertebral arteries which arise from the subclavian arteries. These two circulations communicate with each other at the Circle of Willis and provide backup and cerebral protection in case one gets blocked.
2. **Autoregulation**—The cerebral vessels respond to chemical (hypoxia, hypercarbia), metabolic (hypoglycemia, acidosis), pressure (MAP, ICP), and neural changes, so that a constant blood flow is maintained over a wide range of adverse conditions. However, in neonates, the range of blood pressure over which autoregulation occurs is very narrow, nearing the perfusion pressure itself. Asphyxia itself compromises autoregulation further. The lower limit of autoregulation in age more than 6 months is not reached till blood pressure

decreases by 40% from baseline, but in those under 6 months of age and neonates, it occurs when MAP decreases 20% from baseline. Low cerebral autoregulatory reserve is a risk of both IVH and inadequate cerebral perfusion during periods of hypotension. The period immediately after anesthetic induction, prior to surgical stimulus, is particularly vulnerable.

3. **Cerebrospinal fluid (CSF) buffer**—In newborns, 40–150 mL of CSF is synthesized per day. It contains leukocytes, lymphocytes, protein, electrolytes, and other substances. CSF is incompressible and protects the brain from injury by acting as a buffer. It maintains the water–electrolyte equilibrium of the fluid bathing the intracranial contents, maintaining ICP. Any increase in production or problem in its drainage can alter this equilibrium with rise in ICP, reduction in CPP, cerebral ischemia, and risk of HIE, convulsions, and coma.

4. **Metabolic protection**—Neonates' brain is unique in that in adverse circumstances, it can undergo anerobic metabolism for its energy needs, without undergoing permanent damage.

10.7.5 Intraventricular Hemorrhage (IVH)

The incidence of IVH is up to 50% in LBW and VLBW neonates, due to rupture of fragile capillaries within the germinal matrix, especially within 72 h of birth. This leads to ventricular dilatation, hydrocephalus, parenchymal infarcts, periventricular leukomalacia, cerebral palsy, and permanent CNS deficiency. **Risk factors for IVH include** hypoxia, hypotension, sepsis, toxic injury, RDS, aggressive resuscitation with hypertonic IV fluids, and mechanical ventilation. Presence of PDA also increases the risk of intracerebral bleed. Wide fluctuations in systemic blood pressure may be a contributing factor.

10.7.6 Spine and Spinal Cord

The spinal cord ends at L 3–4 and dura at S 3–4, in neonates. Care should be taken when giving spinal and caudal anesthesia in these neonates. They are at risk of injury to the spinal cord. Intrathecal puncture should be made below L3 and above S3 (Fig. 10.4). Sacrum does not fuse posteriorly until late teens. Sacral hiatus is relatively larger and higher placed. Epidural space has less fat and fibrous tissue.

Pain and pain pathways—Neural mechanisms for pain are present in the fetus by 6 weeks of gestation. The pain pathways are integrated with somatic, neuroendocrine, and autonomic changes early in gestation, and hormonal responses to pain and stress may be exaggerated in newborns.

Anesthetic implications—Brain of a neonate is extremely vulnerable to any hypoxic insult. Maintaining of MAP, CPP, PaO$_2$ and minimizing O$_2$ consumption should be the primary goal during anesthesia management. While both hyper- and hypocapnia are not wanted, controlled permissive hypocapnia may be beneficial. Rise in ICP may not be evident because of open fontanelle, hence due

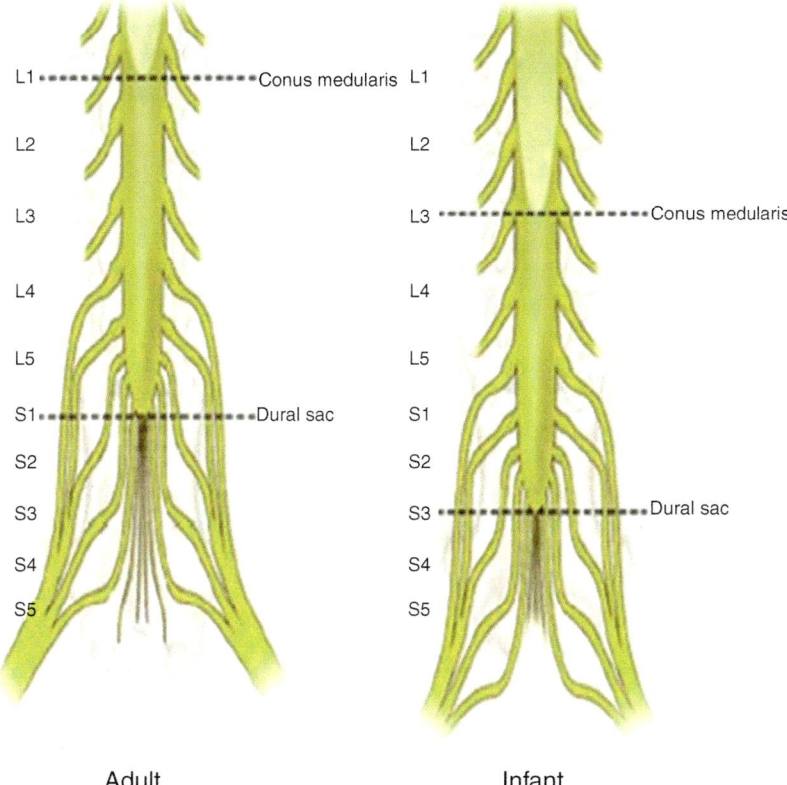

Fig. 10.4 Anatomy of the spine and spinal cord in an infant and adult

precautions must be taken in the perianesthetic care. They are prone to cerebral edema, convulsions, altered requirement of inhalational anesthetics (due to rapid wash in and rapid wash out, higher MAC), and risk of anesthesia neurotoxicity. It is important to maintain MAP within the limits of cerebral autoregulation for cerebral protection.

Special concern is in premature neonates who are very prone to cerebral edema and convulsions, anesthesia neurotoxicity, and greater muscular hypotonia. However, despite their CNS and NM immaturity, premature neonates have a normal response to stress and pain that needs attention during anesthesia and surgery, as in term neonates.

10.8   Thermoregulation, Endocrine, and Metabolic Functions

Newborn babies are prone to various metabolic and endocrinal disturbances. The hypophysial pituitary adrenal axis is immature, and this in turn affects brown fat thermogenesis and temperature control, with risk of hypothermia, and affects hormone releases, response to stress, and glucose and lipid metabolism [33].

Common metabolic disturbances seen in the neonatal period are related to glucose, calcium, magnesium metabolism, and endocrinal disorders (growth hormone, gonadotrophin, thyroid, ACTH, cortisol).

Adverse Effects of Metabolic Immaturity Can Have Long-Term Consequences Because of
- Immature BBB with risk to cerebral edema, raised ICP, and convulsions.
- Acid-base disturbances, because of abnormalities in transition process at birth expose the immature brain of the newborn to early, severe, and extensive hypoxic damage.
- These effects are compounded by the adverse effect of drugs received by the mother in the antenatal or perinatal period, including narcotics, sedatives, anesthetic drugs, maternal drug, and alcohol abuse.
- Additionally, effects of anesthetic drugs and techniques used during operative delivery, complications of anesthesia (airway or hemodynamic related), and indication of Cesarian section itself will add to the newborn risks.

10.8.1 Thermoregulation

A growing fetus produces twice as much heat as an adult, and small amounts dissipate through into amniotic fluid and uterine wall. Core temperature of the fetus is 0.5 °C above the maternal temperature. Fetus does not expend energy to maintain body temperature, and glucose supplied to it is converted to glycogen in the liver and stored for later use. The temperature (axillary) of a newborn is 36.5–37.4 °C, but heat loss starts soon after birth from exposure to external environment. Cutaneous receptors signal the brain to initiate heat production by brown fat metabolism. The newborn utilizes fetal glycogen stores as energy substrate to maintain body temperature and other organ functions.

Thermoneutral temperature is the external temperature at which there is a balance between heat loss and heat gain, while **critical temperature** is that external temperature below which one cannot maintain core body temperature (Table 10.10).

Table 10.10 Thermoneutral and critical temperature °C

	Thermoneutral temperature	Critical temperature
Preterm neonate	34–35	28
Term neonate	32–34	23
Adult	25–28	1

Ideal OT temperature >28 °C
Birth to 1 week age—32 °C and for premature—35 °C

Providing controlled thermal environment improves the chance of survival and quality of outcome, particularly in small (BW <1000 G), premature, and critically ill neonates, by minimizing their O_2 and metabolic demands, and stress responses to cold or overheating. Neonates weighing >1500 g and without respiratory distress or hemodynamic instability can be cared for at 30–32 °C.

10.8.2 Brown Fat Metabolism and Thermogenesis

Hormone surge (cortisol, catecholamines, and thyroid) at birth activates brown fat thermogenesis, alternative to the white fat in adults. Brown fat is about 5% of body weight of a newborn and is abundant around the kidneys, intrascapular, and nuchal areas. It is highly vascular, has higher O_2 consumption, and is rich in iron-containing mitochondria and unmyelinated nerves, providing sympathetic stimulation to the fat cells. It generates heat by uncoupling of oxidative phosphorylation in the mitochondria. When lipid reserves of brown fat are depleted, as on prolonged exposure to cold, it gets darker in color.

Newborns are extremely prone to temperature instability especially in the first few days of life. Both hypothermia and hyperthermia are harmful and should be prevented.

10.8.3 Hypothermia - Causes

1. **Greater heat loss**—Relatively larger body surface-to-body weight ratio.
2. **Poor heat conservation**—Poorly developed thin subcutaneous tissue, and limited fat reserves.
3. **Minimal motor activity**—Inability to generate heat.
4. **Inability to shiver.**
5. **Central thermoregulation**—is immature and there is poor response to hypothermia.
6. **Higher energy utilization** for maintaining body functions.
7. **Anesthesia effects**—Both volatile and intravenous anesthetics depress non-shivering thermogenesis. This contributes to the increased risk of hypothermia in the perioperative period, while heat loss continues with reduced thermogenesis and poor thermal compensation.

Methods by Which Term Neonate Maintains Core Body Temperature:
(a) **Brown fat metabolism** (nonshivering thermogenesis) that produce twice the amount of heat as compared to white fat metabolism.
(b) **Shivering thermogenesis** (from physical activity of kicking and crying)—minor role in heat production, and.
(c) **Peripheral vasoconstriction** secondary to exposure to cold and decreased heat loss from skin surface.

Preterm neonates—While all newborns are at danger of hypothermia, premature and small for date babies are at a greater risk, more so in winters and cold environment, because:

They are poikilothermic—Human beings are homeothermic, i.e., they have the ability to control body temperature independent of ambient temperature, but premature babies lack this feature and they adopt the ambient environment temperature.

(a) They have **less brown fat** as compared to term neonates, so less heat production.

(b) Their BSA:BW:: ↑↑, which allows greater loss of heat from the exposed skin surface.

(c) Their skin is poorly keratinized, thin with less subcutaneous fat, thus poor heat conservation.

(d) Shivering is an important mechanism for production of heat in cold environment in older children and adults. This is absent in premature neonates, so they are unable to generate activity-related heat.

Adverse Effects of Hypothermia— Cold Injury

All newborns, especially premature and small for date neonates, are at risk of hypothermia and its adverse effects. Hypothermia is one of the main causes of neonatal mortality, and special measures must be taken to reduce this risk.

1. **Increase in carbohydrate (CHO) metabolism and glucose utilization,** in an attempt to maintain body temperature. This leads to depletion of already poor glucose stores, increasing the risk of further hypoglycemia.

2. **Cold induces depression of enzymatic and metabolic activity** is proportional to the duration and degree of hypothermia and inversely proportional to the gestational age. Thus, hepatic metabolism of drugs is reduced, with prolongation of their duration of action and effect. Polypharmacy, inherent to general anesthesia, is a cause of concern in babies already suffering from the ill effects of the surgical disease, and slow emergence from anesthesia.

3. **Dosages of anesthetic drugs**—since their ECF volume is more, the Vd of drugs is higher. Initial dose need not be reduced. The serum concentration may be lower but brain and other organ systems being still immature; adequate effect can still be achieved. But care must be exercised with top-up dosages, which must be reduced and have more spacing in-between two.

4. Increase in **cardiovascular stress** because of the stimulation of still immature compensatory mechanisms.

5. **Activation of brown fat thermogenesis** produces twice the amount of heat then from white fat. This consumes more O_2, increasing the metabolic O_2 demand. During hypothermia, neonates need higher FiO2. They are at risk of hypoxemia and metabolic acidosis.

6. **Pulmonary and Intracranial hemorrhages.**

7. Increased risk of **Infections and sepsis** because of immune suppression.

8. **Reduced Bilirubin conjugation and metabolism, causing** hyperbilirubinemia (unconjugated bilirubin), which can easily cross the immature BBB, with occurrence of kernicterus.

9. Hypothermia has a **depressant effect** on medullary respiratory centers and on responses to hypoxia and hypercarbia, with risk of **apnea** or apneic episodes.

Management is preventive and corrective. Prevention and treatment go hand in hand. One need not wait for hypothermia to occur before adopting corrective measures. It is important to maintain thermoneutral environment and prevent reaching critical temperature range in any care setting (ward, NICU, perioperative period, and in the operation room). Measures that must be adopted are:

1. Vigilant monitoring
2. Reduce O_2 consumption—avoid stress, pain, environment temperature fluctuations, hypoxia, respiratory, and hemodynamic disturbances.
3. Reduce heat loss—Maintaining environmental (OT, ward, incubator) temperature to thermoneutral range or at least more than >28 °C (table above), protective wrapping, heat shields, reflective foils, head cover.
4. Provide external heat—use of overhead radiant warmers, forced air heating units, heating mattresses, and blankets. Servo-controlled heat humidifiers are very effective.
5. Avoid transfusing cold intravenous fluids, blood, and blood products. They should be warmed before infusion.
6. Use of warm humidified gases during anesthesia.
7. Use of warm irrigating fluids during surgery.
8. Avoid wide fluctuations in the external temperatures.
9. IV glucose supplement (as a substrate for metabolism).
10. Higher FiO_2, respiratory support, and CPAP.
11. Avoid spontaneous ventilation during anesthesia, except for short procedures. Preferable to use CPAP by mask or secure the airway and use controlled ventilation.
12. Vit K injection (0.25 mg) intravenous, to reduce the risk of spontaneous hemorrhages.
13. Avoid IM and SC injections.

10.8.4 Hyperthermia

Hyperthermia (axillary temperature >37.4 °C or rectal temperature >37.5 °C) can be due to pathological condition (infection, sepsis, septicemia), iatrogenic, or environmental factors.

Effects of hyperthermia are consequent to vasodilatation and increased insensible losses, dehydration, hypovolemia, hypotension, and shock-like state, risk of risk of hypothermia, and secondary cold injury.

Management
(a) Must not lower axillary temperature to normal.
(b) Record skin, axillary, and air or incubator temperature.

  (c) Environmental hyperthermia—reduce environmental heating temperature
      and thermal insulation (blankets or clothing).
  (d) Avoid rebound hypothermia.
  (e) Maintain volume status, renal perfusion, and urine output, and.
  (f) Maintain electrolyte and acid-base balance.

Important Points to Remember
  1. Heat production is an active process needing O_2 and glucose—a newborn
     should be allowed to breathe O_2-rich air for a few hours after birth.
  2. Both hypothermia and hyperthermia are dangerous in the neonatal period
     and should be avoided.
  3. Persistent hypothermia will result in metabolic acidosis, hypoglycemia, and
     decreased surfactant production, hemorrhages—newborn should be kept in
     a warm environment.
  4. Hormonal surge at birth mobilizes glycogen, still glucose levels decline to a
     lowest point at 1 h of age. Newborns should be routinely given dextrose
     water orally or IV until initiation of regular feeds.
  5. Care during anesthetic management and in the perioperative period.

10.9   Endocrine Physiology

Endocrine processes are actively involved in normal fetal growth and development.
Endocrinal physiology is an interplay of several complex processes and disturbances in these can affect fetal growth depending on the stage of development at
which exposure occurs. Clinical manifestations may not be apparent at birth but
predispose the baby for disease at later age. Transient endocrine disorders (adrenal
insufficiency, hypothyroidism) are frequent in the newborn period, but are of not
much physiological consequences in a healthy term newborn. To evaluate suspected
endocrine pathology in a newborn, knowledge of the normal, dynamics, changes,
and maturation of the hormonal function is essential. Special attention must be paid
to thyroid and adrenal gland function, glucose and calcium metabolism, and the
mechanism of switching in energy substrate from CHO to fatty acid oxidation.
Endocrine maturation occurs by 6–12 months of age, but adult hormonal values are
reached by adolescence.

   Physiological endocrinal disturbances at birth—These are mostly related to
the withdrawal from maternal hormones (estrogen, progesterone, and prolactin),
presenting mildly as vaginal discharge or bleeding lasting for 1–2 days in females,
and enlargement of the mammary glands and secretion, in both sexes, by third day
of life, which subsides in 2–3 weeks [34, 35].

10.9.1 Hypothalamic–Pituitary Axis

Hypothalamus arises from neuroblast proliferation in the intermediate zone of the
fore brain, and supraoptic and periventricular nuclei and differentiates into anterior
and posterior pituitary glands. Neurohypophyseal tract is formed by the nerve fibers

between hypothalamus and posterior pituitary. Hypothalamus secretes both stimulatory and inhibitory hormones and regulates the pituitary gland, which becomes functional after 12th week of gestation. Growth hormone-releasing hormone (GHRH), thyrotropin-releasing hormone (TRH), corticotropin-releasing hormone (CRH), and gonadotropin-releasing hormone (GnRH) from the hypophysis stimulate anterior pituitary gland to secrete growth hormone (GH), thyroid-stimulating hormone (TSH), adrenocorticotropic hormone (ACTH), luteinizing hormone (LH) and follicle-stimulating hormone (FSH). The main inhibitory hormones are somatostatin and prolactin inhibitory factor. Somatostatin inhibits GH release and prolactin inhibitory factor inhibits prolactin release. The posterior pituitary secretes vasopressin (ADH) and oxytocin.

Most disorders of the hypothalamic-pituitary axis in the neonate are from insufficient hormone secretion due to genetically inherited disorders, malformations, trauma, and infection.

Anterior pituitary dysfunction is difficult to detect at birth.
1. Presence of malformation (cleft lip and palate, optic nerve atrophy, transsphenoidal encephalocele, holoprosencephaly, anencephaly) is suggestive.
2. Tumors that suggest anterior hyposecretion include hypothalamic hamartoblastoma, Rathke pouch cyst, craniopharyngioma, and glioblastoma.
3. Syndrome of septo-optic dysplasia (SOD) comprises of hypopituitarism, optic nerve hypoplasia, absent septum pellucidum, wandering Nystagmus, and blindness at birth.
4. Hypoglycemia, micropenis, and cholestatic jaundice are indicative. Hypoglycemia is usually severe, and glycemic response to glucagon is brisk, which creates further confusion in diagnosis. Jaundice, initially unconjugated, but later predominantly conjugated, often resolves after hormone replacement therapy.
5. There may be **combined deficiency of multiple pituitary hormones** or **isolated deficiency** of a single hormone.

Posterior pituitary hypofunction (partial to complete panhypopituitarism) includes diabetes insipidus (DI) and SIADH (syndrome of inappropriate secretion of ADH).

10.9.2 Growth Hormone

Growth hormone is important for normal growth in the IU life, but in the early postnatal life, thyroid hormone, insulin, and nutrition are more important growth determinants.
- GH is tonically elevated in the first few days of life and normal serum levels are >10 ng/mL.
- Deficiency of GH (value <10 ng/mL) presents as hypoglycemia and micropenis (stretched penile length <2.5 cm in term infant). GH provocative test with increase in GH value to >25 ng/mL is normal.

- Congenital deficiency of GH—there is no IUGR nor effect on linear growth until 6–9 months.

Family history of short stature indicates familial autosomal dominant GH deficiency.

10.9.3 Gonadotrophins and Gonads

At 5–6 weeks of gestation, there is no sex differentiation of the embryos, and both male and female reproductive components are present. Wilms tumor suppressor gene (WT1) and steroidogenic factor 1 (SF-1) play important role in gonadal development and sex determination. Mutations in these are associated with gonadal dysgenesis. Sexual differentiation is complete by 12 weeks when testes descend into the scrotum and testosterone production increases under pituitary gonadotropin stimulus. At birth, gonadotrophin deficiency may be suspected by micropenis in a male baby, but in female baby, it is not identified until puberty.

10.9.4 ACTH and Adrenocortical Hormone Function

Adrenocorticotropic (ACTH) hormone deficiency rarely presents as acute adrenal crisis. ACTH deficiency causing adrenal insufficiency is unlikely if cortisol level is >20 μg/dL. Cortisol insufficiency is usually mild, with hypoglycemia or hyponatremia, normokalemia, and occasionally hyperbilirubinemia. Combined GH and ACTH deficiency may cause severe hypoketotic hypoglycemia. Isolated ACTH deficiency is extremely rare and is usually in association with multiple pituitary hormone deficiencies. **Adrenal hypoplasia congenita (AHC)** is life threatening. Early diagnosis and treatment with corticosteroid and mineralocorticoid replacement can be lifesaving.

Role of Cortisol at Birth and in Neonates

Adrenocortical hormones and cortisol play an important role in the transitional changes at birth by influencing cardiopulmonary changes, metabolism, and hormonal release. Fetal cortisol synthesis and release are under fetal hypothalamic control; levels are low and increase with the period of gestation (Table 10.11). Fetal adrenal cortex atrophies soon after birth creating a relative cortisol deficiency, and abnormality in transitional process, with persistence of fetal circulation (PFC) and persistent pulmonary hypertension of the newborn (PPHN).

Table 10.11 Cortisol levels

Gestational age	Fetal cortisol levels
30 weeks	5–10 μg/mL
36 weeks	20 μg/mL
40 weeks (prelabor)	45 μg/mL
Few hours postdelivery	200 μg/mL

At birth, normal serum cortisol levels are 2.6–10 μg/dL with no diurnal variation. "Cortisol surge" influences the cardiopulmonary, metabolic adaptations, and hormonal release at birth. Cortisol is responsible for lung maturation and for surfactant production, clearance of lung fluid, for normal transition at birth, thyroid hormone secretion, hepatic gluconeogenesis, catecholamine secretion, production of digestive enzymes, and for temperature regulation. (Box 10.6).

Box 10.6 Role of Cortisol in Newborn

1.	Surfactant production in the fetal lungs
2.	Increase in β-receptor density in the heart and lungs, near term and at birth.
3.	Catecholamine release in response to stress at birth (poor in SFD babies).
4.	Maturation of the thyroid axis and in conversion of T_4 to T_3.
5.	Metabolic and energy substrate metabolism in the liver.
6.	Gut maturation and its digestive capacity.

10.9.5 Catecholamines and Other Vasoactive Substances

Catecholamines and other vasoactive substances (norepinephrine, epinephrine, dopamine, angiotensin II, renin)—In response to stress at birth, there is increase in release of catecholamines. In Cesarean-born babies, catecholamine levels are lower than following labor and vaginal delivery. In premature newborns, catecholamine levels are higher because (1) organs are immature and less responsive, and (2) higher concentration is required to illicit similar response. However, stress response is normal in preterm babies. Catecholamines play a role in adaptation at birth by inducing peripheral vasoconstriction, increasing SVR, closure of extrapulmonary shunts, increase in glucose and fat metabolism after birth, and in brown fat thermogenesis, temperature control, and prevention of hypothermia in newborns.

10.9.6 Thyroid Hormones

There is increase in serum levels of T_3 and T_4 in response to cortisol surge, cord clamping, and cold stimulus at birth. Levels only normalize by the age of 10 years.

Role of Thyroid Hormones in Neonate
- (i) Clearance of fetal lung fluid (by activating Na^+, K^+, ATPase).
- (ii) Congenital hypothyroidism—no abnormality or signs at birth or in neonatal period. Usually presents after 2–3 months of age.
- (iii) Very preterm babies—responses at birth (increase in T_3 and T_4) are blunted with depressed adaptive behavior.

Thyroid-Stimulating Hormone (TSH) deficiency is asymptomatic in the newborn and is usually associated with other pituitary deficiencies. Hormonal screening shows low T_4 concentration with normal TSH value, which can be misinterpreted as euthyroid sick syndrome. In a neonate with any CNS abnormality, secondary hypothyroidism should always be ruled out.

10.10 Metabolism

10.10.1 Carbohydrate Metabolism

Fetal energy needs are met with transplacental transfer of glucose and fetal liver acts as a store for glycogen, fat, and other substrates. The microsomal enzyme system is immature at birth until 3 months of age. In early hours of birth, plasma glucose falls. Catecholamine release, cortisol surge, and decrease in insulin levels help maintain normal levels of plasma glucose and free fatty acids. The normal blood/plasma sugar in a newborn is 50–100 mg% (not on glucose supplement), and caloric requirement is at least 100 kcal/kg/day. A 2.5 kg baby should receive 10% dextrose @ 9–10 mL/h (90–100 mL/kg/day) [5, 6].

Fetal heart is a mere conduit and not much energy is consumed by its myocardial activity. At birth, it assumes its role in maintaining cardiac output and peripheral circulation and tissue perfusion, which are high energy consuming. Availability of substrate for metabolism in the newborn depends on:

(a) Pulmonary gas exchange,
(b) Coronary blood flow,
(c) Nutritional intake, and.
(d) Efficiency in shifting from CHO to fatty acid utilization as substrate.

Neonatal myocardium is capable of anaerobic energy production and can maintain cardiac function even at low PaO_2, protecting the myocardium from ischemic injury. However, persistent hypoxia or asphyxia adversely affects transitional changes much before myocardial effects become apparent.

Important Points that to be Kept in Mind During the Perioperative Period in Neonates Are

1. They have high BMR and glucose utilization.
2. Gluconeogenesis is not active.
3. Glycogen stores from IU period are low and suffice for only 10–12 h of birth,
4. This makes neonates extremely prone to hypoglycemia (blood sugar <40 mg%) even with short periods of starvation. Hence, they should not be kept fasting for long.
5. During fasting or NPO interval, glucose must be supplemented to maintain blood sugar >40 mg% (>2.6 mmol/L) with 0.5–1 mg/kg of dextrose infused @ 5–6 mg/kg/min.
6. AVOID hypoglycemia, hyperglycemia, hypovolemia, and dehydration.

Preterm babies have abnormal response to cortisol and catecholamines. Serum levels are higher and catecholamine release is increased. Their glycogen, fat, and substrate stores are small, which creates difficulty in adaptation at birth. They often need glucose infusion, as substrate for metabolism and energy production, to prevent hypoglycemia, hypothermia and allow normal transitional.

Babies born to diabetic mothers behave differently from those born to non-diabetic mothers:

1. They have lower blood glucose levels.
2. Congenital anomalies—incidence of congenital heart disease (CHD) and CNS anomalies (anencephaly, spina bifida, microcephaly, caudal regression syndrome) is significantly higher.
3. They are at a greater risk for RDS than other newborns of comparable gestational age.
4. Hypoglycemia incidence is high and is proportional to cord plasma glucose value.

Both hypoglycemia and hyperglycemia can have adverse short- and long-term consequences and should be avoided.

Hypoglycemia

Hypoglycemia is defined as plasma glucose of <40 mg% (term and preterm newborns). Maternal, fetal, and postnatal factors can cause hypoglycemia in the newborn baby (Table 10.12).

Diagnosis—The newborn cannot complain hence no symptoms, and diagnosis is based on observation, clinical signs, and laboratory investigations. **Signs** are usually non-specific and include tremulousness, twitching, jitteriness, irritability, exaggerated Moro reflex, high pitched cry, prolonged seizures, apnea, limpness, poor feeding, cyanosis, temperature instability, cerebral damage, and coma. **Screening** for plasma glucose is advised at 1, 2, 4, 8, and 24 h in at-risk newborns, not receiving glucose containing IV fluids, or when exhibiting clinical signs. Newborn hypoglycemia is classified as:

- **Mild**—Plasma sugar levels 20–40 mg% and
- **Severe**—plasma sugar levels <20 mg%

Aim of management (Table 10.4) is to achieve plasma glucose of >40 mg% (2.6 mmol/L) (50–100 mg%), while avoiding over transfusion, using D10% instead of D5%, and maintaining Hct <65%.

(i) **Preventive measures**—during fasting, baby should receive IV glucose (0.5–1.0 mg/kg) @ 5–6 mg/kg/min.

Table 10.12 Newborns at risk of hypoglycemia

Maternal factors	Fetal factors	Postnatal factors
IUGR<10%ile>,	SGA (<10%ie),	Postasphyxia, 5 min APGAR <5,
Diabetic mothers,	LGA) (>90%ile),	Polycythemia, immune hemolytic ds,
Gestational diabetes,	Premature,	Suspected sepsis,
On oral hypoglycemics,	Postmature.	Hypothermia,
Glucose overload prebirth		Congenital anomalies

(ii) **Mild hypoglycemia** (40–50 mg %, asymptomatic)—can be managed with oral feeds and glucose water. If the neonate is NPO, as in the perioperative period, IV glucose can be supplemented as described above.

(iii) **Moderate hypoglycemia** (<40 mg%)—baby should receive 4–8 mg/kg/min dextrose as D10 (plain or in 0.2 NS) @ 100 mL/kg/day or 10 g/kg/day or 7 mg/kg/min.

(iv) **Severe hypoglycemia** (<20 mg%, symptomatic)—D10 bolus (2 mL/kg = 0.2 g/kg) over 1–2 min.

(v) **Continuous infusion:** 90–120 mL/kg/day = (6–8 mg/kg/min) as D10.

Monitoring of plasma glucose (capillary blood from the heel) is done every 2 h after starting treatment, and every 30 min if symptomatic. Infusion is adjusted to maintain plasma glucose >40 mg% (if <40 mg%—increase infusion rate to 10 mg/kg/min). Once normal levels stabilize for 24 h, IV infusion can be tapered off over next 24 h, and oral feeds continued.

While Infusing 10% Dextrose, Care Must Be Taken

- Never give with blood or products in the same line as glucose,
  - Risk of fluid and solute overload, so avoid using D5, and RL solutions, because babies are already in congested states and are at risk of peripheral and pulmonary edema,
  - Volume load causes dilutional hyponatremia, hypokalemia, and hypocalcemia,
  - Hyperglycemia and serum hyperosmolality and intracranial hemorrhage (ICH) especially in VLBW newborns.

Hyperglycemia is defined as plasma glucose >200 mg% in the first few hours to days of life and is usually iatrogenic following IV glucose administration. **Adverse effects** of hyperglycemia are increased risk of IVH, ROP, NEC, BPD, prolonged hospital stay, bacterial and fungal infections, and death. **Neonates at risk** include LBW, VLBW, on IV glucose infusion, and congenital diabetes mellitus. Sudden onset polyuria (plasma glucose >250 mg%) is a sure sign. Abrupt increase in plasma glucose levels (rapid infusion of 25% or 50% dextrose), or unmonitored glucose infusion can result in ICH. **Management** (Table 10.13) is preventive (timely care in

Table 10.13 Plasma glucose levels in newborns and management of hypoglycemia/hyperglycemia

	Plasma Glucose	Management	Screening-capillary sample
Normoglycemia	50–100 mg%	Normal feeds	Once at 2 h
Mild hypoglycemia	20–40 mg%	Enteral glucose	2–4 h until normal for 24 h
Severe hypoglycemia	<20 mg%	Bolus IV D10–2 mL/kg (0.2 g/kg) Infusion at 4–8 mg g/kg/min(90–120 mL/kg/D)	Every 30 min
Hyperglycemia	>200 mg%	Stop IV glucose, IV insulin 0.1 U/kg/h	Every 4 h until normal for 24 h

newborns at-risk and vigilant monitoring) and corrective (plasma glucose >200 mg%), by reducing infusion rate, addition of IV insulin 0.1 U/kg/h, and blood sugar monitoring every 1–4 h until normal for 24 h.

10.10.2 Protein Metabolism

(a) Protein production is slow at birth and normalizes by 1 year of age.
(b) High risk of hypoproteinemia, hypoalbuminemia, fluid overload, peripheral, cerebral, and pulmonary edema.
(c) Reduced drug binding and more of free (active) drug in circulation.
(d) Enzyme system is immature, and different systems mature at different rates.
(e) Drug metabolism is slow—prolonged duration of action of drugs.
(f) They are at risk of adverse drug effects.

Hence, great care must be taken during administration of fluids and electrolytes. It is preferable to use 5% albumin than crystalloids in treatment of hypovolemia and dehydration, avoiding high sodium containing fluids, as well as reducing the doses of drugs administered.

10.10.3 Calcium Metabolism, Neonatal Hypocalcemia, and Osteopenia of Prematurity

A fetus starts to accumulate calcium during the third trimester of pregnancy, and this continues to a peak in early adulthood. Thereafter it begins to decline at a rate of 1% per year. These variations are due to continual remodeling of bone, excess of bone formation during growth spurt in early adulthood, and breakdown in late adulthood. In the newborn, serum calcium levels are low (1.9–2.8 mmol/L), **but become normal by the age of 1 y.** Hypocalcemia is diagnosed when plasma ionized calcium concentration is <0.75 mmol/L (3 mg%). **Neonates at risk** of hypocalcemia include premature, babies born to diabetic mothers, postbirth asphyxia, and congenital, genetic, and hormonal disorders [36].

Categorization of Hypocalcemia by Age of Onset
1. **Early-onset hypocalcemia** is usually iatrogenic. It occurs in preterm newborns who receive sodium bicarbonate for treatment of metabolic acidosis. Risk is greatest at 12–24 h of age. In most asymptomatic babies, it normalizes within 72 h without treatment.
2. **Late-onset hypocalcemia** is seen after 7 days of life in those on formula milk low in calcium and high in phosphorus content. This is not common.
3. **Very late-onset hypocalcemia** (osteopenia or rickets of prematurity) is a relatively frequent in preterm neonates. Large amounts of calcium and phosphorus are transferred from the mother during the third trimester. Hence, in premature newborns, both calcium and phosphorus are reduced. Osteopenia causes weak and brittle bones and often remains silent until signs of rickets or fractures occur at a later age.

Symptoms of hypocalcemia usually occur later in infancy and are nonspecific-jitteriness, seizures, apnea, bleeding, and decreased myocardial contractility. **Management** in symptomatic neonates or hypocalcemia in laboratory report should be instituted immediately. There is no benefit of empirical calcium supplements in all neonates without evidence of hypocalcemia. **Treatment** consists of 10% calcium gluconate administration, starting with 100–200 mg/kg (1–2 mL/kg) as slow IV "push" over 30 min, followed by continuous infusion @ 400 mg/kg/day, or 100 mg/kg every 6 h slowly over 30 min. **Care during calcium infusion** calcium gluconate is preferred and can be given via peripheral line. Do not given with sodium bicarbonate, dioxin, or antibiotics in the same infusion due to risk of precipitation. **Monitoring** of plasma ionized calcium level should be done every 12–24 h. Once calcium level remains normal for 24 h, the infusion is reduced by 50% and discontinues after another 24 h if calcium level is normal and baby is asymptomatic. In neonates on oral feeds, oral calcium supplement is added. To prevent occurrence of late osteopenia, commonly in sickest and least mature premature neonates, long-term enteral and parenteral calcium support must be continued.

10.10.4 Magnesium Metabolism

Magnesium is a trace element, and second most abundant intracellular cation, essential for life [37].

Congenital hypomagnesemia may occur in premature neonates, IUGR, and babies born to Mg-deficient mothers. **Management** is replacement therapy using 50% $MgSO_4$ (0.2 mmol or 0.4 mEq/kg/day = IV 0.1 mL/kg/day) for 5 dose days or oral 1.0 mL of 10% magnesium chloride (0.5 mmol/kg/day Mg).

Hypermagnesemia is more common in newborns, usually from Mg overdose in mother or inadequate renal function in eclamptic mothers. No active **management** is required and Mg normalizes by 48 h. In obtunded and depressed neonates, IV calcium and glucose saline infusion are given. Rarely, dialysis may be needed.

To summarize, metabolic immaturity and imbalance can have greater and long-term adverse effects because of immature BBB and increased risk of cerebral edema, raised ICP, convulsions, and extensive hypoxic damage. Hyperbilirubinemia is common in newborns, but kernicterus occurs at lower bilirubin levels (12–13 mg%); for this reason, exchange transfusion is indicated at serum levels of 15–20 mg% in preterm and at >20 mg% in term neonates. These effects are compounded by the adverse effect of drugs received by the mother in the antenatal or perinatal period, e.g., narcotics, sedatives, anesthetic drugs, maternal drug addictions, and drug and alcohol abuse. Additionally, effects of anesthetic drugs and techniques used during operative delivery, complications of anesthesia (airway or hemodynamic related), and indication of Cesarean section itself will add to the immature newborns' risks.

10.11 Hepatic Anatomy and Physiology

10.11.1 Anatomy

Liver is the biggest gland in the body, with endocrine (secretion of Insulin-like growth factors, angiotensinogen, and thrombopoietin), exocrine (production of Bile), synthetic (protein, carbohydrates, lipids, clotting factors, lymph), metabolic (urea production, drug detoxification), storage, and excretory (bile and products of metabolism) functions. Adult liver is 2.5–3.5% of body weight (1.4–1.6 kg (3.1–3.5 lb). At birth, liver is very small, weighing 120 g (4 oz), but it is 4% of body weight.

10.11.2 Functions of Liver-Fetal Liver Has Two Important Roles Besides Other Functions, Mainly Cardiovascular and Hemopoietic [38–40]

Embryologically, liver appears as a hepatic diverticulum extending out from the foregut at third week of gestation and grows rapidly from fifth to the tenth week. The cells proliferate into hepatocytes and are a rich source of stem cells. As the liver grows, liver sinusoids and bile canaliculi appear. A branch from the diverticulum grows into the gall bladder.

(a) **Cardiovascular (CVS) Function**—Liver occupies major portion of the abdominal cavity of the fetus. It is supplied by the umbilical veins, with Hb saturation of 80%. It acts a conduit between the placental vessels and heart. Blood bypasses the liver via the ductus venosus (shunt between left portal and left hepatic veins) into the IVC, thereby to RA, and to the left side of the heart via Foramen Ovale and Ductus Arteriosus (refer to chapter on fetal circulation and adaptation).

(b) **Haemopoietic function**—Primitive erythropoiesis starts in the yolk sac at around seventh week, and by midterm, liver is the main erythropoietic tissue, producing RBCs before the bone marrow can take over. Hematopoietic stem cells are pluripotent and form all the hematopoietic cells (RBC, WBC, B and T lymphocytes, and platelets). Fetal liver releases blood stem cells that migrate to the fetal thymus, creating T lymphocytes, and by 13th week T lymphocyte production starts in the thymus. By 15th week, erythroid and myelo-lymphoid production moves to spleen and to bone marrow by 16th week. By 32 weeks, bone marrow completely takes over the erythropoiesis. Thrombopoietin, produced in the liver, regulates production of platelets by the bone marrow. The switch mechanism from fetal to adult hemoglobin (Hb) also takes place in the liver. Three hormones play a role at different periods of gestation in production of hemoglobin, **testosterone** (between 10 and 13 weeks), **β-adrenergic stimulation** (between 8–11 weeks), and **erythropoietin** (by late second trimester).

Other activities taking place in the fetal liver are **bile production** (by 12th week), **glycogen storage** (by 30th week) and gradually increase thereafter, and **drug clearance** via P 450 iso-enzymes (reaches 85% of adult levels by 44 weeks and adult levels by 6 months of postnatal age). Within 2–5 days of birth, umbilical vein gets obliterated into round ligament of the liver, while ductus venosus get obliterated into ligamentum venosum. In cirrhosis and portal hypertension, the umbilical vein can reopen. At birth, liver is not mature enough to take over all the functions fully, and special care must be taken in the perioperative period.

(c) **Carbohydrate metabolism**—The microsomal enzyme system matures only by 3 months of age. At birth and during the neonatal period, the basal metabolic rate (BMR) is high and so is glucose utilization:

   (i) Gluconeogenesis is not active. Fetal glycogen stores are low and last only up to 10–12 h. Thus, neonates are prone to becoming hypoglycemic (normal range of blood sugar = 40–60 mg%).

   (ii) They are susceptible to periods of starvation—so minimal duration of fasting in the preoperative period and otherwise.

   (iii) During fasting period, glucose must be supplemented to maintain blood sugar >40 mg% (>2.6 mmol/L) using dextrose infusion of 0.5–1 mg/kg @ 5–6 mg/kg/min.

   (iv) Always avoid hypoglycemia, hyperglycemia, hypovolemia, and dehydration.

(d) **Protein Metabolism**—Protein production is low and becomes normal by the age of 1 year, hence:

   (a) Low drug binding to proteins, and more of free (active) form of in circulation.

   (b) Decreased drug metabolism and prolonged duration of action of drugs.

   (c) Hence, dosages of IV drugs must be reduced, and intervals between supplements prolonged.

(e) **Bilirubin metabolism**—At birth, serum bilirubin is high (17–20 mg%), which normalizes by 1 month of age. This is due to:

   • Deficiency of Vit K-dependent clotting factors (II, VII, IX, X), and 20–60% prolongation in prothrombin time. Hence, all neonates should receive parenteral Vit K for 3 days preoperatively.

   • Liver is unable to conjugate bilirubin. Unconjugated bilirubin can cross the BBB; hence, kernicterus can occur at lower serum bilirubin levels (12–13 mg%).

(f) **Biotransformation of drugs**—The enzyme system is immature, and different systems mature at different rates. Drug metabolism is slow and they are at risk of adverse drug effects. Besides, there is danger of hepatotoxicity of the immature liver by various drugs.

10.12 Neonatal Renal Physiology and Excretory Function

When trying to understand the development and functioning of the renal and the excretory system, it should be done in relation to total body water (TBW), its distribution, expected fluid and electrolyte shifts, and functional capacity of the kidneys. Neonates are already in a delicate state of fluid balance, and these changes become quite relevant in the presence of medical or surgical pathology, and during surgery under general anesthesia [41–43].

Renal system plays a tremendous role in growth and development of a fetus, in maturation and well-being after birth. It maintains body homeostasis and regulates body water, electrolytes, acid-base balance, removal of waste, metabolites, and clearing of drugs from the body. During this time, there is little margin for error especially in the premature and VLBW neonates. Significant risks for all neonates include overhydration, dehydration, electrolyte imbalances, oliguria, and acidosis.

Renal efficacy is a function of GA, total renal mass, renal blood flow, and hemodynamic stability. Abnormal renal functioning in the neonatal period is a predictor of CVS and renal disease risks, though acute renal failure (ARF) may occur in up to 24% of sick neonates in NICU.

Urine formation consists of four processes—glomerular filtration, tubular reabsorption, tubular secretion, and urinary excretion. Fetal kidneys produce urine by late first trimester. Each kidney has about a million nephrons and 60% of nephrogenesis occurs after 20th week, up to 36th week of gestation. At birth, kidneys also undergo transitional changes. Being immature at birth, the excretory system continues to mature over a period of 3 months, attaining full maturity by 2 years of age. The preterm newborns (<36 weeks GA) are especially vulnerable to renal dysmaturity, with prolonged postnatal maturation, up to 7–8 years of age.

Renal blood flow (RBF), glomerular filtration rate (GFR)—Kidneys weigh less than 0.5% of body weight, but they are highly vascular. RBF is 5% of CO at birth, increases to 20% by 1 month, and reaches adult value of 25% by 2–3 years. Effective plasma flow (EPF) is low, 83 mL/min/1.73 m^2 at term, increasing to 650 mL/min/1.73 m^2 by 2 years. At 25 weeks' gestation, GFR is only 10% of adult values, 35% birth, and doubles by second week of life, and continues to increase up to 3 months. (Table 10.14) Various factors affect GFR, such as IUGR, maternal steroids, postnatal high FiO_2, nephrotoxic drugs, stress and sympathetic stimulation, and hypoxic ischemic injury to brain. Clinical conditions associated with renal dysfunction include need for vasopressors in the first week of life, IVH, PDA, NEC, sepsis, and high-frequency ventilation (HFV).

Tubular function is also immature at birth. Renal tubules are insensitive to antidiuretic hormone (ADH), and levels of ADH are high in newborns. **Neonates are obligate salt losers**. They have less ability to excrete sodium load and to concentrate or dilute urine. Their daily requirement of sodium is 2 mmol/kg, and 1 mmol/kg of potassium and calcium, each. They cannot also conserve bicarbonate and are extremely prone to developing metabolic acidosis.

Table 10.14 RBF/EPF, GFR, and urine osmolality in neonates

Age	RBF/EPF	GFR mL/ min/1.73 m^2	Urine Osmolality (mOsm)
TERM			
Newborn	5% of CO/83 mL/ min/1.73 m^2	20–25	525
2–4 weeks	20% of CO	40–60	950 (28 days)
Adult values (by 2 years in term NB),8 years in ELBW)	25% of CO/650 mL/ min/1.73 m^2	100–130	1400
PRETERM			
25 weeks GA		2	
27–31 weeks GA to 7 days age		8–29	
27–31 weeks GA to 21 days age		13–35	

A newborn usually passes hypo-osmolar urine within first 24 h of birth (525 mOsm), which increases to 950 mOsm by 28 days, and 1400 mOsm by 1 year. **Normal urine output is 0.5 mL/day.** They **cannot deal with major volume changes such as overload, dehydration, or solute load.**

Body weight **gain in** the first week of life is due to sodium retention, and once sodium excretion begins, weight gain decreases, rather there may be weight loss, which recovers by 1 month of age. Sodium containing fluids should be avoided in the first week, but need to be given if weight loss is more than 7% of BW.

Hormonal control is inefficient and less effective including renin–angiotensin aldosterone system (RAAS), atrial natriuretic peptides (ANP), vasopressin, and catecholamine system. RAAS plays a role in regulating blood pressure, intrarenal blood flow, and fluid and electrolyte balance.

Sodium balance—Sodium is easily filtered at the glomerulus. Nearly all is reabsorbed (70% in proximal convoluted tubules (pct), 15–20% in ascending loop of Henle, 5% each in the distal convoluted tubules (dct) and collecting tubules), and urine finally formed is hypotonic, very low in sodium content. In premature, sodium losses are high as the immature renal tubules cannot reabsorb. After first week of life, term neonates have a positive sodium balance. Premature neonates are prone to hyponatremia and dilute urine in the first week and later to hypernatremia and increased urinary sodium losses. They require 3–5 meq/kg/d of sodium replacement in the first week of life. Hypoxia, diuretics, jaundice, high fluid load, or salt intake increase sodium excretion and should be avoided.

Potassium balance—Potassium is secreted in the dct. Immaturity of the dct and reduced sensitivity of collecting tubules to aldosterone reduce excretion of potassium in term neonate, with hyperkalemia. In premature neonates, potassium shifts out of the intracellular compartment. With use of diuretics, there is increased loss of potassium. This gradually returns to normal by 2–3 weeks. It is important that

Table 10.15 Acid–base balance

Age	pH	HCO3 mmol/L	PaCO2 mmHg
Birth	7.14–7.34	14–26	29–69
Neonate	7.18–7.5	17–24	27–40
Infant	7.2–7.5	19–24	27–41
Adult	7.37–7.41	20–28	37–45

during perioperative period, meticulous care is taken in fluid and electrolyte therapy, avoid or manage changes in volume status and electrolytes, and prevent acidosis and further deterioration in the already compromised renal function.

Calcium balance—Calcium levels fall soon after birth to about 8 mg% and lower in premature (7 mg%). This usually corrects by 2–3 weeks of age.

Acid-base balance (Table 10.15)—Neonates have poor capacity to conserve bicarbonate. The respiratory buffer has a limited capacity, renal buffer is immature, and remaining buffers (bicarb carbonic acid, oxy Hb, protein, PO4 buffer) are in less quantity. At birth, blood pH is slightly acidic and remains so throughout the neonatal period.

Creatinine is a reliable indicator of renal function. A product of muscle metabolism is secreted into the blood at a steady rate and freely filtered at the glomerulus. It is not affected by weight, gender, or age, but varies with hydration and clinical status.

Serum creatinine (SCr) and GFR are inversely related. High SCr indicates poor renal function. With decline in GFR, creatinine takes 7–10 days to stabilize and hence is a better indicator of chronic renal dysfunction. Higher levels at birth reflect maternal levels (1.1 mg%). Normal values are 0.2–1 mg% on day 1–3 and 0.2–0.5 mg% by 1 year. In VLBW and premature neonates, levels peak by 2–3 days and decrease by 4–5 days, because of tubular reabsorption and leaky renal tubules, which improves by the first week of life.

Accurate measurement of GFR is problematic due to the unavailability of the gold standard inulin for neonates. The traditional use of creatinine to estimate GFR is unreliable in preterm due to its tubular reabsorption and its dependence on muscle mass as an endogenous marker. Alternatively, cystatin C and beta trace protein (BTP) are used. Cystatin C is filtered across capillaries and completely reabsorbed by pct and is a better measure of GFR.

Blood urea nitrogen (BUN) represents urine-concentrating capacity. Urea is formed in the liver from amino acids and ammonia and is filtered in the glomerulus. If GFR decreases, BUN increases. BUN has a wide variation in range, 6–43 mg% (mean 20.9 mg%) on day 1, 8–110 mg% (mean 36 mg %) on day 7, 5–17 mg% at 3 years of age, and 7–20 mg% in adults. It is affected by age, protein intake, and low GFR (dehydration, hypotension) and is not the first choice for estimating renal function in neonates.

Medications and drug clearance—reduced RBF and GFR, and immature tubular function, interferes with clearance of drugs from the body with resultant prolonged action. This also implies that the time interval between two doses of drugs given repeatedly during general anesthesia, such as muscle relaxants and narcotics, is longer.

Drug metabolism is slower in neonates, more so in prematures. Special care is needed in the dosing and monitoring of renal functions when administering drugs that may be nephrotoxic to the developing kidneys, such as antibiotics (aminoglycosides, glycopeptides, amikacin, vancomycin, gentamicin), analgesics (ibuprofen, indomethacin). Ibuprofen, as prophylaxis or treatment of PDA during the neonatal period, reduces GFR significantly, persisting through 1 month of age.

Diuretics are commonly used in a sick neonate, such as lasix, aldactone, and thiazides. Each is associated with several side effects and toxic effects. Furosemide (lasix) inhibits chloride reabsorption in the ascending limb of the loop of Henle, inhibits tubular sodium transport, and leads to increased sodium, potassium, and calcium loss, with severe dyselectrolytemia, ototoxicity, metabolic alkalosis, and renal calcinosis especially in the premature. Lasix dose 1–2 mg/kg once in 12 h in term and once in 24 h in premature. Spironolactone (Aldactone) and aldosterone antagonist (1–3 mg/kg/d in 12 h) is associated with hyperkalemia, lethargy, and GI disturbance in neonates. Chlorothiazide (decreases sodium reabsorption in dct) is associated with dehydration, electrolyte imbalance, metabolic alkalosis, hypercalcemia, hyperglycemia, hyperuricemia, especially in newborns with liver or renal disease. Keeping a check on dosages and intervals in between, aiming to use the least effective dose, at maximum interval, and least number of doses, will help contain these side effects.

10.13 Total Body Water, Body Water Distribution, and Blood Volume

Total body water (TBW) is higher in neonates compared to adults and children. In a full-term neonate, TBW is 80% of body weight and is distributed equally into the intracellular (ICF) and extracellular (ECF) compartments. In preterm neonates, TBW is >80% of body weight, and more than 60% is in the ECF compartment. Adult figures are attained by the age of 4 years, when TBW is 60% body weight, and proportion of ICF volume increases to two times ECF volume (40% is ICF and 20% is ECF) (Table 10.1).

Blood volume is also higher in neonates, 85 mL/kg body weight at term, and 90–100 mL/kg body weight in premature, compared to 60 mL/kg in adults (Table 10.16).

Hemoglobin (Hb) ranges between 16–20 g% in term neonates while it is lower in preterms, with higher hematocrit (Hct) (50–55%). Blood transfusion trigger is

Table 10.16 TBW, distribution, and blood volume

Category	TBW and its distribution (ICF:ECF)	Blood volume
Neonates	TBW 80–85% of body weight	85–100 mL/kg
Full term	80 mL/kg—ICF:ECF::1/1	85 mL/kg
Premature	90 mL/kg—ICF:ECF::1:3.	90–100 mL/kg
4 years	60% of body weight—ICF:ECF::2:1	60–70 mL/kg
Adults	60% of body weight—ICF:ECF::2:1	60 mL/kg

lower in neonates and, more so in the preterm, goal being to maintain the higher Hct except in congenital heart disease, where Hct is kept low.

Two important Anesthetic Implications are relating to:
1. TBW, drug distribution, elimination, and duration of action, and
2. Increased losses and hypovolemia.
    1. Drug distribution, elimination, and duration of action
        (i) Higher TBW and proportion of ECF increase the apparent volume of distribution (Vd) of drugs.
        (ii) Increased Vd acts as a double-edged sword
            a. It will cause greater dilution of drugs given intravenously (induction agents, muscle relaxants, and narcotics), lower serum concentrations and possible inadequate effect, and
            b. Necessitating higher doses for the desired effect, with consequent prolonged duration of action and delayed recovery from anesthesia.
        (iii) Drug dosages administered as per body weight will result in lower plasma concentration, while dosages based on body surface area will result in higher serum concentration.
        (iv) But because of hypoproteinemia and hypoalbuminemia, there is reduced binding of drugs to albumin and α acid-glycoprotein and increased free drug concentration.
        (v) Enzyme systems are immature—poor drug metabolism, impaired renal excretion, and potential hypothermia further slow drug metabolism and excretion.
        (vi) Net effect—increase in elimination half-life, prolonged duration of action, and delayed recovery from anesthesia.

Caution—Care must be taken during drug administration, titrating to the desired effect.

Increased Losses and Risk of Hypovolemia

Larger BSA makes neonates prone to greater loss of water and at risk of developing hypovolemia. Their insensible fluid losses are high (65 mL/kg/day—20 mL by evaporation, 10 mL via GIT, 35 mL by kidneys). Factors that increase losses are as follows:
1. Larger BSA, and thin and less keratinized skin.
2. Higher metabolic (0.2 MJ/kg/day) and respiratory rates, with greater water turnover.
3. Greater ambient temperature and use of radiant warmers.
4. Use of dry inspired O_2 and gases during anesthesia and increased insensible losses.
5. Excretory system is immature at birth and is still in developing phase in the neonates. Glomerular and tubular functions are immature. They have
    (a) Reduced glomerular filtration rate (GFR) at birth. It doubles by second week and reaches adult values by 2 years of age.
    (b) Limited ability to concentrate urine.
    (c) Limited ability to excrete large water load.
    (d) Poor hormonal control—less effective renin–angiotensin mechanism, alpha natriuretic peptide, vasopressin, and catecholamine system.

Table 10.17 Fluid requirements in neonates

Age in days	Fluid requirement mL/kg/day
1	60
2	80
3	100
4	120
5–28	150

Table 10.18 Intraoperative fluid requirement

	Maintenance Fluid	Replacement Fluid
Term neonate	70–80 mL/kg/day	
Preterm neonate	100 mL/kg/day	
Minor loss surgery	4 mL/kg/h	2 mL/kg/h
Moderate loss surgery	4 mL/kg/h	4 mL/kg/day
Extensive loss surgery	4 mL/kg/h	6–8 mL/kg/day

Caution—Meticulous fluid therapy

Hence, neonates are more prone to dehydration and hypovolemia, water and solute overload, and acidosis.

Fluid requirement is high in the newborns and neonates, especially in the first few days of life (Table 10.17), and then remains stable at 150 mL/kg/day throughout the remaining neonatal period.

Intraoperative fluid therapy is provided as 5% or 10% dextrose (D5 or D10) in either Ringer lactate (RL) or normal saline (NS), or as isolyte P. Intraoperative requirement can be calculated as maintenance and replacement fluids. Since neonates requiring surgery are already on IV fluid therapy during fasting, deficit is usually not calculated. The fluid requirement as per the type of surgery is described in Table 10.18.

10.14 Hematopoiesis and Coagulation

10.14.1 Hematopoietic System

RBC production begins in the first week of gestation and proceeds through three phases: mesoblastic (yolk sac), hepatic, and myeloid (bone marrow). **Mesoblastic** (embryonic, primitive) red cells are extremely large, have a short life span, and are insensitive to erythropoietin. They do not mature into RBCs but can differentiate into other cell types. Fetal liver is the major store for iron and main erythropoietic site at midterm **(hepatic phase)**. After 24 weeks, major erythropoiesis shifts to the bone marrow **(myeloid phase)**, but by 36 weeks, bone marrow is the only site.

Three hormonal influences are **testosterone** (in first trimester), **beta-adrenergic activity** (10–13 weeks), and **erythropoietin** (in second trimester) [40, 44].

Hematopoietic system also undergoes transitional changes at birth, namely via circulation and oxygenation. At birth, bone marrow is fully active and only site for hemopoiesis. Postnatal extramedullary hematopoiesis is abnormal, except in premature neonates where a few foci may be seen in the liver, spleen, lymph nodes, or thymus.

10.14.2 Hemoglobin

Hemoglobin types—Abnormalities in embryonic hemoglobin (Hb ε) can lead to a delay in switching from Hb F to Hb A. **Hb F ($\alpha2\ \lambda2$)** has 2 alpha and 2 gamma globin chains and is the major Hb in fetal life. Synthesis of adult Hb (Hb A $\alpha2\beta2$) starts at ninth week and by 21 weeks 14% of total Hb is Hb A. After 34 week, Hb A rises, while Hb F decreases, but even at birth, more than 60% is Hb F. It decreases to less than 2% by 6 months. The switch from Hb F to Hb A is genetically controlled and takes place in the liver. The Hb concentration fluctuates in the early weeks and months after birth and is affected by factors, such as: -

(a) Gestational age (GA) and birthweight (BW),
(b) Time of cord clamping,
(c) Hypoxic stress,
(d) Crying,
(e) Sampling site—Capillary vs venous (higher in capillary sample), warm vs cold limb,
(f) Race—African American—0.5 g% lower than white NN,
(g) Mode of delivery, and.
(h) Genetic defects—Trisomy 13.

The **average Hb** in term newborn is 18–20 g%. Nearly 60% is Hb F with high O_2 affinity, but high blood volume and CO compensate for the decreased release of O_2 from fetal Hb. Hb A levels are achieved by 6 months of age. In preterms, the proportion of Hb F is higher (70–80%) and total Hb is lower (13–15 g%), making them more prone to hypoxemia. By the age of 1 month, Hb decreases to about 14 g% and to 10 g% by 3 months.

Average **Hct** at birth is 55% (45–65%), and more than 65% is abnormal (hyperviscosity). Hct increases by 5% during the first 48 h of life. By 2–4 months, it falls to a mean of 40%.

The total **blood volume** is 85–90 mL/kg for term and 90–100 mL/kg for premature newborn. Adult value of 65 mL/kg is achieved by 4 months of age. Newborns have polycythemia (high RBC count) in the first 24 h due to in utero hypoxia, which triggers erythropoietin production and slowly declines after 2 weeks.

RBCs are macrocytic in the first week of life, whereafter they become normocytic normochromic. In term neonates, 43% RBCs are biconcave disks compared to 78% in adults, 3–5% being dysmorphic (fragments, target cells, distorted).

Table 10.19 Blood cell counts at birth and in neonates

	Newborn	1 Week	4 weeks
BW < 1200 g			
Hb g%	15–16	16–18	11–12
Platelets	1.5–1.6 L	1.5–1.6 L	1.3–1.4 L
TLC	13,000–15,000	12,000–13,000	13,000–14,000
BW 1200–1500 g			
Hb g %	20	18	12
Platelets	1.5 L	1.3–1.4 L	1.7–1.9 L
TLC	10,000–11,000	8000–9000	10,000–12,000
BW >2000–3500 g			
Hb g%	16–20	14–18	12–16 (14)
Hct	45–65 (55)	35–60 (45)	25–45 (40)
TLC	3500–6000	3500–5000	7000–10,000

Reticulocyte count at birth is high (4–6%) and falls to less than 1% by sixth day. Counts are higher and fall is slower in premature. **Leukocytes** (WBC) appear by ninth week and megakaryocytes (platelet precursors) by sixth week of gestation. **Platelet** counts range from 150–400 × 109/L, comparable to adult values. Thrombocytopenia (<100 × 10^9 platelets/L) is associated with birth trauma and high-risk neonates (sepsis, RDS). Normal Hb and cell counts are listed in Table 10.19.

10.14.3 Oxygen Dissociation Curve (ODC)

O2 affinity of Hb F is greater than that of Hb A. Levels of 2,3-DPG (diphosphoglyc-erate) are lower in newborn, HB F has lower affinity for 2–3 DPG, and ODC is shifted to the left. P50 of Hb F (mean PaO2 at which Hb is 50% saturated) is 19 mmHg compared to 26 mmHg of Hb A. Low P50 (and shift of ODC to left) means greater binding of O2 to Hb F. At PaO2 25 mm Hg, 80% O2 is bound to Hb F (Fig. 10.5). Thus, there is decreased O2 release at tissue level. As PaO2 falls <90 mm Hg, 3.0 mL of O2 is released in a newborn, while 4.5 mL is released in an adult, per 100 mL blood (because of higher affinity of Hb F for O2). Adverse effects of leftward shift of ODC in the neonate are offset by high Hb concentration, high Hct, and high cardiac output. Adult values are reached by the age of 1 year.

After birth, the ODC gradually shifts to the right, reaching adult curve morphol-ogy by 6 months. In a premature, 2–3 DPG levels are even less than in term neo-nates, and leftward shift of ODC is more pronounced, requiring greater fall in PaO2 to release equivalent amount of O2. After birth, the rightward shift is also slower. It is important for the neonatal anesthesiologists to be aware of and take special care during peri anesthetic management to avoid factors that may further shift ODC to left, such as hyperventilation, hypocarbia, hypothermia, and alkalosis.

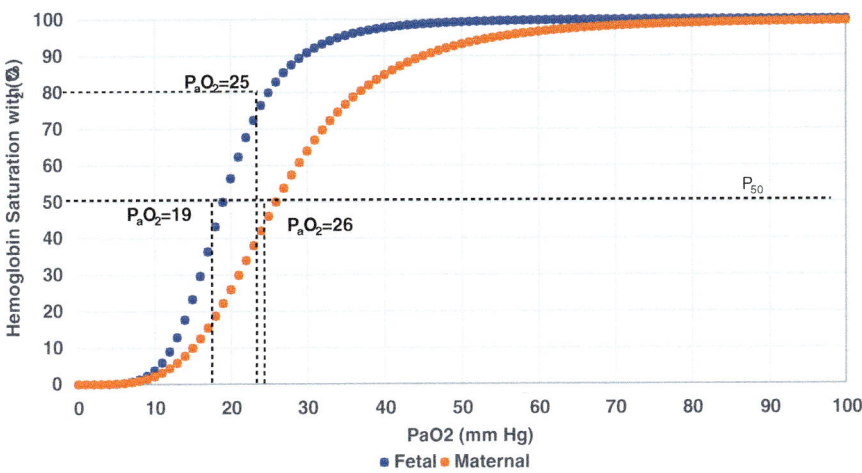

Fig. 10.5 ODC—Oxygen dissociation curve—showing maternal and fetal curves

10.14.4 Physiologic Anemia

Erythropoietin, the primary regulator of erythropoiesis, is present in cord blood and falls to undetectable levels after birth. RBC, Hb, and Hct values decrease slightly in first week, but more rapidly in the second month (physiological anemia) [40].

Causes of Physiological Anemia are:
(a) Changes at birth—increase in PaO2 and decrease in erythropoietin production,
(b) Decrease in Hb production and fall in hematocrit,
(c) Shorter life span of fetal RBC (60–70 days in term, 35–50 days in premature neonates), compared to 120 days in adults, and.
(d) Transmembrane potassium influx is significantly less in neonatal RBC and they are more sensitive to osmotic hemolysis and oxidant injury.

Anemia diagnosis in neonates is difficult because they cannot communicate their symptoms, and clinical signs are non-specific, as they are indicators of other medical conditions also, such as sepsis, apnea, seizures, and growth failure. Hb, Hct, and clinical condition is the only guideline for diagnosis. Hb of less than 13 g% and or Hct of less than 40% is diagnostic of anemia in a neonate.

Perioperative Care in Anemic Neonates –
1. Minimizing losses
   (a) Avoid repeated venous and arterial punctures
   (b) Avoid unnecessary bruising of the skin or hematomas

    (c) Proper stabilization and dressing of indwelling catheters to avoid accidental disconnections or dislodgments.

    (d) Closure of all injection and sampling ports

2. Reducing surgical blood losses,
3. Accurate assessment of blood losses
4. Replacement of losses—Preferably packed red blood cells (PRBC) should be used.
5. Whole blood transfusion is associated with risk of overhydration and early onset of massive blood transfusion problems.
6. Transfusion goal is to maintain high Hct (>45%), or up to 15 mL/kg of PRBC.
7. Rule of thumb—each 1 mL/kg body weight of PRBC transfused, expected rise in Hct is 1%. Hence, to reach the goal of 45% Hct in a newborn with pretransfusion Hb of 10 G% (Hct 30%), will need 15 mL of PRBC/kg. Hence calculate accurately and transfuse appropriately. PRBC has a Hct of 80–90%.
8. Transfuse PRBC Screened for viral pathogens (HIV, hepatitis B, and C, HTLV I/II, and CMV).
9. Extra care in babies who are anemic, congenital heart disease, major surgeries, marked acid-base disturbances, and premature.

10.14.5 Neonatal Homeostasis

Levels of most pro- and anticoagulant proteins are low in the fetus with prolonged PT, TT, APTT. **At birth,** the vitamin K-dependent coagulation factors (II, VII, IX, X) are low (30% of adult values) until 6 months of age. Factors XI and XII are 50% of adult values. Fibrinogen, factor VIII, and von Willebrand factors are normal. There is 30–40% deficiency of physiologic anticoagulants (protein C, protein S, antithrombin) at birth. Fibrinolytics (plasminogen and α2-antiplasmin) are same as in adults. Tissue plasminogen activator (TPa) are low and plasminogen activator inhibitor are increased. Healthy premature neonates over 30 weeks' gestation have slightly lower levels of coagulation factors and longer coagulation tests compared with term neonates. Neonates have a wide "normal" range and the physiological prolongation observed does not indicate a bleeding tendency/need to correct. Low levels of procoagulants are balanced with lower levels of inhibitors and lower activity of the fibrinolytic system.

    Overall, there is no coagulation or bleeding problem in healthy term neonate. But in acutely sick or premature neonates, there is a risk of bleeding diathesis, in the form of pulmonary and intracranial hemorrhages, because of:

    (a) Vit K-dependent factor deficiency is more and prolongation in PT, PTT, and aPTT.

    (b) Thrombocytopenia is more, and.

    (c) Increased capillary fragility and prolonged BT.

High risk and premature newborns must receive 3 doses of vitamin K, as a precaution, especially if these neonates are to undergo surgery.

10.14.6 Anesthetic implications

The aim is to minimize surgical and other blood loss, maintain Hct of 45%, maintain blood volume and CO, by early transfusion. Transfusion trigger is reached early. In neonates with CHD, lower Hct is targeted (35–40%) [45]. Avoidance of hyperventilation, hypothermia, and alkalosis is of paramount significance. Surgical neonates and preterms are at greater risk of bleeding due to low levels of procoagulants and need routine administration of Vit K.

10.15 Neuromuscular System

In the embryonic life, the muscle spindle, NM endplate (NM junction—NMJ), and neural development all complement and facilitate each other, and development occurs as follows:
- 8 weeks—acetylcholine (ACh) receptors appear over the muscle fibers.
- 9–16 weeks—primitive motor-end plates appear.
- 16–24 weeks—transition from polyneuronal to mononeuronal innervation takes place, and
- 24–31 weeks—NMJ matures,
- Growth continues until 1 year postnatal age.

Earlier to 36 weeks of gestation, the fetus is in a state of hypotonia. As maturation progresses, the fetus assumes passive flexor tone which develops in a centripetal direction, i.e., lower limbs earlier than upper limbs, such that, at term the baby is in a flexed posture, while a preterm newborn is in an extended posture. With improving tone, the wrists, hips, and knee joints become more flexible and resistant to extensor stretch.

To assess the maturation of the NM system at birth, Philadelphia Children's Hospital, formulated a method using six evaluations during physical assessment. A score is assigned to each assessment, and all are totalled. Higher score indicates more neurologically maturity. Scores are very low in premature babies. The areas of assessment include **posture** (how does the baby hold his or her arms and legs), **square window** (how far the baby's hands can be flexed toward the wrist. In term baby, the wrists make an acuter angle to the forearm, compared to more flattening in preterm), **arm recoil** (how much the baby's arms "spring back" to a flexed position), and **popliteal angle** (how far the baby's knees extend following gentle extension of the leg and release. Resistance to extension lacks in the preterm newborn, with more obtuse popliteal angle), **scarf sign** (how far the elbows can be moved across the baby's chest), and **heel to ear** (how close the baby's feet can be moved to the ears). By adding the physical assessment and NM scores, one can estimate the gestational age of the baby.

10.15.1 NM Transmission

Two molecules of ACh combine, opening the central pore on the NM end plate, allowing sodium (Na) ions to enter. In the fetus, the pore open time is longer, allowing more Na to enter, thereby generate a larger action potential. This is evident as increased sensitivity to ACh and resistance to d tubocurarine in the newborn baby. There is deficiency of NM transmitters, but increased receptor sensitivity to ACh compensates for this deficiency in the immature nerve endings and facilitates spontaneous fetal movements essential for normal NM development [46, 47].

Fetal receptors are not seen after 31 weeks of gestation, but they may reappear in pathological states with prolonged inactivity (e.g., burns, denervation injury, and prolonged muscle paralysis) at extra junctional sites later in life, with the typical response (hypersensitivity to scoline and resistance to NDMR). Maturation of the myotubules into mature muscle fibers continues for several weeks after birth. Diaphragm and intercostal muscles mature from the initial slow contracting to rapid contracting muscles, with increased force of contraction.

NM transmission is immature at birth. There is less available ACh and increase in sensitivity to NDMR. Maturation of the muscle spindle, NMJ, and NM transmission is slower and delayed in preterm and low birth weight babies.

10.15.2 Features of NM Transmission (NMT) in Neonates

1. Newborns have less NM reserve (less Ach), and muscles are resistant to decamethonium (depolarizing drug), producing nondepolarizing or dual block like features (PTF, improvement after neostigmine).
2. They behave like myasthenics. **Neonatal myasthenia gravis** is a transient disease, due to inherited failure of development of motor-end plates. Clinical implication is that if a baby, after single dose of scoline, does not breathe adequately after a long surgery, reversal with anticholinesterase can improve recovery from dual block.
3. Tetanic stimulation at 50 Hz is poorly tolerated, and following a tetanic stimulation of 15–20 s, there is no fade in twitch height at 1–2 Hz, but significant fade at 20 Hz.
4. In premature newborns, duration of post-tetanic exhaustion (PTE) is longer (15–20 min).
5. Train of four (TOF), degree of PTF (post-tetanic facilitation), and tetanus twitch (TT) ratio improve with age.
6. High CO and faster circulation allow rapid transfer of NM blocking drugs, to and away from the NMJ (faster onset and faster wash out).
7. Larger ECF fraction increases the volume of distribution and dose requirement.
   Clinical Implications—Neonates behave like Myasthenics up to 10 days of life (sensitive NDMR and resistant to DMR) [48–50].

10.15.3 Depolarizing Block and Muscle Relaxants (DMR)

Succinyl choline is the only depolarizing drug approved for clinical use. Newborns are resistant to DMR, arising from the fact that
- They have higher ECF volume and greater volume of distribution,
- Immature NMJ,
- Less Ach stores and less release on stimulation,
- Deficiency of pseudocholinesterase (50% of adult concentration), and
- Persistence of fetal-like NM transmission or desensitization of the motor-end plate.

Features of Depolarizing Block (Scoline) in Neonates
- Rapid onset of action and short duration (6–8 min),
  - Elimination by enzyme hydrolysis (butyrylcholinesterase or pseudocholinesterase),
  - Vagal preponderance and increased risk of bradycardia and arrythmias, especially with second dose. Premedication with atropine (0.1 mg, IV) is advised,
  - No fasciculations or increase in potassium (K) and intragastric pressure (IGP),
  - Rise in intraocular pressure (IOP),
  - They tolerate higher doses (3–4 mg/kg), or 5 mg/kg IM (on body weight basis, calculated dose is higher, but on basis of BSA, the dose is same as in adults),
  - Scoline infusion—Tachyphylaxis occurs before phase 2 block.
  - Phase 2 block is seen with higher dose (4.1 mg/kg) during halothane N2O narcotic anesthesia.

Side effects and disadvantages of DMR are profound bradycardia and arrhythmia, phase 2 block, myoglobinuria, malignant hyperthermia (especially with halothane induction), pulmonary edema, and pulmonary hemorrhage.

10.15.4 Nondepolarizing Block and Drugs (NMB/NDMR)

Increased sensitivity of NMJ to NDMR is due to reduced release of ACh from immature motor nerves. Most studies are using tubocurarine (dTc), but the inferences can be applied to other NDMR keeping each drug's unique properties in mind (authors experience).

10.15.5 Features of NMB in Newborns

- Increased sensitivity to NDMR hence there is need to reduce the dose.
- But because of higher ECF volume and greater volume of distribution—no change in initial loading dose.
- The interval between repeat doses is longer.

- Respiratory depression and NM block both occur at the same time, unlike in adults, where block precedes RESPIRATORY DEPRESSION.
- Mean dTc dose to produce 95% twitch depression, and time to 75% or 50% recovery is same in neonates, children, and adults.
- Reduction in the dose in premature babies, acidosis, hypothermia, concurrent antibiotic therapy, and high concentration of anesthetic drugs in tissues.

NDMR drugs, besides causing muscle relaxation, have other actions that must be kept in mind when evaluating these babies -
  (i) Histamine release (e.g., tubocurarine, atracurium, and some with pancuronium),
 (ii) Vagolytic effect and tachycardia (e.g., with gallamine),
(iii) Risk of bradycardia during intubation in unpremedicated neonates.

Ganglion blocking action and hypotension (d tubocurarine) [50].

Fortified with the knowledge of the effects and side effects of various NM blocking drugs, one can safely use them in neonates, if due precautions are taken regarding the dosages, interval between two doses, avoidance of possible factors which may delay recovery by prolonging their action and having facilities for monitoring and ventilation.

10.15.6 Advantages of Using Muscle Relaxants in Neonates

1. Effective control of ventilation.
2. Relaxed patient for surgical facilitation—a good surgical field.
3. Decreasing the dose of toxic anesthetic agents because in neonates,
4. Availability of a reversal drug.

Vecuronium, Rocuronium, Atracurium, and cisatracurium are safe in all newborns and neonates including premature, low birthweight, and small-for-gestational age babies.

Rate of recovery of NM transmission is slower in neonates compared to in adults.

Elimination rate constant (Kappa) is comparable in infants and children, 0.41/min, 0.38/min respectively, and 0.15–0.17/min in adults.

10.15.7 Antagonism of NM Blocking Drugs

Residual block following NDMR administration should be antagonized by an anticholinesterase. This is especially important in neonates and small infants because of their reduced respiratory reserve. Commonly used anticholinesterases are neostigmine and edrophonium. When administering the reversal drugs, points to be remembered are

- Recovery after edrophonium is significantly faster than after neostigmine.
- Doubling the doses of the antagonists has no significant effect or benefit on recovery.

- Recovery after either antagonist is significantly faster in children than adults.
- Reversal dose in neonates—Atropine 0.03 mg/kg + 0.07 mg/kg neostigmine, or glycopyrrolate 0.01 mg//kg + 0.2 mg/kg pyridostigmine.

10.15.8 Recovery

Adequacy of reversal prior to deciding the extubate are presence of good muscle tone, ability to flex arms legs, ability to sustain tetanus at 50 Hz, and ability to produce inspiratory force of >25 cm H_2O.

Delayed recovery from general anesthesia can be due to several factors, but one most important is **prolongation of NM block.** Premature, LBW, and SGA neonates are more prone to delayed recovery. Causes of delayed recovery from prolongation of NM block are hypothermia, hypotension, acidosis, hypocalcemia, and concurrent use of antibiotics.

10.16 Pharmacology of Drugs in Neonates

Total body water (TBW) in term newborn is almost 75% of body weight and >80% in preterm newborn, with almost 60% in the ECF compartment. Total blood volume is 85 mL/kg and 90–100 mL/kg in a premature newborn. All water-soluble drugs on IV administration get distributed into the ECF volume, the volume of distribution (Vd), and this determines the effective plasma drug concentration.

Fluid requirement increases over the initial days after birth (60, 80, 100,120 mL/kg/day at day 1, 2, 3, and 4, respectively) and then remains at 150 mL/kg/day till throughout the neonatal period.

All drugs undergo metabolism and excretion by the hepatobiliary-renal and respiratory pathways. Hepatorenal function is immature at birth, and respiratory system is still undergoing changes as a part of the adaptation process. Preterm neonates bear greatest brunt of these changes. Complete maturation and normalization of the functions do not occur until the age of 1–2 years. Iso-enzymes P 450 is present at term, but even at 44 weeks, it is still 85% of adult values.

The important **pharmacokinetic variables** in neonates are volume of distribution, renal clearance, and body weight. Vd is important in relation to initial loading doses and clearance determines maintenance dosing and drug infusion rates. These parameters determine the shape of the time-concentration curve and duration of action. Body weight is usually used to calculate drug dosages in all patients including neonates.

10.16.1 Clinical Implications of Altered Pharmacokinetics in the Neonate

(i) Excess ECF volume results in higher Vd of drugs, their dilution, and hence adequacy of effect. **Thus, the initial dose of drugs needs to be higher.**

(ii) Hypoproteinemia, hypoalbuminemia, and low α-1 glycoproteins, from imma- ture hepatic production, lead to reduced drug binding, with increased free drug concentration, risk of adverse drug effects. **Thus, the dose of the drugs needs to be reduced.**

(iii) Most anesthetic drugs are metabolized in the liver. Neonatal hepatic enzyme system, metabolism, and conjugation are immature. **This leads to prolonged effect of drugs.**

(iv) At birth, renal blood flow (RBF) is only 5% of cardiac output (CO) and increases to 20% by 1 month of age. Adult value of 25% is reached by the age of 2 years. Both GFR and tubular reabsorption are immature, leading to slow excretion of drugs, prolonged duration of action, requiring **reduction in drug dosing. In a term newborn, GFR is 35% of mature values (10% at 25 weeks GA), and even at 1 year of age, it is 90% only.** This has implica- tions for drugs chiefly eliminated via renal route, such as aminoglycosides.

(v) Degree of maturation of lung function (alveolar ventilation, FRC, cardiac out- put, and blood/gas solubility) determines absorption and elimination of inhaled anesthetic agents (IAA).

(vi) Hypothermia and hypovolemia compound the hepatic and renal effects, by further affecting drug metabolism and excretion.

(vii) Their BSA to weight ratio is higher than in children and adults. Drugs doses as per body weight may have less than the desired effect.

Taking all above factors into consideration, drugs should be ideally given based on BSA. Commonly drug doses are calculated based on body weight and most often do not require any change in dosing. Special care to be taken is to avoid repeating drugs based on fixed duration or time interval. Continuous monitoring for the waning of the effect and then supplementing will be more prudent, espe- cially for drugs that are repeated during anesthesia, such as muscle relaxants and narcotic analgesics.

10.16.2 Pharmacodynamics

The drug effect on the organs is not merely affected by the absolute dose but also on the gestational age at birth, organ function, and hepato-renal-pulmonary maturation. Effect of anesthetic drugs on the CNS depends on the permeability of BBB and on the brain sensitivity which is a function of its maturation, a function of GA and body weight. Effect on NMJ (neuromuscular junction) and cell membrane is also a func- tion of GA and body weight or size.

Besides, the impact of the surgical condition and critical illness on the already compromised hepato-renal-pulmonary function, thereby on hepatic metabolism, renal clearance, drug effect, and duration of action, in the neonate cannot be ignored.

10.16.3 Inhaled Anesthetic Agents (IAA)

High BMR necessitates high alveolar ventilation, with consequent higher uptake of IAA in neonates as compared to children and adults. High CO also contributes to higher uptake of IAA by the vessel-rich groups, such as brain. They have a greater myocardial depression as compared to adults.

10.16.4 Minimum Alveolar Concentration (MAC)

Minimum alveolar concentration (MAC) or anesthetic vapor potency is low at birth and peaks by 1 month to 6 months age before it decreases to adult values by adolescence. However, MAC of sevoflurane is same in all age groups (3.2%) and is considered safest in neonates and preterms. Safety of IAA may get compromised by the increase in uptake by high alveolar and minute ventilation, as in mechanical or controlled ventilation during surgery, and high CO. This problem was more with the older agents (halothane).

10.16.5 Intravenous Agents (IVA)

Intravenous agents (IVA) are a significant part of modern anesthesia practice in neonates, but requires IV access. This usually does not pose much problem for the anesthetist as most surgical neonates have an already established IV line in situ. There are little data regarding dose-response relationship of drugs in neonates, and whatever knowledge we have is an extrapolation from our experience in adults.

As already stated, neonates have reduced serum proteins, which lead to higher concentration of free (unbound) drug, immature hepatic metabolism, and low renal clearance, that mandate increase in the interval between doses of drugs repeated during anesthesia, e.g., muscle relaxants, and during TIVA.

(a) **Narcotics** are more frequently used in NICU and their pharmacology and side effects are better understood. Morphine, a potent analgesic, is associated with hypotension, prolonged duration of action because of reduced hepatic metabolism and conjugation, and long elimination half-life due to low renal clearance. Morphine went into disfavor with introduction of fentanyl, which is lipophilic, binds to μ receptors with plasma brain equilibration time of 1.5 min, minimum CVS effects, shorter duration of action (terminal elimination—3.1–6.6 h), better safety, and recovery profile. Suppression of stress and reflex responses during laryngoscopy, intubation, and surgery requires higher doses of narcotics. Fentanyl, with its safety profile, suited aptly and with improved outcome too.

(b) **Barbiturates (Thiopentone)** is a time-tested drug used in adults and neonates for more than half century. It is more lipid soluble and gets redistributed into the peripheral lipid stores. Because of higher Vd, induction dose is higher than in adults (4–6 mg/kg). It can be safely used in newborns, neonates, and premature. However, several precautions must be taken when administering thiopentone in neonates, as: a. always use large vein for administration, b. always inject slowly under direct vision because of risk of extravasation, c. in case extravasation occurs, immediately stop and flush with saline, d. use 1.25–2.5% concentration, and e. risk of intra-arterial injection, hence utmost care.

(c) **Propofol** is widely used for induction and tracheal intubation in older children and adults. There is not much literature of its use and safety in neonates, especially newborns and preterm babies, but anesthetist have used it for induction in this very age group. Common unwanted effect reported is hypotension, especially in the critically ill neonate. Its delayed redistribution and clearance lead to prolonged action in neonates as compared to in adults. Chief advantage of propofol is its use as a continuous infusion for sedation, with cessation of action within minutes of stoppage, and no cumulation. Long-term propofol infusion (for hours to days) as in NICU has been associated with metabolic acidosis, organ failure, even death in children and neonates. This warrants careful dosing and duration of infusion in children, and **prohibition of its long-term use in newborns and neonates**. Table 10.20 summarizes the pharmacology of common anesthetic drugs in neonates.

(d) **Neuromuscular blockers (NMB)**—Use of NMB is the mainstay of surgical anesthesia in neonates, to facilitate tracheal intubation and to allow an ideal surgical field. **Neonatal myoneural junction is immature and behaves like myasthenics, i.e., resistant to DMR and sensitive to NDMR.**

Depolarizing NMB (**succinylcholine**) has a rapid onset and short duration of action and provides ideal conditions for laryngoscopy and intubation. It is metabolized by pseudocholinesterase in the plasma. Neonates have 50% concentration of pseudocholinesterase. Being water soluble, scoline has high Vd, and along with the resistance of myoneural junction, higher dose is required for intubation (up to 4 mg/kg), twice as in adults. Despite the large dose, its duration of action is not prolonged because of its rapid clearance. Scoline, like acetylcholine, has parasympathetic effect, and in neonates, with parasympathetic predominance, causes bradycardia. Bradycardia is more severe in combination with halothane induction and can be prevented by pretreatment with anticholinergics (atropine or glycopyrrolate). In modern practice, scoline is reserved for emergency and difficult intubation in neonates.

Non-depolarizing neuromuscular relaxants (NDMR) are more variable in their response in neonates. Being water soluble, they also have a high Vd, decreased hepatic metabolism and renal clearance. Neonatal myoneural junction is more sensitive to NDMR.

Pancuronium has vagolytic property; however, its use was limited by its prolonged duration of action in neonates. **Vecuronium** has no vagolytic property but has shorter duration. **Rocuronium,** also lacking vagolytic action, is the preferred

Table 10.20 Pharmacokinetics/pharmacology of drugs in neonates

	NN Physiology	Effect/Care
General principles	Varied Vd—↑ ECF volume, ↑Vd Hypoalbuminemia - ↓Protein binding Poor peripheral Circulation ↑ free drug Conc Bilirubin displacement by drugs Immature BBB, risk of kernicterus ↓ Hepatic metabolism, oxidation, conjugation ↓Renal clearance - ↓GFR, ↓tubular function	Wide variation in response ↑ dose of H2O soluble drugs (muscle relaxants) Avoid sulfonamides, salicylates Doses as per BSA esp. in first 7 days ↑ Duration of action—narcotics, theophylline, diazepam, phenytoin Delayed recovery from anesthesia
IVA	Thiopentone - ↑sensitivity, safe, dose 4–6 mg/kg (1.25–2.5%) Propofol—safety??? Etomidate—no reports of use Ketamine - ↑O2 consumption & ICP, NDMA receptors absent in neonates—AVOID Diazepam—venous thrombosis, long duration of action—AVOID Midazolam—safe Methohexitone 1% -1.5 mg/kg, fast induction/recovery, muscle movements, pain, respiratory depression Propanidid—anaphylactoid reaction, hypotension, cyanosis, cardiac arrest—AVOID	
IAA	↓MAC at birth—↑ MAC after 1 week ↑ BMR—↑Alveolar ventilation, Rapid Uptake & Washout—rapid induction & recovery Halothane - ↑CBF/ICP, laryngospasm, hypotension, no hepatic failure despite repeated use Methoxyflurane—good analgesia, no renal toxicity, less laryngospasm Enflurane—rapid induction, respiratory irritant and depression, excitatory Isoflurane—Respiratory irritant, involuntary movements (not for induction) **sevoflurane, desflurane safe**	
Opioids	Morphine—↑sensitivity—AVOID in premature Pentazocine −0.5 mg/kg IV—risk of seizures/bronchospasm—AVOID Neurolept analgesia—no role Fentanyl—safe—lipophilic, Sufentanyl, remifentanil—safe Naloxone—keep available, dose 0.01 mg/kg	

drug because of its relative shorter duration of action. **Atracurium** that does not rely on hepatic metabolism or renal excretion is safe in all neonates. **Cis-atracurium** can produce severe hypotension and allergic reactions because of histamine release and should be avoided or used with caution.

However, in combination with IAA and narcotics, their duration of action may remain longer than 60 min in most neonates. Yet, it is beneficial to use NDMR for a good surgical field and also because the effect can be reversed using neostigmine and glycopyrrolate or atropine.

Recovery from anesthesia—The same pharmacological principles that prolong duration of action of anesthetic drugs, also are responsible for delay in recovery after surgery and anesthesia; premature, small for date, and IUGR neonates being more prone, especially for narcotics, theophylline, diazepam, and phenytoin

Other factors contributing to delayed recovery are hypothermia, hypotension, dehydration, shock-like state, acidosis, dyselectrolytemia, hypocalcemia, antibiotics (esp. aminoglycosides), combination of IAA and morphine, poor hepato-renal function, and over dosing.

10.17 Pain Pathways and Development

Pain is a sensation. It is a protective mechanism and is defined **as "An unpleasant sensory and emotional experience associated with actual or potential tissue damage."** Half a century ago, it was believed that neonates, especially newborn and premature babies, did not feel pain, and general anesthesia for surgery in them did not include pain management. Even as late as the 90s, pain management was not always adopted by physicians, but research has proved otherwise, that a baby also feels pain after birth. Prevention of pain is important because of its potential adverse effects on the immature baby and the developing brain [51–56].

10.17.1 Reasons for Poor Pain Management in Neonates

1. Ignorance and belief that neonates do not feel pain!
2. Wrong notion that response to pain is not as much as in adults!!
3. Inadequate knowledge about drugs, their doses, effects, side effects, and safety profile.
4. Difficult to assess pain and its intensity. Crying is the only emotion in these babies whether for Hunger, Cold, Unfamiliar Faces and Surroundings, and PAIN)!
5. Basal heart rate is high (120–160/min). Tachycardia is not a reliable indicator of pain. It can be because of other factors, like effect of the surgical pathology, metabolic, biochemical, acid base and hormonal changes, and effect of anesthesia and drugs administered, anemia, and fluid and blood loss, and underlying congenital diseases.

    Hence neonatal anesthesiologists must have sufficient knowledge of the basic etiopathogenesis of pain if they must prevent long-term adverse effects of pain during surgery. Some knowledge of development of pain pathways is also important as they will be faced with the challenge of anesthesia in the preterm babies too.

10.17.2 Development of Pain Pathways

By late gestation, the fetus has all the anatomic, physiological, and metabolic components for pain perception. Pain receptors are present at 20 weeks and pain pathways by 25th week. Preterm and term infants demonstrate similar or even exaggerated responses to pain. In the fetus and newborn, most fibers are unmyelinated, and nerve transmission is slower than with myelinated fibers. The threshold to stimulation is lower and threshold for sensitization is decreased. Each trauma increases the area of sensitization and is accompanied with structural and chemical changes. The pain pathways are same as in adults:

(i) **Ascending pathway** (Afferent) sends impulses from the peripheral nociceptors in the skin, muscle, and joints via spinothalamic tract in the dorsal root ganglia, to thalamus, hypothalamus, and brainstem.

(ii) **Descending pathway** (Efferent) modulate the response to pain (sympathetic responses and withdrawal).

Density of cutaneous nerve endings is similar or even more than in adults and exposure to prolonged or severe pain may increase neonatal morbidity [56–58].

10.17.3 Anesthetic Implications

1. Even in the intrauterine period, the fetus has the capacity to sense pain and stress and responds accordingly—**fetal distress.** This led to the concept of fetal pain management during fetal surgery [57, 59].
2. **Cutaneous receptors** respond to a stimulus, be it pain, touch or tactile (handling), and temperature.
3. The **effect of pain** may be more profound and more detrimental.
4. Because of the **immaturity of the pathways,** the endogenous response (modulation) to noxious stimulus is erratic.

10.17.4 Pain Assessment in Neonates

Since babies cannot communicate, one must rely on other **indicators** of pain:

1. **Behavioral (specific distress behavior)**—Crying, facial grimaces, rigidity, changes in sleep pattern, and inconsolability.
2. **Physiological**—heart rate, saturation, respiration (rate, pattern), vagal tone, plasma cortisol or catecholamine levels.
3. **Objective indicators or scales—PIPP, CRIES, and NIPS.**
   (a) **Premature Infant Pain Profile (PIPP)**—facial actions—brow bulge, eyes squeezed shut, nasolabial furrow, and physiological indicators—heart rate, and saturation [60, 61].
   (b) **CRIES**—**C**rying, **R**equirement for O2 (for $Sao_2 > 95\%$), **I**ncrease in heart rate and blood pressure, facial **E**xpression and **S**leeplessness [62].
   (c) **Neonatal Infant Pain Scale (NIPS)**—facial expression, cry, breathing pattern, limb movements, and state of arousal [63, 64].

Utility of these scales in a neonate under anesthesia (paralyzed, and with analgesia) is limited. However, CRIES physiological scale may reasonably assess pain in this situation.

Note—A lack of behavioral responses does not indicate a lack of pain.

10.17.5 Clinical Implications During Anesthesia

- All newborns and neonates including premature babies feel pain, like children and adults.
- Surgery is a highly stressful procedure, with major physiological, hormonal, biochemical, and metabolic changes.
- In a developing baby, with added immaturity, pain and stress may affect development and have long-term adverse consequences, unforeseen.
- However, in view of the immaturity of all organ systems, care and precision in type of analgesic used, dosing, and intervals in between repeat doses, must be exercised and tailored to suit each baby depending on the gestational age and pathophysiological status.
- Only essential surgery must be undertaken to avoid adverse effects of drugs.
- Most worrisome adverse effects are on the CNS in the form of memory, and learning deficits.
- Alternative methods of pain management with fewer CNS implications can be used.
- Neonates who have experienced pain during the neonatal period respond differently to subsequent painful events [64, 65].
- Providing analgesia is not only Humane but also decreases morbidity and mortality.
- Not providing pain relief is UNETHICAL and INHUMAN.

10.18 Intestinal Physiology and Feeding

Minimal daily calorie requirement in a neonate is 100 kcal/kg/day. This need is met with by the oral nutrition in the form of breast milk feeds. The capacity of the stomach is small and each feed is of a small volume. Hence, to meet their energy requirement, they need to be fed at more frequent intervals (every 2–4 h in newborns). Larger feeds are associated with the increased risk of regurgitation and aspiration. Formula milk supplementation at very early stage is not advised because of the risk of GI problems (NEC, Sepsis) from hyperosmolarity and bulk, especially in the premature and LBW neonates. Feeding-related problems in the neonate arise from -

1. Weak muscles and poor sucking,
2. Poor swallowing reflex,
3. Early exhaustion,
4. Small gastric capacity,
5. Poorly developed cardiac sphincter and increased risk of regurgitation, and
6. Large hypertonic feeds that increase the risk of necrotizing enterocolitis (NEC)

Parenteral Feeds

Supplemental parenteral feeds must be begun in LBW babies, especially those weighing <1500 g, because these babies have the problems related to feeding, as described above. A suggested method is to start parenteral feeds and continue for first 48 h, followed by addition of enteral feeds @ 60 mL/kg/day, and increased by 10 mL/kg/day to 100–200 mL/kg/day by 10 days, with simultaneous decrease in the quantity or prolonging the in-between interval of parenteral feeds. The goal is that by 10 days the baby should be able to take adequate enteral feeds.

The **intestine physiology** in a neonate is a complex process. It regulates the absorption of essential nutrients for growth and development. Maintenance of normal electrolyte, enzyme, and hormonal homeostasis is essential for adequate intestinal performance. GI diseases, and length and anatomic location of the resected bowel have great physiological impact after intestinal surgery. It can lead to failure of growth and development in the neonate with adverse long-term consequences [66]. When enteral nutrition or intake becomes compromised, parenteral route remains the mainstay of supplying the neonate with nutrition.

10.19   Immune System

The immune system, the network of cells, and proteins that provide defense against infections are immature in the fetus. The hematopoietic progenitor cells are the precursors of the immune system. Early in the embryonic stage, these cells divide rapidly, but with increasing gestational age the speed decreases and specialization increase. Premature newborns have more of the unspecialized progenitor cells than a term newborn. The progenitor cells travel via the blood stream to the three immune organs, liver, spleen, and thymus. By the 13th week, thymus starts producing T cells, though they do not much role in the sterile intrauterine environment. Macrophages appear in the fetal intestines by 12th week and increase rapidly up to 20th week, and B and T cells in the intestine organize into lymph nodes, the Peyer's patches.

Maternal antibodies provide defense from infections in the IU life. IgG can cross the placental barrier unlike Ig M antibodies, and fetus is less prone to infections unless there is a breach in the placental barrier.

1. **Immunity at birth (Innate Immunity)**—At birth, the immune system is still immature, and mature by 3 months of age, making the newborn more vulnerable to infections (ß streptococci, staphylococci, klebsiella, H influenza(b), meningococci, and pneumococci). Neutrophils, the first responders, are limited in quantity and cannot keep pace with overwhelming infections. Their number increases by 2–3 months of age. Newborn baby has three types of immunities:

   (a) **Passive immunity**—is temporary and starts to decrease after the first few months of life, allowing time for baby's immune system to develop.

   (b) **Via the placenta**—IgG antibodies start to cross the placenta by 13th week, but most antibodies cross during the third trimester. Because of this late transfer, premature babies have lower levels of antibodies and are more susceptible to infections than term newborns. At times, these antibodies are directed against the fetal RBC proteins, resulting in anemia and jaundice in the newborn.

   (c) **Via breast milk**—The thick yellowish milk (colostrum) produced in the first few days following birth is particularly rich in antibodies, and breastfed babies have a longer lasting and robust immune system. Breastmilk delivers IgA antibodies (90%), macrophages, and cytokines. IgA antibodies protect intestinal mucosa from gastrointestinal viruses.

2. **Adaptive immunity at birth**

Exposure to any pathogen after birth is a new experience for the newborn and requires specific immune responses. The body responses are slow and B and T cells take longer to develop. Factors that help increase adaptive immunity are skin-to-skin contact (baby is exposed to microorganisms), sleep time (adequate sleep time routine enhances immune development), breastmilk, and vaccination at birth.

10.20 VII. Ophthalmic Effects

Immaturity of the central nervous system also contributes to the development of retinopathy of the premature (ROP). The ophthalmic vessels in the newborn baby have immature musculature and immature vasomotor tone and are extremely sensitive to hyperoxia. They respond to hypoxia and hyperoxia by severe vasospasm, retinal ischemia, and neovascularization at the junction of vascular and avascular zones. This leads to retinal scarring, fibrosis, retinal detachment, ROP, and blindness.

Retinopathy and fibrosis are predominantly seen in premature (<32 weeks gestation) and LBW (<1500 g) newborns. These babies often have low PaO2 and respiratory problems, necessitating O2 therapy with high FiO2, mechanical ventilation, and NICU stay that exposes them to the occurrence of retrolental fibroplasia (RLF) and ROP. Because of the risk of blindness, timely preventive measures must be adopted.

Hyperoxia induces a fall in enzyme superoxide dismutase, which protects against toxic effects of O2 radicals. Tocopherol/vitamin E pretreatment can partially prevent this decrease (Kittens) [67]. O2 induced vasospasm can be prevented by pretreatment with aspirin, which blocks synthesis of prostaglandins, so that retinal damage occurs only where there is inadequate vasomotor tone to protect the immature vessels. Retinal scarring may even occur without exposure to supplemental O2, possibly due to increased blood flow and raised transluminal pressure in the developing retinal vasculature (Beagles) [68].

Anesthesia concerns—During anesthesia management, especially premature, LBW, and with respiratory problems, presenting for surgery under anesthesia, extreme caution must be exerted, like

- Use of minimal FiO2 to maintain target saturation (89–92%),
- Monitoring of preductal SpO2 (ear lobe, upper limb), that reflects retinal perfusion, and postductal SpO2 (lower limb) for effect of PDA, and shunt reversal, and
- Early weaning off O2.

Infants suffering from ROP frequently require anesthetics for ocular examination and potential laser treatment for retinal hemorrhage and RD. While the etiology of

ROP is likely multifactorial, O2 toxicity (perhaps from short-term exposure during brief surgical procedures, and PaO2 >80 mmHg) may be a contributing factor.

10.21   Skin Physiology and Adaptations After Birth

Fetus lies in a bag of fluid, amniotic fluid, throughout the intrauterine period. Whole body is covered with lanugo hairs, denser on face, limbs and trunk, which is shed just before term, at 36–37 weeks of gestation. Babies born before 36 weeks' gestation still have lanugo hair covering.

A term newborn's skin is covered with Vernix Caseosa, formed after shedding of lanugo hair. It is a greasy, grayish white covering of sebaceous secretions, and decomposed epidermis. It is a natural protectant and falls off after birth. Physiological cutaneous change is observed in 100% neonates and number of lesions is more in preterms.

The body surface area-to-weight ratio (BSA:BW) is 5 times as in adults, still higher in preterms, which makes them more prone to heat and water loss, hypothermia, dehydration, electrolyte imbalance, and infections. On exposure to outside dry environment, the skin loses its moisture, becomes dry, is less acidic, nearing neutral pH. It undergoes structural and functional adaptations (moisture retention, acidification) during the first 2 weeks of life until 1 year age.

The skin of a term baby is well developed and thicker and that of a preterm baby is very thin and functionally immature. A post-term newborn skin is thin, wrinkled and has less subcutaneous fat [69, 70].

10.21.1   Functions of the Newborn Skin

Functions of the newborn skin include heat and moisture conservation, protection from light, UV radiations, and trauma, immune barrier and protection from infections, and for tactile sensation essential for baby's growth and bonding.

Premature and VLBW babies are at greater risk of skin damage as their skin is more permeable and deficient in protein and fat. Total epidermal water loss is higher compared to term newborns being 45 $g/m^2/h$ at 26 weeks, 17 $g/m^2/h$ at 29 weeks, and 4-6 $g/m^2/h$ at term.

10.21.2   Physiologic Changes

Newborn skin is subject to cutaneous lesions, more in preterms. **Acrocyanosis** (peripheral cyanosis—palms, soles, around the mouth), no central cyanosis (pink tongue) is present in almost all babies at birth. Some of these are as follows:
1. **Cutis marmorata 5%**—is a bluish mottling over the trunk and extremities. It is a normal response to hypothermia and disappears on rewarming.

2. **Harlequin Color Change**—is deep red coloring on the dependent part of the body while non-dependent part is pale. This is due to poor control vasomotor control and central hypothalamic immaturity, and seen more often in premature babies.
3. **Exfoliation/Physiological scaling 21%**—occurs around the ankles and disappears within a week.
4. **Acne Neonatorum 4.5%**—is benign and self-limiting, seen only in the neonatal period.
5. **Mongolian Spots** (congenital melanocytosis) 56%—are blue–black macular self-resolving lesions over the lumbosacral area, in Asian, black, and Hispanic newborns.
6. **Erythema toxicum Neonatorum 17%**—is blotchy macular rash, over front of the chest, face and limbs, and usually fades away within 1–2 weeks.
7. Sebaceous hyperplasia (6%), Epstein pearl (5%).

10.21.3 Clinical Applications—Care and Precautions During Anesthesia and Clinical Care

Newborn skin being thin and delicate and is prone to various insults and requires care:
1. **Thermal injury/burns**, from being kept in overheated incubators or under radiant heaters or heat blowers or improperly applied cautery plate during surgery,
2. **Dehydration**, from high environmental temperature and increased evaporative water loss from the vasodilated skin,
3. **Chemical burns**, from application of strong cleansing agents and antiseptic solutions. Both alkaline and strongly acidic solutions are harmful. Solutions with neutral pH or mildly acidic should be used.
4. **Injury** from undue pressure, such as tourniquet for placing an IV line, splints, and tight restrainers.
5. **Skin abrasion**—Adhesive tapes are used for securing the vascular lines and thermal probes. At the time of removal of the tapes or of self-adhering ECG electrodes, if care is not taken, skin can easily get abraded.
6. **Ischemic injury** from tight application of a saturation probe on the finger can lead to ischemia of the distal skin.

Precautions—newborn babies should be handled gently with care. Limbs are tiny; circumference is small. When fixing lines with adhesive tape, care must be taken to never cover the entire circumference of the limb or finger. Tape should not cover more than 2/3rds of the circumference. All personnel involved in the care of the neonate should not have long fancy nail. They should remove any sharp finger rings and bangles, because of inadvertent injury to the delicate skin during handling.

10.22 Prematurity

Despite advances in neonatal care, preterm birth remains a leading cause of infant mortality, globally. Due to their LBW and organ immaturity, they may have various problems:

- Their caloric needs are high but due to the lack of sucking and swallowing reflexes, they have difficulty with oral feeding,
- Gastrointestinal immaturity impairs digestion and absorption of carbohydrates and lipids, and increased risk for necrotizing enterocolitis (NEC),
- Pulmonary immaturity makes them prone to apnea, RDS, BPD, HMD, and IRDS.
- Transitional maladaptation at birth exposes them to the risk of persistence of fetal circulation (PFC), PDA, PFO, and elevated PVR.
- Neurological immaturity contributes to the increased risk of CNS insults, which may later manifest as a poor cognitive ability, developmental delays, and other neurological sequelae.
- Visual issues like ROP have to be guarded against,
- They are at increased risk for sudden infant death syndrome (SIDS),
- Metabolic immaturity poor fat insulation, decreased glycogen stores, immature skin with increased water loss, poor vascular control, and lower maximal metabolism, narrows the range of thermal control and makes them prone to hypothermia,
- Immaturity of the immune system places them at high risk for contracting life-threatening infections, and.
- Hepatobiliary immaturity makes biliary atresia more common in them, necessitating surgery, usually by the age of 3–5 months.

Premature newborns need continuous and prolonged specialized care and must be observed for onset of anemia and jaundice and for prompt remedial measures. Round-the-clock, monitoring of blood sugar is essential since hypoglycemia is a potential danger that needs urgent attention.

World Prematurity Day is observed on November 17 each year to increase awareness of preterm birth, its risks and prevention, since 2011. Nearly 10% of all babies born worldwide are born premature (nearly 15 million babies). November is Prematurity Awareness Month. Prematurity is a major contributor to under-five mortality.

References

1. Breschan C, Likar R. Anaesthetic management of surgery in term and preterm infants. Anaesthetist. 2006;55:1087–98.
2. Martin LD. The basic principles of anesthesia for the neonate. Columbian J Anesthesiol. 2017;45(1):54–61.

3. Subramaniam R. Anaesthesia concerns in preterm and term neonates. Indian J Anaesth. 2019;63(9):771–9. https://doi.org/10.4103/ija.IJA_591_19.

4. Lerman J. Neonatal anesthesia; 2016. https://www.springer.com/gp/book/9781441960405. springer.com/referenceworkentry/10.1007/978.

5. Polin R, Abman S. Fetal and neonatal physiology. 4th ed. Expert Consult; 2011.

6. Klein J, Bell F. The Iowa neonatology handbook from the University of Iowa Stead Family Children's Hospital. Online 2018. https://uichildrens.org.

7. Olsson JM. The newborn. Nelson textbook of pediatrics. 21st ed. Philadelphia, PA: Elsevier; 2020; Chap 21.

8. Rozance PJ, Wright CJ. The neonate. Gabbe's obstetrics: normal and problem pregnancies. 8th ed. Philadelphia, PA: Elsevier; 2021; chap 23.

9. Goyal NK. The newborn infant. In: Kliegman RM, St. Geme JW, Blum NJ, Shah SS, Tasker RC, Wilson KM, editors. Nelson textbook of pediatrics. 21st ed. Philadelphia, PA: Elsevier; 2020; chap 113.

10. Gibb CAN, Crosby MA, McDiarmid C, Urban D, et al. Creation of an enhanced recovery after surgery (ERAS) guideline for neonatal intestinal surgery patients: a knowledge synthesis and consensus generation approach and protocol study. BMJ Open. 2018;8(12):e023651. https://doi.org/10.1136/bmjopen-2018-023651.

11. Brindle M, McDiarmid C, Short K, Miller K, et al. Consensus guidelines for perioperative Care in Neonatal Intestinal Surgery: enhanced recovery after surgery (ERAS®) society recommendations. World J Surg. 2020;44(8) https://doi.org/10.1007/s00268-020-05530-1.

12. Subramanian KNS. Extremely low birth weight infant. Chief Editor: Santina A Zanelli; Dec 2020; https://emedicine.medscape.com/article/979717.

13. Ballard JL, Novak KK, Driver M. A simplified score for assessment of fetal maturation of newly born infants. J Pediatr. 1979;95(5):769–74. https://doi.org/10.1016/S0022-3476(79)80734-9.

14. Ballard JL, Khoury JC, Wedig K, et al. New Ballard score, expanded to include extremely premature infants. J Pediatr. 1991;119(3):417–23. https://www.ballardscore.com/Pages/ScoreSheet.aspx. https://doi.org/10.1016/s0022-3476(05)82056-6.

15. Apgar V, Holaday DA, James S, et al. Evaluation of the newborn infant-second report. JAMA. 1958;168(15):1985–8. https://doi.org/10.1001/jama.1958.03000150027007.

16. Fette A. Birth and neonatal care injuries: a special aspect of newborn surgery. Pediat Therapeut. 2012;2:132. https://doi.org/10.4172/2161-0665.1000132.

17. Davis RP, Mychaliska GB. Neonatal pulmonary physiology. Semin Pediatr Surg Nov 2013; 22(4):179–184. doi: https://doi.org/10.1053/j.sempedsurg.2013.10.005.

18. Ahlfeld SK. Respiratory tract disorders. In: Kliegman RM, St. Geme JW, Blum NJ, Shah SS, Tasker RC, Wilson KM, editors. Nelson textbook of pediatrics. 21st ed. Philadelphia, PA: Elsevier; 2020; chap 122.

19. Marcdante KJ, Kliegman RM. Assessment of the mother, fetus, and newborn. Nelson essentials of pediatrics. 8th ed. Elsevier; 2019; chap 58.

20. Keens TG, Bryan AL, Levison H, Ianuzzo DC. Development pattern of muscle fiber types in human ventilatory muscles. J Appl Physiol. 1978;44:909–13.

21. Crowley MA. Neonatal respiratory disorders. In: Martin R, Fanaroff A, Walsh M, editors. Fanaroff and Martin's neonatal-perinatal medicine. 11th ed. Philadelphia, PA: Elsevier Saunders; 2020. p. chap 67.

22. Gregory GA, Steward DJ. Life threatening perioperative apnea in the ex-premie. Anesthesiology. 1983;59:495–8.

23. Segar JL. Pathophysiology of apnea of prematurity. In: Polin RA, Abman SH, Rowitch DH, Benitz WE, Fox WW, editors. Fetal and neonatal physiology. 5th ed. Philadelphia, PA: Elsevier; 2017.

24. Patrinos ME. Neonatal apnea and the foundation of respiratory control. In: Martin R, Fanaroff A, Walsh M, editors. Fanaroff and Martin's neonatal-perinatal medicine. 11th ed. Philadelphia, PA: Elsevier; 2020. p. chap 67.

25. Gregory GA. Respiratory care of the child. Crit Care Med. 1980;8:582–7.

26. Nkadi PO, Merritt TA, Pillers DM. An overview of pulmonary surfactant in the neonate: genetics, metabolism and the role of surfactant in health and disease. Mol Genet Metab. 2009;97(2):95–101. https://doi.org/10.1016/j.ymgme.2009.01.015.

27. Chu J, Clements A, Cotton E, Klaus MH, et al. Neonatal pulmonary ischemia: part 1: clinical and physiological studies. Pediatrics. 1967;40(4):709–82. https://doi.org/10.1542/peds.40.4.709.

28. Huetsch JC, Suresh K, Shimoda LA. Regulation of smooth muscle cell proliferation by NADPH oxidases in pulmonary hypertension. Antioxidants. 2019;8(3):56. https://doi.org/10.3390/antiox8030056.

29. Perkins RM, Anas NG. Pulmonary hypertension in pediatric patients. J Pediatr. 1984;105:511–22.

30. Dwortz AR, et al. Survival of infants with persistent pulmonary without extracorporeal membrane oxygenation. Pediatrics. 1989;84:1–6.

31. Scholz TD, Segar JL. Cardiac metabolism in the fetus and newborn. NeoReviews. 2008;9(3):e109–18. https://doi.org/10.1542/neo.9-3-e109.

32. Tasker RC. Brain vascular and hydrodynamic physiology. Semin Pediatr Surg. 2013;22(4):168–73. https://doi.org/10.1053/j.sempedsurg.2013.10.003.

33. Doherty TM, Hu A, Salik I. Neonatal physiology. Treasure Island (FL): StatPearls Publishing; 2021: Bookshelf ID: NBK539840.

34. Wassner AJ, Modi BP. Endocrine physiology in the newborn. Semin Pediatr Surg. 2013;22(4):205–10. https://doi.org/10.1053/j.sempedsurg.2013.10.010.

35. Feldman PM, Lee MM. Endocrine disorders of the newborn. Obgyn Key. 2016; https://www.obgynkey.com/endocrine-disorders-of-the-newborn.

36. Salle BL, Delvin E, Glorieux F, David L. Human neonatal hypocalcemia. Biol Neonate. 1990;58(1):22–31.

37. Caddell JL. Magnesium in perinatal care and infant health. Magnes Trace Elem. 1991;10(2–4):229–50.

38. Congote LF. Regulation of fetal liver erythropoiesis. J Steroid Biochem. 1977;8(5):423–8. https://doi.org/10.1016/0022-4731(77)90244-8.

39. Giancotti FA, Monti M, Nevi L, et al. Functions and the emerging role of the fetal liver into regenerative medicine. Cell. 2019;8(8):914. https://doi.org/10.3390/cells8080914.

40. Diaz-Miron J, Miller J, Vogel AM. Neonatal hematology. Semin Pediatr Surg. 2013;22(4):199–204. https://doi.org/10.1053/j.sempedsurg.2013.10.009.

41. Balakrishnan M, Tucker R, Stephens BE, Bliss JM. Blood urea nitrogen and serum bicarbonate in extremely low birth weight infants receiving higher protein intake in the first week after birth. J Perinatol. 2011;31:535–9.

42. Sulemanji M, Vakili K. Neonatal renal physiology. Semin Pediatr Surg. 2013;22(4):195–8. https://doi.org/10.1053/j.sempedsurg.2013.10.008.

43. Hunley TE, Kon V, Ichikawa J. Glomerular circulation and function. Philadelphia, PA: Springer Publishing Company; 2009.

44. Esan AJ. Hematological differences in newborn and aging: a review study. Hematol Transfus Int J. 2016;3(3):178–90. https://doi.org/10.15406/htij.2016.03.00067.

45. Widness JA. Transfusion guidelines for preterm and term infants. In IOWA neonatology handbook. https://uichildrens.org/health-library/transfusion-guidelines-preterm

46. Churchill-Davidson HC, Wise RP. Neuromuscular transmission in the newborn infant. Anesthesiology. 1963;24(3) May-June.

47. Glanzman AM, Mazzone E, Main M, Pelliccioni M, et al. The Children's Hospital of Philadelphia infant test of neuromuscular disorders (CHOP INTEND): test development and reliability. Neuromuscul Disord. 2010;20(3):155–61. https://doi.org/10.1016/j.nmd.2009.11.014. Epub 2010 Jan 13.

48. Meakin GH. Neuromuscular blocking drugs in infants and children. Anaesthesia Crit Care Pain. 2007;7(5):143–7. https://doi.org/10.1093/bjaceaccp/mkm032.

49. Cook DR. Muscle relaxants in infants and children. Anesth Analg. 1981;60:335.

50. Bennett EJ, Ignacio A, Patel K, Grundy M, Salem MR. Tubocurarine and the neonate. Br J Anesth. 1976;48:687–9.
51. Perreault T, Fraser-Askin D, Liston R, et al. Pain in the neonate. Paediatr Child Health. 1977;2:201–9.
52. Merskey H, Albe-Fessard DG, Bonica JJ, et al. Pain terms: a list with definitions and notes on usage: recommended by the IASP Subcommittee on taxonomy. Pain. 1979;6:249–52.
53. Prevention and Management of Pain and Stress in the Neonate. Committee on Fetus and Newborn, Committee on Drugs, Section on Anesthesiology, Section on Surgery and Canadian Paediatric Society, Fetus and Newborn Committee. Pediatrics. 2000;105(2):454–61.
54. Anand KJ, Hickey PR. Pain and its effects in the human neonate and fetus. N Engl J Med. 1987;317(21):1321–9. https://doi.org/10.1056/nejm198711193172105.
55. Anand KJ. Clinical importance of pain and stress in preterm neonates. Biol Neonate. 1988;73:1–9.
56. Anand KJ, Carr DB. The neuroanatomy, neurophysiology and neurochemistry of pain, stress, and analgesia in newborns and children. Pediatr Clin N Am. 1989;36:795–822.
57. Fitzgerald M, Millard C, McIntosh N. Cutaneous hypersensitivity following peripheral tissue damage in newborn infants and its reversal with topical anesthesia. Pain. 1989;39:31–6.
58. Fitzgerald M, Beggs S. The neurobiology of pain: developmental aspects. Neuroscientist. 2001;7(3):246–57. https://doi.org/10.1177/107385840100700309.
59. Pacifiers, passive behavior, and pain. Lancet. 1992;339:275–6.
60. Stevens B, Johnston C, Petryshen P, Taddio A. Premature infant pain profile: development and initial validation. Clin J Pain. 1996;12:13–22.
61. Anand KJ, McIntosh N, Lagercrantz H, Pelausa E, et al. Analgesia and sedation in preterm neonates who require ventilatory support: results from the neonatal outcome and prolonged analgesia in neonates trial. Arch Pediatr Adolesc Med. 1999;153:331–8.
62. Krechel SW, Bildner J. CRIES: a new neonatal postoperative pain measurement score: initial testing of validity and reliability. Pediatr Anaesth. 1995;5:53–61.
63. Lawrence J, Alcock D, McGrath P, Kay J, et al. The development of a tool to assess neonatal pain. Neonatal Netw. 1993;12:59–66.
64. Johnston CC, Stevens BJ. Experience in a neonatal intensive care unit affects pain response. Pediatrics. 1996;98:925–30.
65. Grunau RE, Whitfield MF, Petrie J. Children's judgements about pain at age 8–10 years: do extremely low birthweight ($\leq$1000 g) children differ from full birthweight peers? J Child Psychol Psychiatry. 1998;39:587–94.
66. Carlson SJ, Chang MI, Nandivada P, Cowan E. Neonatal intestinal physiology and failure. Semin Pediatr Surg. 2013;22(4):190–4. https://doi.org/10.1053/j.sempedsurg.2013.10.007.
67. Bougle D, Vert P, Reichart E, et al. Retinal superoxide dismutase activity in newborn kitten exposed to normobaric hyperoxia: effect of vitamin E. Pediatr Res. 1982;16:400–2.
68. Flower RW, Blake DA. Retrolental fibroplasia: evidence for the role of the prostaglandin cascade in the pathogenesis of oxygen-induced retinopathy in the newborn beagle. Pediatr Res. 1981;15:1293–302.
69. Fluhr JW, Darlenski R, Lachmann N, Baudouin C, et al. Infant epidermal skin physiology: adaptation after birth. Br J Dermatol. 2012;166(3):483–90. https://doi.org/10.1111/j.1365-2133.2011.10659.x. Epub 2012 Jan 19.
70. Visscher MO, Adam R, Brink S, Odio M. Newborn infant skin: physiology, development, and care. Clin Dermatol. 2015;33:271–80.

The Respiratory System: Development and Physiology in the Neonate

11

Sunil Kumar Sinha

11.1 Introduction

The most common body system invaded and manipulated by the anesthesiologist is the respiratory system. All surgeries are performed under general anesthesia during the neonatal period, and most common technique involves inhalational induction, intubation, and assisted or controlled ventilation. Quite a few babies are already on preoperative respiratory support for alveolar ventilation and oxygenation, which may need to be continued postoperatively.

Ventilation is an important tool in the hands of the anesthesiologist, which when effectively used, can improve the postoperative outcomes. Use of high or low volumes, pressures, and inspired oxygen concentration, can have adverse short- and long-term consequences in these babies. Hence, it becomes imperative for the neonatal anesthesiologist to have a detailed thorough knowledge about the respiratory system, to be able to use it to ones' advantage in the perioperative period, the key to successful anesthetic management and optimum post anesthesia outcomes while avoiding untoward iatrogenic consequences.

This chapter will cover the developmental anatomy and physiology of the respiratory system, lung volumes and capacities, respiratory mechanics, pulmonary compliance and resistance, gas exchange and related problems, breathing patterns, apnea of prematurity and postoperative apnea, respiratory diseases, and clinical implications.

S. K. Sinha (✉)
Department of Anesthesiology, Critical Care, Pain and Palliative Care, Lady Hardinge Medical College, SSk and Kalawati Saran Childrens Hospitals, New Delhi, India

© The Author(s), under exclusive license to Springer Nature Singapore Pte Ltd. 2023
U. Saha (ed.), *Clinical Anesthesia for the Newborn and the Neonate*,
https://doi.org/10.1007/978-981-19-5458-0_11

11.2   Respiratory System

During the intrauterine life, lungs are filled with water and have no function. At birth, the newborn baby undergoes respiratory and cardiovascular adaptations for survival. The maturation of circulatory and respiratory system should be sufficient to withstand these changes which are drastic and occur rapidly within minutes of birth. This requires effective neuronal output and respiratory muscle function to displace the liquid filling the alveoli and airways and breathing in of sufficient air against the surface force so that sufficient alveolar surface for gas exchange is established [1]. Simultaneously, pulmonary blood vessels must dilate rapidly to allow pulmonary blood flow and establish adequate alveolar pulmonary perfusion. The neonatal adaptation of lung mechanics and respiratory control takes several weeks to complete. However, maturation of lungs continues at rapid pace even beyond the first year of life. Respiratory function in infants, especially during the first 6 months of life is both qualitatively and quantitatively different from older children and adults, as is the response to pharmacologic agents and anesthetic drugs.

11.2.1 Anatomical and Physiological Development

The organogenesis is nearly complete after 12 gestational weeks, i.e., end of 1st trimester.

11.2.1.1   Anatomical Development

1. The lungs begin as a bud on the embryonic gut round about 4th week of gestation. Failure of separation of lung bud from gut (later on) gives rise to tracheo-esophageal fistula (TEF) [1].
2. The diaphragm forms during 4th–10th week of gestation dividing abdominal and thoracic cavities:
   (a) If the diaphragm is not completely formed when the midgut reenters the abdomen from the umbilical pouch, the abdominal viscera can enter the thorax leading to congenital diaphragmatic hernia (CDH).
   (b) The presence of abdominal contents within the thorax is associated with arrest of lung growth.
   (c) The lungs of a newborn with CDH are hypoplastic and have decreased number of arterioles. The pulmonary arterioles are abnormally thick, muscular, and highly reactive, resulting in increased pulmonary vascular resistance (PVR).

11.2.1.2   Physiological Development

1. Lung development is not sufficient in a fetus less than 23 week gestation. The alveolar or saccular stage takes place at around 24 weeks, accompanied by thinning of the pulmonary interstitium due to decrease in collagen fiber deposition, increased cellular differentiation, and capillary development, important for gas exchange.

2. Secretion of surfactant, which reduces alveolar wall surface tension and increases alveolar distension and aeration, is often inadequate until last month of gestation (34 weeks):
   (a) Birth before 32 weeks of gestation is associated with respiratory distress syndrome (RDS).
   (b) Glucose metabolism affects lung surfactant maturation, and babies of diabetic mothers are at increased risk of RDS, especially when born premature.
   (c) Antenatal steroid therapy is associated with decreased incidence of RDS and reduced mortality.
3. At birth, the onset of breathing is stimulated by hypoxia, hypercarbia, tactile stimulation, sudden exposure to cold, and decrease in plasma prostaglandin E. After aeration and distention of lungs, PVR decreases, and pulmonary blood flow increases nearly tenfold. Failure of reduction of PVR at birth is associated with extra pulmonary shunting and severe hypoxemia, leading to persistent pulmonary hypertension of newborn (PPHN).

11.2.2 Anatomical Fundamentals of the Neonatal Respiratory Tract and Airways

The neonatal respiratory tract is unique, and its understanding is essential for safe administration of anesthesia:

(a) A neonate's nostril, oropharynx, and trachea are relatively narrow. Breathing can be hindered by irritation of the mucous membrane due to edema building up in this area.
(b) The trachea is short and measures approximately 4 cm from the larynx to the carina. It is also narrow with a diameter of 6 mm.
(c) The tongue is relatively large and tends to fall backwards during sleep and under anesthesia, causing airway obstruction.
(d) Newborns, neonates, infants, and small children have a very soft and short thorax compared to adults. The ribs run horizontally unlike diagonally as is adults. The intercostal muscles are immature and do not have rigidity of adults.
(e) The salivary secretions are more pronounced.
(f) The larynx is more ventrally located, at the level of the 3rd and 4th cervical vertebrae, a whole vertebra higher than that in adults (cervical 4–6).
(g) Until the age of 8–10 years, the narrowest area of the lower airway is the very sensitive mucous membrane at the level of the cricoid cartilage and not glottis, as in adults.
(h) The epiglottis is relatively large, floppy, and U shaped, overhanging the glottis.
(i) Small babies breathe through their nose until they reach an age of 5 months (**obligatory nose breathers**). Inserting a stomach tube through the nose can be a massive respiratory hindrance. Hence, all nasal manipulations should be avoided.

11.2.3 Upper Airway Muscles and Anesthesia

The genioglossus, geniohyoid, and other pharyngeal and laryngeal abductor muscles have phasic inspiratory activity synchronous with diaphragmatic contraction. Their tonic activity maintains the patency of the upper airway [2]. The genioglossus and geniohyoid muscles increase the caliber of the pharynx by displacing the hyoid bone and tongue anteriorly. They are the most important muscles for the maintenance of oro-pharyngeal patency. The tone of all the laryngeal and pharyngeal muscles, including the abductors, is depressed during general anesthesia with resultant upper airway obstruction.

In neonates, under GA and inhalational anesthesia, the work of breathing (an index of the degree of upper airway obstruction) is significantly increased when breathing by mask, without an oral airway in place, even when partial upper airway obstruction is not clinically apparent. An addition of CPAP (5–6 cm of H_2O) opens-up the pharynx and improves airway patency as shown by a significant decrease in the work of breathing.

11.2.4 Controlling the Respiratory Process

Control of breathing in the neonates evolves gradually during the first month of extrauterine life and beyond and is different from that in older children, especially in response to hypoxia. Inspiration is an active process, initiated by contraction of the diaphragm, which creates negative intrathoracic pressure that allows air to be drawn into the lungs. Expiration, on the other hand, is passive, due to the elastic recoil of the lungs and thorax. It may be increased actively by contraction of abdominal and thoracic expiratory muscles during exercise.

The respiratory process in both premature and term newborns, and neonates is controlled by changes in $PaCO_2$, PaO_2, and pH. At birth the breathing regulation and response to hypoxia is not fully developed. The $PaCO_2$ and PaO_2 values of newborns and neonates are lower than those of adults until the end of the first year of life. (Table 11.1)

Table 11.1 Normal range of arterial blood gas values*

	ELBW (<1000 g)	VLBW (<1500 g)	Term infant36.–toddler	Child–adult
Parameters	**<28 weeks of GA**	**28–40 weeks of GA**	**Up to 2 years age**	**2 years**
pH	≥7.25 (≥7.20)	≥7.25 (≥ 7.20)	7.3–7.4	7.35–7.45
$PaCO_2$ (mm of Hg)	45–55 (60)	45–55 (60)	30–40	35–45
PaO_2 (mm of Hg)	45–65	50–70	80–100	80–100
HCO_3 m Eq/L	15–18	18–20	20–22	22–24

ELBW Extremely low birth weight, *GA* Gestational age, *VLBW* Very low birth weight. Values in parenthesis for lung protection strategies.
*Pagtakhan RD, Pasterkamp H, Intensive care for respiratory disorders. In Chernick V, editor: Kendig's disorders of respiratory tract in children, ed 5. Philadelphia: WB Saunders, 1990:205–224 and Durand DJ, Philips P, Boloker J: Blood gases; technical aspects and interpretation. In Goldsmith JP, Karotkin EH, editors: Assisted ventilation of the neonate, ed 4, Phiadelphia: WB Saunders/Elsevier Science, 2003

11.2.5 Response to Hypoxemia

During the first 2–3 weeks of age, both term and preterm neonates, in a warm environment, show a biphasic response to hypoxemia (FiO_2—15%). There is an initial transient (30 s) increase in ventilation followed by sustained ventilatory depression or apnea [3]. If hypothermia or hypoglycemia occurs simultaneously, the initial period of transient hyperpnea is abolished; hypoventilation is the immediate result, indicating the importance of maintaining a neutral thermal environment and prevention of hypoglycemia. By 3 weeks after birth, hypoxemia induces sustained hyperventilation, as it does in older children and adults.

11.2.6 Response to CO_2

Neonates responds to hypercapnia by increasing ventilation but less so than in infants. The slope of CO_2 response curve increases appreciably (response becomes more vigorous) with postnatal age, independent of postconceptual age (PCA) [4].

11.3 Patterns of Breathing in Neonates

The respiratory control mechanism and O_2 receptors are immature and still developing in neonates. Premature babies often experience respiratory arrest (apnea) either at regular (**periodical breathing**) or irregular intervals. Periodical breathing is considered as an episode of 3 or more respiratory pauses of at least 3 s (usually 5 to 10 sec) with normal breathing periods of less than 20 s. Apnea phases can be due to a central cause (no physical breathing exertion) or less often caused by an obstruction (no airflow despite physical breathing exertion). Most commonly, apnea of the prematurity is usually of the mixed type, i.e., central and obstructive. Periodical breathing is seen in all babies during the neonatal age and is not usually dangerous. The clinically relevant forms of apnea are discussed below.

11.3.1 Clinical Importance of Severe Forms of Apnea in Neonates

11.3.1.1 Apnea is defined as cessation of respiration for more than 15 s, or less than 15 s if associated with bradycardia (HR<100/min), cyanosis or pallor [5]

1. **Central apnea**

    The control of breathing and oxygenation even in healthy term newborns is not precise, because respiratory center is immature, more so in preterm neonates. 2–3% of term newborns commonly have prolonged apnea (explained below) lasting 30 s, associated with desaturation, with a central, obstructive, or mixed cause. The risk of having such episode is 20–30 times higher among preterm than term newborns, before 43 week PCA. Central apnea occurs more frequently in the in-hospital neonates due to depression of respiratory center by sedatives and narcotics, and exacerbated by metabolic disturbances such hypoglycemia, hypocalcemia, hypothermia, and sepsis. Central apnea is treated with methyl xanthenes, such as caffeine citrate [especially in premature born (<34 week gestation age)].

Apparent life-threatening events (ALTE) are characterized by an episode of sudden onset apnea, color changes (pallor, cyanosis) tone changes (limpness or rarely stiffness) which require immediate resuscitation for revival and restoration of normal breathing pattern. Treatable pathologic conditions are found in about 30% of neonates, while in others, no cause may be found.

2. **Obstructive apnea**

This occurs due to inconsistent maintenance of a patient airway. It can result from incomplete maturation and poor coordination of upper airway musculature. This form of apnea may respond to changes in head position, insertion of oral/ nasal airway or placing the baby in prone position, occasionally administration of CPAP or high flow oxygen nasal cannula may be beneficial. This therapy is effective in neonates with large tongue, such as with trisomy 21.

3. **Mixed apnea**

This represents a combination of both central and obstructive apnea.

11.3.1.2 Postoperative Apnea

Life threatening apnea is a serious postoperative event in prematurely born babies and may occur up to 60 week PCA. Though it is more frequent following general anesthesia, apnea may occur even after regional or local anesthesia, up to 12–24 h postoperatively. Postoperative hypoxemia, hypothermia, and anemia (Hct <30%) are significant risk factors regardless of gestational or PCA [6]. Both theophylline, and especially caffeine, are effective in reducing apneic spells in preterm neonates.

If it is not possible to delay surgery until the baby is more mature, it is mandatory to use postoperative apnea monitoring in neonates who undergo anesthesia at less than 60 week PCA, for at least 24 h.

11.4   Respiratory Mechanics

11.4.1 Characteristics of Neonatal Lungs and Thorax

The development and growth of lungs and surrounding thorax continue with fast pace during the first year of life. At birth the number of terminal sacs (most of which are saccular) are 20–50 million only, one tenth of fully grown lungs of a child during the first year, and is essentially completed by 18 months of age [7].

11.4.2 Compliance of Lungs

In neonates, static (elastic) recoil of lungs is very low (i.e., compliance normalized for lung volume is unusually high or highly compliant), because elastic fibers do not develop until postnatal period [8]. The elastic fibers in lungs give shape to alveoli and respiratory bronchioles and do not allow them to collapse as it gives outward

Table 11.2 Relationship between age and compliance

	Newborn	Infants	Small child	School aged
Age	1–28 days	Up to 1 year	2–5 years	6–14 years
Weight	2.5–5 kg	5–10 kg	10–20 kg	>20 kg
Compliance mL/mbar	5	10–20	20–40	100

traction to these structures. Since elastance is proportional to elastic fibers present and compliance is inverse of elastance ($C = 1/$elastance) the compliance of neonate lungs is high (also called that elastic recoil pressure of neonatal lungs is very low).

11.4.3 Compliance of Neonatal Thorax (Chest Wall)

The elastic recoil pressure of neonate's thorax (chest wall) is extremely low (highly compliant) because of its compliant cartilaginous ribcage and poorly developed thoracic muscle mass, which does not add rigidity. As neonate's thorax is more compliant than adults' it offers little resistance to over inflation. As the child grows older and the size also continuously grows; in absolute terms the total compliance (i.e., compliance of lung and chest wall) increases, as shown in Table 11.2.

11.4.4 Clinical Implications

The low lung compliance means more pressure or energy is required to provide the normal amount of air volume brought into the neonate lungs with each breath. The neonate chest wall is more compliant as explained above. With significant lung disease, the chest wall may actually be more compliant than the lungs, causing retractions, in which the ribs and sternum distort inward during inspiration instead of expanding the lungs.

Because of high lung and thoracic compliance, both lungs and thorax have a tendency to collapse; in other words, negative intrathoracic pressure is poorly maintained. Therefore, each tidal breath is accompanied by functional airway closure. In addition, adults have high proportion of slow-twitch, high oxidative, fatigue-resistant fibers in their diaphragm and intercostal muscles. Whereas adults have 65% of these fibers in the intercostal muscles and 60% in the diaphragmatic muscles, neonates have only 19–46% of these fibers in their intercostal muscles and 10–25% in the diaphragm. Consequently, neonates are more vulnerable to muscles fatigue and decreased stability of the chest wall. These unique characteristics make neonates more prone to lung collapse, especially under general anesthesia when inspiratory muscles are markedly relaxed.

In neonates, because of the horizontal placement of ribs and consequent inability to increase the transverse diameter of the thorax, the diaphragm does almost all the work expended for breathing. Abdomen hindrances, for example splinting of the diaphragm from raised intra-abdominal pressure, can lead to insufficient spontaneous breathing.

11.5 Surface Activity and Pulmonary Surfactant

The alveolar surfaces in human lungs are lined with surface active material that decreases the surface tension of gas fluid interface in the alveoli and is responsible for the stability of the air spaces in the lungs. This surfactant is secreted by Type II pneumocytes in the alveolar lining. The relationship among pressure (P), surface tension (T), and radius of a sphere, such as soap bubble, is expressed by the Laplace equation as follows:

$$P = 2T / r$$

It can be seen from this equation that if surface tension is constant in a number of connected spheres, the pressure is inversely proportional to the radius of the sphere, smallest sphere has the highest pressure. Thus, the smallest spheres would empty their gas contents into the larger ones, during the emptying phase. If this concept is applied to lung units, the lungs would be unstable, with most units collapsing into several large ones, as seen in the lung of a neonate with RDS, a condition deficient in the amount of surfactant. Surfactant consists of mainly lipids (90%), 10% protein and minimal carbohydrates (0.1%). The lipids lower the surface tension, but proteins allow absorption and dispersion of the lipids in the air liquid interface. They become more concentrated, i.e., greater reduction in alveolar surface tension, when the alveoli are smaller, as during expiration, and become less concentrated during inspiration, when alveoli expand and become larger. Therefore, in normal lungs, the surface tension decreases as the alveolar radius decreases (during exhalation) and vice versa and ratio T/r in above equation remains same, in other words the pressure of the alveoli remains same during exhalation and inhalation. Thus, physiologically the stability of air spaces is maintained regardless of the size of each alveolus or lung unit.

11.6 Pulmonary compliance

Pulmonary compliance can be reduced from various causes in neonates, chiefly, due to parenchymal damage, surfactant disorders or from reduced lung volume. The following are relevant to anesthetist:

1. **Parenchymal damage:** bronchopneumonia, pulmonary edema, RDS, and pulmonary fibrosis.
2. **Functional surfactant disorders**: alveolar pulmonary edema, atelectasis, aspiration, and RDS.
3. **Reduced volume**: pneumothorax, raised diaphragm.

11.7 Pulmonary Volumes

Relative to its size, the volume of a baby's lung is equivalent to that of an adult's. A term newborn has a total lung capacity (TLC) of approximately 160 mL, a functional residual capacity (FRC) of 80 mL and a tidal volume (Vt) of approximately

16 mL. One-third of the Vt is equal to dead space (Vd) volume. The proportion of Vd to Vt remains constant for spontaneously breathing children; it can, however, increase during controlled ventilation. In order to keep total Vd volume to minimum, accessories of anesthetic system should be operated using the smallest possible dead space available, especially when ventilating a neonate with a Vd of only 5 ml.

The following four static volumes and 4 static capacities (values in neonates) can be distinguished:

1. Tidal volume (Vt): is the volume normally expired and inspired. (4–6 mL/kg).
2. **Residual volume (RV)**: is the volume remaining in the lungs after a maximal expiration.
3. **Expiratory reserve volume (ERV)**: is the additional volume which can be exhaled after a normal expiration.
4. **Inspiratory reserve volume (IRV):** is the additional volume which can be inspired after a normal inspiration.
5. **Total lung capacity (TLC):** includes total air volume in the lungs after a maximal inspiration (FRC + IC) (63 mL/kg).
6. **Vital capacity (VC):** is the maximum volume which can be exhaled after a maximal inspiration (ERV + IC) (40 mL/kg).
7. **FRC:** is the volume remaining in the lungs after normal expiration (RV + ERV) (30 mL/kg).
8. **Inspiratory capacity (IC)**: is the maximum volume which can be inspired after maximal expiration (Vt + IRV).

In addition to the above volumes and capacities, closing volume is a very important parameter. Although all respiratory paths (airways) are open in a completely filled lung, decreasing expiatory volume may cause peripheral paths to become blocked, as peripheral paths easily collapse in neonate because of lack of elastic fibers that gives outward traction to peripheral airways and keep it open in older child and adults. The closing volume of neonates and small children is rather large compared to that of adults, and may exceed the FRC during normal ventilation, and impair or encroach normal Vt.

Intubation eliminates physiologically intrinsic PEEP in the larynx. The larynx undergoes some adduction which acts as an expiratory retard normally in neonates due to tonic activity of these mussels during expiration which counteracts peripheral respiratory path blockage. Autogenic PEEP can be compensated for in most anesthetic machines or ventilators using slightly extrinsic PEEP (3–5 mbar).

The alveolar ventilation (ventilation of the alveoli for the purpose of blood gas exchange) of a neonate, 100–150 mL/kg/min, is twice that of an adult. This is achieved mainly through an increase in respiratory rate and not through increase in TV. As pulmonary blood flow is continuous, the O_2 present in the lungs in form of FRC provides oxygenation of the blood during expiratory phase, expiratory pause or apnea. The ratio of alveolar ventilation to FRC is 5:1 for neonates and 1.5:1 for adults (i.e., the 'Buffer' or reserve of FRC of total alveolar ventilation in adults is much larger compared to neonates). As a result, the FRC of a neonate is only a slight or small "buffer" against fluctuations in the volumes and

Table 11.3 Average respiratory rates, tidal volumes and resistance values as per age

	Neonate	Infants	Small children	School age
Age	1–28 days	Up to 1 year	2–5 year	6–14 year
Weight	2.5–5 kg	5–10 kg	10–20 kg	>20 kg
RR/min	40–60	30–60	30–40	12–20
Vt (mL/kg)	7–10	7–10	7–10	7–10
Resistance (mbar/L/s)	40	20–30	20	1–2

concentrations of the inspiratory gases and anesthetic agents so that changes in anesthetic agent concentrations are reflected very quickly in the arterial blood gas values. Any reduction in FRC, e.g., by anesthetics or muscle relaxant, can lead to blockage in the smaller airways, uneven gas distribution, and consequent hypoxemia.

11.8 Airway Size and Resistance to Flow

The actual size of airway from nose to larynx to bronchioles in neonates is much smaller than in children and adults, and therefore, the flow resistance in absolute terms is extremely high. When normalized for body size, however, neonates' airway size is relatively much larger, airway resistance much lower than adults.(Table 11.3) Infants and toddlers, however, are prone to severe obstructions of the upper and lower airways, because their absolute (not relative) airway diameters are much smaller than those in adults; resistance to air flow increases by fourth power of radius with any decrease in airway diameter. Consequently, mild airway inflammation, edema or secretions can lead to far greater degree of airway obstruction in neonates than in adults (e.g., subglottic croup of laryngotracheobronchitis or accumulation of secretions).

Similarly, during surgery and anesthesia, significant fluctuations in respiratory resistance can occur. For example, bronchial dilatory effect of inhalational anesthesia reduces respiratory resistance while even a slight swelling or accumulation of secretion in the respiratory tract or tiniest obstruction in the tube area, can increase total flow resistance greatly.

11.9 Oxygen Requirements

At 7 mL/kg/min the O_2 needs of a neonate are twice as high as that of an adult. At the same time, the level of O_2 consumption depends on the baby's state of health, bodily maturity and stress due to cold, e.g., postoperative hypothermia doubles the O_2 requirement (15–16 mL/kg/min), whereas under general anesthesia it decreases as the body temperature falls. The O_2 consumption according to body weight is shown in Table 11.4.

Neonates are significantly more susceptible to hypoxia than adults because of higher O_2 consumption (twice that of adult), higher alveolar ventilation (twice that of adults), and in addition, less surface area for gas exchange (as alveoli are still developing and far less in number) and small FRC. The ventilatory requirement per

Table 11.4 Interdependency of O_2 consumption and FRC to body weight

Body weight kg	O_2 consumption	FRC
5	9 mL/kg × min	10 mL/kg
10	7 mL/kg × min	15 mL/kg
20	6 mL/kg × min	30 mL/kg
Adults	3.5 mL/kg × min	

unit of lung volume in neonate is markedly increased. The FRC is reduced even more after anesthetics have been administered (60% reduction of FRC in neonates vs. 30% reduction in adults after anesthesia from awake level). The small O_2 reserve available to a newborn or small child is quickly used up during hypoventilation or apnea of short duration, and therefore, they desaturate rapidly; hypoxia can occur within 10–20 s of apnea. For comparison, a healthy adult has apnea tolerance of 2–3 min.

Premature and low birth weight newborns (<1500 gm) do not react to hypoxia, such as an adult, with tachycardia, but rather with a reduced heart rate (bradycardia). This state is not remedied by administering medication such as atropine but responds only to increasing the O_2 supply.

The use of pulse oximetry routinely has improved ability to monitor and properly maintain oxygenation during the care of the neonate in the NICU or the OT. This is especially true in premature neonates who are susceptible to O_2 toxicity and retinopathy (ROP). The risk of retinopathy increases with the degree of immaturity, the duration of O_2 application, and the height of partial pressure. Babies in acute danger of developing ROP are premature babies born before the 44th week of pregnancy and exposed to:

(a) PaO_2 of more than 80 mmHg for more than 3 h or
(b) PaO_2 of more than 150 mm of Hg for more than 2 h

The risk of damaging the retina by excessive partial pressure of O_2 depends on the postnatal age and is practically nonexistent when premature neonate reaches the infant stage.

In neonate, whose P50 is 18–20 mmHg, the range of SaO_2 to maintain adequate PaO_2 (60–80 mmHg) is 97–98%. At PaO_2 value more than 80 mm of Hg the manifestation of ROP increases as saturation drops, PaO_2 also decreases significantly, at 1-day age, SaO_2 of 91% corresponds to PaO_2 of 41 mmHg, and at 2-week age it is 50 mmHg, which is dangerously low. Hence, FiO_2 should be such that it maintains SaO_2 at 97–98% (PaO_2 targeted at 70 mmHg) [1]. Table 11.5 shows the relationship between O_2 saturation values and corresponding PaO_2 values. (Note - as the baby desaturates, rate of decrease in PaO_2 is significant, reaching hypoxic levels).

Under anesthesia hyperventilation induced respiratory alkalosis, shifts the oxygen dissociation curve (ODC) curve to further left with further decrease in P50 value. This is hazardous in neonate whose P50 is unusually low even without respiratory alkalosis. Hence, maintenance of normal $PaCO_2$ by monitoring $EtCO_2$ under anesthesia is prudent.

Table 11.5 Relationship between P_{50}, SaO_2 and corresponding PaO_2

	1 day	2 weeks	6–9 weeks	Adult
P50 (mm of Hg)	19	22	24	27
SaO₂ (%)	**Estimated PaO₂ mm of Hg**			
99%	108	130	143	156
98%	77	92	101	111
97%	64	77	84	92
96%	56	68	74	82
95%	52	62	68	74
92%	43	52	57	62
91%	41	50	55	60

11.10 Functional Residual Capacity (FRC) and Anesthesia

The main mechanism that maintains FRC is the tonic contraction of both diaphragm and intercostal muscles throughout respiratory cycle (inspiration + expiration) in awake neonates. This mechanism effectively stiffens the chest wall. This intrinsic tone of inspiratory muscles maintains the outward recoil and rigidity of thorax and maintains a higher end expiratory lung volume. Anesthesia and paralysis would abolish this muscle tone reducing thoracic compliance (outward movement of thorax is reduced), while elastic recoil of lungs is not altered. This change alters the balance between elastic recoil of lungs and thorax in opposite direction and consequently diminished FRC. The compliance of the lungs decreases shortly thereafter with resultant airway closure (in matter of few minutes) from reduced FRC. The average decrease in FRC is 46–70% under anesthesia (while in adults this varies 9–25%).

The compliance of respiratory system as a whole (Crs, or total compliance) under general anesthesia decreases to about 35% (a value comparable with adult). The reduction in Crs occurs both during spontaneous and manual ventilation with low Tv and after muscle relaxant administration. When Vt is doubled, however, Crs returns to preanesthetic control levels. Hence, higher Tv is maintained under anesthesia depending on SaO_2, and $PacO_2$ values. It is explained more later.

11.11 Mechanical Modes of Ventilation

All known ventilation modes used in pediatric anesthesia come from adult anesthesia. These modes include the conventional modes of anesthesia, volume control mode (VCM), synchronized intermittent mandatory ventilation (SIMV), and pressure controlled ventilation (PCV).

11.11.1 Volume Control Mode (VCM)

VCM is a time cycled volume-controlled ventilation mode. The ventilator delivers a preset volume at a constant inspiratory flow rate. Time and frequency are set or given. The patient does not breathe on his/her own. The pressure which develops inside the breathing system and the lungs is derived from both set parameters, and pulmonary resistance and compliance. Pressure monitoring is of great importance in order to avoid high peaks of pressure. The anesthetist must set a maximum pressure limit, Pmax, which cannot be exceeded. IPPV is primarily used on those babies with healthy lungs and ensures that the patient constantly receives a defined minute volume.

11.11.2 Synchronized Intermittent Mandatory Ventilation (SIMV)

SIMV is a mixture of both spontaneous and controlled ventilation, in which the inspiratory strokes of the respirator are synchronized with those of the patient. The patient is able to breathe spontaneously at regular, predetermined intervals. Mandatory ventilatory strokes ensure the minimum ventilation within these intervals. Mechanical respiratory strokes triggered by the patient means they take place within a time frame anticipated by the patient and his or her inspiratory efforts, not during the unsynchronized delivery of respiratory strokes. SIMV is a useful mode in pediatric anesthesia, for instance, during the recovery phase.

11.11.3 Pressure Controlled Ventilation (PCV)

PCV is ideal for general use in pediatrics anesthesia. The lungs of children are susceptible to over inflation during anesthesia. Reasons for this are insufficient flexibility of the alveoli, shallow breaths and highly compliant thorax.

Having set maximum pressure, which makes it possible to limit the pressure at which the gases are delivered into the respiratory tract, minimizes the risk of barotrauma and helps avoid high pressure peaks. Barotrauma can also occur during VCM secondary to very high inspiratory flows, secretions, mucus deposits, or bronchospasm. In these situations of blockade of airways, where resistance becomes too high, in VCM, the ventilator increases the peak flow to reach a set TV.

The major advantage of PCV over VCM is in being able to use uncuffed endotracheal tubes (ETT) in neonates, which allows large amounts of leakage (>20% of minute volume). By increasing the flow to maintain the set pressure, loss caused by leakage is automatically compensated to a certain degree. However, not only is ETT leakage counteracted, leakages caused by lungs (e.g., lung fistulas) are also counteracted. In IPPV mode the leakages will initiate low pressure alarm and prevent the Tv to be achieved.

In addition, gas distribution disorders within the lungs can be better compensated for in PCV than in VCM. For example, if the lungs are nonhomogeneous, conventional volume-controlled ventilation, overinflates the healthy lung areas and under inflates the obstructed lung areas. This results in temporary pressure differences and different volume throughout the lungs, which are exposed to great mechanical loads. PCV ensures that the lungs fill more evenly and that the healthy lung is not damaged by excess pressure.

Table 11.6 Initial respirator settings in Volume and Pressure Control Modes

Initial respirator settings in VCM

	Neonates (5 kg)	Small children
Respiratory rate	20–30/min	15–20/min
I:E Ratio	1:2	1:2
Inspiratory pressure limit	<20 mbar	<20 mbar
PEEP	3 mbar	3–5 mbar
FiO$_2$	0.5	0.5
Tidal volume	10–15 mL/kg	10–15 mL/kg
Initial Respirator Setting in PCV		

	Premature (2 kg)	**Neonate (5 kg)**	**Small children**
Pressure Limit (mbar)	16–18	25	25
RR/min	30–60	20–30	15–25
I:E	1:2	1:2	1:2
PEEP (mbar)	2	2	2
Inspiratory flow (L/min)	4–6	4–8	4–12

11.11.4 Clinical Implications

The initial ventilation parameters are shown in Table 11.6 for both VCM and PCV modes.

(a) **Tidal Volume**

The anesthesiologist often controls a neonate or pediatric ventilation manually or mechanically during general anesthesia, because most anesthetics techniques cause spontaneous ventilation to decrease or cease. This is because most anesthetics are potent respiratory depressants, and because the ETT and anesthesia circuits add elastic and resistive loads to breathing. Because anesthesia causes a decrease in FRC, the uneven distribution of ventilation and an increase in physiological Vd, the Tv must be increased. The mechanical Vd and internal compliance of anesthetic equipment must also be taken into account for proper estimation of ventilatory requirement. Physiological Vd is further increased in patients with preexisting lung dysfunction. Therefore, it is practical to start with Tv of 10-/kg body or roughly 1.5–2 that is required in awake individual. In awake individuals Vt of 4–6 ml/kg for premature neonates and 6–8 mL/kg for term neonates, are taken as normal.

In VCM, tidal volume can be set directly, while in PCM, the desired tidal volume is influenced by patient's respiratory characteristics (compliance) and by pressure settings of the ventilator. Tidal volumes settings are monitored by the resulting EtCO$_2$ and capillary CO$_2$ values.

(b) Respiratory Rate

Neonates are ventilated with a frequency of 30–60/min.

(c) The I:E Ratio

It should be between 1:1 and 1:2 for uncomplicated cases during mechanical ventilation. If O$_2$ exchange disorders are present (e.g., RDS), neonates can be ventilated such as adults using an inverted I:E ratio and low inspiratory flow (inverse ratio ventilation). In this case, a change in the I:E ratio affects the mean airway pressure and, in conjunction with FiO_2, oxygenation. A short inspiratory phase with high peak pressure of up to 35 mbar are less likely to cause barotrauma than long inspiratory phases (>0.6 s).

(d) PEEP

Physiologically, premature neonates and newborns build up a physiological PEEP in the larynx area during expiration which is eliminated by intubation. By setting the PEEP the risk of bronchial and alveolar collapse, which is easily triggered by high closing volume of neonate, is reduced. PEEP helps keeping the alveoli open throughout the respiratory phase and also increases the FRC. Ventilating the neonate with a PEEP of 5 mbar increases the FRC of intubated or anesthetized neonate by 28%.

Depending on the patient's oxygenation level, PEEP pressure is set to 4–8 mbar. Higher levels are not well-tolerated by neonates. Changing the setting should take place in increments of 1–2 mbar. One side effect of PEEP is the disruption of cardiac and circulatory systems, e.g., a decrease in cardiac output due to a lessening in venous return flows and cardiac compression.

(e) Peak Pressure

Peak pressure affects alveolar ventilation via $PaCO_2$ during artificial respiration and depends on resistance, compliance, inspiratory flow and tidal volume. Pressure limiting is of utmost importance in VCM to reduce the risk of alveolar overinflation. Peak pressure should not be set higher than 20–25 mbar. Peak pressure of >35 mbar should be avoided altogether, since the risk of brain hemorrhage increases. Peak pressure between 6 and 8 mbar are usually sufficient for ventilating premature and low birth weight neonates (<1000 g). Changes is the setting should be made in increments of 2 mbar.

(f) Inspiratory Flow

While the inspiratory flow is regulated directly in PCV modes, it can only be indirectly regulated in VCM through I:E ratio, Tip (inspiratory plateau time), inspiratory time and the respiratory rate. If, during PCV mode the inspiratory flow chosen is too low, the desired volume cannot be delivered in the preset time and ventilation will be insufficient. The steepness of the rise in pressure increases in VCM as the inspiratory flow increases, and peak pressure increases simultaneously. In order to protect the airway, alarm is triggered whenever the respiratory pressure reaches the set upper limit. Standard flow rates are 6–10 L/min for neonates. Much of this is not delivered to the to the baby, rather is used to drive the ventilator. Babies on PIP more than 20 cm H_2O and respiratory rates more than 60/min, may require higher flow rates (12–16 L/min) so as to achieve the peak pressure and deliver a larger tidal volume.

(g) Inspiratory O_2 (FiO_2) on ventilator

The following dictum supports the theory about maintaining he FiO_2 in neonates:

Keep it as low as possible, but as high as necessary.

The FiO_2 should be set so that PaO_2 value is less than <70 mmHg (higher PaO_2 promotes ROP).

(h) $EtCO_2$ or $PaCO_2$ monitoring

Once the mechanical ventilation is established, RR and Tv can be decreased and refined with the aid of capnography. The changes in $PaCO_2$ reflect alveolar ventilation, thus $EtCO_2$, PCO_2 or capillary $paCO_2$ is useful for adjusting and monitoring alveolar ventilation and it is targeted at 30–40 mmHg. In patients with lung disease, time constant duration (inspiratory time and inspiratory pause), should be increased to allow sufficient time for passive lung gas diffusion. The addition of low level of PEEP (5–7 cm H_2O) restores the volume (FRC) lost from relaxation of inspiratory muscles and helps prevent end expiratory airway closure.

The various parameters that need to be considered for improving oxygenation (PaO_2) and ventilation ($PaCO_2$) are shown in Box 11.1

Box 11.1 Parameters That May Need a Change to Improve Oxygenation (PaO_2) and Ventilation ($PaCO_2$)

1. Improving oxygenation ($\uparrow PaO_2$) by
    (a) Increasing the Inspiratory O_2 concentration (FiO_2)
    (b) Increasing Mean Airway Pressure by
        – Increasing PEEP in PCV/VCV modes
        – Lengthening the Inspiratory phase in PCV/VCV modes
        – Increasing plateau pressure in PCV mode
        – Increasing Inspiratory flow in IPPV mode
2. Improving ventilation ($\downarrow PaCO_2$) by
    (a) Increasing Minute Volume (MV) by
    (b) Increasing frequency
    (c) Increasing tidal volume
    (d) Optimizing form of ventilation
    • Adequate I:E ratio
    • Adequate Inspiratory flow

11.12 Considerations in Neonatal Respiratory Diseases

11.12.1 Clinical Presentation

Signs of respiratory distress are tachypnea, grunting, nasal flaring, intercostal and subcostal retractions, rales, rhonchi, asymmetry respiratory sounds on auscultation, and apnea. Pulse oximetry (SpO_2) is a useful noninvasive tool to screen systemic oxygenation in neonates. Blood gas tension (PaO_2 and $PaCO_2$), the invasive monitoring tool, is essential for suspected pulmonary and cardiopulmonary abnormalities.

Various disease states that present similarly as parenchymal diseases should be considered when evaluating neonates with respiratory distress:

1. **Airway obstruction**: choanal atresia, vocal cord palsy, laryngomalacia, laryngeal stenosis, compression of trachea by external masses, such as cystic hygroma, hemangioma, and vascular rings.
2. **Developmental Anomalies**: TEF, CDH, congenital lobar emphysema, pulmonary sequestration, bronchial cysts, congenital pulmonary airway malformations.
3. **Non pulmonary diseases:** cyanotic heart disease, persistent pulmonary hypertension of neonate, congestive heart failure, metabolic disturbances.

11.12.2 Laboratory Studies

For a neonate in respiratory distress, laboratory studies should include arterial blood gas, pre and post ductal O_2 saturation by SpO_2, hemoglobin, 12 lead ECG, and chest X ray.

If these results are abnormal, potential cardiac disease should be re-evaluated by ABG, while neonate breathes 100% O_2 (**Hyperoxia test**). This is used in cyanotic babies to rule out cardiac cause.

11.12.3 Hyperoxia Test Methodology

1. Pre-oxygenation PaO_2. Baby allowed to breathe 100% O_2 for 10 min in a hood or via ETT. Repeat PaO_2 (right radial artery). There should be an increase in PaO_2 of 30 mmHg or more from the pretest value. If not, then most probable cause of cyanosis is cardiac (intracardiac shunt of >30%).
2. In terms of absolute PaO_2 values after breathing 100% O_2 for 10 min:
   (a) If PaO_2 is >150 mmHg, cyanosis is of pulmonary etiology, and if less than 150 mmHg, cyanosis is of cardiac origin.
   (b) PaO_2 of 50–150 mmHg is seen in cardiac disease without restriction of pulmonary blood flow (single ventricle with PDA, Truncus arteriosus), and
   (c) PaO_2 less than 50 mmHg—indicative of cardiac disease with restricted pulmonary blood flow (TOF Tetralogy of Fallot's, TA Tricuspid Atresia, TGA Transposition of great arteries).

However, echocardiography and cardiac consultation will be needed for further evaluation and management.

11.13 Respiratory Distress Syndrome (RDS)

11.13.1 Pathophysiology

RDS results from physiologic surfactant deficiency. Surfactant is essential for normal alveolar development in the intrauterine life, and expansion after birth. Surfactant deficiency causes decrease in lung compliance, alveolar instability, progressive atelectasis, intrapulmonary shunting and hypoxemia.

Premature babies have increased incidence of RDS and can be identified prenatally by amniocentesis and measuring lecithin to sphingomyelin ratio (>2), and saturated phosphatidyl choline levels (>500 μg).

Causes of RDS in a neonate, beside surfactant deficiency, include Bronchopulmonary dysplasia (BPD), and Hyaline membrane disease (HMD), and Meconium Aspiration Syndrome (MAS). *(These are discussed in the chapter on transitional changes in the newborn).* However, presentation, diagnosis and management is similar in all four conditions.

Antennal Glucocorticoid (betamethasone) treatment (once a day for 2 days to the mother), at least 48 h prior to premature delivery, decreases the incidence and severity of RDS in the newborn baby.

Clinically tachypnea, nasal flaring grunting and retraction is seen. Cyanosis appears soon after birth. Because of large intrapulmonary shunt due to atelectatic lung units, newborn remains hypoxic despite high FiO_2.

11.13.2 Initial Treatment

Symptomatic newborns should be kept in a warm humidified hood. O_2 can be provided in the hood or via nasal catheter:

- FiO_2 should be adjusted to maintain PaO_2 of 50–80 mmHg ($SaO_2 = 88$–92%).
- If FiO_2 >60% is required, nasal CPAP or even intubation may be indicated.
- Endotracheally given exogenous surfactant decreases morbidity and mortality.
- High frequency oscillation ventilation (HFOV) is helpful in decreasing air leaks and chronic lung disease.

11.14 Pneumothorax

Pneumothorax is a very serious condition which if undiagnosed can be fatal.

11.14.1 Causes of Pneumothorax

(i) **Iatrogenic Pneumothorax** can occur in neonates requiring positive pressure ventilation in ICU or intraoperatively during anesthesia.

(ii) **Spontaneous pneumothorax** can occur in 1–2% of otherwise healthy term neonates who often remain asymptomatic or mildly symptomatic and require no intervention.

11.14.2 Clinical Features

The diagnosis should be considered in any neonate with acute deterioration in clinical condition, such as sudden cyanosis and hypotension. Occasionally asymmetric chest movements and asymmetric breath sounds may be appreciated. However, endobronchial intubation should be ruled out.

11.14.3 Laboratory Studies

Transillumination of the thorax with strong light usually will show hyperlucent hemithorax. If the patient is stable, chest X ray can be done to confirm the diagnosis, but those in distress and are hemodynamically unstable, need immediate intervention.

11.14.4 Treatment

Immediate aspiration of the air with an IV catheter must be performed. Puncture is done in the 2nd intercostal space of the affected side, remembering that the neonates' chest wall is very thin, and the depth of insertion is not more than 0.5–1 cm (to avoid injury to the lung and heart). A three-way stopcock should be attached to the needle. At no time should the need be left open to the air. Once confirmed (by air gushing out, and improvement in the clinical condition), a chest tube drain will need to be inserted under LA at the same site, with a continuous draining tube and underwater seal attached, under all aseptic precautions, at the bed side, as re-accumulation is a potential occurrence, until the air leak gets sealed off.

11.15 Conclusion

This chapter covers the developmental anatomy and physiology of the lung, normal parameters, gas exchange, importance of FiO_2, ventilatory patterns and problems of ventilation in the newborn and the neonate, various ventilatory modes commonly used, and ventilatory parameters, and concerns regarding neonates with respiratory diseases and surfactant deficiency. Fortified with this knowledge, the anesthesiologist will be able to better understand and manage neonates during and after surgical procedure, according to the probable lung pathology or disease. Importance of keeping FiO_2, airway pressures and volumes, to the minimal, but enough to maintain parameters within normal range, should be the prime concern. Maintenance of PaO_2 and $PaCO_2$ are the two main goals of ventilation and these can be easily monitored noninvasively using pulse oximetry and capnography, without the need of repeated arterial punctures, which are reserved for those with major cardiac defects and major shunt fractions. Apnea of prematurity is a real threat and must be anticipated and prevented in the immediate postoperative period, though the risk may persist up to 12–24 h. Pneumothorax is a potential cause of sudden deterioration in the clinical condition and must always be kept in mind as timely air aspiration may save the baby.

References

1. Motoyama EK, Finder JD. Chapter 3, Respiratory physiology in infants and children. Davies PJ, Cladis FP, Motoyama EK (eds): Smith's anesthesia for infants and children. 8th edition. Mosby Elsevier Inc, Philadelphia, USA. 2011;22–79.
2. Brouillette RT, Thatch BT: A neuromuscular mechanism maintaining extra-thoracic airway patency. J. Appl Physiol 1979;46:772.
3. Rigatto H, BradyJP, de La Torre Verduzco R: Chemoreceptor reflexes in preterm infants. I. The effect of gesttional and post natal age on ventilatory responses to inhalationof 100% and 15% oxygen. Pediatrics. 1975(b);55:604.
4. Frantz ID III, Adler SM, Thach BT, Taeusch HW Jr: Maturational effects of respiratory responses to carbon dioxide in premature infants. J Appl Physiol. 1976;41:634.
5. Brooks JG: Apnea of infancy and sudden infant death syndrome. Am J Dis Child. 1982;13b: 1012.
6. Cote CJ, Zaslavsky A, Downes JJ et al: Post operativeapnea in former preterm infants after inguinal herniorrhaphy. A combined analysis. Anesthesiology. 1995;82:809–22.
7. Langston C, Kida K, Reed M, Thurlbeck WM: Human lung growth in late gestation and in the neonate. Am Rev Respir Dis. 1984;129:607.
8. Fagan DG: Shape changes in static V-P loop for children's lung related to growth. Thorax. 1977;32:193.

Further Reading

1. Neumann R, et al: Chapter 7 - Developmental physiology of respiratory system; In Andropoulos DB, Gregory GA, editors: Gregory's Pediatric anesthesia, 6th edition, Wiley Blackwell, Hoboken, New Jersey. 2020;120–40.
2. Morton NS, et al: Chapter 23 - Anesthesia for the full term and expremature infant: In In Andropoulos DB, Gregory GA, editors: Gregory's Pediatric anesthesia, 6th edition, Wiley Blackwell, Hoboken, New Jersy. 2020;524–47.
3. Walsh BK, Crezee KL: Chapter 17 - Invasive mechanical ventilation of the neonate and pediatric patient: In editors Walsh BK: Neonatal and pediatric respiratory care: 4th edition, Saunders Elsevier Inc, St Louis, Missouri. 1995;300–41.
4. Gregory AG, Brett C. Chapter 17 - Neonatology for Anesthesiologists: In editors Davis PJ, Cladis FP, Motoyama EK,: Smith's anesthesia for infants and children, 8th edition. Elsevier Mosby, Philadelphia USA. 2011;512–53.
5. Robert D, Courtney SE. Chapter 17 - Non invasive respiratory support: In editors Goldsmith JP, Karotkin EH, Keszler M, Suresh GK: Assisted ventilation of the neonate. An evidence-based approach to newborn respiratory care, 6th edition, Elsevier, Inc., Philedelphia, PA, USA. 2017;162–79.

The Neonatal Airway

12

Rashmi Ramachandran, Bhavana Kayarat, and Vimi Rewari

12.1 Introduction

Neonates and their anaesthetic problems are not just equivalent to smaller adults, and definitely not smaller children. This statement is most prominently visible in neonatal airway. The difference in the airway between the neonates and adults/older children encompasses the anatomical, physiological as well as pharmacological aspects of airway management. Effective and safe airway management of neonates requires understanding how these differences can possibly alter and affect the neonatal airway management. A detailed knowledge of the neonatal airway anatomy and a thorough understanding of the respiratory physiology is important to understand their associated clinical implications. The knowledge about the various equipment and procedures used for neonatal airway management related to the anatomy and physiology of the neonate is the key to successful and uneventful airway management in neonates. Prematurity and its potential sequalae come with its own set of problems related to airway management. Wherever needed, the problems of prematurity have been emphasised in the relevant segments. This chapter has following sections under which neonatal airway will be discussed:

1. **Anatomical and physiological aspects**
2. **Airway assessment**
3. **Neonatal airway management: procedures and equipment**
4. **The difficult airway**
5. **Anaesthetic considerations and management in difficult airways**

R. Ramachandran (✉) · B. Kayarat · V. Rewari
Department of Anaesthesiology, Pain Medicine and Critical Care, AIIMS, New Delhi, India

© The Author(s), under exclusive license to Springer Nature Singapore Pte Ltd. 2023
U. Saha (ed.), *Clinical Anesthesia for the Newborn and the Neonate*,
https://doi.org/10.1007/978-981-19-5458-0_12

12.2   Anatomical and Physiological Considerations

12.2.1 Anatomical Considerations

Anatomically, the neonatal airway will include nose, nasal passages, mouth, oral cavity, pharynx, larynx and finally the glottis, subglottis, and the trachea. Apart from this, the nonairway part of the neonate, i.e., the head, neck, cheeks, and the face may cause problems in airway management.

(a) **The head and neck**: the brain of the foetus grows disproportionately rapidly in-utero and causes a relatively larger head than the body. Proportion of the head compared to the rest of the body is 19% in a neonate compared to 9% in an adult [1]. Also, the neuro-cranium (cranial vault) is larger than the viscero-cranium (face). This makes the skull shape elongated with a prominent occiput. In supine position, the relatively long and prominent occiput causes the head to flex over the neck, an extremely unfavourable position of the airway axis, causing the airway to obstruct easily (Fig. 12.1). Keeping a small roll under the shoulders, with the head in a neutral or minimally extended position, achieves the nearly sniffing position, guaranteeing airway patency. Failure to ensure this leads to a situation of difficult airway, i.e., difficult mask ventilation and poor direct laryngoscopic view. The newborn also has a short neck which makes the head seemingly sitting right over the shoulders. This means there is less length available for flexion of the neck over shoulders, and this makes attaining of the sniffing position more difficult in neonates. Neonates have hypoplastic jaw, small mouth, and small intraoral and pharyngeal spaces. All these peculiarities contribute to the difficult airway in the neonate.

(b) **Small nasal airway**: neonates are preferential or obligate nose breathers. The small intraoral space and large tongue, makes the tongue, in its entire length, nearly in apposition with the hard and soft palates, occluding the passage of air through the mouth. Due to the high position of the larynx (at the level of C3–4 vertebrae compared with C5–6 vertebrae in adults) the resistance to the air flow in the oral airway to reach the glottis is increased. The narrow nasal airways are

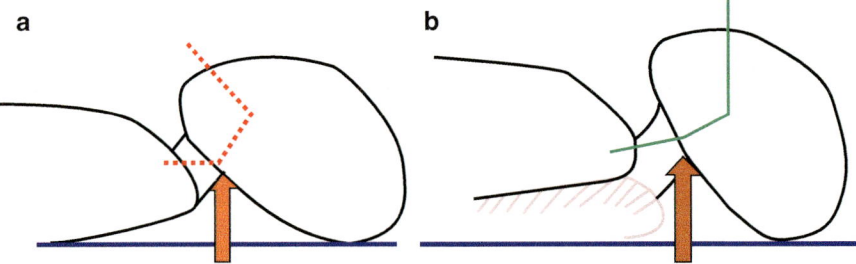

Fig. 12.1 Positioning for airway management in neonates and infants. The orange arrow shows the site of potential obstruction (**a**) relieved by keeping a soft pillow under the shoulders (**b**)

prone to obstruction by secretions or inflammation and can lead to significant respiratory difficulty.

(c) **Tongue and oral cavity**: the large tongue in proportion to the oral cavity can obstruct the airway following loss of muscle tone after induction of anaesthesia, especially with use of muscle relaxants, in the supine position, and difficult mask ventilation and, spontaneous breathing. Recent imaging studies have demonstrated that a major proportion of airway obstruction is also due to the nasopharyngeal and epiglottic collapse [2].

(d) **Larynx**: larynx is more cephalad (C3–4) and descends to adult level with age. This contributes to difficult visualisation of vocal cords during direct laryngoscopy as the angle between the pharyngeal and the laryngeal axis increases (Fig. 12.1). In adults, the angle between the vocal cords and trachea is almost 90° in the antero-posterior direction, while in neonates, it is more oblique and slant, thus hampering glottic view at laryngoscopy [3].

(e) **Epiglottis and laryngeal cartilages**: the epiglottis in neonates is narrow, omega shaped, stiff, proportionally longer and angled away from the axis of the trachea. Other laryngeal cartilages, the arytenoids, corniculate and cuneiform are also proportionally larger compared to the laryngeal inlet. The aryepiglottic folds are closer to midline. All these factors further obscure the glottic view. The large, floppy epiglottis is difficult to be raised on the glosso-epiglottic fold by the curved McIntosh blade. This explains why the glottis is easier visualize by lifting the epiglottis with the straight Miller blade. In a neonate, the hyoid bone is ossified only in the central part, while lateral part is still cartilaginous. Hyoid is the main support for the muscles that hold the cartilages of the larynx in its resting position. During direct laryngoscopy, the traction force applied over the base of the tongue (or vallecula) doesn't lift the unossified hyoid bone effectively and doesn't modify the laryngeal view to aid glottic visualization. To visualise the entire glottic opening the blade of the laryngoscope needs to lift the epiglottis. The unique anatomy of the newborn airway along with the low muscle tone makes it more vulnerable to collapse during inspiration. Use of some continuous positive airway pressure (CPAP) by keeping the pressure-limiting valve or the expiratory port partially closed at induction of anaesthesia and during sedation, helps to keep the airway patent.

(f) **Shape of the neonatal airway**: the paediatric larynx is thought to be funnel shaped as compared to the cylindrical shape in adults. Traditional teaching is that the subglottis is the narrowest part of the neonatal airway. However, some newer MRI studies have demonstrated that narrowest portion of the airway might be glottis and the subglottis may be elliptical rather than cylindrical [4]. This encouraged the use of cuffed tubes in neonates as uncuffed tubes would produce excessive pressure on one side and excessive leak on the other side of a supposedly elliptical sub glottis, leading to suboptimal ventilation and increased chance of aspiration. Recent CT-based studies (CT is considered better than MRI for airway imaging) have shown that cricoid (which is subglottic) is indeed round shaped in neonates, with a smaller diameter than the anteroposterior diameter of the glottis and is, thus functionally and anatomically the narrowest part of the larynx [1].

12.2.2 Physiological Considerations

(a) **Preferential nasal breathers:** neonates are obligate nasal breathers. Therefore, obstruction to the anterior or posterior nares by congenital (choanal atresia) or acquired (nasal congestion, secretions) condition, could cause obstruction and severe asphyxia.

(b) **Lung volumes and capacities,** especially the functional residual capacity (FRC), are disproportionately low relative to their body size. Their metabolic rate and oxygen requirement is (7–9 mL/kg/min) almost twice that of an adult. This results in a greatly increased ventilatory requirement per unit lung volume for the neonate. During periods of apnea, both these factors, i.e., low FRC and high O_2 requirement, lead to early desaturation, thus complicating the control of an already compromised airway. Use of CPAP and positive end expiratory pressure (PEEP) prevents alveolar collapse and improves FRC during ventilation.

(c) The proportional **airway resistance** is greater in neonates, even at the same airway generations as compared to children and adults due to their small calibre. Application of Poiseuille's law makes this clear. The pressure difference across a lumen change inversely to the power of four with change in radius of the lumen. This means that the relative increase in work of breathing is immensely more when the already small radius of the airways is further decreased by inflammation, edema or secretions.

(d) **Muscles of respiration:** the percentage of **type I muscle fibres** (slow-twitch, high-oxidative fatigue resistant) and the type II (fast-twitch, low-oxidative and fatigue prone) in the diaphragm and intercostal muscles vary with age in infants. The intercostal muscle maturity is achieved by 2 months of age, while diaphragmatic muscles mature by 8 months. The diaphragm, in premature neonates (<37 week gestation) has only 10% type I fibres, compared to 25% in full-term neonates and 55% in older children. The intercostal muscles, in premature neonates have 20% type I fibres versus 45% in full-term neonates and 65% in older children [5]. Increase in work of breathing from any cause is poorly tolerated by neonates as their ventilatory muscles are more prone to fatigue, and this is more pronounced in premature neonates. The need for ventilatory support requirement is earlier in neonates, especially premature, and early ventilatory decompensation should always be anticipated.

(e) The **protective airway reflexes,** coughing and swallowing are not well-developed in neonates. They are extremely sensitive to any stimulation of the airway (secretions and/or mechanical irritants), to which they usually respond with breath holding and laryngospasm and bradycardia. In the premature babies the additional cause of apnea is the nondeveloped or poorly developed brain centres for regular and cyclic breathing and may occur even without airway irritation.

12.3 Airway Assessment

No clear-cut measurements or predictors of difficult airway exist in neonates. Airway evaluation involves mainly history and physical examination, along with evaluation for comorbid conditions.

12.3.1 History

The medical history should include history of snoring or noisy breathing which may indicate potential obstruction of upper airway, difficulty in breathing while feeding which may indicate a nasal obstruction and any coexisting congenital or acquired medical conditions. Any extra thoracic intraluminal (as in upper trachea or above) will cause inspiratory stridor as the airway lumen will constrict due to the negative intrathoracic pressures generated during inspiration, e.g., in conditions such as extra-thoracic foreign body, laryngomalacia, macroglossia and laryngeal web. Obstruction of the lower trachea or bronchi will lead to exaggerated stridor during expiration as the obstruction increases during forced expiration due to compression of intrathoracic airways.

Relevant medical comorbidities related to prematurity such as bronchopulmonary dysplasia, apnoeic spells, or intraventricular haemorrhage relevant to airway management should also be sought out. History of recent or ongoing upper respiratory tract infection is important to assess the risk of complications, such as laryngospasm, bronchospasm, and desaturation during and post anaesthesia.

12.3.2 Physical Examination

The physical examination should include observation of head contour, shape, facial expression, size of mouth, size and configuration of the palate and mandible as well as features of respiratory obstruction and distress, such as presence of nasal flaring, mouth breathing and presence of retractions (suprasternal, intercostal, and subcostal). A baseline room air SpO_2 should always be a part of neonatal airway examination. Features suggestive of difficult airway include reduced mouth opening during crying, restricted neck mobility, hypoplasia of mandible or maxilla or both, dysmorphic features of the face, abnormalities of ear, facial cleft, cleft lip and palate, and abnormalities or mass of the neck. These are usually quite evident on the examination and should not be missed. Intraoral, pharyngeal, and laryngeal masses may, however, be missed if not given enough thought during airway examination. Some obvious signs of congenital disease with airway implications should be looked for. Bilateral microtia has been shown to be associated with difficulty in visualising the

Table 12.1 Syndromes associated with airway problems

Syndrome	Associated airway abnormalities
Achondroplasia	Midfacial hypoplasia, small nasal passage, and mouth
Congenital hypothyroidism	Large tongue
Crouzon syndrome	Maxillary hypoplasia with V shaped palate, large tongue, OSA
Goldenhar syndrome	Hypoplastic zygomatic arch, mandibular hypoplasia, macrostomia, cleft palate, tracheoesophageal fistula
Hurler syndrome	Coarse facial features, short neck, tonsillar hypertrophy, narrowing of laryngeal inlet and tracheobronchial tree
Hunter syndrome	Coarse facial features, tracheomalacia, macrocephaly, macroglossia
Pierre Robin sequence	Hypoplastic mandible, high arched cleft palate
Treacher Colins syndrome	Malar and mandibular hypoplasia, cleft lip, choanal atresia, macrostomia or microstomia
Down syndrome	Small mouth, hypoplastic mandible, protruding tongue
Charge Syndrome	Coloboma of the eye, Heart disease (TOF), Atresia of choanae. Retarded growth or development, Genital and Ear abnormalities

laryngeal inlet and may be associated with mandibular hypoplasia [6]. Facial hae-mangioma is associated with Sturge–Weber syndrome and may be indicative of an airway haemangioma as well. A list of syndromes with associated airway problems is provided in Table 12.1.

Presence of encephalocele, hydrocephalus and meningomyelocele can interfere with optimal positioning for airway management. Presence of a coexisting medical disease can affect drug choice during airway management. Hemodynamic instability and/or congenital heart disease may preclude use of certain premedicants and other anaesthetic agents that may need to be provided for hemodynamic management during airway control. Neonates with necrotizing enterocolitis, omphalocele, and gastroschisis have a high risk of aspiration and have significantly diminished FRC, making them more susceptible to hypoxemia and desaturation [7].

12.3.3 Diagnostic imaging

Diagnostic imaging is usually not possible as the procedure itself may need sedation and anaesthesia, thus mandating airway management. Imaging studies are under-taken only if the need for airway management is not imminent and appropriate personnel and equipment needed to manage airway are available. ***Radiographs*** of the soft tissue of head and neck may provide insight about the aetiology and site of airway obstruction if present/suspected. ***Endoscopic evaluation*** of the airway with mucosal local anaesthetic application can be useful in neonates if a glottic pathology is being investigated. The spatial resolution of airway structures is best with ***computed tomography*** due to its superior discrimination of the air/tissue interface.

12.4   Neonatal Airway Management: Procedures and Equipment

12.4.1 MASK Ventilation (MV)

The practice and technique of mask ventilation in neonates differs slightly from that in adults because of the anatomical and physiological challenges as described previously. While choosing a mask for a neonate it is important to choose one with minimal external dead space, ease of application on slightly flat facial contours and ability to see the underlying face of the baby.

Face masks of various sizes and shapes for neonatal airway management are available (Fig. 12.2) (Table 12.2). Commonly used face masks are the anatomical face mask, plastic transparent anaesthesia face mask with syringe adjustable air-cushioned rim, which on inflation/deflation can be altered to match the contour of the patient's face, and the Rendell–Baker–Soucek (RBS) mask. The use of clear plastic mask allows visualisation of the mouth, vapours of the expired air, secretions, vomitus, and lip colour. The RBS mask was specifically designed for children under 10 years of age and is especially suited for neonates. It is made of malleable rubber or silicone and allows a proper face seal and can fit a variety of facial configurations. Its triangular shaped body minimises the dead space (3 mL in size 0 and 4 mL in size 1).

12.4.1.1   Technique of Mask Ventilation:

The objective of a good mask ventilation is to ventilate the patient effectively, with minimal inflation pressure, reflected by adequate chest expansion and absence of gastric insufflation The commonly used techniques for mask ventilation include (Fig. 12.3):

i. **One hand technique (E–C clamp technique):** the thumb and the index finger are placed on the body of the mask to form a C, while the remaining three fingers are placed on the inferior surface of the mandible to form an E.

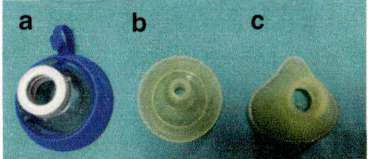

Fig. 12.2 Face masks for neonates. (**a**) Plastic transparent mask with syringe adjustable air-cushioned rim. (**b**) Anatomical face mask. (**c**) RBS mask

Table 12.2 Types and sizes of face masks in neonates and infants

	Anatomical mask	Transparent plastic mask	Rendell-Baker-Soucek mask
Preterm	–	00	0
Infant	0	0	1
Small child	1	1	2

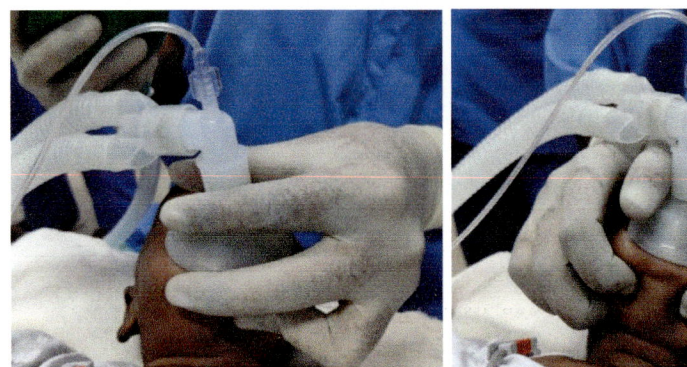

Fig. 12.3 Mask ventilation techniques—one hand and two hand holding mask holding

ii. ***Two handed jaw thrust technique:*** this technique is employed if ventilation is not possible by single hand. In this, both the thumbs are placed over the mask, while index and middle fingers are used to lift the mandible.

iii. ***Claw hand technique:*** the anaesthesiologist stands by the side of the patient, instead of the head end. The facemask is applied with right hand with the palmar surface facing slightly upwards and to the left side of the anaesthesiologist. The ring finger and the middle finger are placed under the right and left side of the angle of the mandible, respectively. The index finger and thumb encircle the body of the mask on the face with a tight grip. This technique has been suggested for babies undergoing short ophthalmological procedures as the head-end of the table is occupied by the ophthalmologist [8].

The commonest error during mask ventilation is compression of soft tissue in the submental triangle with the fingers of proceduralist, partially occluding the airway. Care should be taken that the fingers rest on the bony ridge of the mandible and not on the soft tissue. During mask ventilation, the mouth of the neonate should always be kept open, and mandible translocated anteriorly to lift the tongue away from the posterior pharyngeal wall and palate.

12.4.2 Oropharyngeal Airways (OPA)

The large tongue and the collapsible oropharynx predispose the obstruction of oropharynx during induction of anaesthesia. If optimal ventilation is not possible despite a good technique, an OPA of appropriate size can be used to relieve the obstruction. The size needed corresponds to the distance between the angle of the mouth and the angle of the mandible. Usually, size 00 for pre-term and 0 for term babies is appropriate. The tip of an inappropriately small OPA will push against the base of the tongue further aggravating the obstruction, while a longer OPA may push the epiglottis onto the glottis, worsening the obstruction. Care should always be taken to avoid trauma to the lips, tongue, and palate during insertion of the OPA.

12.4.3 Supraglottic Airway (SGA) Devices

With advancements in the design, multiple SGA devices are now available for use in neonates and infants. The functional elegance of the SGA is its ease of insertion while providing adequate airway patency. SGAs have found a unique place in the management of already difficult neonatal airway. However, the success rate of placement of SGAs in neonates is less than that in adults, and skills and equipment for alternative methods to secure the airway should always be available.

Indications for SGA: indications include elective airway management in diagnostic procedures, short surgical procedures, as a rescue device for managing difficult mask ventilation and intubation, and for preoxygenation in neonates, where low lung compliance and poor cardiopulmonary reserves prevent effective preoxygenation with face mask. SGAs are now increasingly being used for neonatal resuscitation in delivery rooms and for surfactant administration. An advantage is that it can be inserted in an awake neonate after intraoral local anaesthetic application.

Currently, the following SGAs are available for use in neonates: (Fig. 12.4)

i. LMA Classic™, LMA Proseal™: Size 1(<5 kg)
ii. i-gel™: Size 1 (2–5 kg)
iii. Ambu AuraOnce™: Size 1 (<5 kg)
iv. Air-Q™ LMA (laryngeal mask airway): Size 0.5 (<4 kg)

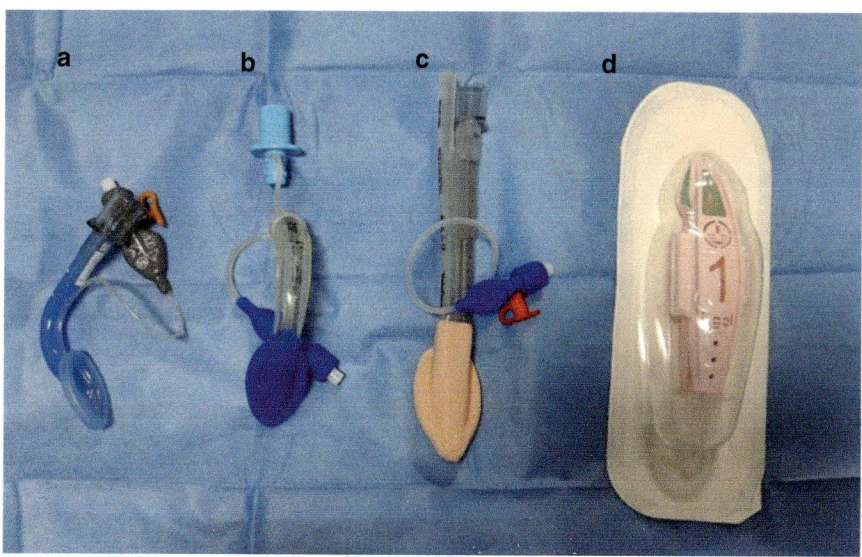

Fig. 12.4 Supraglottic airway devices. (**a**) Ambu AuroOnce™. (**b**) Air-Q™ LMA. (**c**) LMA Proseal™. (**d**) i-gel™ LMA

Use of SGAs in Neonates: troubleshooting

- If the SGA is inserted too far (which can be easily done by novices) it can easily enter the oesophagus. The oesophagus can get intubated and distended by the SGA tip. This can be diagnosed immediately due to lack of signs of lung ventilation despite easy and smooth placement. This happens if the size of SGA is too small and can be resolved by slight withdrawal of the device or choosing one size larger.
- The SGA may bend the epiglottis over the laryngeal inlet causing airway obstruction. The large and floppy neonatal epiglottis is more prone to cause glottic obstruction Repositioning of the SGA may help, but if ventilation is unsatisfactory, endotracheal intubation may be required [9].
- The tip of the SGA can fold on itself during insertion and can be resolved by withdrawing and repositioning or by gently sweeping on the dorsal surface of SGA with the finger.
- The SGAs can get displaced while in use, in a neonate, and cause stomach distension and impedance to lung expansion. This is common with 1st generation SGAs (without gastric drainage tube). A correctly sized 2nd generation SGA, e.g., LMA Proseal and i-Gel, form a better seal with the peri glottic tissues and may be safer in neonates. In addition, the in-built drainage tube aids in venting of gastric air thus preventing gastric distension. They can be used as a conduit for endotracheal tube (**ETT**). A 3 mm ETT can usually be passed through the i-Gel, LMA classic and Air-Q SGAs.

12.4.4 Endotracheal Intubation

a. Technique of Endotracheal Intubation

Optimal Positioning and Selection of Laryngoscope Blade

Unlike adults, oral, pharyngeal, and laryngeal axes in infants are better aligned by simple extension of the head rather than sniffing position. Neonates due to their larger occiput obstruct the airway when placed on a pillow, due to flexion of head. Hence, optimal position for laryngoscopy will be a slight head extension (without using pillow) and placing a small roll beneath the shoulders (please see the section on Anatomy).

The laryngoscope blades commonly used in neonates are straight Miller, Oxford or curved Mcintosh blades (Fig. 12.5). A straight blade is more suitable in neonates because of its more efficient elevation of the epiglottis, giving a clearer view of the glottis. Miller's straight blade sizes 0 and 1 are used in term babies, while size 00 is reserved for extreme premature (<27 weeks of gestation) or low weight <750 g. Based on their experience, some anaesthesiologists prefer the curved MacIntosh type blades 00, 0 and 1 (Table 12.3).

b. Size of Endotracheal Tube (ETT)

ETT sizing in the neonatal population is largely predetermined. Ideally, for any age group, the largest sized ETT should be chosen to minimise airway resistance while limiting undue pressure on the subglottis and trachea. The general

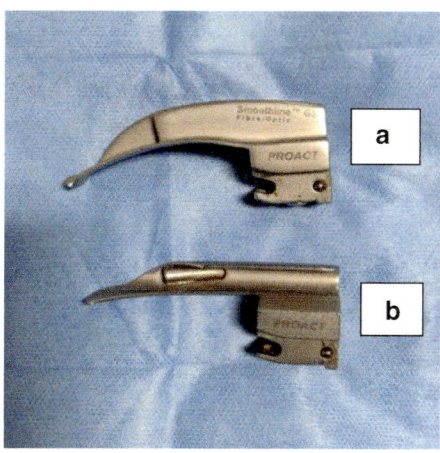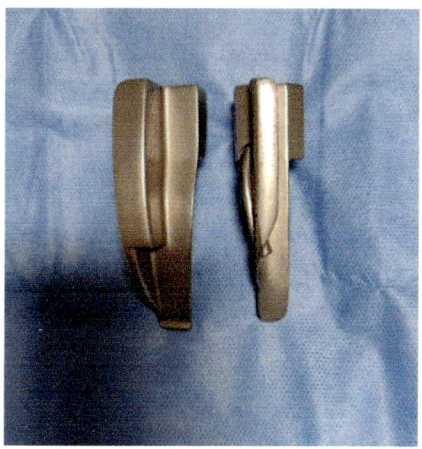

Fig. 12.5 Laryngoscope blades size 0. (**a**) McIntosh. (**b**) Miller

Table 12.3 Sizes and length of miller and mcintosh blade for use in neonates

	Miller blade		McIntosh blade	
	Size	Length(mm)	Size	Length(mm)
Premature neonate	00	62	–	–
Term neonate	0	77	0	83
Infant	1	102	1	92

Table 12.4 Endotracheal tube size (ID mm) and distance for insertion in neonate by age

Age	ET Uncuffed	ET Cuffed	Distance of insertion (cm)
Preterm			
1000 g	2.5	–	6–7
1000–200 g	3.0	–	7–9
Term	3.0–3.5	3.0–3.5	9–10

recommendation is to use an uncuffed 2.5 mm ID ETT for preterm weighing up to 1000 g, 3 mm ID for preterm ranging in weight from 1000 to 2500 g and 3.0 to 3.5 mm ID cuffed or uncuffed ETT for term neonates (Table 12.4).

During intubation, ETT size of 0.5 mm ID smaller or greater than the anticipated size should always be available. Neonates with Down syndrome may require a smaller ETT than predicted. The length of the trachea (vocal cords to carina) in neonates and infants up to 1 year of age varies between 5 and 9 cm [10]. In preterm neonates, trachea is shorter. Therefore, it is important to observe for symmetry of the chest expansion and equality of breath sounds on auscultation in the axillae and apices as well. Auscultation on the anterior chest wall may not be reliable as the breath sounds may reverberate across the precordium in small children. The popular rule of 7–8–9 gives a guide on the depth of insertion of the **ETT** (Table 12.4). Babies weighing 1 kg are intubated to a depth of 7 cm, 2 kg at 8 cm and 3 kg at 9 cm

Table 12.5 Implications of uncuffed and cuffed tubes

Uncuffed tubes	Cuffed tubes
Greater internal diameter (id), Lower resistance	Lower exchange rate
In elliptical epiglottis can produce pressure on one side and excessive leak on the other	Less laryngeal oedema and post extubation stridor
Leakage, suboptimal ventilation	Leaks can be adjusted ensuring adequate ventilation
Increased OT pollution	Allow less fresh gas flow (FGF)
Inaccurate control of $EtCO_2$	Accurate control of $PaCO_2$
Increased chance of aspiration	Less OT pollution
Increased tube exchange rate	Needs cuff pressure monitoring (<20–25 cm H_2O)

c. Choice of ETT: Cuffed vs Uncuffed

The essential differences between uncuffed and cuffed tubes are highlighted in Table 12.5.

12.4.4.1 Microcuff ETT

These are high-volume low-pressure cuffed ETTs made of ultrathin polyurethane of 10 μm thickness (compared to 50–70 μm in PVC tubes). The cuff is short and more distally placed along the shaft as the Murphy's eye has been removed. On inflation, the cuff expands below the subglottis in the upper trachea, providing a seal with low cuff pressure, usually less than 20 cm H_2O. The trachea is sealed at upper trachea (rather than at sub glottis), where the posterior membranous wall can stretch and produce a complete seal. The pressure over the cricoid ring and the risk of subsequent subglottic stenosis is also reduced. The thin cuff allows complete and uniform surface contact with minimal folds. The risk of endobronchial intubation is reduced with these tubes. The cuff should be inflated to minimal pressure that seals the air leak. Microcuff ETT are available from size 3 onwards and can be used in term neonates >3.0 kg (Figs. 12.6).

12.4.5 Video Laryngoscopy (VL)

VL has revolutionised airway management. Surprisingly very little high-quality evidence is available regarding its superiority to traditional laryngoscopy when used for endotracheal intubation in neonates. One reason for this is the lack of well-controlled studies in this population due to multiple ethical reasons, and the few available studies do describe its superior image quality compared to traditional laryngoscopic view. However, this has not been correlated with the success rate of intubation or to time to intubate.

VL can be used as the primary device or as a rescue/back up device for direct laryngoscope. They are of two types, channeled and nonchanneled. The nonchanneled VL are equipped with an optical system in the blade with either an inbuilt or a stand-alone viewing window, and include C-MAC® VLS, GlideScope®, Multiview Scope®, and Truview PCD™ Pediatric. The channeled VL has an optical system with

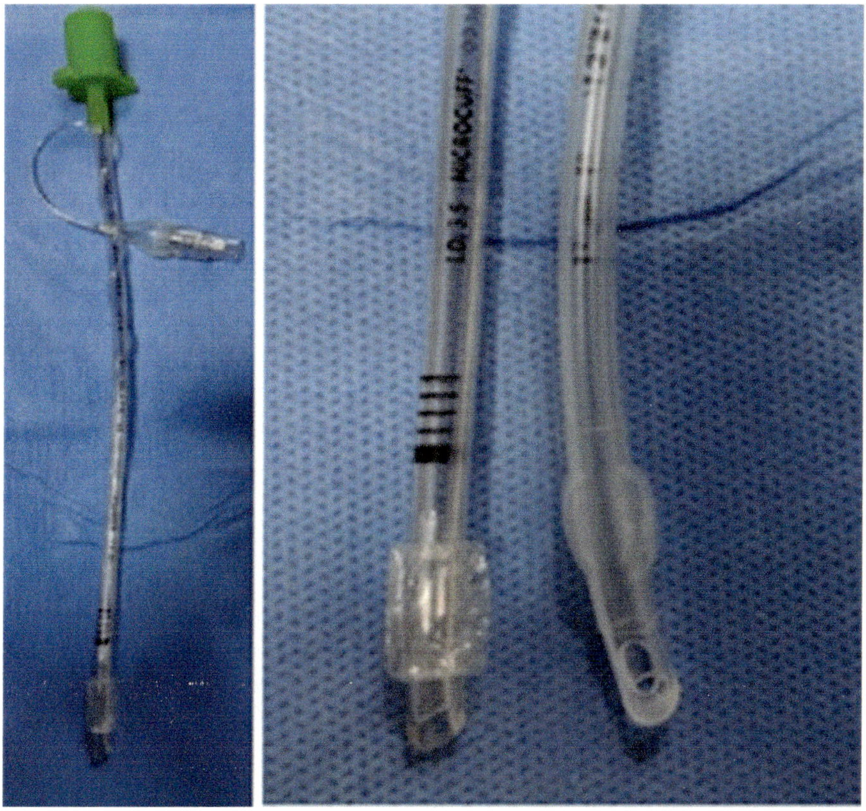

Fig. 12.6   Microcuff endotracheal tube - absence of Murphy eye and distally placed cuff

Fig. 12.7   Video laryngoscope (C-MAC) blades size 0: Macintosh and Miller

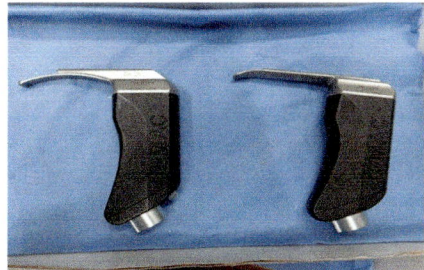

a viewing window as well as an inbuilt channel in the blade for preloading an ETT. These include the King Vision®, AirTraq™, and AirWay Scope® [11]. The blade designs include Miller, McIntosh, hyper angulated D-blades or customised blades which are used when optimal neck extension is not achievable. In neonates, Miller 0,1 or McIntosh 0 size may be used (Fig. 12.7). The method of laryngoscopy

Table 12.6 Various sized fibre optic bronchoscope available in neonate

Outer diameter (mm)	Working channel (mm)	Suction Channel mm)	ET size (minimum)	
2.2	Yes	No	3.0	<6 months age
2.8	1.2	1.2	4.0	Any Pediatric age

is similar as in direct laryngoscopy. In some, the manufacturer recommendations describe midline insertion of the blade without sweeping the tongue and is useful for those not proficient with neonatal intubations.

The greatest advantage of VL is as a good teaching and training tool, since the laryngoscopic view is visible to all, and can even be projected to a larger screen for greater viewability, while at the same time, the teacher can help the performer with the intubation as well [12].

12.4.6 Fibreoptic bronchoscope (FOB)

FOB may be required for airway management in babies with diagnosed cervical inflexibility (Klippel–Feil syndrome) or cervical instability (Achondroplasia, Down Syndrome, and rarely trauma). Many reports of use of FOB for oral and nasal intubation in neonates are available for various congenital conditions, such as syngnathia, Pierre Robin Syndrome, oral and pharyngeal tumours. Any condition where neck movements or intraoral/pharyngeal space is restricted, the flexibility of the FOB is advantageous. Various sized FOBs are available for intubation in neonates (Table 12.6).

The oral approach may be less stimulating than the nasal and better tolerated in neonates but is more difficult to negotiate. On the other hand, the nasal route may be technically easier but can cause nasal trauma and bleeding. A gentle jaw thrust is helpful in opening the posterior pharyngeal and supraglottic spaces and in the negotiation of the FOB. The size for neonates lacks a working channel and suction port, and so neither secretions can be cleared nor O_2 can be administered. This necessitates administration of O_2 using alternative device during the procedure. Another problem encountered is the resistance to the passage of ETT. This can be overcome by withdrawing the ETT a few millimetres, changing the direction of the bevel and reinserting. Usually, a bevel facing up for nasal intubation and the bevel facing down for oral intubation is helpful. FOB guided intubations can be difficult in neonates not just due to an anatomically difficult airway but also due to the minimal O_2 reserve. Methods of continuous O_2 insufflation as well as maintenance of spontaneous respiration should be actively followed during FOB guided oral and nasal intubations both in awake as well as sedated neonates. In difficult cases, LMA guided FOB aided endotracheal intubation can be done.

12.4.7 Rapid Sequence Induction (RSI) and Intubation (RSII) in Neonate

Rapid Sequence Induction and Intubation (RSII) describes a coordinated, sequential process of preparation, anaesthesia, and paralysis to facilitate emergency tracheal intubation in patients who are at high risk for regurgitation and aspiration. Classic RSII puts paediatric patients at risk of complications, such as desaturation, traumatic intubation, and hemodynamic morbidity. Neonates, especially, may not allow complete preoxygenation, may be difficult to intubate and with decreased apnoea time available, may quickly decompensate to hypoxia and bradycardia. A 'controlled' RSII (cRSII) technique has been described for paediatric patients and may be suitable for neonates rather than the classic RSII used in adults [13]. The changes in RSII protocol for neonates may include all or some of the following modifications:

- Use of opioids and/or benzodiazepines to decrease induction drug dosages and decrease stress response to intubation
- Avoiding cricoid pressure altogether or releasing just before intubation
- Gentle face mask ventilation during the time waiting for peak effect of muscle relaxants to occur

The equipment and methods for intubation essentially remain the same with use of cuffed ETT.

12.5 The Difficult Neonatal Airway

Airway management in neonates is categorized as being difficult even without any anticipated or unanticipated added medical, anatomical, or physiological challenges.

12.5.1 Definition

Difficult intubation (DI) is defined as endotracheal intubation requiring three or more laryngoscopy attempts by an experienced performer. A multicentric retrospective review reported DI in 14% of the neonates with a fourfold increased odds for severe desaturation [14]. DI was more common in premature neonates (<32 week gestational age) and weighing <1500 g.

12.5.2 Identifying of Difficult Airway

Incidence of tracheal intubation associated adverse events is approximately 20–40% of all neonatal intubations. It is important to recognize circumstances that can cause airway obstruction or difficulty. Upper airway obstruction, a known history of

Table 12.7 Causes of difficult airway encountered in neonate and infants

Craniofacial abnormalities	Compromised airway	Cervical spine anomalies
Pierre Robin sequence	Bilateral choanal atresia	Down syndrome
Treacher Collin syndrome	Subglottic stenosis	Klippel Feil malformation
Goldenhar syndrome	Tracheomalacia	Goldenhar syndrome
Mucopolysaccharidosis	Ludwig s angina	Mucopolysaccharidosis
Achondroplasia	Acute epiglottitis	–
Crouzon syndrome	Foreign body	–
–	Trauma	–

difficult airway, micrognathia, limited mouth opening, limited neck extension, cleft palate and short thyromental distance are generally indicative of a difficult airway. Neonates belonging to a syndrome/sequence which involves airway anomalies along with other systemic involvement need to be identified. A list of syndromes and conditions associated with features leading to difficulty in airway management is provided in Table 12.7. Careful preanesthetic evaluation and clinical assessment and recognition of possible signs and symptoms of these conditions will reduce airway management-related complications.

12.5.3 Approach to Difficult Airway

The safest approach to manage a difficult airway is to formulate a plan that includes several contingencies for failure or loss of airway, a clear communication between the members of the team and specific details to facilitate the process. All equipment should be checked to ensure good working condition and all the resuscitation drugs should be prepared in appropriate dilutions and dosages. Equipment in appropriate sizes should include, but may not be restricted to, tracheal tubes and SGA devices, laryngoscope blades, stylets, facemasks, OPA, suction devices, reliable O_2 source, and vascular access equipment.

12.5.4 Management Nonsurgical

Nonsurgical: A reasonable principle in the management of difficult airway is to maintain spontaneous ventilation. Topical anaesthesia can be used in conjunction with sedation or general anaesthesia to blunt airway reactivity in whom spontaneous ventilation is to be preserved. Decision-making must start with the choice of sedation management. A predetermined place in the continuum of anaesthesia ranging from awake, semiawake, sedative/local anaesthesia, or general anaesthesia has been described in literature for the management of a neonate with difficult airway. Adequate visualisation of the vocal cords is a mandatory step for successful intubation. A recently conducted trial demonstrated that the early use of VL with standard blade improved the first-attempt success rate with reduced complications in anaesthetised neonates [15]. The advantages of VL are obvious and useful in difficult neonatal airway. It can facilitate intubation in most cases, while SGA and FOB may be useful for cases with

Table 12.8 Various tracheostomy tubes (TT) and sizes (mm) available for neonates

TT	ID	OD	Distal length	Cuff	Material
Bivona (NEO)	2.5	4	30	Y	Silicone
	3	4.7	32	Y	
	3.5	5.3	34	Y	
	4	6	36	Y	
Shiley (NEO)	2.5	4.2	30	Y	PVC
	3.0	4.8	30	Y	
	3.5	5.4	32	Y	
	4.0	6.0	34	Y	

anticipated difficult mask ventilation. Patients with anatomical anomalies above the larynx can be managed with SGA, FOB, or combination of the two.

In case of unanticipated difficult airway, call for help immediately. The goal will be to maintain oxygenation and ventilation. Consider an early use of VL. In case of failed intubation, ventilation should be attempted by facemask or SGA, and if possible, then intubation may be attempted via SGA and FOB. In case of failed intubation and inadequate ventilation, proceed to rescue techniques, such as surgical tracheostomy.

Surgical airway–tracheostomy: invasive airway access is particularly challenging in neonates. The diameter and length of the subglottic airway varies with gestational age. The internal diameter of subglottis in a newborn is 3.5–4 mm, 3 mm or less in premature newborn [16], and tracheal length (glottis to carina) is about 40 mm (4 cm). It is thus important to use an appropriate size of tracheostomy tube (TT) in neonates. Needle cricothyroidotomy may not be a practical approach as the cricothyroid membrane is difficult to locate and too small to accommodate even an appropriate tube.

Paediatric TTs are usually single lumen without inner canula. Currently, fenestrated TTs for neonates are not available. Paediatric tubes are manufactured in standard neonatal and paediatric sizes (Table 12.8). For children up to 5 kg neonatal sizes are used. It is important to be ensure that the tip of TT is not endobronchial. A common way to determine the correct placement of the tube is by performing a flexible tracheoscopy through the tube, after the procedure itself.

The common indications for tracheostomy in neonates include the need for prolonged ventilation, facilitation of ventilator weaning and upper airway obstruction (Table 12.9). In preterm neonates, BPD requiring ventilatory support is a common indication for tracheostomy [17]. The procedure and care during and after neonatal tracheostomy are same as standard paediatric tracheostomy. The neonatal physiology and anatomy should always be under consideration while performing them. The tracheal incision for the tracheostomy is vertical. Stay sutures are used which are useful for rapid identification of the newly created stoma in case of accidental decannulation.

Complications: neonatal tracheostomies have high morbidity and mortality (1.5–8.9%) especially in the presence of cardiac risk factors [18].

a. Short-term complications
b. Long-term complications

Table 12.9 Indications for tracheostomy in a neonate

i.	Craniofacial disorders with upper airway obstruction
ii.	Cardiopulmonary disease requiring long term positive pressure ventilation
iii.	Neurological disorders, congenital and acquired
iv.	Acquired or congenital glottic, subglottic or tracheal stenosis
v.	Acute airway infections (epiglottitis, tracheitis, croup)
vi.	Congenital high airway obstruction syndrome (CHAOS)

Short-Term Complications
- Bleeding
- Thyroid gland injury
- Skin pressure necrosis
- Accidental decannulation
- Creation of a false track
- Blockage by mucous plug or clot
- Tracheal ulceration

Long-term complications
- Granulation tissue formation
- Ulceration/erosion: anteriorly leading to trachea-innominate fistula and posteriorly leading to tracheoesophageal fistula
- Tracheal stenosis

The management of these complications, as with the management of tracheostomy is complicated in neonates and expert help should be called for as soon as feasible. All care should be taken to prevent the occurrence of these complications.

12.6 Anesthetic Considerations of Difficult Airway

Two conditions deserve special mention which may prove fatal if not identified and managed early.

12.6.1 Choanal Atresia (CA)

Congenital CA is the complete blockage of the posterior nasal opening. This anatomical deformity occurs due to enlargement of the vomer bone and medialization of the pterygoid plate during the intrapartum growth. The atresia can be categorised as membranous or bony, and unilateral or bilateral, with majority being unilateral. Bilateral posterior CA is associated with high mortality, especially in neonates with congenital heart disease and tracheoesophageal fistulas.

Preoperative considerations: bilateral CA is detected soon after birth due to early symptoms associated with severe respiratory distress. Unilateral CA is often

Table 12.10 Anatomical mechanism of upper airway obstruction in laryngomalacia

Type 1	Cuneiform cartilages are drawn inwards during inspiration
Type 2	Long tubular epiglottis curls on itself
Type 3	The arytenoids collapse inwards
Type 4	The epiglottis is displaced against the posterior pharyngeal wall or vocal folds
Type 5	Short aryepiglottic folds
Type 6	Overly acute angle of the epiglottis at the laryngeal inlet

not detected until adolescence when patients present with nasal congestion. Association with CHARGE syndrome is observed in 75% of the patients with bilateral CA. Other congenital anomalies associated with CA include humeroradial synostosis, mandibulofacial synostosis, microcephaly, micrognathia, palatal defects, Treacher–Colin syndrome and other craniofacial dysmorphisms [19]. They are also at increased risk of laryngomalacia. Bilateral CA is an emergency and need immediate airway management, often tracheostomy. Preparation for the difficult airway and considerations for the associated anomalies remain the chief concerns.

Intraoperative considerations: mask ventilation may be difficult. The protocols and practices for difficult airway should be followed. The presence of surgical team is desirable in the event of emergency tracheostomy. Muscle relaxants may be used to facilitate surgery after securing airway.

Postoperative considerations: patients with CHARGE syndrome are at increased risk for airway events and should be watched closely. Neonates should be extubated in controlled setting, either in the theatre with all preparations for reintubation or in NICU.

12.6.2 Laryngomalacia

Congenital laryngomalacia is the most common cause of stridor in neonates, usually presenting within 2 weeks of birth. The neonates present with inspiratory stridor that worsens with feeding and in supine position. The anatomical mechanisms for the upper airway obstruction in laryngomalacia are enumerated in Table 12.10 [20]. Only 5–10% require surgical treatment involving division of the aryepiglottic folds, resection of excess arytenoid tissue, and suspension of the prolapsing epiglottis. Supra glottoplasty is the most common procedure performed in neonates with severe laryngomalacia in stridor.

Preoperative considerations: severe laryngomalacia can cause upper airway obstruction, cyanotic spells, feeding difficulties, failure to thrive, corpulmonale, and developmental delay. Neonates may present with cardiorespiratory failure. The spectrum of signs suggestive of cardiorespiratory failure ranges from nasal flaring to chest retraction, tachypnoea, tachycardia, and cyanosis. Feeding difficulties occur because of gastro-oesophageal reflux secondary to upper airway obstruction. The diagnosis of laryngomalacia is usually made by flexible nasal endoscopy. The use of antisialogogue, such as atropine (20 mcg/kg), prior to induction of anaesthesia can be considered.

Intraoperative considerations: babies with laryngomalacia frequently have easily recognizable difficult airway features, making the conventional methods of securing the airway difficult. The altered anatomy may sometimes require urgent tracheostomy. Intubation is usually difficult due to the associated large overhanging epiglottis, redundant arytenoid tissue, and the inspiratory positional stridor. Inhalational induction in the lateral position while maintaining spontaneous respiration is a safer option. Intubation with VL or FOB is the gold standard. Supra glottoplasty necessitates an obstructed airway, clear view of the structures and use of laser for excision. Considering a shared airway by the surgeon and anaesthesiologist and risk of airway fire and trauma, a well-charted airway plan is required. The options for ventilation include spontaneous ventilation, intermittent positive pressure ventilation, apnoeic ventilation, and jet ventilation depending on the experience of the anaesthesiologist and availability of the equipment.

Postoperative considerations: tracheal extubation should also incorporate an effective comprehensive plan to prevent cannot intubate and cannot ventilate situation. The neonate should be monitored and closely watched for signs of airway obstruction preferably in NICU. Humidified O_2, racemic epinephrine and dexamethasone may be required in the event of airway obstruction.

12.7 Summary

Neonates form a unique subset of paediatric patients with significant differences in their anatomy and physiology and these differences have a huge impact on the airway management and its outcome. Neonatal anatomy predisposes to airway obstruction. The "anterior airway" mandates modification of intubation technique. Failure to modify medical management appropriate to the neonate can lead to complications, such as loss of airway with failed ventilation. There are guidelines for difficult airway management in paediatric patients, while none specifically exists for neonates. Therefore, it is of utmost importance to formulate a plan that includes several contingencies for failure or loss of the airway including a clear communication between the members of the team. Early usage of SGA and VL should be considered in the airway management plan. Neonatal airway management is required at birth for resuscitation or subsequently for elective or emergency surgical procedures. It is a core skill in neonatology and proficiency in managing the difficult airway may be lifesaving in an acute emergency.

12.8 Conclusion

Airway management in neonates requires a thorough knowledge of airway anatomy, respiratory physiology as well as familiarity with the equipment available for the procedure. Knowledge and competence in basic airway management skills such as mask ventilation, laryngoscopy, SGA placement, and endotracheal intubation is acquired with experience. Successful management of difficult airway in a neonate is a multidimensional challenge to the anaesthetist and is to be approached with caution, and requisite preparation to face unanticipated problems.

References

1. Park RS, Peyton JM, Kovatsis PG. Neonatal airway management. Clin Perinatol. 2019;46(4):745–63.
2. Litman RS, Wake N, Chan LML, McDonough JM, etal. Effect of lateral positioning on upper airway size and morphology in sedated children. Anesthesiology. 2005;103(3):484–488.
3. Cote CJ, Lerman J, Anderson BJ. Cote and Lerman's a practice of anesthesia for infants and children. 5th ed. Elsevier Saunders.
4. Litman RS, Weissend EE, Shibata D, Westesson PL. Developmental changes of laryngeal dimensions in unparalyzed, sedated children. Anesthesiology. 2003;98(1):41–5.
5. Lavin T, Song Y, Bakker AJ, McLean CJ, etal. Developmental changes in diaphragm muscle function in the preterm and postnatal lamb. Pediatr Pulmonol 2013;48(7):640–648.
6. Uezono S, Holzman RS, Goto T, Nakata Y, etal. Prediction of difficult airway in school-aged patients with microtia. Paediatr Anaesth 2001;11(4):409–413.
7. Palahniuk RJ. Anaesthesia for neonatal surgical emergencies. Can J Anaesth. 1989;36(1 Supplement):49–52.
8. Podder S, Dutta A, Yaddanapudi S, Chari P. Challenges in paediatric mask holding; the 'claw hand' technique. Anesthesia. 2001;56:697–9.
9. Trevisanuto D, Micoglio M, Ferrarese P, Zanardo V. The laryngeal mask airway: potential applications in neonates. Arch Dis Child Fetal Neonatal Ed. 2004;89(6):485–9.
10. Saddawi-Konefka D, Hung SL, Kacmarek RM, Jiang Y. Optimizing mask ventilation: literature review and development of a conceptual framework. Respir Care. 2015;60(12):1834–40.
11. Sawa T, Kainuma A, Akiyama K, Kinoshita M, Shibasaki M. Difficult airway management in neonates and infants: knowledge of devices and a device-oriented strategy. Front Pediatr. 2021;9(May):1–9.
12. Moussa A, Luangxay Y, Tremblay S, Lavoie J, etal. Videolaryngoscope for teaching neonatal endotracheal intubation: a randomized controlled trial. Pediatrics 2016;137(3).
13. Neuhaus D, Schmitz A, Gerber A, Weiss M. Controlled rapid sequence induction and intubation—an analysis of 1001 children. Paediatr Anaesth. 2013;23(8):734–40.
14. Sawyer T, Foglia EE, Ades A, Moussa A, Napolitano N, etal. Incidence, impact and indicators of difficult intubations in the neonatal intensive care unit: a report from the National Emergency Airway Registry for Neonates. Arch Dis Child Fetal Neonatal Ed 2019;104(5):F461–F466.
15. Garcia-Marcinkiewicz AG, Kovatsis PG, Hunyady AI, etal. First-attempt success rate of video laryngoscopy in small infants (VISI): a multicentre, randomised controlled trial. Lancet 2020;396(10266):1905–1913.
16. Watters KF. Tracheostomy in infants and children. Respir Care. 2017;62(6):799–825.
17. Walsh J, Rastatter J. Neonatal tracheostomy. Clin Perinatol. 2018;45(4):805–16. https://doi.org/10.1016/j.clp.2018.07.014.
18. Isaiah A, Moyer K, Pereira KD. Current trends in neonatal tracheostomy. JAMA Otolaryngol Head Neck Surg. 2016;142(8):738–42.
19. Yildirim ZB, Akdağ M, Çelik F, Baysal E. Anesthesia management in patients with choanal atresia. J Craniofac Surg. 2016;27(8):1991–4.
20. Baxter MRN. Congenital laryngomalacia. Can J Anaesth. 1994;41(4):332–9.

Autonomic Nervous System in the Neonate

13

Sakshi Arora

13.1 Introduction

The autonomic nervous system (ANS) is an important system of the body, essential for maintaining cardiovascular (CVS), respiratory and higher cortical functions. At birth, the central ANS is immature, and vulnerable to adverse environmental and physiologic influences [1].

The central ANS has two major components, the **Sympathetic nervous system** responsible for the well-known "fight-or-flight" response activated from a sense of danger or stress, and the **Parasympathetic nervous system**, involved in vegetative functions, and moderating sympathetic activity. This relationship is not so simple, but is more complex, with multiple interconnections and modulations by higher centers. The nucleus of the solitary tract and the paraventricular hypothalamic nucleus are the principal regulators. Critical connections are formed early in development between the ANS and limbic system that modulate psychological and physiological responses. Autonomic responses play an important role in anesthesia and surgery in the neonates.

13.2 Developmental Neuroanatomy of the ANS

Early in gestation, fetal heart rate is high, under control of sympathetic nervous system and peripheral chemoreceptors. As the fetus grows, parasympathetic system matures, heart rate (HR) decreases and its variability becomes more pronounced [1].

S. Arora (✉)
Dr Baba Saheb Ambedkar Medical College and Hospital, New Delhi, India

© The Author(s), under exclusive license to Springer Nature Singapore Pte Ltd. 2023
U. Saha (ed.), *Clinical Anesthesia for the Newborn and the Neonate*,
https://doi.org/10.1007/978-981-19-5458-0_13

247

13.2.1 The Limbic System Includes the Amygdala, Thalamus, Fornix, Olfactory Cortex, Hippocampus, Hypothalamus, and Cingulate Gyrus

During early gestation, these structures develop multiple interconnections, and connections to the medullary ANS center, thereby modulating changes in the cardio vascular system, respiratory system, and gastrointestinal systems. The development of the limbic system is influenced by the "intrauterine milieu," including maternal health and stress hormone levels before and during pregnancy.

Throughout the life, connections of the limbic system strengthen or weaken in response to the environment, stress, and other exposures. This plasticity plays an important role in life.

13.2.2 Amygdala

The amygdala is related to the neuropsychiatric development, memory associations, survival instincts, and mood. It receives sensory inputs from both thalamus and cerebral cortex and records the emotional responses to an exposure, enabling a beneficial response in the event of re-exposure. Memory of a stressor or negative event activates medullary sympathetic center and responses [increase in heart rate, blood pressure, and muscle responsiveness]. Parasympathetic center (nucleus ambiguus) puts a "vagal brake" dampening the sympathetic physiologic responses [1].

13.2.3 Hippocampus

Hippocampus is important for memory and mood regulation and can shut off the stress response when needed. Chronic stress is associated with mood disorders and aggression. Depression is associated with activation of amygdala and hypothalamus, and inhibition of hippocampus, mediated through cortisol release [1].

13.2.4 Primitive Unmyelinated Vagal Nerve

The primitive unmyelinated vagal nerve develops first but has not much influence prior to 25 weeks of gestation. Maturation occurs in the 3rd trimester with a steep increase in vagal tone near term, that continues during the infancy period [2–4].

Under conditions of fetal stress and hypoxia, bradycardia is the primary response, as nucleus ambiguus may not be mature enough to provide the 'vagal brake', depending upon the gestational age. The normal parasympathetic tone is evidenced as increased HR variability (HRV) in term newborns. With increasing postnatal age, there is progressive parasympathetic influence on the resting HR.

13.2.5 Sympathetic System

The sympathetic system grows steadily and matures earlier than the parasympathetic nervous system and plays an important role in maintaining heart rate and blood pressure during the fetal life.

In premature newborns the increase in parasympathetic tone gets dampened, and there is sympathetic predominance, with potential short- and long-term health implications.

13.2.6 Development Milestones of the ANS: [1]

1. Towards the end of 2nd trimester, parasympathetic maturation occurs, with differentiation of the lateral zone of the hypothalamus and increasing myelination of vagal nerve fibers.
2. 32 weeks onwards, vagal modulatory capacity enhances, seen as baroreflex responsiveness and occurrence of sinus arrhythmias. Simultaneous sympathetic maturation is evidenced by the HR accelerations in response to fetal movements.
3. Late 3rd trimester is characterized by increase in HR patterns (sinus arrhythmia from fetal thoracic movements) and synchronization of accelerative HRV with increasing fetal activity.
4. During its development the ANS is highly vulnerable to various exposures, affecting its growth and maturation trajectory, limiting its responsive capacity. Prematurity, growth restriction, and environmental stress cause dysmaturation of the ANS and resultant autonomic imbalance.

13.3   Evaluation of the ANS Using HR

Autonomic function can be measured noninvasively from physiologic signals of heart rate, respiratory rate, and blood pressure. Heart Rate Variability (HRV) (fluctuation in R–R intervals), provides a measure of sympathetic and parasympathetic interplay, and ANS maturity. High-frequency HRV reflects parasympathetic function and is influenced by the respiratory rate, while low-frequency HRV is due to a combination of sympathetic and parasympathetic inputs and baroreflex-induced changes. Atropine blocks almost all HRV.

With maturation of the parasympathetic function (vagal myelination), there is greater high-frequency HRV, and hence is a reliable marker for ANS function in the newborn. This is an indicator of sinus arrhythmia, i.e., beat-to-beat HRV in response to the amplitude of chest wall movements with respiration [5, 6].

13.4   Impaired Vagal Balance: Polyvagal Theory

The polyvagal theory was first proposed by Stephen Porges in 1995 and relates the development of the vagal system to social and emotional development. It focuses on the role of two efferent branches (old and new) of the vagal nerve from the medulla. The older branch (unmyelinated) arises from the dorsal motor nucleus of the vagus and the newer (myelinated) from the nucleus ambiguus. The social responses (social behavior and mood regulation) are mediated either by vagal input or withdrawal through the components of the limbic system. This Social Engagement System ('face-heart' connection) develops only by 6 months of age and is immature in preterm infants. It has no role in a neonate [7].

Vagal imbalance influences a broad range of neuropsychiatric disorders later in life. Decreased parasympathetic tone is implicated in anxiety, depression, post-traumatic stress disorder and schizophrenia, with unopposed sympathetic responses to fear or stress. In prematurely born neonates, the Social Engagement System remains immature, with lack of proper social cues to trigger normal coregulation with the parent or care-giver.

13.5   Impact of Maternal Factors on ANS Maturation

Maternal stress during pregnancy has significant effects on fetal development and neonatal outcome, depending on the timing and severity of stress. Stress results in increase in cortisol, norepinephrine and inflammation, affecting fetal environment and its growth and maturation, in the form of increased risk of preterm birth and neonatal morbidity, and low birth weight [8]. Studies have shown that:

- Premature babies born to mothers who smoked during pregnancy had higher sympathetic and lower parasympathetic function, and less cardiac autonomic adaptability compared to babies of nonsmoking mothers [9].
- Neonates exposed to opioids prenatally had higher HRV, sympathetic and parasympathetic tones compared to nonexposed newborns [10].
- Children exposed to opiates in utero have reduced social maturity at 3 years of age, compared to those not exposed. Children born to opiate-addicted mothers have increased incidence of hyperactivity, aggressiveness, and ADHD at schoolage.

Important Points for the Caretaker:
- First 6 months of age are fundamental for maturation of the parasympathetic nervous system.
- Noise, light, pain, and hypoxia, common stimuli in the neonatal period, are associated with increased sympathetic activity and physiological instability.
- Premature newborns have greater difficulty decelerating their accelerated heart-beat.
- Proper body positioning is necessary especially in premature neonates who are unable to resist the force of gravity to maintain a midline body alignment or

physiologic flexion position on their own, all of which are fundamental to adequate neurological development.
- Improper positioning is a source of stress affecting autonomic control and behavior.
- Prone position is associated with least stress, as evidenced by lowest salivary cortisol levels in this position in preterm babies [5].
- In NICU, body positioning, autonomic control and environmental stress occur simultaneously.

13.6 Adrenergic and Cholinergic Receptors

13.6.1 Adrenergic Receptors [11]

These mediate the effects of epinephrine and nor epinephrine and have an important role in regulation of myocardial function. Adrenoceptors are divided into three major classes: alpha-1 (1A, 1B, 1D), alpha-2, and beta (β1, β2).

alpha-1 receptors are in the blood vessels (vasoconstriction) and cardiac muscles (contraction) and alpha-2 in cerebral cortex and regulate central sympathetic activity.

β1 are mainly found in the cardiac muscles and pacemaker fibers and have inotropic and chronotropic effect. β2 are found in the smooth muscles of blood vessels, bronchi and bronchioles, myometrium, GIT. urinary bladder muscles, and pupils and stimulation causes relaxation or dilatation. They also reduce platelet aggregation and increase hepatic glycogenolysis. The β2 mediated cAMP dependent myocardial contractility is only seen in neonates. β3 are found in the adipose tissue and cause lipolysis.

13.6.2 Muscarinic Receptors [6]

Muscarinic receptors are widely distributed throughout the human body. They mediate distinct physiological functions according to their location and subtype (five subtypes—M1–M5). M1, M2 and M4 are prejunctional receptors. M2 and M4 inhibit the release of Ach, whereas M1 facilitates the release:

1. Urinary bladder: detrusor muscle is predominantly under parasympathetic control (M1 receptors). Anticholinergics (atropine) inhibit its contraction.
2. Salivary glands have M1 and M3 receptors and parotid glands have M3 receptors.
3. GIT: gut smooth muscles have all five muscarinic receptor subtypes in differing proportions. M2 receptors contribute to GI muscles contractility.
4. Brain: muscarinic receptor activation modulates neuronal excitability, synaptic plasticity and regulation of Ach release. All five muscarinic receptor subtypes are present.
5. Eye: all five subtypes exist (in ciliary muscles, iris sphincter, trabecular meshwork). 60–75% are M3.
6. Heart has M1, M2 and M3 receptors (effect on HR, pacemaker activity, AV conduction and in the coronaries.

Nicotinic Acetylcholine Receptors (nAChRs) Sites:
1. **Nervous system**: central and peripheral ANS signal transmission.
2. **Neuromuscular junction**: control muscle contraction.
3. **Immune system**: regulating inflammatory process.

13.7 Stress Response in Neonates

Fetal parasympathetic (nicotinic and muscarinic) receptors mature with gestational age. By the 3rd trimester, cholinergic mechanisms are functional and control vascular tone. The central cholinergic system is well-developed by the time of birth.

In utero, stress initiates pulmonary vasoconstriction (and increase in R–L shunting through Foramen Ovale and Ductus arteriosus), and dilatation of ductus venosus, directing blood away from the liver to the vital organs (heart, brain and placenta).

At birth, stress creates abnormalities in the adaptation process with persistent fetal circulation (PFC) and/or persistent pulmonary hypertension of newborn (PPHN), effect of pulmonary vasospasm.

Hormonal response in neonates is different from adults. Stress induced increase in serum cortisol and growth hormone levels is much higher and slow to return to baseline levels, in neonates (24–48 h postoperatively). The neuroendocrine reflex is mediated through the afferent arc (nociceptors, chemoreceptors and baroceptors) that signal the CNS, and the efferent arc from the hypothalamus (release of catecholamines, adrenocorticoids, vasopressin and prolactin) that produce the response.

In neonates, with already immature body systems, and high energy consuming growth, maturation and metabolism, the nutrient reserves are already limited. They are unable to meet the further increase in demand following stress of surgery or illness, with higher morbidity and mortality, compared to children and adults, in similar circumstances.

The metabolic response to surgery in neonates is evident with decrease in plasma values of zinc, copper and magnesium when measured postoperatively. The fall is due to increased urinary losses, that continues up to 24 h.

Fetal stress (fetal distress) can be diagnosed by measuring ß-endorphins and ACTH levels in the amniotic fluid, and in cord blood (at birth) which are elevated. These hormones also increase following stress in neonates (surgery, septic shock).

Norepinephrine is the dominant catecholamine secreted by fetal and neonatal chromaffin tissue in times of stress. Changes in norepinephrine levels is similar to as in adults, but epinephrine levels may fall during surgery, only to rise in the postoperative period [12, 13].

Halothane and fentanyl-based anesthesia can ablate these responses, suggesting pain to be the chief cause.

Epinephrine stimulates the metabolic response in the form of hepatic gluconeogenesis and decreased peripheral utilization of glucose, increased glucagon secretion, and decreased insulin release, and consequent hyperglycemia. Glycogenolysis in the skeletal muscles produces lactate and pyruvate. Normal response to hyperglycemia is by release of endogenous insulin to maintain glucose homeostasis as seen in term neonates but lacking in preterms because of decreased responsiveness of pancreatic ß cells or due to direct inhibition of insulin secretion by epinephrine released during surgery. Poor insulin response explains the development of greater hyperglycemia and rapid increase in plasma osmolality during and after surgery, unopposed catabolism in the postoperative period in preterm neonates. There is also decreased release of corticosteroid hormones, and increased secretion of steroid precursors [14].

13.8 Key Features of Autonomic Nervous System

1. Neonates do not have the adult circadian cycle of plasma cortisol levels (neuroendocrine immaturity).
2. Cortisol and ACTH responses to stress (surgical, biochemical) is less in neonates than infants.
3. Within 9 days of birth, the response is more rapid, but amounts of cortisol released following surgical stress is much less.

After surgery, trauma or stress, a brief period of reduction in metabolism is followed by increase in metabolism and O_2 consumption. Similar response is seen in neonates, but increased metabolism is not related to the intensity of stress unlike in adults; rather it is a function of the caloric intake.

In healthy term neonates, O_2 consumption increases with postnatal age in the first few weeks of life. Fetal energy requirement is met with carbohydrate utilization and post birth 80% calories come from fat (fat depots are 10–15% of neonatal body weight). This is of significance, because newborn baby has glycogen reserves for only 10–12 h and whenever fasted, must be provided with parenteral glucose supplements to maintain normal blood sugar level. Immature hepatic glycogenolysis, insulin secretion, hormone induced reduced glucose utilization, and altered GI function, are responsible for hypoglycemia in a starving baby, and in the preoperative period [7].

13.9 Clinical Implications of Stress-Related Hyperglycemia in Neonates

Catecholamines play an important role in stress response modulation by affecting hormonal and metabolic changes, inhibiting release of insulin, causing hyperglycemia, and inducing catabolic responses (lipolysis, proteolysis).

Plasma osmolality: XE "Plasma osmolality" : increase of >25 mOsm/kg over a short period (3–4 h) can adversely affect renal and cerebral cortex and precipitate intracranial hypertension (ICH).

- Hyperglycemia provides additional glucose as energy substrate to meet the increased metabolic demands in the postoperative period, with better outcome.
- Stress induced proteolysis provides amino acid for healing and reparative process in the injured tissues.
- Brain and skeletal muscles can utilize ketone bodies as alternative metabolic substrate. Stress induced lipolysis and ketone bodies production, serves the purpose, allowing available glucose as substrate for organs dependent on glucose only.

Note: Hypermetabolic response can have adverse effects in the surgical neonate by increase in oxygen consumption, increased oxygen and energy requirement, hyperthermia, increased cardiac output to meet the demand, and altered inflammatory and immune response.

13.10 Separation Anxiety

This is a developmental stage in which the child gets anxious on separation from the caretaker or mother. The response occurs in three phases—protest, despair, and detachment. This can progress on to separation anxiety disorder (SAD) which is a serious emotional disorder characterized by extreme distress on separation from the mother [15, 16]

Adverse Effects of Separation Anxiety:
- Higher postoperative pain and analgesics requirement
- Prolonged postoperative stay
- Higher incidence of emergence delirium, sleep disturbances maladaptation and behavioral changes, lasting from days to weeks after surgery

Separation Anxiety in Neonates:
- Separation anxiety develops by 3–4 months of age when the child begins to recognize faces and is not seen or evident in neonates.
- However, child may develop long term behavioral problems later in life from effects of separation from the mother or care giver [16].
- Even though not supported by scientific literature, neonates should be handled with utmost care in the perioperative period, taking into consideration the postoperative and long term sequelae of separation anxiety.

13.11 Pain Stress

Neonates have well-developed neural pathways for pain. The density of cutaneous nociceptive receptors is equivalent to that in adults. The cutaneous nociceptors are present throughout the skin and mucosal surfaces by 20th week and neural connections by the 25th week of gestation. At birth, the pain inhibitory pathways are immature suggesting greater pain sensation in neonates than older children and adults.

Poor pain management in the neonates has been associated with various short- and long-term negative physiological and psychological consequences. Preterm (<32 weeks) neonates display blunted HR response to acute pain in the first week of life due to poor responsiveness of the immature CVS system and parasympathetic predominance. By 3 weeks, the neonate begins to exhibit tachycardic response to pain. Response is normal in neonates born after 32 weeks of gestation right since birth [17, 18]

13.12 ANS Concerns During Surgery and Anaesthesia

1. **Bradycardia and HR related**:

   Baseline HR in neonates is high 140–160/min. It increases further in the pre-operative period due to stress. Response to any stressor is predominantly parasympathetic, and bradycardia. Stressors include sepsis, hypoxia, pain, any procedure performed, placement of IV line, laryngoscopy, intubation, any other airway manipulation, surgical pathology and surgery, fluid losses and shifts, blood loss and anemia, etc.

   Neonates cannot increase myocardial contractility, and their cardiac output is HR dependent. Bradycardia is poorly tolerated and is always accompanied by hypotension, and poor tissue perfusion, altered drug kinetics and dynamics, and delayed recovery after anesthesia.

   Primary goal is to maintain HR (120–160/min) while suppressing detrimental stress responses during surgery and anesthesia. This goal can be achieved using anticholinergic drugs pre induction, balanced anesthesia with adequate depth and analgesia (narcotics, NSAIDs, regional techniques), and avoiding or use with caution drugs and techniques that cause bradycardia (propofol, succinylcholine, vecuronium) laryngoscopy and tracheal intubation, maintaining oxygenation, intravascular volume, hemoglobin and O_2 carrying capacity with timely blood transfusion, reducing the surgical stress, and vigilant monitoring.

   Equally important is prevention of tachycardia (>180/min) which increases O_2 and metabolic demand in babies already under stress or deficiency.

2. **Respiratory related**

   Neonates have low O_2 reserves, low FRC, basal tachypnea (RR 40–60/min) and poor tolerance for apnea. The initial response is bradycardia. They desaturate very fast. The muscles of respiration are immature with less contractile element and fatigue easily. Central compensatory responses to hypoxia and hypercarbia are not fully functional. Anesthetic drugs further cause suppression of respiration. Always assist or control ventilation during general anesthesia. Trachea and airway are narrow, prone to edema, spasm and further narrowing with increased work of breathing and O_2 demand. Always secure the airway, using appropriate sized supraglottic device or tracheal tube.

Maintenance of oxygenation is of paramount importance. Low FiO_2 may be associated with risk of hypoxemia and desaturation, while high FiO_2 is associated with the risk of BPD and ROP. Use minimum FiO_2 to maintain saturation more than 90%.

3. **Transitional changes related**

Babies are at risk of reverting to fetal circulation and reopening of shunts in the neonatal period. Avoiding factors that increase the risk (high pulmonary vascular resistance) and adopting those that prevent decrease in peripheral vascular resistance is advocated.

Note:

(i) Only essential surgeries should be conducted in this age group of patients and that too by experienced staff so as to reduce unnecessary high morbidity and mortality.

(ii) Vigilance monitoring and knowledge is the key to success by avoiding all risk factors and undue autonomic responses.

13.13 Conclusion

The most important actions of the ANS of concern to the anesthesiologists, are the effects on the CVS hemodynamics (via modulation of HR and vascular tone), maintaining vascular tone and cardiac activity, on the pulmonary vasculature, bronchi and bronchioles, on the GI smooth muscles, detrusor muscles in the bladder and on the metabolism. Most abnormalities relating to these systems become evident by the changes in HR and Blood pressure, two most important basic parameters monitored intraoperatively. Drugs acting on the sympathetic and parasympathetic receptors can be used for maintaining normality during anesthesia. Immaturity of the ANS at birth and in the neonatal period, may not always produces predictable effects of the hyper or hypoactivity of the components of ANS, and also of the drugs so used. Continuous monitoring and vigil, while using ones knowledge, can aid the anesthetist in improving outcome from anesthesia and surgery in the neonates, especially the preterm, small birth weight and those critically ill babies.

References

1. Mulkey SB, et al. Autonomic nervous system development and its impact on neuropsychiatric Outcome. Pediatr Res. 2019;85(2):120–6.
2. Porges SW, Furman SA. The early development of the autonomic nervous system provides a neural platform for social behavior: a polyvagal perspective. Infant Child Dev. 2011;20:106–18.
3. Reed SF, Ohel G, David R, Porges SW. A neural explanation of fetal heart rate patterns: a test of the Polyvagal Theory. Dev Psychobiol. 1999;35:108–18.
4. Clairambault J, et al. Heart rate variability in normal sleeping full-term and preterm neonates. Early Hum Dev. 1992;28:169–83.

5. Cardoso S, Silva MJ, Guimaraes H. Autonomic nervous system in newborns: a review based on heart rate variability. Childs Nerv Syst. 2017;33(7):1053–63. https://doi.org/10.1007/s00381-017-3436-8. Epub 2017 May 13.

6. Young HA, et al. Heart-rate variability: a biomarker to study the influence of nutrition on physiological and psychological health? Behav Pharmacol. 2018;29:140–51.

7. Porges SW. The polyvagal theory: New insights into adaptive reactions of the autonomic nervous system. Cleve Clin J Med. 2009;76(Suppl 2):S86–90. https://doi.org/10.3949/ccjm.76.s2.17.

8. Su Q, Zhang H, Zhang Y, Zhang H, Ding D, et al. Maternal stress in gestation: birth outcomes and stress-related hormone response of the neonates. Pediatr Neonatol. 2015;56:376–81.

9. Gomes ELFD, Santos CM, Santos ACS, et al. Autonomic responses of premature newborns to body position and environmental noise in the neonatal intensive care unit. Rev Bras Ter Intensiva. 2019;31(3):296–302. Epub Oct 14, 2019. https://doi.org/10.5935/0103-507x.20190054.

10. Mao C, Lv J, Li H, Chen Y, et al. Development of fetal nicotine and muscarinic receptors in utero. Braz J Med Biol Res. 2007;40(5):735–41.

11. Bevan JC. Metabolic response to surgery in children. Baillieres Clin Anaesthesiol. 1989;3(2):349–64.

12. Fifer WP, Fingers ST, Youngman M, Gomez-Gribben E, Myers MM. Effects of alcohol and smoking during pregnancy on infant autonomic control. Dev Psychobiol. 2009;51(3):234–42.

13. Abrams P, Andersson KE, Buccafusco JJ, Chapple C, et al. Muscarinic receptors: their distribution and function in body systems, and the implications for treating overactive bladder. Br J Pharmacol. 2006;148(5):565–78.

14. Spiss CK, Maze M. Adrenoreceptors. Rev Anaesthesist. 1985;34(1):1–10.

15. Milosavljevic SB, Pavlovic AP, Trpkovic SV, Ilic AN, et al. Influence of spinal and general anesthesia on the metabolic, hormonal, and hemodynamic response in elective surgical patients. Med Sci Monit. 2014;20:1833–40.

16. Eisen AR, Schaefer CE. Separation anxiety in children and adolescents: an individualized approach to assessment and treatment. Psychology. Guilford Press; 2007.

17. Anand KJS, Hansen D. Hormonal-Metabolic stress responses in neonates undergoing cardiac surgery. Anesthesiology. 1990;73:661–70.

18. Prevention and Management of Pain and Stress in the Neonate. American Academy of Pediatrics Committee on Fetus and Newborn Committee on Drugs Section on Anesthesiology Section on Surgery, Canadian Paediatric Society Fetus and Newborn Committee. Pediatrics 2000; 105 (2). Downloaded from www.aappublications.org/news on August 7, 2021.

Ventilation and Ventilatory Modes in Neonates

14

Deepanjali Pant and Jayashree Sood

14.1 Introduction

Incredible advances in neonatal intensive care and appearance of neonatal intensive care units (NICU), over the last few decades, have allowed survival of extremely premature as well as critically ill neonates. In this context, neonatal mechanical ventilation (MV) is an integral component in the respiratory care continuum for their survival. In June 2020, the world's tiniest baby, 212 g, 25 week gestation, was delivered by cesarean section at National University Hospital, Singapore. Her chances of survival were grim. After great care for 13 months, she was discharged, weighing 6.3 kg, in August 2021, though she does have pulmonary hypertension (PHT) and chronic lung disease [1].

In the last three decades, the role of MV in NICU has evolved from the phase of restricted or no access to ventilator, to the use of paediatric volume ventilation with adult ventilators, to the present day of highly sophisticated dedicated neonatal ventilators. In the USA, there has been a remarkable decrease in respiratory distress syndrome (RDS)-related infant mortality from 268 to 98 per 100,000 live-births from 1971 to 1985, and to 17 per 100,000 live-births in 2007. The reasons are multi-factorial, but improvement in ventilator technology, its understanding and application by the concerned caretakers, is a major game changer [2, 3].

Thus, it is essential for the health professionals involved in the neonatal care (neonatologist, anesthesiologist, trainees, nurses, technical staff), both in OT and in NICU, to have the basic and the updated knowledge about essentials of ventilation to support the neonate's respiratory system during period of compromise while limiting long-term complications, as well as in the care and maintenance of the sophisticated, expensive ventilators and other related equipment.

D. Pant (✉) · J. Sood
Institute of Anaesthesiology, Pain and Perioperative Medicine, Sir Ganga Ram Hospital, New Delhi, India

© The Author(s), under exclusive license to Springer Nature Singapore Pte Ltd. 2023
U. Saha (ed.), *Clinical Anesthesia for the Newborn and the Neonate*, https://doi.org/10.1007/978-981-19-5458-0_14

This chapter will cover the understanding of the basic principles of neonatal ventilation, the range of existing ventilatory modes and the decision-making strategies, for their suitable application in the critically sick term and preterm newborns and neonates. Also included are ventilatory requirement during newborn resuscitation and during transport of sick neonates for surgical emergencies to the operating room and to and from the NICU.

Note: Since the neonatal physiology has been covered in detail in previous chapters, this section will only stress on the respiratory physiology and mechanics of clinical relevance for respiratory support.

14.2   Relevant Terminologies

1. **Compliance (C)** is the change in volume (ΔV) per unit of change in pressure (ΔP) and is expressed in mL/cm H_2O (volume/pressure = $\Delta V/\Delta P$). It is a measure of elasticity or distensibility of respiratory structures, both the pulmonary parenchyma and the chest wall. Low compliance means reduced distensibility or stiffness and will need a higher pressure gradient to bring about the same change in volume or for pushing the air inside. Volume–Pressure curves graphically display this relationship.

    Surfactant deficient lungs as in the prematures creates a condition of low compliance, whereas BPD has areas of both low (under distended) and high compliance (over distended).

2. **Airway resistance (R_{aw})** is the change in pressure per unit change in flow and is expressed in cm $H_2O/L/s$ (Pressure/Flow). R_{aw} is the opposition to gas flow, which depends on the radius and the length the airway, the type of flow (laminar or turbulent) and density and viscosity of the gas. Resistance is usually lower during inspiration when the lung distending forces increase the diameter of tracheobronchial tree [4]. During MV, endotracheal tube (ETT) is the most important contributor to R_{aw} and is displayed by Flow–Volume curve.

3. **Elastance (E)** is the measure of the ease of the recoil tendency and is the reciprocal of compliance. The low compliant alveoli inflate with difficulty but deflate easily, and such alveolar units are prone to atelectasis.

4. **FRC** is the volume of gas that remains in the lung after normal expiration. Low FRC impinges on to closing volume and affects optimum gaseous exchange.

5. **Time constant (T = tau—Greek letter)** is used in engineering and physics. It is time taken for the system response to decay to zero if the initial rate of decay was maintained. In one **tau**, the function reaches 37% of its initial value and after 5 time constants, it reaches a value of less than 1%. When applied to respiratory physiology it measures how quickly the lungs inflate or deflate and is a factor of both compliance and resistance (Compliance x Resistance). One **tau** is the time taken to empty 63% of its initial volume, and in 3 time constants, 95% emptying of the lungs takes place. Inspiratory **tau** is shorter than expiratory **tau** because of airway distension during inspiration. Graphic display of flows help to judge the appropriateness of the chosen inspiratory (T_I) and expi-

ratory (T_E) times for the given clinical situation [5]. For example, in RDS, stiff lung with low compliance and low resistance has a short **tau**, thus will empty quickly, and can be ventilated with high respiratory rates (RR). Conversely, in BPD, the highly compliant lung and high resistance has a long **tau**, and needs a longer time to fill and empty, thus needing lower RR.

6. **Physiological dead space (V_{DS})** consists of anatomical and alveolar dead space (Vd) gases that do not take part in gas exchange. Anatomical Vd is the volume of air within the conducting airways and is approximately 1.5 mL/kg. During MV, the mechanical Vd (tube connector, flow sensor, Y-piece) is fixed, and total Vd (anatomical + mechanical) is proportionally larger in preterm neonates than in term neonates [6]. Minimal mechanical Vd is desirable as excessive Vd can cause rebreathing and CO_2 retention. Alveolar Vd is constituted by the gas in the areas of underperfused alveoli.

7. **Wasted ventilation,** ratio of V_{DS} to V_T (V_{DS}/V_T), is the proportion of tidal volume that does not participate in gas exchange. A high V_{DS}:V_T ratio as in rapid shallow breathing is clinically relevant.

8. **Work of breathing (WOB):** the transdiaphragmatic pressure–time product estimates WOB and energy expenditure of diaphragmatic muscles.

9. **Fraction of inspired oxygen** (FiO_2) is expressed as in fraction of 1 or %, where FiO_2 of 1 = 100% O_2.

10. **Flow of gas** (L/min) is the flow of the delivered gas, that generates the inflating pressure during inspiration. The ventilator measures both inspiratory and expiratory flows.

11. **Peak inspiratory pressure/peak inflating pressure (PIP)** is the peak pressure reached during inspiration and ideally should be <20 cm H_2O. It affects both oxygenation and alveolar ventilation.

12. **Positive end-expiratory Pressure (PEEP),** the pressure at the end of expiration, maintains FRC by preventing the alveolar collapse. PEEP can be minimal, optimal or maximal. Normal range should be 4–6 cm H_2O (optimal PEEP).

13. **Pressure gradient (Δ P) (PIP–PEEP)**, between the mouth (airway opening) and the alveoli drives the gas flow during inspiration and expiration and is a function of C and R_{aw}. Tidal volume (V_T) is proportional to ΔP [7].

14. **Mean airway pressure (MAP)** is the average airway pressure during the entire respiratory cycle and is determined by PIP, PEEP, inspiratory and expiratory times, and gas flows. MAP influences the adequacy of alveolar recruitment and oxygenation. MAP = (RR × Ti/60) × (PIP–PEEP) + PEEP. During MV, MAP is measured by the ventilator, whereas in HFOV, it is a ventilator setting.

15. **Oxygenation index (OI)** determines the O_2 demand (FiO_2 (%) × MAP/PaO_2). As the oxygenation improves, higher PaO_2 can be achieved with a lower FiO_2. OI is a criterion for nitric oxide (NO) therapy and/or ECMO in sick neonates and assesses the severity of respiratory failure and persistent PHT of newborn (PPHN).

16. **Noninvasive O_2 saturation index (OSI)** can be used instead of OI. It is calculated as MAP × FiO_2/SpO_2.

17. **Tidal volume (V_T)** is the volume of air/gas inspired or delivered per breath (range 4–6 mL/kg).
18. **RR** is the number of breaths taken or delivered in a minute.
19. **Minute volume** is the total volume of air/gas inspired or delivered to the lungs per minute (L/min) = V_T(mL) × RR. It quantifies CO_2 elimination. The average value is 0.2–0.3 L/min/kg in healthy neonates. The alarm limits are set 10–20% above and below this range during MV.
20. **Inspiratory time (T_I)** is the duration of inspiration (0.30–0.40 s). Increasing Ti can improve oxygenation in stiff lungs [5].
21. **Expiratory time (T_E)** is the duration of expiration. Normally T_E is twice T_I.
22. **I:E ratio** is the ratio of T_I to T_E and should be set as I:E::1:2. It is determined by RR and T_I.
23. **Trigger threshold** is the sensitivity of the ventilator to patient's inspiratory gas flow rate, to initiate a ventilator breath.
24. **Leak (L)** is the gas lost from the ventilatory circuit. It is the difference between inspired and expired volumes.
25. **Frequency (f)** is measured in hertz (Hz) in high-frequency ventilation (HFV). 1 Hz = 60 oscillations. Normal range: 8–10 Hz.
26. **Amplitude/Delta P/power** is the variation in pressure generated across the MAP and affects chest wiggle/bounce and controls CO_2 levels in HFOV.

14.3 Major Indications for Mechanical Ventilation

Despite the growing interest in non-invasive respiratory support strategies traditional MV (invasive) remains the cornerstone of advanced respiratory support for the critically ill neonates in NICU. Approximately 60–80% of very premature neonates require MV at some point during their hospital stay [8]. The common indications are:

(a) **Apnea of prematurity**: poor respiratory drive leading to multiple apneic episodes (≥6 episodes/min requiring stimulation) associated with bradycardia and desaturation or more than one episode requiring positive pressure ventilation (PPV) within a 6 h period.
(b) **Inadequate gas exchange** (oxygenation and CO_2 elimination) indicated as acidosis (pH <7.2) with hypercarbia ($PaCO_2$ >65 mmHg) or requiring high FiO_2 (>0.4–0.5) to achieve target SpO_2.
(c) **Overwhelming WOB** and **hemodynamic instability.**
(d) **Need for surfactant replacement.**

14.4 Potential Risks of Mechanical Ventilation

Though MV is a life-saving intervention, it can be associated with acute or chronic injury to the respiratory tract, brain, and other organ systems. Ventilator induced lung injury (VILI) can result from excessive pressure (**barotrauma**), over distension of alveoli (**volutrauma**), cyclic collapse and reopening of alveoli (**atelectrauma**) and use of high FiO$_2$ (**biotrauma**) [9]. Macroscopic mechanical lung injury manifests as air leaks such as pneumothorax, pneumomediastinum, pulmonary interstitial emphysema and microscopic as increased leakage of fluid into alveolar space and impaired gas exchange. The most critical determinant of VILI appears to be the end-inspiratory lung volume. Volutrauma has gained a larger role than barotrauma in neonates [10, 11]. Volutrauma results in endothelial and peripheral airway injury, hypocarbia, and increased likelihood of periventricular leukomalacia (PVL) in low birth weight (LBW) neonates [12].

Neonates, especially preterm, are at risk of O$_2$ toxicity due to their immature antioxidative system [13]. In addition, high FiO$_2$ can promote absorption atelectasis, reduction in FRC, contributing to development of BPD and ROP [14]. Recent large, randomized trials suggest that pre-ductal SaO$_2$ of 90–95% vs. 85–89% increases survival without increased risk of necrotizing enterocolitis (NEC) [15].

14.5 Broad Principles of Neonatal Ventilation

The goal of neonatal ventilation is to facilitate gas exchange, without causing lung injury, hemodynamic instability and secondary injury to the brain and other organs.
The strategic principles to achieve this include:

- Preferential and early use of non-invasive respiratory support so as to avoid need of MV
- Irregular respiratory pattern leads to ventilator asynchrony, high airway pressure, poor oxygenation, and fluctuation in intracranial pressure (ICP). Hence. synchronized or patient triggered ventilation should be preferred [16]
- Lung protective strategies should be used for invasive MV [17]
- Preferential use of volume targeted ventilation (VTV) with low TV (4–6 mL/kg) minimizes volutrauma. However, too less or suboptimal TV, consequent hypoventilation, hypercapnia and hypoxemia should be avoided [18]
- Adequate PEEP maintains lung recruitment, avoids atelectasis, and acts as a stent to collapsed airways in tracheobronchomalacia [19, 20]
- Avoid high FiO$_2$ [21]
- Gas exchange targets should not aim for normal PaCO$_2$ level, modest permissive hypercapnia is acceptable [22]
- Increase in use of HFV as a primary mode in neonates at risk of VILI, or as a rescue mode for neonates with refractory respiratory failure while on CMV [23]

14.6 Modes of Mechanical Ventilation (MV)

There are various modes of MV with different terminologies in different models. Thus, it is essential to have a thorough knowledge of the ventilators in clinical practice. Broadly, MV can be categorized as conventional MV (CMV) or high frequency ventilation (HFV), with distinct subcategories in each. Adjunct therapies such as inhaled nitric oxide (iNO) and ECMO are used as rescue therapies for specific cases.

(i). **Conventional** MV **(CMV)** is used more frequently than HFV. The common feature of different subtypes of CMV is intermittent gas exchange with normal physiological settings. Various CMV modes such as IMV, SIMV, ACV, PSV are available in almost all ventilators and two neonatal modes have been added, VTV and NAVA. The appropriate ventilation mode and settings are individualized based on the clinical condition, the disease process, response to previous ventilator support, availability of equipment and user expertise. CMV modes are categorized based on three factors:

(a) **Initiation of breath—controlled:** breath is initiated by a timing mechanism unrelated to spontaneous inspiratory effort, or **Synchronized:** breath triggered by patient inspiratory effort.
(b) **Control of gas flow—pressure controlled**: delivers a predetermined pressure, or **Volume controlled**: delivers a predetermined tidal volume.
(c) **Limitation of each breath—time-cycled**: inspiration is terminated at a preset time, or **flow-cycled**: inspiration is terminated with cessation of inspiratory flow.

(ii). **Volume control ventilation (VCV)** is not suitable in neonates. In VCV the ventilator delivers a constant flow of gas into the ventilator circuit. Pressure rises passively and reaches the peak just before expiration which occurs as soon as the set V_T is delivered. V_T is the primary control variable and inflation/airway pressure is a derived variable. The set V_T is measured at the proximal (ventilator) end of the circuit. In older children with cuffed ETT the correlation between the set V_T and the V_T reaching the lungs is quite reasonable. In neonates and especially ELBW babies, much of the set V_T is lost to gas compression in the ventilator circuit and leak around uncuffed ETT. Thus, to deliver the required V_T; higher V_T needs to be set. However, since ETT leak and degree of loss of volume to compression varies with PIP, the relationship between set V_T and delivered V_T is not constant. Use of a separate flow sensor to measure exhaled V_T at the airway opening may allow frequent manual adjustments of set V_T to deliver the desired amount. However, variable ETT leak makes it an unreliable approach and clinical assessment of chest rise and breath sounds auscultation for selecting V_T is not reliable [24, 25].

(iii). **Pressure control ventilation (PCV)/pressure limited ventilation (PLV)**: the primary control variable is the inflation pressure and V_T is a dependent variable and changes with compliance. The ventilator delivers a decelerating flow pattern. When the circuit is pressurized, the gas enters the lungs in proportion to the inflation pressure and respiratory compliance. PLV is the standard approach for neonatal MV, but its main disadvantage is the tidal volume variability due to changes in lung dynamics and ventilator circuit mechanics, such as in post-surfactant status, partially blocked ETT and positional leak [26]. Either unacceptably large or small V_T can contribute to volutrauma and atelectrauma, respectively, and $PaCO_2$ fluctuation may contribute to unstable cerebral perfusion and brain injury. However, because it is more widely available, less costly, easier to use, less prone to inadequate tidal delivery and errors from ETT leaks, PLV has become the standard ventilatory mode for neonates, by providing more consistent V_T and reduction in WOB.

(iv). Intermittent mandatory ventilation (IMV) delivers a set number of mandatory breaths at a predetermined rate regardless of neonate's spontaneous respiratory cycle. The spontaneous breaths in between ventilatory breaths can lead to asynchrony between the neonate and the ventilator. IMV is used for neonates requiring maximum respiratory support with minimal spontaneous efforts.

(v). Patient triggered ventilation (PTV), synchronized intermittent mandatory ventilation (SIMV): a set number of mandatory breaths, triggered and synchronized with the neonate's spontaneous breaths, are delivered. The neonate can take additional unassisted spontaneous breaths in between the ventilator delivered breaths. If a breath is not sensed in the set-time period, the ventilator delivers a breath at the end of the set time interval. This mode is extensively used in neonates both for ventilatory and weaning mode [27].

(vi). Patient triggered ventilation (PTV), assist control ventilation (ACV): each spontaneous breath triggers the ventilator to deliver a set time-cycled and pressure-limited breath. A background back up rate is set for the event of apnea with the same settings. Breath limitation is the same regardless of whether a control or assist breath. By reducing the pressure, ACV mode can be used as a weaning mode, while the rate is controlled by the neonate [16].

(vii). Patient triggered ventilation (PTV), pressure support ventilation (PSV) (Fig. 14.1): in this mode, neonate's spontaneous breathing efforts are supported by the ventilator to a preset pressure and breath termination is flow cycled (time cycled in ACV mode). The flow termination sensitivity is set so that the Ti will terminate when neonate's inspiratory flow declines to a predetermined percentage of the peak inspiratory flow. The V_T delivered may vary with each pressure supported breath.

(viii). Pressure support ventilation (PSV) mode is available in newer anaesthesia ventilators, and is commonly used in conjunction with SIMV (SIMV + PSV) to ensure that every spontaneous breath beyond the set SIMV rate is supported to a predetermined fraction of PIP set for the mandatory breaths. This imparts greater support for a neonate who may not be able to manage on SIMV alone. This is an useful weaning mode [28, 29].

Fig. 14.1 Pressure support monitoring

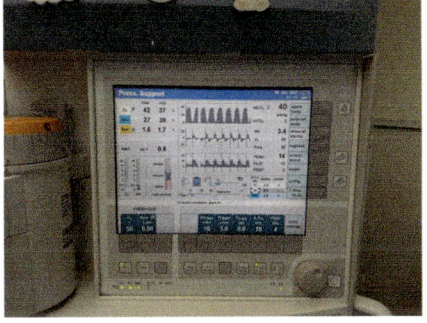

(ix). Volume guarantee ventilation (VGV)/volume targeted ventilation (VTV) is used in PCV modalities and is specifically designed for neonatal ventilation. Failure to distinguish between adult VCV and neonatal VTV has been a major hindrance to its wider acceptance in neonates. VTV targets a user set V_T measured at airway opening with automatic adjustment of PIP in accordance with the changes in pulmonary compliance. It can be used in conjunction with SIMV, ACV or PSV, but synchronized modes that support patient's spontaneous breath (ACV/PSV) are preferred to SIMV. VTV provides a constant flow of gas throughout inspiration producing the characteristic 'square wave' pattern on flow-time graph. The peak pressure and volume delivery occur at the end of inspiration resulting in slower and more uniform lung inflation. This delivery of optimal V_T at the lowest possible pressure avoids the risk of volutrauma, barotrauma and possible hypocarbia [30]. The measured PIP may vary with each breath as the lung compliance changes. VTV may be useful in neonates recovering from respiratory distress and being weaned off ventilation, where the desired V_T will be delivered at a lower PIP.

The algorithm is meant for slower adjustment for low V_T and faster response to potentially dangerous excessive V_T. The recommended V_T targets are based on ACV mode, as with SIMV mode a slightly larger V_T is required for the same alveolar minute ventilation as only a few breaths are supported and volume targeted.

On the contrary, if the lung compliance worsens, the desired V_T may be difficult to deliver at a lower pressure, so the maximum set PIP will be reached. Therefore, it is very important to set an approximate maximum pressure limit in deteriorating lung conditions to avoid lung injury. This ability to deliver a guaranteed and consistent V_T at the lowest pressure and signaling changes in lung compliance is one of the main benefits of this ventilation mode. This autoregulation of inflation pressure leads to automatic weaning too and is considered as a closed-loop ventilation technology [31–33].

The choice of appropriate V_T is the key to success and depends on size, postnatal age and underlying disease process. The largest V_T/kg requirement in the smallest neonates is due to the proportionally larger impact of instrumental dead space (especially 0.7–1 mL for the flow sensor).

(x). Neurally adjusted ventilatory assist (NAVA) is a novel mode of ventilation, is designed to reduce neonate–ventilator asynchrony. Gas delivery from the ventilator is triggered and cycled by interpreting neural signals from the electrical activity of the diaphragm. A specialized nasogastric tube with EMG electrodes is placed in the lower esophagus to receive diaphragmatic EMG signal. NAVA reduces trigger delay, ventilator response time and WOB, and is used as an adjunct to CMV modes (SIMV, SIMV–PS, PSV). Smaller crossover trials have reported lower PIP level with NAVA, but improvement in gas exchange was inconsistent [34, 35]. Its drawback is the need of specialized equipment and clinical expertise.

(xi). High-frequency ventilation (HFV) delivers sub tidal breaths at frequencies much greater than normal physiological range, with a sustained MAP. It can be used as a rescue modality in persistent poor gas exchange despite maximum conventional lung protective strategies or primarily in neonates who require high settings to achieve adequate gas exchange. The two principal forms of HFV are High frequency oscillatory ventilation (HFOV) and High frequency jet ventilation (HFJV).

a. In **HFOV** the positive and negative pressure oscillations are generated by an oscillating linear motor piston or vibrating electromagnetic diaphragm or a combination of servo controlled inspiratory valve and an expiratory venturi jet at a frequency of 8–15 Hz (480–900 bpm) to deliver a small volume (V_T 1.5–2.5 mL/kg) of vibrating gas towards the lungs during inspiration and away during expiration [36]. Expiration is an active process unlike in CMV/HFJV, where it is passive [23].

b. In **HFJV** the gas flow is interrupted by a pneumatic valve to produce short, rapid, high velocity pulses delivered through a port on a specialized ETT adaptor into the inspiratory circuit creating very small V_T (1 mL/kg) at a rate of 4–11 Hz. This is most effective where major problem is CO_2 elimination, as with HFJV it can be achieved more readily at a lower peak and MAP than with HFOV [37]. This is applied parallel to conventional ventilator that provides PEEP and delivers optimal intermittent sigh breaths at 2–10/min, when additional lung recruitment is desired. This differs from low frequency jet ventilation which uses a manually triggered hand-held device. HFOV is more commonly used than HFJV.

(xii). Permissive hypercapnia: Lowering the magnitude of MV while accepting a $PaCO_2$ of more than 40 mmHg is called permissive hypercapnia. Both hypocapnia and hypercapnia as well as $PaCO_2$ fluctuations in initial days of life were associated with IVH in preterm babies. Retrospectively, it was observed that a $PaCO_2$ <30 mmHg before the first dose of surfactant is associated with increased risk of BPD in preterms. Even mild hypocapnia may be deleterious ($PaCO_2$ 35 mmHg) and is reported as main factor for development of PVL [38, 39]. It is prudent to avoid large fluctuations in $PaCO_2$ levels which may be associated with PVL (following hypocapnia) or IVH (following hypercapnia) in preterm neonates. Mild permissive hypercapnia (45–55 mmHg) in VLBW neonates is a suggested ventilation strategy for its safety and protectiveness to reduce pulmonary morbidity. Buffering the acidosis should be restricted when optimal lung protection is desired as many of the biochemical benefits of hypercapnia are mediated by acidosis [40–42].

(xiii). Volume targeted ventilation (VTV) vs Pressure limited ventilation (PLV): the use of VTV in neonates has increased over time as technical advances have allowed more accurate measurement of small V_T and better compensation for ETT leaks. Still, many vulnerable extremely preterm babies continue to be exposed to traditional PLV despite level 1 evidence for safety and efficacy of VTV [43]. Volutrauma (overdistension) caused more lung inflammation and injury than barotrauma (high pressure with excessive stretch) and superiority of VTV over PLV was confirmed in various meta-analyses of clinical trials, which demonstrate improved short term outcomes, but little data on long term neurodevelopmental outcome [44].

A Cochrane systemic review and meta-analyses (2017) of 20 RCTs in 977 neonates, predominantly preterm babies, concluded that VTV offered more benefits than PLV, such as shorter duration of MV, lower incidence of pneumothorax, BPD at 36 weeks, hypocapnia, PVL or grade 3/4 IVH and trends of lower mortality. However, all these trials had considerable heterogeneity with respect to the specific modes used in each arm [29]. During VTV, arterial blood gases were maintained at lower airway pressure, but because of a greater contribution to minute ventilation, their WOB increases, which may delay weaning and extubation [18].

(xiv). **Volume targeted ventilation (VTV) with Patient triggered ventilation (Synchronized intermittent mandatory ventilation (SIMV)/Assist control ventilation (ACV)):** the maximal (set) PIP should be used only if V_T is not achieved. In addition, the inflation is terminated once V_T is achieved, with shorter Ti (<0.2 s) than that preset. This alters the waveform to give a shallower upstroke to the inflating pressure to prolong the inflation time.

Use of smaller V_T (4–6 mL/kg) is the key strategy for protective ventilation in neonates, but higher V_T may be required in conditions such as pneumonia, BPD or other lung pathology that results in increased resistance to airflow. In PLV group 61% breaths fall outside the range (4–6 mL/kg) vs. 37% in babies receiving VTV [45, 46].

14.7 Selection of Mode

Though the components of gas exchange may be explained simplified by ventilation referring to CO_2 clearance and oxygenation as uptake of O_2 in lungs, each ventilation mode and setting can impact both the components as they interact and work together to achieve optimum blood levels of O_2 and CO_2. A very low V_E may result in poor oxygenation and extremes of PEEP can impair ventilation. Selection of modes and settings must be tailored to the needs of individual neonates as gas exchange needs differ not only between patients but also in the same patient over time, especially in ELBW and severely preterm babies.

Primarily, CO_2 clearance is determined by minute ventilation, and oxygenation by FiO_2 and MAP. During CMV, MAP is determined largely by the set PEEP (since the expiratory phase predominates respiratory cycle), and to a lesser extent by V_T, PIP and Ti.

14.8 Non-invasive Ventilation (NIV)

NIV is a recent trend as a primary and superior mode of respiratory support before proceeding to intubation and invasive ventilation in neonates. It provides a gentle way of delivering continuous pressure to keep the alveoli open, allowing sufficient gas exchange [47].

Different methods of NIV are:

1. **Nasal continuous positive airway pressure (nCPAP)**
2. **Nasal high flow therapy (nHFT).**
3. **Nasal intermittent positive pressure ventilation (nIPPV)**
4. **Bi-level continuous positive Airway pressure (BiPAP)**
5. **Nasal high-frequency oscillatory ventilation (nHFOV)**

Feeding intolerance is a frequent complication in preterm babies receiving NIV as the pressurized or high flow of gases causes bowel distension or an effect on the mesenteric blood flow and gastric emptying. However, maintain adequate enteral nutrition has several beneficial effects on improving growth and reducing the need for parenteral nutrition, thus decreasing the risk of infections, shortening the length of hospital stay, reducing cost and improving quality of life.

14.8.1 Nasal Continuous Positive Airway Pressure (nCPAP) (Fig. 14.2)

The most common clinical indications of nCPAP are:

- Newborn resuscitation,
- Prophylactic and in early management in RDS,
- Post-extubation
- Apnea of prematurity
- Tachypnea and labored breathing
- Respiratory acidosis
- Atelectasis

Early nCPAP in the delivery room reduces the need for surfactant administration and invasive MV [48].

The American Academy of Pediatrics (AAP) recommends that the early application of CPAP with subsequent selective surfactant administration vs. prophylactic surfactant therapy in extremely premature newborns results in lower rates of BPD and death. At the same time, it is important to determine when CPAP administration cannot be effective alone and the objective measures of CPAP failure should be interpreted in conjunction with other clinical findings. Complications with CPAP include skin reactions, air leak, over or underventilation and pneumonia [49–51].

The threshold of transition to invasive MV is lower in most preterm babies. Usually, CPAP is titrated up to 8 cm H_2O to optimize FRC and lung compliance. Clinically most apneas are mixed apneas due to immature central respiratory control system with poor respiratory drive along with reduced pharyngeal muscle tone in very

Fig. 14.2 Nasal CPAP

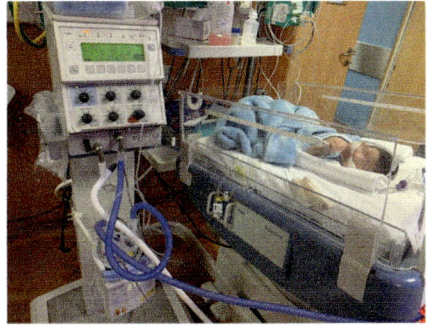

preterm neonates, especially during sleep [52]. CPAP increases pharyngeal cross-sectional area, thereby decreasing airway resistance and WOB. Before decision to commence weaning from CPAP, parameters such as CPAP pressure, FiO_2, respiratory distress and apnea frequency must be satisfactory for at least 12 h prior.

14.8.2 Nasal High Flow Therapy (nHFT)

nHFT is being increasingly used in preterm neonates in NICUs worldwide. It delivers heated humidified blended O_2 and air via bi-nasal cannulas at high flow rates of 2–8 L/min. The cannulas are 2–4 mm external diameter and occlude approximately half the diameter of external nares. The physiological effects of nHFT include improved alveolar ventilation (VA) by reducing dead space ventilation and generation of end-expiratory airway pressure; improved oxygenation by lowering RR and reduction in the WOB [53]. It is used as a primary mode post-extubation, and for weaning from nCPAP. The advantages of nHFT over nCPAP are ease of use, less nasal trauma, and more patient comfort. There are a few systematic reviews and meta-analyses showing its effectiveness over nCPAP in preterm babies and in post-extubation cases. It was found to be inferior to nCPAP when used as a primary support in RDS [54].

Implementation of a standardized weaning protocol from nHFT is essential to decrease weaning failure rates and the time to reach full enteral feeding in preterm babies. Unnecessarily slow weaning may cause nasal trauma, nosocomial sepsis, pulmonary air leak, increased NICU stay and cost of care.

Weaning Criteria from nHFT:
  i. Stable hemodynamic parameters
 ii. FiO_2 <0.25 and SpO_2 90–95%
iii. No apneic episodes requiring bag and mask ventilation (BMV) and not more than 6 episodes requiring stimulation during 24 h
 iv. RR <60/min
  v. No significant chest recession
 vi. Satisfactory blood gases (pH >7.25, $PaCO_2$ <60 mmHg, base deficit <8)

Weaning should be done in decrements of 0.5–1 L/min every 12–24 h as tolerated until a flow of 2 L/min, then discontinued. Monitoring during weaning includes clinical assessment, SpO_2 (target of 90–95%) and analysis of blood gases 12 hourly. The neonates should be observed up for 72 h after discontinuation of nHFT.

Weaning failure criteria:
  i. Increase in FIO_2 >0.4 to maintain SpO_2 >90 (90–95%)
 ii. Frequent apnea, ≥6 episodes requiring intervention in 24 h-period or ≥1 episode requiring BMV

iii. Respiratory acidosis: pH <7.2 and $PaCO_2$ >60 mmHg

iv. Increased WOB (RR >70/min, chest recession, expiratory grunt)

14.9 Neonatal Resuscitation

Seconds matter during neonatal resuscitation. Inadequate oxygenation can lead to permanent neurological deficits in the form of hypoxic ischemic encephalopathy (HIE), cerebral palsy, PVL and IVH. Preterm newborns are more likely to require prolonged and advanced resuscitation, intubation, and ventilation, and develop complications than term babies [55]:

- **Ventilation**: babies at birth not breathing or struggling to breathe after initial stabilization should be oxygenated and/or ventilated depending on the circumstances. If the newborn is cyanotic with labored breathing and HR >100 bpm, supplemental O_2 and CPAP may be considered, but if HR <100 bpm with apnea or gasping breathing, proceed with PPV.
- **Suction**: only babies with obvious airway obstruction (mucus secretion or meconium aspiration) are immediately suctioned. The risks involved with airway suctioning are bradycardia, hypoxemia, hypotension, pneumothorax and reduced O_2 availability [56].
- **Oxygen**: blended O_2 or room air should be used. The recommended initial FiO_2 for PPV is 21% for ≥35 weeks of gestational age (GA) and 21–30% for <35 week GA [57]. SpO_2 guides FiO_2 to achieve the target saturation.
- **CPR**: before cardiac compression is started the baby should be intubated and ventilated with FiO_2 of 1.

A few large breaths (35–40 mL/kg) administered at birth to immature lung are sufficient to cause lung injury and inhibit the effect of surfactant. Therefore, lung protective ventilation should be initiated in the delivery room itself, especially in preterm babies. In newborns <32 week GA, 5 cm H_2O CPAP should be considered as an alternative to routine intubation and surfactant administration. PPV can be administered via face mask or ETT or SGA with a self-inflating bag or a T-piece resuscitator (gas-powered resuscitator that delivers controlled, consistent and precise pressure, independent of operator expertise) (Fig. 14.3) [58]. Complications of PPV in newborns include leaks, ineffective ventilation, gastric inflation, aspiration, hyperventilation, pulmonary barotrauma, BPD and ROP [59].

Fig. 14.3 T-piece
resuscitator

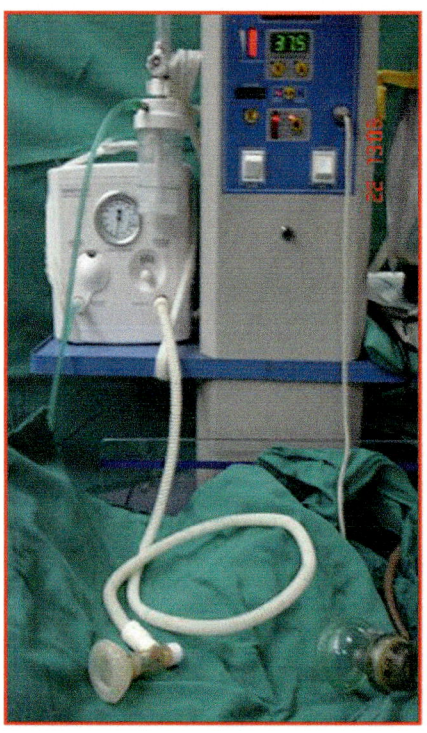

14.10 Mechanical Ventilation

14.10.1 How to Initiate Invasive Mechanical Ventilation (MV)

Evidence-based practices guide the initial settings with subsequent titration according to the clinical progress. There is no standardized practice, it varies from center to center according to the GA, underlying lung condition, available ventilator and user expertise:

- Initiate with CMV. Reserve HFV for selected high-risk or refractory respiratory failure babies who cannot be optimized by CMV.
- Synchronized patient triggered modes such as SIMV+ PS or ACV with both mandatory and spontaneous breaths are preferred.
- Preferentially use VTV in all preterms (except in cases with large ETT leak).
- Settings: V_T = 4–6 mL/kg, Ti = 0.35–0.4 s, PIP: BW <1500 g (16–28 cm H_2O) and BW ≥1500 g (20–30 cm H_2O).
- Since PIP is a reflection of anticipated lung compliance, set PIP is based on adequate chest movement. A subsequent change in PIP is determined by blood gases, pH values and the clinical course.
- PEEP = 4–6 cm H_2O (higher PEEP if FiO_2 is high). During MV the presence of an ETT eliminates the laryngeal control of expiratory flow, thus PEEP of a few cm

H_2O is necessary to counteract the otherwise unavoidable drop in end-expiratory volume [19]. It becomes still more significant in lung diseases with low compliance.

- Pressure support: 4–6 cm H_2O (minimal). Usually start PS at PIP–PEEP/2 (cm H_2O), measured over PEEP.
- VCV (rarely used): V_T = 5–10 mL/kg (premature), 7–10 mL/kg (term), RR: 30–40/min
- HFV settings: frequency (Hz), amplitude or power, PEEP or MAP (cm H_2O), and FiO_2.

14.10.2 How to Assess Adequacy of MV

1. Continuous SpO_2 monitoring (target SpO_2 90–95%).
2. Blood gases (capillary/venous/arterial): An arterial line is placed if blood sampling is advised more frequently than 6 hourly or hemodynamic instability requiring active titration of vasoactive drugs. Blood gases are analysed within a few hours of initiation of assisted ventilation. During the acute phase of the disease process, ABG and pH must be checked at 15–30 min after a significant change in ventilator settings due to change in neonate's condition.
3. TCOM (Transcutaneous CO_2 monitoring): is done in select cases, e.g., neonates with severely compromised ventilation or where $PaCO_2$ fluctuations are anticipated, or transition to or titration of HFOV.
4. Target $PaCO_2$ in preterm babies in the first few weeks of life is 40–65 mmHg (modest permissive hypercapnia). In older preterm with evolving BPD, higher $PaCO_2$ can be allowed as long as pH >7.25.
5. Ventilator monitor displays set and measured parameters, and graphic display of real-time curves.
6. Chest X-ray is ordered judiciously only for decisions about ventilation settings and to identify accurate changes, such as a leak or ETT malposition.
7. If PaO_2 or SaO_2 is below the standard limit, FiO_2 can be raised gradually to a maximum of 1.0, under SpO_2 or TcO_2 monitoring. If still low, MAP can be raised by increasing PIP, PEEP, Ti or RR.
8. When RR is reduced without a concomitant decrease in I:E ratio, Ti can become quite prolonged. Total Ti should never exceed 0.6 s. Similarly, when RR is increased to >60/min, I:E ratio should be 1:1. If $PaCO_2$ is high, RR or PIP can be increased.
9. The breath sounds should be auscultated in the upper and lower lung fields bilaterally to evaluate for the quality of uniform aeration and presence of adventitious breath sounds, and in the epigastric region to rule out esophageal intubation (5 point auscultation).
10. Chest wall vibration is an indicator of lung compliance, airway patency and appropriate ventilator settings. A sudden decrease in chest wall vibration may indicate a blocked ETT or pneumothorax. The vital signs and cardiopulmonary stability should be evaluated. The ventilator alarm status should be checked and ventilatory parameters reviewed. For CMV mode, check for FiO_2, ventilatory

rate, PIP, PEEP, V_T, I: E, flow rate, MAP, and for HFV mode, check for FiO_2, amplitude, frequency, MAP).

11. Always an appropriate size self-inflating resuscitation bag with mask should be available.
12. A functioning suction apparatus should always be at the bed-side.
13. The head end of the bed is elevated, unless contraindicated, to reduce the incidence of aspiration for prevention of ventilator associated pneumonia (VAP) and to reduce the risk of IVH.
14. Sedation may be necessary to achieve ventilator synchrony.
15. Routine scheduled tube suctioning should not be done as it is associated with adverse consequences, especially in the preterms. Signs that indicate need for suctioning are visible secretions in the ETT, decreased breath sounds or increased adventitious sounds, desaturation, reduced chest wall movement or vibration and changes in vital parameters.
16. Respond immediately to audible or visual alarms which may be associated with a need for suctioning, draining out water from tubing or circuit disconnection.
17. The neonate should be routinely examined for signs and symptoms of hypoxemia and ventilation failure, such as desaturation, pallor or cyanosis, tachypnea, agitation, tachycardia, bradycardia, increased WOB, chest wall retraction, hypercarbia, and acidosis.
18. Changes in compliance may occur, requiring ventilator setting adjustments.
19. Signs of accidental extubation should be kept in mind for early detection, such as sudden deterioration in clinical status, abdominal distension, audible crying, decrease in chest wall movement, breath sounds in the abdomen, agitation, cyanosis and or bradycardia.

14.11 Weaning Off Mechanical Ventilation

14.11.1 How to Wean

The goal is to wean the neonate from the ventilator as soon as possible to minimize VILI. During weaning, transfer of WOB from the ventilator to the neonate, must be gradual, without being excessive increase. Premature weaning is associated with extubation failure and poor outcomes [60]. For the smooth weaning process, three factors are essential:

1. **Criteria for readiness to wean**
2. **Standard weaning techniques or protocols**
3. **Recognize weaning failure**

14.11.2 Criteria for Weaning

Review of neonate's clinical status, blood gases and radiographic findings indicate when weaning can be initiated. The outlines are:

(a) Clinical improvement of the original disease process
(b) Presence of adequate cough reflex
(c) Adequate spontaneous respiratory effort
(d) Hemodynamic stability for more than 24 h
(e) Ventilator settings reduced to RR <25/min and PIP of 16–18 cm H_2O with adequate chest expansion
(f) Acceptable ABG–PaO_2 ≥60 mmHg on PEEP <5 cm H_2O and FiO_2 ≤0.4 and PaO_2: FiO_2 ≥150–300
(g) GCS ≥13 without sedation.

14.11.3 Weaning Protocol Principles

(a) In VTV, weaning occurs in real-time rather than intermittently in response to ABG values, thus faster weaning. During weaning, a volume targeted level of 6 mL/kg rather than a lower level (4–5 mL/kg) could be used in conjunction with patient triggered mode to avoid increase in WOB [18]. Switch settings to PTV modes, if not on already. Stop sedation.
(b) On SIMV mode, reduce the ventilator RR (never <20/min). Reduce PIP gradually according to ABG.
(c) The back-up rate during ACV and PSV should remain constant.
(d) Caffeine is used as a loading dose of 20 mg/kg followed by a maintenance dose of 5 mg/kg/day for apnea of prematurity and in the peri-extubation period [61].

O_2 consumption, which is an indicator of WOB, was 30% lower and the duration of weaning was less prolonged with ACV vs. slow rate SIMV (14/min). An increase in WOB prolongs duration of weaning and also contributes to growth failure. Thus, in preterm neonates, excessive WOB predisposes them to fatigue, adversely affecting their ability to trigger the ventilator, and prolonged or weaning failure [48].

14.11.4 Weaning Failure

In the post-extubation period the neonates are put on nasal NIV or nasal O_2 therapy according to RR and pattern of breathing (WOB).

Lung ultrasonography (LUS) is a rapid, non-invasive, repetitive, reliable and a safe bedside technique to predict weaning success of the critically ill ventilated neonates [62]. LUS calculations based on aeration for each hemithorax were significantly higher in neonates with extubation failure than those weaned successfully. This validated score enables a dynamic assessment of aeration changes in lungs unlike chest X ray [63].

Neonates should be followed for 48 h post-extubation for extubation failure, which is more common in extremely premature and LBW babies, and after prolonged duration of MV [59].

14.12 Surfactant Administration

Immature lungs are stiff, thick-walled, surfactant-deficient, and particularly suscep-tible to lung injury. Prophylactic surfactant in very immature babies is superior to its use as a rescue therapy [64, 65].

- **<24 week GA:** The babies are intubated immediately after birth and prophylac-tic surfactant is administered within first 30 min of life. Between intubation and surfactant administration, these babies should be ventilated with low V_T and air-way pressures.
- **≥24 week GA:** For babies intubated immediately after birth, surfactant should be given early (within 2 h of birth) except if on room air and minimal ventila-tory support at NICU admission. They should be immediately extubated to nCPAP.

14.12.1 In Case a Newborn is Initially Treated with NIV–Intubation and Surfactant May Be Required If:

(a) High FiO_2 (>0.5) is necessary to maintain SpO_2 >88% or PaO_2 >45 mmHg, or and
(b) persistent low PaO_2 (55–60 mmHg) with a pH <7.25, or and
(c) Apnea requiring BMV, or and
(d) >6 episodes of apneas in 6 h, or and
(e) Evidence of significant WOB (retraction, grunting),

14.12.2 Required Interventions Before Surfactant Delivery

- Preoxygenate to achieve SpO_2 >95%
- Suction ETT and check air entry
- Lung recruitment maneuver: provide 5–10 inflations with pressure 1–2 cm H_2O above previous ventilator settings to assure alveolar recruitment to facilitate sur-factant distribution
- Record vital signs (HR, BP, SpO_2, $TcCO_2$)

14.12.3 Risk of Surfactant Administration

Though surfactant therapy is very beneficial in many newborns and Bradycardia, hypoxemia, pulmonary hemorrhage.

14.13 High-Frequency Oscillatory Ventilation (HFOV)

HFOV is an advanced and useful ventilator modality that can provide lung-protective ventilation/ oxygenation to correct refractory hypoxia and/or hypercarbia with

Fig. 14.4 HFOV

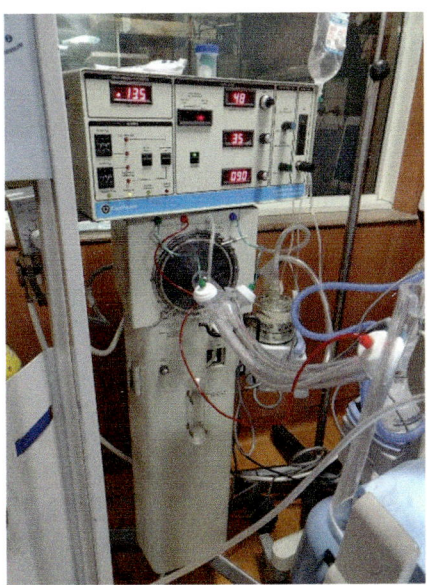

respiratory acidosis in some severe lung conditions especially when CMV fails (Fig. 14.4). Most evidence of the effectiveness of HFOV is available in neonatal population only. It can be described under four main headings:

1. **Working principle**
2. **Clinical applications**
3. **How to do the settings**
4. **How to wean**

14.13.1 Working Principle

HFOV uses a constant distending airway pressure (=MAP) over which small V_T are superimposed with oscillating pressure variations (delta P/power/amplitude) at a very high frequency (Hz). MAP is equivalent to CPAP, that inflates the lungs to a constant and optimal volume maximizing the area for gas exchange and preventing alveolar collapse in the expiratory phase. The amplitude setting controls the distance the diaphragm travels from its resting position. Gas exchange during HFOV occurs by molecular diffusion, dispersion, turbulence, pendelluft, cardiogenic mixing and collateral ventilation [66–69]. The details of these mechanisms are beyond the scope of this chapter.

14.13.2 Clinical Applications

(a). **HFOV is used mainly as a rescue therapy when CMV fails in term or pre-term neonates in situations like:**

(a) Air leak syndromes, such as pneumothorax, pulmonary intestinal emphysema
(b) Persistent PHT of newborn (PPHN)
(c) Obstructive disorders such as meconium aspiration syndrome (MAS)
(d) Severe atelectatic disorders such as RDS
(e) Pulmonary hypoplasia

(b). The important characteristics of HFOV are:
- Low V_T (1.5–2.5 mL/kg)
- Supraphysiological RR (10–15 Hz) (600–900/min)
- Active expiration to prevent gas trapping due to high RR
- Small ΔP (1–2 cm H_2O): decrease of ΔP during passage from proximal airway to the alveoli

(c). Limits to Detect Failure of CMV and Oxygenation:
- Inspiration pressure $\geq$ to 30 to 35 cm H_2O
- V_T: 5–7 mL/kg
- Severe respiratory acidosis: pH <7.1
- Oxygenation parameters: SpO_2 <90%, PaO_2/FiO_2 <150 despite FiO_2 >0.6, optimal PEEP, OI >15

(d). Relative Contraindications to HFOV:
- Obstructive airway disease as it may lead to severe air trapping with improper use.
- Traumatic brain injury or raised ICP as high MAP can reduce venous return and cerebral perfusion.
- Hemodynamic instability, especially unresponsive to fluids and vasopressors. These are the situations when CMV fails and ECMO needs to be considered.

14.13.3 How to Set

In HFOV, oxygenation and ventilation are not so inter-dependent as in CMV. Oxygenation depends on MAP and FiO_2, whereas ventilation (CO_2 elimination) depends on amplitude than on frequency (Hz).

(a) Bias flow allows further increase in MAP when needed. It is usually set at 20 L/min.
(b) Starting FiO_2 should be 1 (100%). SpO_2 can change in the first 30 min of initiation of HFOV. If SpO_2 falls, it is because the set MAP may not be high enough. Once that is corrected, FiO_2 should be slowly reduced to a target SaO_2 of 88–92%.
(c) MAP should be set at 2–3 cm H_2O above the previous MAP on CMV. When starting as a primary mode, set MAP should be 8–10 cm H_2O. Later increments should be of 1 cm H_2O to avoid barotrauma.
(d) The starting amplitude should be 50 cm H_2O and adjusted afterwards until chest wall motion from nipple line to umbilicus (chest wiggle factor) is perceived.
(e) The initial frequency (f) should be set at 12–15 Hz (720–900/min) for preterm and 10–12 Hz (600–720 bpm) for term neonates.
(f) Ti is normally set at 30–33% of the cycle time (Ti 0.33) corresponding to I:E ratio of 1:2. A lower frequency causes increase in Ti. If I:E ratio is fixed, at any

given power and MAP, lower frequency will deliver a larger Vt because of higher Ti, which carries the risk of air tapping and massive air leak.

(g) Alveolar ventilation = $V_T \times F$. Bias flow or Ti are usually not adjusted [67].

Initiating HFOV may reduce venous return and affect blood pressure, it is prudent to infuse 5–10 mL/kg fluid boluses. The neonate should be oxygenated using hand ventilation, ETT clamped at inspiration, and then attached to HFOV to avoid derecruitment. Blood gases should be monitored at 30 min to check $PaCO_2$, and chest X-ray at 4 h to look for hyperinflation. TCOM can help to monitor the trend in CO_2.

14.13.4 How to Wean:

(a) Switching from CMV may be tolerated if HFOV settings are MAP <16–17 cm H_2O, FiO_2 <0.4, and power <40 cm H_2O.
(b) Set MAP 3–4 cm H_2O less than on CMV and amplitude of 20–25 cm H_2O.
(c) Reduce FiO_2 to <0.4 before weaning MAP except in radiological evidence of overinflation or pulmonary air-leak syndrome, where reduction in MAP as a low volume strategy takes priority over weaning from FiO_2.
(d) Reduce MAP by 1–2 cm H_2O increments to around 15 cm H_2O.
(e) Amplitude should be weaned in 2–4 cm H_2O decrements.
(f) Do not wean frequency (Hz).

14.13.5 Troubleshooting Situations with Possible Solutions

(a) **Poor oxygenation**: increase FiO_2 and MAP (1–2 cm H_2O increments) + recruitment maneuver
(b) **Over oxygenation**: decrease FiO_2 and MAP (1–2 cm H_2O decrements)
(c) **Under ventilation**: increase amplitude, decrease frequency (1–2 Hz) if amplitude maximal
(d) **Over ventilation**: decrease amplitude, increase frequency (1–2 Hz) if amplitude minimal

14.13.6 Limitations

- HFOV needs user **expertise.**
- **De-recruitment** is a potential problem if the circuit gets disconnected for any reason.
- **Suctioning** should be avoided in first 24 h unless specifically indicated, and never as a routine, and using in-line suctioning only. Indications include diminished chest wobble, elevated $PaCO_2$, obvious visible/audible secretions in the ETT. Some ventilators have a stop button to use briefly while quickly inserting and withdrawing the suction catheter.
- There is no sigh benefit for alveolar recruitment and requires heavy sedation and neuromuscular blockade.

- There is a higher risk of hemodynamic instability due to higher MAP.
- There is no feed-back from the ventilator regarding lung volume or compliance for HFOV adjustments. The clinical examination of respiratory sounds is difficult, the only finding being a wobble. Hence, regular chest X-ray is needed to avoid lung hyperinflation. It is important to be aware of changes in lung compliance due to secretions and inadequate neuromuscular blockade.
- HFOV may not always benefit. This may be because of inappropriate set up, very bad lung condition, or another co-existing lung condition, such as pneumothorax.

There is no statistical evidence of benefit of HFOV in terms of reducing mortality [23, 70].

14.14 Significance of Humidification and Flow Sensor Location

Humidification of inspired gases should never be underestimated as the respiratory system of the neonate is very sensitive. Dry (0% relative humidity) and cold (15 °C) medical gases must be conditioned to water-saturation (47 mmHg 100% relative humidity) and warmed to 37 °C to contribute significantly to the success of ventilatory therapy. Humidifying and heating the inspired gas increases its volume, ensures physiological conditioning of airways and improves drainage of secretions. It is achieved with the use of HME or servo controlled heated humidifiers in the inspiratory limb of the circuit (Fig. 14.5).

The best position for measurement of airflow, volume and pressure should be as close to the patient as possible. The modern neonatal ventilators have the proximal flow sensor at the distal end (patient end) of the breathing circuit as it relies on accurate measurement of very small flows and the effects of circuit composition is minimal (Fig. 14.6). The additional advantage of proximal flow measurement is the ability for instant detection of respiratory signals to which the ventilator can respond faster. Reusable flow sensors should be cleaned by autoclaving. Transport and anaesthesia ventilators lack proximal sensors.

14.15 Choice of Endotracheal Tube: Cuffed vs Uncuffed ETT

Contrary to the traditional approach of using uncuffed ETT in children under 8 years of age, availability of recently developed high-volume low-pressure Microcuff ETT has changed the trend even in neonatal anesthesia practice in most set-ups.

The major disadvantage of a potential ventilatory leak around the uncuffed ETT leads to inaccurate monitoring of tidal volume and capnography and thereby inappropriate ventilation settings. On the other hand, the cuffed tubes when used appropriately with close monitoring of cuff pressure (<20 cm H_2O) are quite safe even during longer periods of intubation of several weeks [71, 72].

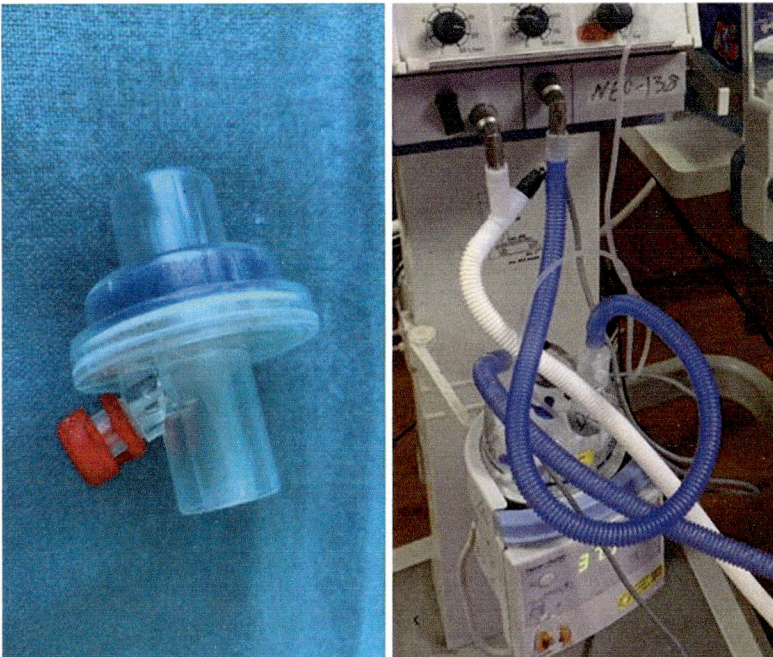

Fig. 14.5 Humidification devices

Fig. 14.6 Proximal flow
sensor

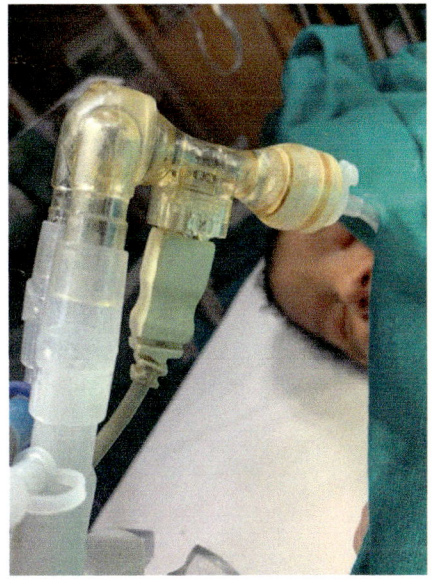

Fig. 14.7 Micro-cuff endotracheal tube with cuff pressure monitor

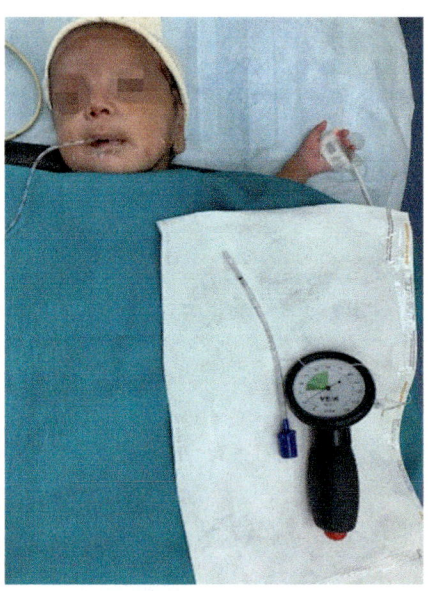

In our setup, the use of cuffed ETT is not a routine practice in NICU, but Microcuff tubes are routinely employed in all neonates (except TEF repair) undergoing anaesthesia, with an intermittent cuff pressure monitoring at around 11–12 cm H_2O. Continuous cuff pressure monitoring is a routine when N_2O is used in babies older than neonatal age group (Fig. 14.7).

In addition, in the anaesthesia setting, uncuffed tubes have been associated with a significantly increased risk of perioperative respiratory complications including postoperative stridor. Avoiding cuff hyperinflation with close monitoring avoids the potential damage to the tracheal mucosa due to hypoperfusion, leading to subglottic oedema and injury [73–75].

14.16 Concerns During Transport

The transfer of ventilated extremely premature or very unstable neonates to the OR is associated with a long list of avoidable critical situations, such as accidental extubation, ventilatory circuit disconnection, equipment failure, desaturation, and cardiac arrest. The risk–benefit analysis of operating a critically ill neonate in NICU or OR should be a joint decision of the team comprising of the anesthesiologist, surgeon, and neonatologist [76–78] (Fig. 14.8).

Points in favor of surgery in NICU include better temperature control, optimized ventilation with NICU ventilators and the maintained hemodynamics with fluids and inotropes with invasive monitoring.

The beneficial effects of surgery in OR include the comfort of space, equipment, sterility, lighting, handling any unanticipated emergency and complex surgeries.

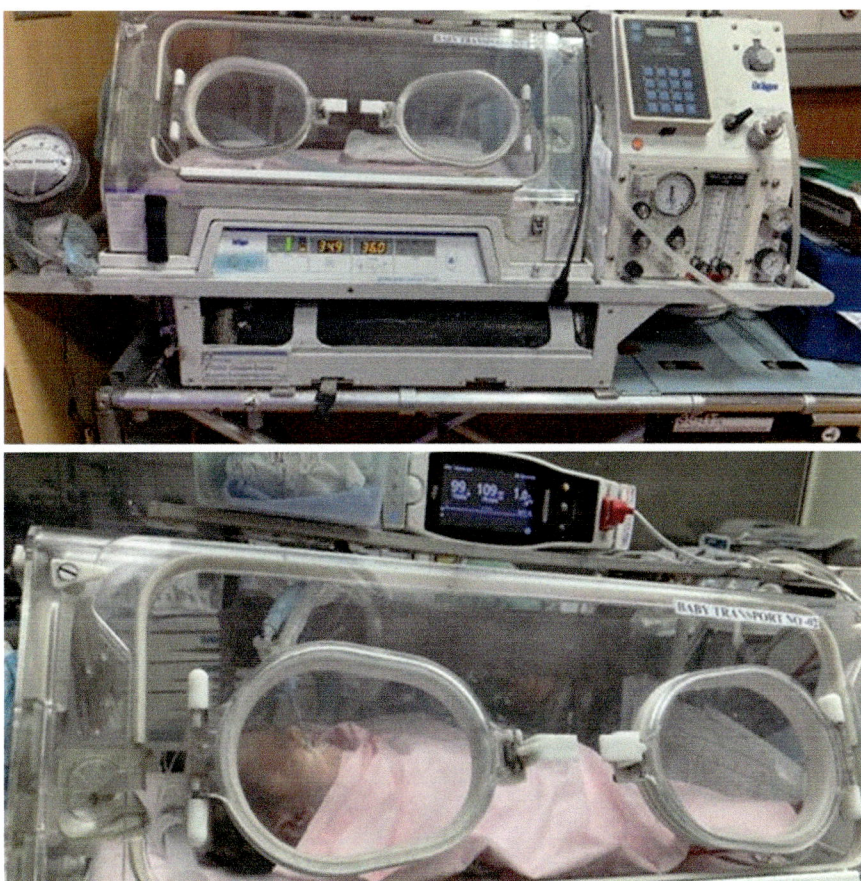

Fig. 14.8 Transport ventilator incubator

The de-recruitment episodes with the potential loss of FRC associated with disconnection from NICU ventilator to transport ventilator or manual ventilation during transport and reconnection to anaesthesia ventilator with limited modes may lead to requirement of escalated ventilatory support and O_2 requirement. Moreover, the babies on HFOV, iNO or ECMO cannot be transported to OR.

14.17 Ventilatory Considerations in the Operation Room (OR)

General anaesthesia and surgery impose a considerable risk of atelectasis and V/Q mismatch in neonates as they are critically dependent on dynamically elevated FRC to maintain their lung volume above the closing volume during tidal breathing. The increasing trend of laparoscopic surgery in neonates, effect of various anaesthetic drugs, management of airway and hemodynamic parameters, may all affect FRC, ventilation homogeneity and V/Q mismatch [79–83].

14.17.1 Management Strategies

- Electronic pre-use self-test of anaesthesia machine should be done with the breathing circuit tubing expanded to the anticipated length required during surgery for the measurement of circuit compliance, and to incorporate and calculate the expired tidal volume. The circuit should be neither compressed nor overexpanded after the self-test to avoid erroneous V_T delivery, based on previously measured compliance [84].
- Continuous PEEP of 4–6 cm H_2O is needed to maintain normal FRC and prevent atelectasis during anaesthesia. PEEP is particularly helpful after surgical closure of abdominal wall defects along with intra-abdominal pressure (IAP) monitoring to prevent abdominal compartment syndrome and respiratory failure [22].
- Intraabdominal pressure during CO_2 pneumoperitoneum in laparoscopic surgery should be <6 mmHg [85].
- For minor cases, use of SGA/LMA is recommended, due to less risk of respiratory complications and requirement for postoperative ventilation than with ETT.
- Optimise V_T using VTV mode or by adjusting PIP.
- Adjust the RR between 40 and 60/min to maintain normocapnia to mild hypercapnia (35–55 mmHg). Sampling for $EtCO_2$ should be as close as possible to the ETT to exclude V_D of the HME filter and Y-piece. However, $EtCO_2$ may be a poor measure of $PaCO_2$, leading to overestimation of real $PaCO_2$, and failure to recognize hypocarbia which can be detrimental for cerebral perfusion. Blood gas analysis should be helpful, though of limited significance in dynamic setting of sudden changes in compliance and resistance during anaesthesia and surgery.
- Optimise FiO_2 to achieve target SpO_2 level (preterm: 90–95%, term: 94–98%) during maintenance of anaesthesia. Higher FiO_2 may be required during induction and extubation.
- For neonates, who are already being ventilated prior to surgery, NICU ventilator settings are used as a guide to continue ventilation during anaesthesia (Fig. 14.9).

Fig. 14.9 Anaesthesia ventilation with monitor

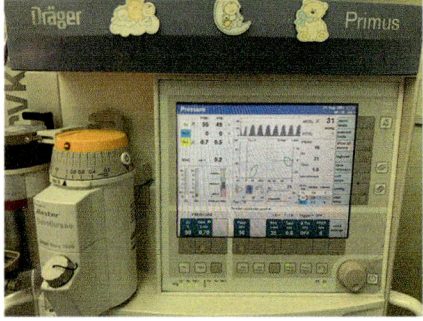

- Use of a NICU ventilator in OR is extremely useful in very small or critically ill neonates for delivering and monitoring required V_T and minute ventilation using flow sensors. Even if volatile anaesthetic administration is not feasible in such a situation with ICU ventilator, opioid-based anaesthesia is a recognized alternative in this group of patients.
- Plan for early extubation after minor and short-duration procedures. CPAP is useful postoperatively to overcome obstructive apnea or respiratory distress by decreasing WOB. Recent trends are towards slightly delayed extubation in NICU, while allowing safety during transport to NICU.

14.18   Inhaled Nitric Oxide (iNO)

Nitric oxide is an endogenous signaling molecule which regulates vascular flow, angiogenesis, inflammatory and oxidative stress. It is a potent and selective pulmonary arterial vasodilator, thus has a major role in developing lung by regulating pulmonary vascular tone. Its use is evidence-based and FDA approved for treatment of PPHN, improves oxygenation and decreases the need for ECMO. In congenital diaphragmatic hernia (CDH), the key factor for response to iNO is the presence and degree of left ventricular dysfunction (Fig. 14.10). In the setting of LV dysfunction

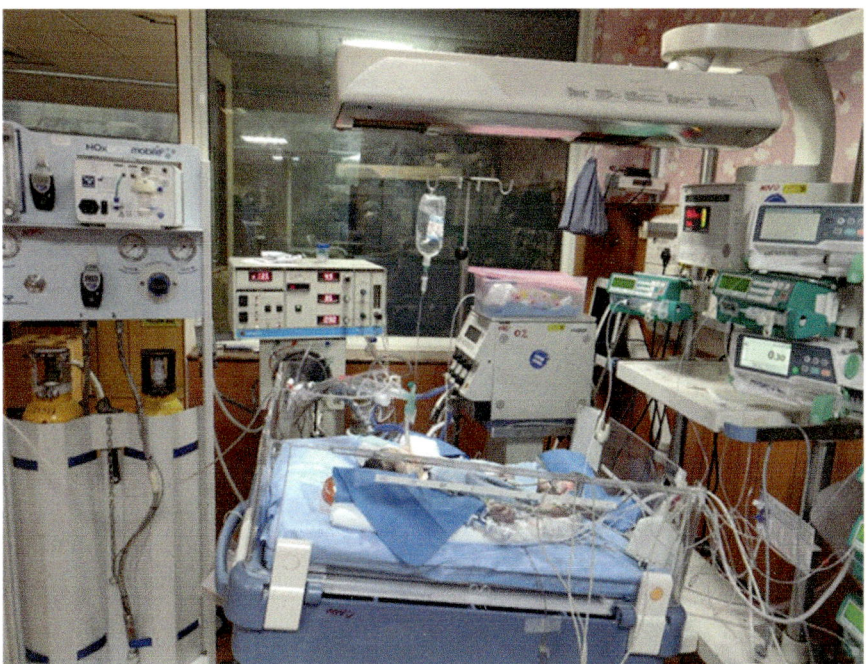

Fig. 14.10   Inhaled nitric oxide therapy

and consequent pulmonary venous hypertension, use of NO (pulmonary arterial dilatation) may be detrimental and lead to pulmonary hemorrhages. Clinical trials do not support nitric oxide's role in prevention of BPD in preterms [86–88].

14.19 Conclusion

A clear understanding of the concepts of neonatal lung physiology and mechanics is of paramount importance for successful respiratory support. There is a growing evidence in the provision of "lung protective ventilation" in neonates for the optimal benefits of MV without its associated risks. Combining a low tidal volume with sufficient PEEP and a high ventilatory rate with permissive hypercapnia may be an optimal strategy. In a nutshell, patient triggered ventilation, volume monitoring at proximal airway and new ventilation modes such as volume targeted ventilation and HFOV are the recent advances in neonatal ventilation practices which are to be embraced as well as explored further in due course of clinical research for the ultimate effectiveness to reduce mortality and long term consequences, such as chronic lung disease.

Clinical Pearls
1. Management of respiratory support should always be tailored to the needs of each individual neonate, which may differ between patients and even within the same neonate over time.
2. Although MV can be life-saving, its contribution to VILI, hemodynamic instability and secondary injury to brain and other organ systems need to be overemphasized, especially in neonates.
3. Understanding the sophisticated technology and capabilities of the available ventilator is essential. Extensive education and planning for a new sophisticated approach to ventilation can be challenging. It is best to gain experience with the newer ventilatory modes in adults and older children, relatively straightforward patients, to gain confidence in managing difficult neonates effectively in due course.
4. Individualized assessment and frequent reassessment of the adequacy of ventilation setting is critical.
5. In terms of patient ventilator interaction and clinical outcomes, synchronised ventilation is superior to CMV modes, such as IMV. Neonate's spontaneous respiratory efforts should be encouraged using PTV modes with optimum back-up rate, allowing full control of baby's own breathing in due course.
6. Various "lung-protective" strategies should be utilized for neonates with respiratory failure to support gas exchange while minimizing VILI, such as VTV, use of optimal or minimal PEEP, avoidance high FiO_2, moderate permissive hypercapnia, and early use of HFV, where indicated.
7. Caffeine and synchronised or VTV have a positive effect on respiratory muscle function.
8. Since the structural abnormalities of BPD are irreversible, it is essential to take preventive measures.

9. Limiting the duration of MV is crucial. Choosing the optimal time for weaning and predicting post-extubation distress is of great clinical significance.
10. Premature weaning and extubation can be as harmful as leads to unnecessary prolonged invasive ventilation.

References

1. Picheta R. World's smallest known baby at birth, who weighed 7.5 ounces, leaves hospital; August 2021. https://edition.cnn.com/2021/08/10/asia/kwek-yu-xuan-baby-leaves-hospital-scli-intl/index.html
2. Singh GK, Yu SM. Infant mortality in the United States: trends, differentials, and projections, 1950 through 2010. Am J Public Health. 1995;85(7):957–64.
3. Heron M, Sutton PD, Xu J, Ventura SJ, et al. Annual summary of vital statistics. Pediatrics. 2010;125(1):4–15.
4. Pillow JJ, Stocks J, Sly PD, Hantos Z. Partitioning of airway and parenchymal mechanics in unsedated newborn infants. Pediatr Res. 2005;58(6):1210–5.
5. Chakkarapani AA, Adappa R, Mohammad Ali SK, et al. "Current concepts of mechanical ventilation in neonates"—Part 1: Basics. Int J Pediatr Adolesc Med. 2020;7(1):13–8.
6. Montazami NS, Abubakar KM, Keszler M. The impact of instrumental dead-space in volume-targeted ventilation of the extremely low birth weight (ELBW) infant. Pediatr Pulmonol. 2009;44(2):128–33.
7. Martin K, Abudakar KM. Physiologic principles. In Assisted ventilation of the neonate 2011, pp. 19–46.
8. Brown MK, DiBlasi RM. Mechanical ventilation of the premature neonate. Respir Care. 2011;56(9):1298–313.
9. Attar MA, Donn SM. Mechanisms of ventilator-induced lung injury in premature infants. Semin Neonatol. 2002;7(5):353–60.
10. Dreyfuss D, Saumon G. Ventilator-induced lung injury: lessons from experimental studies. Am J Respir Crit Care Med. 1998;157(1):294–323.
11. Protti A, Andreis DT, Milesi M, Iapichino GE, etal. Lung anatomy, energy load, and ventilator-induced lung injury. Intensive Care Med Exp 2015;3(1):34.
12. Resch B, Neubauer K, Hofer N, etal. Episodes of hypocarbia and early-onset sepsis are risk factors for cystic periventricular leukomalacia in preterm infant. Early Hum Dev. 2012; 88(1):27-31.
13. Saugstad OD, Sejersted Y, Solberg R, Wollen EJ, Bjørås M. Oxygenation of the newborn: a molecular approach. Neonatology. 2012;101(4):315–25.
14. Baraldi E, Filippone M. Chronic lung disease after premature birth. N Engl J Med. 2007;357(19):1946–55.
15. Stenson BJ, Tarnow-Mordi WO, Darlow BA, Simes J, etal, BOOST II United Kingdom Collaborative Group; BOOST II Australia Collaborative Group; BOOST II New Zealand Collaborative Group, Oxygen saturation and outcomes in preterm infants. N Engl J Med 2013; 30;368(22):2094-2104.
16. Vervenioti A, Fouzas S, Tzifas S, Karatza AA, Dimitriou G. Work of breathing in mechanically ventilated preterm neonates. Pediatr Crit Care Med. 2020;(5):430–6.
17. Ozer EA. Lung-protective ventilation in neonatal intensive care unit. J Clin Neonatol. 2020;9:1–7.
18. Patel DS, Sharma A, Prendergast M, Rafferty GF, Greenough A. Work of breathing and different levels of volume-targeted ventilation. Pediatrics. 2009;123(4):e679–84.
19. Sternberg UBS, Regli A, Schibler A, Hammer J, etal. The impact of positive end-expiratory pressure on functional residual capacity and ventilation homogeneity impairment in anesthetized children exposed to high levels of inspired oxygen. Anesth Analg. 2007; 104(6):1364-1368.

20. Mok Q, Negus S, McLaren CA, etal. Computed tomography versus bronchography in the diagnosis and management of tracheobronchomalacia in ventilator dependent infants. Arch Dis Child Fetal Neonatal Ed 2005;90(4): F290-F293.
21. Sola A. Oxygen in neonatal anesthesia:friend or foe? Curr Opin Anaesthesiol. 2008;21(3):332–9.
22. Thome UH, Ambalavanan N. Permissive hypercapnia to decrease lung injury in ventilated preterm neonates. Semin Fetal Neonatal Med. 2009 Feb;14(1):21–7.
23. Meyers M, Rodrigues N, Ari A. High-frequency oscillatory ventilation: a narrative review. Can J Respir Ther. 2019;55:40–6.
24. Herber-Jonat S, von Bismarck P, Freitag-Wolf S, etal. Limitation of measurements of expiratory tidal volume and expiratory compliance under conditions of endotracheal tube leaks. Pediatr Crit Care Med 2008; 9:69–75
25. Singh J, Sinha SK, Clarke P, etal. Mechanical ventilation of very low birth weight infants: is volume or pressure a better target variable? J Pediatr 2006; 149:308–313.
26. Chow LC, Vanderhal A, Raber J, etal. Are tidal volume measurements in neonatal pressure-controlled ventilation accurate? Pediatr Pulmonol 2002; 34:196–202
27. Greenough A, Rossor TE, Sundaresan A, etal. Synchronized mechanical ventilation for respiratory support in newborn infants. Cochrane Database Syst Rev 2016; 9(9):CD000456.
28. Patel DS, Rafferty GF, Lee S, Hannam S, Greenough A. Work of breathing during SIMV with and without pressure support. Arch Dis Child. 2009;94(6):434–6.
29. Claure N, Bancalari E. New modes of mechanical ventilation in the preterm newborn: evidence of benefit. Arch Dis Child Fetal Neonatal Ed. 2007;92(6):F508–12.
30. Klingenberg C, Wheeler KI, McCallion N, etal. Volume-targeted versus pressure limited ventilation in neonates. Cochrane Database Syst Rev 2017; 10:CD003666.
31. Grover A, Field D. Volume-targeted ventilation in the neonate: time to change? Arch Dis Child Fetal Neonatal Ed. 2008;93(1):F7–F13.
32. Klingenberg C, Wheeler KI, Davis PG, Morley CJ. A practical guide to neonatal volume guarantee ventilation. J Perinatol. 2011;31(9):575–85.
33. Keszler M. Update on mechanical ventilatory strategies. NeoReviews. 2013;14:e237–51.
34. Stein H, Firestone K, Rimensberger PC. Synchronized mechanical ventilation using electrical activity of the diaphragm in neonates. Clin Perinatol. 2012;39(3):525–42.
35. Breatnach C, Conlon NP, Stack M, Healy M, O'Hare BP. A prospective crossover comparison of neurally adjusted ventilatory assist and pressure-support ventilation in a pediatric and neonatal intensive care unit population. Pediatr Crit Care Med. 2010;11(1):7–11.
36. Lee SM, Namgung R, Eun HS, Lee SM, etal. Effective tidal volume for normocapnia in very-low-birth-weight infants using high-frequency oscillatory ventilation. Yonsei Med J. 2018; 59(1): 101-106.
37. Watkins PL, Dagle JM, Bell EF, Colaizy TT. Outcomes at 18 to 22 months of corrected age for infants born at 22 to 25 weeks of gestation in a center practicing active management. J Pediatr. 2020;217:52–8.
38. Fabres J, Carlo WA, Phillips V, Howard G, Ambalavanan N. Both extremes of arterial carbon dioxide pressure and the magnitude of fluctuations in arterial carbon dioxide pressure are associated with severe intraventricular hemorrhage in preterm infants. Pediatrics. 2007;119(2):299–305.
39. Garland JS, Buck RK, Allred EN, Leviton A. Hypocarbia before surfactant therapy appears to increase bronchopulmonary dysplasia risk in infants with respiratory distress syndrome. Arch Pediatr Adolesc Med. 1995;149(6):617–22.
40. Wiswell TE, Graziani LJ, Kornhauser MS, Stanley C, etal. Effects of hypocarbia on the development of cystic periventricular leukomalacia in premature infants treated with high-frequency jet ventilation. Pediatrics 1996; 98(5):918-924.
41. Ryu J, Haddad G, Carlo WA. Clinical effectiveness and safety of permissive hypercapnia. Clin Perinatol. 2012;39(3):603–12.
42. Laffey JG, Engelberts D, Kavanagh BP. Buffering hypercapnic acidosis worsens acute lung injury. Am J Respir Crit Care Med. 2000;161(1):141–6.
43. Keszler M. Volume-targeted ventilation: one size does not fit all. Evidence-based recommendations for successful use. Arch Dis Child Fetal Neonatal Ed. 2019;104(1):F108–12.

44. McCallion N, Davis PG, Morley CJ. Volume-targeted versus pressure-limited ventilation in the neonate. Cochrane Database Syst Rev. 2005;(3):CD003666.
45. Abubakar K, Keszler M. Effect of volume guarantee combined with assist/control vs synchronized intermittent mandatory ventilation. J Perinatol. 2005;25:638–42.
46. Szakmar E, Morley CJ, Belteki G. Leak compensation during volume guarantee with the Dräger Babylog VN500 neonatal ventilator. Pediatr Crit Care Med. 2018;19(9):861–8.
47. Moss ML. The Velo epiglottic sphincter and obligate nose breathing in the neonate. J Pediatr. 1965;67(2):330–5.
48. Wheeler CR, Smallwood CD. Year in review: neonatal respiratory support. Respir Care. 2019;65(5):693–704.
49. Fischer HS, Bührer C. Avoiding endotracheal ventilation to prevent bronchopulmonary dysplasia: a meta-analysis. Pediatrics. 2013;132(5):e1351–60.
50. Moya FR, Mazela J, Shore PM, Simonson SG, Segal R, etal. Prospective observational study of early respiratory management in preterm neonates less than 35 weeks of gestation. BMC Pediatr 2019;19(1):147.
51. Polin RA, Carlo WA. Committee on Fetus and Newborn; American Academy of Pediatrics. Surfactant replacement therapy for preterm and term neonates with respiratory distress. Pediatrics. 2014;133(1):156–63.
52. Dransfield DA, Spitzer AR, Fox WW. Episodic airway obstruction in premature infants. Am J Dis Child. 1983;137(5):441–3.
53. Nielsen KR, Ellington LE, Gray AJ, Stanberry LI, etal. Effect of high-flow nasal cannula on expiratory pressure and ventilation in infant, pediatric, and adult models. Respir Care 2018;63(2):147-157.
54. Lavizzari A, Colnaghi M, Ciuffini F, etal. Heated, humidified high-flow nasal cannula vs nasal continuous positive airway pressure for respiratory distress syndrome of prematurity: a randomized clinical noninferiority trial [published online ahead of print, 2016 Aug 8]. JAMA Pediatr 2016;10.1001
55. Fernandes CJ. Neonatal resuscitation in the delivery room. UPTODATE 2019 [URL: https://www.uptodate.com/contents/neonatal-resuscitation-in-the-delivery-room]
56. Gonçalves RL, Tsuzuki LM, Carvalho MG. Endotracheal suctioning in intubated newborns: an integrative literature review. Rev Bras Ter Intensiva. 2015;27(3):284–92.
57. Carlo WA, Finer NN, Walsh MC, Rich W, Gantz MG, etal, SUPPORT Study Group of the Eunice Kennedy Shriver NICHD Neonatal Research Network. Target ranges of oxygen saturation in extremely preterm infants. N Engl J Med 2010; 362(21):1959-1969.
58. Aziz K, Lee CHC, Escobedo MB, etal. Part 5: Neonatal resuscitation 2020 American Heart Association Guidelines for cardiopulmonary resuscitation and emergency cardiovascular care. Pediatrics 2021;147(Suppl 1):e2020038505E.
59. Fraser D. 10 Complications of positive pressure ventilation. [URL: http:// www. academyof-neonatalnursing. org/NNT/Respiratory_ARC3_10ComplicationsPPV.pdf]
60. Kavvadia V, Greenough A, Dimitriou G. Prediction of extubation failure in preterm neonates. Eur J Pediatr. 2000;159(4):227–31.
61. Williams EE, Hunt KA, Jeyakara J, Subba-Rao R, etal. Electrical activity of the diaphragm following a loading dose of caffeine citrate in ventilated preterm infants. Pediatr Res. 2020; 87(4):740-744.
62. El Amrousy D, Elgendy M, Eltomey M, Elmashad AE. Value of lung ultrasonography to predict weaning success in ventilated neonates. Pediatr Pulmonol. 2020;55(9):2452–6.
63. Soummer A, Perbet S, Brisson H, Arbelot C, etal; Lung Ultrasound Study Group. Ultrasound assessment of lung aeration loss during a successful weaning trial predicts postextubation distress*. Crit Care Med. 2012; 40(7):2064-2072.
64. Frank L, Socenko ID, Gerdes J. Pathophysiology of lung injury repair; special features of the immature lung. In: Polin RA, Fox WW, editors. Fetal and neonatal physiology. Philadelphia: WB Saunders; 1998. p. P1175–88.
65. Soll RF, Morley CJ. Prophylactic versus selective use of surfactant in preventing morbidity and mortality in preterm infants (Cochrane Review). The Chochrane Library; 2002.

66. Cools F, Offringa M, Askie LM. Elective high frequency oscillatory ventilation versus conventional ventilation for acute pulmonary dysfunction in preterm infants. Cochrane Database Syst Rev. 2015;(3):CD000104.

67. Tana M, Lio A, Tirone C, Aurilia C, Tiberi E, etal. Extubation from high-frequency oscillatory ventilation in extremely low birth weight infants: a prospective observational study. BMJ Paediatr Open. 2018; 2(1):e000350.

68. Chang HK. Mechanisms of gas transport during ventilation by high-frequency oscillation. J Appl Physiol: Respirat Exercise Physiol. 1984;56:553–63.

69. Ganguly A, Makkar A, Sekar K. Volume targeted ventilation and high frequency ventilation as the primary modes of respiratory support for elbw babies: what does the evidence say? Front Pediatr. 2020;8:27.

70. Aurilia C, Ricci C, Tana M, Tirone C, Lio A, etal. Management of pneumothorax in hemodynamically stable preterm infants using high frequency oscillatory ventilation: report of five cases. Ital J Pediatr. 2017; 43(1):114.

71. Mahmoud RA, Proquitté H, Fawzy N, Bührer C, Schmalisch G. Tracheal tube airleak in clinical practice and impact on tidal volume measurement in ventilated neonates. Pediatr Crit Care Med. 2011;12(2):197–202.

72. Newth CJ, Rachman B, Patel N, Hammer J. The use of cuffed versus uncuffed endotracheal tubes in pediatric intensive care. J Pediatr. 2004;144(3):333–7.

73. Calder A, Hegarty M, Erb TO, von Ungern-Sternberg BS. Predictors of postoperative sore throat in intubated children. Paediatr Anaesth. 2012;22(3):239–43.

74. Ong M, Chambers NA, Hullet B, Erb TO, etal. Laryngeal mask airway and tracheal tube cuff pressures in children: are clinical endpoints valuable for guiding inflation? Anaesthesia. 2008; 63(7):738-744.

75. Keszler M. Leaks cause problems not only in Washington politics! Has the time come for cuffed endotracheal tubes for newborn ventilation? Pediatr Crit Care Med. 2011;12:231–2.

76. Wallen E, Venkataraman ST, Grosso MJ, Kiene K, Orr RA. Intrahospital transport of critically ill pediatric patients. Crit Care Med. 1995;23(9):1588–95.

77. McKee M. Operating on critically ill neonates: the OR or the NICU. Semin Perinatol. 2004;28(3):234–9.

78. Wolf AR. Ductal ligation in the very low-birth weight infant: simple anesthesia or extreme art? Paediatr Anaesth. 2012;22(6):558–63.

79. Sternberg BS, Boda K, Chambers NA, Rebmann C, etal. Risk assessment for respiratory complications in paediatric anaesthesia: a prospective cohort study. Lancet. 2010;376(9743):773-783.

80. Dewhirst E, Naguib A, Tobias JD. Chest wall rigidity in two infants after low-dose fentanyl administration. Pediatr Emerg Care. 2012;28(5):465–8.

81. Bannister CF, Brosius KK, Wulkan M. The effect of insufflation pressure on pulmonary mechanics in infants during laparoscopic surgical procedures. Paediatr Anaesth. 2003;13(9):785–9.

82. Sternberg BS, Hammer J, Schibler A, etal. Decrease of functional residual capacity and ventilation homogeneity after neuromuscular blockade in anesthetized young infants and preschool children. Anesthesiology 2006; 105(4):670-675.

83. Mansell A, Bryan C, Levison H. Airway closure in children. J Appl Physiol. 1972;33(6):711–4.

84. Glenski TA, Diehl C, Clopton RG, Friesen RH. Breathing circuit compliance and accuracy of displayed tidal volume during pressure-controlled ventilation of infants: a quality improvement project. Paediatr Anaesth. 2017;27(9):935–41.

85. Truchon R. Anaesthetic considerations for laparoscopic surgery in neonates and infants: a practical review. Best Pract Res Clin Anaesthesiol. 2004;18(2):343–5.

86. Barrington KJ, Finer N, Pennaforte T, Altit G. Nitric oxide for respiratory failure in infants born at or near term. Cochrane Database Syst Rev. 2017;1(1):CD000399.

87. Kinsella JP, Steinhorn RH, Mullen MP, Hopper RK, etal; Pediatric Pulmonary Hypertension Network (PPHNet). The left ventricle in congenital diaphragmatic hernia: implications for the management of pulmonary hypertension. J Pediatr 2018; 197: 17-22.

88. Sherlock LG, Wright CJ, Kinsella JP, Delaney C. Inhaled nitric oxide use in neonates: Balancing what is evidence-based and what is physiologically sound. Nitric Oxide. 2020;95:12–6.

Hematological Diseases and Syndromes in the Neonate: Haemoglobin, Haemoglobinopathies, and Oxygen Therapy

Udeyana Singh

15.1 Introduction

The study of Haemoglobins (Hb) is fascinating as it provides basic insight into the transport of oxygen (O2) in the blood, and has the greatest role in the growth, development, both physical and mental, and functioning of all organ systems. Proteins with function such as haemoglobin (Hb motifs) were found in ancient unicellular plants and animals (Hemocyanin, Erythrocruorin). Over millions of years, these bioproteins have evolved to give rise to the Hb molecule which provides oxygen to various parts of the complex multicellular organism. The evolution process has caused Hb gene clusters to accumulate on two separate chromosomes whose expression is developmentally regulated [1–3]. Amazingly, in humans, haemoglobin in the fetus and newborns is different from that in adults, with several unique properties suitable for both intra uterine and extra uterine life.

15.2 Haemoglobin

Adult haemoglobin (HbA), a protein hetero tetramer (64.4 kd), consists of two pairs of polypeptide chains, alpha and nonalpha. In adults, it is nearly 96% of total Hb. Hb molecule exists as a globular molecule in its quaternary structure. The four haem groups lie in clefts between the folded polypeptide chains. The alpha globin chains contain 141 amino acid residues, while the nonalpha (beta) chains contain 146 amino acid residues. Greek letters are used to name the globin chains Adult Hb (HbA $\alpha 2\beta 2$), i.e., two chains each of α- and β-globin [4].

The α-globin genes (two copies each) are located on chromosome 16. α-chains are essential component of normal Hb (HbA, HbA_2, and HbF), and progressive loss

U. Singh (✉)
DMC, Ludhiana, Punjab, India

© The Author(s), under exclusive license to Springer Nature Singapore Pte Ltd. 2023
U. Saha (ed.), *Clinical Anesthesia for the Newborn and the Neonate*,
https://doi.org/10.1007/978-981-19-5458-0_15

of α-alleles leads to increasing severity of **haemolytic anaemias**, such as **thalassemia**. When all the four α-globin genes are inactive or deleted, extrauterine life is not possible (**hydrops fetalis**).

β-Globin gene (one copy each) is present on chromosome 11. This cluster contains other genes too (embryonic β-globin, fetal gamma, epsilon, and delta globin). Both α- and β-chains are essential for life.

The haem molecule has a single ferrous (Fe^{++}) bound to protoporphyrin IX. The haem iron (Fe) is linked to histidine residues between the α- and β-chains. Oxidation of Fe^{++} to ferric (Fe^{+++}) changes Hb into **methaemoglobin**. Charged side groups (lysine, glutamic acid, and arginine) cover the surface of Hb molecule making it hydrophilic and preventing its precipitation.

The HbA carries and delivers O2 to the tissues for aerobic metabolism. This is its most important life sustaining function. It also carries nitric oxide (NO), thus regulating vasomotor tone throughout the body. The uptake and release of O2 by the Hb occur at the haem Fe. Each globin chain is bound to one haem Fe, so each Hb molecule can carry four O2 molecules when fully saturated. With deoxygenation, there is a change in configuration of Hb molecule. β-Chains rotate apart and the deoxy Hb stabilises in a tense (T, constrained) form by change in inter- and intrasubunit bonds. As O2 gets added, the bonds are broken and fully oxygenated Hb assumes a relaxed (R) configuration. There is less bonding energy between the subunits in an oxygenated molecule, thus leading to the formation of two alpha–beta dimers [5]. When the oxygenation of Hb is expressed as a function of O2 concentration, a sigmoid-shaped O2 dissociation curve is formed.

15.2.1 Oxygen Dissociation Curves (ODC)

The sigmoid shape of ODC is due to a phenomenon known as '**cooperativity**', whereby the addition of the first molecule of O2 to Hb increases the affinity of the remaining haems for O2. Other haem proteins such as Bart's (gamma 4) and HbH do not show this phenomenon, thereby exhibiting a hyperbolic ODC. This affinity of Hb for O2 can be increased or decreased (ODC shift to right or left) by various exogenous factors, such as temperature, pH, and 2,3-bisphosphoglycerate (2,3-BPG). Figure 15.1 shows the ODC of Hb A, fetal Hb, myoglobin, and of carboxyhaemoglobin.

15.2.2 O2 Affinity

This is defined by $P_{50,}$ which is the partial pressure of O2 in arterial blood (PaO2) at which Hb is 50% saturated. Under normal physiological conditions (37 °C, pH 7.4), P_{50} of HbA is 27 mm Hg. A right shift of ODC (higher P_{50}) implies that a higher PaO2 is needed to saturate HbA passing through the pulmonary circulation at the level of lungs, reduced affinity of Hb for O2, and higher O2 delivery to the tissues. Conversely, a left shift of ODC (lower P_{50}) implies greater saturation of HbA at lower PaO2, increased affinity of HbF or O2 and lower O2 delivery to the tissues.

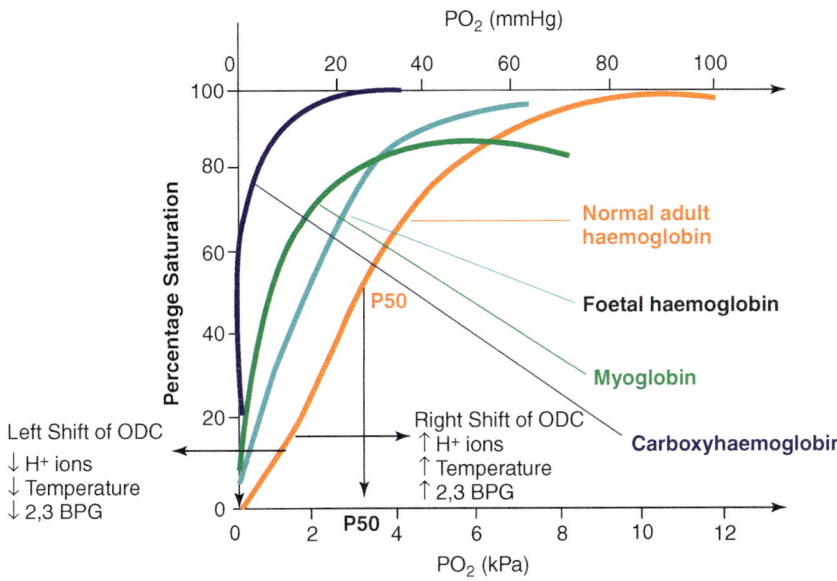

Comparison of Oxygen Dissociation Curves

H+ ions : Hydrogen ions
2,3 BPG : 2,3 Bis Phospho Glycerate

Fig. 15.1 Comparison of oxygen dissociation curves

Bohr effect: the change in affinity of Hb for O2 as a function of pH (6.0–8.5) is described by the Bohr effect. This has two important physiologic consequences.

1. Ready release of O2 at tissue level where PaCO2 is high and pH is low. This is important in the body's adaptability to stress.
2. This also means that O2 is more easily taken up by Hb in the pulmonary circulation where the efflux of CO2 causes pH to rise [6].

2,3-BPG is a potent modulator for O2 affinity. It is synthesized in the glycolytic pathway and is normally present in the red cells in low concentration. 2,3-BPG is strongly bound to deoxy HbA and weakly to oxy Hb. Its binding to deoxy Hb helps in stabilization of the T form of Hb, thus decreasing O2 affinity. Therefore, increased 2,3-DPG decreases O2 affinity (ODC shift to right) promoting tissue O2 delivery to the tissues.

O2 affinity has an inverse relationship with temperature. At high body temperatures, O2 is unloaded to the tissues, at a time when metabolic demand of O2 is probably high.

Hb is also proposed to be a transporter of NO, a potent vasodilator. It binds to the Cys-SH group of HbF forming S-nitrosothiol (SNO) derivative. As blood reaches the tissues and releases O2, NO is also released from Hb, diffusing into the lumen of capillaries and arterioles, causing local vasodilatation [7–10].

15.2.3 HbA2

HbA2 ($\delta 2\alpha 2$) has two delta and two alpha chains and comprises 2–3% of total Hb in adults. Its concentration is increased in β-thalassemia trait and megaloblastic anaemia. Decreased levels are found in α-thalassemia, iron deficiency, and sideroblastic anaemias. Although it has higher O2 affinity than HbA, it exhibits similar responses to changes in pH, temperature, and 2,3-BPG. Higher concentrations of HbA2 decrease the polymerization of HbS (i.e., it protects against sickling) [12].

15.2.4 Fetal Hb (HbF) [11]

HbF is the major Hb in fetal life and comprises of 2 alpha and 2 gamma ($\alpha 2 \lambda 2$) chains. Synthesis of HbA starts at eighth week of gestation and levels of HbF start to rise till 20 weeks of gestation. At 21st week, it is 14% of total Hb and increases to nearly 90% by 23 weeks. After 34th week, HbA levels start to rise, while HbF decreases. At birth, more than 60% of the haemoglobin is HbF and it decreases to less than 2% by 6 months of age. The switch from HbF to HbA is genetically controlled. Babies born at 28 week gestation have 90% HbF. HbF has unique properties. It has higher O2 affinity than HbA as it poorly binds 2,3-BPG. This is helpful to the fetus as it ensures O2 delivery at the expense of maternal HbA helping transplacental O2 transfer. [13, 14] As with HbA2, high concentrations of HbF retards sickling in patients with sickle cell disease.

15.2.5 Embryonic Haemoglobins [15]

These are formed from the yolk sac erythroblasts and can be detected only in the early stages of embryogenesis except for traces in patients of severe α-thalassemia. They are synthesized between 4 and 14 weeks of gestation. After that, erythropoiesis starts in the liver and spleen, and gradually, the embryonic haemoglobins are superseded by HbF.

Embryonic/fetal haemoglobins have increased O2 affinity (P_{50} 4–12 mm Hg) which helps in transport of O2 in a low O2 environment characteristic of early embryogenesis [16]. Abnormalities in Embryonic Hb epsilon (Hb ε) can lead to a delay in switching from HbF to HbA. The different types of embryonic Hb are:

1. **Hb E Gower 1,** the primary Hb in a young embryo (<5 weeks) has two zeta and two epsilon chains. It is unstable and breaks down easily.
2. **Hb E Gower 2,** in embryos less than 13 weeks, has two alpha and two epsilon chains, is more stable than Gower 1, and has a role in management of β-thalassemia and β-chain hemoglobinopathies.
3. **Hb E Portland I** has two zeta and two gamma chains and is present in α-Thalassemia.

4. **Hb E Portland II** is composed of two zeta chains and two beta chains, is very unstable, and has a role in management of α-hemoglobinopathies and α-thalassemia.
5. **Hereditary persistence of fetal haemoglobin (HPFH)** is a rare group of disorders with abnormally high expression of λ globin gene well into adulthood. It is usually asymptomatic or presents with mild anaemia.
6. **HbA1c** is formed by glycosylation of HbA and normally accounts for 3% of total Hb. Its levels are increased in diabetic patients with uncontrolled blood sugar levels.

15.3   Sickle Cell Disease (SCD)

SCD results from the inheritance of a mutant ß-globin gene that codes for HbS, a variant of HbA. It has an autosomal recessive inheritance. The basic defect is the substitution of thymine for adenine on chromosome 11 and of valine for glutamic acid on the sixth position of the β-globin gene [17]. Various genotypes produce disease states:

1. **Sickle cell anaemia:** paired inheritance of the mutant gene results in exclusive expression of HbS and the most severe form of disease.
2. **Sickle cell trait**: the heterozygous inheritance of a mutant and a normal gene results in a carrier state (trait), with RBCs containing both HbS and HbA.
3. The **co-expression of HbS and C**.
4. **Co-inheritance of HbS with other rare mutants**: HbO-Arab, HbD-Punjab, and Hb Lepore-Boston [18].
5. The term **SCD** encompasses many genotypes, such as SS, SC, SE, Sβ°, and Sβ+ thalassemias [19].
6. The most common type **(SS)** is typically called **SCD** and has HbS content of 80–95%.

SCD has a worldwide existence especially with increasing number of cross-cultural marriages and worldwide migration. **Population at risk, includes**:

1. African Americans
2. Mediterranean countries
3. Africa
4. Middle East
5. Asian Subcontinent

15.3.1 Pathophysiology of SCD

The young RBCs containing HbS have normal biconcave shape. On exposure to adverse conditions, such as hypoxia, acidosis, dehydration, hypothermia, and mechanical distortion, HbS molecule gets deoxygenated. The deoxygenated HbS is insoluble, and precipitates out of solution into the cytosol, distorting the RBC's (sickling) and exposing them to mechanical damage during circulation. Initially, this is reversible, but with repeated episodes of sickling, extensive cell membrane damage occurs, leading to an irreversible damage and haemolysis. Free iron is released into the circulation. There is with widespread oxidative damage to the vascular endothelium with inflammatory changes. This leads to deficiency of nitric oxide because of its impaired transport within the RBC, adding on to inflammatory vasculopathy [20]. The lifespan of the RBCs in SCD is reduced, and HbA is low (5–8 G %). There is increased expression of HbF which provides some protection from sickling.

15.3.2 Clinical Presentation

Clinical manifestations include:

1. **Anaemia**: chronic haemolytic anaemia and aplastic anaemia.
2. **Infarctions**: splenic, pulmonary, CVA, bone infarcts, papillary necrosis, and renal failure.
3. **Infections**: meningitis, osteomyelitis, pneumonia, and genitourinary.
4. Some patients may just present with **cholelithiasis, cholestasis, and jaundice**, to be later diagnosed as SCD.

Most common presenting feature is pain and "**Painful episodes**", due to tissue ischaemia following sickling, severity ranging from mild to crippling. Coexistence of a painful episode with a life-threatening event can lead to **Sickle Cell Crisis.** The four main **"crisis"** situations are:

1. **Splenic sequestration**
2. **Acute chest syndrome**
3. **Right upper quadrant syndrome**
4. **Aplastic crisis**

1. **Splenic sequestration** is due to erythrocyte trapping and destruction, splenomegaly, and auto infarction, often necessitating splenectomy in early childhood [21, 22]. This presents as a precipitous fall in haematocrit level, severe hypovolemia, pain, and shock. Management includes infusion of IV fluids and blood products, and pain management.
2. **Acute chest syndrome** is characterised by development of fever, respiratory distress, chest pain, and new infiltrates on chest radiograph. This syndrome accounts for almost 25% of sickle cell deaths [23, 24]. Management includes supplemental O_2, antibiotics, and bronchodilators. Transfusions/exchange transfusions may be needed to maintain the haematocrit at 30%.

3. **Right upper quadrant syndrome**: fever, jaundice, liver failure, and pain indicate the onset of this syndrome. It may be due to hepatic ischemia, cholecystitis, cholangitis, or ischemia of other abdominal organs. IV fluids, analgesics, antibiotics, and supplemental O_2 are the mainstay of treatment.
4. **Aplastic crisis**: failure of reticulocyte formation leads to severe anaemia and aplastic crisis. Supplemental O_2 and transfusions are needed to maintain haematocrit and tissue oxygenation.

15.3.3 Medical Management of SCD

Prenatal and neonatal screening, early detection, and early referral to a centre that provides multidisciplinary approach for routine and emergency care of these patients are paramount:

(i) **Bone-marrow transplantation** may be curative when performed early, especially in severe cases.
(ii) **Hydroxyurea therapy** to increase HbF formation and thus amelioration of symptoms.
(iii) Use of a **viral vector**, based on the human immunodeficiency virus to insert gene therapy modified stem cells, is a novel promising approach for treatment of these patients [25].

15.3.4 Anesthesia Considerations and Management

Preoperative assessment: since SCD can affect multiple organ systems, preoperative assessment should be aimed at determining risk of complications specific to SCD as well as other nonspecific complications with the intention of anticipating and preventing these problems. Assessment relates to the type of procedure, disease activity/severity, and previous exacerbations. Pre-existing organ dysfunction greatly increases perioperative complication rate.

Neonatal concerns - in babies born to parents who are symptomatic or have milder heterozygous variants of SCD, preoperative evaluation depends on the type of procedure, duration of surgery, and expected perioperative fluid shifts. The importance of a thorough clinical examination cannot be overemphasised.

Relevant investigations include:

- Hemoglobin, haematocrit, blood crossmatch (including minor antigens)
- Hemoglobin electrophoresis
- Echocardiogram
- Chest radiograph
- BUN, creatinine, and serum electrolytes
- Platelet count
- PT/PTTK and INR

- MRI/transcranial Doppler in neonates exhibiting neurological signs
- Preoperative pulse oximetry
- ABG

During the early neonatal period, the high concentration of HbF is extremely beneficial and promotes optimal O_2 delivery.

Preoperative blood transfusion: given the wide variation in clinical picture of SCD and lack of any information from the patient and parents, decision for preoperative transfusion is based on neonate's clinical status, complexity and duration of surgery, and risk of surgical haemorrhage. Literature does recommend preoperative transfusion to achieve a haematocrit of 30% and to decrease HbS to <30% [26], but guidelines for prophylactic transfusion are not well-established. Current evidence supports avoiding transfusion in low-risk cases, and should it be necessary, then detailed cross-matching for minor blood groups is mandatory, because of high incidence of alloimmunization, which can lead to life threatening transfusion reactions [27].

15.3.5 Intraoperative Management

Both **general and regional anaesthesia** can be used if care is taken to avoid sickling. Earlier literature reported a higher incidence of postoperative complications with regional anaesthesia, but present-day practice supports the use of neuraxial anaesthesia and regional blocks successfully. Prevention of conditions that promote sickling is the cornerstone of anaesthetic management. All throughout the perioperative period, it is imperative to maintain:

- (i) **Adequate oxygenation**
- (ii) **Adequate O_2 carrying capacity**
- (iii) **Avoiding excessive O_2 consumption**
- (iv) **Avoiding hypovolemia, acidosis, hypothermia**
- (v) **Localized stasis of circulation**

Factors to be kept in mind during anaesthetic management of such neonates:

- **Oxygenation**: hypoxia is a potent trigger for exacerbation of sickling, and **avoidance of hypoxia is the basic standard of anaesthetic care** [28, 29]. Neonates already have limited O_2 reserves and high metabolic consumption of O_2 for growth and maturation. This is further increased with the stress from surgical condition and pain, and any further perioperative hypoxic stress should be avoided. Hyperoxygenation or prolonged O_2 supplementation is not indicated. Pulse-oximetry underestimates true SpO_2 by 2%, due to coexisting methaemoglobin, so attention must be paid when interpreting these values [30].
- **Acid–base balance**: maintenance of normal acid–base balance is equally important. Avoid hypercarbia and accumulation of H+, since acidosis promotes sick-

ling. Uncontrolled acidosis (from underlying surgical condition) can contribute to perioperative hemodynamic instability.

- **Thermoregulation**: normothermia minimizes O_2 consumption and should be maintained. Hypothermia induced peripheral vasoconstriction and localised stasis can induce sickling. A warm ambient temperature, use of forced air warming devices, warm intravenous fluids, and inhaled gases are recommended [29].
- **Hydration and electrolyte balance**: optimum perioperative hydration is imperative to maintain volume status of various compartments. Along with normal electrolyte balance, it helps maintain intracellular volume and osmotic gradients. Cellular dehydration can produce cell membrane damage, so should be avoided. Dehydration will also increase blood viscosity and cause vascular stasis. Thus, intravenous hydration should be guided by clinical signs. Invasive intravascular monitoring should be used only when significant fluid shifts are expected.
- **Use of tourniquet/blood pressure cuff** [31], even while inserting peripheral lines should be avoided as it may promote local stasis and sickling which may degenerate into a generalized phenomenon. Careful positioning and padding is necessary to prevent venous stasis and consequent ischemia.
- **Congenital cardiac anomalies,** need a special mention regarding correction of the anomaly and use of cardiopulmonary bypass. The use of exchange transfusions to reduce HbS concentration to <5% used to be the norm. Recently, reports of bypass without this are available. The pump prime dilutes HbS concentration and the circuit preferentially filters out the sickle cells [32, 33].

15.3.6 Postoperative Care

The same care and considerations must continue into the postoperative period.

- **Control of pain** is paramount as uncontrolled pain can start the cascade of a pain crisis. Pain estimation can be difficult in neonates. Multimodal analgesia and neuraxial and regional blocks provide good pain relief [34–36].
- Untiring **vigilance** is required to keep physiological parameters within normal limits
- The lungs should be regularly examined to detect the development of **acute chest syndrome**. Early detection and management can prevent postoperative adverse events in these neonates.
- Eternal vigilance for development of new signs and effective communication between the treating team (neonatologist, surgeon, anaesthesiologist, nursing team) are indispensable for optimal outcomes.

15.4 Thalassaemia

Thalassaemia's comprise an expansive group of inherited blood disorders characterised by defective synthesis of globin chains of Hb bioprotein. The term 'thalassaemia' originates from the Greek words meaning 'sea' and 'blood'. This was due to the geographical association of the early reported cases with regions around the Mediterranean Sea, as reported by Cooley and Lee in 1925. They described children from Italy presenting with splenomegaly and bone deformities [37, 38]. Due to worldwide travel and interracial marriages, thalassaemia has become a disease with a global burden and anaesthesiologists need to be familiar with this group of diseases.

15.4.1 Pathophysiology

The human body produces various types of haemoglobins over the period of intra- and extra-uterine life to cover the variable O2 demands. The basic common feature is the tetrameric structure of this bioprotein with two different pairs of polypeptide chains (globin) combined with an iron containing molecule (haem).

In the normal adult, HbA is the predominant Hb (96%) and comprises of two α-globin and two β-chains ($\alpha_2 \beta_2$). HbA2 is a normal variant (2–3%) containing two α and δ chains ($\alpha_2\delta_2$). HbF ($\alpha_2 \gamma_2$) is the predominant Hb during fetal life. In term neonate, 60–80% is HbF, decreasing to less than 1% by adulthood. Other less common embryonic Hb are Hb-Gower1 ($\zeta_2\epsilon_2$), Hb-Portland ($\zeta_2\gamma_2$), and Hb-Gower 2($\alpha_2\epsilon_2$) [39].

Each chromosome 16 has two α-globin genes and each chromosome 11 has one non α-globin gene. Normally, six alleles code for globin chains. The α-chains are controlled by four codominant alleles and β-chains by two codominant alleles [37].

Decreased production of α-chains leads to **α-thalassaemia**, which further has two types—α or α^0, characterised by decrease or complete absence of α-chains [40]. There is an abundance of β-like chains to compensate for the decrease in α-chains:

- Individuals with 'α α /α-' genotype have only one nonfunctional allele and are thus silent carriers of the disease.
- Individuals with ($-\alpha/-$ α or $\alpha\alpha/--$) present with mild anaemia and jaundice [40].
- Serious variants include HbH disease ($--/\alpha$-) with only one functional allele leading to formation of tetramers of β-chains (HbH), Bart's hydrops fetalis syndrome with formation of tetramers of γ chains (Hb Bart's) and no functional allele ($--/--$). Hb Barts and HbH have infinite O2 affinity, thus provide no O2 to the fetus, leading to fetal demise or early neonatal death despite aggressive intrauterine transfusions [40].
- Similarly, in β-thalassemia, there exist β and β^0 types with decreased or absent β-globin chain production. The α-like chains are in excess causing them to precipitate inside the erythrocytes resulting in haemolysis and ineffective erythropoiesis.

Clinical symptoms can be characterised into three phenotypes according to the severity of the disease and need for early blood transfusion [39]:

(i) **The minor (trait)**

(ii) **The intermedia**
(iii) **The major (traditionally known as Cooley's anaemia)**

Abnormalities of δ-globin and β-globin genes sometimes lead to increased γ-globin expression moderately (δβ-thalassemia with Hb-Lepore) or severely leading to a condition known as hereditary persistence of fatal haemoglobin (**HPFH**).

Another common type is the HbE/β-thalassaemia which occurs due to co-expression of genes for HbE and β-thalassemia [39].

The disease is found in the Mediterranean areas and south–east Asia as heterozygous individuals are resistant to Plasmodium falciparum malaria by mechanisms not yet understood [41]. Tropical and subtropical areas shown endemicity for α-thalassemia [39, 42]. Thalassemia show an autosomal recessive inheritance, thus homozygous individuals show complete expression of the phenotype. However, coexpression off other genes plays a vital role in the clinical expression [43].

Clinical spectrum results from ineffective erythropoiesis leading to extramedullary erythropoiesis, iron overload due to chronic haemolysis, and the side effects of chelation therapy. This enhanced erythropoiesis cannot compensate for the lack of normally functioning Hb and the relative excess of α-chains is responsible for many of the detrimental effects. Thalassemia are multisystem disorders involving all systems of the body:

1. **The cardiovascular system**: the disease may present as severe biventricular cardiomyopathy with pulmonary hypertension and congestive heart failure. Conduction abnormalities with an increased risk of Torsade's de Pointes, ventricular tachycardia, and sudden death have been reported. These are more prevalent in thalassemia intermedia and major [44, 45].
2. **The respiratory system** shows restrictive lung dysfunction with a reduced total lung capacity and lung fibrosis, more severe in thalassemia major and progress with increasing duration of the disease. Pulmonary hypertension may be present in 50–75% of the cases. Free Hb released during haemolysis causes nitric oxide scavenging and reduced bioavailability of nitric oxide is the proposed mechanism for the same [46–48].
3. **The renal system** shows abnormalities of glomerular filtration, renal tubular function in the form of high creatinine clearance and increased loss of urinary electrolytes (calcium, phosphate, magnesium), and uric acid. These are exacerbated by the direct nephrotoxicity of iron chelators, such as desferrioxamine. Low molecular weight protein urea is the most common abnormality seen in β-thalassaemia [49–51].
4. The most prominent of the **endocrine disorders** such as anterior pituitary dysfunction, hypogonadism, hypothyroidism, and hypoparathyroidism is due to chronic iron overload and can usually be reversed partially by intensive chelation. With aggressive medical management, patients exhibit growth retardation (resistant to growth hormone), fertility problems, and glucose intolerance as they reach puberty and early adulthood [52, 53].

5. **Ineffective erythropoiesis** leads to erythropoiesis in extra-medullary areas causing craniofacial abnormalities such as fronto-parietal bossing, prominent zygomatic bones, and maxillary over growth with dental malocclusion giving rise to characteristic 'chipmunk face'. In the spine, expansion of marrow cavities may lead to spinal deformities along with compression of neural structures leading to cauda equina syndrome. Visual abnormalities and hearing loss may occur due to neural compression by the expanding skull. Osteopenia, osteomalacia, and microfractures may occur. This **osteopathy** progresses with inadequate transfusion and chelation therapy [54–56].

6. Patients exhibit an **increased thrombotic tendency**, probably due to platelet and endothelial activation due to chronic haemolysis and decreased levels of antithrombin-III, and deficiency of protein C and S. The chronic endothelial oxidative injury leads to ischemia–reperfusion and is a cause of pulmonary hypertension and thromboembolic events. The incidence of silent cerebral infarctions is quite high in β-thalassaemia intermedia and major. Regular transfusions decrease the risk of cerebral thrombosis.

7. **Haemochromatosis** results from repeated blood transfusions, and increased intestinal iron absorption and release of iron from the reticuloendothelial system. This iron deposition is responsible for many of the systemic abnormalities.

8. **Infections:** multiple transfusions also lead to a higher rate of hepatitis B and C, HIV, West Nile virus, and babesiosis [57, 58].

15.4.2 Clinical Presentation of α-Thalassemia Varies

- Asymptomatic: patients with trait (2/4 functional alleles) are symptom free and are diagnosed during routine screening either antenatal or during evaluation for the cause of microcytic hypochromic anaemia.
- Patients with **HbH disease** (high O2 affinity) present with jaundice, stunted growth, and splenic enlargement with intermittent haemolytic episodes. They may require urgent blood transfusion [40].
- Fetus with **Hb Bart's (γ_4)** receive almost no O2 at the tissue level. Severe haemolytic anaemia ensues with abnormal brain development, congenital cardiac abnormalities, heart failure, pleural and pericardial effusions, ascites, hepato-splenomegaly, and other associated defects [59]. These neonates usually have an early postnatal death. This syndrome also causes preeclampsia and edema in the mother (known as **mirror syndrome**) along with dystocia and increased chance of retained placenta (due to enlarged placental size) and postpartum haemorrhage [59].

Diagnosis: early diagnosis of these conditions is vital for preventing end organ damage and for a healthy neurological outcome. Along with a blood picture of microcytic hypochromic anaemia, a blood film and reticulocyte count are performed when haemolysis is suspected. High-performance liquid chromatography (HPLC), isoelectric focusing, and microcolumn chromatography help in identification of various of Hb fractions. Serum ferritin levels are the standard routine test in case iron loading is suspected. Recently MRI has been suggested as an alternative to liver biopsy to evaluate iron accumulation.

Medical management: significant progress has been made over the last few decades and now effective treatment strategies and supportive care exists for these patients:

- **β-Major type** requires regular blood transfusions (many times a month) for optimal growth and suppression of ineffective erythropoiesis.
- Hydroxycarbamide (hydroxyurea) promotes the production of γ-chains and HbF, thus reducing transfusion requirements. Desferrioxamine is the traditionally used chelating agent which is administered IV or subcutaneously (5–7 times/week) to transfusion dependent patients. It has multiple side effects including pulmonary fibrosis, teratogenesis and as yet no safety profile exists for possible risks to breastfed neonates.
- Orally administered chelating agents are now available (deferiprone, deferasirox and deferitin) with better compliance and reduce side effects [60].
- Stem cell transplantation offers only hope of a permanent cure. Stem cells can be sourced from bone marrow, peripheral blood, and cord blood. Disease-free survival rates of 80–97% have been reported [58].

15.4.3 Perioperative Management

Preoperative assessment: thalassemia, due to multisystem involvement, warrants a thorough evaluation prior to surgery. Clinical assessment should guide the way to relevant laboratory and radiographic analysis. Investigations should include:

- Complete hemogram with peripheral blood film
- Coagulation profile
- Renal function tests
- Liver function tests
- Echocardiogram

Because of the neonatal age group of our patients, airway assessment may be difficult and the typical features seen in thalassemia patients have not yet developed. Nevertheless, we should always be prepared to encounter a difficult airway scenario while handling this group of patients. Standard operating room procedure should be followed as in the case of all neonates with thermal control, adequate warm IV fluids, avoidance of stress, vasoconstriction, stasis, and acidosis.

Both general and regional anaesthesia can be safely used, keeping these general principles in mind. Before using regional anaesthesia, care should be taken for documentation of any pre-existing neurological compression or deficit.

During the neonatal period, the high concentration of HbF is helpful in ensuring adequate O2 supply to the tissues. Though HbF has a higher O2 affinity than HbA, the ODC is predictable, and safe anaesthesia can be conducted using slightly higher FiO_2, correlating them to SpO2 and serial ABG estimations.

Careful assessment of the neonates should be done throughout the perioperative period by a team consisting of a neonatologist, haematologist, anaesthesiologist, and a paediatric surgeon. Optimal communication and cooperation between the team is necessary for a good clinical outcome.

15.4.4 Monitoring and Care

- Usually, noninvasive vital monitoring is sufficient in such neonates undergoing surgery, however, those with cardiomyopathy and pulmonary hypertension, may need **invasive monitoring,** for careful perioperative management.
- **Cardiovascular depression** should be avoided and the use of volatile anaesthetics should be at low concentrations.
- **Pulmonary arterial catherization** might be needed in selected high-risk cases. The several haemodynamic parameters derived from it may help guide therapy in these cases. The risk of adverse events and complications should always be taken into consideration when pulmonary artery catherization is being contemplated.
- Diuretics, angiotensin converting enzyme inhibitors, and Prostaglandin E_1 maybe helpful in guiding therapy and managing cardiac workload.
- Avoidance of nitrous oxide should be considered in such cases [61, 62].
- Haematocrit should not be allowed to fall below 30%.
- Maintenance of intravascular volume is of paramount importance.
- Steps to minimise intraoperative bleeding should be used.
- Blood scavenging may be considered to prevent alloimmunisation. During the use of cell salvage, suction pressures should be kept low and a continuous check on the effluent line for excess haemolysis, and blood should be leukodepleted when it is returned to the patient [63, 64].
- As these neonates are immune compromised, appropriate broad-spectrum antibiotics should be used to minimise perioperative infections.
- Careful screening should be done to prevent and treat hypercoagulability, although no formal guidelines exist as of now.

Postoperative care: the postoperative period should be a continuation of the intraoperative care with prevention of hypothermia, hypoxia, hypercarbia, and acidosis. Neonates should be closely monitored for the development of hypertension as it may herald impending seizures.

15.4.5 Mutant Haemoglobins and Anesthesia

In addition to thalassemia and sickle celled disease, more than 1000 different mutations of the globin chains in the human Hb molecule have been identified [65, 66]. Some of the more common mutant haemoglobins are as follows:

Haemoglobin E: a mutation in the beta-globin chain is associated with clinical disease leading to mild anaemia with a thalassaemic blood picture. Heterozygotes have up to 30% HbE while homozygotes may have more than 90% HbE and no HbA. It is commonly found in India and South East Asia as HBE gives resistance to *P. falciparum* [67, 68].

Haemoglobin C: in addition, a beta globin chain mutation commonly found in Atlantic West Africa. Affected individuals have a mild degree of haemolysis with mild-to-moderate anaemia and splenomegaly [69]. This mutation protects against severe forms of malaria.

Haemoglobin D: its most common variant is HbD–Los Angeles (also called Hb Punjab). Individuals with trait are symptomatic, and homozygous individuals have only mild features. Inheritance with HbS can result in disease with features similar to homozygous sickle cell anaemia.

Haemoglobin M: in this Hb, the haem iron is oxidised to ferric (Fe^{+++}). Patients may present with cyanosis, especially on exertion, caused by high levels of methaemoglobin.

Other common variants include **Hb Lepore, Hb Constant Spring, Hb O-Arab** which may be identified on haemoglobin electrophoresis.

Pathophysiology: these abnormal haemoglobins may behave as either of the following:

(i) **Hb with high O2 affinity:** are associated with decreased tissue O2 delivery and compensatory erythrocytosis. They can be identified through P50 estimation and genetic testing [70].

(ii) **HB with low O2 affinity**: release O2 readily to the tissues, and Hb may be so unsaturated as to cause visible cyanosis.

Anaesthetic implications: when there is a suspicion that we are dealing with an abnormal Hb variant, it would be prudent to form an estimation of ODC by correlating different FiO_2 values, SpO2 and ABG estimations. Thereby, safe FiO_2 values can be applied during the perioperative period to prevent hypoxia. Often, the first indication of a mutant Hb maybe abnormal SpO2 readings which do not correlate with the clinical picture. Hence, after ruling out cardiovascular and respiratory disease, a haematological evaluation would be in order for this subset of patients.

15.5 Oxygen Therapy for Preterm and Term Neonates

Prematurity can be defined on the basis of two parameters, gestational age (GA) as calculated from the first day of the mother's last menstrual period, and birth weight (BW):

1. Based on **GA**:
   (a) Extremely preterm (EPT)—≤28 weeks
   (b) Very preterm (VPT)—≤32 weeks
   (c) Moderate preterm—32–33 weeks ± 6 days
   (d) Late preterm—34–36 weeks ± 6 days

2. According to **BW**:
    (a) Extremely low BW (ELBW)—<1000 g
    (b) Very low BW (VLBW)—<1500 g
    (c) Low BW—<2500 g

Oxygen is one of the most commonly administered drugs either in hospital settings, in the delivery room, or in the NICU. A very fine balance needs to be maintained while administering O2, as both hypoxia and hyperoxia are dangerous to neonates.

(i). Clinical Indicators of Hypoxia in the Neonate:

- **Cyanosis**: the development of bluish discoloration of hands and feet is a normal phenomenon at birth (acrocyanosis) which eventually disappears. Peripheral cyanosis is also normal on exposure to cold. Cyanosis (central) occurring around the lips or tongue is a cause of concern and should be investigated and treated.
- **Heart rate**: a fixed heart rate ≤ 120 beats/min or decreasing trend is a common accompaniment of hypoxia.
- **Motor activity**: initial restlessness followed by lethargy and unresponsiveness should also send up a red flag.
- **Respiratory**: hypoxia leads to anaerobic metabolism. The onset of acidosis is heralded by rapid breathing followed by cardiopulmonary depression.

(ii). Common indications for O2 supplementation are:

   (i) Birth asphyxia
  (ii) Hypoxemia (SpO_2 <87%, PaO_2 <50 mmHg on room air)
 (iii) Cyanosis
  (iv) Respiratory distress
   (v) Hypothermia
  (vi) Apneic spells
 (vii) Pneumothorax/pneumomediastinum

(iii). In a breathing neonate, supplemental O2 may be provided by a hood, nasal cannula (low for high flow), nasal prongs, continuous positive airway pressure (CPAP), and nasal intermittent positive pressure ventilation (NIPPV) systems.

In a neonate who is either in respiratory distress/fatigue or not breathing at all, IPPV with tracheal intubation is the only option.

(iv). The recommended target SpO2 levels for various premature neonates are as follows [71, 72]:

- <32 weeks—88–92% (PaO_2 50–70 mmHg)
- 32–36 weeks—90–95% (PaO_2 60–80 mmHg)
- ≥ 37 weeks—90–98% (PaO_2 60–90 mmHg)

These target pulse oximetry saturation ranges have been suggested as a result of evidence gathered after multiple meta-analysis, so that the metabolic demands of the preterm neonates are met without causing hyperoxia and its consequences, such as bronchopulmonary dysplasia (BPD) and retinopathy of prematurity (ROP) [73–75].

Checking for the attainment of these target levels is usually done by the use of pulse oximeters which are convenient to use while being noninvasive. They have their inherent drawbacks such as inability to interpret the data with motion artifacts and are perfusion dependent:

- Neonates are continuously moving/crying making motion artefacts common place.
- Unless maintained in a thermoneutral environment their peripheries might be cold.
- At saturations above 96%, PaO_2 values may continue to increase with little if any further increase in the SpO_2 value. This is due to the flat portion of the ODC at PaO_2 above 60 mmHg.
- HbF has high O2 affinity shifting the ODC to the left, which may result in O2 saturation values being around 85–90%, while the PaO_2 may be at or below 45 mmHg.
- As neonates may have Hb variants or abnormal Hb, whose absorption properties may be different, this can interfere with pulse oximetry readings [76].
- Rapidly changing hemodynamics.

Measures to be taken for a better idea of the actual metabolic picture of the neonate:

(a) Always look for the presence of good oximetric wave form, and the pulse rate corresponds to the neonate's actual heart rate.
(b) Get periodic ABG estimations through an indwelling catheter or periodic pricks.

15.5.1 O2 Delivery Devices

O2 hood: these are high flow (7–15 L/min) high concentration systems that utilize either a hard plastic or soft tent-like structure that fits over the neonate's head or entire body. High FiO_2 of 80–90% can be obtained. O2 enters the hood through a gas inlet and exits around the patient's neck. A pass over system may be used to humidify the gas. Due to limited accessibility to the neonate, these are not preferred. An O2 analyzer should periodically be used to test the O2 concentration within the hood.

Nasal cannula: these deliver O2 through two soft prongs inserted into the anterior nares. These can be used to deliver low flows or high flows. The O2 entering the patients' nasopharynx through the cannula mixes with the air being taken in through the mouth and nose; therefore, a variable concentration of O2 is delivered depending on the respiratory rate, tidal volume, amount of mouth breathing, and O2 flow rate.

Low flow nasal cannula (LFNC): usually, flow rates of 1–2 L/min are used. This flow rate provides minimal positive pressure. A variable concentration of inspired O2 is delivered sometimes equivalent to room air. These gases tend to dry the airway and may lead to crusting, mucosal injury and cannula blockade [77, 78].

High flow nasal cannula (HFNC): these deliver humidified and heated O2 at flow rates varying from 4 to 8 L/min. The proposed benefit of using this is that the high gas flows wash out the end expiratory and dead space gases to replace it with fresh gas in the upper airway, while also providing some positive airway distending pressure [79, 80]. This benefit is seen in term neonates, but studies fail to support its use in VPT babies in whom nCPAP is preferred. It is to be noted that some amount of gastric distension will occur as a consequence of high flows used. The size and diameter of the HNFC prongs are smaller than those used for CPAP, so that there is sufficient leak in the nares to protect the mucosa from the high pressure which very rarely has led to traumatic air dissections [81].

Continuous positive airway pressure (CPAP): when additional respiratory support is needed, CPAP can be used both as primary respiratory support and for post extubation respiratory aid. The lung recruitment caused by the positive pressure and splinting of the airway reduces the airway collapse and work of breathing. nCPAP is the preferred noninvasive ventilatory support for VPT babies who are risk for RDS [82, 83]. Post-extubation, its application decreases the incidence of apnea, need for reintubation and for ventilation.

CPAP systems may be administered either through nasal prongs or mask. Various CPAP systems available are: constant flow systems, bubble CPAP systems, and fluidic CPAP (variable flow CPAP). The most preferred is the fluidic CPAP system specially for smaller neonates. This system has two flow paths, one for inspiration and the other for expiration. This reduces the work of breathing and improves lung compliance and hypopharyngeal function [84].

Nasal intermittent positive pressure ventilation (NIPPV): this provides respiratory support to preterm neonates who would otherwise require intubation and mechanical ventilation. It delivers positive pressure from a ventilator through nasal prongs or mask, and both synchronized and nonsynchronized breaths can be delivered, though synchronization is difficult to achieve in neonates. This mode is costly and the safety profile is as yet unknown, and abdominal distension is a known complication [81, 85].

Most clinicians still prefer CPAP over NIPPV as long-term results of NIPPV therapy are still unknown.

Noninvasive neurally adjusted ventilatory assist (NIV–NAVA): this is a synchronized mode of NIPPV. Ventilator breaths are triggered by diaphragmatic contraction. This method is least affected by leaks around the interface as the patient's own inspiratory effort and breathing pattern regulate the breathing activity. Limited data are available about its beneficial effects [86, 87].

Other modes of respiratory support with little data comparing them with other traditional modes of ventilation are:

Noninvasive high-frequency oscillatory ventilation: some clinicians have used it in preterm neonates and reported lower rates of intubation and mechanical ventilation. More clinical trials are needed to determine its safety profile.

Bilevel nasal CPAP: it provides breaths at lower pressures, lower cycle rates with longer inflation times than NIPPV. As a result, two alternating levels of CPAP pressures are generated. Little evidence exists as to its superiority over the standard CPAP.

15.5.2 Oxygen Toxicity

Excess oxygen in the body causes increased production of oxygen free radicals. These are highly reactive and cause lipid peroxidation, DNA damage, and degradation of proteins in multiple organ systems. Our body normally has antioxidants (vitamins A, C, E) and free-radical scavengers, such as superoxide dismutase and glutathione peroxidase. Prolonged administration of high FiO2 can overwhelm the body's natural defense. O2 free-radical damage is believed to be a cause of retinopathy of prematurity (ROP), bronchopulmonary dysplasia (BPD), necrotising enterocolitis (NEC), and patent ductus arterioles (PDA).

15.5.3 Retinopathy of Prematurity (ROP)

It is a proliferative vascular disorder of the retinal vessels seen in preterm babies. The incidence and severity increase with decreasing GA and BW. The disease develops in two stages. The initial insult, caused by hypotension, hypoxia, or hyperoxia, damages the newly forming blood vessels in the eye. After this, the vessels may regrow normally or abnormal new vessels may grow into the retina or the vitreous cavity. These new vessels are prone to edema and hemorrhage, which heals by fibrosis, and later causes retinal distortion or detachment. While prematurity is the most important risk factor, others include prolonged ventilatory support, multiple blood transfusions, surfactant therapy, and prolonged illness [88, 89].

Screening for ROP is recommended in all babies with BW <1500 g or GA ≤30 weeks. Screening in selected babies with BW >1500 g is recommended when they have more than one of the above-mentioned risk factors.

15.5.4 Bronchopulmonary Dysplasia (BPD)

It is a condition of chronic lung disease due to interruption of normal lung development and lung injury in preterm babies. It is defined as the need for oxygen supplementation either at 28 days postnatal or 36 weeks postmenstrual age. The disease pathology consists of decreased alveolar septation, alveolar hypoplasia, dysregulation of pulmonary vasculature leading to pulmonary hypertension, and thickening of interstitium leading to defective gas exchange. The etiology is multifactorial and includes intrauterine growth retardation, maternal smoking, mechanical ventilation, oxygen toxicity, and infections [90, 91].

Babies with severe BPD become hypoxemic and hypercapnic due to cardiopulmonary abnormalities. Most improve gradually over 2–4 months, while those with severe disease may develop heart failure.

In addition NEC, with a multivariate etiology and PDA have also been linked to oxygen toxicity, though more research is needed to conclusively prove the same. Nevertheless, all these data prove that oxygen administration is a double-edged sword. Levels in the body needs to be exquisitely titrated to clinical and laboratory preset end points.

References

1. Schechter AN. Hemoglobin research and the origins of molecular medicine. Blood. 2008;112:3927.
2. Hardison RC. Evolution of hemoglobin and its genes. Cold Spring Harb Perspect Med. 2012;2:a011627.
3. Hardison R. Hemoglobins from bacteria to man: evolution of different patterns of gene expression. J Exp Biol. 1998;201:1099.
4. Perutz MF. Molecular anatomy, physiology, and pathology of hemoglobin. In: Stamatoyannopoulos G, Nienhuis AW, et al., editors. The molecular basis of blood disorders. Philadelphia: WB Saunders; 1987. p. 127.
5. Shibayama N. Allosteric transitions in hemoglobin revisited. Biochim Biophys Acta Gen Subj. 2020;1864:129335.
6. Bohr C, Hasselbalch K, Krogh A. Ueber einen in biologischer Beziehung wichtigen Einfluss. den die Kohlen- sauerespannung des Blutes auf dessen Sauerstoffbinding ubt. Skand Arch Physiol. 1904;16(402)
7. Jia L, Bonaventura C, Bonaventura J, Stamler JS. S-nitrosohaemoglobin: a dynamic activity of blood involved in vascular control. Nature. 1996;380:221.
8. Stamler JS, Jia L, Eu JP, et al. Blood flow regulation by S-nitrosohemoglobin in the physiological oxygen gradient. Science. 1997;276:2034.
9. Gow AJ, Stamler JS. Reactions between nitric oxide and haemoglobin under physiological conditions. Nature. 1998;391:169.
10. Crawford JH, Isbell TS, Huang Z, et al. Hypoxia, red blood cells, and nitrite regulate NO-dependent hypoxic vasodilation. Blood. 2006;107:566.
11. Bunn HF, Forget BG. Hemoglobin: molecular, genetic and clinical aspects. Philadelphia: WB Saunders; 1986.
12. Nagel RL, Bookchin RM, Johnson J, et al. Structural bases of the inhibitory effects of hemoglobin F and hemoglobin A2 on the polymerization of hemoglobin S. Proc Natl Acad Sci U S A. 1979;76:670.
13. Tyuma I, Shimizu K. Different response to organic phosphates of human fetal and adult hemoglobins. Arch Biochem Biophys. 1969;129:404.
14. Adachi K, Konitzer P, Pang J, et al. Amino acids responsible for decreased 2,3-biphosphoglycerate binding to fetal hemoglobin. Blood. 1997;90:2916.
15. Hofmann O, Mould R, Brittain T. Allosteric modulation of oxygen binding to the three human embryonic haemoglobins. Biochem J. 1995;306(Pt 2):367.
16. Manning LR, Popowicz AM, Padovan JC, et al. Gel filtration of dilute human embryonic hemoglobins reveals basis for their increased oxygen binding. Anal Biochem. 2017;519:38.
17. Honig GR. Hemoglobin disorders. In: Behrman RE, Kliegman RM, Jenson HB, editors. Nelson textbook of pediatrics. 18th ed. Philadelphia, PA: WB Saunders Company; 2007. p. 2026–31.

18. Firth PG, Head CA. SCD and anesthesia. Anesthesiology. 2004;101(3):766–85.
19. Maxwell LG, Goodwin SR, Mancuso TJ, et al. Systemic disorders in infants and children. In: Motoyama EK, Davis PJ, editors. Smith's anesthesia for infants and children. 7th ed. Philadelphia, PA: Mosby Elsevier, Inc.; 2006. p. 1060–4.
20. Gladwin MT, Vichinsky E. Pulmonary complications of SCD. N Engl J Med. 2008;359(21):2254–65.
21. Al-Salem AH. Indications and complications of splenectomy for children with SCD. J Pediatr Surg. 2006;41(11):1909–15.
22. Marchant WA, Walker I. Anaesthetic management of the child with SCD. Paediatr Anaesth. 2003;13:473–89.
23. Vichinsky EP, Styles LA, Colangelo LH, et al. Acute chest syndrome in SCD: clinical presentation and course. Blood. 1997;89(5):1787–92.
24. Vichinsky EP, Neumayr LD, Earles AN. Causes and outcomes of the acute chest syndrome in SCD. National Acute Chest Syndrome Study Group. N Engl J Med. 2000;342(25):1855–65.
25. Pawliuk R, Westerman KA, Fabry ME, Payen E, et al. Correction of SCD in transgenic mouse models by gene therapy. Science. 2001;294:2368–71.
26. Vichinsky EP, Haberkern CM, Neumayr L, et al. A comparison of conservative and aggressive transfusion regimens in the perioperative management of SCD. The Preoperative Transfusion in SCD Study Group. N Engl J Med. 1995;333(4):206–13.
27. Petz LD, Calhoun L, Shulman IA, et al. The sickle cell hemolytic transfusion reaction syndrome. Transfusion. 1997;37(4):382–92.
28. Shapiro ND, Poe MF. Sickle-cell disease: an anesthesiological problem. Anesthesiology. 1955;16(5):771–80.
29. Barash PG, Cullen BF, Stoelting RK. Clinical anesthesia. Philadelphia: Lippincott; 1989.
30. Fitzgerald RK, Johnson A. Pulse oximetry in sickle cell anemia. Crit Care Med. 2001;29(9):1803–6.
31. Adu-Gyamfi Y, Sankarankutty M, Marwa S. Use of a tourniquet in patients with SCD. Can J Anaesth. 1993;40(1):24–7.
32. Metras D, Coulibaly AO, Ouattara K, et al. Open-heart surgery in sickle-cell haemoglobinopathies: report of 15 cases. Thorax. 1982;37(7):486–91.
33. Frimpong-Boateng K, Amoah AG, Barwasser HM, et al. Cardiopulmonary bypass in sickle cell anaemia without exchange transfusion. Eur J Cardiothorac Surg. 1998;14(5):527–9.
34. Camous J, N'da A, Etienne-Julan M, et al. Anesthetic management of pregnant women with SCD—effect on postnatal sickling complications. Can J Anaesth. 2008;55(5):276–83.
35. Yaster M, Tobin JR, Billett C, et al. Epidural analgesia in the management of severe vaso-occlusive sickle cell crisis. Pediatrics. 1994;93(2):310–5.
36. Finer P, Blair J, Rowe P. Epidural analgesia in the management of labor pain and sickle cell crisis—a case report. Anesthesiology. 1988;68(5):799–800.
37. Firth PG. Anesthesia and hemoglobinopathies. Anesthesiol Clin. 2009;27:321–36.
38. Cooley TB, Lee P. A series of cases of splenomegaly in children with anemia and peculiar bone changes. Trans Am Pediatr Soc. 1925;37:29–30.
39. Higgs DR, Weatherall DJ. The alpha thalassaemias. Cell Mol Life Sci. 2009;66:1154–62.
40. Harteveld CL, Higgs DR. Alpha-thalassemia. Orphanet J Rare Dis. 2010;5:13.
41. Weatherall DJ. Common genetic disorders of the red cell and the 'malaria hypothesis'. Ann Trop Med Parasitol. 1987;81:539–48.
42. Weatherall DJ. The inherited diseases of hemoglobin are an emerging global health burden. Blood. 2010;115:4331–6.
43. Higgs DR, Engel JD, Stamatoyannopoulos G. Thalassaemia. Lancet. 2012;379:373–83.
44. Hahalis G, Alexopoulos D, Kremastinos DT, Zoumbos NC. Heart failure in b-thalassemia syndromes: a decade of progress. Am J Med. 2005;118:957–67.
45. Aessopos A, Farmakis D, Deftereos S, et al. Thalassemia heart disease: a comparative evaluation of thalassemia major and thalassemia intermedia. Chest. 2005;127:1523–30.
46. Du Z-D, Roguin N, Milgram E, Saab K, Koren A. Pulmonary hypertension in patients with thalassemia major. Am Heart J. 1997;134:532–7.

47. Grisaru D, Rachmilewitz EA, Mosseri M, et al. Cardiopulmonary assessment in beta-thalassemia major. Chest. 1990;98:1138–42.
48. Morris CR, Kuypers FA, Kato GJ, et al. Hemolysis-associated pulmonary hypertension in thalassemia. Ann N Y Acad Sci. 2005;1054:481–5.
49. Ponticelli C, Musallam KM, Cianciulli P, Cappellini MD. Renal complications in transfusion-dependent beta thalassaemia. Blood Rev. 2010;24:239–44.
50. Yacobovich J, Stark P, Barzilai-Birenbaum S, et al. Acquired proximal renal tubular dysfunction in b-thalassemia patients treated with deferasirox. J Pediatr Hematol Oncol. 2010;32:564–7.
51. Quinn CT, Johnson VL, Kim H-Y, et al. Renal dysfunction in patients with thalassaemia. Br J Haematol. 2011;153:111–7.
52. Toumba M, Sergis A, Kanaris C, Skordis N. Endocrine complications in patients with thalassaemia major. Pediatr Endocrinol Rev. 2007;5:642–8.
53. Delvecchio M, Cavallo L. Growth and endocrine function in thalassemia major in childhood and adolescence. J Endocrinol Investig. 2010;33:61–8.
54. Abu Alhaija ESJ, Hattab FN, Al-Omari MAO. Cephalometric measurements and facial deformities in subjects with beta thalassaemia major. Eur J Orthod. 2002;24:9–19.
55. Zafeiriou DI, Economou M, Athanasiou-Metaxa M. Neurological complications in b-thalassemia. Brain Dev. 2006;28:477–81.
56. Orvieto R, Leichter I, Rachmilewitz EA, Margulies JY. Bone density, mineral content, and cortical index in patients with thalassemia major and the correlation to their bone fractures, blood transfusions, and treatment with desferrioxamine. Calcif Tissue Int. 1992;50:397–9.
57. Jain R, Perkins J, Johnson ST, et al. A prospective study for prevalence and/or development of transfusion-transmitted infections in multiply transfused thalassemia major patients. Asian J Trans Sci. 2012;6:151–4.
58. Rachmilewitz EA, Giardina PJ. How I treat thalassemia. Blood. 2011;118:3479–88.
59. Chui DHK, Waye JS. Hydrops fetalis caused by a-thalassemia: an emerging health care problem. Blood. 1998;91:2213–22.
60. Prabhu R, Prabhu V, Prabhu RS. Iron overload in beta thalassemia—a review. J Biosci Technol. 2009;1:20–31.
61. Kitoh T, Tanaka S, Ono K, Hasegawa J, Otagiri T. Anesthetic management of a patient with b-thalassemia intermedia undergoing splenectomy: a case report. J Anesth. 2005;19:252–6.
62. Katz R, Goldfarb A, Muggia M, Gimmon Z. Unique features of laparoscopic cholecystectomy in beta thalassemia patients. Surg Laparosc Endosc Percutan Tech. 2003;13:318–21.
63. Perez Ferrer A, Ferrazza V, Gredilla E, et al. Bloodless surgery in a patient with thalassemia minor. Usefulness of erythropoietin, preoperative blood donation and intraoperative blood salvage. Minerva Anestesiol. 2007;73:323–6.
64. Waters JH, Lukauskiene E, Anderson ME. Intraoperative blood salvage during cesarean delivery in a patient with b thalassemia intermedia. Anesth Analg. 2003;97:1808–9.
65. Hardison RC, Chui DH, Riemer C, et al. Databases of human hemoglobin variants and other resources at the globin gene server. Hemoglobin. 2001;25:183.
66. Hardison RC, Chui DH, Giardine B, et al. HbVar: a relational database of human hemoglobin variants and thalassemia mutations at the globin gene server. Hum Mutat. 2002;19:225.
67. Macdonald VW, Charache S. Differences in the reaction sequences associated with drug-induced oxidation of hemoglobins E, S, A, and F. J Lab Clin Med. 1983;102:762.
68. Lachant NA, Tanaka KR. Dapsone-associated Heinz body hemolytic anemia in a Cambodian woman with hemoglobin E trait. Am J Med Sci. 1987;294:364.
69. Agarwal A, Guindo A, Cissoko Y, et al. Hemoglobin C associated with protection from severe malaria in the Dogon of Mali, a west African population with a low prevalence of hemoglobin S. Blood. 2000;96:2358.
70. Yudin J, Verhovsek M. How we diagnose and manage altered oxygen affinity hemoglobin variants. Am J Hematol. 2019;94:597.
71. Quine D, Stenson BJ. Arterial O2 tension (PaO2) values in infants <29 weeks of gestation at currently targeted saturations. Arch Dis Child Fetal Neonatal Ed. 2009;94:F51.

72. Castillo A, Sola A, Baquero H, et al. Pulse O2 saturation levels and arterial O2 tension values in newborns receiving O2 therapy in the neonatal intensive care unit: is 85% to 93% an acceptable range? Pediatrics. 2008;121:882.

73. Brockmann PE, Poets A, Urschitz MS, et al. Reference values for pulse oximetry recordings in healthy term neonates during their first 5 days of life. Arch Dis Child Fetal Neonatal Ed. 2011;96:F335.

74. Harigopal S, Satish HP, Taktak AF, et al. O2 saturation profile in healthy preterm infants. Arch Dis Child Fetal Neonatal Ed. 2011;96:F339.

75. Greenspan JS, Goldsmith JP. O2 therapy in preterm infants: hitting the target. Pediatrics. 2006;118:1740.

76. Jennis MS, Peabody JL. Pulse oximetry: an alternative method for the assessment of O2ation in newborn infants. Pediatrics. 1987;79:524.

77. Benaron DA, Benitz WE. Maximizing the stability of O2 delivered via nasal cannula. Arch Pediatr Adolesc Med. 1994;148:294.

78. Walsh M, Engle W, Laptook A, et al. O2 delivery through nasal cannulae to preterm infants: can practice be improved? Pediatrics. 2005;116:857.

79. Yoder BA, Manley B, Collins C, et al. Consensus approach to nasal high-flow therapy in neonates. J Perinatol. 2017;37:809.

80. Manley BJ, Dold SK, Davis PG, Roehr CC. High-flow nasal cannulae for respiratory support of preterm infants: a review of the evidence. Neonatology. 2012;102:300.

81. Cummings JJ, Polin RA. Committee on Fetus and Newborn, American Academy of Pediatrics. Noninvasive respiratory support. Pediatrics. 2016;137

82. Verder H, Albertsen P, Ebbesen F, et al. Nasal continuous positive airway pressure and early surfactant therapy for respiratory distress syndrome in newborns of less than 30 weeks' gestation. Pediatrics. 1999;103:E24.

83. Aly H, Milner JD, Patel K, El-Mohandes AA. Does the experience with the use of nasal continuous positive airway pressure improve over time in extremely low birth weight infants? Pediatrics. 2004;114:697.

84. Diblasi RM. Nasal continuous positive airway pressure (CPAP) for the respiratory care of the newborn infant. Respir Care. 2009;54:1209.

85. Claure N, Bancalari E. New modes of mechanical ventilation in the preterm newborn: evidence of benefit. Arch Dis Child Fetal Neonatal Ed. 2007;92:F508.

86. Gibu CK, Cheng PY, Ward RJ, et al. Feasibility and physiological effects of noninvasive neurally adjusted ventilatory assist in preterm infants. Pediatr Res. 2017;82:650.

87. Rosterman JL, Pallotto EK, Truog WE, et al. The impact of neurally adjusted ventilatory assist mode on respiratory severity score and energy expenditure in infants: a randomized crossover trial. J Perinatol. 2018;38:59.

88. Pierce EA, Foley ED, Smith LE. Regulation of vascular endothelial growth factor by O2 in a model of retinopathy of prematurity. Arch Ophthalmol. 1996;114:1219.

89. Sood BG, Madan A, Saha S, et al. Perinatal systemic inflammatory response syndrome and retinopathy of prematurity. Pediatr Res. 2010;67:394.

90. Baraldi E, Filippone M. Chronic lung disease after premature birth. N Engl J Med. 2007;357:1946.

91. Eriksson L, Haglund B, Odlind V, et al. Perinatal conditions related to growth restriction and inflammation are associated with an increased risk of bronchopulmonary dysplasia. Acta Paediatr. 2015;104:259.

Thermoregulation in Newborns, Neonates, and Premature

16

Shilpa Goyal

16.1 Introduction

Human beings are homeothermic organisms, being able to maintain their body temperature within normal range by thermoregulatory defences, that are limited in neonates especially in preterms. Fluctuations in body temperature can significantly alter function at cellular and tissue level.

The axillary temperature of a newborn ranges between 36.5 and 37.4 °C (term and preterm), but heat loss starts soon after birth from exposure to external environment. Signals from cutaneous receptors signal the brain to initiate heat production by brown fat metabolism. In early days, baby utilizes fetal glycogen stores as energy substrate to maintain body temperature and other organ functions.

Thermoneutral temperature is the external temperature at which there is a balance between heat loss and heat gain, while **critical temperature** is that external temperature below which one cannot maintain core body temperature. Normal temperature zone is the range of temperature at which the metabolic need is at the minimum and temperature regulation is maintained through physiological process, such as vasodilation and vasoconstriction [1]. The **"upper critical temperature"** is that above which evaporative heat losses are initiated, and **"lower critical temperature"** is that below which heat generation through metabolism is initiated, such as shivering and nonshivering thermogenesis (NST) [2].

In a naked full-term neonate, this range is 32–35 °C at 50% humidity, but is >35 °C in preterm neonates and critical temperature is 23 °C and 28 °C, respectively. Neonates weighing more than 1500 g and without respiratory distress or hemodynamic instability can be cared for at incubator temperature of 30–32 °C.

S. Goyal (✉)
Department of Anesthesiology and Critical Care, AIIMS, Jodhpur, Rajasthan, India

U. Saha (ed.), *Clinical Anesthesia for the Newborn and the Neonate*, https://doi.org/10.1007/978-981-19-5458-0_16

Table 16.1 WHO definition of temperature range [1]

Normothermia	36.5 °C–37.5 °C
Hypothermia	<36.5 °C
Mild Hypothermia	<36.0 °C–36.5 °C
Moderate Hypothermia	32.0 °C–36.0 °C
Severe Hypothermia	<32.0 °C
Hyperthermia	>37.5 °C

Hypothermia is the single most risk factor for predicting morbidity and mortality in neonates [3]. WHO defines different temperature ranges in neonates (Table 16.1) [1].

16.2 Physiology of Brown Fat Metabolism and Thermogenesis

Thermoregulatory defence mechanism plays a primary role in maintaining the temperature intraoperatively. Even though anaesthesia and the surgical procedure contribute to hypothermia, but the final thermoregulation depends on the effective thermoregulatory defences [4]. Neonates have thin skin with minimal subcutaneous tissue and large body surface area-to-mass ratio along with low glycogen stores. This causes lot of difference between heat production and heat loss thus making them prone to hypothermia.

A newborn baby's skin is wet and smeared with amniotic fluid and covered with vernix. The surroundings are cold as compared to warm uterine temperature, so the baby loses heat by evaporation, dropping the core temperature, which is difficult to measure. The head accounts for 85% of the total heat loss. The skull bones are thin with scanty hair, and brain is highly perfused and metabolically active [2]. Insulating the neonate's head is a prerequisite before any surgical procedure to minimise intraoperative heat loss.

Shivering is an important mechanism for production of heat in cold environment in older children and adults. This is absent in premature neonates and they are unable to generate activity-related heat. Neonates try to compensate for hypothermia by heat production by **NST or Brown fat metabolism, and increased cellular metabolism** [5].

NST: Shivering is a mechanism to increase heat production seen in older children and adults, on exposure to cold. Newborns and neonates cannot shiver because of immature musculature. Heat is produced by brown fat metabolism, present in the nape of the neck, and interscapular and perirenal regions.

Hormone surge (cortisol, catecholamines, and thyroid) at birth activates brown fat thermogenesis, alternative to the white fat of adults. Brown fat is about 5% of body weight of a newborn and is abundant around the kidneys, intrascapular and nuchal areas. It is highly vascular, has higher O_2 consumption, and is rich in iron containing mitochondria and unmyelinated nerves, providing sympathetic stimulation to the fat cells. It generates heat by uncoupling of oxidative phosphory-lation in the mitochondria. This is a high O_2 and glucose consuming process and continuous cold stress results in hypoxia and hypoglycemia [6]. Anesthesia and anesthetic drugs inhibit brown fat thermogenesis, thereby increasing the risk of intraoperative and postoperative hypothermia after general anesthesia in neonates.

16.3   Mechanisms of Heat Loss

Body loses heat by four mechanisms:

1. **Radiation**: bare skin is exposed to the surroundings which is colder, but there is no direct contact between the two. It depends on the temperature gradient, the area exposed and the distance between the child and the object.
2. **Evaporation**: skin is wet with amniotic fluid making the newborn baby prone to heat loss to the surroundings. It depends on surface area of the baby exposed to the environment and the air velocity [7]. The heat loss is greatest by this route in a newborn.
3. **Conduction**: contact with a cool surface, such as tray or weighing machine. The amount of heat loss depends on the area in contact with cooler objects and the temperature gradient between the two.
4. **Convection**: flow of cooler ambient air of the surroundings carries heat away from the neonate (a fan).

Causes of Hypothermia in Neonates Can Be Enumerated as Due To:

1. **Greater heat loss:** relatively larger body surface-to-body weight ratio
2. **Poor heat conservation**: poorly developed thin subcutaneous tissue, and limited fat reserves
3. **Decreased heat production:** minimal motor activity, inability to shiver
4. **Immature central thermoregulatory control**
5. **High metabolic rate and energy needs**
6. Anesthesia-induced inhibition of the central control and on brown fat metabolism

16.4   Preterm Neonates

While all newborns are at danger of hypothermia, preterm and small for date babies are at a greater risk, more so in cold environment, because:

i. **They are poikilothermic**, i.e., they do not have the ability to control body tem-perature and adopt the ambient temperature.
ii. They have **less Brown Fat** as compared to term neonates and less heat produc-tion. Brown fat is deposited only after 28 weeks of gestation, so there will be no

developed NST in babies born earlier than 28 weeks. SGA neonates have NST mechanism but at a minimum level [8].

iii. Their body surface area-to-weight ratio is more (**BSA: BW:** ↑↑) which allows greater loss of heat from the exposed skin surface.

iv. Their **skin is poorly keratinized**, and thin with less subcutaneous tissue and fat, thus poor heat conservation.

16.5   Complications of Hypothermia (Cold Injury)

Hypothermia significantly increases morbidity and mortality, particularly after heat losing surgeries, such as exploratory laparotomy and thoracotomy. Compensatory brown fat metabolism escalates O_2 consumption, and proves to be deleterious in newborns, preterms, and those with respiratory insufficiency, with consequent tissue hypoxia, hyperkalaemia, metabolic acidosis, hyperbilirubinemia, and neurological damage. Extreme and prolonged hypothermia can cause life-threatening complications, such as DIC, RDS, sepsis, pulmonary and intracranial haemorrhage, and difficult resuscitation [3]. Effect of anesthetic drugs is more pronounced affecting recovery from anesthesia in hypothermic babies.

16.6   Temperature Monitoring

16.6.1 Core Versus Peripheral Temperature Monitoring

Temperature monitoring is essential in surgeries lasting for more than 30 min. Providing controlled thermal environment improves the chance of survival and quality of outcome, particularly in small (BW <1000 G), premature and critically ill neonates, by minimizing their oxygen and metabolic demands, and stress responses to cold or overheating.

Core temperature (Fig. 16.1a) depicts the thermoregulatory status of the body and is preferable for intraoperative monitoring. It best reflects the body temperature changes as it is maintained even with extremes of environmental temperature fluctuations and is not much influenced by thermoregulatory defences and vasomotor mechanisms. Core temperature is 2–4 °C higher than the peripheral temperature and is measured deep thoracic, abdominal or from CNS, the vessel rich organs.

<u>Monitoring sites:</u> core temperature measurement is an invasive technique and can be done by various routes, each with its own advantages and complications:

1. **Pulmonary artery catheter:** this is the gold standard for measuring core temperature, but is not feasible in all the cases. This is usually used in cardiac surgeries (especially open-heart procedures) and in very sick neonates in NICU settings.

2. **Tympanic:** the probe is placed in the middle ear and sealed. For accurate measurement of core temperature, there should be no air leak around the probe.

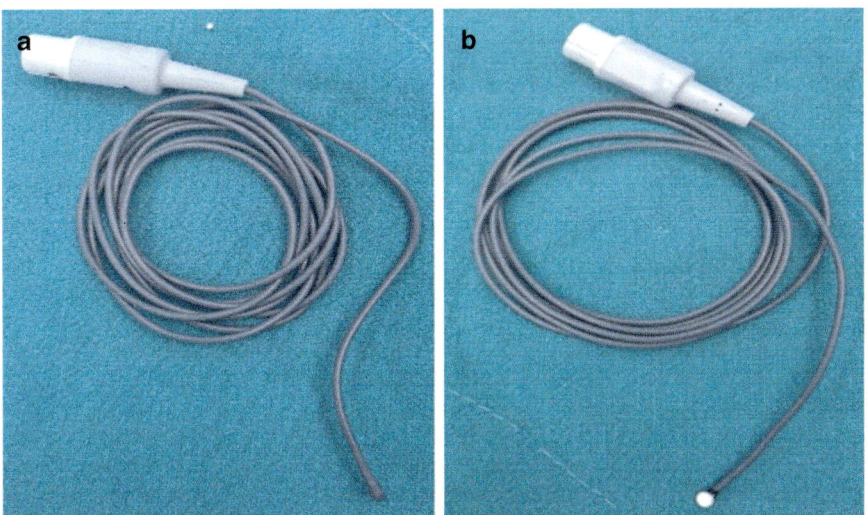

Fig. 16.1 (**a**) Core temperature probe. (**b**) Peripheral temperature probe

Besides, this is associated with a high risk of tympanic membrane perforation, and so is not used routinely in the OT in neonates.

3. **Lower oesophagus**: this measures the core temperature when the probe is put in lower 1/3rd of oesophagus. Readings are unreliable if the probe remains in the upper oesophagus when it will be affected by the temperature of the air leaking from around the uncuffed endotracheal tube (ET). Besides, there is risk of esophageal injury by improper insertion of the probe. The advantage is that there is less chance of dislodgment of a properly placed and strapped probe, and no interference with temperature monitoring. The probe should be introduced under direct vision during laryngoscopy, care being taken not to force it if resistance is felt.

4. **Nasopharyngeal**: it fairly represents the core temperature. It is put through the more spacious nostril and introduced up to the nasopharynx, but is influenced by expired warm gases leaking around the ET or LMA. Because of ease of access in any intraoperative position of the baby, this is used quite commonly. Complications associated are damage the nasal mucosa, nasal septum, and cribriform plate, and creation of false passage in the nasopharynx.

5. **Oropharyngeal**: the probe is placed in oropharynx through the oral route, and reflects core temperature, but this also is affected by the expired gases leaking around the ET.

6. **Rectal:** it truly reflects the core temperature, but is associated with the risk of damage to the rectal mucosa, and readings may be altered by soiling with faeces. Besides, it is not always feasible to place a probe in the rectum, as in intestinal, colonic, and rectal surgeries.

7. **Bladder**: this also reflects the core temperature but only when the urine output is adequate or high. If urine output is less, it will give falsely low readings.

Fig. 16.2 Zero heat flux
(ZHF) Sensor

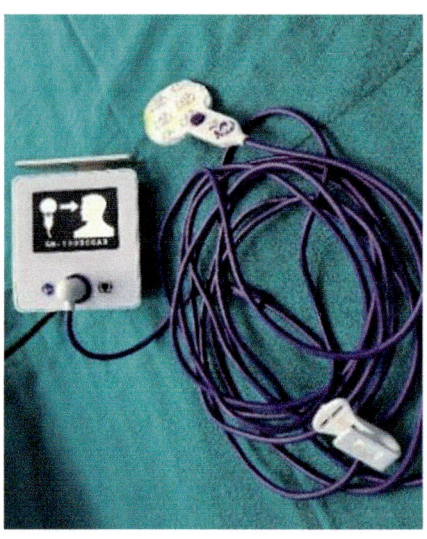

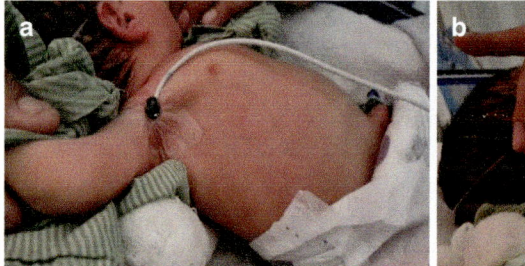

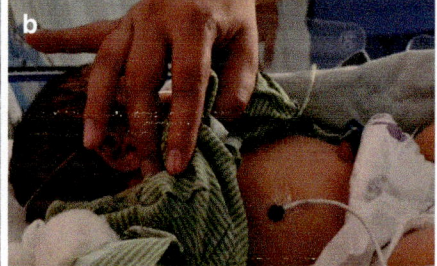

Fig. 16.3 (**a**) probe at axilla. (**b**) probe over right hypochondrium

8. **3M spot on sensor**: this is a new modality to measure core temperature through **zero heat flux principle** [9] (Fig. 16.2). An electrode is placed on the forehead and the skin underneath the electrode gets heated up by heat transfer from the core body heat. As the temperature equalises between the body and electrode, an isothermic tunnel is created. As the point of zero heat flux is reached (no more heat is transferred from core to skin), the temperature beneath the sensor represents the core temperature. This is noninvasive and an attractive option for measuring core temperature in neonates and small babies.

Peripheral temperature monitoring (Fig. 16.1b): peripheral temperature is dependent on the duration and area of exposure of peripheries or the external monitoring site to atmosphere, the temperature of the OT or environment and by the thermoregulatory mechanisms affecting heat distribution. This is usually 2–4 °C lower than the core temperature. Sites most used are axillary (Fig. 16.3a), temporal, and chest or hypochondrium (Fig. 16.3b):

1. **Axillary** site is the most convenient, but for accuracy, the probe must be kept over the axillary artery with the arm adequately adducted. It will not take correct readings in case of displacement.
2. The other site most used in neonates is **right hypochondrium** (Fig. 16.3b) as underlying is liver which is a highly perfused organ. There is a high likelihood of getting dislodged from the placement site, the position can get altered under the drapes, and the site may be exposed to ambient OT temperature, influencing the final readings.
3. **Chest:** it may get affected by exposure of the chest to the surroundings with no proper drapes over the chest.

The placement of peripheral probes at different sites does not show significant difference in hemodynamically stable neonate [10].

16.7   Hyperthermia

Passive hyperthermia: this **is** a rare entity in newborns and prematures due to the different thermoregulatory physiology as compared to infants and children. Hyperthermia (axillary temperature >37.4 °C or rectal temperature > 37.5 °C) can be due to pathological condition (infection, sepsis, and septicemia) or iatrogenic, from environmental factors. It may sometimes result intraoperatively due to active warming and excessive prolonged insulation by drapes.

Effects of Hyperthermia
- Vasodilatation and dehydration due to excessive insensible heat losses and hypotension shock, such as state, apnea, seizures, and neurological damage [11].
- It may also result in hyperkalaemia from increased muscle damage [7].
- Heat loss by radiation and secondary cold injury.

Associated excessive fluid losses should be supplemented and replaced adequately by Ryle's tube or intravenously (IV) [7].

Management: Methods to Lower Increased Body Temperature:
- **Stop active warming,** turning off heating devices and remove heating blankets.
- **Remove drapes** and expose baby to the surrounding OT temperature after the surgery is over.
- **Antipyretic** medications such as paracetamol may be given but not always be effective.
- While lowering temperature, **do not reduce lower axillary temperature to normal.**
- Avoid rebound hypothermia and **secondary cold injury**.
- **Maintain volume status, renal perfusion, electrolytes, acid base balance, and urine output.**

16.8   Effects of Anaesthesia

The core temperature is comprising of vessel rich organs receiving major part of cardiac output (75%) and is 22% of body weight in neonates. Mildly low core temperature (1–3 °C) is common and quite well-tolerated by them.

16.8.1 General Anesthesia (GA):

Induction of GA leads to vasodilation and thermal dysregulation by the following methods:

(a) Reduced metabolic heat production by 30% under anaesthesia.
(b) Thermal imbalance: occurs as heat loss to the surrounding atmosphere exceeds the heat production on exposure to surroundings. This process may last for 2–3 h.
(c) Central inhibition of thermoregulatory defences by GA.
(d) Internal redistribution of heat: from core to periphery and decrease in core temperature. GA causes loss of autonomic thermoregulation, with marked loss of cold response thresholds as compared to warm responses which are better preserved.
(e) Thermal steady state: this is reached when metabolic heat production is comparable to heat lost to the atmosphere. Either the heat production is increased, or the loss is reduced by vasoconstriction, thus striking the balance between the two.

Intraoperative blood sugar and SpO_2 must be monitored in neonates. Dextrose should be adequately supplemented intravenously in case of hypoglycemia and to maintain blood sugar >40–50 mg% [12] and adequacy of oxygenation maintained by adequate FiO_2 and assisted ventilation, to maintain the metabolic triangle of hypoxia, hypothermia, and hypoglycaemia and prevent related adverse consequences [13].

16.8.2 Regional anaesthesia (RA)

It is exceedingly difficult to determine hypothermia under RA as it is not possible to measure core temperature during these procedures (invasive monitoring), so it may go unnoticed and can be lethal. Prolonged RA, especially those surgeries having large evaporative losses, may lead to peripheral distribution of heat. RA per se contributes to heat loss and hypothermia by causing peripheral vasodilation. Caudal blocks do not alter thermoregulatory responses and can be used in premature and SGA neonates also.

Surgeries in newborns such as gastroschisis or omphalocele, neural tube defects, and exomphalos have high evaporative losses through the exposed gut and mucosa due to loss of skin integrity, with high chances of hypothermia [9]. Therefore, maintaining normothermia is a real challenge. Warming the IV fluid, use of warm humidified inspired gases, and covering the exposed gut with warm sterile gauzes or plastic sheets helps in reducing the heat loss. The gut should also be washed with, and abdomen irrigated with warm saline, keeping the duration of exposure to minimum.

16.9   Mechanism to Maintain Normothermia in the Perioperative Area

Main aim is to reduce heat loss, provide external heat, and reduce body energy consumption, by adopting following methods:

(a) **Reduce O$_2$ consumption:** avoid stress, pain, environment temperature fluctuations, hypoxia, respiratory, and hemodynamic disturbances.

(b) **Warm IV fluids** to be given through fluid warmers set at 37 °C (Fig. 16.4). They have complete casing for the IV set to prevent heat dissipation to the surroundings. They are electrically heated devices with integrated temperature sensors. Adequate temperature will be maintained only if fluid is given at a rate of 750 mL/h with a length of tubing ≤25 cm from the warmer to patient. However, this amount of flow is too high for a neonate, so length of the tubing should be kept to minimum. The diameter of the extension tube if used should be minimum; hence, pressure monitoring line should be preferred.

(c) **Forced air warming device/blanket**: (Fig. 16.5) this is an active warming device in which air is entrained through surroundings and heated through elec-

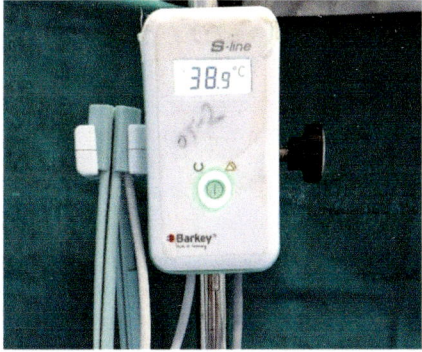

Fig. 16.4 Fluid warmer (Make: Barkey)

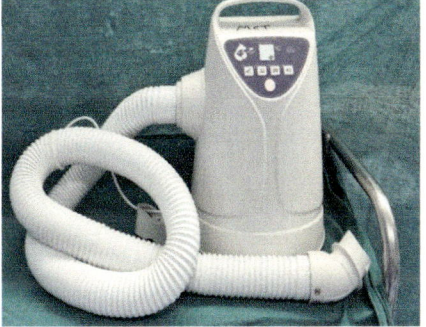

Fig. 16.5 Forced air warmer (Make: Bayer Hugger)

Fig. 16.6 Incubator

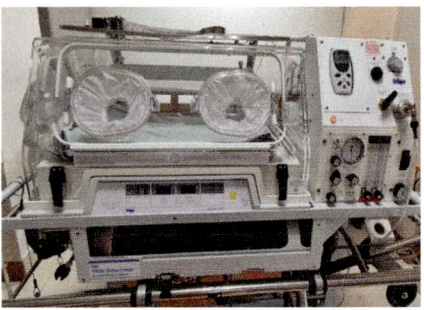

Fig. 16.7 Cling foil wrap
in postoperative patient
in NICU

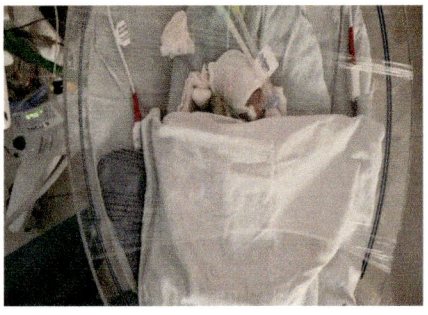

tric coils. The blower delivers heat through a hose pipe either under sterile sheets or through blankets. It keeps the child warm through convection [14]. They have the risk of causing thermal burns if kept in close contact with the fragile skin of the neonate.

(d) **Radiant warmer/incubator**: incubators minimise the temperature gradient between the baby and the surroundings by maintaining adequate temperature of the air around. This minimises evaporative heat loss and metabolism as well. Double-walled incubators can prevent radiant heat losses. Prewarmed incubators are used during transport from OT to ward/ICU (Fig. 16.6). Radiant warmers increase convective and evaporative heat losses, but maintains radiant one, thus conserving net heat. It increases loss of insensible heat which proves to be the greatest disadvantage.

(e) **Occlusive plastic wrapping** (Fig. 16.7): neonates and preterms requiring NICU admission are transported with cling foil wrapped around their body below the shoulders or those needing ventilator support are kept in NICU postoperatively with cling foil wrap over their cradle to prevent heat loss. This prevents evaporative heat losses from the thin skin of neonates, especially preterms.

(f) **Exothermic warming mattresses:** these are gel-based mattresses which are thermostatically controlled and deliver heat through conduction [14].

(g) **Heated and humidified air/gases** in the breathing circuit are provided to minimise heat losses. Active humidification is done through heated humidifier in the anaesthesia workstation or the ventilator in NICU. They add heat and moisture in the inspired gases. Passive humidification can be provided through heat and moisture exchanger (HME). They conserve the heat and moisture of the exhaled air from the patient and transferring to inhaled air.

(h) **Warm polythene caps** to minimise loss of heat from large surface area of the head and thin skin of the scalp over the whole perioperative period of the baby, particularly in preterm babies. Use of cling foil wrap in the postoperative period. (Fig. 16.7)

(i) **Ambient OT temperature** [15] should be maintained >28 °C (term neonates), 32 °C (birth–1 week), and 35 °C (premature neonates).

(j) **Supplement dextrose as energy substrate.**

A combination of these techniques should be used judiciously to prevent hypothermia, but at the same time, hyperthermia becomes a concern with the overzealous use of these modalities.

Pearls of Wisdom

1. Keep the OT adequately warmed before the neonate is taken in for surgery.
2. Keep OT table warm by forced air warmer set at normal body temperature.
3. Keep the neonate, particularly head adequately covered with warm blankets or plastic hats before beginning induction.
4. Always do temperature monitoring in surgeries of duration >30 min.
5. Give IV fluids or blood through fluid warmer.
6. Give dextrose containing IV fluids and high FiO2 with assisted ventilation in babies at risk of hypothermia.
7. Coordinate with surgeons to use warm saline for washing body cavities.
8. Always transport the neonates to and from the OT in prewarmed incubator.

16.10 Conclusion

Newborns and neonates require special care to prevent hypothermia in the intraoperative period and also postoperatively. Prolonged and extreme hypothermia can have several metabolic effects, complications of cold injury, and even life-threatening complications. Various modalities are available and can be used according to the patient anesthesia and surgical requirements. Intraoperative temperature monitoring is necessary to maintain body temperature and detect impending hypothermia so that preventive and corrective measures can be taken.

References

1. Smith J, Usher K, Alcock G, Buettner P. Application of plastic wrap to improve temperatures in infants born less than 30 weeks gestation: a randomized controlled trial. Neonatal Netw. 2013;32(4):235–45. https://doi.org/10.1891/0730-0832.32.4.235.

2. Luginbuehl I, Bissonette B, and Davis PJ. Chapter 6: Thermoregulation: Physiology and Perioperative Disturbances. Smith's anesthesia for infants and children. 9th ed; 2016. Elsieveier Health Sciences, Philadelphia.

3. Perlman J, Kjaer K. Neonatal and maternal temperature regulation during and after delivery. Anesth Analg. 2016;123:168–72.

4. Sessler DI. Temperature monitoring and perioperative thermoregulation. Anesthesiology. 2008;109:318–38.

5. Cınar ND, Filiz TM. Neonatal thermoregulation. J Neonatal Nursing. 2006;12(2):69–74. ISSN 1355-1841. https://doi.org/10.1016/j.jnn.2006.01.006.

6. Waldron S, Mackinnon R. Neonatal thermoregulation. Infant. 2007;3(3):101–4.

7. Newborn thermoregulation: developed by the Interprofessional Education and Research Committee of the Champlain Maternal Newborn Regional Program (CMNRP) June 2013.

8. Cannon B, Nedergaard J. Brown adipose tissue: function and physiological significance. Physiol Rev. 2004;84:277–359.

9. Carvalho H, Najafi N, Poelaert J. Intraoperative temperature monitoring with cutaneous zero-heat- flux-thermometry in comparison with oesophageal temperature: a prospective study in the paediatric population. Paediatr Anaesth. 2019;29(8):865–71.

10. Schafer D, Boogaart S, Johnson L, Keezel C, etal. Comparison of neonatal skin sensor temperatures with axillary temperature: does skin sensor placement really matter? Adv Neonatal Care 2014;14(1):52-60.

11. Gunn AJ, Gluckman PD. Should we try to prevent hypothermia after cardiac arrest? Pediatrics. 2000;106:132–3.

12. WHO. Thermal control of the newborn: a practical guide. World Health Organization. WHO/RHT/MSM/97.2; 1997.

13. Aylott M. The Neonatal energy triangle part 2. Thermoregulatory and respiratory adaptation. Paediatric Nursing. 2006;18(7):38–43.

14. Ackermann W, Fan Q, Parekh AJ, Stoicea N, et al. Forced-air warming and resistive heating devices. updated perspectives on safety and surgical site infections. Front Surg. 2018;5(64)

15. Sultan P, Habib AS, Carvalho B. Ambient operating room temperature: mother, baby or surgeon? Br J Anaesthesia. 2017;119(4):839.

Clinical Pharmacology of Anesthetic Drugs in Neonates

Nisha Kachru

17.1 Introduction

Neonates include preterm, term, and former preterm neonates (who may now be older than 28 days in age). This heterogenous group of patients consists of newborns with postmenstrual age (PMC) ranging from 22 weeks (severe preterm) to 50 weeks (post term), and birth weight ranging from 500 g to 5000 g. The leading indication for surgery is correction of congenital defects or malformations (seen in nearly 3% of newborns and occurring due to defective embryogenesis). These congenital defects contribute to around 15% of the perinatal mortality in India [1].

The neonatal period is characterised by immaturity and underdevelopment of all organ systems, affecting drug pharmacokinetics, pharmacodynamics, drug responses, and long-term effects. Effective and safe administration of drugs in the neonate depends on their evolving physiological characteristics, such as age, weight and size, comorbidities, coadministration of other drugs, genetic susceptibilities, and pharmacokinetics and pharmacodynamics of the drug being used.

Since neonates are a vulnerable population and, therefore, not usually added to studies by pharmaceutical companies for ethical or logistical reasons, such as technical issues, lack of self-reporting, lack of specific formulations etc., there is limited drug data in neonates. Outcome measures are also difficult to assess. Many of the medications are used 'off label', with only three anesthetic drugs; sevoflurane, remifentanil, and rocuronium having received food and drug administration (FDA) approval for use in neonates and none for preterm neonates born before 30 weeks of gestation [2].

This chapter will take the reader through the pharmacological principles of drug action in neonates, such as developmental pharmacology, neurodevelopmental

N. Kachru (✉)
ABVIMS & Dr. RML Hospital (Atal Behari Vajpayee Institute of Medical Sciences and Dr. Ram Manohar Lohia Hospital), New Delhi, India

© The Author(s), under exclusive license to Springer Nature Singapore Pte Ltd. 2023
U. Saha (ed.), *Clinical Anesthesia for the Newborn and the Neonate*,
https://doi.org/10.1007/978-981-19-5458-0_17

effects, pharmacokinetics and pharmacodynamics, body composition (plasma protein, Fetal Hb), cardiac output and regional blood flow, drug elimination (hepatic and extrahepatic), anesthetic drugs, local anesthetic, miscellaneous and resuscitative drugs, their doses, and anesthetic implications or considerations.

Note: Oxygen, nitrous oxide. Air, IV fluids, Blood and blood products, also are drugs in technical terms, as they deserve same care, precautions and considerations, as all chemical drugs, because low and high doses will have less or more effect, side effects and adverse or toxic effects on the developing organs, especially the brain. These are discussed elsewhere in this book.

17.2 General Pharmacological Definitions and Terms

17.2.1 Pharmacology

Pharmacology is a branch of medicine that is concerned with drug or pharmacon defined as any artificial, natural, or endogenous molecule with biochemical or physiological effects. It studies the interactions between living being and chemicals, and includes neuro, renal, cardiovascular, endocrine, and immune pharmacology, central and peripheral nervous system, and drug metabolism and regulation. This requires intimate knowledge of the biological system affected, and cell biology and biochemistry.

The two main areas of pharmacology are:

(a) Pharmacodynamics (effect of a drug on biological systems)
(b) Pharmacokinetics (effects of biological systems on the drug)

17.2.2 Clinical pharmacology

Clinical pharmacology is application of pharmacological principles to patient care, and **posology** is the study of medicine dosing. Modern pharmacology is a biomedical science that uses genetics, molecular biology, biochemistry, and other advanced tools to understand molecular information which is transformed into therapies directed against disease and pathogens or for diagnostic, preventive, and therapeutic care [3].

17.2.3 Therapeutic index

Therapeutic index describes the safety profile of a drug. It is the ratio of the desired to the toxic effect. A narrow therapeutic index (close to one) means that the desired effect of a drug occurs at a dose close to the toxic dose, while a wide therapeutic index (>5) means that the desired effect occurs at a dose much below the toxic dose.

17.2.4 Drug approvals

In the US, the FDA is responsible for creating guidelines for approval and use of drugs, with the condition that all approved drugs fulfill two requirements:

1. **Efficacy**: must be effective against the disease for which it is seeking approval
2. **Safety**: must meet safety criteria (animal and controlled human testing)

17.3   Developmental Pharmacology

The major reasons for pharmacokinetic variabilities in neonates are due to age, weight, and organ function. Although the most common variable used to calculate drug requirement is weight, it is not sufficient to predict drug clearance, which is important for drug infusion or maintenance rates. The gestational age/maturity plays a significant role in determining metabolism and clearance from the body. Compromised organ (liver and kidney) development and function due to illness may further impact drug clearance.

17.4   Pharmacokinetics

Pharmacokinetics describe the effect of the body or the biological systems on the drug or chemical (e.g., half-life and volume of distribution). **LADME** describes the pharmacokinetic properties of the API (active pharmaceutical ingredient), i.e., Liberation (for oral drugs), Absorption, Distribution, Metabolism and Excretion. The pharmacokinetics of drugs is very different in neonates when compared to infants and older children [4, 5].

17.4.1 Drug Absorption

Drug absorption and its effects depend on the route of administration.

Most anesthetic drugs are administered through the intravenous or the inhalational route.

17.4.1.1 Oral

Oral route is employed for premedication (in liquid form), and for postoperative analgesia. The absorption of oral medications is slow due to reduced gastric emptying and poor GI motility, especially if associated with abdominal pathologies, such as duodenal atresia and necrotising enterocolitis (NEC) or due to coadministration of opioids. Slow gastric emptying and absorption means inadequate or delayed desired effect. This, along with delayed clearance means that both onset of action and excretion will be slow, and hence, the interval between doses must be increased and frequency reduced, e.g., the dose of paracetamol ranges from 25 mg/kg/day in a preterm neonate to 60 mg/kg/day in a term neonate, at 8–12 h interval instead of 4–6 h interval in older children and adults.

17.4.1.2 Rectal

Rectal route has been frequently used for agents such as thiopentone and methohexitone for induction of anesthesia in the pediatric age group. In neonates, rectal administration of anesthetics can also lead to speedy induction; however, due to variability in absorption, altered bioavailability, and gastrointestinal diseases, this is not a very suitable route for administration of drugs.

17.4.1.3 External Application

A relatively large body surface area, thinner stratum corneum layer of skin, and more vascularity, predispose neonates to greater absorption of local anesthetics applied to the skin as compared to older children. EMLA ointment (eutectic mixture of lignocaine and prilocaine) applied before placement of intravenous (IV) or intra-arterial cannulae has a quicker onset of action, but is associated with risk of methemoglobinemia because of prilocaine. Higher amounts of fetal hemoglobin (fHb) with reduced methemoglobin reductase activity mean that neonates have a higher tendency to form methemoglobin. Hence, use of this ointment is better avoided. A study by Shahid et al. on 907 infants under the age of 3 months, published in 2019, reported minimal benefits of EMLA in terms of reduction of venipuncture pain and no benefit in comparison with sucrose and/or breastfeeding. Moreover, it produced elevation in methemoglobin levels and skin blanching [6].

17.4.1.4 Inhalation Route

Absorption of inhaled anesthetics and speed of induction depends on functional residual capacity (FRC), alveolar ventilation, cardiac output, and tissue blood solubility of the agent. It is more rapid in neonates because of higher alveolar ventilation-to-FRC ratio, higher cardiac output, lower blood gas solubility, and lower tissue solubility of volatile anesthetics. Even while FRC is small, but because of increased alveolar ventilation, pulmonary absorption is rapid, with faster induction of anesthesia.

This is further facilitated by high cardiac output, better distribution of blood to highly vascular areas, such as brain, and lower tissue blood solubility. In neonates suffering from cyanotic heart disease or lung diseases, or in conditions with greater right to left (R–L) shunt, induction may be slowed, while left to right (L–R) shunt has minimal impact.

17.4.1.5 Intravenous Route

Intravenous route: IV route is a sure and direct method of drug administration, that bypasses hurdles faced by other routes in drug absorption. The onset of action is quick, effect is more predictable and clearance is also faster. In neonates with R–L intracardiac shunt, the onset of action is faster, because it bypasses the pulmonary circulation and reaches the brain earlier, compared to L–R shunt, where onset is slower and effect is less because of greater dilution of the drug in the heart.

17.4.2 Drug Distribution

Distribution of drugs in the body compartments depends on the **body composition, protein binding, and regional blood flow.**

17.4.2.1 Body Composition

Neonates have relatively higher total body water (TBW) and larger extracellular fluid (ECF) volume, lower muscle mass and less fat as compared to older children. This affects their volume of distribution (V_D) for drugs. Distribution is also affected by the nature of the drug, whether hydrophilic or lipophilic. The V_D of hydrophilic drugs is greater (higher TBW and ECF) than that in older children and adults. Hence, the initial dose of **polar (hydrophilic) molecules and drugs** (Table 17.1) (such as neuromuscular blocking (NMB) agents, which are rapidly distributed in the ECF and have slow cellular uptake), will be higher than in older children or adults on per kg body weight basis. In some cases, this leads to larger volume of free drug, which can increase risk for toxicity, especially that of local anesthetics, especially because of their slow metabolism and poor clearance. Premature babies have even greater body water and lower fat content as compared to term neonates, and all these effects are more pronounced in them, requiring greater care and precision during IV drug administration.

Termination of action of drugs such as **thiopentone** and **propofol** is by redistribution rather than clearance. The lesser fat and muscle content in neonates means that they have a lower volume for redistribution into the tissues, and CNS concentration remains high for a longer period of time. Thus, they have prolonged duration of action and delayed awakening as compared to older children.

Fentanyl has a higher volume of distribution, so initially, there is less respiratory depression with the standard dose. However, since clearance by redistribution is reduced higher or repeated dosing can lead to a prolonged effect and greater or delayed respiratory depression.

Table 17.1 Polar and nonpolar molecules

Polar molecules	Nonpolar molecules
• Water—H_2O	• Noble gasses: He, Ne, Ar, Kr, Xe
• Ammonia—NH_3	• Homonuclear diatomic elements: H_2, N_2, O_2, Cl_2
• Sulfur dioxide—SO_2	• Carbon dioxide—CO_2
• Hydrogen sulfide—H_2S	• Benzene—C_6H_6
• Ethanol—C_2H_6O	• Carbon tetrachloride—CCl_4
• NaCl (sodium chloride)	• Methane—CH_4
• Neuro muscular blockers	• Ethylene—C_2H_4
	• Hydrocarbon liquids, such as gasoline, toluene
	• Most organic molecules
	• Volatile anaesthetic agents
	• Opioids

17.4.3 Plasma Proteins and Protein Binding

Changes in concentration and composition of circulating plasma proteins also influence the distribution of highly protein bound drugs. Total serum proteins and albumin fraction are low in neonates and reach adult values by 6 months of age. They also tend to have metabolic acidosis which can affect the ionization and binding of drugs to plasma proteins. The ability to bind to drugs can take from 6 months to 1 year to reach adult values. This implies that the loading dose of drugs has to be modified accordingly. Diazepam and barbiturates bind to albumin, and lignocaine binds to alpha-1 acid glycoprotein, and will have higher free level and greater effect.

The presence of fetal albumin, which is functionally immature, has been postulated to explain the **reduced ability of newborn plasma to bind bilirubin and various drugs,** resulting in higher free fraction of protein bound drugs.

For hydrophilic drugs, higher dose by body weight is required to reach therapeutic levels. This leads to more free form of drugs with increased risk of toxicity, especially that of local anesthetics.

Highly lipophilic drugs such as propofol have a lower volume of distribution potentially resulting in a higher drug concentration because of limited distribution in the reduced fat tissue. The free level of thiopentone is higher in neonates (13%) as compared to older children and adults (7%); hence, induction dose should be reduced.

Fetal albumin also affects binding of bilirubin and fatty acids. These also compete with drugs for binding sites on albumin and further increase the free drug levels. Besides, displacement of bilirubin from protein binding sites increases the risk of kernicterus, especially in sick neonates.

Protein binding has a significant effect on drug clearance. The desired effect of a drug is proportional to its free form in the plasma, and that bound to plasma proteins acts as a reservoir. Clearance occurs of the free ionized form in the plasma. Because of high protein binding of some drugs, though the plasma concentration may be low, it will continue to be maintained as more and more drug is released from the binding site to replace that cleared. This causes prolongation of effect. However, high protein binding may also be beneficial by maintaining clearance by keeping plasma concentration constant.

17.4.3.1 Regional Blood Flow

Distribution of regional blood flow to the brain determines the onset of action, whereas redistribution to tissues such as the skeletal muscle determines the termination of action of many drugs. This distribution can be further affected by persistence of embryonic circulation, such as a patent ductus arterioles (PDA). The brain in neonates is large in relation to the total body weight, but receives a relatively lesser proportion of cardiac output. Redistribution is also limited. Hence, onset as well as termination of IV induction agents is slower than older children.

The blood–brain barrier (BBB) is a network of junctions that limit diffusion of compounds between the blood and the brain. It is underdeveloped at birth and more immature in preterm babies. The transport of water soluble and lipophilic drugs (such as morphine) across the BBB depends on its maturation. Protein bound drugs usually cannot cross the BBB in term neonates, while unbound lipophilic drugs can cross over easily. The higher brain concentrations of morphine and greater respiratory depression seen with it in neonates are explained by the higher permeability of the BBB to morphine. Pathological conditions of the CNS, fever or other drugs may alter the permeability of the BBB and modify the responses to drugs, such as opioids.

Bupivacaine, similar to lignocaine, also binds to alpha 1 acid glycoprotein, which is low in neonates, and hence results in higher free concentration of this drug. Due to its lipophilic nature, bupivacaine can cross the immature BBB, with tendency to cause seizures in the neonate.

17.4.4 Drug Elimination

Elimination of drugs from the body depends on their clearance and excretion. A few definitions are important to understand elimination of drugs from the body, and will help the reader understand how this affects the neonate. **Clearance** is defined as the volume of plasma from which a substance is completely removed per unit time (L/h or ml/min) and **excretion** is the amount of substance removed from the body per unit time, expressed in mg/min, µg/min. The sum of clearance of a substance by all the routes must be considered for calculating **total body clearance.** It must be kept in mind that while a constant amount of drug is eliminated per unit time, this amount keeps changing with the changes in the blood levels of the drug. Another important term is **intercompartmental clearance** which refers to the redistribution of drug or substance between body compartments, e.g., plasma, muscle, and fat.

The primary routes of elimination of all compounds, substance, drugs, and their metabolites, whether exogenous or endogenous, are through the **hepatic (hepatobiliary) and extrahepatic (renal, pulmonary, and enzymatic)** routes. At birth, especially in premature babies, these are immature and adult levels are not achieved until the age of 2 years.

17.4.4.1 Hepatic Elimination

Liver is the primary organ for inactivation and metabolic clearance of drugs and substances. Most compounds are usually metabolized by more than one enzyme systems. The presence of genetic polymorphism is responsible for variations in drug metabolism in different individuals. Chromosomal and genetic abnormalities in a neonate increase chances of this polymorphism and affect drug metabolism. Drug metabolism occurs in two phases: **Phase 1 reactions** (oxidation, reduction, and hydrolysis) and **Phase 2 reactions** (conjugation–sulphuration, glucuronidation, and acetylation). While some substances undergo either one of the two reactions, others undergo both reactions, one after the other.

Plasma clearance of drugs metabolized in the liver is age dependent, such that drug elimination by biotransformation is slower in neonates than in infants and older children. Phase II sulfate conjugation is fully developed at term, but glucuronidation and acetylation are not. Anesthetic drugs such as propofol, dexmedetomidine, morphine, and paracetamol depend on glucuronidation for their clearance. Their duration of action is prolonged in newborns, especially the preterm neonate, and only nears adult values after the first year of life. Nondepolarizing muscle relaxants (NDMR)s, vecuronium, and rocuronium are also metabolized in the liver and excreted in the bile. Enzyme systems, cytochrome P 450 and noncytochrome P 450, both are involved in metabolism and these too are immature at birth, but by 44 weeks of postmenstrual age, their activity reaches 85% of adult values. Hence, less frequent dosing and lower infusion rates must be used soon after birth and in premature neonates.

17.4.4.2 Extrahepatic Drug Elimination

17.4.4.2.1 Renal Elimination

Renal elimination of drugs and their metabolites occurs through two mechanisms: **glomerular filtration or tubular secretion.** Almost all substances pass through the kidneys for elimination by filtration, secretion or for reabsorption. Besides, kidneys also have enzymes that metabolize many substances.

Renal function in the neonates is lower than expected on basis of the body weight or body surface area, due to reduced renal blood flow and GFR, decreased capacity of the renal tubules to concentrate or acidify urine, and poor transport of organic ions for active tubular secretion.

Glomerular filtration is the main mechanism by which substances are removed from circulation. At birth, GFR is only 35% of adult values in a term newborn and much lower in a preterm newborn. It attains 90% of adult activity by 1 year of life. This influences clearance of drugs excreted via the kidneys, with increase in the half-life and duration of action of drugs principally eliminated by renal clearance, in neonates, and especially in preterm. Anesthetic drugs eliminated through the kidneys include milrinone, which is commonly used after congenital cardiac surgery in neonates, theophylline, antibiotics (aminoglycosides, penicillin, cephalosporin, and tetracycline), cardiac drugs (beta-blockers, digoxin, procainamide, and diuretics), lithium, antacids (cimetidine, ranitidine), and phenobarbital.

Urinary pH, by influencing the ionization of compounds excreted, affects their renal elimination. Many drugs are weak acids or bases, and are in both ionized and nonionized forms. The ionized component, being water soluble or hydrophilic, is easily cleared. Phenobarbital is a weak polar acid, and moderately binds to proteins, but instead of being eliminated, it is reabsorbed in the renal tubules, with low clearance and prolonged duration of action. Morphine and paracetamol are metabolized by the kidneys.

Several drugs can themselves cause renal damage, such as antibiotics (ciprofloxacin, methicillin, vancomycin, and sulphonamides) and NSAID analgesics (aspirin, naproxen, and ibuprofen). They can reduce the GFR by nearly 20%, especially in the preterm neonate, and reduce renal elimination of other drugs so should be administered with care.

All these factors affect drug excretion in the neonates and the premature. This necessitates a change in drug schedules, dosing intervals and infusion rates.

17.4.4.2.2 Pulmonary Elimination

Alveolar ventilation, FRC, cardiac output, and blood gas solubility are the main factors that affect anesthetic drug absorption through the lungs, and these are the very factors that also affect their elimination and washout. The increase in alveolar ventilation, high alveolar ventilation-to-FRC ratio, reduced solubility of volatile anesthetics, and higher percentage of the cardiac output being delivered to the brain leads to higher uptake of volatile agents, in neonates as compared to older children and adults. The minimum alveolar concentration (MAC) of inhalation agents is characteristically reduced in preterms, peaks at 1–6 months of age and then falls to reach adult values by adolescence. Lower concentration of inhalational agents is also required, because they produce greater myocardial depression in the neonate. However, the MAC of sevoflurane (3.2%) is not reduced in preterm or neonates, and is comparable to older children.

17.4.4.2.3 Enzymatic Metabolism/Hydrolysis

Many drugs are not metabolized in the liver nor cleared by the kidneys and lungs. They undergo hydrolysis in the plasma by esterases, leading to the termination of their effect, and hence their elimination depends on the maturity and concentration of esterases. Esterases are of two types: **acetyl or erythrocyte or true cholinesterase (ACHE) and pseudo or plasma or butyryl or false cholinesterase or cholinesterase2 (BCHE). Colloquially, cholinesterase refers to pseudocholinesterase.**

(a) **ACHE** is present at the neuromuscular junction (NMJ), in the RBC membrane, and at other neural sites. It hydrolyses acetylcholine more quickly into choline and acetic acid. High levels in amniotic fluid are predictive of abdominal wall and neural tube defects. Drugs such as **atracurium, succinylcholine, and remifentanil** are metabolized by ACHE and are not dependent on the liver or kidney for their elimination. Since these enzymatic reactions are mature at birth, even in preterm neonates, dose modification is not required, rather clearance of these drugs may be increased as compared to adults.

(b) **BCHE** is present in the plasma, and it hydrolyses butyrylcholine more rapidly. It is synthesized in the liver and immediately released into the plasma, with a half-life is 10–14 days. It hydrolyses succinylcholine, atracurium, and cis-atracurium (benzylisoquinoline diesters).

Pseudocholinesterase deficiency occurs in 1:3,200–5,000 people, and may be genetic (gene mutation) or acquired. Deficiency or reduced activity of BCHE results in significant prolongation of effect of ester local anaesthetics (procaine, chloroprocaine, and tetracaine) and increases in sensitivity of muscles to scoline- and mivacurium-induced neuromuscular blockade. In neonates, BCHE is deficient because of immature hepatic production. Pseudocholinesterase deficiency is silent and is not discovered until an abnormal drug reaction occurs.

Causes of BCHE Deficiency:
  i. **Genetic** or inherited—BCHE gene mutation
 ii. **Acquired**—neonates, elderly individuals, and pregnancy, chronic infections (tuberculosis), extensive burns, liver and kidney disease, uraemia, heart failure, malignancy, malnutrition, organophosphate poisoning, collagen diseases, hypothyroidism, plasmapheresis, and **medications** like cholinesterase inhibitors—chlorpromazine, cyclophosphamide, ecothiophate eye drops, esmolol, glucocorticoids, and pancuronium, and benzodiazepines (temazepam).

Clinical Implication in Neonates:
 (a) **Dose of scoline** in neonates is higher than in children (3–4 mg/kg), but caution needs to be exercised because of inability to establish the deficiency of BCHE. Neonates have low plasma levels of BCHE because of reduced hepatic production. Because of potential risk of prolonged duration, Phase 2 block, and availability of shorter acting nondepolarizing muscle relaxants (**NDMR**), anaesthetists are moving away from using scoline for intubation.
 (b) **Avoid use of ester local anaesthetics** as prilocaine has an additional risk of causing methemoglobinemia. It is preferred to use amide local anaesthetics in this age group.

17.5 Pharmacodynamics

Pharmacodynamics is defined as how the body reacts to the drug or the effect of the drug on the body (desired or toxic).

Pharmacodynamics of drugs is altered in neonates, but there are large gaps in our knowledge about the pharmacodynamics of anesthetic drugs in neonates. Outcome measures such as effect on circulation, respiration, and neuromuscular blockade can be assessed, but variables such as pain, memory, and unconsciousness are hard to evaluate:

   i. The MAC of **inhalational agents** is less in neonates than that in infants.
  ii. Their brain is more sensitive to the effects of **sedatives**.
 iii. There is increased sensitivity to depolarizing **drugs**.
  iv. Reduced duration of regional block with **amide local anesthetics**.
   v. Prolonged effect with **ester local anesthetics**.
  vi. For **spinal anesthesia**, the weight to dose requirement of local anesthetics is more and the duration of action is shorter. This might be due to incomplete myelination.
 vii. Some drugs are **ineffective** in neonates, e.g., bronchodilators, due to underdeveloped bronchial smooth muscle or drugs that affect intestinal motility.

17.6 Anesthetic Agents

17.6.1 Inhaled Anesthetic Agents

Inhalation induction is commonly used technique for neonates due to its rapid onset. The absorption as well as elimination of drugs via the respiratory system depends on many factors, such as inspired concentration, alveolar ventilation, FRC, cardiac output, and blood gas solubility. Neonates have a high alveolar ventilation to FRC ratio of 5:1 which is nearly three times that of adults. The increase in alveolar ventilation in neonates leads to a higher volatile agent uptake. The solubility of volatile anesthetics is reduced in the newborn, so there is less uptake of anesthetic by the tissues, allowing partial pressures in the FRC to rise rapidly. Furthermore, a higher percentage of the cardiac output is delivered to vessel rich organs, especially brain, allowing rapid equilibration of alveolar and cerebral partial pressures of the agent. All these factors lead to rapid inhalational induction in newborns. In neonates with cyanotic heart disease or lung diseases, where there is a greater right to left shunt, induction may be slowed, while left-to-right shunts have a minimal impact.

The MAC of inhalational anesthetic agents in children is age dependent. (Table 17.2) It is lower in preterm than term neonates [7, 8]. Lower concentration of inhalational agents must be used in newborns as they produce greater depression of myocardium, greater hypotension, and depression of respiration, with inhibition of the ventilatory response to CO_2. This requires respiration to be assisted early during induction, which increases the potential for overdose of inhalation agent, while attempts are being made to establish an IV line. While myocardial depression is most often seen with halothane, it can occur with sevoflurane also. Recovery from inhalation agents is slower than expected. The effect of inhalational anesthetics on various organ systems in the neonate has not been studied but is thought to be similar to those seen in infants and older children.

a. **Halothane:** Before sevoflurane, halothane was the agent of choice for induction of anesthesia in neonates. It is a relatively potent agent, but because of its higher blood gas solubility, induction and recovery are slower as compared to sevoflurane. Its MAC is low in neonates, and causes profound myocardial depression, hypotension, with sensitization of the myocardium to both exogenous and endogenous catecholamines, and high risk of arrythmias, especially if accom-

Table 17.2 Comparative MAC for modern inhalational agents [10]

	Sevoflurane	Desflurane	Isoflurane	Nitrous oxide
MAC adult	2.05%	7.0%	1.2%	104%
MAC neonate (full term)	3.2%	9.2%	1.6%	–

panied with hypoxemia and hypercarbia. This is believed to be due to lesser number of myocardial contractile elements, less sensitivity of the myocardium to calcium, and incomplete cardiac sympathetic innervation. Cardio depressant effects of halothane can be attenuated by maintaining the heart rate and preload; hence, atropine is frequently used at induction, more so if scoline is used for intubation [9].

b. **Sevoflurane:** Sevoflurane is less pungent than isoflurane and desflurane, has low blood solubility, hence causes rapid induction and emergence from anesthesia. It is the anesthetic agent of choice for induction in neonates. It is not associated with vomiting or emergence delirium seen in children. Unlike other agents, the MAC of sevoflurane (3.3%) is the same in term, preterm neonates and infants under 6 months of age.

c. **Isoflurane:** Isoflurane has blood solubility intermediate of halothane and sevoflurane. It is more potent than sevoflurane, but its unpleasant smell leads to a higher risk of airway complications, such as breath holding, laryngospasm, and bronchospasm, thus making it unsuitable for induction. However, it can be used for maintenance of anesthesia.

d. **Desflurane:** Just like the other agents, MAC of desflurane is low in neonates. Its blood solubility is lower than isoflurane and sevoflurane, which facilitates rapid induction and emergence from anesthesia. It is suitable for maintenance. It is not suitable for induction due to its noxious smell, high incidence of laryngospasm, and high cost.

e **Nitrous oxide:** Nitrous oxide has low solubility, low potency and is a weak analgesic. It can be used along with other inhalational agents for increasing the speed of induction and to reduce their requirement during maintenance. Neonates, especially preterm, are at high risk of O_2 toxicity and retinal damage and use of N_2O avoids high oxygen tensions. However, any difficulty with the airway can lead to rapid desaturation so, air is a better option than N_2O and should be preferred if available.

17.6.2 Intravenous Anesthetic Agents

The dose–response relationship for intravenous agents has not been well-studied in neonates; thus, dosage guidelines are generally extrapolated from adult data or that from older children. In neonates, there is delayed awakening from IV induction, and termination of action is by redistribution which is slow due to less fat and muscle mass. Hence, brain concentration stays high for a longer period.

a. **Propofol:** Although there is paucity of literature regarding neonates, propofol has been used in them. The induction dose is less than that for older children (1–2 mg/kg) and clearance is longer. It tends to cause profound myocardial depression which leads to hypotension, especially in sick neonates, so should be used with caution. Furthermore, as an infusion, there is a risk of metabolic acidosis, organ failure, and death. Though the induction dose of propofol in neonates is relatively higher than in adults/kg body weight due to a larger volume of distribution, but the dose and duration of propofol need to be limited, especially in early postnatal life. Reduction in systemic vascular resistance, caused by propofol in acidotic or hypoxemic newborns, can cause return of circulation to fetal type transiently.

b. **Thiopentone:** Dose requirement of thiopentone is much lower in neonates than in infants. There are many reasons postulated. It crosses the BBB more easily and its clearance by redistribution is also slower hence causes prolonged effect. The cerebral cortical function is more immature with fewer synapses, making the brain more susceptible to the action of thiopentone. It may be used for induction in a reduced dose (2–4 mg/kg).

c. **Ketamine:** Ketamine is used very infrequently for induction in neonates. Since it does not cause myocardial depression and maintains systemic vascular resistance, it has been used for premedication and induction in neonates with cyanotic congenital heart disease. It is a potent analgesic, but is considered controversial, because ketamine has been shown to cause neuronal apoptosis in newborn rats. The initial requirement is higher than in older children, and clearance is also reduced. There is no merit in routine use of ketamine in neonates, except in very sick, hemodynamically unstable, and bradycardic neonates.

d. **Etomidate:** Etomidate suppresses adrenal function and corticoid secretion, and has limited indication in neonates. Its volume of distribution is large, so initial dose requirement is high.

17.6.3 Analgesics

17.6.3.1 Alpha 2 Agonists

a. **Clonidine:** An increase in clearance time has been observed with clonidine in neonates, which reaches adult levels by 1 year of age. Clonidine has been used for sedation in the NICU, for management of neonatal abstinence syndrome, and as an additive to caudal and epidural anesthesia. It prolongs the duration of analgesia in children, but not much data is available in neonates [11]. It can lead to apnea in neonates [12, 13], has not received FDA approval.

b. **Dexmedetomidine:** There has been limited use of this agent in neonates. As with many other agents, it shows reduced clearance. It has been used as an additive to neuraxial block and though it has still not received FDA approval for use in neonates. Its uses in children include procedural sedation, opioid withdrawal, prevention of emergence delirium, and postoperative analgesia, but studies in neonates are limited.

17.6.3.2 Opioids (Table 17.3)

a. **Morphine:** Morphine is a long-acting opioid which has been used in neonates, for both intraoperative and postoperative analgesia, as bolus or infusion, especially in those requiring assisted ventilation. Apart from the IV route, oral, rectal, and caudal routes have also been used. It is metabolized in the liver and is eliminated after glucuronidation and sulfonation. Although sulfonation plays a minor role in adults, it is an important pathway for drug clearance in neonates.

Table 17.3 Recommended analgesic dosing for neonates

Medication	Intermittent dose	Infusion dose	Adverse effects
Acetaminophen	10 mg/kg IV/ PO	N/A	None reported[a]
NSAIDS	Not recommended	N/A	Unwanted ductal closure, gastropathy, nephropathy, NEC, IVH, surgical bleeding
Morphine	0.05–0.1 mg/ kg IV	0.005– 0.03 mg/H	Respiratory depression, decreased gastrointestinal motility, hypotension, urinary retention
Fentanyl	1 mcg/kg IV	0.5–2 mcg/ kg/H	Respiratory depression, hypotension, muscle rigidity, hypothermia
Ketamine	0.5–2 mg/kg IV	0.5–1 mg/ kg/H	Respiratory depression, increased secretions

[a]No reported adverse effects in therapeutic doses. Known hepatotoxicity with overdosing. *NSAIDS* Nonsteroidal anti-inflammatory drugs, *NEC* Necrotizing enterocolitis, *IVH* Intraventricular hemorrhage

The metabolites of morphine are dependent on renal elimination. Hence, prolongation of action of morphine is seen due to immature liver function and reduced renal excretion. Furthermore, it causes severe respiratory depression, especially in preterm, probably due to immaturity of the BBB. It is, therefore, better to avoid morphine in this age group or to use it with extreme caution.

b. **Codeine:** Codeine, especially in combination with paracetamol or NSAIDS, has been used in infants. Its analgesic effect is due to its metabolism to morphine. It can be used in term neonates, but is not useful in preterm neonates as its conversion to morphine is limited. Intravenous use can lead to hypotension and is not recommended. It can be used orally, rectally or intramuscularly [14].

c. **Pethidine:** Pethidine is more lipophilic than morphine and lesser amounts cross the BBB, so it can be used in newborns. Even though it is less metabolized in neonates than adults, it should not be used for long periods or repeated administration due to risk of accumulation of its toxic metabolite norpethidine, which can lead to seizures. Elimination of pethidine is greatly reduced in neonates with prolongation of its action.

d. **Fentanyl:** The introduction of fentanyl has allowed safer and more effective pain management in the neonates. Its advantages include rapid onset due to high penetration of BBB, short duration of action, hemodynamic stability, suppression of neonatal stress response and better outcome after surgery. The volume of distribution is high, clearance is reduced, elimination half-life is longer, compared to older children and adults. Hence, the dose needs to be modified accordingly. It has a short duration of action is due to redistribution. In high doses, it behaves like a long-acting narcotics, producing respiratory depression, muscle rigidity, cholinergic effects and bradycardia, and mild vasodilatation leading to hypotension. The dose is 1–3 µg/kg, but higher doses have been used in cardiac surgery. Common routes of administration are intravenous and caudal, and there are hardly any studies about transdermal and transmucosal use in neonates.

e. **Alfentanyl and sufentanyl**: have a similar profile to fentanyl. Alfentanil causes muscle rigidity and is recommended to be used with muscle relaxants in newborns.

f. **Remifentanil:** Remifentanil has very favorable pharmacokinetics in neonates. It is degraded by plasma and tissue esterase, which are mature even in preterms and hence its metabolism is independent of hepatic or renal functions. It has a very short half-life and neonates can clear the drug more rapidly than older children. Hence, it has a higher safety profile than any other narcotic agent, and can be safely used in neonates without risk of cardiovascular or prolonged respiratory depression. Side effects such as respiratory depression and muscle rigidity are seen at higher concentrations.

g. **Tramadol:** Tramadol is a weak opioid with less chances of respiratory depression. However, it has reduced clearance and is not of much use in neonates.

Respiratory depression due to narcotics can be treated with naloxone 0.1 mg/kg.

17.6.3.3 Other Analgesics

a. **Paracetamol** (acetaminophen) has a central analgesic effect, mediated through activation of descending serotonergic pathways. In neonates, it has a higher volume of distribution. The metabolism is different from adults, the major pathway being sulphate conjugation and limited metabolism by glucuronidation. Thus, it has a lower initial peak concentration with less effective analgesia, but repeated administration can lead to accumulation. There are no known adverse effects at therapeutic dosing. Hepatotoxicity is rare, probably due to decreased activity of cytochrome P-450. It can be used intravenously in small doses. Although rectal bioavailability is higher than in children, oral and rectal routes do not provide adequate postoperative analgesia.

(b) **NSAIDS** are effective analgesics in children; however, not much data is available for neonates. They have been used for ductal closure. Side effects such as gastropathy, nephropathy, necrotising enterocolitis and intraventricular haemorrhage and surgical bleeding are similar as in older children.

17.6.4 Muscle Relaxants

At birth, the neuromuscular junction (NMJ) is immature, muscle mass is less, and volume of distribution is high due to higher ECF volume. Muscle relaxants behave differently in newborns than in adults.

a. **Succinylcholine (scoline):** The only depolarizing muscle relaxant in clinical use is scoline. It was very popular as a component of rapid sequence intubation (RSI), but its side effects such as arrythmias, hyperkalemia and risk of malignant hyperthermia have led to its disrepute. Scoline has a very high volume of distribution and the recommended dose is 3 mg/kg as compared to older children, where it 2 mg/kg. However, its action is not prolonged due to rapid clearance by plasma esterase. Malignant hyperthermia is not generally seen, and increase in potassium is not significant to warrant being termed hyperkalemia, which in neonates is defined as serum potassium more than 6 mEq/L. Adequate relaxation for intubation can be obtained without using muscle paralysis, by deepening the plane of anesthesia with inhalational anesthetics or propofol use of opioids (fentanyl or remifentanil), and assisted ventilation.

(b) **Nondepolarizing muscle relaxants (NDMR):** The response to NDMRs is more unpredictable in neonates, The NMJ is very sensitivity to NDMRs, even though their volume of distribution is high. The duration of action is prolonged due to slow metabolism and poor elimination due to immature hepatic and renal function. **Atracurium** and **cisatracurium** are not dependent on the kidney or liver for excretion, (they undergo ester hydrolysis and Hofmann elimination), hence are preferred in newborns and neonates [15]. **Rocuronium** behaves similar to adults in neonates. **Vecuronium** is metabolized in the liver, which is still immature, prolonging the duration of action: 0.1 mg/kg dose of vecuronium and 1 mg/kg of rocuronium maintain paralysis for almost an hour in neonates [16]. Pancuronium is a long acting nondepolarizing neuromuscular blocking agent, with a prolonged duration of action. It has a sympathomimetic effect and causes tachycardia, which is beneficial to neonates, but prolonged duration of action with delayed excretion precludes its use in neonates [17]. Mivacurium is a NDMR which is administered in doses of 0.1–0.2 mg/kg with rapid onset of blockade, lasting 15–30 minutes. It undergoes ester hydrolysis and is ideal for short surgical procedures. In plasma cholinesterase deficiency, duration of action of mivacurium is prolonged.

Reversal of NM blockade: Neuromuscular blockade should always be antagonized in neonates, even if they appear to have completely recovered, because the smallest increase in work of breathing can cause fatigue and respiratory failure. **Neostigmine** and **atropine** or **glycopyrrolate** combination is commonly used. Data regarding **sugammadex** are limited.

17.6.5 Sedatives

a. **Benzodiazepines:** It is difficult to quantify sedation in neonates. Benzodiazepines have an increased half-life due to reduced drug clearance and can result in prolonged sedation.

b. **Midazolam** is the only benzodiazepine approved by FDA for use in neonates, with a half-life of 6–12 h. The IV dose is 0.05–0.10 mg/kg. When given in combination with fentanyl, it can cause severe hypotension and respiratory depression. Discontinuation of midazolam after long use in the ICU can cause withdrawal symptoms, such as agitation in children, though difficult to quantify in neonates.

c. **Diazepam** has an extremely long half-life (80 h) in neonates and should not be used.

17.6.6 Anticholinergic Drugs

The decision whether to routinely premedicate neonates with anticholinergics (**atropine**, **glycopyrrolate**) is controversial and this use is declining. Current use is limited to treatment of bradycardia or sometimes to reduce secretions, e.g., in oral surgeries. Hypoxia is the most common cause of bradycardia and should be managed by ensuring oxygenation, and not by anticholinergics, which will induce tachycardia at the expense of increase in myocardial O_2 consumption and myocardial damage. However, anticholinergics must always be given with neostigmine at the time of reversal of NM blockade. Clearance of both atropine and glycopyrrolate is reduced due to hepatic and renal immaturity.

17.6.7 Local Anesthetics (Table 17.4)

Both lignocaine and bupivacaine can be used in neonates and help to reduce the dose of opioids given to them. Lignocaine is used for local anesthesia in reduced doses of 1–1.5 mg/kg, since its clearance is reduced and there is risk of accumulation. Cardiac toxicity is more common that neurotoxicity, though that could be due to masking of symptoms during anesthesia. In addition, unlike adults, toxicity manifests less as cardiac arrest and more in the form of arrythmias, convulsions, and respiratory arrest [14].

Bupivacaine is usually bound to alpha 1 acid glycoprotein, which is low in neonates, and hence the free level of drug is high. Due to its lipophilic nature, it can cross the underdeveloped BBB and hence can cause seizures in the neonate. For local anesthesia, it is used up to a maximum dose of 1 mg/kg. The dose of bupivacaine for spinal anesthesia in infants is 0.6–1 mg/kg which is higher than the adult requirement because of a larger CSF volume of circulation, myelination, and rapid drug clearance due to higher heart rate and cardiac output. Use of

Table 17.4 Commonly used local anaesthetics and doses in neonates

S no.	LA drug	Maximum dose[a]	Neonatal dose	Use/Comments
1	Bupivacaine	2.5 mg/kg	1 mg/kg	Field block, wound infiltration
2	Ropivacaine	3 mg/kg	1.5 mg/kg	Less motor block and cardiotoxicity than bupivacaine
3	Lidocaine	5 mg/kg	2.5 mg/kg	Avoid digital and penile blocks with addition of vasoconstrictor
4	Prilocaine	Not recommended		Risk of methemoglobinemia
5	Chloroprocaine	14 mg/kg	7 mg/kg	Short T1/2, no accumulation
6	EMLA	1 g/5 kg	1 g	Maximum skin contact—1 h, risk of methemoglobinemia

[a]Maximum doses are additive and not independent of each other; local anaesthetic dosing should be decreased by 50% in neonates [10].

adjuvants such as fentanyl or clonidine can result in respiratory depression and apnea and is not recommended. Ropivacaine may be used as a local anesthetic up to a dose of 1.5 mg/kg. It has less chances of cardiotoxicity and motor block. If given as an infusion, ropivacaine can also accumulate and cause seizures in neonates due to low clearance.

When EMLA is used in neonates, due to higher body surface area compared to body weight, and high skin permeability, there is higher absorption of the local anesthetics. Since they have high amounts of fetal hemoglobin and reduced methemoglobin reductase activity, these children have a higher tendency to form methemoglobin. Hence, the use of this ointment is better avoided in neonates.

17.6.8 Miscellaneous Drugs

a. **Calcium** has a greater impact on myocardial contractility as their endogenous calcium stores are low.
b. **Catecholamine:** Response to catecholamines in the neonates is variable and depends on the myocardial structure, number of contractile elements, sympathetic innervations, and development of adrenergic receptors which are underdeveloped, and on noradrenaline stores which are low. Alpha receptors get stimulated at lower doses compared to beta receptors, because they develop earlier.
c. **Dopamine** infusion is accepted in neonates especially after cardiac surgery or in pulmonary hypertension as it causes more systemic than pulmonary vasoconstriction. The initial requirement may be higher. However, the action is usually prolonged due to reduced metabolism.

Some drugs are ineffective in neonates such as drugs affecting **intestinal motility or bronchodilators** and **xanthines**, as neonates have underdeveloped smooth muscle [18, 19].

Neonates have a developing brain and the impact of anesthesia and possibility of neurodevelopmental harm is a topic of active research especially in premature babies and those needing multiple surgeries. This topic is discussed in a separate chapter.

17.7 Anesthetic Implications of Clinical Pharmacology in Neonates

Note: An important point to be kept in mind while diluting drugs for neonates is that the volume of drug which is given contributes to the total volume replacement with intravenous fluids during surgery.

Both general anesthesia and spinal anesthesia have been successfully used in neonates and former premature infants, who are at risk of postoperative apnea, bradycardia, and desaturation [20, 21].

Premedication: the decision whether to routinely premedicate neonates with **anticholinergic drugs** are controversial [22]. Many anesthetists have abandoned routine premedication with no negative consequences, pointing out that bradycardia is almost always due to hypoxia, for which the treatment is O_2 and not drugs. However, advocates of routine premedication with anticholinergics believe that since the parasympathetic system is fully developed, incidence of bradycardia, especially with scoline is high. In addition, delivery of IV medication is delayed during bradycardia and hence must be given in advance. **Benzodiazepines** have an increased half-life due to reduced drug clearance and can result in prolonged sedation and must be avoided in neonates. However, the role they play as anxiolytic and sedative is debatable and cannot be quantified. (Table 17.5)

As regards **intravenous agents,** the dose response relationship has not been well-studied in neonates, and dosage guidelines are extrapolated from adult data. Although **propofol** has been used in neonates, it leads to hypotension, especially in sick patients. In addition, its redistribution and delayed clearance leads to prolonged recovery. Furthermore, its use as an infusion has been shown to cause metabolic acidosis and organ failure leading to death, so the dose and duration of propofol need to be limited.

NMB **agents** are commonly used during surgery. In general, the NMJ in neonates is resistant to depolarizing NMBs, and sensitive to nondepolarizing NMBs. Their response is similar to myasthenia gravis patients. All relaxant drugs are polar and water soluble, and hence have a high volume of distribution. This means that the initial dose must be high to achieve a target effect, but supplements will be smaller in dose or at longer intervals. Depolarizing NMBs are hydrolyzed by plasma cholinesterase and so there is not much prolongation of effect, unless there is deficiency of the enzyme. Nondepolarizing NMBs are metabolized in the liver and excreted in urine, hence will have prolonged action, even in absence of hepatic or renal disease.

The pharmacology and side effects of **narcotics** are better understood than that of induction agents. Morphine is generally avoided as it causes hypotension and prolonged respiratory depression due to its dependance on renal metabolism and elimination. Fentanyl, introduced in the 1980s, with its better safety profile and shorter duration of action has replaced morphine and pethidine in neonates for

Table 17.5 Preoperative medications, routes, and doses in neonates

Drug	PO	Nasal	IV	IM
Midazolam	0.5–1.0 mg/kg (max 15 mg)		0.05–0.1 mg/kg	No
Fentanyl			1–3 µg/kg	No
Morphine			0.05–0.10 mg/kg	No
Sufentanil		0.25–0.5 µg/kg		No
Ketamine	2–4 mg/kg		1–2 mg/kg	8–10 mg/kg
Methohexital	25–30 mg/kg per rectal (max 500 mg)		1–2 mg/kg	No

surgical analgesia. It has a minimal cardiovascular effect, is able to suppress the stress response, with improved outcome. However, prolonged use and in high doses, it can cause respiratory depression, bradycardia (cholinergic action), and hypotension (vasodilator effect). Because of its potential to cause rigidity, monitoring of respiration is essential in neonates on spontaneous respiration. Though morphine has limited use in neonates, but its potent analgesic effect is most beneficial in and after major surgeries, with large volume shifts, long duration (>2 h), and where postoperative ventilatory support may be anticipated or planned.

Paracetamol has a higher volume of distribution with limited metabolism (immature glucuronidation). Thus, it has a lower initial peak concentration with less effective analgesia, and repeated administration can lead to accumulation (Table 17.3).

Bupivacaine has lower protein binding capacity and clearance which leads to increased free form in the plasma, with risk of adverse effects. The dose for spinal anesthesia is 0.6–1 mg/kg, higher than in adults, because of a larger CSF volume (4 mg/kg vs 2 mL/kg in adults). **Adjuvants** (fentanyl, clonidine) should be used cautiously because of risk of delayed respiratory depression and apnea, and are best avoided in neonates not on respiratory support.

EMLA has been used in neonates, but due to larger body surface area and high skin permeability, LA absorption is high, with risk of LA-induced seizures and methemoglobinemia.

The possibility of neurodevelopmental harm by anesthetics is a topic of active research, to the developing brain of the neonate. This can influence long term neurological outcome especially in premature babies and those needing multiple surgeries and anesthesia exposures.

Resuscitation medications: (Box 17.1) all resuscitative medications should be kept available when anesthetizing neonates. They should be diluted appropriately and loaded in syringes, labelled for use in an emergency intraoperatively. Their volume adds on the IV fluid volume, and should be considered when calculating fluid requirements.

Box 17.1 Resuscitation medication in children

Epinephrine = 10–100 µg/kg for arrest (100 µg/kg in ETT), 1–4 µg/kg for hypotension
Atropine = 0.01–0.02 mg/kg (0.3 mg/kg in ETT)—actual dose 0.1–1 mg
Adenosine = 0.1 mg/kg (max 6 mg)
Lidocaine = 1–1.5 mg/kg
Scoline = 2–3 mg/kg
Rocuronium 1 mg/kg
Calcium chloride = 10–20 mg/kg (dilute to 10 mg/cc or else veins will sclerose, prefer central vein)
Bicarbonate = 1 mEq/kg (dilute to 1 mEq/cc or else veins will sclerose)
Naloxone = 0.1 mg/kg
DEFIBRILLATION = 2 J/kg (can increase up to 4 J/kg)

17.8 Conclusion

Anaesthetising the neonate is fascinating, but challenging even for experienced anaesthesiologists. Neonates differ from other paediatric patients not only anatomically and physiologically but also pharmacologically. For successfully managing this group of patients, it is essential to have knowledge about their pharmacological variations and exercise extra caution while anaesthetising them, keeping in mind their developing physiology, coexisting pathologies and pharmacokinetics and pharmacodynamics of any given drug.

References

1. Thaddanee R, Patel HS, Thakor N. A study on incidence of congenital anomalies in newborns and their association with maternal factors: a prospective study. Int J Contemp Pediatr. 2016;3:579–82. https://doi.org/10.18203/2349-3291.ijcp20161042. ISSN: 2349-3283. http://www.ijpediatrics.com, (https://ijpediatrics.com/index.php/ijcp/article/view/290/285).
2. Nasr VG, Davis JM. Anesthetic use in newborn infants: the urgent need for rigorous evaluation. Pediatr Res. 2015;78(1):2–6. https://doi.org/10.1038/pr.2015.58. https://www.ncbi.nlm.nih.gov/pmc/articles/PMC4471569/).
3. Rang HP, Dale MM, Ritter JM, Flower RJ. Pharmacology. Elsevier; 2007. ISBN 978-0-443-06911-6.
4. Ruggiero A, Ariano A, Triarico S, et al. Neonatal pharmacology and clinical implications. Drugs Context. 2019;8:212608. https://doi.org/10.7573/dic.212608. Published online 2019 Oct 14. (https://www.ncbi.nlm.nih.gov/pmc/articles/PMC6821278/)
5. Besunder JB, Reed MD, Blumer JL. Principles of drug bio-disposition in the neonate. A critical evaluation of the pharmacokinetic-pharmacodynamic interface (Part I). Clin Pharmacokinet. 1988;14(4):189–216. https://doi.org/10.2165/00003088-198814040-00001. (https://pubmed.ncbi.nlm.nih.gov/3292100/)
6. Shahid S, Florez ID, Mbuagbaw L. Efficacy and safety of EMLA cream for pain control due to venipuncture in infants: a meta-analysis. Pediatrics. 2019;143(1):e20181173. https://doi.org/10.1542/peds.2018-1173.
7. Nickalls RWD, Mapleson WW. Age-related iso-MAC charts for isoflurane, sevoflurane and desflurane in man. Br J Anaesth. 2003;91(2):170–4. https://doi.org/10.1093/bja/aeg132.
8. Rosenfeld DM, Warner DO. Clinical Anesthesia, 5th ed. Anesthesiology. 2006;105:1284–5. https://doi.org/10.1097/00000542-200612000-00044.
9. Lerman J, Robinson S, Willis MM, Gregory GA. Anesthetic requirements for halothane in young children 0–1 month and 1–6 months of age. Anesthesiology. 1983;59:421–4.
10. Vadi M, Nour C, Lieter P, Carter H. Anesthetic management of the newborn surgical patient. Pediatric and neonatal surgery. Joanne Baerg: IntechOpen; 2017. p. 10.5772/66932. https://www.intechopen.com/chapters/53583.
11. Rochette A, Troncin R, Raux O. Clonidine added to bupivacaine in neonatal spinal anesthesia: a prospective comparison in 124 preterm and term infants. Paediatr Anaesth. 2005;15:1072–7.
12. Fellmann C, Gerber AC, Weiss M. Apnoea in a former preterm infant after caudal bupivacaine with clonidine for inguinal herniorrhaphy. Paediatr Anaesth. 2002;12:637–40.
13. Breschan C, Krumpholz R, Likar R, et al. Can a dose of 2 microg.kg (-1) caudal clonidine cause respiratory depression in neonates? Paediatr Anaesth. 1999;9:81–3.

14. Haidon JL, Cunliffe M. Analgesia for neonates. Continuing Education in Anaesthesia Critical Care & Pain. 2010;10(4):123–7. https://doi.org/10.1093/bjaceaccp/mkq016. (https://academic.oup.com/bjaed/article/10/4/123/380855).

15. Kisor DF, Schmith VD. Clinical pharmacokinetics of cisatracurium besilate. Clin Pharmacokinet. 1999;36:27–40.

16. Meretoja OA. Is vecuronium a long-acting neuromuscular blocking agent in neonates and infants? Br J Anaesth. 1989;62(2):184–7.

17. Cabal LA, Siassi B, Artal R, Gonzalez F, et al. Cardiovascular and catecholamine changes after administration of pancuronium in distressed neonates. Pediatrics. 1985;75(2):284–7.

18. Henderson-Smart DJ, Steer P. Methylxanthine treatment for apnea in preterm infants. Cochrane Database Syst Rev. 2001;(3):CD000140. https://doi.org/10.1002/14651858.CD000140.

19. McNamara DG, Nixon GM, Anderson BJ, et al. Methylxanthines for the treatment of apnea associated with bronchiolitis and anesthesia. Paediatr Anaesth. 2004;14(7):541–50.

20. Krane EJ, Haberkern CM, Jacobson LE. Postoperative apnea, bradycardia, and oxygen desaturation in formerly premature infants. prospective comparison of spinal and general anesthesia. Anesth Analg. 1995;80(1):7–13.

21. Cote CJ, Zaslavsky A, Downes JJ, Kurth CD, et al. Postoperative apnea in former preterm infants after inguinal herniorrhaphy: a combined analysis. Anesthesiology. 1995;1995(82):809–22.

22. Jöhr M. is it time to question the routine use of anticholinergic agents in paediatric anaesthesia? Editorial. Paediatr Anaesth. 1999;9(2):99–101.

For Further Reading

Barash PG, Cullen BF, Stoelting RK. Clinical Anesthesia. 5th ed. Philadelphia: Lippincott Williams & Wilkins; 2006.

Lerman J. Neonatal anesthesia. Springer; 2015.

Miller RD. Miller's anesthesia. New York: Elsevier/Churchill Livingstone; 2005.

Neuromuscular Disorders in Neonate

18

Anita Malik and Namisha Goyal

18.1 Introduction

Neuromuscular (NM) disorders comprise of abnormalities of any component of the peripheral nervous system or the lower motor neuron system, composed of the anterior horn motor neurons, nerve roots and plexus (motor, sensory, and autonomic), NM junction (NMJ), and the skeletal muscles [1, 2]. These are mostly due to genetic mutations and are inherited disorders. Hundreds of genetic loci responsible for the molecular basis of NM disorders have been identified in the last two decades [3–5].

Presentation of NM disorders is different in neonates than in adults. Most common manifestation in the newborn is profound hypotonia, severe but transient weakness, poor reflexes, contractures (focal or generalized), seizures, and perinatal asphyxia. Brain and spinal cord can also be affected [2].

Babies with severe hypotonia but minimal weakness usually do not have lower motor neuron disease and other conditions, such as genetic, metabolic, congenital heart disease, hypothyroidism, and sepsis must be ruled out [1, 6].

Parents may observe limpness and flaccidity or even rigidity of limb muscles, weakness, weak cry, inadequate respiration (slow and shallow), feeding problems, swallowing difficulty (inadequate sucking, regurgitation, and drooling from mouth and nose), and risk of pulmonary aspiration. As per a study in 2005, Clinical signs that may indicate NM disorders in neonates are absent or extremely reduced antigravity movements, severe muscle weakness, and contractures due to peripheral nerve or muscle involvement [7].

A. Malik (✉)
Department of Anesthesiology & Critical Care, King George's Medical University (KGMU), Lucknow, India

N. Goyal
Department of Anesthesiology, National University Hospital (NUH), Singapore, Singapore

© The Author(s), under exclusive license to Springer Nature Singapore Pte Ltd. 2023
U. Saha (ed.), *Clinical Anesthesia for the Newborn and the Neonate*,
https://doi.org/10.1007/978-981-19-5458-0_18

In case these neonates require surgery for related [e.g., muscle biopsy, electro-myography (EMG) studies] or unrelated diseases, they are at high risk of periopera-tive complications and delayed recovery after anesthesia. A thorough knowledge of the causes of hypotonia, there presentation, infirmity caused, and how it interacts with the physiologic, metabolic, and biochemical changes due to the surgical condi-tion, is essential for the neonatal anesthesiologists to be able to course these babies safely through the difficult perioperative period, preventing complications and other catastrophic consequences [8]. An intensive, dedicated, dynamic, multidisciplinary perioperative approach is required for a better outcome.

18.2   Neuromuscular Disorders

The common types of NM disorders that may be seen in neonates, depending on the level of involvement, fall under four categories: [1, 2]

1. **Disorder of the anterior horn motor neurons/motor neuron disorders**—e.g., spinal muscular atrophies (5q Spinal Muscular Atrophy, Non-5q Spinal Muscular Atrophies, Spinal Muscular Atrophy with Respiratory Distress, X-Linked Infantile Spinal Muscular Atrophy, Pontocerebellar Hypoplasia Plus Spinal Muscular Atrophy)
2. **Disorders of peripheral nerves**—e.g., peripheral neuropathies, brachial plexus neuropathy.
3. **Disorders of NM junction (NMJ)**—e.g., myasthenia gravis (MG syndrome, transient MG), congenital myasthenic syndromes.
4. **Disorders of muscle cell**—e.g., congenital myopathies [Nemaline Myopathy, Core Myopathies, Myotubular (Centronuclear) Myopathy] and muscular dystrophies.

Muscular dystrophy includes wide group of diseases that cause muscle weakness and loss of muscle mass, due to abnormal gene mutations that interfere with produc-tion of muscle protein. There are several types of MD and symptoms usually begin in childhood, mostly in boys. There is no cure except for symptomatic management. Though the main feature is progressive muscle weakness, specific signs and symp-toms appear at different ages and in different muscle groups, depending upon the involvement [9]. The most common types of dystrophies are Duchenne MD (DMD), Becker MD, myotonic, limb girdle (Erb's), and facioscapulohumeral dystrophy. These present in childhood or later and will not be discussed in this chapter. Often, it is difficult to differentiate between myopathies and neuronal disorders in neo-nates, based on the clinical presentation, but the degree of care in the perioperative period and need of postoperative ventilation is similar in both.

Nerve conduction studies, EMG, electroencephalography (EEG), cerebrospinal fluid (CSF) analysis, and magnetic resonance imaging (MRI) play an important role in differentiation of NM disorders in neonates with a wide range of presenta-tion [10].

This chapter will cover these NM disorders along with their anesthetic implications in a neonate.

18.2.1 Motor Neuron Disorders

1. **Spinal muscular atrophy (SMA)** is a relatively common autosomal recessive, progressive degenerative disease affecting the motor neurons.
   (a) **SMA type 0** presents prenatally with weak fetal movements. Hypotonia, areflexia, and respiratory failure are present at birth, and is fatal without respiratory support [11, 12].
   (b) **SMA type 1** (Werdnig–Hoffman disease) manifests with profound hypotonia, severe weakness more in the legs than arms, proximal muscles are weaker than distal ones, and without facial weakness. Chest is bell-shaped because of the involvement of the intercostal muscles. The breathing pattern is paradoxical due to weak intercostal muscles but intact function of the diaphragm. The chest configuration can contribute to the impairment of lung development. Gastrointestinal dysmotility presents with constipation and delayed gastric emptying [13]. Tongue fasciculations are often present. Bulbar weakness manifests with swallowing difficulties, choking due to pooling of secretions in the hypopharynx, and poor feeding. Babies are prone to recurrent respiratory infections due to regurgitation and aspiration. Cardiac malformations (hypoplastic left heart, atrial and ventricular septal defects) may be present [1].
2. **Spinal muscular atrophy with respiratory distress (SMARD)** [1]
   Sudden and severe respiratory insufficiency is an indication for ventilatory support. Diaphragmatic weakness manifesting as eventration of diaphragm is characteristic. The distal rather than proximal muscles are more affected in SMARD unlike SMA. Swallowing difficulties, aspirations, and poor caloric intake are also common.
3. **X-linked infantile spinal muscular atrophy (XL-SMA)** [1]
   Hypotonia, proximal weakness, facial weakness, arthrogryposis or deformities of the limbs and joints at birth, and respiratory failure at birth are features of this type of SMA.
4. **Pontocerebellar hypoplasia plus spinal muscular atrophy** [1]
   Pontocerebellar hypoplasia is a degenerative disease of the motor neurons, neurons of the brainstem and cerebellum. Hypotonia, weakness, contractures, respiratory distress, and encephalopathy may be present in the neonatal period.

18.2.1.1 Anesthesia Considerations
Pulmonary involvement and bulbar dysfunction are the most common anesthetic risks. High prevalence of cardiac malformations in cases of SMA 0 and severe SMA I requires preoperative cardiac evaluation. The gastroesophageal reflux and aspiration risk must be evaluated. Hypoglycemia is reported in patients with low muscle mass and fat content [14]. As during fasting, skeletal muscles and fat are an

important source of gluconeogenic substrates, hypoglycemia is a concern in the perioperative period.

Anesthetic approach to these patients must be individualized depending upon the severity of the disease. Succinylcholine should be avoided to prevent hyperkalemia [15]. Due to variable sensitivity, nondepolarizing muscle relaxants should be avoided or dose reduced. NM monitoring is essential. Proper reversal of the muscle relaxant is required at the end of surgery. Postoperative ventilatory support may be required.

18.2.2 Peripheral Neuropathies

Congenital peripheral neuropathies are a rare cause of neonatal hypotonia. If present the hypotonia and weakness are associated with feet abnormalities. Electrophysiologic studies will demonstrate neuropathic findings and genetic testing is oriented by subdividing them into axonal vs demyelinating [16].

18.2.3 Neuromuscular Junction (NMJ) Disorders

(a) **Transient Neonatal Myasthenia Gravis (MG)**

A transient form of MG in neonates results from passive placental transfer of acetylcholine receptor antibodies (AChR) from a mother with autoimmune MG [17] and leads to generalized hypotonia and weakness including facial involvement in the newborn. Respiratory dysfunction or feeding difficulties may be present [18]. The diagnosis is confirmed by administration of anticholinesterase and is based on the presence of AChR antibodies (rarely muscle-specific kinase antibodies) in newborn serum.

(b) **Congenital Myasthenic Syndromes (CMSs)**

Congenital myasthenic syndromes is a heterogeneous group of disorders secondary to a genetic defect, manifested by failure of NM transmission at the NMJ. Neonates may present with fatigable muscle weakness of bulbar, extraocular, respiratory and limb muscles in different combinations [19].

In the neonatal period choline acetyltransferase mutations may lead to hypotonia with marked bulbar symptoms and respiratory dysfunction followed by life-threatening episodes of apnea in infancy [20]. Certain unusual patterns may appear sometimes, like in patients of Dok7 CMS (downstream of tyrosine kinase 7 CMS) in the neonatal period, presenting with stridor due to bilateral vocal cord paralysis, respiratory distress, feeding difficulties, requiring intubation, and ventilatory support [21].

18.2.3.1 Anesthesia Considerations

Preoperative documentation of the severity of the muscle weakness and the muscle groups affected by the disease is required (respiratory and bulbar function). During the perioperative period, the primary concern for patients with myasthenic syndromes is to avoid respiratory compromise from weakened respiratory muscles or upper-airway muscles [22, 23].

NM transmission is affected by inhalational anesthetic agents, and in MG, these effects may be exaggerated. However, Sevoflurane has been used in pediatric myasthenic patients [24]. Succinylcholine is best avoided. Due to high sensitivity to non-depolarizing muscle relaxants, intubation of the trachea is best performed without muscle relaxants [25]. To avoid use of reversal with acetylcholinesterase inhibitors, rocuronium-induced NM blockade can be reversed by Sugammadex along with NM monitoring [26, 27].

18.2.4 Muscle Disorders

In neonates with hypotonia or weakness, disorders of the muscle can be subdivided into muscular dystrophies and congenital myopathies. In general, the muscular dystrophies are characterized by severe disruption of muscle architecture on tissue biopsy, whereas congenital myopathies show a relative preservation of muscle cell structure and fiber type proportion.

18.2.4.1 Congenital Muscular Dystrophies (CMD)

The actin–myosin filaments contract, but due to the dissociation of contractile force to the surrounding connective tissue, they are no longer connected well to the cell membrane or the surrounding tissue and so fail to generate effective mechanical force [28].

(a) **α-Dystroglycanopathies:** dystroglycanopathies are caused by defects in connective tissue glycoproteins which form the contractile element and extracellular matrix connection. Abnormal glycosylation of α-dystroglycan disrupts the link between inside the cell and components of extracellular matrix. Walker–Warburg syndrome, muscle–eye–brain (MEB) disease, and Fukuyama congenital MD are the three severe forms of presentations [1].

- **Walker–Warburg syndrome:** this is the most severe form and central nervous system involvement is present. Neonatal hypotonia and severe weakness are accompanied by hydrocephalus, lissencephaly and cerebellar malformations. Ocular involvement includes microphthalmia, retinal dysgenesis, and anterior chamber malformations [29]. Respiratory and cardiac involvement is also common. Cleft lip and palate may be sometimes. Creatine phosphokinase (CPK) is markedly elevated.

- **Muscle–eye–brain disease:** hypotonia, weakness, and hydrocephalus is accompanied with milder form of ocular abnormalities and distinctive facial features, sometime with cleft lip and palate. Respiratory and cardiac involvement is common [1].

- **Fukuyama congenital muscular dystrophy:** this is a rare, with autosomal recessive pattern of inheritance, 2nd most common form of MD in Japan (1960), where one in every 90 is a heterozygous carrier. It affects brain, eyes, skeletal muscles, leading to weakness, hypotonia, swallowing difficulty, deformed appearance, blunted brain development (cerebral and cerebellar dysplasia), affecting cognitive and social skills, hydrocephalus, seizures, and ocular manifestations. Joint contractures, respiratory and cardiac involvement are common. There is no cure, except symptomatic (ACEI, beta blockers, antiepileptics, physical therapy, muscle stretching). Surgical release of contractures and skeletal abnormalities may be required. Prognosis is poor and proves fatal by age 20 years [30–32].

(b) **LAMA2-related muscular dystrophy:** LAMA2 extracellular matrix protein (primary merosin deficiency) mutations should be suspected in neonates with significant hypotonia, respiratory insufficiency, sometimes arthrogryposis (multiple congenital joint contractures) without significant encephalopathy or ocular abnormalities. CPK levels are raised, often four to five times above normal limits [33]. Diagnosis is based on clinical assessment, elevated CPK levels, molecular analysis, muscle biopsy, and genetic testing.

(c) **Congenital myotonic dystrophy:** myotonic dystrophy type 1 (DM1) presents in neonatal period with hypotonia, impaired swallowing, characteristic triangular open mouth (inverted V/cupid's bow/carp appearance), bell-shaped chest, clubfoot deformities and arthrogryposis may be present. Respiratory failure is common due to pulmonary hypoplasia and poor intercostal muscle development. Cardiomyopathy and pulmonary hypertension have also been reported [34].

18.2.4.1.1 Anesthesia Considerations

Careful cardiac monitoring is needed in all DM1 neonates for their high risk of arrhythmic events. Succinylcholine, and anticholinesterase agents can precipitate myotonia. Hypothermia should be avoided. Sevoflurane for induction has been used uneventfully. Patients are sensitive to IV hypnotics and sedatives. Smaller doses of nondepolarizing agents are advised along with NM monitoring. The ultrasound-guided nerve blocks are helpful, but dystrophy may increase muscular echogenicity making nerve identification a problem [35].

18.2.4.2 Congenital Myopathies

Congenital myopathies are neonatal muscle disorders without dystrophic changes on muscle biopsy. Generalized hypotonia with hyporeflexia, prominent facial weakness with or without ptosis, weakness and dysfunction of the respiratory and bulbar muscles are present. Risk for respiratory failure persists. Histology can demonstrate nemaline myopathy, and Core myopathy (Central Core disease (CCD) and Multiminicore disease (MmD)). Of these, CCD and MmD are of particular interest to anesthesiologists due to their susceptibility to MH: [36]

(a) **Nemaline myopathy:** two types of presentations may be seen in neonates. Generalized weakness involving facial, axial, bulbar muscles with feeding and respiratory difficulty, requiring support, and a more severe form with history of polyhydramnios and reduced fetal movement, and severe weakness, feeding difficulties, arthrogryposis, and respiratory failure postnatal [37]. Serum CPK levels may be normal or slightly elevated. No susceptibility to MH is documented. Due to the potential for hyperkalemia, depolarizing relaxants should be avoided.

(b) **Central Core disease (CCD):** there is loss of myofibrils, mitochondria, and glycogen in the central core area (area of central clearing in the muscle. Proximal muscle weakness is more than distal weakness, with variable bulbar involvement [37]. Scoliosis and contractures may be present. They may need respiratory support. Fetal akinesia syndrome may result in the most severe CCD [38]. Ryanodine receptor gene (RYR1) gene, the most common gene associated with CCD encodes the ryanodine receptor (calcium channel on the sarcoplasmic reticulum) [39, 40]. The ryanodine receptor and mutations in RYR1 may also result in malignant hyperthermia (MH). MH has been frequently associated with CCD [41].

(c) **Multi minicore Disease (MmD):** this presents with axial muscle weakness, myopathic facies, and respiratory dysfunction. Because of decreased fetal movement due to muscle weakness in the antenatal period, arthrogryposis multiplex congenita may manifest in the neonatal period.

18.2.4.3 Mitochondrial Myopathies

Tochondria within the nerves and muscle cells. Abnormalities in mitochondrial function is manifested as mitochondrial myopathies. Due to lack of ATP in the muscle, weakness and wasting results. Mutations in mitochondrial proteins lead to myopathy, cardiomyopathy, encephalopathy, and seizures. Inadequate ATP levels during stress, further aggravate the condition [42].

18.2.4.3.1 Anesthesia Considerations in Congenital and Mitochondrial Myopathies

A nontriggering anesthetic should be given in CCD and MmD (RYR1 variant) due to known association with MH syndrome in children. It is advisable to avoid inhalational anesthetics. Elevated CK values are more consistent with a dystrophic disease suggesting avoidance of inhalational anesthetics. In all myopathic patients' succinylcholine should be avoided and dose of nondepolarizing relaxants should be reduced [42].

Respiratory failure, cardiac conduction defects, cardiac depression and dysphagia are the concerned problems of mitochondrial myopathy and stress of surgery and anesthesia increase the risk further [8, 43]. Preoperative evaluation of cardiac, respiratory, and metabolic status (glucose, lactate, serum creatinine, and liver enzymes) should be done. ECG and Echocardiography may reveal cardiomyopathy or conduction deficits.

The perioperative period is a stressful period when ATP production is insufficient for the metabolic demands and leads to metabolic (lactic) acidosis. Prolonged fasting, hypoglycemia, hypothermia, and hypovolemia should be avoided. To avoid anaerobic metabolism, intravenous fluids with glucose should be considered. Intravenous anesthetics are dependent on energy requiring metabolism but volatile anesthetics, removed by ventilation is an advantage, though they affect the muscles. Succinylcholine should be avoided. Due to an increased sensitivity, nondepolarizing relaxants should be given in titrated doses under NM monitoring. Postoperative respiratory support must be kept ready [44]. As the response to pain may increase the risk of lactic acidosis from increased O2 demand and depletion of energy stores, perioperative pain management is essential.

18.3 Malignant Hyperthermia

MH, a disorder of the skeletal muscle, manifests in response to anesthetic triggering agents. Core myopathies and MH are both involved in the dysfunction of calcium regulation in skeletal muscle and are closely associated. RYR1 (Ryanodine receptor 1) mutation is responsible for susceptibility to MH [45].

Calcium buildup due to alterations in calcium inactivation by abnormal RYR1 leads to excessive skeletal muscle contraction. Anaerobic and aerobic metabolism is affected because of reduced level of ATP leading to acidosis. Hypercarbia, tachypnea, and tachycardia result initially followed by fever, sympathetic nervous system activation, hyperkalemia, muscle rigidity, myoglobinuria, disseminated intravascular coagulation and multiorgan dysfunction and failure if treatment is delayed [25].

A lower susceptibility to MH in infants under 2 months of age may be due to lack of case reports, but if core myopathy is a certain diagnosis in neonate, volatile agents should be avoided [42].

Careful monitoring for signs of rhabdomyolysis (serial plasma CK, myoglobin and urine myoglobin), EtCO$_2$, and temperature monitoring are essential.

In acute crisis, inhalational agents should be discontinued. Active cooling, changing the breathing circuit, hyperventilation with 100% O$_2$, to remove trigger anesthetic agent, should be instituted. Dantrolene, loading bolus of 2.5 mg/kg IV followed by 1 mg/kg every 6 h is given till signs of MH subside [46]. acidosis and hyperkalemia should be taken care of. Survival without dantrolene has been reported in children, with early recognition and appropriate management [47, 48].

Sinus tachycardia and hypercapnia are two most reliable early clinical signs in children [49].

Early recognition and early treatment is the key to successful management of MH.

18.4 Approach to Neonatal NM Disorders

A good history and detailed physical and neurologic examinations are important. Pregnancy history of decreased fetal movement, polyhydramnios and previous pregnancy losses is often available. Hypoxic–ischemic injury (HIE) as a cause for hypotonia and weakness may be detected in obstetric history and family history of neurologic disorders and unexplained death under general anesthesia, should be enquired. Physical and neurologic examination of the floppy neonate should depict weakness (proximal vs distal vs diffuse), hypotonia (axial vs proximal vs distal vs diffuse), presence or absence of deep tendon reflexes, resting position and spontaneous movements [1].

Poor spontaneous movements and the frog-like posture (hip abduction, knee flexion) due to poor antigravity movement are characteristic of lower motor neuron conditions. Excessive head lag on traction of the arms, inverted U position when held prone (rag doll) and slipping through the hands when held upright testing, are elicited. Anterior horn cell involvement is suggested by tongue fasciculations (not during cry) and generalized weakness with sparing of the diaphragm, facial muscles, pelvis, and sphincters. Facial diplegia (myopathic facies) along with respiratory and bulbar weakness suggests congenital structural myopathy or MG (h/o fatigue on continuous sucking, drooping of eye lids). Mitochondrial defect is suspected if myopathy is associated with lactic acidosis.

All muscle diseases are multiorgan diseases. Respiratory function is affected as the diaphragm and intercostals are weak. Pharyngeal muscle tone is decreased, gastrointestinal dysfunction complicates dystrophinopathy, myotonic dystrophy type 1, and some mitochondrial diseases. Brain anomalies are present in muscle–eye–brain disease and myotonic dystrophy type 1.

Transient hypotonia may result from systemic infection, electrolyte disorders, hypermagnesemia, seizures or drugs administered to the baby or mother. Preterm babies have reduced tone and strength compared to term infants.

Significantly elevated CPK values (>5 times normal) will point toward a muscle disorder, more likely a CMD. Normal or mildly elevated values can be seen in congenital myopathies and SMA. EMG can be of immense help though difficult to perform in newborns for the diagnosis of a neurogenic process vs myopathic process vs NMJ defect. Despite advances in genetic diagnosis, muscle biopsy identifies and differentiate specific types of congenital myopathy or CMD. In the last decade availability of genetic testing has increased. A clinicopathologic diagnosis is no longer sufficient, and every effort should be made for genetic confirmation [1].

Blood glucose, calcium, magnesium and lactate, acid–base status, urine and plasma amino acids, urine organic acids, plasma ammonia, acylcarnitines, thyroid function tests are also helpful. ECG and ECHO can exclude conduction defects, arrhythmias, and cardiomyopathy.

Anesthesia must be provided either to confirm the diagnosis (muscle biopsy, MRI), for palliative purpose (gastrostomy), or for any unrelated surgical emergency. The diagnosis of NM disorder is usually unknown at the time when anesthesia is required [8].

In the presence of a suspected or diagnosed muscle disease and elevated CK, halogenated agents must be avoided, but the use of inhalation agents for induction of anesthesia until venous access is obtained is acceptable [50, 51]. Care should be taken to avoid use of triggering agents related complications. Avoid using succinylcholine, as it can trigger MH, produce rhabdomyolysis in fragile muscles and life-threatening hyperkalemia in situations, where acetylcholine nicotinic receptors are spread outside the NMJ [52]. Succinylcholine can be replaced with a nondepolarizing muscle relaxant even if a (modified) rapid sequence induction is necessary. Sensitivity to nondepolarizing muscle relaxants makes NM monitoring mandatory.

Various metabolic stress creating conditions such as prolonged fasting, hypothermia, hypoglycemia, acidosis, and hypovolemia should be avoided. The combination of muscle weakness of a myopathy and anesthetics can result in severe respiratory depression easily. These babies should be closely monitored during the perioperative period and be cared for in the NICU in the postoperative period, even if not on ventilatory support.

Due to scarcity of evidence-based data on the perioperative anesthetic management of neonatal patients with a variety of NM disorders, anesthesiologist's knowledge, and experience in adult and pediatric patients, is the best guide to management in neonates, keeping in mind their unique physiology and pharmacological requirements

Key Points

(a) CPK levels, lactic acidosis, weak cry, poor respiration, muscle weakness after birth, are indicators for more detailed assessment for NM disorders in neonates.

(b) Dystrophinopathy is the most frequent diagnosis if CK is elevated and Mitochondrial disease if lactates are elevated.

(c) Involvement can be focal or generalized, hypotonic or contractures (poor muscle relaxation).

(d) Cardiac involvement is usually present, EKG and Echo to exclude conduction defects, arrhythmias, and cardiomyopathy

(e) Respiratory muscles are weak with poor airway tone, poor secretion clearance. Oropharyngeal weakness, incoordination, failure of protective laryngeal closure, abdominal muscle weakness with ineffective cough increases the risk of aspiration.

(f) Risk of anesthesia-induced rhabdomyolysis, avoid halogenated agents [53].

(g) Inhalation induction until venous access is obtained is acceptable [50, 51].

(h) Myopathic muscles are at risk of rhabdomyolysis as chronic accumulation of ionized Ca modifies the normal RYR1 receptor and reduces the metabolic capacity of mitochondria [54].

(i) Succinylcholine is avoided as it can trigger MH, produce rhabdomyolysis in fragile muscles.

(j) Increased sensitivity to nondepolarizing relaxants, hence reduced doses. NM monitoring is mandatory to titrate the dosage and for adequate recovery of NM transmission at the end.

(k) Respiratory insufficiency can be unmasked by the surgical procedure, stress and pain, in the postoperative period, especially in babies who are not on preoperative respiratory support.

18.5 Conclusion

Diagnosing muscular dystrophies in a newborn and neonates, including premature, is not easy. Concerns arise because of the high morbidity and mortality in such babies, especially in the perioperative period. They may be hypotonic at birth, with muscle weakness, poor respiration, poor reflexes, difficult swallowing, weak crying, and seizures. These may be because of underlying MD or because of genetic, metabolic, and developmental abnormalities. Transient hypotonia may result from systemic infection, electrolyte disorders, seizures or drugs administered to the baby or mother. Babies may need respiratory support soon after birth or any time later on. Facilities for ventilation should be available

In case of suspicion, diagnosis is made by blood levels of CPK and Lactate, genetic studies, muscle biopsy, EMG, and MRI. These are often not available especially in case of a surgical emergency in the neonate. Neonatal screening is the only way to detect these disorders early. They may require anesthesia for diagnostic purposes and for the surgical condition.

In any case, it is advisable to treat all neonates, whether diagnosed or not for MD, with caution, and avoid use of halogenated agents, scoline and care with nondepolarizing relaxants. Besides vitals, intake output and temperature monitoring, NM monitoring is mandatory so as to titrate the dose of muscle relaxants and allow good recovery at the end. Anesthesia and triggers such as hypothermia, acidosis, pain, stress, infections, and prolonged fasting, should be avoided as they can induce rhabdomyolysis and acute renal failure, and MH, which if not diagnosed and treated, can be fatal.

There is no cure, only symptomatic management is done, along with stretching and physical therapy.

Maintenance of volume and acid base status, adequate gas exchange, prevention of hypothermia, prolonged fasting, pain, and surgical stress, avoidance of triggering agents, and vigilant vital and NM monitoring can result in good postoperative outcome in neonates with NM disorders. An intensive, dedicated, dynamic, multidisciplinary perioperative approach is required for a better outcome.

References

1. Natarajan N, Ionita C. Neonatal neuromuscular disorders. Avery's diseases of the newborn. 10th ed.; 2018. chapter 64, pp. 952–960.e2. doi: https://doi.org/10.1016/B978-0-323-40139-5.00064-4
2. Fay AJ. Neuromuscular diseases of the newborn. Neonatal Neurology. Ed Donna Ferriero. Semin Pediatr Neurol. 2019;32:100,771. https://doi.org/10.1016/j.spen.2019.08.007.
3. Bharucha-Goebel DX, Santi M, Medne L, et al. Severe congenital RYR1-associated myopathy: the expanding clinicopathologic and genetic spectrum. Neurology. 2013;80(17):1584–9.
4. Shieh PB. Muscular dystrophies and other genetic myopathies. Neurol Clin. 2013;31(4):1009–29.
5. Laing NG. Genetics of neuromuscular disorders. Crit Rev Clin Lab Sci. 2012;49(2):33–48.
6. Darras BT. Neuromuscular disorders in the newborn. Clin Perinatol. 1997;24(4):827–44. https://doi.org/10.1016/S0095-5108(18)30152-0.
7. Vasta I, Kinali M, Messina S, Guzetta A, et al. Can clinical signs identify newborns with neuromuscular disorders? J Pediatr. 2005;146(1):73–9. https://doi.org/10.1016/j.jpeds.2004.08.047.
8. Ross AK. Muscular dystrophy versus mitochondrial myopathy: the dilemma of the undiagnosed hypotonic child. Paediatr Anaesth. 2007;17:1–6.
9. Roland EH. Neuromuscular disorders in the newborn. Clin Perinatol. 1989;16(2):519–47.

10. Darras BT, Jones RH, jr. Neuromuscular problems of the critically ill neonate and child. Semin Pediatr Neurol. 2004 Jun;11(2):147–68. https://doi.org/10.1016/j.spen.2004.04.003.
11. MacLeod MJ, Taylor JE, Lunt PW, Mathew CG, et al. Prenatal onset spinal muscular atrophy. Eur J Paediatr Neurol. 1999;3(2):65–72.
12. D'Amico A, Mercuri E, Tiziano FD, Bertini E. Spinal muscular atrophy. Orphanet J Rare Dis. 2011;6:71.
13. Wang CH, Finkel RS, Bertini ES, et al. Consensus statement for standard of care in spinal muscular atrophy. J Child Neurol. 2007;8:1027–49.
14. Bruce AK, Jacobsen E, Dossing H, et al. Hypoglycaemia in spinal muscular atrophy. Lancet. 1995;346:609–10.
15. Islander G. Anesthesia and spinal muscle atrophy. Paediatr Anaesth. 2013;23(9):804–16.
16. Baets J, Deconinck T, De Vriendt E, et al. Genetic spectrum of hereditary neuropathies with onset in the first year of life. Brain. 2011;134(Pt 9):2664–76.
17. Berrih-Aknin S, Frenkian-Cuvelier M, Eymard B. Diagnostic and clinical classification of autoimmune myasthenia gravis. J Autoimmun. 2014;48–49:143–8.
18. Dubowitz V. Myasthenia gravis. In: Dubowitz V, editor. Muscle disorders in childhood. Philadelphia: WB Saunders; 1978. p. 191–201.
19. Engel AG. Current status of the congenital myasthenic syndromes. Neuromuscul Disord. 2012;22(2):99–111.
20. Ohno K, Tsujino A, Brengman JM, et al. Choline acetyltransferase mutations cause myasthenic syndrome associated with episodic apnea in humans. Proc Natl Acad Sci USA. 2001;98:2017–22.
21. Jephson CG, Mills NA, Pitt MC, et al. Congenital stridor with feeding difficulty as a presenting symptom of Dok7 congenital myasthenic syndrome. Int J Pediatr Otorhinolaryngol. 2010;74:991–4.
22. Blichfeldt-Lauridsen L, Hansen BD. Anesthesia and myasthenia gravis. Acta Anaesthesiol Scand. 2012;56:17–22.
23. Mahfouz AK, Rashid M, Khan MS, Reddy P. Late onset congenital central hypoventilation syndrome after exposure to general anesthesia. Can J Anaesth. 2011;58:1105–9.
24. Rocca DG, Coccia C, Diana L, et al. Propofol or sevoflurane anesthesia without muscle relaxants allow the early extubation of myasthenic patients. Can J Anaesth. 2003;50:547–52.
25. Crean PM, Tirupathi S. Essentials of neurology and neuromuscular disorders, Ch 24. In: Coté CJ, Lerman J, Anderson BJ, editors. Coté and Lerman's a practice of anesthesia for infants and children. 6th ed. Elsevier; 2019.
26. Casarotti P, Mendola C, Cammarota G, Corte DF. High-dose rocuronium for rapid-sequence induction and reversal with sugammadex in two myasthenic patients. Acta Anaesthesiol Scand. 2014;58:1154–8.
27. Boer HD, Shields MO, Booij LH. Reversal of neuromuscular blockade with sugammadex in patients with myasthenia gravis: a case series of 21 patients and review of the literature. Eur J Anaesthesiol. 2014;31:715–21.
28. Vincent CH, Morgan PG. Genetic muscle disorders. Ch 49. In: Davis PJ, Cladis FP, editors. Smith's anesthesia for infants and children. 9th ed. Elsevier; 2017.
29. Dobyns WB, Pagon RA, Armstrong D, et al. Diagnostic criteria for Walker-Warburg syndrome. Am J Med Genet. 1989;32:195–210.
30. Fukuyama Y, Kawazura M, Haruna H. A peculiar form of congenital progressive muscular dystrophy. Paediat Univ Tokyo. 1960;4:5–8.
31. Lopate G. Congenital muscular dystrophy treatment & management. Medscape. Accessed 30 November 2012.
32. Sato T, Murakami T, Ishiguro K, et al. Respiratory management of patients with Fukuyama congenital muscular dystrophy. Brain Dev. 2016;38(3):324–30.
33. Oliveira J, Santos R, Soares-Silva I, et al. LAMA 2 gene analysis in a cohort of 26 congenital muscular dystrophy patients. Clin Genet. 2008;74:502–12.
34. Schara U, Schoser BG. Myotonic dystrophies type 1 and 2: a summary on current aspects. Semin Pediatr Neurol. 2006;13(2):71–9.

35. Santareas T. Limitations in ultrasound imaging techniques in anesthesia: obesity or muscle atrophy? (letter). Anesth Analg. 2009;109:993.
36. Jungbluth H, Sewry CA, Muntoni F. Core myopathies. Semin Pediatr Neurol. 2011;18:239–49.
37. Romero NB, Sandaradura SA, Clarke NF. Recent advances in nemaline myopathy. Curr Opin Neurol. 2013;26:519–26.
38. Romero NB, Monnier N, Viollet L, et al. Dominant and recessive central core disease associated with RYR1 mutations and fetal akinesia. Brain. 2003;126:2341–9.
39. Ferreiro A, Monnier N, Romero NB, et al. A recessive form of central core disease, transiently presenting as multi-minicore disease, is associated with a homozygous mutation in the ryanodine receptor type 1 gene. Ann Neurol. 2002;51:750–9.
40. Jungbluth H, Muller CR, Halliger-Keller B, et al. Autosomal recessive inheritance of RYR1 mutations in a congenital myopathy with cores. Neurology. 2002;59:284–7.
41. Jungbluth H. Central core disease. Orphanet J Rare Dis. 2007;2:25.
42. Vincent H, Morgan PG. Myopathies of the newborn Ch 11. In: McCann ME, editor. Essentials of anesthesia for infants and neonates. 1st ed. Cambridge University Press; 2018.
43. Muravchick S, Levy RJ. Clinical implications of mitochondrial dysfunction. Anesthesiology. 2006;105:819–37.
44. Niezgoda J, Morgan PG. Anesthetic considerations in patients with mitochondrial defects. Paediatr Anaesth. 2013;23:785–93.
45. Wu S, Ibarra MC, Malicdan MC, et al. Central core disease is due to RYR1 mutations in more than 90% of patients. Brain. 2006;129(Pt 6):1470–80.
46. Racca F, Robba C. Perioperative care of children with neuromuscular disease. In: Marinella AG, Salvo AI, editors. Perioperative medicine in pediatric anesthesia. Springer; 2016; chapter 12.
47. Liu ST, Liu LF, Wang S, Chin Y. Treatment of malignant hyperthermia without dantrolene in a 14-year-old boy. Med J (Engl). 2017;130(6):755–6.
48. Sami Menasri RS, Grainat N, Brinis N, et al. Successful management of malignant hyperthermia without dantrolene in paediatric anaesthesia. Update Anesthesia. 2019;33:70–2.
49. Nelson P, Litman RS. Malignant hyperthermia in children: an analysis of the North American malignant hyperthermia registry. Anesth Analg. 2014;118:369–74.
50. Litman RS, Rosenberg H. Malignant hyperthermia-associated diseases: state of the art uncertainty (editorial). Anesth Analg. 2009;109:1004–5.
51. Gurnaney H, Brown A, Litman RS. Malignant hyperthermia and muscular dystrophies. Anesth Analg. 2009;109:1043–8.
52. Naguib M, Flood P, McArdle JJ, et al. Advances in neurobiology of the neuromuscular junction. Anesthesiology. 2002;96:202–31.
53. Brandom BW, Veyckemans F. Neuromuscular diseases in children: a practical approach. Pediatric Anesthesia. 2013;23:765–9.
54. Bellinger AM, Reiken S, Carlson C, et al. Hypernitrosylated ryanodine receptor calcium release channels are leaky in dystrophic muscles. Nat Med. 2009;15:325–30.

Part III

Special Aspects of Neonatal Anesthesia

Preoperative Workup, Perioperative NPO, and ERAS

19

Sudakshina Mukherji and Anisha De

19.1 Introduction

The role of a surgeon has always been targeted toward radical cure, but the quality of the road travelled to achieve it including patient's safety has always been put in the hands of an anaesthesiologist. In addition, this responsibility is increased by several manifolds in case of a neonate. Neonates, especially premature, are different from their 'born at term' counterparts in various aspects. They are unique with vulnerable and dynamic physiology, immature anatomy, at higher risk of anesthesia related adverse effects and with higher age group mortality. Therefore, a detailed understanding of the baby as a whole is essential to successful and safe neonatal anesthesia.

With the development of specialised incubators, provision of mechanical ventilation, high frequency ventilators and introduction of artificial pulmonary surfactants to reduce neonatal respiratory distress syndrome (RDS) there has been a significant improvement in the NICU care facility resulting in significant decrease in mortality of premature babies. This requires expertise and skill to handle such neonates, perioperatively for a favourable outcome after surgery. The risk of prematurity, presence of congenital syndromes, the particular ongoing disease process such as necrotising enterocolitis (NEC) and patent ductus arteriosus (PDA) with a very narrow margin of safety in this group of patients makes it an extremely challenging task for the attending anaesthesiologist [1]. the reader should familiarize with some terms important when defining neonates (Box 19.1).

S. Mukherji (✉)
Department of Anaesthesiology, Medical College, Kolkata, India

A. De
Department of Paediatric Anaesthesiology, Institute of Child Health, Kolkata, India

© The Author(s), under exclusive license to Springer Nature Singapore Pte Ltd. 2023
U. Saha (ed.), *Clinical Anesthesia for the Newborn and the Neonate*,
https://doi.org/10.1007/978-981-19-5458-0_19

> **Box 19.1 Definition as Per Gestational Age (The American Academy of Paediatrics)**
>
> **Gestational Age (GA)** as the time elapsed between the first day of the last menstrual period and the day of delivery.
> **Chronological age (CA)** as time elapsed from birth.
> **Post menstrual age (PMA)** as GA+ CA.
> **These definitions replace older definitions, such as Post conception age (PCA).**

In depth discussion on neonatal anatomy, physiology and pharmacology will be dealt in the respective sections of this book. This chapter will essentially highlight the key factors necessary for perioperative workup of a neonate undergoing surgery.

19.2 Terminology

1. **In 2010, WHO** published its premature birth fact sheet stating that more than 1 in 10 infants (>15 million children or 10%) were born prematurely, worldwide [2]. WHO defines:
   (a) **Preterm birth**—birth <37 weeks which can again be subdivided into three:
      i. Extremely Preterm (<28 weeks),
      ii. Very preterm (28–32 weeks), and
      iii. Moderate to late preterm (32–37 weeks).
   (b) **As per birth weight (BW), preterm babies can also be classified as:**
      i. **Low birth weight (LBW)** (<2500 g),
      ii. **Very low birth weight (VLBW)** (<1500 g), and
      iii. **Extremely low birth weight (ELBW)** (<1000 g).
   (c) **Two other important definitions are:**
      i. **Small for gestational age (SGA)**—babies weighing below 10th percentile for the GA.
      ii. **Large for gestational age (LGA)**—babies weighing more than 90th percentile for the GA.
2. **Newborn**—babies younger than 72 h (3 days).
3. **Neonate**—babies older than 72 h but less than 28 days.

19.3 Prematurity and Its Implications

Incidence of premature birth is 18% of live births in India and other South–East Asian countries. Extreme prematurity often presents with significant medical issues and complications, with higher perinatal mortality, inversely proportional to GA. Recent studies show greater survival of extremely premature, VLBW and ELBW babies, because of availability of newer prenatal testing, marked development and improvement in antenatal care, and better NICU facilities.

The first few weeks of life are most crucial especially in a preterm baby, during which mortality and morbidity is maximum, necessitating longer hospital stay, repeated admissions, with risk of developing chronic lung disease (CLD) later in life. Whenever a neonate or premature requires surgery, one must keep in mind the physiological consequences that determine the outcome. A British study reported that among extremely premature neonates, 83% required ICU admission for survival. Major morbidities such as bronchopulmonary dysplasia (BPD), intraventricular haemorrhage (IVH), retinopathy of prematurity (ROP), NEC, cardiac anomalies, hearing impairment and cognitive developmental delays were reported in 59% of survivors. Extremely premature infants and children especially those with neonatal brain injury are more likely to have neurodevelopmental disabilities, such as impaired cognitive skills, motor deficits, cerebral palsy, severe visual and hearing impairment, and behavioural and psychological problems, which become prominent and persist as the child develops. In spite of all advancements in technology, more trained and skilled personnel handling these babies, extremely premature infants still have 30–50% mortality and 20–50% risk of long-term disability [3–6].

19.4 Understanding a Newborn

19.4.1 Newborn Apnoea

Apnea of prematurity is defined as cessation of respiration of more than 20 s duration, and is replaced by normal biphasic response to hypoxaemia, i.e., initial hyperventilation followed by hypoventilation, pallor, bradycardia, and cyanosis. Post anesthesia apnea with bradycardia and cyanosis occurs in 20–30% of preterms, mostly in the first 12 h of surgery. Chronic apnoea and recurrent hypoxaemia yield free radicals which are responsible for long term adverse outcome.

Babies under 38 week GA are very prone to developing apnoea. The respiratory system is mainly controlled by the central respiratory rhythmogenesis, and central and peripheral chemoreception, both of which are underdeveloped. It takes weeks to months to reach the adult stage thereby resulting in higher incidence of apnea. The production of surfactant is inadequate prior to 32–34 weeks of gestation, hence babies born prior to 32–34 weeks are very much susceptible to RDS. A compliant rib cage, paradoxical chest movements, reduced FRC, higher closing capacity and relatively fewer slow twitch Type 1 fibres in the diaphragm result in easy fatigability in neonates which is further accentuated in preterms. Common triggers for apnea in the premature are Hypoxia, Hypoglycemia, Hypothermia, Hypercarbia, Anemia, and Hypocalcaemia [7–9].

Clinical Pearls

- It is advisable to postpone any elective or nonemergent surgery in babies under 38 week GA.
- All semi urgent or urgent cases should be admitted at least two days prior to and for 12–48 h after surgery.

- Exogenous surfactant administration, antenatal steroids, continuous positive airway pressure (CPAP), all contribute to improved and favourable outcome.
- Avoidance of spontaneous respiration during anesthesia, especially in preterms as they have increased work of breathing and easy fatigability.

19.5 Upper Airway Assessment

It is already evident from the previous chapters that the anatomy of a neonatal airway is different and presents with variations in size, shape, position and surrounding structures along with important physiological differences when compared to an adult. There may be associated congenital defects and syndromes, such as Pierre–Robin, Treacher Collins, Downs, Klippel Feil or Goldenhar, with craniofacial abnormalities. Neonates are obligate nose breathers; hence it is essential to maintain the patency of their small nares. Any additional airway compromise, anatomical (choanal atresia, laryngeal web, subglottic stenosis, tracheomalacia, occipital encephalocele, cystic hygroma), physiological (sleep or factors reducing muscle tone and relaxing the airways) or pathological (edema, inflammation) can lead to severe compromise and affect normal gas exchange leading to cardiac arrest [10].

Clinical Pearls

1. Preoperative identification of an anticipated difficult airway; timely detection and prompt interventions of hypoxic event can prevent airway catastrophe in the perioperative period.
2. To aid the attending anaesthesiologist to be well-prepared for any airway adversities, a concise preoperative airway assessment should include:
    (a) Documentation of any birth complications, prior airway manipulations, airway trauma
    (b) History of apnea, stridor, snoring or signs of upper airway obstruction.
    (c) General inspection, preferably in a crying or feeding baby to exclude gross craniofacial abnormalities involving the airway or presence of postnatal teeth.
    (d) Relying on positive predictor tools such as protrusion of mandible, atlanto-occipital joint movement, submandibular space and tongue thickness, in absence of specific neonatal assessment scale.

19.6 Lower Respiratory System

Surfactant production increases after 34 weeks of gestation thereby predisposing premature newborns to RDS. Besides, the physiological development of lungs in the postnatal period is disrupted by inflammation, infection, volutrauma and barotrauma which may finally lead to pathological lung changes such as reduced alveolar surface area and impaired gas exchange. These patients are more prone to develop CLD, the most prevalent sequelae of prematurity. The incidence of pulmonary hypertension (PAH) is nearly 40% which contributes significantly to increased morbidity and mortality. Persistent raised pulmonary vascular resistance (PVR) eventually leads to impaired right ventricular (RV) function and a low cardiac output state, pulmonary edema and sudden death. Moderate to very preterm neonates are prone to BPD, especially those who require FiO_2 >0.3 after 36 week postmenstrual age.

Clinical Pearls

- During preoperative preparation, symptoms such as noisy breathing or wheeze should be treated with bronchodilators, anti-inflammatory drugs, and antibiotics.
- They should be cared for in thermo-controlled humidified incubator.
- Hydration should be maintained by oral or gastric feeds or IV fluids.
- Newer ventilator modes, high-frequency ventilation (HFV) and nasal CPAP (nCPAP), may reduce the incidence of BPD.
- Consequences of prolonged intubation, tracheomalacia, subglottic stenosis, must be borne in mind.

19.7 Cardiovascular System (CVS)

There is higher incidence of CVS malformations in preterm (12.5/1000 preterms) vs 5.1/1000 (term) neonates, which puts them at higher risk of CVS compromise during surgery and anaesthesia. Moreover, they have highly variable biological parameters. Cardiac output is rate dependent with limited capacity to increase the stroke volume. Immature and noncompliant left ventricular muscle mass results in poor diastolic function. Minimal blood loss may lead to hypovolemia, hypotension, and shock. The autonomic system is underdeveloped, with parasympathetic preponderance, making these babies prone to bradycardia in response to stressors, and even with hypovolaemia there is no reflection in heart rate.

Clinical Pearls

- Understanding the basic correct **age specific** normal values of all biological parameters (e.g., heart rate, blood pressure (systolic/diastolic/mean).
- Accurate measurement of fluid and blood loss and its replenishment.
- They are prone to sudden bradycardia and cardiac arrest in response to any stressor hence strict monitoring, prompt detection and swift interventions is the thumb rule.
- Prophylactic atropine (20 µg/kg iv) prior to intubation is standard.
- MAP of more than 35 mmHg in anaesthetised infants under 6 month age is necessary for preservation of cerebral oxygenation as measured by near infrared spectroscopy (NIRS).

19.8 Other Systems at a Glance

The haemoglobin (Hb) level (mainly HbF) of a term baby is about 18–20 g/dL, whereas extremely premature newborns have comparatively lower level (13–15 g/dL). They often present with vitamin K deficiency and Vitamin K dependent coagulation factors (II, VII, IX, X) often resulting in haemorrhagic disease of the newborn. Moreover, when associated with a lower platelet count, this increases the chance of excessive bleeding from the surgical sites leading to hypovolemia. Estimated blood volume (EBV) and haematocrit (Hct) values vary with GA (100–120 mL/kg in preterm and 90 mL/kg in term neonate). The normal and acceptable Hct, respectively, is (40–50; 35) in preterm and (45–65;30–35) in term neonates.

Neonates have delayed gastric emptying time and reduced lower esophageal sphincter tone which may be lower in those with surgical condition.

Clinical Pearls

1. Supplementation of Vitamin K (0.5 and 1 mg IM/IV in <1.5 and >1.5 kg, respectively) along with fresh frozen plasma @ 12–15 mL/kg to control Vit K deficiency bleeding is recommended.
2. Blood transfusion to maintain target Hct (30–35%).
3. Preoperative Platelet transfusion is indicated with:
   (a) **Counts <100,000/cumm** in neonates undergoing major surgery or having major bleeding disorders,
   (b) **Counts <50,000/cumm** in neonates with bleeding, established coagulopathy, and
   (c) **Count <25,000/cumm** in neonatal alloimmune thrombocytopenia, babies having siblings with IVH, in neonates with no bleeding.

Proper adherence to the recommended fasting guidelines and suitable interventions to reduce gastroesophageal reflux, vomiting and pulmonary aspiration syndrome is advocated.

19.9 Fluid and Electrolytes [11, 12]

With the upcoming recent controversies regarding the practice of the age-old Holliday Segar's formula using glucose containing hypotonic maintenance fluids, we need to move on and through a continuous process of learning, unlearning, and relearning, reconsider fluid administration with new insights.

The intracellular (ICF) and extracellular fluid (ECF) comprises the total body water (TBW). ECF includes intravascular (IV—plasma, lymph) and interstitial (IS) fluid. Water loss is mainly by sensible (urine, stool, CSF, drains) and insensible (evaporation through skin, respiratory tract) losses. Insensible water loss is more in preterms. Moreover, neonates have reduced capacity to concentrate or dilute urine in response to volume changes, and kidney maturation takes several weeks to reach adult state.

Table 19.1 Common consequences of injudicious use of fluids

Too little—dehydration	Too much—fluid overload
Dehydration	Pulmonary edema
Poor tissue perfusion	Congestive cardiac failure
Acidosis	Opening of ductal shunt
Hypernatremia	IVH
Hypotension, CVS collapse	BPD

Table 19.2 Assessment of a newborn before fluid administration

1. Maternal history	Oxytocin or excessive hypotonic fluids—hyponatremia
	Poorly controlled diabetes—renal vein thrombosis
	Use of drugs such as ACE inhibitors—affects the kidney of the newborn
	Use of antenatal steroids—early skin maturation and hyperkalaemia
	Oligohydramnios—renal disorders
2. Birth history	Birth weight (BW)
	Gestational age (GA)
	Presence of posterior urethral valve, bladder exstrophy, omphalocele, etc
3. Physical examination	Body weight
	Baseline parameters—pulse rate and volume, blood pressure, capillary-skin refill (not specific and may also be abnormal in cold stress or acidosis), core or skin temperature.
	Any sudden changes in weight
	Sunken anterior fontanelle
	Increased 3rd space collections in surgical neonates (in peritoneal and pleural cavities)

The ratio of TBW to fat-muscle mass is 70–75% in term neonates and higher in preterms (80–90%). Large fluid shifts at birth result in salt water diuresis in the first 2–3 days of life, explaining the physiological weight loss (about 5–15%). In its absence, the baby may present with multiple comorbidities such as NEC, symptomatic PDA, tissue and pulmonary edema and CLD. Hypovolemia and low cardiac output is generally compensated by increasing heart rate due to limited ability to increase in stroke volume. Hence, maintenance fluid in the first few weeks should be adjusted to maintain normal intra vascular volume and tonicity as emulated by heart rate, urine output, acid–base and electrolyte status. The choice of fluid should be individualized and is largely determined by the disease pathology and surgery type.

The goals of fluid administration are Maintenance of optimum tissue and organ perfusion, Adequate O2 delivery, Normovolemia, Normoglycemia and Electrolyte balance. Administration of fluids should be judicious as these babies have very narrow safety windows (Table 19.1).

19.9.1 Assessment of Fluid and Electrolyte Status

Prior to initiation of IV fluids, proper assessment of fluid and electrolyte status is necessary. Neonatal period marks the transition between in-utero and ex-utero life, hence assessment (Table 19.2) should always begin from obtaining proper antenatal and birth history as these have various implications on fluid status.

19.9.2 Investigations

Few investigations can be performed to correlate with clinical findings. These include baseline values of

1. Complete blood count (CBC) especially Hb, Hct and TLC
2. Serum electrolytes
3. Blood gas values
4. Serum creatinine
5. Urine volume, Specific gravity, urine electrolytes and fractional excretion of sodium.

Moreover, it is essential to exclude any concurrent use of diuretics. Urine output is almost negligible on day 1, and thereafter it increases to reach normal of 2–4 mL/kg/h within a few days.

The newer assessing modalities include trans-esophageal echocardiography (TEE) to measure ventilation induced variation in aortic flow velocity (best dynamic measure) and stroke volume (best static measure). NIRS to measure end organ perfusion aids in titrating fluid requirements, but their reliability in preterms and newborns are still inconsistent.

19.9.3 Special Considerations

Some amount of dehydration and electrolyte imbalance is always associated with few surgical conditions:

(a) **TEF/EA**: mild dehydration and hyponatremia are common due to low intake and salivary losses.
(b) **Pyloric stenosis:** vomiting leads to loss of gastric secretions, dehydration, hypokalaemia, hypochloraemia and metabolic alkalosis, along with paradoxical aciduria.
(c) **Intestinal obstruction:** presents with acid–base disturbance depending on the level of obstruction.
(d) **Perforated viscus**: usually accompanied by hyperkalaemia, metabolic acidosis, high BUN.
(e) **Abdominal wall defects**: present with severe dehydration, dyselectrolytemia, and hypothermia.

Hence adequate identification, resuscitation, volume, electrolyte and acid–base optimization, is vital to have hemodynamically stable baby in the OR.

19.9.4 Three Pillars of Fluid Administration [13, 14]

(a) **Replacement of pre-existing deficits and dehydration**: reduced fasting periods and early initiation of IV fluids results in fewer episodes of dehydration, hypoglycemia or hypovolemia in term and healthy neonates. However, a critically ill, sick or premature baby may present with associated dehydration due to vomiting /diarrhoea, early cord clamping, repeated blood sampling in NICU and SIADH due to sepsis or renal failure. Assessing the grade of dehydration and correction over 24 h is recommended (Table 19.3).

(b) **Maintenance fluid** in NICU is directed toward supporting adequate nutrition for growth and vital functions, electrolyte homeostasis while avoiding fluid overload. However, during surgery, focus shifts to maintaining a stable intravascular volume, replenishing ongoing losses, and restoring anesthesia induced hypotension and increase in volume capacity. The current recommendation regarding type of fluids and rate of administration for a healthy term baby are summarized in Table 19.4.

   In preterm babies weighing less than 1 kg and not receiving feeds by 3rd day, parenteral nutrition via central venous access should be started. In extremely premature babies, fluid requirements are higher in the 1st week (Table 19.5).

Table 19.3 Assessment of dehydration and its management

Grade of dehydration	Signs	Management
10% dehydration (100 mL/kg)	Depressed fontanelle, sunken eyes, poor capillary skin refill, oliguria	50% of total maintenance dose over 8 h, rest over next 16 h + maintenance fluid
15% dehydration (150 mL/kg) or more	Hemodynamic instability, features of shock along with the above findings	10–20 mL/kg NS over 1–2 h, followed by 50% correction over 8 h and remaining over 16 h + maintenance fluid

Table 19.4 Maintenance fluid type and rate of administration in healthy term baby

Age (days)	Type of fluid	Rate
1	10% dextrose	@ 2–3 mL/kg/h (60–80 mL/kg/day)
2	10% Dextrose ± sodium/potassium supplement	@ 4 mL/kg/h (100–120 mL/kg/day) + sodium (2–3 mEq/dL) + potassium (1–2 mEq/dL) once urine output is stabilized
3–7	0.18% NaCl (N/5) in 10% dextrose	@ 4 mL/kg/h (100–150 mL/kg/day)
>7	Isotonic fluids + electrolytes + glucose	@ 4 mL/kg/h (150–160 mL/kg/day)

Table 19.5 Fluid requirement (mL/kg/day) during 1st week of life (BW in grams)

Age (day)	BW 751–1000 g	BW 1001–1250 g	BW 1251–1500 g	BW 1501–2000 g
1	85	75	70	60
2–3	105	95	80	75
4–7	130	120	105	95

Priority should always be to minimize insensible water loss by taking simple measures such as using plastic sheets (heat shields are ineffective) and double walled incubators.

The fluid rates may further need to be increased in conditions such as pyrexia, hypermetabolic states, such as burns, use of radiant heaters (increased loss when compared to incubators by about 0.94 mL/kg/h), or phototherapy, (rates should be increased by 10 mL/kg/day in term and to 20 mL/kg/day in LBW newborn). The rates need to be reduced in presence of cardiac lesions and in cases of inappropriate ADH secretion. However, infusion rates must always be customised as per GA, associated pathology and patient requirements.

(c) **Replacement of ongoing or 3rd space loss:** Both fluids and blood components need to be replaced during surgery. Ongoing fluid losses should be replaced with an isotonic fluid, such as 0.9% sodium chloride or ringer lactate [15]. Ongoing blood loss should be replaced with crystalloids (1:2), or colloids/blood (1:1). Maximum allowable blood loss (MABL) is calculated by the formula:

$$MABL = \frac{EBV \times (\text{Starting Hct} - \text{Target Hct})}{\text{Starting Hct}}$$

EBV and Hct values vary with GA. However, in the setting of continued hemodynamic instability, ongoing blood loss and cyanotic heart disease (CHD), blood replacement needs to be initiated earlier.

The 3rd space loss is defined as sequestered fluid from IV space into the tissues and around the surgical site. It is less in laparoscopic surgeries. It is replaced with isotonic fluids. Although it is difficult to quantify, a rough estimate of replacement of losses can be made. (Table 19.6)

Table 19.6 Estimates of replacement rates of 3rd space losses

Type of surgery	Replacement rates
Superficial surgery (minimal loss)	@ 1–2 mL/kg/h
Thoracotomy (moderate loss)	@ 4–7 mL/kg/h
Abdominal surgery (major loss)	@ 5–10 mL/kg/h

Table 19.7 Neonatal hypoglycemia—cutoff values

Time after birth	Serum glucose levels (mg/dL)	
	Term	Preterm
<24 h	<40	<45
> 24 h	<60	<50

19.10 Glucose Homeostasis

Glucose handling is immature in neonates. A term baby has a significant level of hepatic glycogen store (5% of body weight) most of which gets depleted by the first 48 h of life through glycogenolysis. However, it gets repleted by feed initiation and gluconeogenesis in absence of any stressful conditions. The level may go down to 30 mg/dL in the first few hours of life but gradually rises to 45 mg/dL by 12 h. The cut off values for neonatal hypoglycemia varies among institutions around the globe, but commonly acceptable values are given in Table 19.7.

The symptoms of hypoglycemia include apathy, apnea, weak or high-pitched cry, cyanosis, hypotonia, hypothermia, tremors and convulsions. While managing such cases it is prudent to know that both hypoglycemia and hyperglycaemia are detrimental in newborns. Management includes initial bolus of 2.5–5 mL/kg 10% Dextrose/1–2 mL/kg of 25% Dextrose followed by maintenance @ 5–8 mg/kg/min in term and 8–10 mg/kg/min in preterm neonate with periodic monitoring. In absence of IV-line, buccal dextrose gel can be used in severe hypoglycemia.

Glucose is recommended usually in all babies less than 48 h of age. However, it is also recommended after 48 h in:

- Those who are already on parenteral nutrition or dextrose containing solutions,
- Those with less than third percentile body weight planned for prolonged surgery, and
- Those having reduced sympathetic response to regional anesthesia.

Monitoring should be done every 4–6 h and a target glucose level of > 45 mg% (2.5 mmol/L) is to be maintained to avoid neurological damage. Deleterious effects of hyperglycaemia include hyperosmolality, osmotic diuresis, dehydration and dyselectrolytemia, and it worsens neurological outcomes during cerebral ischemia [16].

19.11 Electrolytes

In healthy term newborns, electrolytes are rarely required to be replaced on day one of life. Thereafter, replacement is only initiated once urine output is established. The recommended maintenance electrolyte therapy is given in Table 19.8.

Table 19.8 Maintenance electrolytes in the newborn

Electrolytes	Normal range	Maintenance dose in healthy term newborn (D 2 onwards)
Sodium	135–145 mEq/L	2–4 mmol/kg/day
Potassium	3.5–5.8 mmol/L	1–2 mmol/kg/day
Calcium (ionized)	1–1.25 mmol/L (4–5 mg/dL)	200–400 mg/kg/day of 10% calcium gluconate

Table 19.9 Common causes of Sodium and Potassium Imbalances

Electrolytes	Decreased (<135 mEq/L)	Increased (>145 mEq/L)
Sodium	1. Increased tubular losses—extreme prematurity, Polyuric renal failure, diuretic therapy 2. Dilutional hyponatremia—increased ADH secretion, CHF 3. Salt wasting syndromes—hypoadrenalism 4. Maternal hyponatremia 5. Laboratory errors	1. Inadequately replenished excessive urine or insensible water loss 2. Maternal hypernatremia 3. ADH deficiency 4. Laboratory errors
Potassium	1. Alkalosis causes intracellular shifting of potassium thereby hypokalaemia, but does not affect total body potassium. 2. Polyuric renal failure 3. GI losses—diarrhoea, vomiting, third space loss 4. Intake deficiency 5. Diuretic therapy 6. Laboratory errors	1. Severe metabolic acidosis (0.6 mmol/L rise in K per 0.1 pH drop) 2. Cellular death 3. Acute renal failure 4. VLBW 5. Severe haemolytic anaemia 6. Adrenal insufficiency 7. Laboratory error/haemolysed sample

It is essential to rule out common causes of dyselectrolytemia in the preoperative workup (Table 19.9)

19.11.1 Sodium

Neonatal hyponatremia is corrected with 5% dextrose in 0.45–0.9% saline. In severe cases 3% saline may be required. Hypernatremia correction should be slow and under monitoring of body weight, serum electrolytes, urine output and specific gravity. In both cases target correction should not exceed a change of 10–12 mEq/L/day to avoid neurological complications.

19.11.2 Potassium

Potassium imbalance leads to life threatening arrhythmias. Low potassium results in paralytic ileus, abdominal distension, urinary retention, and respiratory muscle paralysis. Hence, it should always be corrected before surgery. Hyperkalaemia accentuates bradycardia responses with risk of cardiac blocks and arrest. Both hypo and hyperkalaemia should be avoided

19.11.3 Calcium

Normally, calcium is lowest in the first 2 days of life and reaches normal values by day three, and preterms are at greater risk of hypocalcaemia. Neonatal hypocalcaemia is defined as total serum calcium <8 mg/dL (<2 mmol/L) in term newborns and <7 mg/dL (<1.74 mmol/L) in preterms, and or ionized calcium <4 mg/dL (<1 mmol/L) in both. Symptomatic hypocalcaemia presents with jitteriness, seizures, lethargy, poor feeding, vomiting, and prolonged Q-Tc interval, and should be immediately corrected with elementary calcium of 10–20 mg/kg (1–2 ml/kg/dose 10% calcium gluconate over 30 minutes) under cardiac monitoring, followed by 80 mg/kg/day in first 2 days, and 40 mg/kg/day on 3rd day and then stopped. Care must be taken to avoid extravasation. Overcorrection is hazardous and in resistant cases, magnesium levels need to be checked and corrected.

19.12 Acid–Base Balance

This is another pillar in fluid and electrolyte homeostasis. Although pH values do not vary much but $PaCO_2$ and bicarbonate levels are lower in newborns. Hence prompt correction of any metabolic acidosis or alkalosis is necessary.

Postoperatively, IV fluids should be continued till oral intake approximates maintenance rate. Record should be maintained of all intake and output on the fluid balance sheet. Fluid restriction in the immediate postoperative period is recommended due to raised ADH levels. Isotonic fluids with required electrolyte supplements should be given to replace on going losses, and additional in case of fever, use of radiant warmers, and GI losses from drains and orogastric tube, at half the recommended rate (2:1:0.5 instead of 4:2:1) in first 12 h, and thereafter at full rate.

Clinical Pearls

– Identification and correction of electrolyte imbalance prior to surgery
– Monitoring once a day or twice daily in ELBW babies
– Daily acid–base status in case of electrolyte imbalance.

19.13 The Perioperative Workup

19.13.1 Preparing the Parent or Caregiver

The birth of a preterm baby or a term baby with comorbidities requiring immediate surgical intervention is itself an emotionally difficult situation for the parents. In

addition, the feeling of helplessness, anxiety and lack of control and trust complicates the matter further. Hence empathy, compassion and communication skills are
pertinent to get well cooperative parents. Parents should be adequately counselled
regarding the planned conduct of anesthesia, pain relief options, blood transfusion,
invasive monitoring or post operative ventilation and HDU/NICU support [17].

19.13.2 Preparing the Baby

Neonates are trust seekers, and they adapt to any unfamiliar environment by their
emerging sensory and motor abilities. Hence positive sensory stimulus, protection
from loud noise, bright light, supportive and comfortable bedding that allow them
to use their own movements, and touch that has a calming effect, are beneficial.

19.13.3 History and Physical Examination

An accurate estimate of body weight, BW, GA (to rule out prematurity) and APGAR
score (indication of how newborn adapts after birth) should be obtained. Trends of
baseline heart rate, blood pressure, SpO_2, temperature, fluid input, urine output,
ventilatory and acid–base status, ongoing medications, feeding and nil per oral status must be noted. Antenatal history, birth events (asphyxia, meconium aspiration),
and immunization status, needs to be recorded in order to anticipate any perioperative crisis.

19.13.4 Fasting Guidelines

In absence of any specific guidelines for newborn, the same regime as advocated by
ASA /APA for pediatric patients is followed: 2 h for clear fluids, 4 h for breast milk
and 6 h for non human milk in neonates. Keeping in mind that any surgery undertaken in the neonatal period falls under the category of an emergency, the NPO
status will have to be modified accordingly. Concomitant initiation of dextrose containing IV fluids is recommended during fasting to prevent hypoglycemia.

19.13.5 Preoperative Investigations

Latest investigations should be well within 24 h to reflect an accurate picture.
Investigations include complete blood count (Hb, Hct, TLC, platelets), serum glucose and electrolytes, coagulation studies, blood grouping and cross matching, and
echocardiography. Only indicated investigations must be advised and blood sampling be kept to minimum to reduce the risk of additional anaemia and hypovolemia. In cases, where neonatal screening for metabolic disorders and other congenital
and genetic defects has been undertaken, anaesthetist must make a note and

accordingly modify anesthetic management. In the first 2–3 days of life, babies may be hypothyroid, because of presence of maternal Thyroid stimulating hormone, but this does not need any treatment. Other investigations such as radiographs, renal and liver profile or any specific tests should be supplemented based on disease profile and clinical suspicion.

19.13.6 Intravenous Access

Since most surgical neonates are NPO for longer durations, early commencement of IV maintenance fluids is vital to maintain normal hemodynamics and uneventful induction. Proper IV access in neonates and preterms is often difficult and the procedure deserves extreme care, as without a proper IV line it will not be possible to initiate surgery. For successful venous cannulation, one must be able to see or palpate the veins which are small, fragile, and hard to locate. If the neonate is very sick and has undergone multiple previous IV insertions, cannulation becomes more difficult for the anaesthesiologist. Before attempting cannulation, ensure that the room has adequate lighting and all necessary equipment and infusion fluids in appropriate volume and combinations are ready at hand. The classic rubber tourniquet should not be used, instead light pressure over the vein by the index finger or assistant encircling the wrist or ankle, are enough to allow vein visualisation, with just light compression, as too much pressure can collapse the vein and jeopardize distal arterial supply. Warming the extremity by gentle massaging between two hands helps dilating the veins and in successful cannulation. In difficult cases transillumination or ultrasound scanner may become necessary.

Peripheral sites, such as dorsum of hand or foot, palmar surface of the wrist, ankle, scalp, are preferred, using 26 G/24 G cannula. In cases, where peripheral access fails, a central venous catheter may be placed via the internal jugular (IJV), subclavian or femoral routes. It may also be indicated for total parenteral nutrition (TPN), drug administration and CVP monitoring. Extreme caution should be taken to avoid air bubbles and drugs should be adequately diluted and pushed cautiously. Umbilical vein is usually avoided because of portal vein thrombosis and any way is not available after 72 h of life.

In critically ill babies, for sampling and hemodynamic monitoring, intra-arterial access can be achieved via the right radial or posterior tibial artery. Umbilical arteries should be avoided after the 2nd day. Heparin should be diluted in 0.45% saline (0.1–1 U/mL) and rate should not be more than 0.5–1 mL/h. Heparinized solution should be changed every 24 h. Intraosseous route is generally reserved for emergency life threatening conditions. (Refer to the Chap.4 for further details).

19.13.7 Skin and Eye Care

This is of utmost importance as there is greater risk of skin breakdown in premature babies while preparing and transporting to the operating room (OR). Skin care requires gentle techniques and careful selection of prepping agents play a vital role for prevention of skin damage. Extreme care should be taken while attaching the monitors such as blood pressure cuff, pulse oximeter probe, ECG leads, introduction of nasogastric tube, etc. to prevent skin abrasion and injury. Use of hydrocolloid dressing (duraplast) or leukoplast is preferred. Their handling should be minimal and gentle, using fingertips and not whole hand. Care should be taken to avoid pressure complications on eyes, occiput and heel. Hands should be cleaned before touching and protective non allergic gloves should be worn.

19.14 Preparing the Environment

19.14.1 Transportation

Transportation related neonatal mortality in India approximates 15–36%. Hence special precautions need to be taken during the transit to the OR and back to the ward or NICU. Attempts should be taken to minimize the travelling distance and time. Transport should be in heated incubator or isolette with uninterrupted monitoring and continuation of ongoing fluids, drugs, and respiratory supports, and always accompanied by expert medical and nursing personnel [18].

19.14.2 The Operation Theatre

19.14.2.1 Personnel

All neonatal surgeries, however, trivial, should be undertaken at a place, where all the technical facilities for neonatal anaesthesia, surgery, and provision of NICU are available. The availability of well-trained, skilled, and experienced personnel is of immense value for proper care of the newborn and premature neonates undergoing surgery. The role of nurse in the perioperative period is vital who becomes the surrogate parent. For healthy term newborn, holding, rocking, and swaddling may provide comfort and the nurse should use soothing voice and positive facial expression, and must be quick in keeping the baby warm while changing diapers. However, this comforting mechanism may not be possible in premature babies who may be intubated and on ventilator. However, presence of and close contact with the parents is of great comforting value. At least two trained and experienced pediatric anaesthesiologists along with trained circulating and scrub nursing staff should be available.

19.14.2.2 Temperature Regulation

In premature babies, newborns and neonates, the difficulty in regulating body temperature and prevention of hypothermia is a significant concern for the anaesthesiologist. Their large head size relative to their body size, lack of subcutaneous fat, increased thermal conductance and increased permeability of the epidermis, all result in increased evaporative water losses (15-fold increase) predisposing them to hypothermia accompanied by dehydration. The mechanism of thermoregulation is immature with decreased ability to produce heat, and the only way to heat production is by brown fat thermogenesis (cold stress activates brown fat lipolysis), with conversion of brown fat to glycerol and fatty acids. In prolonged conditions glucose stores get depleted. Neonates lose heat by four processes, namely, conduction (cold surfaces in contact), convection (body to air), radiation (hot body to cooler objects without contact), and evaporation (wet body to air and depends on ambient humidity). Premature babies have thinner epidermis hence are more vulnerable to insensible fluid and temperature losses [19, 20].

Hypothermia in newborn is defined as:

- Mild—35–36.3 °C
- Moderate—32–34.9 °C
- Severe—<32 °C

Hence, the room should be warmed to 25–28 °C and ensuring baby's temperature to be at least 36 °C (96.8 °F). Commonly used methods for prevention of hypothermia include:

1. Passive insulation
2. Forced air-warming devices
3. Circulating water mattress
4. Hot air drapes /garments
5. Incubator
6. Warming and humidification of inspired gases, IV fluids, blood, skin preparation and irrigation fluids to 36 °C.

19.14.2.3 Equipment

All equipment should be pretested for its workability and must be of suitable size. Breathing systems which are light weighted with minimal resistance, reduced dead space and which allow for warming and humidification are preferred. While the old school still prefers the valveless modified Jackson Rees circuit which is assumed to be capable of sensing minute changes in compliance and airway, the modern school proposes the use of neonatal ventilators with pressure control mode. Heat moisture exchangers should always be used. Suction catheters (5–8 F), Suction apparatus (wall suction with maximum pressure of 100 mmHg, Feeding tubes (6–8 F), oral airways, Face masks, Miller 0, 1, blades and handle, Uncuffed (ID 2.5, 3.0, 3.5, 4.0 mm) and cuffed Micro ETT (ID 3.0, 3.5 mm), SGA devices (size 1) including I-gel and disposable AirQ, IV fluid warmer, Infusion pumps for both drugs and fluid, emergency crash trolley with functional and appropriate defibrillator and drugs should be kept at hand.

19.14.2.4 Drugs and Blood Products

Preoperative cross matched and typed blood along with FFP/cryoprecipitate should be transfused (if needed) and reserved for intraoperative use during major surgeries. All necessary medications should be diluted to relevant concentrations and aptly labelled prior to the surgery. Adequately sized syringes and infusion pumps should be made available to inject calculated aliquots of the drugs. All medications, fluids, blood products (preferably in Pedi pack) should be prechecked for expiry dates, and infusion devices for their workability and functionality. The timing and choice of antibiotics should be discussed with the consulting neonatologist.

19.14.2.5 Monitors

Clinical skill, judgement and evaluation are still the time-tested age-old reliable monitors such as colour of the skin, chest mobility and palpation. Other prechecked mandatory monitors include:

- **Precordial/esophageal stethoscope**—indispensable, simple, effective method to assess HR, rhythm, and respiration.
- **ECG**—to detect arrhythmias, bradycardia, changes from electrolyte imbalance.
- **SpO2**—appropriate fitting, highly sensitive, preferably two (one preductal in right hand; another post ductal in lower extremity). It is ideal to maintain SpO_2 of 83–95% to avoid oxidative stress. In critically ill babies or for intrathoracic or intraabdominal surgeries, higher FiO_2 may be needed because of lung pathologies and absence of recruitment manoeuvres.
- **NIBP** with appropriate neonatal cuff (4 cm) and minimum cycling set at 3–4 min to prevent limb ischemia is advocated. In critical cases invasive BP or Doppler ultrasonic transducers may be used.
- **EtCO₂**—correlates well with $PaCO2$; however, in emergency scenarios, neonates are at higher risk of large dead space in addition to small tidal volumes, which may not be reflected in $EtCO_2$. Hence it is crucial to limit the dead space by shortening the ventilator circuit and eliminating the elbow.
- **Urine output**—although challenging, it is still a simple tool to assess the hydration status and should be maintained between 0.5 and 2 mL/kg/h, using a correct sized feeding tube.
- **Temperature monitoring** is mandatory via rectal/esophageal/skin probe.
- **Newer monitors**—NRS, Invasive cardiac output monitoring are needed for cardiac cases.

19.15 Enhanced Recovery After Surgery (ERAS) [21, 22]

The ERAS plays a significant role in improving patient recovery after anesthesia. Though the concept is somehow different from traditional postsurgical care, it has a growing influence on the low to middle income than the developed countries, as it seems to confer quantitative benefits in the perioperative period such as hospital length of stay (LOS), time to enteral feeding, opioid consumption and related adverse events, and early postsurgical mobility. However, these parameters are applicable to adult postsurgical patients, and little is known in paediatric surgical patients, more so in neonates or preterms. The first paediatric ERAS protocol was reported in 2009 by Ure et al., it is still in a nascent stage of how to implement this in neonates and preterms. The purpose of ERAS protocol in children is to advocate less invasive operation, prevention of complications, promotion of recovery after surgery, and good mental as well as physical development.

Four important factors play a pivotal role in ERAS in neonates:

1. **Avoidance of prolonged fasting** (2 h for clear fluids, 4 h for breast milk, 6 h for nonhuman milk)
2. **Nonroutine use of tubes and drains** after giving a proper peritoneal lavage as avoidance of drainage tube leads to physical reduction in intraperitoneal bacteria count, resulting in faster wound healing, early recovery and shorter hospital stay.
3. **Early oral nutrition**—though there is recommendation of early oral nutrition in LBW babies as it can minimize atrophy of bowel mucosa, normalization of intestinal flora and intestinal peristalsis, thereby preventing the post operative infection, but it increases the risk of NEC [23].
4. **Mobilization** (not applicable for neonates).

A careful patient selection is very important for early recovery but a consistent policy from the preoperative period has not yet been established as clinical conditions vary depending on the wide variety of individual diseases which further influences the perioperative outcome. Social and communication issues of neonatal surgery are also unique in nature. Despite these major differences, neonates may be well-suited for ERAS approach provided proper guidelines will come into practice which will offer tremendous opportunities to improve postsurgical care. There is a vast category of neonatal surgeries and different approaches are followed in different centres by the attending neonatologist, surgeon, nursing staff and the parents.

Development of the first neonatal surgical ERAS protocol is ongoing but as this group of patients are totally different, the recommendation should include some of the important points of ERAS, but more attention is to be given to the unique needs of these patients. Some recommendations are:

1. The importance of early oral feeding with breast milk to improve the nutritional status which can improve intestinal immunity, shorten time to feed and hospital stay.
2. Previously it was assumed that the newborns do not feel pain. However, it has now been well-documented that these neonates do feel pain such as adults, and adequate analgesia must be provided in the perioperative period. Multimodal analgesia is a good choice early recovery. Caudal analgesia provides excellent pain relief with low complication rate and can be applied easily in neonates. The use of oral sucrose is also advocated during minor procedures.

A highly effective multidisciplinary ERAS team consisting of well-aligned surgeons, anaesthesiologist, neonatologist, paediatric intensivists, pain management physicians, nurses and advanced practice providers are to be formed who will work hand in hand to make the pathway successful and sustainable. The active participation of parents and preoperative education in the child's recovery process plays a pivotal role in the recovery process and positive outcome [21, 24]. Paediatric ERAS became more widely utilised from 2010 to 2019, but neonatal ERAS represents a radically different approach than most paediatric ERAS guidelines. Any neonatal surgery presents the extreme end of physiologic challenges, so while contemplating neonatal ERAS guidelines certain points need to be addressed:

1. Nutritional requirement is very important as there is a higher energy requirement for growth and wound healing.
2. Neonates show exquisite sensitivity to fluid overload as well as under resuscitation as both have detrimental effects in the perioperative period.
3. Temperature instability is to be controlled correctly for a favourable outcome.
4. Neonates show a markedly different immune response to surgical stress.

In population-based studies, surgical site infection (SSI) rate is more in neonates than in adults. SSI will lead to poor growth, longer hospital stay, and need for re-exploration which will ultimately lead to increased morbidity and mortality. To get a success in neonatal ERAS the parents are to be included in the process of hospitalization of their baby by properly educating them about the procedures and management. They also will get confidence, satisfaction and by increasing their knowledge and taking active part in their child's postoperative course of treatment, more favourable outcome can be expected. It also reduces urgent emergency room visits after discharge and readmissions which ultimately improve the developmental outcome of the neonates.

19.16 Conclusion

Caring for the neonates and specially the premature needs a special skill to be developed by the attending nurse, surgeons and anaesthesiologists. Neonates are unique in character and differ from the adults in every aspect, be it anatomical or physiological, pharmacological or pathological, ethical or equipment related. The anaesthesiologist has to face a variety of challenges. It is a formidable task to detect the problems or complications in time and to take active measures to correct as quickly as possible, as the margin of safety is very narrow. One has to formulate a plan of care for every individual needing surgery from the preoperative period and continued up to the discharge of the patient from hospital. Neonatal ERAS is still in a very nascent stage, further evidence is needed to formulate it in practical life. Though there is profound advancement in technology, high quality care is available in many advanced centres, still surgery in neonates and premature babies carries a high risk of morbidity and mortality.

References

1. Frawley G. Special considerations in the premature and ex-premature infant. Anesth Intensive Care Med. 2017;18:79–83.

2. World Health Organization. Premature birth fact sheet No 363. Available at http://www.who.int/mediacentre/factsheets/fs363/en/.

3. Taneja B, Srivastava V, Saxena KN. Physiological and anaesthetic considerations for the preterm neonate undergoing surgery. J Neonat Surg. 2012;1(1):14–9.

4. Glass HC, Costarino AT, Stayer SA, etal. Outcomes for extremely premature infants. Anesth Analg 2015;120(6):1337-1351.

5. Varghese E. Extremely premature infants and anesthesia; chapter 15. In: Yearbook of anesthesiology. 7 JP Brothers Medical Publishers (P) Ltd; 2018, pp. 168–78.

6. Taneja B, Srivastava V, Saxena KN. Physiological and anaesthetic considerations for the preterm neonate undergoing surgery. J Neonatal Surg. 2012;1(1):14.

7. Thomas J. Reducing the risk of neonatal anesthesia. Pediatric Anesth. 2013;24:106–13.

8. Derieg S. An overview of perioperative care for pediatric patients. AORN J. 2016;104(1):4–10.

9. Morriss F, Saha S, Bell E, et al. Surgery and neurodevelopmental outcome in very low birth weight infants. J Am Med Assoc Pediatr. 2014;168:746–54.

10. Vashist M, Miglani HPS. Approach to difficult and compromised airway in neonatal and pediatric age group patients. IJA. 2008;52(3):273–81.

11. Chawla D, Agarwal R, Deorari AK, Paul VK. Fluid and electrolyte management in term and preterm neonates. Indian J Pediatr. 2008;75:255–9.

12. Murat I, Humblot A, Girault L, Piana F. Neonatal fluid management. Best Pract Research Clin Anaesthesiol. 2010;24:365–74.

13. APA consensus guideline on perioperative fluid management in children v 1.1 September 2007 © APAGBI Review Date August 2010.

14. Murat I. Perioperative fluid therapy in pediatrics, edited by Hahn RG, Prough DS, Svensen CH. Informa Healthcare; 2007. p. 425.

15. New HV, Berryman J, Bolton-Maggs PH, et al. Guidelines on transfusion for fetuses, neonates and older children. Br J Haematol. 2016;175:784–828.

16. Hays SP, Smith EO, Sunehag AL. Hyperglycemia is a risk factor for early death and morbidity in extremely low birth-weight infants. Pediatrics. 2006;118:1811–8. 26.

17. Franck LS, Mcnulty A, Alderdice F. The perinatal –neonatal care journey for parents of preterm infants. J Perinat Neonatal Nurs. 2017;31(3):244–55.

18. Roy MP, Gupta R, Sehgal R. Neonatal transport in India: $rom public health perspective. Med J DY Patil Univ. 2016;9:566–9.

19. Bazwa SJS, Swati MD. Perioperative hypothermia in pediatric patients: diagnosis, prevention and management. Anaesth Pain Intensive Care. 2014;18(1):97–100.

20. Sultan P, Habib AS, Carvalho B. Ambient operating room temperature: mother, baby or surgeon? BJA. 2017;119(4):839–20.

21. Gibb ACN, Croshy MA, McDiarmid C, et al. Creation of an Enhanced Recovery After Surgery (ERAS) Guideline for neonatal intestinal surgery patients: a knowledge synthesis and consensus generation approach and protocol study.BMJ. Open. 2018;8(12):e023651.

22. Franclin AD et al. Pediatric enhanced recovery after surgery. https://doi.org/10.1007/978-3-030-33443-7_58.

23. Prasad GR, Rao JVS, Aziz A, Rashmi TM. Early enteral nutrition in neonates following abdominal surgery. J Neonatal Surg. 2018;7:21.

24. Brindle ME, McDiarmid C, Short K, et al. Consensus guidelines for perioperative care in neonatal intestinal surgery: Enhanced Recovery After Surgery (ERAS®) Society recommendations. World J Surg. 2020;44:2482–92. https://doi.org/10.1007/s00268-020-05530-1.

Central Venous and Peripheral Arterial Access in Neonates

20

Shilpa Agarwal

20.1 Introduction

Vascular access is a major life saving procedure, especially in critically ill and preterm neonates. It is an essential component of patient care, and surgical and anesthetic management of any neonate. With improvement in perinatal care, greater proportion of premature babies are surviving, and requiring surgical interventions. Various techniques and sites are used for securing an intravenous (IV) line in these babies, but it can be extremely challenging. This is one of the most common simple procedures that can make even the expert very anxious for success in first attempt in these tiny babies. Usually, peripheral lines suffice, which are safer, and easier to access and maintain.

Open surgical venous cut down and cannulation was the usual procedure in babies in whom percutaneous venous access was difficult. Today, ultrasound guided approach as the "standard of care" has made this procedure easier and with less complications. Small size of the baby, and even smaller size of the blood vessels and smaller catheter diameter, increases the technical difficulty. Problems may be encountered at the initial insertion, during its maintenance and even at the time of removal, necessitating extra care. Central venous cannulation is not a routine procedure in newborns and neonates because of technical difficulties, lack of expertise, problems in its maintenance, and higher complication rates. Therefore, central venous cannulation (CVC) must be done only if it is unavoidable, absolutely essential, and if benefits outweigh the risks [1–3].

S. Agarwal (✉)
Department of Anesthesiology, Chacha Nehru Bal Chikitsalya, New Delhi, India

© The Author(s), under exclusive license to Springer Nature Singapore Pte Ltd. 2023
U. Saha (ed.), *Clinical Anesthesia for the Newborn and the Neonate*,
https://doi.org/10.1007/978-981-19-5458-0_20

20.2   Central Venous Cannulation (CVC)

The purpose of CVC is the cannulation of a central vein, whereby the catheter tip is threaded so as to lie in the lower SVC (superior vene cava), and has several benefits over the peripheral IV cannulation [2–4]. CVC can be done by the peripheral or central routes:

i. Percutaneous inserted central catheter (PICC line)
ii. Centrally inserted venous catheter (CICC)

PICC is preferred over CICC. In specific circumstances, PICC is also used for arterial access. Examples of CVC include implantable ports (portacath) and central lines. Portacath is a thin, soft, plastic catheter, whose injection port remains under the skin. The catheter line can be tunneled under the skin and subcutaneous tissue or nontunneled. This is a short procedure, usually of 30–60 min duration, and can be done on outpatient basis or by the bed side. It should be carried out under all aseptic precautions, with or without sedation, depending on the neonates' clinical condition. In critically ill neonates, it is often undertaken in the operation theatre, under sedation or anesthesia. The success of cannulation is highest if it is carried out under fluoroscopy guidance.

a. Indications of CVC
   i.   Failure to secure a peripheral IV line
   ii.   Need of a reliable IV access for a longer time
   iii. For resuscitation: CICC more quickly accessed
   iv.   For postresuscitation management of preterm neonates (PICC preferred)
   v.   Large volume fluid resuscitation
   vi.   Infusion of Irritant drugs, antibiotics, hyperosmolar fluids (25% dextrose), and packed RBC
   vii. For long-term total parenteral nutritional support (TPN)
   viii. As a route for diagnostic procedures, e.g., prior to open heart surgery
   ix.   For chemotherapy
   x.   For hemodynamic monitoring [5]

b. Benefits of CVC
   • Provides a reliable IV access.
     – Can be inserted and removed without anesthesia.
     – Less chance of fluid extravasation.
     – Allows for minimal handling of sick neonates.
     – Has low complication rate (lowest with smaller catheter with least number of lumens).
     – Avoids frequent needle stick punctures and pain.
     – Smaller catheter more likely to get blocked.
     – In situ (dwell) time is >1 to 4–8 weeks for PICC and <7 days for CICC.

- Any IV infusate can be given through it, including 25% dextrose and sodium bicarbonate.
- "Power-injectable' PICC lines can withstand high pressure allowing radiological contrast injection.

20.2.1 Site for Central Venous Canulation

a. **Site of PICC:** The site most appropriate is determined by the ease of access, and duration for which the line is required. Common sites are in the **upper arm** (basilic, cephalic, medial cubital, and brachial veins), **lower limb** (saphenous, femoral, and popliteal veins), and **others** (temporal, and postauricular veins—for short term). **Upper arm veins are preferred**. Cephalic vein is laterally placed. It makes an acute angle at its junction with subclavian vein in the neck, which makes threading of the catheter difficult. It is also more prone to vasospasm, and hence unsuitable. Brachial vein is more central and deeper and in close proximity with the Brachial artery and Median nerve. Its cannulation is associated with risk of injury to these structures. **Basilic vein is medially placed above the cubital fossa, is larger in size and more superficial in location. By virtue of this, it is the most preferred site in neonates.**
b. **Site for CICC:** commonly used sites are in the neck, the internal jugular vein (IJV), subclavian vein and femoral vein (for short-term <7 days).

20.2.2 The Size and Length of Catheter

The **size and length of catheter**: the size of the catheter is determined by the size of the vein and therapy required. Several height, weight, and surface-landmark-based formulas guiding the length of catheter insertion are available. In practice, 4–5 Fr catheter (5 cm long is suitable for IJV cannulation), while 1 Fr catheter is used for PICC line in neonates. In general, catheter bore size is wider for CICC and smaller for PICC with the disadvantage of slower infusion rates. When selecting the catheter, following points should be kept in mind:

- Catheter diameter should be < 1/3rd the vein diameter.
- Smaller catheter with least number of lumens is associated with less complications.
- Too small a catheter is more likely to get blocked.
- For frequent or repeated blood sampling through PICC line, at least 3 Fr size should be placed.
- Catheter should be pre heparinized.

20.2.3 Technique

Technique of insertion of PICC and CICC are similar as in children and adults, using Seldinger technique, under ECG monitoring. Right IJV is preferred because of its short and straight course. Procedure should be done under all asepsis, and care taken to prevent air embolism and injury to carotid vessels and right atrium.

20.3 Umbilical Vein Cannulation

Umbilical vein catheter (UVC): umbilical vein remains patent for a short period after birth, up to 1 week, but is never the first choice for venous access in newborns and neonates. It can be cannulated for emergency resuscitation when a peripheral vein may be difficult to cannulate, and can be used for drugs and fluid administration, blood sampling and exchange transfusion [6, 7]. It has the advantage of being a bed side procedure, with no need for sedation/anesthesia. After initial use, it can be replaced by PICC/CICC/surgical line, if it is necessary to keep it for a longer than 10–14 days (maximum duration it can stay viable). However, it is contraindicated in neonates with NEC, abdominal wall defects, omphalitis and peritonitis.

Technique of UVC: a single or double lumen catheter (3.5–5 Fr G:: preterm–term) is threaded in, such that its tip comes to lie in the IVC above the level of diaphragm. Successful cannulation is confirmed by the free flow of blood and when it can be aspirated easily. UVC should be done under all aseptic conditions in a warm comfortable environment. An umbilical tape or purse–string suture is applied to the base of the umbilical stump as an anchor and for hemostasis. The end of the stub is freshened with a scalpel and umbilical vein identified (it remains patent and continues to ooze, whereas the two arteries are thick walled and go into spasm). The vein is cleared of any clot or thrombus, using a fine forceps, and cannulation done with a preheparanized cannula with the stopcock attached. The catheter is threaded in the direction of the baby's right shoulder until free flow of blood ensues and 1–2 cm more (usually at 4–5 cm). This is enough in an emergency. However, if required for longer duration, catheter should be threaded to reach its final destination, i.e., the tip in the IVC, above the ductus venosus, below the level of right atrium (10–12 cm). (Correct length can be calculated by dividing the shoulder to umbilicus length by 0.6, in cm). No force should be used, and if resistance is felt, the suture/tape should be released to reduce obstruction or kinking. During insertion, care must be taken to prevent air embolism during insertion and at the time of removal.

20.4 Intraosseous/Intramedullary Access (IO)

Intraosseous access can be rapidly achieved with a high success rate and provides direct, noncollapsible access to venous circulation. Fluids and medications administered, drain via the venous sinusoids into the emissary veins, and from there into the systemic circulation. Any drug or fluid which can be given intravenously can be infused IO but must be delivered under pressure to overcome the intrinsic resistance of the medullary cavity and bone marrow. Though not a routine method, it can be lifesaving when peripheral venous line is not available or possible, as it can be accessed rapidly even in critically ill, hypovolemic and dehydrated neonates [8]. (Pediatric resuscitation guidelines 9th ed of ATLS manual) [9].

a. **Sites for Intraosseous Access and Needle Size:**

- Most common in neonates: anteromedial aspect of proximal tibia (1–3 cm below and medial to tibial tuberosity)
- Other sites: proximal humerus and distal femur
- IO needle size for manual insertion: 18–14 G, 3–4 cm long
- Spinal needles and IV cannula may be used if IO needle is not available (but not recommended).
- Correct placement is confirmed with the aspiration of marrow and with the easy infusion of fluid.
- This is only a temporary route 12–24 h. IO should be removed early [8].

b. **Contraindications:**

  i.   Bone disease, such as osteoporosis or osteogenesis imperfecta
  ii. Infection at the insertion site
  iii. Site used for IO insertion within prior 24 h
  iv. Fractured bone (risk of compartment syndrome due to leak from previous cortex breach)

20.5 Complications

20.5.1 Complications of CVC

Complications of CVC can be acute (at insertion) and late (during its maintenance). Complications are less with PICC than CICC [10, 11].

(a) **Phlebitis** can occur in the first few days of insertion. This is a normal response to a foreign body. Management consists of dry compresses and limb elevation. If not resolved or becomes severe, PICC should be removed.
(b) **Catheter migration or malposition and vessel erosion**: can occur during insertion or anytime later. Outcome depends on the tip site, leading to pericardial, pleural, or peritoneal effusions, cardiac arrhythmias, and extravasation.
(c) **Catheter dysfunction**: leads to inability to infuse fluids, withdraw blood, or leakage of fluid. Causes are malposition, occlusion, presence of clots, precipitates, lipid deposits, or tight splinting.

(d) **Catheter breakage** is a serious complication leading to embolization of the intravascular catheter segment. Catheter can get severed at the time of introduction or because of excessive pull or pressure or at the time of removal when a fibrin sheath around it makes removal difficult. Broken part if visible outside, must be grasped and pulled out using a fine-toothed surgical forceps and apply dressing. If fail to pull out the catheter, apply pressure over catheter tract, get an X-ray and do surgical removal.

(e) **Damage to the artery, nerve or thoracic duct** and bleeding, at the time of insertion or later due to catheter migration or embolization.

(f) **Thrombosis** occurs when infusion fluid is not heparinized, at low flow rate, or long standing PICC.

(g) Air embolism.

(h) Pneumothorax.

(i) Cardiac arrhythmias, and

20.5.2 Complications of UVC

Complications of UVC are malposition (risk of hepatic necrosis if tip lies in portal vein and hyperosmolar fluids are injected), infection [12, 13], vessel injury and formation of false tract [14], liver abscess or necrosis [15] air or catheter tip embolism, portal vein thrombosis [16], and arrhythmias and pericardial tamponade [17–19] Important precaution is to check for free flow of blood before use.

20.5.3 Complications of IO

Complications of IO are rare, such as osteomyelitis, fracture, leakage, extravasation (vasopressors/irritant/hyperosmolar infusions), compartment syndrome, and failure of infusion.

20.6 Arterial Cannulation (IA)

a. Indications

Peripheral arterial lines are commonly indicated for (i) Hemodynamic monitoring and (ii) Blood sampling for arterial blood gases (ABG). (iii) Other indications are [20]:

- Failure of umbilical artery cannulation (UAC), and
- During exchange blood transfusion.

Decision to cannulate an artery in newborns and neonates should be taken with extreme caution as this is a very high-risk procedure, and complication rate is greatest in this age group. Complication rates are less with distal arterial cannulation and highest with femoral art cannulation [21]. Parental consent is mandatory.

20.6.1 Special Considerations in Newborns and Neonates

- **Basic consideration** is to choose an artery, where there is collateral circulation to the area affected by the cannulated artery [22].
- **Common site** within 48–72 h of birth is the Umbilical artery.
- **Other sites** are: radial, ulnar [23], brachial [24], temporal [25], femoral, posterior tibial, dorsalis pedis arteries. Radial arterial cannulation is the most common site because of the ease of access and maintenance (caution in premature and LBW neonates).
- Cannula size: 24 G Fr is appropriate for a neonate
- Arterial cannulation is painful and some sedation/pacifying is required.
- Local xylocaine infiltration must always be done to prevent arterial spasm [8].
- Rarely, surgical cutdown may be needed.

20.6.2 Contraindications [20]

- Failed Allen's test, recent cannulation or attempt of another artery in the same limb
- Local skin infection
- Bleeding disorder, and
- Malformation of limb

20.6.3 Technique of Radial Artery Cannulation

Technique of radial artery cannulation: a 24G cannula is inserted at an angle of 30–45 °. Once blood is visible at the hub, the stylet is withdrawn, while cannula is gently advanced. The artery may go into spasm, with delay in blood appearance. Once confirmed, a three-way stopcock is attached and closed (cannula and stopcock must be primed with heparinized solution), cannula flushed with heparinized saline, and firmly secured, taking care not to encircle the entire wrist, and that fingers are visible.

20.6.4 Complications of Arterial Cannulation: [20, 26]

- Thromboembolism/vasospasm/thrombosis, distal hypoperfusion, blanching, ischemia, tissue necrosis/gangrene, digit loss (radial artery)
  - Infection
  - Hemorrhage/hematoma
  - Air embolism.

Management is by immediate catheter removal, limb elevation, warming the contralateral extremity, topical vasodilators (NTG), anticoagulation, and thrombolysis.

20.7 Precautions and Care at Insertion and Maintenance of Vascular Lines:

   i. Do not insert if neonate has sepsis with positive blood culture report
  ii. Always obtain informed consent from parents
 iii. Minimum handling of the catheter, procedure done under strict asepsis, and site covered with sterile dressing
  iv. Heparinize the cannula and line before use and ensure all heparin is aspirated before insertion
   v. Flushing: use 10 mL syringes to flush the lines. Smaller syringes generate higher injection pressure which can damage the catheter or blood vessel. Do not to inject large volumes of flushing fluid.
  vi. Heparinized solution for flushing: 50 mL normal saline + 100 units heparin @ 0.3–0.5 mL/h [20].
 vii. Confirmation of catheter tip position by ultrasound, fluoroscopy, chest X-ray (upper limb lines) and X-ray abdomen (lower limb lines). Repeat weekly to detect catheter migration/damage.
viii. Tip position: for upper limb or neck lines is in the distal 3rd of SVC or at Cavo-atrial junction, and for lower limb lines in the IVC above the ductus venosus, below the level of RA.
  ix. Upper limb lines move an average of 2.2 rib spaces with arm movements, so may not always remain in position. Therefore, it should be fixed with the baby's arm in natural position.
   x. Where high flow rates are required, wide bore (hemodialysis/plasmapheresis) catheters are used.
  xi. IV fluids should be heparinized (0.25 μ/mL of fluid if rate >2 mL per hour, or 0.5 μ/mL if rate <2 mL/h). Maximum daily heparin dose should be <100 μ/kg/day. Change solution daily.
 xii. Check for manufacturer recommended maximum fluid rates on each catheter.
xiii. Avoid using for blood sampling, and packed cell transfusion (risk of infection, clotting of the line, hemolysis).
xiv. CVC must be removed at the earliest, once peripheral routes are appropriate or fluid and drug requirement has reduced.
 xv. Documentation: day, date, time, what procedure, details of cannula size, line insertion mark, number of flushing and volume used each time, local condition of skin, name of the operator, any difficulty met, etc.
xvi. If anticipating difficulty, blood grouping and cross matching must be done.

20.8 Anesthesia for Vascular Cannulation

Some sort of sedation or analgesia or even anesthesia must be provided for CICC, IA and IO placement, as:

(a) These are painful and time-consuming procedures.
(b) Baby needs to be immobile to avoid multiple attempts, failure, and complications.

(c) Technical difficulty arises from the small diameter of vessels, small catheter size, and location of blood vessel. Ultrasound improves visualisation and success rate.

(d) In critically ill neonates with gross coagulopathy, hypovolemia or hypotension, CVC is extremely difficult and should be done in the OT, under sedation or anesthesia or comfort swaddling method, or under ultrasound/fluoroscopy guidance.

Neonate should be provided comfort swaddling method to tolerate the procedure: swaddling, thermoneutral environment, shielding the baby's eyes from bright light used during cannulation, allowing baby to suck on a pacifier during the procedure. In preterm and low birth weight neonates, glucose sweetened pacifier provides comfort.

20.8.1 Anesthesia Techniques

Goal of anesthesia care is to maintain hemodynamic stability, adequate gas exchange, provide enough relaxation to allow positioning of the neonate for the procedure, and prompt recovery at the end. The total duration is usually 15–30 min:

i. **If no peripheral IV line present**: oral sedation by syrup Phenargan, Midazolam or Ketamine along with comfort swaddling technique.
ii. **If peripheral line is in situ**: IV Midazolam/Ketamine.
iii. Either IV or inhalational induction using Sevoflurane can be used. Usually, face mask or LMA suffices (tracheal intubation is reserved for difficult cannulations, congenital distortion of the site, or for IJV cannulation), with retaining spontaneous respiration, baby breathing O_2, N_2O and Sevoflurane mixture and assisted ventilation. There is no need for muscle relaxant. Analgesia using Fentanyl or Remifentanyl must be provided.

References

1. Krishnamurthy G, Keller MS. Vascular access in children. Cardiovasc Intervent Radiol. 2011;34:14–24.
2. Insertion, management and removal of central venous devices. Royal Children's Hospital, Melbourne. https://www.rch.org.au/.../CVAD_procedure_revision_2020_FINAL_V6... · PDF file. Approved 21 Dec 2020.
3. Scott-Warren VL, Morley RB. Paediatric vascular access. BJA Educ. 2015;15:199–206.
4. Larson SD, Hebra A, Raju R, Lee S. Vascular access in children. Medscape; 2020.
5. Othersen HB Jr, Hebra A, Chessman KH, et al. Central lines in parenteral nutrition. In: Baker Jr RD, Baker SS, Davis AM, editors. Pediatric parenteral nutrition. New York: Chapman and Hall; 1997. p. 254–71.
6. Butler-O'Hara M, Buzzard CJ, Reubens L, McDermott MP, DiGrazio W, D'Angio CT. A randomized trial comparing long-term and short-term use of umbilical venous catheters in premature infants with birth weights of less than 1251 grams. Pediatrics. 2006;118(1):e25–35.
7. Murki S, Kumar P. Blood exchange transfusion for infants with severe neonatal hyperbilirubinemia. Semin Perinatol. 2011;35(3):175–84.
8. Smith R, Davis N, Bouamra O, Lecky F. The utilisation of intraosseous infusion in the resuscitation of paediatric major trauma patients. Injury. 2005;36(9):1034–8; discussion 1039. [Medline].

9. American College of Surgeons Committee on Trauma. Advanced trauma life support student course manual. 9th ed. Chicago: American College of Surgeons; 2012.

10. Bagwell CE, Salzberg AM, Sonnino RE, Haynes JH. Potentially lethal complications of central venous catheter placement. J Pediatr Surg. 2000;35(5):709–13. [Medline].

11. Chiang VW, Baskin MN. Uses and complications of central venous catheters inserted in a pediatric emergency department. Pediatr Emerg Care. 2000;16(4):230–2. [Medline].

12. Mutlu M, Aslan Y, Kul S, Yılmaz G. Umbilical venous catheter complications in newborns: a 6-year single-center experience. J Matern Fetal Neonatal Med. 2016;29(17):2817–22. [Medline].

13. Mileder LP, Pocivalnik M, Schwaberger B, Pansy J, Urlesberger B, Baik-Schneditz N. Practice of umbilical venous catheterization using a resource-efficient 'blended' training model. Resuscitation. 2018;122:e21–2. [Medline].

14. Costa S, De Carolis MP, Savarese I, Manzoni C, Lacerenza S, Romagnoli C. An unusual complication of umbilical catheterisation. Eur J Pediatr. 2008;167(12):1467–9. [Medline].

15. Moens E, Dooy JD, Jansens H, Lammens C, Op de Beeck B, Mahieu L. Hepatic abscesses associated with umbilical catheterisation in two neonates. Eur J Pediatr. 2003;162(6):406–9. [Medline].

16. Sakha SH, Rafeey M, Tarzamani MK. Portal venous thrombosis after umbilical vein catheterization. Indian J Gastroenterol. 2007;26:283–4. [Medline].

17. Hermansen MC, Hermansen MG. Intravascular catheter complications in the neonatal intensive care unit. Clin Perinatol. 2005;32(1):141–56, vii. [Medline].

18. Onal EE, Saygili A, Koç E, Türkyilmaz C, Okumus N, Atalay Y. Cardiac tamponade in a newborn because of umbilical venous catheterization: is correct position safe? Paediatr Anaesth. 2004;14(11):953–6. [Medline].

19. Sehgal A, Cook V, Dunn M. Pericardial effusion associated with an appropriately placed umbilical venous catheter. J Perinatol. 2007;27(5):317–9.

20. Hafez M, Robertson SJ. Peripheral arterial access in neonates. Ashford and St Peter's Hospitals, NHS Foundation Trust; 2019.

21. Gleich SJ, Wong AV, Handlogten KS, Thum DE, Nemergut ME. Major short-term complications of arterial cannulation for monitoring in children. Anesthesiology. 2021;134(1):26–34. https://doi.org/10.1097/ALN.0000000000003594.

22. Irwin RS, Rippe JM. Manual of intensive care medicine. Lippincott Williams & Wilkins; 2010. p. 15. ISBN: 9780781799928.

23. Nicol M, Bavin C, Cronin P, et al. Essential nursing skills e-book. Elsevier Health Sciences; 2012. p. 125. ISBN: 978-0723437772.

24. Schindler E, Kowald B, Suess H, Niehaus-Borquez B, Tausch B, Brecher A. Catheterization of the radial or brachial artery in neonates and infants. Paediatr Anaesth. 2005;15(8):677–82. https://doi.org/10.1111/j.1460-9592.2004.01522.x.

25. Nobuo J, Tsunehiko S. Cannulation of the temporal artery in neonates and infants. Paediatr Anaesth. 2007 Jul;17(7):704–5. https://doi.org/10.1111/j.1460-9592.2006.02188.x.

26. Mosalli R, Elbaz M, Paes B. Topical nitroglycerine for neonatal arterial associated peripheral ischemia following cannulation: a case report and comprehensive literature review. Case Rep Pediatr. 2013;2013:608516. https://doi.org/10.1155/2013/608516. Epub 2013 Oct 23.

Ultrasound Guided Vascular Access in Neonates

21

Chitra Garg

21.1 Basic Principle of US Guided Vascular Access

Maintaining good body ergonomics is the key. It means the operator; the patient and ultrasound machine are positioned in straight line. This allows operator to perform without turning and leads to more logical orientation of the USG screen, such that structures appearing on left side of screen corresponds to left side of the patient, when performing across the visual axis. Always rest the ulnar border of hand holding the probe on patient's body to allow fine manoeuvres.

Vessels appear nonechoic (black) on ultrasound. Veins are compressible with light pressure and are nonpulsatile unlike arteries. Flow can be confirmed with colour Doppler, if there is a confusion with any other nonechoic structure. Always identify the anatomy around the vessel to avoid any damage to surrounding structures, such as nerves or pleura.

Good probe selection is important. High frequency linear probe (7–10 MHz) and hockey stick probe (13 MHz) are most suitable in neonates and small children.

At the outset, it is necessary to state that USG cannulations must be carried out under all aseptic precautions.

21.1.1 Advantages of Ultrasound Over Traditional Landmark Insertion:

(a) Clear demonstration of anatomy, diameter, and patency of vessels
(b) Real-time guidance of needle tip and angle of approach
(c) Real-time placement of guidewire and confirmation of catheter placement into the vessel
(d) Immediate recognition of complications, as hematoma and pneumothorax

C. Garg (✉)
Royal Victoria Infirmary, Newcastle upon Tyne, UK

21.1.2 Disadvantages of Ultrasound

(a) Needs experienced and skilled practitioner
(b) Steep learning curve especially if handling small babies
(c) Large equipment size in comparison to size of patient may be limiting

21.1.3 Possible Vascular Access Sites

1. **Peripheral arterial catheterisation**
2. **Peripheral venous catheterisation**
3. **Central venous catheterisation**

21.2 Arterial Cannulation

The indications, techniques and sites for arterial access are same as that of older kids, except that in newborns, the umbilical artery may be used for cannulation.

As mentioned earlier there is a higher chance of failure and complications when using landmark techniques over ultrasound. In neonates 24–22 G nonported cannula-over-needle devices (e.g., Jelco) are commonly used. In addition, standard 0.018 inches diameter guidewires will not pass through less than 22 G needle, so 0.012 inches baby wires are alternatives for arterial cannulation.

Usually, radial, brachial, and posterior tibial arteries are preferred due to their larger calibre, straighter course, less anatomical variation and low incidence of complications.

21.3 Peripheral Venous Cannulation

The most common peripheral intravenous (IV) access site is dorsum of hands and feet. Ultrasound can be useful in up to 50% of kids, where veins can be difficult to visualise and are not palpable. Vein diameter is important independent predictor of successful cannulation. Therefore, saphenous vein, cephalic and basilic veins have higher chance of successful cannulation than veins at dorsum of hand and feet. In addition, these veins are slightly deeper, so less prone for collapse by US probe pressure.

21.4 Determination of Optimal Catheter Size

Catheter or cannula size is determined by two factors:

1. Relation between the vessel and catheter diameter
2. Catheter travel distance from skin to vessel

In general, catheter diameter should be less than 20% of arterial lumen and less than 30% of venous lumen. In paediatric patients, 24G catheter with diameter around 0.7 mm is commonly used. Assuming that the artery is round, a minimum diameter of 1.57 mm is required to not to exceed 20% of arterial lumen when using 24G catheter. Thus, measuring internal diameter of artery before cannulation will ensure more appropriate selection of catheter size and decrease the chances of complications.

Similar to venous cannulation, there is increase chances of extravasation and infiltration when using larger size of catheter.

In addition, a longer catheter travel distance from skin to vessel increases the chance of catheter dislodgement, meaning shorter intravascular length. There is increased chance of catheter failure if <30% of the entire catheter length is in the vein. 32.4% of IV catheters failed when 30–64% of the catheter length was inside the vein and no failure when >65% of the catheter length was in the vein.

21.5 Central Venous Access

Most common sites are femoral and internal jugular veins, as it is easily done at these places with decreased chance of complications.

21.5.1 Internal Jugular Vein (IJV)

Compared to adults IJV cannulation in neonates can be difficult due to a short neck, shallow, small and mobile structures and reduced space for ultrasound probe. IJV is mostly placed anterolaterally to carotid artery (CA). Variations in anatomy can be there in up to 18% children under 6 years of age.

Optimum positioning includes neck extension and in neutral position. Rotation of head to the other side can increase IJV overlap with CA, so more neutral position is useful. In addition, head down position and liver compression are not of benefit to increase vein diameter in neonates.

Choosing correct length and size of the cannula is vital to minimise the complications, and the length of cannula is based on height and weight or using surface landmark. In general, 5 cm, 3 to 5 Fr G cannula are suitable for most newborns, with number of lumens restricted to minimum as per the need. It is useful to have both straight wires and J-wires while attempting central cannulation. Straight wires may fail to pass sharp turns and increase the chance of perforation, while J-wires are easier to pass sharp turns but are of larger diameter, it is important to choose the correct size of the wire that will pass through the IV cannula.

21.5.2 Femoral Vein (FV)

This is the most favoured site for venous cannulation in small kids as it avoids potential intrathoracic complications of IJV and **subclavian vein** (SCV) cannulations. Disadvantages of femoral venous cannulation include higher risk of kinking (groin site), less accurate filling pressures, infection, and thrombosis.

FV lies superficially in the femoral triangle, medial to the femoral artery. Femoral artery may completely or partially overlap the FV in nearly 10–12% young children. Hence care must be taken to prevent arterial puncture.

The FV is usually cannulated close to the inguinal ligament but not above it as external compression may not be possible there. It is easier to cannulate the FV if a small towel or roll is placed under the hip and leg is slightly externally rotated or slight abduction at the thigh.

Cannula size is similar to as for IJV cannulation, and length is less of an issue.

21.5.3 Subclavian Vein (SCV)

SCV is formed as a continuation of axillary vein and runs between the clavicle and first rib. It is less mobile and less likely to collapse as compared to IJV. It is not the common choice for central venous access in neonates due to significant risks of complications (3–34%). With ultrasound results are better, but there is paucity of literature for the same.

SCV can be visualised and cannulated with in plane or out of plane technique either above or below the clavicle depending on the expertise of the operator. Slight head rotation to the opposite side and a small roll under the ipsilateral shoulder provide optimal position for SCV cannulation.

21.6   USG Guided Vascular Access Technique and Approaches

Long-axis in-plane view (LAX-IP) and short-axis out-of-plane view (SAX-OOP) are the two main approaches that are used to cannulate a vessel using US. In a recent systematic review of adult patients and phantoms, SAX-OOP approach had a higher success rate than LAX-IP approach. This is controversial in paediatric patients; therefore, operator should be familiar with the advantages and disadvantages of each approach and pursue with the one he or she is most familiar and experienced with.

21.6.1 LAX-IP Approach

In this approach, sound waves from US intersect the vessel in longitudinally. The whole shaft of the needle and longitudinal view of the target vessel are visualised in real time (Fig. 21.1a). However, when approaching small vessels, it is difficult to maintain the probe along the best plane in which largest diameter is visualised along its course (Fig. 21.1c). Thus, this may be of disadvantage in paediatric settings [1–4].

Fig. 21.1 Schematic and ultrasound views. (**a**) LAX-IP—whole shaft of needle is visualised. (**b**) SAX-OOP—the target vessel is visualised in transverse orientation and needle tip is visualised as hyper echoic bright dot. (**c**) In paediatric setting when approaching small vessels, the probe is easily moved away from the plane of largest diameter in LAX [1–4]

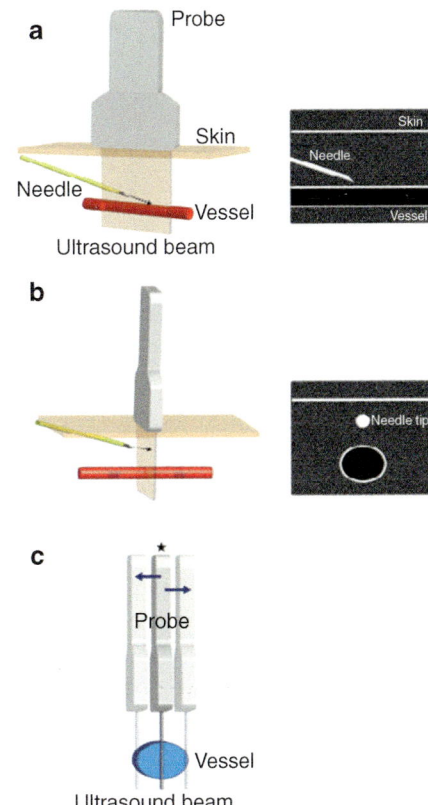

In LAX-IP approach especially cannulating smaller vessels, needle tip sometimes leaves the US plane as it advances. Certain manoeuvres can be done to bring needle tip back into US plane. Therefore, we can either rotate the probe towards the needle or needle towards the probe or withdraw and redo the cannulation (Fig. 21.2) [5, 6]. Sometimes even when entire catheter looks to be rightly placed, there is no back flow at the catheter hub. This may happen because of side lobe or slice thickness artefact (Fig. 21.2e, f) [5, 6]. In this situation, it is better to withdraw the needle till skin, realign the probe to get the best view and retry cannulation again.

21.6.2 SAX-OOP Approach

In this approach, ultrasound beam intersects the vessel transversally, such that only the needle tip is visualised as an echogenic dot and rest of the shaft is off screen (Fig. 21.1b) [1–4]. The advantage of SAX-OOP approach, especially in paediatric patient is that the maximum vessel diameter can be always visualised.

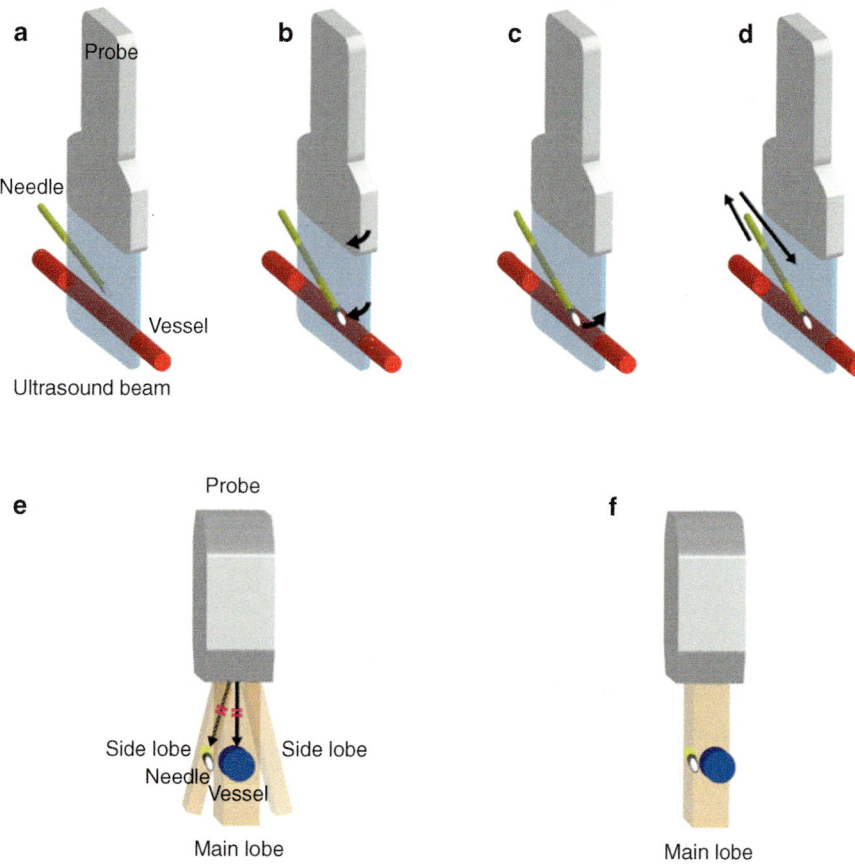

Fig. 21.2 Schematic representation of manoeuvers to bring needle tip back in best plane when using LAX-IP technique. (**a**) Needle tip is in USG plane. (**b**) Probe is rotated towards the needle tip. (**c**) Needle tip moved towards the centre of the beam. (**d**) Withdraw the needle till skin and restart the procedure. (**e**) Side-lobe artefact—when there is a strong reflection from the side lobe, the ultrasound machine mixes the reflected signals from main and side-lobe beam into same image. (**f**) Slice-thickness artefact—when needle and vessel are in the same beam width, even if the needle is not in the vessel, they are structure into the same image [5, 6]

21.6.3 Dynamic Needle Tip Positioning (DNTP)

It is possible to track needle tip in SAX-OOP approach and increase success rate using DNTP (Fig. 21.3) [7]. In DNTP technique

1. The needle tip is seen as bright echogenic dot between skin and anterior vessel wall.
2. While holding the needle in the dominant hand, slide the transducer probe slightly forwards such that needle tip disappears from the ultrasound image.

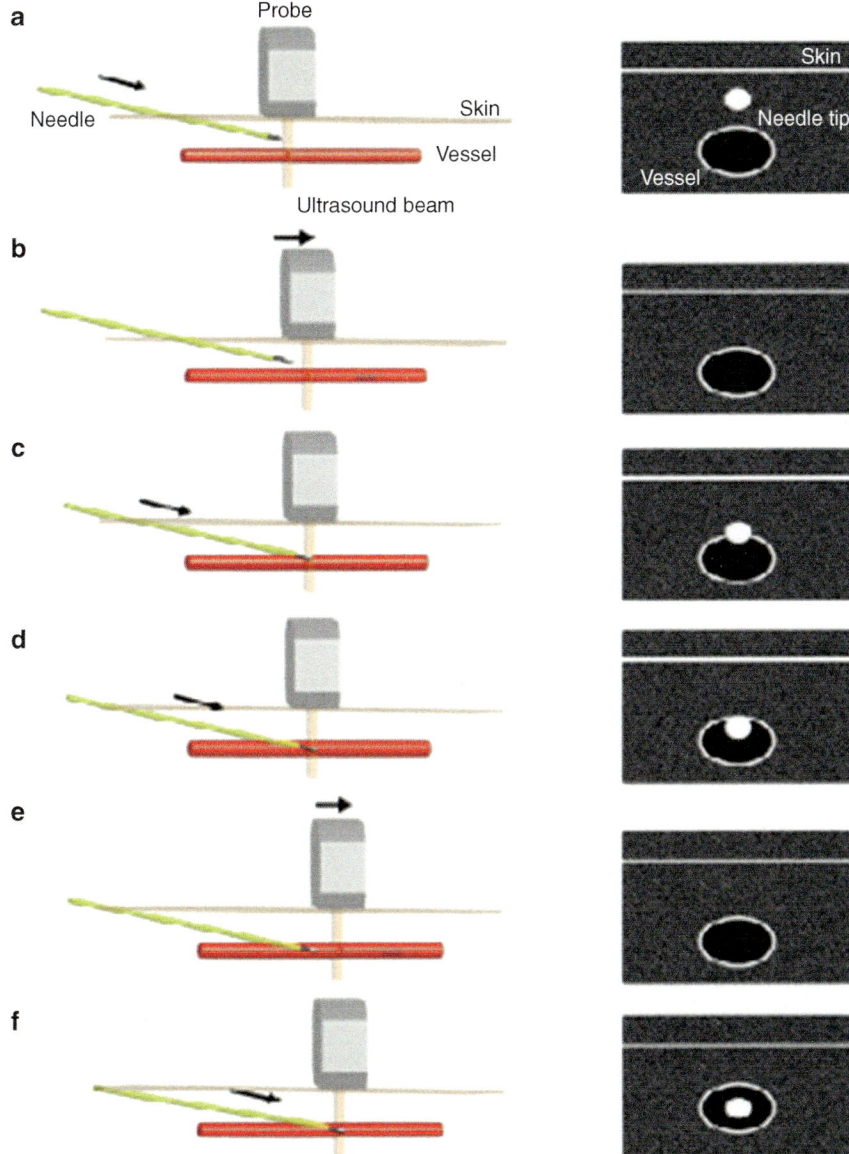

Fig. 21.3 Schematic and ultrasound representation of dynamic needle tip positioning (DNTP). (**a**) Needle tip is seen as a bright echogenic dot in subcutaneous tissue above anterior vessel wall. (**b**) Probe is advanced slightly forwards such that echogenic needle tip disappears from the image. (**c**) Needle is advanced such that needle tip is seen on top of the vessel wall. (**d**) Needle tip penetrates vessel wall and needle tip is seen inside vessel wall. (**e**) Probe is further advanced until echogenic point disappears from the image. (**f**) Needle is advanced till echogenic tip appears in the centre of the vessel [7]

3. Now keep holding the probe in that position and advance needle gradually till needle tip reappears in the image.
4. Repeat steps 1–2–3 until needle is inside the vessel. When needle has entered adequate depth, withdraw the stylet and thread in the catheter.

DNTP has better success rate than static SAX-OOP approach. However, sufficient experience in ultrasound is required to successfully perform this procedure in smaller children and neonates as it involves series of fine and precise movements.

21.6.4 Techniques Aiding USG Vascular Access

In paediatric population, where radial artery is located at a depth <2 mm. Increasing the depth to 2–4 mm by subcutaneous saline injection improves success rate in SAX-OOP approach. Saline injection also provides anechoic area on top of vessel wall which enhance USG signals and improves visibility of needle tip.

21.7   Complications

Complications of USG vascular access are same as in the non-USG cannulations. Some complications relating to the equipment and probe failure, electric or battery failure, and guidewire breakage etc. are unique to the USG approach. All the complications of vascular cannulation are listed in Box 21.1.

Box 21.1 Complications of vascular access

On insertion	Postinsertion
Air embolism	Dislodgement
Arrhythmias	Catheter-associated infection, sepsis
Arterial puncture	Catheter malfunction
Nerve injury	Device occlusion
Cardiac tamponade	Extravasation
Failure	Thrombosis
Guidewire fracture	Right atrial perforation
Haematoma at insertion site	Cardiac tamponade
Haemorrhage	Hydrothorax
Haemothorax	Chylothorax
Pneumothorax	At the time of removal—vascular tear, catheter breakage, bleeding
Vascular damage	
Tricuspid valve damage	
Chylothorax	

21.8 Conclusion

There is increasing evidence supporting utility of ultrasound for vascular access. Understanding of appropriate techniques and operator experience is key for successful vascular catheterisation and avoidance of complications

References

1. AIUM practice guideline for the use of ultrasound to guide vascular access procedures. J Ultrasound Med. 2013;32:191–215.
2. Gottlieb M, Holladay D, Peksa GD. Comparison of short- vs long-axis technique for ultrasound-guided peripheral line placement: a systematic review and meta-analysis. Cureus. 2018;10:e2718.
3. Quan Z, Tian M, Chi P, Cao Y, Li X, Peng K. Modified short-axis out-of-plane ultrasound versus conventional long-axis in-plane ultrasound to guide radial artery cannulation: a randomized controlled trial. Anesth Analg. 2014;119:163–9.
4. Song IK, Choi JY, Lee JH, Kim EH, Kim HJ, Kim HS, et al. Short-axis/out-of-plane or long-axis/in-plane ultrasound-guided arterial cannulation in children: a randomised controlled trial. Eur J Anaesthesiol. 2016;33:522–7.
5. Takeshita J, Yoshida T, Nakajima Y, Nakayama Y, Nishiyama K, Ito Y, et al. Superiority of dynamic needle tip positioning for ultrasound-guided peripheral venous catheterization in patients younger than 2 years old: a randomized controlled trial. Pediatr Crit Care Med. 2019;20:e410–e4.
6. Takeshita J, Yoshida T, Nakajima Y, Nakayama Y, Nishiyama K, Ito Y, et al. Dynamic needle tip positioning for ultrasound-guided arterial catheterization in infants and small children with deep arteries: a randomized controlled trial. J Cardiothorac Vasc Anesth. 2019;33:1919–25.
7. Clemmesen L, Knudsen L, Sloth E, Bendtsen T. Dynamic needle tip positioning - ultrasound guidance for peripheral vascular access. A randomized, controlled and blinded study in phantoms performed by ultrasound novices. Ultraschall Med. 2012;33:E321–5.

Monitoring During Anaesthesia in the Newborn and Neonate

Archna Koul and Jayashree Sood

22.1 Introduction

Neonatal period is a highly vulnerable age in the life of a person. This vulnerability increases in babies who are born premature, low birth weight, with genetic and congenital deformities, defects and medical diseases. Surgical condition adds on the risk to their lives. Though many elective surgeries can be postponed in the neonatal age, especially to the 60 week postconceptual age, when the risk is less, many surgeries need to be undertaken in the neonatal period itself, often in the early days of life and within hours of birth. It is this time when the baby is struggling to cope with the extra uterine environment. Provision of anesthesia is essential for the surgery but has its own adverse affects.

The basic aim of monitoring during anaesthesia in neonates is to ensure the safety of the baby while not compromising with the quality of anaesthesia. The anaesthesiologist, through monitoring, should strive for prevention of occurrence of critical events during surgery and early detection of such events, if they occur, so that prompt measures can be instituted. Guidelines for intraoperative monitoring during anaesthesia were published by the American Society of Anaesthesiologists in 1986, amended in 2010 and reaffirmed on December 13, 2020 [1]. They recommend the presence of a qualified anaesthesiologist throughout the surgery to monitor oxygenation, ventilation, circulation and temperature of the patient (Fig. 22.1).

22.2 Various Monitoring Modalities Are as Follows

1. General examination

A. Koul (✉) · J. Sood
Institute of Anaesthesiology, Pain & Perioperative Medicine, Sir Ganga Ram Hospital, New Delhi, India

© The Author(s), under exclusive license to Springer Nature Singapore Pte Ltd. 2023
U. Saha (ed.), *Clinical Anesthesia for the Newborn and the Neonate*, https://doi.org/10.1007/978-981-19-5458-0_22

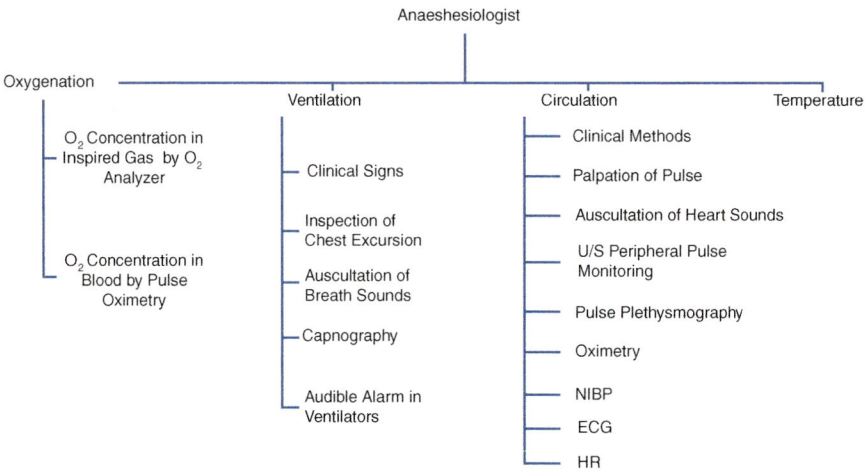

Fig. 22.1 Standards for basic anaesthetic monitoring developed by the Committee on Standards and Practice Parameters (CSPP)

    (a) Inspection
    (b) Palpation
      (c) Auscultation
          i. Precordial stethoscope
          ii. Oesophageal stethoscope
2. Systemic arterial blood pressure monitoring
    (a) Noninvasive blood pressure (NIBP)
    (b) Invasive blood pressure (IBP)
3. Central venous pressure (CVP)
4. CO2 measurement - End-tidal CO_2 (EtCO$_2$), Transcutaneous partial pressure of CO_2 (TcPCO$_2$)
5. Pulse oximetry (SpO2)
6. Electrocardiography (ECG)
7. Temperature
8. Near-infrared spectroscopy (NIRS)
9. Neurophysiological monitoring
    (a) Electroencephalography (EEG)
    (b) Evoked potential
    (c) Bispectral index (BIS)
10. Neuromuscular transmission (NMT)
11. Urine output Monitoring (UO)
12. Arterial Blood gases (ABG)

22.2.1 General Examination

Besides monitoring modalities, evaluation of qualitative clinical signs is very important as monitors can fail but anaesthesiologist can still rely on clinical assessment.

However, positioning and draping can make access to the baby difficult. If feasible, the following steps should be followed:

1. **Inspection**
    (a) Colour
        i. Cyanosis (lip, tongue, nail bed)
        ii. Pallor (conjunctiva, skin)
        iii. Mottling (trunk, extremities)
    (b) Respiration
        i. Rate and pattern
2. **Palpation**
    (a) Peripheral pulses
        i. Presence or absence
        ii. Capillary refilling time
    (b) Compliance of reservoir bag
3. **Auscultation** of heart and lung sounds is recommended by ASA guidelines. Precordial and oesophageal stethoscopes were important monitoring devices in the 1970s but these are less used nowadays, since advanced monitoring devices such as pulse oximetry and capnography are available for use [2]. These devices use sound waves for measurements and so are less prone to equipment malfunction:
    (a) **Precordial stethoscope** consists of the chest piece strapped on to baby's chest, which is then connected to an earpiece through an extension tubing. It can be placed at the apex of the heart, suprasternal notch or left sternal border, close to the left axilla above the nipple line. It went into disuse because of its bulkiness, liability of displacement, pressure injury in prone position and hindrance to intraoperative radiological assessment, when required the most [3].
    (b) **Oesophageal stethoscope** is a soft, plastic catheter (8–24F) with a distal opening covered by a balloon, passed through the mouth of the neonate (nasal route avoided) after tracheal intubation. It is passed down the oesophagus till the maximum intensity of heart and breath sounds is heard. However, being invasive, it carries the risk of esophageal injury and can be easily displaced into the stomach, and cannot be used during esophageal and tracheal surgeries, and neck dissection [4]. It is useful in cases, where a precordial stethoscope cannot be used.

22.2.2 Systemic Arterial Pressure Monitoring

This can be done by invasive and noninvasive means.

1. Noninvasive Blood Pressure (NIBP)

Monitoring of blood pressure is important under anaesthesia, because hypotension and hypertension in premature and newborn babies are risk factors that increase mortality and morbidity [5]. Conditions such as periventricular haemorrhage, encephalopathy, and long term neurodevelopmental defects can be avoided by proper management of perfusion to vital organs. Systolic blood pressure correlates with circulating blood volume, and can guide volume resuscitation, blood transfusion, administration of inotropes and vasopressors.

Measurement of blood pressure by an oscillometric method is preferred over the auscultatory method in preterm and newborn babies, because it is difficult to hear Korotkoff sounds in them [6]. However, the disadvantage of NIBP in neonates is that the systolic blood pressure is overestimated and diastolic blood pressure is underestimated [7] especially during hypotension. **Therefore, the reliability of NIBP is questionable in this age group.** In newborns, systolic pressure in the arms and legs is same; if leg systolic pressure is lower, then coarctation of the aorta must be suspected [6]. NIBP in the leg is usually lower than that in the arm in children as compared to adults probably due to soft compliant arteries, lower sympathetic tone and lower blood volume in legs [8, 9]. Right upper arm is the preferred site for NIBP as it best reflects the pressure in the ascending aorta, and is beneficial in neonates with coarctation of the thoracic aorta [10]. In preterm neonates (body weight <1.0 kg), blood pressure in the calf can also be recorded, but values are more variable and less accurate than those in the arm.

Precautions
1. The width of the cuff should be at least 40% of the arm circumference (arm circumference ratio close to 0.5). A too narrow cuff will overestimate and too wide a cuff will underestimate the blood pressure recording. In newborn and premature babies cuff size of 4.3 × 8 cm (Fig. 22.2) is usually used.

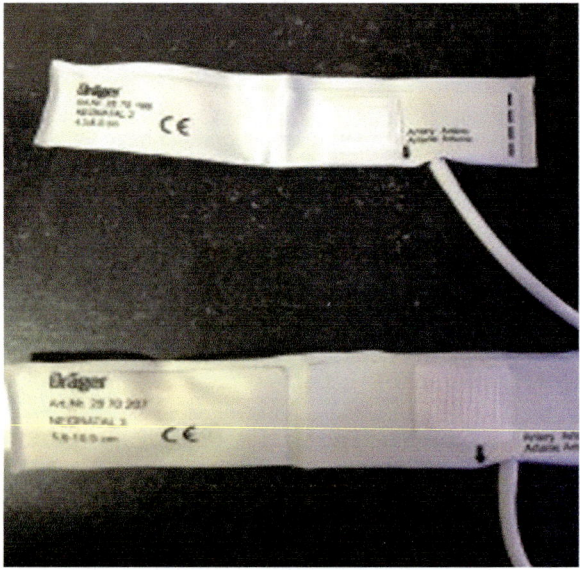

Fig. 22.2 Neonatal blood pressure cuffs

2. The cuff cycling time should not be less than 3–5 min to avoid any probability of limb ischemia. Repeated NIBP measurements may even fracture the bones in premature low birth weight babies as their bones are poorly ossified and calcium deficient.
3. The length of the cuff should cover 80% of the upper arm circumference [11]. it should not be so long as to completely encircle the arm, and the ends should never overlap. Thigh BP does not correlate well with arm or calf, so should be avoided in neonates [12, 13].
4. If BP does not correlate with the clinical condition of the neonate or if MAP <30 mmHg, then oscillometric devices are not reliable, and IBP is preferred.

Blood pressure in neonates is affected by gestational age and weight at birth, and postnatal age [14]. However, the most important endpoint of adequate blood pressure is end-organ perfusion.

Earlier, hypotension in newborn babies was defined as MAP less than gestational age in weeks, or MAP less than 30 mmHg [15]. During the first postnatal week, regardless of gestational age, blood pressure values vary each hour [16]. Hypotension is defined as any value that falls below the 5th percentile for gestational age or 10th percentile for postnatal age.

Neonatal hypertension is systolic blood pressure of at least 95th percentile for gestational age, birth weight and postnatal age [5]. Tables and charts are available that display blood pressure values based on sex, age and height percentile.

2. Invasive Blood Pressure/Intra-arterial Pressure (IBP)
IBP is the gold standard and provides accurate and continuous measurement of blood pressure, and is preferred choice in high-risk sick neonates [17]. In extreme preterm babies, NIBP values tend to be higher than IBP [18]. However, cannulation of arteries in this age group is technically challenging because of the small size of vessels and increased risk of complications.

Indications for IBP Monitoring:
1. Major surgery when excessive blood loss is anticipated.
2. When repeated arterial blood gas (ABG) analysis is required.
3. When NIBP monitoring is not possible or not reliable to guide fluid management.

Favoured sites: sites that have good collateral flow are preferred. In neonates, radial artery is preferred for cannulation (Fig. 22.3) [19]. Other sites are posterior tibial artery, ulnar artery, dorsalis pedis and femoral artery. The brachial artery does not have collaterals and is close to the median nerve, so is not advocated.

Umbilical Artery Cannulation is done usually in NICU in the first week of life. The tip of the catheter is placed in the inferior vena cava (IVC), at a level where it does not affect renal blood flow, i.e., either above T10 or below L5 [20], and confirmed radiologically. A disposable pressure transducer connected to the UAC is used for BP recording.

Fig. 22.3 Radial artery cannulation for IBP monitoring

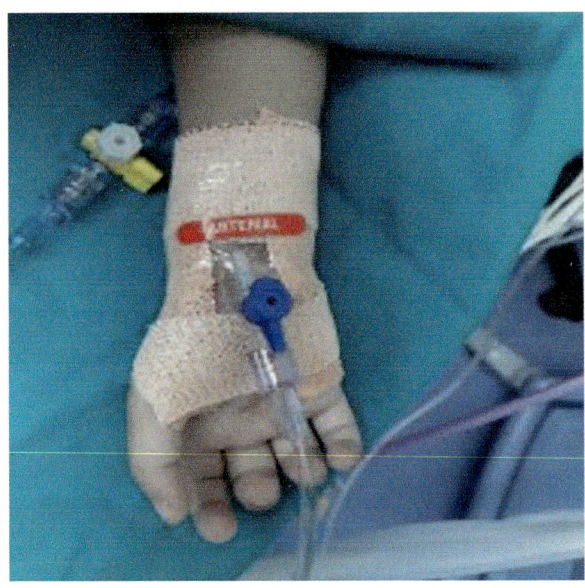

Size of cannula: the size of the arterial lumen occupied by the cannula should not be more than one-third of the internal diameter of the artery [21]. For term neonates (birth weight <1.2 kg) 24G IV cannula or UAC (2.5F size) with an outer diameter of 0.75 mm can be used. UAC (5F size) is used for babies with birth weight >1.2 kg.

Complications: the risk of complications is higher in premature and low birth weight babies, because the catheter-to-vessel size ratio is high, and technically difficult, involving multiple attempts, and adverse events. Minor complications (20%) include blanching due to temporary ischemia [22]. Thromboembolic events are the most common cause of limb ischemia in neonates [23]. Other complications include local hematoma, infection and nerve damage. Systolic and diastolic readings are affected by excessive damping caused by the mechanical properties of the intra-arterial catheter or transducer system and the presence of air bubbles. MAP is more reliable as it is not affected by damped traces [24].

Precautions: in extremely low birth weight babies the flush volume should be included in the fluid intake chart, 0.1–0.5 U/mL of heparin is used at the rate of 0.5 mL/h for babies <1 kg and 1 mL/h for >1 kg. Pressurized bags should be avoided and infusion pumps with low volume tubings and closed sampling lines should be used to minimize the risk of infection and loss of blood volume [25]. Flushing a blocked arterial line at high pressure can lead to cerebral artery embolization due to retrograde flow especially in babies with patent foramen ovale or patent ductus arteriosus. The use of ultrasound has improved the success rate [26]. Arterial cannulation should be avoided in the same limb, lower or higher, than the previous attempt [27].

22.2.3 Central Venous Pressure (CVP)

There is no absolute indication for CVP monitoring in neonates, as it is not practical and does not give much information about excessive afterload. CVP does not reflect accurate right atrial pressure in newborns due to shunts and transitional circulation [28]. The trends in CVP monitoring are more important than an absolute value to guide fluid replacement [29]. It is important to consider risk–benefit analysis before embarking on CVP catheterization in this vulnerable population. Global assessment of the CVS along with various signs of poor perfusion (skin colour, capillary refilling time, temperature, urine output, lactate and HCO_3 values) may have a better clinical outcome [30, 31].

Recommendations for CVP Monitoring:
- During surgeries, where major fluid shifts are anticipated
- Major blood loss of >50% of blood volume
- Cardiac surgeries
- Deliberate hypotension technique is used

Sites: for monitoring of CVP, central veins (internal jugular, subclavian) are preferred over peripheral veins (femoral). The umbilical vein is the preferred in babies weighing <800 g, best within 48 h of birth (maximum up to 1 week). An umbilical vein catheter must pass through the ductus venous and lie in the IVC, above the liver. Multiple lumen catheter is preferable in infants <1000 g or in those who are extremely sick, while single lumen catheter is preferred in others, size 3.5F for babies with birth weight <1.5 kg and 5F for birth weight >1.5 kg.

Normal CVP is usually between 2 and 6 mmHg (Fig. 22.4). CVP more than 7 mmHg is indicative of cardiac dysfunction or persistent pulmonary hypertension or respiratory embarrassment due to increased intrathoracic pressure, such as pneumothorax. The younger the patient, greater is the prevalence of anatomical variation in the landmarks, smaller is the size of the veins, with increased collapsibility during puncture [32, 33]. Use of ultrasound for localization and insertion increases the success rate. Infection, venous thrombosis, catheter obstruction, technical difficulties during insertion and maintenance are commonly encountered complications in neonates.

Fig. 22.4 Monitoring of
ECG, SpO$_2$, NIBP, IBP,
CVP and temperature

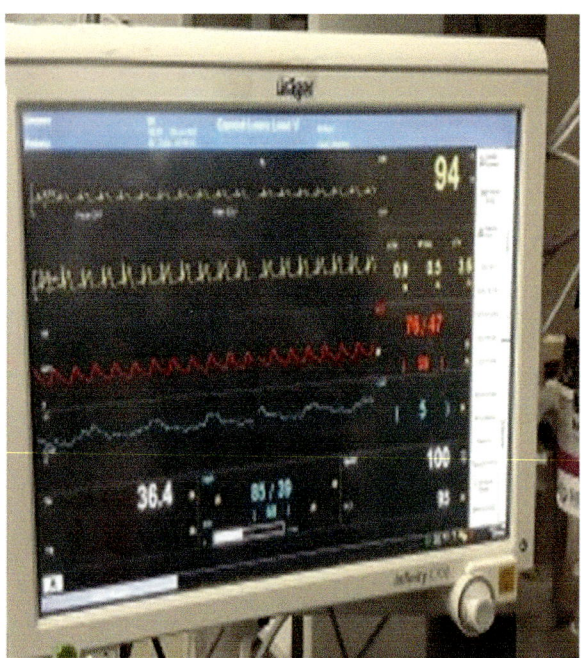

22.2.4 CO$_2$ Monitoring

22.2.4.1 End-Tidal CO$_2$ (EtCO$_2$)

ABG is the standard for evaluation of arterial CO$_2$ levels with limitations of being invasive and noncontinuous. During general anaesthesia, continuous, noninvasive measurement of CO$_2$ in expired gas is done by sampling expired CO$_2$ using either a mainstream or side stream sampling line [34, 35]. Monitoring of EtCO$_2$ is important for prevention and detection of hypocarbia and hypercarbia as these can lead to adverse neurological [36] outcomes such as intracranial haemorrhage, periventricular leukomalacia [37] and diffuse white matter injury. Capnography allows rapid detection of unintended oesophageal intubation, and is a useful to confirm correct placement of ETT.

Limitations of Capnography in Neonates and Preterm:

1. Analyser dead space can lead to rebreathing of expired CO2, especially in low weight babies.
2. CO2 production is low (15 mL/min) and can lead to sampling errors and erroneous readings.
3. An exaggerated phase II and or absence of alveolar plateau in Phase III in the capnographic trace may be seen, with wide variation in EtCO2, contributory factors being low tidal volume, higher respiratory rate and low maximum expiratory flow rates [3, 38].
4. Leakage around uncuffed tubes and loss of expired gases, also gives lower EtCO2 values.

5. In preterm neonates with significant lung disease, EtCO2 poorly correlates with PaCO2 [39].
6. Right-to-left shunt (decreased pulmonary blood flow) affects accuracy of $EtCO_2$ estimation [40].

22.2.4.1.1 Mainstream Analyzers vs Side Stream Analyzers

In the mainstream analyzers, the infrared light source and a detector are located in the analyzer itself, the sample chamber is inline and close to the endotracheal tube (ET). The response is fast and reliable at the respiratory rates of neonates. However, the chamber dead space may be more than the tidal volume and its weight may kink or dislodge the ET or breathing circuit [41]. The $EtCO_2$ values may not be precise especially in babies <1.4 kg, being nearly 13 mmHg lower than $PaCO_2$ [42].

Sidestream analyzers receive expired gases via a long tube attached to a T piece adaptor in the breathing system. They are lighter and have low dead space; however, their response time is longer and the sampling line can get blocked due to kinking or secretions. A sampling flow rate (expired gas flow) of 150 mL/min is appropriate for neonates, and if the flow rate is less, it underestimates the CO_2 values [35].

In preterms with tidal volume <5 mL, a side stream analyzer is preferred with a shorter sampling line [34, 35, 43]. New microstream capnometers with small chamber and low suction rate (30 mL/min) [44], and lightweight infrared mainstream sensors (dead space <1 mL) are available [41].

22.2.4.1.2 Advantages of Capnography

It is a useful to detect failed intubation and ventilation, anaesthesia machine/circuit failure and failed circulation before any fatal damage occurs [45]. Updated ASA Standard for monitoring (2005) recommend capnography in children both during spontaneous and controlled ventilation [46].

In spontaneously breathing babies, $EtCO_2$ monitoring is a predictor of $PaCO_2$ thus avoiding arterial puncture. It also acts as an apnea monitor, and detects airway obstruction in conditions, such as bronchial asthma and laryngotracheobronchitis and can also help detect conditions, such as bronchopulmonary dysplasia, where the arterial-to-end-tidal CO_2 gradient can rise [45].

An ABG is invasive, intermittent and requires repeated blood sampling which may not be feasible in premature and low birth weight babies.

Monitoring $EtCO_2$ is the standard of care for indirect estimation of $PaCO_2$ in OT, because it confirms the correct placement of the ET, detects disconnection and dislodgement of ETT and identifies apnoea or airway obstruction even before a pulse oximeter can [45].

Correlation of $EtCO_2$ and $PaCO_2$ may be affected by factors, such as sampling errors, patient positioning, V/Q mismatch, small tidal volume and presence of congenital cyanotic heart disease [47, 48]. Noninvasive, continuous monitoring of transcutaneous partial pressure of carbon dioxide ($TcPCO_2$) can be used as an adjunct with $EtCO_2$ monitoring [34]. Various causes of abnormal $EtCO_2$ measurements in the neonate are listed in Table 22.1.

Table 22.1 Common causes of abnormal EtCO$_2$ values in preterm, neonates and newborns

	Increased EtCO$_2$	Absent or decreased EtCO$_2$
Respiratory related	Hypoventilation, Rebreathing Endobronchial intubation, Partial airway obstruction, Aspiration, pneumothorax	Hyperventilation, Apnoea, Total airway obstruction
CVS related	Increase in CO or BP	Decrease in CO or BP, Pulmonary embolism, Hypovolemia, Left to Right shunt, Cardiac arrest
Equipment related	Exhausted soda-lime, machine Ventilator–valve dysfunction, Kinks in the breathing circuit, ET obstruction, Increase in apparatus dead space, HME filter, Long ET, Mainstream capnometer	Accidental extubation or disconnection of the tube from the circuit
Others	Hyperthermia, Administration of NaHCO3	Hypothermia

22.2.4.2 Transcutaneous Partial Pressure of CO$_2$ (TcPCO$_2$)

Noninvasive continuous monitoring of TcPCO$_2$ can be used as an adjunct to EtCO$_2$ monitoring [34]. It measures skin surface partial pressure of CO$_2$ and O$_2$. An electrochemical or optical sensor is placed on any flat skin surface such as chest, abdomen or forehead. It increases the skin temperature of the skin up to 42–43 °C causing vasodilatation and arterialisation of capillaries, improving CO$_2$ diffusion through the skin and to the membrane of the monitor [49]. The thin skin of preterm neonates may facilitate better diffusion of CO$_2$ compared to adults and so the measured values of TcPCO$_2$ are more reliable. TcPCO$_2$ gives a better reflection of PaCO$_2$.

Advantages
- Is noninvasive.
- Can be used in cases, where EtCO$_2$ in monitoring is not reliable.
- Can be used for continuous CO$_2$ monitoring in un-intubated babies [43, 50, 51].
- Can be used during airway endoscopic procedures and procedural sedation.

Disadvantages
- Requires local preheating, calibration and equilibration of the sensor, so a 10 min time lag after application of the sensor to the skin [52].
- Accuracy of measurement is affected by many factors, such as skin thickness, edema, poor tissue perfusion, scarring, acidosis, and vasoconstrictors (dopamine, epinephrine).
- Heat-induced skin damage and burns is a probability [53]. The sensor position should be changed at regular intervals, with recalibration each time, which is not be feasible in a draped and inaccessible baby.

- For every 1 °C increase in temperature, there is 4–5% increase in local CO_2 production from the epidermal cells. This may overestimate CO_2 values, so temperature correction is required [54].

Hence, $TcPCO_2$ is only a complementary tool along with $EtCO_2$ monitoring in critically ill babies.

22.2.5 Pulse Oximetry (SpO₂)

SpO_2 is the standard of care for monitoring of proper oxygenation during surgery under anaesthesia. Continuous oximetry is included in the basic monitoring standards of ASA that can detect hypoxia before occurrence of cyanosis [55]. Foetal and adult Hb have similar absorption characteristics, so there is no interference in accuracy of measurement.

SpO_2 is based on the principle of differential absorption and transmission of red and infrared light by oxy and deoxygenated haemoglobin in the blood, and measures the amount of light transmitted. The ratio of red light to infrared light transmitted is processed into SpO_2 value (Beer–Lambert law). The equipment also displays a plethysmographic trace that reflects the pulse volume (Fig. 22.5a)

Preterm infants are susceptible to the harmful effects of hypoxia (NEC, death) and hyperoxia (ROP, BPD), thus, there is an oxygen dilemma as both hypoxia and hyperoxia are detrimental [56]. The European guidelines recommend SpO_2 target between 90 and 95% and alarm limits of 89–95% [57]. In

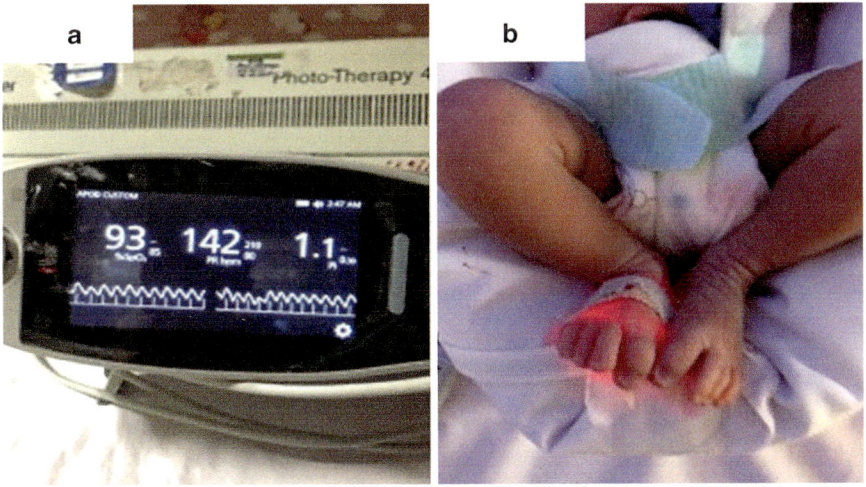

Fig. 22.5 (**a**) Pulse oximeter showing SpO₂, HR and perfusion index along with plethysmographic trace. (**b**) Pulse oximeter probe placed on the sole

clinical practice, SpO_2 of 95–97% corresponding to PaO_2 of 50–70 mmHg in neonates should be safe under anaesthesia. After 1st week of life, SpO_2 <94% is inadequate for tissue perfusion. In extremely low birth weight babies target range of SpO_2 depends on gestational age, postnatal age, Hb and underlying disease [56]. A difference of more than 5–10% in preductal (right hand) and postductal (foot) should raise an alarm. In neonates with congenital heart disease (CHD), pulse oximetry has a screening role (before the onset of symptoms) [58, 59] (Fig. 22.5b).

Limitations with Pulse Oximeters

1. *Accuracy:* there is some discrepancy between the values of SpO_2 and saturation of arterial blood (SaO_2) in neonates. SaO_2 measures O_2 saturation of both functional and nonfunctional Hb but SpO_2 measures the oxygen saturation of only functional Hb. SpO_2 overestimates saturation especially at values <91% (range 85–89%) [60]. Pulse oximeters are only calibrated down to 80%, and values <80% may not be a predictor of accurate PaO_2 [61]. In babies with cyanotic heart disease, pulse oximeters exhibit a positive bias, thus decreasing their accuracy.
2. *Averaging times:* most devices have a lag time of 12–16 s before they interpret the information, averaging over several heartbeats. Long averaging times can lead to delay in the detection of desaturation.
3. *Relationship between PaO_2 and SaO_2:* this is linear at SaO_2 <80% [62]. At SaO_2 >80%, small change in SaO_2 results in a large change in PaO_2. This is due to fetal Hb which shifts oxygen dissociation curve (ODC) to left. Therefore, at high levels, SpO_2/SaO_2 becomes less reliable predictor of PaO_2; this is crucial in neonates receiving supplemental O_2.
4. *Pretem babies:* accuracy of measurement of light absorbed by the pulsatile arterial component is disturbed by motion artifacts, presence of vernix, lower perfusion pressure, peripheral edema, high ambient light (headlamps, phototherapy), hypothermia, Hemoglobinopathies [63], skin wrinkles or cracks and acrocyanosis. The dermis is thin and liable to injury (pressure, burn) if the probe is applied for prolonged period. Probe site should be changed every 2 hourly. A too tight probe can even cause limb ischemia [50].

New pulse oximeters based on **signal extraction technology (SET),** that measures composite of arterial and nonarterial pulsatile signals, overcomes the interference caused by low perfusion and motion [64]. They detect desaturation more efficiently with fewer incidences of false alarms [65]. **SET technology** measures composite of arterial and nonarterial pulsatile signals. **Reflectance pulse oximeters** measure reflected rather than transmitted light and might be less affected by motion artifacts and low perfusion, so SpO_2 is measured from the core body (chest, back wrist, forehead). However, this is sensitive to noise, pressure and ambient light [66].

22.2.6 ECG

The basic goal of ECG monitoring in neonates is to estimate heart rate and rhythm so that intraoperative arrhythmias are managed before any irreversible damage is done. ECG can detect hypoxia-induced bradycardia much before SpO_2 detected desaturation.

ECG of Infants and Preterm Babies is Different from the Adults:

1. Since, the right ventricle is thicker than the left ventricle in newborns and neonates as compared to adults, right ventricle predominance is noted in precordial leads with right axis deviation. In premature babies (<35 week gestation) have relatively less right ventricular dominance [67].

2. A neonatal heart is small with few myocardial contractile element (depolarization and repolarization), so PR interval, QRS duration and QT intervals are shorter compared to adults. In adults QRS width is <0.12 s and in children it is <0.08 s [68].

3. The appearance of arrhythmias is also different due to elevated basal heart rate, small size of the heart, autonomic denervation and sinus and AV nodal function immaturity.

4. Normal heart rate range varies with the age. Day 1 (94–155/min), 1–3 days (91–158/min), and 7–30 days (106–182/min) [68]. At rapid heart rates it is difficult to diagnose arrhythmias [69].

5. ST-segment changes are rare in children and are difficult to interpret at rapid heart rates. Lead II is recommended for intraoperative monitoring as it provides more information regarding the atrial activity for diagnosis of arrhythmia [70].

6. Common arrhythmias encountered introperatively are sinus tachycardia, sinus bradycardia and supraventricular tachycardias (SVT). For proper diagnosis, assessment of rate, regularity and length of ORS complex is very important and a correction factor added for tachycardia. The most common cause of sinus bradycardia is hypoxia, while sinus tachycardia is caused by pain, fever, hypovolemia and light plane of anaesthesia. SVT are commonly seen during intubation or light plane of anaesthesia [71].

7. CHD: cardiac monitoring is for babies with CHD undergoing noncardiac surgery or those who have undergone repair of the defect. These babies are extremely prone to develop arrhythmias (atrial flutter, junctional ectopic tachycardia) [72].

8. Electrolyte abnormalities: hyperkalemia and hypocalcemia following rapid blood transfusion intraoperatively can also be detected by the ECG.

22.2.7 Temperature

Hypothermia is an important risk factor for mortality in premature and newborn babies. Uncorrected thermal stress is a cause of cerebral, circulatory and respiratory depression in neonates [73]. Hypothermia initiates a vicious cycle; thermal stress causes compensatory release of norepinephrine which leads to pulmonary and peripheral vasoconstriction. Pulmonary vasoconstriction facilitates the right to left intracardiac shunting, while peripheral vasoconstriction can cause anaerobic metabolism leading to acidosis, hypoxia and further right to left shunt, reversal to fetal circulation (PFC), increased O_2 demand, depletion of nonprotein-energy stores, reduction in surfactant production and respiratory distress [3, 74]. Besides, hypothermia can also cause delayed wound healing, surgical infections, coagulation abnormalities (from platelet dysfunction), diminished metabolism of drugs leading to delayed recovery from anaesthesia [75].

Temperature monitoring is very important during anaesthesia and surgery. Normal body temperature is 37 ± 0.2 °C. Preterm and newborn babies are highly susceptible to hypothermia.

Ambient temperature in newborns should not be less than 22 °C, because

- They have a large surface area to body mass ratio, enhancing heat loss by evaporation.
- Thin fat devoid tissue layers and reduced stratum corneum provide poor or no insulation, and facilitate insensible water losses, while structural and functional immaturity of the skin causes high transepidermal water loss [76].
- The head occupies almost 20% of body surface area, skull bones are thin, hair is sparse and vessels are in proximity to the scalp, further promoting heat loss.
- The preterm neonates are deficient in brown adipose tissue making them more vulnerable to hypothermia [77].
- Thermoneutral temperature, i.e., the temperature at which O_2 demand is minimal is 32–35 °C for neonates and >35 °C in small premature babies. The difference between environmental (32–34 °C) and the skin temperatures (36 °C) should be 2–4 °C in newborns [78]. Hypothermia is classified as Mild (core temperature 36 °C–36.4 °C), Moderate (35.9 °–32 °C) and Severe (<32 °C) [79].

a. Heat Loss Mechanisms in OR and Under GA

Under GA, first hour following induction, there is internal redistribution of heat from the core to periphery and ultimately to the environment, by radiation (39%), convection (34%), evaporation (24%) and conduction 3% [80]. Heat production is also reduced due to decreased metabolic rate, absent muscle activity, and inhibition of nonshivering thermogenesis (NST) along with inhibition of central thermoregulation.

Anaesthesia lowers the threshold temperature at which the body initiates a compensatory mechanism. NST is the main mechanism of heat production in premature babies (26–30 week gestational age). Anesthesia abolishes NST because of opioids, propofol and inhalational anaesthesia [81, 82].

b. Temperature Monitoring Devices in OR

Mercury in glass thermometers have been replaced by thermocouples and thermistors which can give continuous recording of temperature. Infrared scanners and thermometers are used for intermittent temperature monitoring in NICU.

c. Temperature Monitoring Sites

Ideally, the temperature monitoring site should reflect core temperature. Site chosen depends on the surgical procedure, duration of surgery and ease of placement of the probe [83].

The various temperature probes commonly used in OR are:

Nasopharyngeal probe: it should be placed in the posterior nasopharynx in contact with the soft palate. The low temperature of cold respiratory gases leaking around the uncuffed tube can interfere with its accuracy (Fig. 22.6a).

Esophagal temperature probe: can measure core temperature accurately if the tip of the probe lies in the distal third of the oesophagus. In premature and newborns, its accuracy may be reduced by the closeness to cold gases in the tracheobronchial tree.

Tympanic membrane: though an ideal monitoring site is not used much due to the risk of perforation of tympanic membrane if the probe touches it.

Axillary temperature: is commonly used and is convenient. The probe should be on the skin over the axillary artery and arm adducted.

Rectal and bladder temperature: probes have also been used. However, they are not used very frequently due to the risk of infection, interference by faeces and quantity of urine.

Skin temperature: is least indicative of core temperature especially if the sensor is placed more peripherally [84]. However, skin temperature over carotid has been found to accurately reflect core temp with a minor correction factor of 0.52 [85].

Prevention of hypothermia:

1. Operating room temperature should be 29 °C for premature and 27 °C for term babies.
2. Relative humidity of operation theatre should be 40–60%.

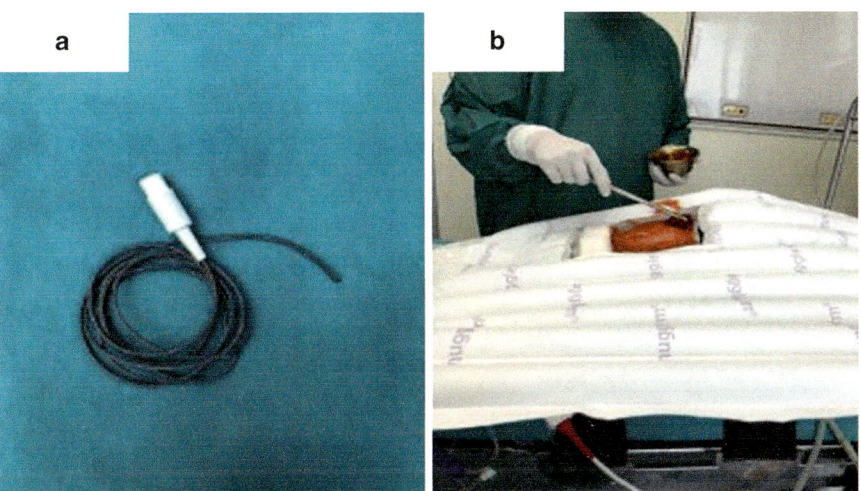

Fig. 22.6 (a) Nasopharyngeal temperature probe. (b) Convective forced air warmer

3. Baby should not be left exposed before and after induction of anaesthesia, radiant heaters can be used. However, their prolonged use must be avoided to prevent insensible heat loss and burns [86].
4. The baby's skin should not be in contact with any metallic surfaces to prevent heat transfer and thermal injuries.
5. The body and head should be covered during preinduction and induction of anaesthesia, as a simple single layer of covering also reduces heat loss by convection and radiation.
6. Convective forced-air warmers are most effective skin surface warming devices (Fig. 22.6b) [87].
7. Warming mattress is quite effective in very low birth weight and preterm babies with body surface area <0.5 sqm [88].
8. IV fluids and blood must be prewarmed. Length of tubing distal to warmer should be short [89].
9. All irrigation fluids should be warmed.
10. Circulating water mattresses and energy pads are also used occasionally.
11. Neonates have high minute ventilation per kg of body weight. Heat and humidity can be added to inspired gases using ultrasonic heated humidifiers or heat and moisture exchanging filters. Inspiratory gases should be heated only to normal temperature, and dead space of the exchanger should be small [90]. Small filters are also prone to occlusion, obstruction and increased work of breathing. Extreme vigilance is mandatory when using these devices [91].

Hyperthermia: anaesthesia increases the threshold temperature for compensatory mechanisms which are sweating and vasodilation. Neonatal hyperthermia (in OR, temp >37.5 °C) is usually secondary to overheating or sepsis or hypermetabolism. If untreated can lead to seizures, coma and death.

22.2.8 Near-Infrared Spectroscopy (NIRS)

Protection of cerebral function in premature and expremature neonates during anaesthesia and surgery is important because of their vulnerability due to physiological factors. NIRS is a noninvasive, portable, continuous monitoring device that can detect hypoxic or ischemic changes in organs, such as the brain, muscles, kidney and intestine.

It was originally used for estimation of cerebral oxygenation during deep hypothermic circulatory arrest during cardiopulmonary bypass in neonates with CHD [92], and since has gained popularity for use in noncardiac surgeries, congenital diaphragmatic hernia (CDH) and esophageal atresia [93].

a. Principle
It works on the same principle as the pulse oximeter, except that it is nonpulsatile venous oximeter. It applies infrared light of wavelength (650–1100 nm range) that can penetrate tissue and bone. The emitted photons are differentially absorbed by

oxy and deoxyhaemoglobin and reflected photons are returned to the detector on the tissue surface [94]. NIRS does not require pulsatile flow, measures arterial (16%) and venous (84%) components alike, is reliable and works even in circulatory arrest states. It measures the regional O_2 saturation (**rSO$_2$**) and can be used to measure cerebral regional O_2 saturation (**C-rSO$_2$**), that reflects changes in blood pressure, arterial O_2 saturation and PaO_2 [95]. It can detect hypoperfusion regardless of the cause, and can help predict the long term postoperative neurological outcome. Apart from neuro and cardiac surgeries, it has a potential for detecting intra-abdominal hypertension and compartment syndrome after abdominal surgeries in neonates [92, 96].

b. Normal Values and Anesthesia
C-rSO$_2$ reference range is ±65% to ±70% and is same for term, preterm and SGA babies [97]. As validated lower safety margins are not available, awake value is taken as baseline to predict trends (Fig. 22.7b). To ensure safety under anaesthesia, target for C-rSO$_2$ values is higher than baseline.

A fall of 20% in rSO$_2$ from baseline or an absolute value of 50% indicates hypoxic injury, and an absolute value of <30% signifies severe ischemia (below 40%, brain injury increases hourly) [98–101].

c. Placement of Sensors:
Sensors are placed on the skin over the area of interest (cerebral sensors on forehead) (Fig. 22.7a, b), and renal sensors on the lower back between T_{10}–L_2. Currently available sensors may not be reliable in neonates <2.5 kg as its tiny head will detect oxygenation of white matter rather than the cortical trace [97, 102].

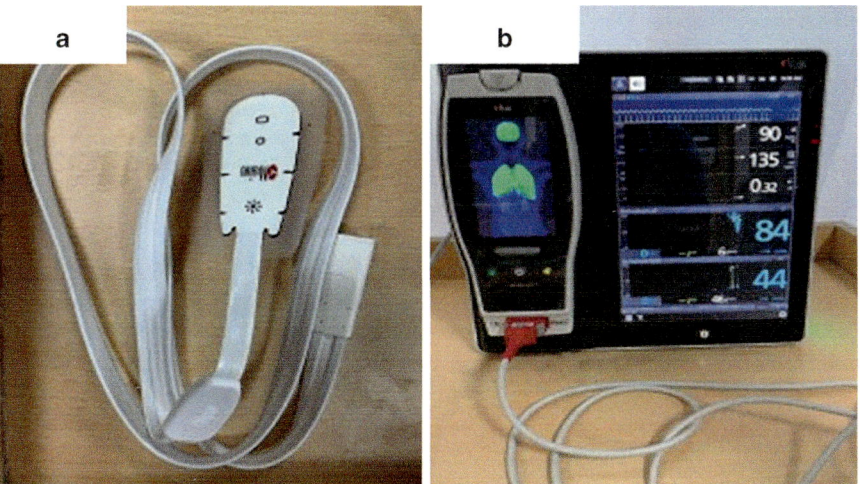

Fig. 22.7 (**a**) Sensor for NIRS monitoring. (**b**) NIRS monitor

At induction, after the sleep dose of hypnotics, there is 5–10% increase in C-rSO$_2$ due to decrease in cerebral metabolic rate (CMRO$_2$). Decreased C-rSO$_2$ indicates inadequate ventilation and hypotension.

During maintenance, C-rSO$_2$ will be less than that at induction due to reduction in FiO$_2$ than at induction, but should still be more than the baseline. Hypotension is the most common cause of low C-rSO$_2$, while sedatives and hypnotics (decrease CMRO$_2$) increases C-rSO$_2$. Blood glucose and body temperature by affecting cerebral perfusion may also affect C-rSO$_2$ value

Limitations
- Baseline awake C-rSO$_2$ is mandatory to interpret intraoperative measurements.
- Very high and very low values are easy to interpret.
- The intermediate values may create difficult interpretation.
- It gives an idea about cerebral perfusion and oxygenation while simultaneous evaluation of vitals (BP, HR, PaCO$_2$, SpO$_2$) which contribute to cerebral perfusion, enable safety in OR.
- The information provided by NIRS cannot be extrapolated to indicate global hypoperfusion.
- There can be interference due to scalp, skull, dura, skin, hyperbilirubinemia and melanin.
- The forehead sensor cannot detect changes in posterior circulation.
- NIRS is frequently monitored in NICU, but its use in OR needs to be widened.

22.2.9 Neurophysiological Monitoring

This is used to detect any insult during surgery so that prompt remedial steps can be taken before any irreversible damage occurs. Commonly used methods are electroencephalography (EEG), bispectral index (BIS), and evoked potentials.

22.2.9.1 Electroencephalography (EEG)
Preterm and neonates are extremely vulnerable to brain insults during anaesthesia and surgery secondary to potential hemodynamic disturbances, ventilation and gas exchange issue and increase in ICP, especially during the surgical repair of CHD requiring deep hypothermic circulatory arrest. EEG can be used to interpret the exact time and severity of brain insult [103–105].

Conventional EEG is the gold standard for evaluating neurological well-being of sick neonates in NICU. It records the electrical activity of the brain through a number of electrodes (9–40) attached to the scalp and face. Limitations to its routine use arise from its technical complexity, time demands, requirement for exact interpretation and cost. Amplitude-integrated EEG (aEEG) is now being used instead of conventional EEG, which is based on single or double channel for recording EEG using 3–5 scalp electrodes. The signals are filtered, rectified, time-compressed and displayed on a semi-logarithmic scale [106, 107].

22.2.9.1.1 How EEG is Evaluated:

The background activity: major part of the EEG trace is occupied by the background activity. In very preterm babies background activity is discontinuous, with increased amplitude waves alternating with low amplitude activity. In term, late preterm and near term neonates, the background activity is continuous and of low amplitude waves. With the increase in gestational age, EEG becomes more continuous. Burst suppression (high-voltage bursts alternating with suppressed background) and continuous low voltage or flat trace are pathological. In babies with intraventricular haemorrhage and periventricular leukomalacia, there is an acute disturbance in background activity [108].

Sleep–wake cycling: there is a cyclical fluctuation in amplitude and degree of discontinuity in various phases of sleep and wakefulness. The absence of sleep awake cycling is a predictor of poor motor and cognitive outcome.

Seizures: usually present as spike and slow-wave complexes.

Artifacts: may be physiological (myogenic potentials, ECG artifacts, respiratory artifacts) or nonphysiological (electrical or device-related).

Anesthesia: factors such as oxygen saturation, changes in CO_2 levels, depth of anaesthesia, blood pressure and temperature can all affect EEG but the changes are slow in onset in contrast to ischemic changes which occur within seconds. Opiates and benzodiazepines decrease the amplitude of waves, and discontinuity increases with level of sedation.

Hypoxic–ischemic encephalopathy (HIE): *mild HIE* (hypoxia, ischemia, hypoglycemia) is reflected as discontinuous EEG with absence of cyclicity with increased amplitude, while **Severe HIE** is reflected as low voltage complexes, absent sleep–wake cycling followed by burst suppression.

22.2.9.2 Evoked potentials

Somatosensory evoked potentials (**SSEP**) assess the integrity of the sensory dorsal column or ascending tract on the spinal cord. Stimulation sites are the median or ulnar nerve in the upper limb or posterior tibial or common peroneal nerve in the lower limb and recording is done by the electrodes placed over the scalp or spine.

Motor evoked potentials (**MEP**) assess the integrity of descending spinal motor tracts through transcranial, electrical or magnetic stimuli. Motor area in brain or spinal cord is stimulated and the response is recorded at the level of the muscle or the efferent nerve. Intraoperatively, if MEP is maintained at a baseline level and if it deteriorates temporarily and recovers before the end of the surgery, chances are that no new motor deficit will occur [109].

Besides SSEP and MEP, brain stem auditory evoked potential and visual evoked potentials aid in checking the functional integrity of cranial nerves.

22.2.9.2.1 Anesthesia, Neonate and Evoked Potential Monitoring

Salient features in neonates

(a) MEP can be recorded in all age groups as suggested by many studies and case reports [110–112].

(b) Due to slower conduction velocity, the display windows should be kept between 200 and 300 ms; the baseline kept at 100 m/s and if the responses are absent they are increased up to 300 m/s to check for delayed responses.

(c) Inhalational agents and neuromuscular blocking drugs should be avoided as they interfere with the monitoring.

(d) Hypothermia, very common in neonates, significantly affects the latency and morphology of evoked potentials.

(e) Neonates require higher intensities for stimulation, intensities for more than 500 V are often needed for MEP. Neonates also require longer interstimulus intensity (5ms) train and or double train stimulation [113].

(f) Evoked potentials are assessed in terms of latency, amplitude and interpeak latencies. More than a 50% decrease in the amplitude and a 10% increase in the latency during spinal surgery may represent injury.

Challenges in neonates during evolved potential monitoring

1. In neonates, there is incomplete myelination of the corticospinal tract [112]. Although myelination begins in the second trimester, yet this process is not complete at birth. This may lead to the desynchronisation of MEP.

2. At birth, the conduction velocity of motor neurons in the spinal cord is less (approximately 10 m/s) as compared to adults (50–70 m/s) [114]. Therefore, lesser the age, higher the threshold voltage required for eliciting the muscular activity.

3. Due to the high stimulation intensity required, neonates can be more prone to risks and injuries [115].

4. It is not always possible to use TIVA in the neonatal age group so monitoring can become challenging [116].

22.2.9.3 Bispectral Index (BIS)

BIS is an EEG-guided tool that uses an algorithm to estimate the depth of anaesthesia. It integrates the algorithm to arrive at a number between 0 and 100, where 0 represents electrical silence and 100 represents wakefulness. BIS is commonly used in adults to prevent awareness during anaesthesia, as a guide to titrate drug dosages, preventing overdosage and allowing rapid recovery from anesthesia. A few studies reported its utility in children, but its use and reliability in neonates was questioned because of age-related and higher interindividual variations in its value [117, 118].

Depth of anaesthesia is a theoretical construct and there is no gold standard for clinical measurement of sedation or hypnosis [119].

The clinical usefulness of BIS can only be established after it is validated for use in neonates. Extrapolating adult data may not be ideal because of a dynamic brain state under general anaesthesia in these babies. Ethical concerns regarding recruitment of neonates and infants for the research purpose is a big limitation [120].

So at present, there is a paucity of data regarding the clinical utility of BIS in neonates and preterm babies.

22.2.10   Neuromuscular Transmission (NMT) Monitoring

The monitoring of NMT aims to improve the safety in neonatal anaesthesia as it facilitates the detection of residual NM blockade, helps to titrate the dose of muscle relaxants and enables documentation of the presence and degree of NM blockade. The incidence of residual NMB in children is high.

a. Site and Patterns of Stimulation

The ulnar nerve is most commonly preferred and the response is observed in the adductor policis muscle. Other sites such as posterior tibial and facial nerve are less commonly used in children [121]. Maturation of NMT occurs in the first 2 months of age, newborns have less neuromuscular reserve than older children. The clinician can obtain adequate information by stimulating at 0.25 Hz, 2 Hz for 2 s and 50 Hz for 5 s.

- **Train-of-four (TOF) stimulation** (2 Hz for 2 s every 15 s) is the most widely used method. TOF ratio is a good predictor of recovery from NMB in neonates, as TOF numerical values will be small in under 2 months of age. TOF ratio of 0.9 is the goal for tracheal extubation.
- In neonates, tetanic stimulation is not informative, because fatigue is observed even in absence of NMB [122]. If tetanic stimulation is given, 50 Hz is preferable to 20 Hz (less fatigue at 50H).
- Supramaximal stimulation can be achieved using 40–70 mA current. The ground electrode is placed between the stimulating and recording electrode after cleaning the skin.

For analyzing subtle changes in NMT, recording is more important than observing the events.

b. Recording Methods

Electromyography (EMG) and acceleromyography (AMG) are the frequently used recording methods in small infants [mechanomyography (MMG) is too cumbersome]. AMG devices are small portable and can be used in OR. In a study, 28% of paediatric patients were found to have residual block (TOF ratio <0.90), while 6.5% had severe block (TOF ratio <0.70) [123].

Recent consensus guidelines for the use of muscle relaxants in critically ill children in ICU recommend the use of TOF monitoring at least once every 24 h [124]. AMG devices are small portable and can be used in OR.

c. Controversies

- Results of the three recording methods are not interchangeable as different mechanisms are employed
- AMG is easy to use, but tends to underestimate partial NMB, shows reverse fade and staircase phenomenon.
- Lower body weight implies lower muscle mass and less strength to overcome the weight of the acceleration transducers, so there can be a discrepancy in the recording method.
- Prolonged NM monitoring (>48 h) has been associated with prolonged weakness that could last up to 6 months [125].
- Hypothermia interferes with AMG recording [126].
- Altered response to nondepolarising neuromuscular blocking drugs in neonates records lower baseline TOF ratio [127].
- Validation of NMT monitoring and clinical parameters in neonates is difficult and complicated.

22.2.11   Urine Output Monitoring

Intraoperative urine output measurement is important as it is an indirect evaluation of the renal perfusion and cardiovascular status. The colour and hourly estimation of the volume of urine intraoperatively has been most widely used as an indicator of intravascular volume status, because preterm and term infants generally do not maintain an adequate urine output if there is intravascular volume depletion [128].

The kidneys of a neonate have decreased GFR and renal plasma flow, limited ability to concentrate urine or handle an excess of intravascular volume.

Normal urine output is age dependant, in newborns and infants up to 1 year normal urine output is 2 mL/kg/h, while in toddlers, the normal urine output is 1.5 mL/kg/h.

To avoid renal hypoperfusion, minimum urine output of 0.5 mL/kg/h is required [129]. However, some studies recommend that urine output less than 1 mL/kg/h in neonates indicates a reduction in urine output [130].

Indications of monitoring urine output:

- Any surgery of prolonged duration
- Surgeries, where large blood loss >20% of estimated blood volume is anticipated [3]
- Surgeries, where major fluid shifts (75% of EBV) are expected, such as complex cardiac surgeries, neurosurgeries, and major abdominal surgeries.
- Planed use of diuretics

A 6Fr-Foley's catheter can be inserted in a newborn, which is then connected 100–200 cm long PVC tube which is attached to a calibrated urometer of 100 mL capacity for closed collection system or can be vented to 10–20 mL syringe.

Drawbacks of monitoring:

- In a neonate, less than 1 week, urine output alone is not a sensitive indicator of the adequacy of intravascular volume status.
- There is always a risk of introducing bacterial sepsis.
- The feeding tube should be avoided for catheterization as their rigid material and long length increases the risk of trauma and knotting.

However, sometimes it is difficult to measure urine output due to the large dead space of the tube and sometimes the weight of the urometer can cause traumatic pull at the catheter leading to injury.

22.2.12 Arterial Blood Gases (ABG)

ABG analysis is the gold standard monitoring modality for the evaluation of oxygenation and ventilation. An indwelling arterial catheter in the radial or umbilical artery is a practical, reliable and accurate method of neonatal blood gas sampling.

Indications of ABG Intraoperatively:
- In babies with severe respiratory, metabolic or circulatory disorders
- Suspicion of hypoxia and hypercarbia
- Shock
- Sepsis
- Massive blood transfusion
- Electrolyte abnormality
- Renal disturbances

Precautions
- Strict asepsis should be maintained to prevent the introduction of organisms into the bloodstream.
- Universal precautions should be taken.
- Heparination of the syringe should not involve large volumes, since heparin is acidic and lowers the pH and dissolved oxygen in heparinized saline can increase PaO_2.
- So use a lower strength of heparin or hep-lock solution.
- Let the syringe fill spontaneously and avoid air bubbles
- There should not be a delay of more than 30 s in the processing of the sample as cells consume O_2 and produce CO_2.

a. Clinical Significance
Uncorrected severe acidosis (pH 7.20) results in myocardial depression with arrhythmias, hypertension and hyperkalemia, while uncorrected severe alkalosis causes muscle irritability arrhythmias, tissue hypoxia and hypokalemia. Therefore, in order to prevent intraoperative morbidity and mortality, monitoring of ABG is essential during major surgical procedures in newborns and neonates.

Box 22.1 Causes of acid–base disturbances in neonates

Increased Anion Gap	Normal Anion Gap
1. Lactic acidosis	1. Pre-existing diarrhoea
(a) Shock, sepsis	2. Renal tubular acidosis
(b) Hypoxia	3. Excessive loss of HCO_3 in urine or gut
(c) hypothermia	4. Exogenous chlorides
2. Ketoacidosis	
(a) Diabetes	
(b) Starvation	
3. Other acids	
(a) Renal failure	

Metabolic acidosis is the common disorder encountered in neonates. Common causes of acid–base disturbances encountered intraoperatively may be with increased or normal anion gap. (Box 22.1).

If an increased anion gap is evident, treat the cause, since the administration of HCO_3 may be hazardous. The use of HCO_3 for treatment of normal anion gap acidosis should be done judiciously, since HCO_3 is hypertonic and hyperosmolar and if given rapidly particularly in premature babies may cause intraventricular haemorrhage. Besides extra CO_2 produced can worsen intracellular acidosis, can shift the O_2–Hb dissociation curve to the left, precipitate hypokalemia and hypocalcemia.

So, the correction is advised only when the HCO_3 falls below 15 mEq/L.

Required HCO_3 can be calculated by the formula:

$$0.3 \times \text{Base deficit} \left(\text{mmol} / \text{L} \right) \times \text{Weight} \left(\text{kg} \right)$$

- Half of the HCO_3 correction can be done immediately via slow intravenous administration after diluting with 5% dextrose and the rest can be administered in the maintenance fluid over 24 h.

b. Metabolic Alkalosis

Common intraoperative causes

- GIT losses
  - Vomiting
  - NG tube aspiration
- Rapid HCO_3 correction
- Massive blood transfusion
- Massive diuresis

- Correction of the cause will restore the normal status

c. Respiratory Acidosis

Common intraoperative causes

- Pre-existing respiratory, thoracic or neuromuscular disorder
- Aspiration pneumonitis
- Pleural effusion, pneumothorax
- Pneumoperitoneum during laparoscopic surgeries not compensated by increased minute ventilation
- Inadequate alveolar ventilation
- ET block, tube dislodgement and increased dead space
- Pulmonary oedema, lung collapse
- Surgeries involving one-lung ventilation

- CO_2 should be eliminated by increasing the mechanical ventilatory support

d. Respiratory Alkalosis
- A common intraoperative cause of respiratory alkalosis is hyperventilation which can be managed by adopting a correct ventilatory strategy. Hypocarbia and severe respiratory alkalosis should be avoided whenever possible as the neurological outcome is poor in neonates and preterm babies.

22.3 Conclusion

Goal of intraoperative monitoring is prevention of morbidity in the patients, while not compromising quality of anaesthesia care. There are innumerable equipments and monitors available and choice of the device depends upon the complexity of the surgery, patient's age and disease. Monitoring devices should only supplement the anaesthesiologist's clinical observation and judgement, they are not replacement for clinical skill. Constant surveillance and vigilance during the intraoperative period is mandatory for a successful outcome following surgery in term and preterm newborns and neonates.

References

1. Guideline on Standards for Basic Anesthetic Monitoring. Approved by the ASA House of Delegates on October 21, 1986, last amended on October 20, 2010, reaffirmed December 13, 2020. [file:///C:/Users/nurse/Desktop/standards-for-basic-anesthetic-monitoring.pdf].
2. Watson A, Visram A. Survey of the use of oesophageal and precordial stethoscopes in current paediatric anaesthetic practice. Paediatr Anaesth. 2001 Jul;11(4):437–42.
3. Motoyama E. Smith's anesthesia for infants and children. 8thed. Peter Davis Franklyn Cladis (Editor). Mosby; 2010.
4. Kugler J, Stirt JA, Finholt D, Sussman MD. The one that got away: misplaced esophageal stethoscope. Anesthesiology. 1985;62(5):643–5.
5. Giri P, Roth P. Neonatal hypertension. Pediatr Rev. 2020;41(6):307–11.
6. Parkm M. Park's pediatric cardiology for practitioners. 6th ed. Mosby; 2014.
7. König K, Casalaz DM, Burke EJ, Watkins A. Accuracy of non-invasive blood pressure monitoring in very preterm infants. Intensive Care Med. 2012;38(4):670–6.

8. Greaney D, Nakhjavani S, Desmond F, et al. Suitability of the forearm for non-invasive blood pressure measurement in children. Paediatr Anaesth. 2017;27(11):1125–30.

9. Short JA. Noninvasive blood pressure measurement in the upper and lower limbs of anaesthetized children. Paediatr Anaesth. 2000;10(6):591–3.

10. Shimokaze T, Akaba K, Saito E. Oscillometric and intra-arterial blood pressure in preterm and term infants: extent of discrepancy and factors associated with inaccuracy. Am J Perinatol. 2015;32(3):277–82.

11. Flynn JT, Kaelber DC, Baker-Smith CM, et al. Clinical practice guideline for screening and management of high blood pressure in children and adolescents published correction appears in Pediatrics. Pediatrics. 2017;140(3):e20171904; Correction in Pediatrics. 2018;142(3).

12. Zubrow AB, Hulman S, Kushner H, Falkner B. Determinants of blood pressure in infants admitted to neonatal intensive care units: a prospective multicenter study. Philadelphia Neonatal Blood Pressure Study Group. J Perinatol. 1995;15(6):470–9.

13. Dionne JM, Bremner SA, Baygani SK, et al. Method of blood pressure measurement in neonates and infants: a systematic review and analysis. J Pediatr. 2020;221:23–31.e5.

14. Cayabyab R, McLean CW, Seri I. Definition of hypotension and assessment of hemodynamics in the preterm neonate. J Perinatol. 2009;29(Suppl 2):S58–62.

15. Batton B, Li L, Newman NS, et al. Use of antihypotensive therapies in extremely preterm infants. Pediatrics. 2013;131(6):e1865–73.

16. Batton B. Neonatal blood pressure standards: what is "Normal"? Clin Perinatol. 2020;47(3):469–85.

17. Dempsey EM, Barrington KJ, Marlow N, et al. Management of hypotension in preterm infants (The HIP Trial): a randomised controlled trial of hypotension management in extremely low gestational age newborns. Neonatology. 2014;105(4):275–81.

18. Zhou J, Elkhateeb O, Lee KS. Comparison of non-invasive vs invasive blood pressure measurement in neonates undergoing therapeutic hypothermia for hypoxic ischemic encephalopathy. J Perinatol. 2016;36:381–5.

19. Schindler E, Kowald B, Suess H, Niehaus-Borquez B, et al. Catheterization of the radial or brachial artery in neonates and infants. Paediatr Anaesth. 2005;15(8):677–82.

20. Imamura T, Momoi N, Go H, Ogasawara K, Kanai Y, et al. Evaluation of arterial catheter management in very preterm neonates: peripheral artery versus umbilical artery. Fukushima J Med Sci. 2012;58(1):1–8.

21. Varga EQ, Candiotti KA, Saltzman B, Gayer S, Giquel J, et al. Evaluation of distal radial artery cross-sectional internal diameter in pediatric patients using ultrasound. Paediatr Anaesth. 2013;23(5):460–2.

22. Breschan C, Kraschl R, Jost R, Marhofer P, Likar R. Axillary brachial plexus block for treatment of severe forearm ischemia after arterial cannulation in an extremely low birth-weight infant. Paediatr Anaesth. 2004;14(8):681–4.

23. Słowińska-Klencka D, Klencki M, Sporny S, Lewiński A. Fine-needle aspiration biopsy of the thyroid in an area of endemic goitre: influence of restored sufficient iodine supplementation on the clinical significance of cytological results. Eur J Endocrinol. 2002;146(1):19–26.

24. Suman RP, Udani R, Nanavati R. Kangaroo mother care for low birth weight infants: a randomized controlled trial. Indian Pediatr. 2008;45(1):17–23.

25. Scott-Warren VL, Morley RB. Paediatric vascular access. BJA Educ. 2015;15(4):199–206.

26. Gao YB, Yan JH, Gao FQ, Pan L, et al. Effects of ultrasound-guided radial artery catheterization: an updated meta-analysis. Am J Emerg Med. 2015;33(1):50–5.

27. Karacalar S, Ture H, Baris S, Karakaya D, Sarihasan B. Ulnar artery versus radial artery approach for arterial cannulation: a prospective, comparative study. J Clin Anesth. 2007;19(3):209–13.

28. Soleymani S, Borzage M, Seri I. Hemodynamic monitoring in neonates: advances and challenges. J Perinatol. 2010;30(Suppl):S38–45.

29. Gan H, Cannesson M, Chandler JR, Ansermino JM. Predicting fluid responsiveness in children: a systematic review. Anesth Analg. 2013;117(6):1380–92.

30. Yager P, Noviski N. Shock. Pediatr Rev. 2010;31(8):311–9.
31. Ahn SY, Kim ES, Kim JK, Shin JH, Sung SI, Jung JM, et al. Permissive hypotension in extremely low birth weight infants (≤1000 gm). Yonsei Med J. 2012;53(4):765–71.
32. Detaille T, Pirotte T, Veyckemans F. Vascular access in the neonate. Best Pract Res Clin Anaesthesiol. 2010;24(3):403–18.
33. Brasher C, Malbezin S. Central venous catheters in small infants. Anesthesiology. 2018;128(1):4–5.
34. Kugelman A, Zeiger-Aginsky D, Bader D, Shoris I, Riskin A. A novel method of distal end-tidal CO2 capnography in intubated infants: comparison with arterial CO2 and with proximal mainstream end-tidal CO2. Pediatrics. 2008;122(6):e1219–24.
35. McEvedy BA, McLeod ME, Kirpalani H, Volgyesi GA, Lerman J. End-tidal carbon dioxide measurements in critically ill neonates: a comparison of side-stream and mainstream cap-nometers. Can J Anaesth. 1990;37(3):322–6.
36. McKee LA, Fabres J, Howard G, Peralta-Carcelen M, Carlo WA, Ambalavanan N. PaCO2 and neurodevelopment in extremely low birth weight infants. J Pediatr. 2009;155(2):217–21.
37. Giannakopoulou C, Korakaki E, Manoura A, Bikouvarakis S, et al. Significance of hypo-carbia in the development of periventricular leukomalacia in preterm infants. Pediatr Int. 2004;46(3):268–73.
38. Hochwald O, Borenstein-Levin L, Dinur G, Jubran H, et al. Continuous noninvasive carbon dioxide monitoring in neonates: from theory to standard of care. Pediatrics. 2019;144(1):e20183640.
39. Hagerty JJ, Kleinman ME, Zurakowski D, Lyons AC, Krauss B. Accuracy of a new low-flow sidestream capnography technology in newborns: a pilot study. J Perinatol. 2002;22(3):219–25.
40. Whitesell R, Asiddao C, Gollman D, Jablonski J. Relationship between arterial and peak expired carbon dioxide pressure during anesthesia and factors influencing the difference. Anesth Analg. 1981;60(7):508–12.
41. Harigopal S, Satish HP. End-tidal carbon dioxide monitoring in neonates. Infant. 2008;4(2):51–3.
42. Karlsson V, Sporre B, Hellström-Westas L, Ågren J. Poor performance of main-stream capnography in newborn infants during general anesthesia. Paediatr Anaesth. 2017;27(12):1235–40.
43. Tingay DG, Stewart MJ, Morley CJ. Monitoring of end tidal carbon dioxide and trans-cutaneous carbon dioxide during neonatal transport. Arch Dis Child Fetal Neonatal Ed. 2005;90(6):F523–6.
44. Hagerty JJ, Kleinman ME, Zurakowski D, Lyons AC, Krauss B. Accuracy of a new low-flow side stream capnography technology in newborns: a pilot study. J Perinatol. 2002;22:219–25.
45. Bhavani-Shankar K, Moseley H, Kumar AY, Delph Y. Capnometry and anaesthesia. Can J Anaesth. 1992;39(6):617–32.
46. Eipe N, Doherty DR. A review of pediatric capnography. J Clin Monit Comput. 2010;24(4):261–8.
47. Short JA, Paris ST, Booker PD, Fletcher R. Arterial to end-tidal carbon dioxide tension differ-ence in children with congenital heart disease. Br J Anaesth. 2001;86(3):349–53.
48. Badgwell JM, Heavner JE, May WS, Goldthorn JF, Lerman J. End-tidal PCO2 monitoring in infants and children ventilated with either a partial rebreathing or a non-rebreathing circuit. Anesthesiology. 1987;66(3):405–10.
49. Tobias JD. Transcutaneous carbon dioxide monitoring in infants and children. Paediatr Anaesth. 2009;19(5):434–44.
50. O'Connor TA, Grueber R. Transcutaneous measurement of carbon dioxide tension dur-ing long-distance transport of neonates receiving mechanical ventilation. J Perinatol. 1998;18(3):189–92.
51. van Wijk JJ, Weber F, Stolker RJ, Staals LM. Current state of noninvasive, continuous moni-toring modalities in pediatric anesthesiology. Curr Opin Anaesthesiol. 2020;33(6):781–7.

52. Nosovitch MA, Johnson JO, Tobias JD. Noninvasive intraoperative monitoring of carbon dioxide in children: endtidal versus transcutaneous techniques. Paediatr Anaesth. 2002;12(1):48–52.

53. Eberhard P. The design, use, and results of transcutaneous carbon dioxide analysis: current and future directions. Anesth Analg. 2007;105(6):S48–52.

54. Hochwald O, Borenstein-Levin L, Dinur G, Jubran H, Ben-David S, Kugelman A. Continuous noninvasive carbon dioxide monitoring in neonates: from theory to standard of care. Pediatrics. 2019;144(1):e20183640.

55. Committee on Hospital Care of the American Academy of Pediatrics and Pediatric Section of the Society of Critical Care Medicine. Guidelines and levels of care for pediatric intensive care units. Pediatrics. 1993;92(1):166–75.

56. Saugstad OD. Oxygenation of the immature infant: a commentary and recommendations for oxygen saturation targets and alarm limits. Neonatology. 2018;114(1):69–75.

57. Sweet DG, Carnielli V, Greisen G, Hallman M, Ozek E, Plavka R, Saugstad OD, Simeoni U, Speer CP, Vento M, Halliday HL; European Association of Perinatal Medicine. European consensus guidelines on the management of neonatal respiratory distress syndrome in preterm infants—2013 update. Neonatology 2013;103(4):353-368.

58. Koppel RI, Druschel CM, Carter T, et al. Effectiveness of pulse oximetry screening for congenital heart disease in asymptomatic newborns. Pediatrics. 2003;111(3):451–5.

59. Ewer AK, Martin GR. Newborn pulse oximetry screening: which algorithm is best? Pediatrics. 2016;138(5):e20161206.

60. Wackernagel D, Blennow M, Hellström A. Accuracy of pulse oximetry in preterm and term infants is insufficient to determine arterial oxygen saturation and tension. Acta Paediatr. 2020;109:2251–7.

61. Cummings JJ, Polin RA, Committee on Fetus and Newborn. Oxygen targeting in extremely low birth weight infants. Pediatrics. 2016;138(2):e20161576.

62. Gupta S, Jawanda MK. The impacts of COVID-19 on children. Acta Paediatr. 2020;109(11):2181–3.

63. Dawson JA, Davis PG, O'Donnell CP, Kamlin CO, Morley CJ. Pulse oximetry for monitoring infants in the delivery room: a review. Arch Dis Child Fetal Neonatal Ed. 2007;92(1):F4–7.

64. Goldman JM, Petterson MT, Kopotic RJ, Barker SJ. Masimo signal extraction pulse oximetry. J Clin Monit Comput. 2000;16(7):475–83.

65. Malviya S, Reynolds PI, Voepel-Lewis T, Siewert M, Watson D, Tait AR, Tremper K. False alarms and sensitivity of conventional pulse oximetry versus the Masimo SET technology in the pediatric postanesthesia care unit. Anesth Analg. 2000;90(6):1336–40.

66. Polin RA, Bateman DA, Sahni R. Pulse oximetry in very low birth weight infants. Clin Perinatol. 2014;41(4):1017–32.

67. Tipple M. Interpretation of electrocardiograms in infants and children. Images Paediatr Cardiol. 1999;1(1):3–13.

68. Davignon A, Rautaharju P, Boiselle E, Soumis F, Megelas M, Choquette A. Normal ECG standards for infants and children. Pediatr Cardiol. 1979;1:123–31.

69. Schwartz PJ, Garson A Jr, Paul T, Stramba-Badiale M, Vetter VL, Wren C, European Society of Cardiology. Guidelines for the interpretation of the neonatal electrocardiogram. A task force of the European Society of Cardiology. Eur Heart J. 2002;23(17):1329–44.

70. Johnsrude CL, Perry JC, Towbin JA. Myocardial infarction in children. Primary Cardiol. 1994;20:23–32.

71. Doniger SJ, Sharieff GQ. Pediatric dysrhythmias. Pediatr Clin North Am. 2006;53(1):85–105.

72. Drew BJ, Califf RM, Funk M, et al. Practice standards for electrocardiographic monitoring in hospital settings: an American Heart Association scientific statement from the Councils on Cardiovascular Nursing, Clinical Cardiology and Cardiovascular Disease in the Young: endorsed by the International Society of Computerized Electrocardiology and the American Association of Critical-Care Nurses [correction in Circulation. 2005;25;111(3):378]. Circulation. 2004;110(17):2721–46.

73. Nilsson K. Maintenance and monitoring of body temperature in infants and children. Paediatr Anaesth. 1991;1:13–20.
74. Perlman J, Kjaer K. Neonatal and maternal temperature regulation during and after delivery. Anesth Analg. 2016;123(1):168–72.
75. Russo A, McCready M, Torres L, et al. Reducing hypothermia in preterm infants following delivery. Pediatrics. 2014;133(4):e1055–62.
76. Manchanda V, Sarin YK, Ramji S. Prognostic factors determining mortality in surgical neonates. J Neonatal Surg. 2012;1(1):3.
77. Waldron S, MacKinnon R. Neonatal thermoregulation. Infant. 2007;3(3):101–4.
78. Kumar V, Shearer JC, Kumar A, Darmstadt GL. Neonatal hypothermia in low resource settings: a review. J Perinatol. 2009;29(6):401–12.
79. World Health Organization. In: World Health Organization, editor. Maternal and newborn health/safe motherhood. Thermal protection of the newborn: a practical guide; 1997. https://apps.who.int/iris/handle/10665/63986] assessed on 27th August 2021.
80. Thomas K. Thermoregulation in neonates. Neonatal Netw. 1994;13(2):15–22.
81. Plattner O, Semsroth M, Sessler DI, Papousek A, et al. Lack of nonshivering thermogenesis in infants anesthetized with fentanyl and propofol. Anesthesiology. 1997;86(4):772–7.
82. Russo A, McCready M, Torres L, Theuriere C, Venturini S, et al. Reducing hypothermia in preterm infants following delivery. Pediatrics. 2014;133(4):e1055–62.
83. Cork RC, Vaughan RW, Humphrey LS. Precision and accuracy of intraoperative temperature monitoring. Anesth Analg. 1983 Feb;62(2):211–4.
84. Bissonnette B, Sessler DI, LaFlamme P. Intraoperative temperature monitoring sites in infants and children and the effect of inspired gas warming on esophageal temperature. Anesth Analg. 1989;69(2):192–6.
85. Jay O, Molgat-Seon Y, Chou S, Murto K. Skin temperature over the carotid artery provides an accurate noninvasive estimation of core temperature in infants and young children during general anesthesia. Paediatr Anaesth. 2013;23(12):1109–16.
86. Dewar DJ, Fraser JF, Choo KL, Kimble RM. Thermal injuries in three children caused by an electrical warming mattress. Br J Anaesth. 2004;93(4):586–9.
87. McCarthy LK, O'Donnell CP. Warming preterm infants in the delivery room: polyethylene bags, exothermic mattresses or both? Acta Paediatr. 2011;100(12):1534–7.
88. Negishi C, Hasegawa K, Mukai S, Nakagawa F, Ozaki M, Sessler DI. Resistive-heating and forced-air warming are comparably effective. Anesth Analg. 2003;96(6):1683–7.
89. Sessler DI. Complications and treatment of mild hypothermia. Anesthesiology. 2001;95(2):531–43.
90. Lawes EG. Hidden hazards and dangers associated with the use of HME/filters in breathing circuits. Their effect on toxic metabolite production, pulse oximetry and airway resistance. Br J Anaesth. 2003;91(2):249–64.
91. Whitelock DE, de Beer DA. The use of filters with small infants. Respir Care Clin N Am. 2006;12(2):307–20.
92. Desmond FA, Namachivayam S. Does near-infrared spectroscopy play a role in paediatric intensive care? BJA Educ. 2016;16(8):281–5.
93. Costerus S, Vlot J, van Rosmalen J, Wijnen R, Weber F. Effects of neonatal thoracoscopic surgery on tissue oxygenation: a pilot study on (neuro-) monitoring and outcomes. Eur J Pediatr Surg. 2019;29(2):166–72.
94. Marin T, Moore J. Understanding near-infrared spectroscopy. Adv Neonatal Care. 2011;11(6):382–8.
95. Weber F, Scoones GP. A practical approach to cerebral near-infrared spectroscopy (NIRS) directed hemodynamic management in noncardiac pediatric anesthesia. Paediatr Anaesth. 2019;29(10):993–1001.
96. Steppan J, Hogue CW Jr. Cerebral and tissue oximetry. Best Pract Res Clin Anaesthesiol. 2014;28(4):429–39.

97. Alderliesten T, Dix L, Baerts W, Caicedo A, van Huffel S, Naulaers G, Groenendaal F, van Bel F, Lemmers P. Reference values of regional cerebral oxygen saturation during the first 3 days of life in preterm neonates. Pediatr Res. 2016;79(1-1):55–64.

98. Kurth CD, McCann JC, Wu J, Miles L, Loepke AW. Cerebral oxygen saturation-time threshold for hypoxic-ischemic injury in piglets. Anesth Analg. 2009;108(4):1268–77.

99. Moerman A, Wouters P. Near-infrared spectroscopy (NIRS) monitoring in contemporary anesthesia and critical care. Acta Anaesthesiol Belg. 2010;61(4):185–94.

100. Tortoriello TA, Stayer SA, Mott AR, McKenzie ED, et al. A noninvasive estimation of mixed venous oxygen saturation using near-infrared spectroscopy by cerebral oximetry in pediatric cardiac surgery patients. Paediatr Anaesth. 2005;15(6):495–503.

101. Scott JP, Hoffman GM. Near-infrared spectroscopy: exposing the dark (venous) side of the circulation. Paediatr Anaesth. 2014;24(1):74–88.

102. Wallin M, Lönnqvist PA. A healthy measure of monitoring fundamentals! Paediatr Anaesth. 2018;28(7):580–7.

103. Hellström-Westas L. Amplitude-integrated electroencephalography for seizure detection in newborn infants. Semin Fetal Neonatal Med. 2018;23(3):175–82.

104. Liu W, Yang Q, Wei H, Dong W, Fan Y, Hua Z. Prognostic value of clinical tests in neonates with hypoxic-ischemic encephalopathy treated with therapeutic hypothermia: a systematic review and meta-analysis. Front Neurol. 2020;11:133.

105. Fogtmann EP, Plomgaard AM, Greisen G, Gluud C. Prognostic accuracy of electroencephalograms in preterm infants: a systematic review. Pediatrics. 2017;139(2):e20161951.

106. Bruns N, Felderhoff-Müser U, Dohna-Schwake C. EEG as a useful tool for neuromonitoring in critically ill children—current evidence and knowledge gaps. Acta Paediatr. 2021;110:1132–40.

107. Gucuyener K. Use of amplitude-integrated electroencephalography in neonates with special emphasis on hypoxic-ischemic encephalopathy and therapeutic hypothermia. J Clin Neonatol. 2016;5:18–30.

108. Hellström-Westas L, Klette H, Thorngren-Jerneck K, Rosén I. Early prediction of outcome with aEEG in preterm infants with large intraventricular hemorrhages. Neuropediatrics. 2001;32(6):319–24.

109. Oria M, Duru S, Scorletti F, Vuletin F, Encinas JL, et al. Intracisternal Bio Glue injection in the fetal lamb: a novel model for creation of obstructive congenital hydrocephalus without additional chemically induced neuroinflammation. J Neurosurg Pediatr. 2019;24(6):652–62.

110. Yi YG, Kim K, Shin HI, Bang MS, Kim HS, Choi J, et al. Feasibility of intraoperative monitoring of motor evoked potentials obtained through transcranial electrical stimulation in infants younger than 3 months. J Neurosurg Pediatr. 2019;15:1–9.

111. Aydinlar EI, Dikmen PY, Kocak M, Baykan N, et al. Intraoperative neuromonitoring of motor-evoked potentials in infants undergoing surgery of the spine and spinal cord. J Clin Neurophysiol. 2019;36(1):60–6.

112. Flanders TM, Franco AJ, Hines SJ, Taylor JA, Heuer GG. Neonatal intraoperative neuromonitoring in thoracic myelocystocele: a case report. Childs Nerv Syst. 2020;36(2):435–9.

113. Fulkerson DH, Satyan KB, Wilder LM, Riviello JJ, Stayer SA, Whitehead WE, Curry DJ, Dauser RC, Luerssen TG, Jea A. Intraoperative monitoring of motor evoked potentials in very young children. J Neurosurg Pediatr. 2011;7(4):331–7.

114. Vecchierini-Blineau MF, Guiheneuc P. Vitesses de conduction nerveuse motrice chez l'enfant: valeurs normales et applications à quelques cas pathologiques [Motor nerve conduction velocity in children: normal values and application to a few pathologic cases]. Rev Electroencephalogr Neurophysiol Clin. 1984;13(4):340–8.

115. Chen X, Sterio D, Ming X, Para DD, Butusova M, Tong T, Beric A. Success rate of motor evoked potentials for intraoperative neurophysiologic monitoring: effects of age, lesion location, and preoperative neurologic deficits. J Clin Neurophysiol. 2007;24(3):281–5.

116. Baang HY, Swingle N, Sajja K, Madhavan D, Shostrom VK, Taraschenko O. Towards successes in the management of nonconvulsive status epilepticus: tracing the detection-to-needle trajectories. J Clin Neurophysiol. 2020;37(3):253–8.

117. Ganesh A, Watcha MF. Bispectral index monitoring in pediatric anesthesia. Curr Opin Anaesthesiol. 2004;17(3):229–34.

118. Sciusco A, Standing JF, Sheng Y, Raimondo P, Cinnella G, Dambrosio M. Effect of age on the performance of bispectral and entropy indices during sevoflurane pediatric anesthesia: a pharmacometric study. Paediatr Anaesth. 2017;27(4):399–408.
119. Lu H, Rosenbaum S. Developmental pharmacokinetics in pediatric populations. J Pediatr Pharmacol Ther. 2014;19(4):262–76.
120. O'Connor MF, Daves SM, Tung A, Cook RI, Thisted R, Apfelbaum J. BIS monitoring to prevent awareness during general anesthesia. Anesthesiology. 2001;94(3):520–2.
121. Withington DE, Davis GM, Vallinis P, Del Sonno P, Bevan JC. Respiratory function in children during recovery from neuromuscular blockade. Paediatr Anaesth. 1998;8(1):41–7.
122. Goudsouzian NG. Maturation of neuromuscular transmission in the infant. Br J Anaesth. 1980;52(2):205–14.
123. Ledowski T, O'Dea B, Meyerkort L, Hegarty M, von Ungern-Sternberg BS. Postoperative residual neuromuscular paralysis at an Australian Tertiary Children's Hospital. Anesthesiol Res Pract. 2015;2015:410248.
124. Playfor S, Jenkins I, Boyles C, Choonara I, Davies G, Haywood T, et al. A United Kingdom Paediatric Intensive Care Society Sedation, Analgesia and Neuromuscular Blockade Working Group. Consensus guidelines for sustained neuromuscular blockade in critically ill children. Paediatr Anaesth. 2007;17(9):881–7.
125. Wokke JH, Jennekens FG, van den Oord CJ, Veldman H, van Gijn J. Histological investigations of muscle atrophy and end plates in two critically ill patients with generalized weakness. J Neurol Sci. 1988;88(1-3):95–106.
126. Saldien V, Vermeyen KM. Neuromuscular transmission monitoring in children. Paediatr Anaesth. 2004;14(4):289–92.
127. Goudsouzian NG, Crone RK, Todres ID. Recovery from pancuronium blockade in the neonatal intensive care unit. Br J Anaesth. 1981;53(12):1303–9.
128. Makaryus R, Miller TE, Gan TJ. Current concepts of fluid management in enhanced recovery pathways. Br J Anaesth. 2018;120(2):376–83.
129. Chappell D, Jacob M, Hofmann-Kiefer K, Conzen P, Rehm M. A rational approach to perioperative fluid management. Anesthesiology. 2008;109(4):723–40.
130. Walters S, Porter C, Brophy PD. Dialysis and pediatric acute kidney injury: choice of renal support modality. Pediatr Nephrol. 2009;24(1):37–48.

Perioperative Fluid Management and Blood Transfusion in Newborns and Neonates

23

Pratibha Jain Shah

23.1 Introduction

A newborn baby's body weight is mostly from its water content. The proportion of body weight, that is body water, is more than 80% in term and about 85% in preterm (<32 week GA) newborns. This decreases to about 80% at 1 week, 75% at 1 month, and to 65% by 3 months of age. Neonates are extremely susceptible to changes in body water content and electrolytes. In a surgical neonate, the surgical condition, its physio-biochemical changes, insensible losses, and the surgical losses, add on to the adverse consequences.

Fluid homeostasis in neonates is special, suiting the unique physiological demands of transition at birth, followed by a period of spurt in growth and development in the early postnatal period. Immature organ systems, different body fluid composition, need of different quantity and volume of fluids at different phases of growth, and an extremely limited margin for error, makes fluid and electrolyte therapy a challenging component of perioperative management in the neonate. Errors in fluid management may lead to serious complications and negative long-term effects. Prematurity, critical illness, and major surgical interventions impose additional challenges. Each baby requires an individualized approach and meticulous care in perioperative fluid administration, according to the adequacy of cardiopulmonary adaptation, and time of onset of postnatal diuresis.

The volume and composition of intravenous (IV) fluids administered during anesthesia has been a subject of debate in all ages. Literature related to fluid therapy in neonates is quite limited, hence, most of the knowledge is extrapolated from anesthesiologist's experience in adult and pediatric populations.

This chapter reviews the basics of physiology of adaptation in neonates related to body water distribution, concept of perioperative fluid therapy, calculation of

P. J. Shah (✉)
Pt JNM MC, Raipur, Chhattisgarh, India

© The Author(s), under exclusive license to Springer Nature Singapore Pte Ltd. 2023
U. Saha (ed.), *Clinical Anesthesia for the Newborn and the Neonate*,
https://doi.org/10.1007/978-981-19-5458-0_23

type, volume, and rate of fluid infusions, blood transfusion (BT) triggers, and nutritional requirements.

23.2 Anatomical and Physiological Developmental Changes at Birth

The anatomical and functional maturation of organ systems is proportional to the gestational age (GA) at birth. The immediate postnatal period is marked by dramatic changes in almost all organs of the body that determine newborn's viability and ability to grow properly, especially the cardiovascular, pulmonary, renal systems, and fluid distribution. These changes are interdependent, such that inadequacy in one can affect the changes and maturation in the other. Therefore, understanding of these physiological changes is crucial for a successful postoperative outcome:

1. **Transitional changes:** Fetal circulation is a parallel system, where both ventricles pump blood into the systemic circulation via three shunts: ductus venosus, foramen ovale and ductus arteriosus. In the fetal life, flow to pulmonary circulation is restricted by pulmonary vasoconstriction and high PVR, secondary to hypoxemia, and acidosis. After birth, with initiation of breathing, functional closure of shunts occurs in response to fall in PVR, increase in PaO_2 and SVR. The muscular ductus arteriosus goes into spasm and closes at a PaO_2 of 50 mmHg in a term baby, while in preterm it is slower, delayed and occurs at a higher PaO_2.

Clinical significance:

   (a) Increase in PVR (in response to hypoxia, acidosis, sepsis, high prostaglandin levels, fluid overload) can delay functional closure of the shunts, reverting to fetal circulation (PFC), R →L shunting and cyanosis.

   (b) The same adverse exposure any time later can reopen these shunts with L→R flow. This is acyanotic but is associated with pulmonary overperfusion and hyperemia, with high risk of NEC, BPD, and poor long term outcome.

   (c) Ductus remains patent (PDA) in almost 50% of preterm babies, especially in LBW (<800 g).

2. **Fluid compartment:** the fluid and electrolyte homeostasis is maintained by a fine balance between intake and losses regulated by rennin–angiotensin–aldosterone system (RAAS), antidiuretic hormone (ADH) and atrial natriuretic peptide (ANP). Thirst, an important symptom in adults, is absent in neonates.

   (a) **Total body water (TBW)** and its distribution in various body compartments varies with GA. (Table 23.1) The extracellular fluid (ECF) compartment is subdivided into interstitial (IS 35%), transcellular (CSF, vitreous, aqueous humor, synovial, pleural, and peritoneal fluid 1%), and intravascular fluid (IVF–5%). Remaining (55–60%) fluid is in intracellular fluid (ICF) compartment. With age, TBW and ECF gradually reduce due to diuresis and natriuresis, and ICF increases due to cell growth. In premature and LBW newborns, both TBW and ECF component are higher than in term newborns.

Table 23.1 Distribution of body water according to Gestational age and body weight

Age/body weight	TBW %	ECF (% of TBW)	ICF %
16–27 week GA/BW 0.5–1 kg	>90	60 (66)	30
28–34 week GA/BW 1–2 kg	>85	45–50	35
Term/BW >2.5 kg	>80	40 (50)	35
1 week	80	40 (50)	35
1 month	75	40 (50)	35
3 months	70	35 (50)	35
12 months and more	60	20 (33)	40

Clinical significance:

    i. ICF acts as a reservoir that mobilizes fluid to replenish in case of low volume states, such as during fasting, fever, vomiting, and diarrhea. This reservoir is not available in neonates, because the ICF compartment is already small.

    ii. IVF is 10% in preterm and 5% in term neonates compared to 35% IS fluid. In neonates, protein and albumin levels are low, with low oncotic and higher hydrostatic pressures in the IVF compartment. This causes fluid to translocate from the IVF into the interstitium. Lower serum albumin, as in hepatorenal disease states, further lowers the oncotic pressure, while heart failure and fluid overload increase hydrostatic pressures. These create a situation of low intravascular volume, and significantly compromises organ perfusion.

(b) **Capillary endothelial integrity**: the movement of water and solutes from IVF to IS compartment depends on endothelial glycocalyx layer (EGL). This comprises of capillary endothelium and overlying glycocalyx on the luminal side. EGL is fragile and requires normal levels of plasma albumin to be stable. It plays an important role in homeostasis, inflammation, and regulation of vascular tone. It is freely permeable to water and sodium, semipermeable to albumin and impermeable to large molecules (>70 kDa). Higher hydrostatic pressure (outward) and smaller colloid osmotic pressure (inward) in the IVF compartment, allows net outward movement of water and sodium from the capillary into the interstitium. IS oncotic pressure has minimum effect on transcapillary fluid filtration. Injury to EGL results in increased capillary permeability, loss of plasma proteins and IS oedema.

Clinical significance:

    i. Keeping in mind the low serum albumin content, both crystalloids and colloids, are similarly effective in hypovolemic states in neonate, in contrast to 3:1 volume ratio used in adults. After infusion they are retained in the IVF compartment until hydrostatic pressure rises and filtration into IS compartment occurs. However, colloids do increase the osmotic pressure and are retained in plasma with less transcapillary filtration of fluid.

    ii. As there is no reabsorption of fluid at the venous end of the capillaries, colloids cannot reverse existing IS edema regardless of integrity of EGL. Thus, colloids should be used in neonates only when indicated.

    iii. Various factors in the perioperative period can damage the EGL, such as over transfusion of IV fluids, surgery, hypoxia, ischemia, sepsis, inflammation, release of cytokines, acute hyperglycemia, and shock.

    iv. Once EGL is damaged, it takes 5–7 days to get repaired. Albumin and plasma infusions, Sevoflurane for induction and maintenance, hydrocortisone and antithrombin III are protective to the EGL.

  (c) **Total Blood volume** in term is 85 ml/kg compared to 90–100 ml/kg in preterm.

3. **Cardiovascular system:** neonates have limited cardiovascular reserve in response to high preload and afterload because of limited myocardial contractility, relatively noncompliant myocardium, and already high resting cardiac output (CO). (Table 23.2) Resting CO is already near its maximum capacity to allow for high metabolic rate and O2 consumption, and HbF.

4. **Renal system:** neonatal renal system is adapted to cope with liquid diet with low Na^+ content. Fetal kidneys are passive and nonfunctional. They receive little blood flow (RBF 3% vs 25% of CO in adults) due to high renal vascular resistance and low SVR. Nephron development is complete by 34 week GA, but tubules are short and immature. Glomerular filtration rate (GFR) is low due to low RBF and low glomerular permeability. (Table 23.3)

At birth, rise in SVR and aortic pressure, and fall in renal vascular resistance, increases RBF and GFR. Renal system is functionally 25% mature at birth and 60% by 1 month of age.

5. **Neuroendocrine control:** circulating vasopressin level is high during first 24 h of life. Continual fall in PVR and increase in pulmonary venous return, in 72 h in term and a week in preterm neonates, is accompanied by release of ANP. (Table 23.4) ADH, esp on day 1, is high, probably to maintain TBW and blood volume. In some babies, there may be persistent increase in ADH (Box 23.1).

6. **Central Nervous System:** cerebral autoregulation is immature, and the range of blood pressure is narrow (adult 50–150 mmHg) Cerebral autoregulation is the vital cerebral protective mechanism that develops in the 3rd trimester. Impaired autoregulation increases the risk of brain injury and persistent neurological disability.

Table 23.2 Cardiovascular physiology

Neonatal CVS physiology	Clinical significance
↓ contractile mass/g cardiac tissue, Immature sarcoplasmic reticulum, ↓ Ca^{++} ATP activity	↓ effective increase in SV to fluid overload:↑pre/afterload ↓ or minimal response to inotropes
CO is HR dependent: resting CO close to maximum	Cannot maintain CO during bradycardia ↓reserves (30%↑CO compared to 300% in adults
Parasympathetic influence > Sympathetic	Limited stress response (prone for bradycardia)
Immature Baroreflex	↓ ability to compensate for hypotension: no ↑HR to ↓BP ↑depression of baroreceptors to↑ depth of anaesthesia

Table 23.3 Renal physiology

Renal changes	Response	Clinical significance
Shorter loop of Henle ↓ tonicity of medullary interstitium Immature tubular function Insensitivity of Conducting tubules to ADH	↓ tubular reabsorption: water, Na, HCO_3 ↓ ability to concentrate urine (1st 7 days)	Easily dehydrate with conservative fluid regimes, NB conserve Na^+ better than excrete, Risk of hypernatremia on excess Na^+ administration esp on D1, ↓ serum HCO_3: metabolic acidosis mild hyperkalemia
RAAS Immature feedback mechanism ↓ response to aldosterone	↓ reabsorption of H_2O, Na in dct, Urine osmolality: low Preterm: 50–600 mmol/L Term: 800 mmol/L	Easily dehydrated High risk of hyponatremia after 24 h
↓Low RBF: Term-80–85 mL/min LBW-45 mL/min VLBW-20 mL/min	↓ GFR (double by 2nd week) ↓ clearance of free H_2O and Na^+ ↓ UO ↑ to 2–3 mL/kg/h after D1	Poor response to fluid or Na load Prolong $t\frac{1}{2}$ of drugs ↓ UO after D1 = ↓ IVF/↓renal function
↓ threshold for glucose	Glycosuria	Osmotic diuresis

Table 23.4 Neuroendocrine Physiology

Neuroendocrine changes	Response	Clinical significance
High ADH in 1st 24 h	Low urine output	↓fluid requirement Excessive fluids before postnatal diuresis leads to adverse outcome esp. in ELBW
High ANP – at 72 h in term – at 1 week in preterm	– Postnatal diuresis – Weight loss (5–10% in term, 10–15% in preterm) – Peak weight loss at D 5, return to BW by 7–10 D in term & longer in preterm	Fluid/Na^+ supplement as per weight loss
Limited capacity of RAAS, Immature feedback mechanism	Slow aldosterone secretion	↓ reabsorption of Na^+ from dct Supplement once diuresis begins

Clinical significance:

   (a) It is easily disrupted by hypoxia, acidosis, seizures, prematurity, and low diastolic BP.
   (b) Hypovolemia leads to cerebral ischemia.
   (c) Hypervolemia increases BP and leads to rupture of fragile immature brain vessels.
7. **Fluid losses:** apart from sensible water losses from kidney and intestines, neonates have additional insensible water losses (IWL) due to evaporation from skin and respiratory tract. 70% (2/3rd) of IWL is from skin (perspiration) and 30% (1/3rd) from respiration. IWL is inversely proportion to birth weight. (Table 23.5) Full maturation of epidermis takes more than 28 days.

Table 23.5 IWL and birth weight

Birth weight	<1 kg	1–1.25 kg	1.25–1.5 kg	1.5–1.75 kg	1.75–2 kg
IWL (mL/kg/day)	60–70	60–65	30–45	15–30	15–20

Table 23.6 Factors affecting insensible water loss

Increased loss	Decreased loss
• ↑ RR	• Humidified incubator
• Hyperthermia (↑ 30 %/°C)	• Humidification of inspired gases
• ↑ Ambient temp. (↑ 30%/°C)	• Plexiglas heat shields
• ↓Ambient humidity	• ↑ Ambient humidity
• Motor activity (crying ↑50–70%)	• Protective cover: thin transparent
• Radiant warmer/Phototherapy (50%↑)	plastic barrier (30% ↓)
• Surgical conditions: gastroschisis, omphalocele, neural tube defects	

Clinical significance:

(a) Various factors that affect IWL should be considered when calculating fluid requirement in neonates. (Table 23.6)

(b) Adopt measures to reduce IWL by maintenance of OT temperature, humidity, supplementation of humidified O2, use of heated incubator, and cover head and body during transportation and operation.

(c) IWL is higher in preterm and small for date neonates, due to larger body surface area to weight ratio, high respiratory rate and thin, fragile, poorly keratinized skin.

Box 23.1 Causes of Persistent High ADH in Newborn

1. Early cord clamping,
2. Repeated blood sampling,
3. Volume depletion,
4. Hypoxia,
5. Acidosis,
6. Hypercarbia
7. Assisted ventilation (IPPV)
8. Sepsis

23.3 Nutrition Requirements

Requirement of water, electrolytes and calories varies with GA and BW. While calculating nutritional requirement, volume of fluid that may be used, must also be considered.

Table 23.7 Water and Electrolytes requirement as per postnatal age and BW

Water (mL/kg/day)	D 1	D 2	D 3	D 4	D 5	D 6	D 7–28
Term/Preterm BW >1500 g	50–60	70–80	100–120	120–150	140–160	140–160	150–180
Preterm BW<1500 g	80–90	100–110	120–130	130–150	140–160	150–180	150–180
Electrolytes							
Na (mEq/kg/D)	–	1–3 (high in preterm/BW<1000 g)					3–5
K (mEq/kg/D)	–	1–2 (high in preterm/BW<1000 g)					2–3
Cl (mEq/kg/D)	–	1–3					3–5
Ca	0.8–1 (mmol/kg/D)						
HCO₃	1–2 mmol/kg/D in extremely preterms due to poor reabsorption of bicarbonate.						

1. **Calorie/glucose requirement** in a term newborn is 32 kcal/kg with rapid increase in 1st week of life. Thereafter, it increases linearly with growth. Preterm neonates are more prone to hypoglycemia due to limited glycogen stores. The developing brain of a neonate is relatively protected from damage secondary to hypoglycemia, as it can use both ketones and glucose as energy substrate, but prolonged hypoglycemia (<2.6 mmol/L or < 40 mg%) may lead to adverse neurological outcome. Hence, glucose should be administered at 3–5 mg/kg/min in term and 5–7 mg/kg/min in preterm with blood glucose monitoring, especially during periods of starvation.
2. **Water requirement** in neonate is to compensate for losses both sensible and insensible. Neonates are born waterlogged and have high ADH in first 24 h. They then start losing weight until 1 week. Therefore, water requirement is less on 1st day of life. Insensible losses are more in the premature and so is the maintenance fluid requirement. (Table 23.6)
3. **Electrolyte requirements:** supplementation of sodium, potassium and chloride is not required in 1st 24 h, because term neonates conserve Na⁺ better. Extremely LBW and premature babies require Na⁺ at 12–24 h because of high fractional extraction of Na⁺, with a daily requirement of 3–5 mmol/kg, preferably as sodium acetate (risk of hyperchloremic metabolic acidosis with sodium chloride). With growth spurt, need for potassium increases to 2–3 mEq/kg/day, and of sodium and chloride to 3–5 mEq/kg/day each, after the 1st week. Preterm neonates require more potassium because of high aldosterone, high postnatal diuresis and high prostaglandin excretion after completion of postnatal volume contraction (Table 23.7).

Goal of Perioperative Fluid Management:
1. to ensure smooth transition from aquatic in-utero environment to dry ex-utero environment
2. to ensure adequate organ perfusion, oxygenation and nutrition without any electrolyte disturbances or increasing lung water or tissue oedema or hypoglycemia.

23.4   Components of Perioperative Fluid Therapy

23.4.1 Intraoperative Fluid Requirement

Intraoperative fluid therapy in neonates should provide basal metabolic requirements (maintenance), compensate for preoperative deficit (fasting and other losses),
replace losses during surgery and support systemic blood pressure. The goal is to
provide just adequate, not too much fluid (Box 23.2). The evidence regarding intraoperative fluid therapy in neonates is limited, so it is difficult to give accurate
guidelines.

Box 23.2 Adverse Outcome of Excessive IVF

1. Generalized tissue edema,
2. Abnormal pulmonary function,
3. CCF,
4. PDA,
5. NEC,
6. BPD.

There are three components of fluid therapy that determine the type and volume
of fluid to be administered, namely, **maintenance, deficit, and replacement**:

1. **Maintenance fluids:** this compensates for ongoing losses due to basal body
   metabolism, and sensible and insensible losses. The term neonates require fluid
   @ 60, 75, 90, 105, 120, 135 and 150 mL/kg/24 h for initial 7 postnatal days,
   and thereafter 150 mL/kg/24 h for rest of the neonatal period. Premature neonates require more fluid.
   (a) While choosing type of maintenance fluid, following points should be
       kept in mind:
       i. **Age, weight, and maturity**: on 1st postnatal day, neonates need glu-
          cose but not Na^+, until diuresis starts.
       ii. Avoid hypotonic solutions due to risk of hyponatremia. Use isotonic
          crystalloids with sodium in the range of 131–154 mmol/L.
       iii. If neonate is stable on a particular fluid, continue same fluid at
          that rate:
   (b) **Type of fluid**: on D 1: 5%/10% dextrose; D 2 onward: 0.45% saline with
       10% dextrose.
   (c) Measure plasma electrolytes and glucose when starting IVF for mainte-
       nance (except for elective surgery) and every 24 h thereafter.
   (d) In case of risk of water retention (secondary to high ADH secretion): a
       50–80% restriction in routine maintenance fluids (based on insensible
       losses within 300–400 mL/m^2/24 h) + urine output.
2. **Deficit fluid therapy:** this compensates for any losses prior to medical care; GI
   loss (diarrhea, vomiting); significant blood loss in trauma; and inadequate
   intake during prolonged fasting. Clinical features of dehydration are given in
   Table 23.8:

Table 23.8 Clinical features of dehydration

Signs/Symptoms	No clinical S/S	Clinically detectable	Shock
GC, Appearance	Alert, normal responsiveness	Looks unwell, irritable, lethargic/deteriorating	Altered consciousness
Eyes	Not sunken	Sunken	–
Mucus membranes	Moist	Dry	–
BP	Normal	Normal	↓↓
RR	Normal	↑	↑↑
Capillary refill time	Normal	Normal	Prolonged
HR	Normal	↑	↑↑
Peripheral pulses	Normal	Normal	Weak
Skin turgor	Normal	Reduced	-
Skin color	Normal	Normal	Pale, mottled
Extremities	Warm	Warm	Cold
Urine output	Normal	↓	↓↓/Anuria

(a) Preoperative fasting fluid deficit is minimal in most neonates following the modern liberal NPO guidelines and continuous IV infusion in critically ill babies.

(b) Continuous clinical and laboratory assessment to determine presence of dehydration, its severity (mild, moderate, severe as per the % of IVF loss <5%, 5–10% or > 10%, respectively), and the type (isotonic, hypotonic, hypertonic according to serum Na levels 130–150 mEq/L, <130 mEq/L or 150 mEq/L, respectively). (Table 23.8)

(c) Laboratory investigations include serum Na, K, urea, creatinine, and glucose.

(d) ABG and serum chloride in case of shock.

(e) Any fluid deficit should be corrected before induction of anaesthesia.

Type of fluid for dehydration: isotonic salt solution (Hartmann's, Plasmalyte, NS) or blood, FFP or platelets as required. All fluid types are listed in Appendix 1.

(f) Measure BW daily: <5% loss in BW—increment of 10 mL/kg fluid, and >5 % loss in BW: increment of 15–20 mL/kg/day.

3. **Replacement fluid therapy:** this replaces ongoing losses during medical care, such as bleeding, loss through drains including NG drain, shunts, continuing diarrhea, vomiting, etc.:

(a) **Type of fluid for Resuscitation in Hypovolemic shock:** glucose-free crystalloids containing 131–154 mmol/L of sodium in a bolus of 10–20 mL/kg over 10 min, and smaller volume in cases of cardiac or renal dysfunction.

    i. Reassess after each bolus and decide on the need of next bolus.

    ii. If >40–60 mL/kg fluid is needed during initial resuscitation—investigate further.

    iii. Inotropes should be started if there are signs of poor perfusion or fluid unresponsiveness.

(b) In case Hypernatremia/Hyponatremia develops, manage as per Algorithm 23.1.

23.4.2 Postoperative Fluid Therapy

This should be continued as maintenance fluids until the neonate is able to take orally. Ongoing losses should be measured and replaced.

Algorithm 23.1 Management of hypernatremia/Hyponatremia during fluid therapy

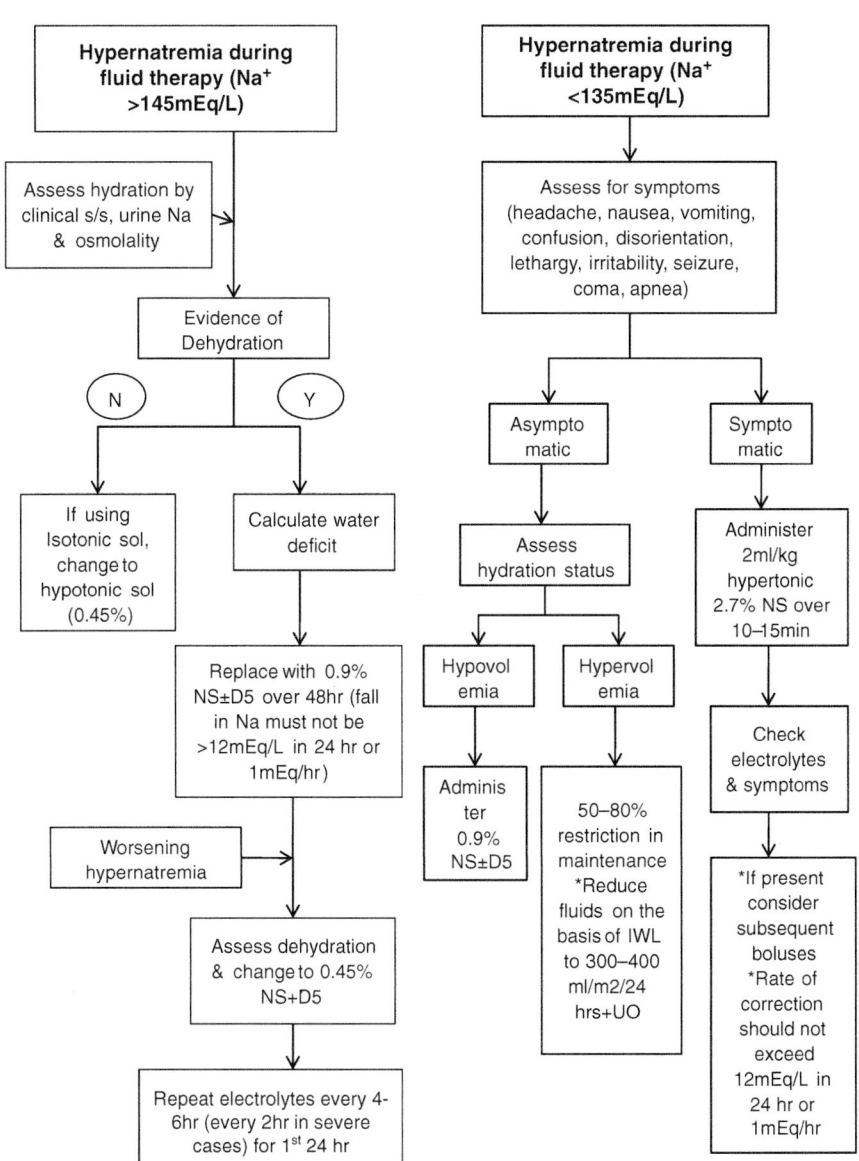

23.4.3 How to Measure Fluid Responsiveness in Neonates

The clinical and laboratory findings (changes in BP, HR, capillary refill time, core-peripheral temperature gradient, urine output, blood lactate and base deficit etc.) do not reliably predict fluid responsiveness in neonates. Central venous pressure (CVP) and pulmonary artery wedge pressure (PCWP) are also unreliable.

Dynamic parameters based on arterial pressure waveform and contour analysis in response to ventilation also has a limited predictive value because of:

1. First, more compliant vasculature, lungs and chest wall that alters respiratory–cardiovascular relationship.
2. Second, high tidal volume (>10 ml/kg) is required to produce ventilation induced CVS changes, and lung-sparing ventilation technique (low tidal volume with high PEEP) limits use of dynamic parameters.
3. Third, the variation of pulse oximetry waveform with ventilation is also unreliable due to difficulty in establishing a constant trace during surgery.
4. The most reliable dynamic measure in neonates is variation in aortic flow velocity with ventilation, measured by transthoracic (TT) or transesophageal (TE) Echocardiogram.
5. Stroke volume index (SVI 33–47 mL/m^2/beat) measured by TEE Doppler is the best static parameter to predict fluid responsiveness in neonates.

23.4.4 Care During IV Fluids Administration

1. IV fluid should be given through burette set or infusion pump because of narrow margin of safety.
2. Always consider fluid used for flushing and administering drugs during fluid calculation.
3. Fluid boluses are recommended in hypovolemic, not in euvolemic neonates.
4. As far as possible, use separate IV line for maintenance fluid at set rate and for replacement fluids, because administration of two different types of fluids is required at two different rates.
5. Hypotonic fluids should be used with caution and must not be infused in large volumes.
6. Correction of Hypovolemia should be done with rapid infusion of isotonic saline (NS), and of dehydration more slowly over 14–72 h.
7. Administer D 5% or D 10% @ 120 mg/kg/h in malnourished or neonates with low blood sugar levels.
8. Measure serum electrolytes and glucose regularly in all who require large volumes of IVF for more than 24 h.

23.5 Blood Transfusion

The principles of blood component therapy in neonates are same as in older children and adults, i.e., ensuring adequacy of intravascular volume, with components added as indicated.

Few differences that should be considered while planning for BT in Neonates are small intravascular volume; high O_2 consumption; higher CO to blood volume ratio; significantly high Hb level at birth and of HbF, and immature immune system.

(i). Neonates are usually anemic from several causes:

1. Transition from Hb F to Hb A
2. Limited responsiveness to Erythropoietin
3. Rapid growth
4. Early umbilical cord clamping
5. Repeated blood sampling
6. Sepsis
7. Surgical intervention

(ii). Consequences of untreated anemia:

- associated with apnea
- Poor weight gain
- Poor neuro-developmental outcome

(iii). BT is associated with risk of:

- Necrotizing enterocolitis (NEC)
- Retinopathy of prematurity (ROP)
- Bronchopulmonary dysplasia (BPD)

Need for BT can be reduced by delayed umbilical cord clamping, minimal blood sampling, optimum nutrition, selection of lower transfusion triggers and use of Pedi packs.

(iv). **Massive Transfusion** in neonates is defined as:

1. Infusion of blood equivalent to a single circulating volume within 24 h or
2. Equivalent to 50% of circulating volume in 3 h or
3. BT @ 50 mL/kg/min or more.

One mL/kg of packed red blood cells (PRBC) will increase hematocrit (Hct) by 1% after 15 min for up to 24 h, if no ongoing bleeding occurs. Massive BT is associated with risk of hyperkalemia, hypocalcemia, and hypothermia. Therefore, blood should be administered through a warmer, followed by monitoring of electrolytes and with calcium replacement.

Table 23.9 Transfusion trigger in term neonates

Indications	Transfusion trigger Hb
Anemia in first 24 h	12 g/dL
Receiving intensive care	12 g/dL
Chronic O_2 dependency	11 g/dL
Late anemia, stable, no respiratory support	7 g/dL
Acute blood loss	10% of blood volume[a]
Posted for major surgery	10 g/dL
Moderate cardiopulmonary disease	10 g/dL
Severe cardiopulmonary disease	13 g/dL

[b]ABL calculation: ABL = BW × EBV × $[(H_o – H_1)/H_m]$; where H_o = initial Hct, H_1 = target Hct, H_m = avg Hct

The volume of PRBC (mL) transfused is calculated as: required increase in Hb (g/dL) × BW (kg) × 4.8 (4 mL/kg PRBC raises Hb by 1 g/dL)

[a]Estimated blood volume (EBV): 80–90 mL/kg in term, 90–100 mL/kg in preterm

Table 23.10 Transfusion threshold for preterm neonates (< 32 week GA)

Postnatal age	Transfusion threshold (Hb g/dL)		
	On IPPV	On O_2/CPAP	None
First 24 h	<12	<12	<10
1–7 days	<12	<10	<10
8–14 days	<10	<9.5	<7.5–8.5
>15 days	<8.5	<8.5	<8.5

(v) **Transfusion Triggers:** the main indication of BT in neonates is to maintain O_2 carrying capacity and O_2 delivery to tissues. Transfused blood contains Hb A, which allows better O_2 delivery at tissue level. BT also reduces CO in anemic patients. Various transfusion triggers along with calculation of allowable blood loss (ABL) and volume of packed red cells transfused to achieve target Hb are shown in Tables 23.9 and 23.10. Losses below the maximum allowable blood loss (MABL) are managed by crystalloids or colloids, while once blood loss exceeds MABL, it must be replaced with blood.

(vi) **Precautions During BT:**

(a)	Use Pedi-pack (35–66 mL) to minimize donor exposure.

(b)	Use fresh (usually within 5 days of donation) because of low K+ content.

(c)	Use γirradiated blood that destroys lymphocytes in neonates with immune deficiency (preterm to avoid graft vs host reaction). Lymphocytes in donor blood attack recipient bone marrow and other tissues, causing fever, pancytopenia, hepatitis, diarrhea etc., though rare but is a deadly complication. (use within 24 h of irradiation for suspected or known T-cell immunodeficiency)

(d)	Some centers use leuco-depleted blood to reduce alloimmunization, febrile hemolytic transfusion reactions and risk of NEC, ROP and BPD.

Table 23.11 Prophylactic platelet transfusion threshold

Platelet count (×10⁹/L)	Indications
<30	Transfuse all even in absence of bleeding
30–49	BW <1500 g & ≤7 days, Clinically unstable, Concurrent coagulopathy, Previous significant hemorrhage (grade 3 or 4 IVH), Prior to planned surgery, Post-operative (72 h)
50–100	Active bleeding, Neonatal alloimmune thrombocytopenia (NAIT) with IC bleed, Before or after neurosurgical procedures

(e)   Neonates have weak expression of ABO antigen at birth. Therefore, cross matching is not always needed, but prior ABO, Rh typing, and initial antibody screening is required.

(vii) Platelet Transfusion:

- Majority of platelet transfusions are given 'prophylactically' in absence of bleeding.
- Threshold for prophylaxis in major surgery is 100×10^9/L. (Table 23.11)
- Platelets should be ABO and Rh compatible, cytomegalovirus negative and of single donor.
- Recommended dose: 10–20 mL/kg.

23.6   Fresh Frozen Plasma

Indications for FFP transfusion is coagulopathy, but its diagnosis is uncertain in neonates because of different age-related values for common coagulation screening tests such as prothrombin time, thrombin time, and activated partial thromboplastin time which are prolonged without any associated risk of bleeding, even in healthy term newborns. At birth, vitamin-K-dependent clotting factors are 40–50% of adult levels and are lower in preterms.

Indication: Vitamin K deficiency with bleeding, DIC, coagulation factor deficiencies.

Recommended dose: 12–15 mL/kg

It should not be used as volume replacement and is not superior to crystalloid or colloid infusion.

23.7   Cryoprecipitate

A more concentrated source of fibrinogen than FFP that is indicated when fibrinogen level is <0.8–1.0 g/dL in the presence of bleeding from acquired or congenital hypofibrinogenaemia.

Indication: major hemorrhage, bleeding after cardiac surgery or DIC.

Recommended dose: 5–10 mL/kg; higher volume in case of active bleeding.

Aim is to achieve Fibrinogen concentration >1 g/dL, and >2 g/dL in case of continued bleeding.

23.8 Conclusion

Neonates are not a miniature of adults. Their fluid and electrolyte requirements are unique due to major fluid shifts after birth, varying water requirements, high insensible losses and limited cardiac and renal function. Frequent clinical and laboratory monitoring are prudent to ensure proper fluid therapy because of narrow margin of safety.

Pearls of Wisdom

- TBW is 80% in term neonates. As ECF is more than ICF, water requirement is more and tolerance to dehydration is poor.
- Movement of water and solutes from IV to IS compartment depends on EGL. Damage to EGL results in increase capillary permeability, loss of plasma proteins into IS, and subsequent IS oedema.
- Neonates have limited ability to handle both volume over and under load due to immature cardiac and renal functions.
- They easily dehydrate with conservative fluid therapy.
- They are prone for hypernatremia in first 24 h if excess sodium is infused and for hyponatremia after 24 h with initiation of diuresis. Avoid Na on 1st day of life.
- They are prone for hypoglycemia due to limited glycogen stores, so administer D 5–10%. One should balance hypoglycemia with potential augmentation of ischemic injury from iatrogenic hyperglycemia.
- Standard maintenance fluid: 1st day: D 5–10%; 2nd day onward: 0.45% saline in D10%
- Standard deficit and replacement fluid is isotonic salt solution (RL, Plasmalyte) or blood.
- Crystalloids and colloids are equally effective in hypovolemic state in contrast to 3:1 ratio in adults.
- Administer glucose-free crystalloids that contain 131–154 mmol/L sodium, as 10–20 mL/kg bolus, over 10 min for resuscitation in hypovolemia, repeat as per response.
- Clinical and laboratory parameters unreliable to assess fluid responsiveness.
- Avoid colloids (except 4.5% albumin) due to insufficient safety data in neonates owing to immature renal and coagulation functions.
- 4.5% albumin is iso-oncotic to plasma and can be used.
- In absence of active bleeding, 4–5 mL/kg PRBC raise Hb by 1 g/dL in neonates.

Appendix 1: Composition of Crystalloids and Colloids

Fluid (1 L)	Osmolality mOsm/L	Tonicity	Na mEq/L	K mEq/L	Ca mEq/L	Cl mEq/L	Others/L	pH	Uses
Saline 0.9%	308	Isotonic	154			154		5	Brain injury, hypochloremic metabolic alkalosis, hyponatremia
Hartmann's	281	Isotonic	131	5	2	111	Lactate 29	6.5	ECF replacement
Plasmalyte	294	Isotonic	140	5		98	Acetate 27, Gluconate 23, Mg 3 mEq	4-6.5	ECF replacement
Dextrose 5%	252	Hypotonic					Glucose 50 g	4	Hypernatremia, hypoglycemia
Saline 0.45%	154	Hypotonic	77			77		4-5	Hypernatremia, hypovolemia
4% Dextrose + 0.18% saline	284	Hypotonic	31			31	Glucose 40g	4-5	Maintenance fluid
5% Dextrose + 0.45% saline	432	Hypertonic	75			75	Glucose 50g		Maintenance fluid
5% Dextrose + 0.9% saline	560	Hypertonic	154			154	Glucose 50g		Replacement
4.5% albumin in saline	270-300	Isotonic	100-160	<2		100-160	Albumin 45g	7.4	Plasma vol expander
20% albumin in saline	270-300	Isotonic	50-120	<10		140	Albumin 200g	7.4	Plasma vol expander
Gelofusine MW 30000	274	Isotonic	154	0.4	0.4	125	Gelatin 40 g, Mg 0.4	7.4	Plasma vol expander
Haemaccel MW 30 000	301	Isotonic	145	5.1	6.25	145	Gelatine 35g	7.3	Plasma vol expander
Dextran 70 (mol wt 70,000) in D 5/NS	287	Isotonic					Dextran 60g, Glu 50g or Na 154	5-6 4-5	hyperviscosity, vol expander
Hespan 6% (mol wt) 2,00,000)	310	Isotonic	154			154	Citrate < 15 Starch 60g	5.5	Volume expander
Voluven (mol wt 1,30,000)	307	Isotonic	154			154	Starch 60g	4-5.5	Plasma vol expander
NS 3%	1026	Hypertonic	513			513		5	Hyponatremia
NaHCO3 7.5%	1786	Hypertonic	893				HCO3 893	8	Acidosis

Further Readings

Barash PG. Clinical anesthesia, 7th ed. Chapter 48. Neonatal anaesthesia.

Bhardwaj N. Perioperative fluid therapy and intraoperative blood loss in children. Indian J Anaesth. 2019;63(9):729–36.

New HV, Berryman J, Bolton-Maggs PHB, et al. Guidelines on transfusion for fetuses, neonates, and older children. Br J Haematol. 2016;175(5):784–828.

Murat I, Humblot A, Girault L, Piana F. Neonatal fluid management. Best Pract Res Clin Anaesthesiol. 2010;24(3):365–74.

NICE Guideline No. 29. Intravenous fluid therapy in children and young people in hospital. London: National Institute for Health and Care Excellence (UK); 2020; ISBN-13: 978-1-4731-1576-7.

O'brien F, Walker I. Fluid homeostasis in the neonate. Pediatric Anaesthesia. 2013;24(1):49–59.

Sparger K, Deschmann E, Visner MS. Platelet Transfusions in the NICU. Clin Perinatol. 2015;42(3):613–23.

Stendal AC, Visram AR. Management of fluids in neonatal surgery. BJA Education. 2018;18(7):199e203.

Visram AR. Intraoperative fluid therapy in neonates. South Afr J Anaesthesia Analg. 2016;22(2):46–51.

Central Neuraxial Blocks in Neonates

24

Chitra Garg

24.1 Introduction

The nervous system of neonates is immature and has absence of full myelination and poorly myelinated thalamocortical radiation but that does not indicate lack of function. Recent studies have shown that both neonates and premature babies do possess the neuroanatomical and synaptic prerequisites to perceive nociceptive stimulus. Painful experience due to insufficient pain relief is associated not only with negative short-term effect but also with long-term effects.

Regional anaesthesia is commonly used as adjuvant to general anaesthesia (GA) as a part of multimodal perioperative pain relief. The small size of neonate does not preclude the use of local (LA)/regional anaesthesia (RA) techniques. However, it must be carried out with extreme precision and care.

The aim of this chapter is to provide clinical information on safe use of central neuraxial block in neonates and premature babies.

24.2 Anatomy

Knowledge of the anatomy of the spine and spinal cord, and anatomical differences between a neonate and older child, is essential to perform a successful spinal block with minimal complications in this age group. Some of the significant differences are as follows (Fig. 24.1, Table 24.1):

1. The **spinal cord ends** at a lower caudad level in neonates (at L3 in newborns and at L1 by the age of one year (Fig. 24.1). To avoid injury to the spinal cord during dural puncture for subarachnoid block (SAB), dural puncture should be attempted below L3.

C. Garg (✉)
Royal Victoria Infirmary, Newcastle upon Tyne, UK

© The Author(s), under exclusive license to Springer Nature Singapore Pte Ltd. 2023
U. Saha (ed.), *Clinical Anesthesia for the Newborn and the Neonate*,
https://doi.org/10.1007/978-981-19-5458-0_24

Fig. 24.1 Diagrammatic representation of anatomical difference between neonate and infant

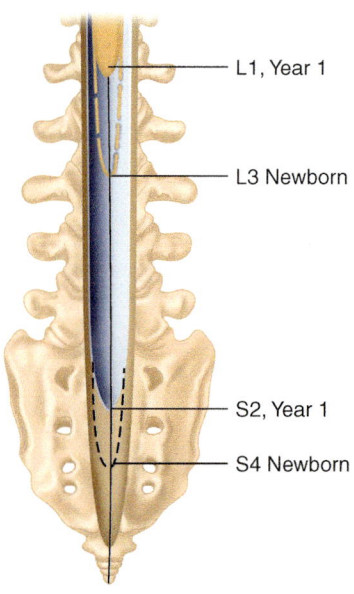

L1, Year 1

L3 Newborn

S2, Year 1

S4 Newborn

Table 24.1 Anatomical and physiological considerations in neonates and children

	Neonates	Children more than 1 year
Dural sac ends	S4	S2
Spinal cord ends	L3	L1
Intercristal space	L5-S1	L5
Lumbar lordosis	Absent	Present (acquired upright position)
Plasma albumin/alpha 1 glycoprotein	Very low	Low

2. Due to proportionately smaller pelvis and more cephalad placement of sacrum, the **intercristal line (Tuffier's line or Jacoby's line),** the horizontal line across the highest point of both iliac crests in anteroposterior lumbar radiograph, crosses at L5-S1 in neonates, and anywhere in between inferior end plate of L4 to superior endplate of L5 in adults (lower level in neonates).

3. The **dural sac** also terminates at more caudad location in neonates (S4 in newborn and S2 at 1 year of age). This position of dural sac makes it more likely to have inadvertent dural puncture while performing caudal block in neonates; therefore, extra precaution is warranted.

4. **Cerebrospinal fluid volume (CSF)** is larger in neonates on ml/kg basis (4 mL/kg) as compared to older children and adults (2 mL/kg). This may account for larger dose requirement and shorter duration of action of the LA drugs in newborns and neonates.

24.3 Spinal Anesthesia (SAB)

24.3.1 Indications of Spinal Anaesthesia

Spinal anaesthesia or Sub Arachnoid Block (SAB) has been found to offer special advantage in preterm babies (newborns, neonates, and ex-premature infants), who are at greater risk of apnea after GA. Spinal anesthesia technique may reduce but does not eliminate the risk of postoperative apnea. Careful assessment and consideration of additional risk factors must be made, such as:

1. History of previous episodes of apnea
2. Post conceptual age less than 48 weeks
3. Use of sedatives
4. Inadequate or nonavailability of monitoring facilities

Table 24.2 Indications for spinal anaesthesia

Inguinal hernia repair
Circumcision
Laparotomy
Meningomyelocele repair
Lower limb surgery
Cardiac surgery
Thoracic surgery
Urogenital procedures
Colostomy and colostomy closure

Note – spinal anesthesia term is commonly used for SAB

Table 24.2 lists common neonatal surgeries performed under spinal anaesthesia, with or without GA.

24.3.2 Technique for SAB in Neonates

Besides the type of surgery, neonate's age, medical status, duration of surgery, and experience of anesthesiologist dictate the indication for spinal or sub arachnoid block (SAB). If being used as a sole technique, it can be used for surgeries of short duration, usually under 60 minutes, but if combined with GA, time factor does not matter.

Preparation

1. Procedure should be carried out in an operation room apt for neonates, especially regarding temperature management (warm blankets, heated mattresses, and radiant lamps).
2. It should be performed where surgery is likely to be undertaken, so as to reduce transfers after drug has been administered, to prevent ascent of block.
3. To reduce the pain of the spinal needle puncture, EMLA cream can be applied locally, 30–40 min before the procedure. After application of EMLA cream, the site can be covered with a dressing to prevent it from getting wiped off (with the baby in supine position), or baby is kept prone with area uncovered.
4. SAB is usually done without sedation keeping in mind the indication in premature and ex-preterm neonates, and the risk of sedation induced apnea and bradycardia.
5. Make sure that a working IV canula is in place.
6. Appropriate informed consent must be taken from the parents or caretakers.
7. The procedure should be carried out under careful vigilant monitoring (ECG, HR, color, Saturation, respiration, RR, and temperature), with emergency drug tray available, and ensuring patient safety.

Position and Care During SAB

(a) Usually, lateral flexed but also with baby held in sitting position.
(b) Neck flexion should be avoided to prevent airway obstruction.
(c) L4-5, L5-S1 interspinous spaces should be identified.
(d) All aseptic precautions must be taken during the procedure.
(e) If EMLA was not applied earlier, then LA should be administered before the skin puncture in an awake neonate.
(f) A short 22 or 25 G needle is used, especially designed for neonates.
(g) The pop of dural puncture not perceived because the ligamentum flavum is soft.
(h) Only when CSF is seen at the end of the spinal needle, confirming needle tip position in the intrathecal space, LA drug should be injected.
(i) The barbotage method is not recommended as this may result in high levels of block and even total spinal.
(j) Caudad end of the baby should never be elevated for positioning and placement of cautery pads due to risk of ascent of block and high or total spinal blockade. Allow adequate time for the fixation of LA drug before any manipulation.

24.3.3 Assessment of Block

This is often difficult in neonates and infants, particularly in sedated and anaesthetized babies. Generally, pinprick, cold stimuli (alcohol swab), rate and pattern of ventilation in awake babies can guide as to the level of block. Bromage scale (Box 24.1) for assessing the level of block is validated for more than 2 years of age as it requires voluntary movements, but may be helpful in a healthy awake neonate to some extent.

Box 24.1 Bromage scale

No block—full flexion of knees and feet possible

Partial block—just able to flex knees, full flexion of feet possible

Almost complete block—unable to flex knees, flexion of feet possible

Complete block—unable to move legs or feet

24.3.4 Adverse Effects

Hypotension, bradycardia, PDPH, and transient radicular symptoms seen in adults are less common in neonates. Complications of high or total spinal block are seen in the form of apnea, bradycardia, hypotension, desaturation, and even cardiac standstill. Risk of these complications is more in presence of hypothermia, anaemia, acid base, electrolyte disturbances, and associated congenital anomalies, especially cardiac.

24.3.5 Local Anaesthetics and adjuvants

Use of tetracaine, bupivacaine, Lidocaine, L-bupivacaine and ropivacaine have been described in the literature. Commonly 0.5–1 mg/kg of **L-bupivacaine** is used for SAB. Dilution of the drug should be avoided as it can lead to incomplete or partial effect or requiring greater volume.

Additive, such as **Clonidine,** in a dose of 1 mcg/kg added along with bupivacaine, prolongs duration of block. Higher doses of clonidine are associated with hypotension and sedation during intraoperative (if used as a sole technique) and postoperative period and apnea, negating one of the benefits of SAB. It may be advisable to use caffeine (10 mg/kg) intravenously to prevent potential apnea in the postoperative period, especially if clonidine is used in SAB.

Morphine may be used in a dose of 10 mcg/kg intrathecally, in cardiac patients who would be ventilated postoperatively. Otherwise, intrathecal morphine must be avoided in neonates because of the potential risk of postoperative apnea.

Table 24.3 Contraindications to SAB in neonates

1	Spine abnormalities
2	Allergy to LA
3	Family's refusal/no consent
4	Coagulopathy
5	Raised intra-cranial pressure
6	Infection at spinal puncture site
7	Sepsis
8	Presence of a VP shunt
9	Neuromuscular disorders -myopathy, degenerative NM disease, etc.

24.3.6 Contraindications

Contraindications to use of spinal anaesthesia in children are similar to as in adults. Table 24.3 lists the contraindications to SAB in neonates.

24.4 Epidural Block

Since the popularization of this technique in paediatric patients in the late 1980's, epidural block has become a standard procedure in children to provide intra- and postoperative analgesia. In neonates undergoing major abdominal surgery, use of epidural block results in significantly better modification of the neuroendocrine surgical stress response than postoperative intravenous morphine infusion, besides shortening the period of postoperative paralytic ileus also. Although use of epidural blockade in neonates and infants has been questioned by some, this method represents one of the cornerstones of high-quality analgesia for neonates undergoing more extensive surgical interventions. Caudal epidural is the most common technique used in neonates.

24.4.1 Caudal Epidural Block

This is one of the most common and routinely used regional anaesthetic techniques in paediatric population and is also well suited to the smallest patient category. It is one of the easiest blocks to learn. With caudal block, adequate anaesthesia can be achieved up to the mid-thoracic region, thus can be used either alone as an awake anaesthesia technique, or as a supplement (anaesthesia/analgesia) to GA for surgical procedures down below mid-thoracic level.

With ultrasound, it is now possible to visualize the injection of LA in the caudal space as well as monitor the cranial spread. The use of ultrasound is highly

Table 24.4 Caudal block- levels of surgical anaesthesia and LA volume. Modified Armitage formula

Volume of injectate (mL/kg)	Surgical procedure
0.5	Urogenital, club foot surgery
1.0	Sub umbilical surgery
1.25	Surgeries below mid-thoracic level

recommended in neonates who receive concomitant GA. It is much more difficult to use in the awake and mobile baby. Although this block can be used for almost all surgical interventions below the level of the umbilicus, the use of this technique in association with neonatal inguinal hernia and hypospadias repair is by far the most common one. By applying Modified Armitage formula, one can achieve different levels of block by injecting different volumes of LA caudally (Table 24.4).

The awake caudal technique is a useful alternative to GA in ex-premature neonates who often suffer from various degrees of bronchopulmonary dysplasia (BPD). Such babies often have had great difficulties in weaning from mechanical ventilation. Parents, neonatologist, and anaesthesiologists want to avoid the risks involved with GA, delayed recovery, tracheal re-intubation, and need for mechanical ventilation.

24.4.2 Care During Awake Caudal Block in Ex-Premature Neonates

The use of the awake caudal technique will also limit the risk for postoperative apnoea in this specific patient category. To fulfil this requirement, precautions to be adopted are as follows:

- The block must be carried out without the use of adjunct sedatives (e.g., midazolam, ketamine, and low-concentrations inhalational anaesthetic by nasal prongs) or else the risk for postoperative apnoea will not be reduced as expected.
- Even in the case of a **"pure" awake** caudal technique, these neonates cannot be transferred to an ordinary ward after surgery but must remain in NICU/HDU environment overnight. This is particularly true if supplemental drugs such as ketamine or clonidine have been used as adjuncts to LA solution.
- The use of supplemental sedation is often not necessary since the systemic absorption of the LA together with loss of sensory input from the lower body usually make the child sedated, sleepy and still, within 15–20 min of injection.
- Care must be taken not to exceed the maximum recommended dosage of LA and additive drugs (they do not receive any sedative drugs that increase the seizure threshold).
- Administration of oral sucrose can help in neonates with awake caudal anaesthesia. It not only alleviates the discomfort of preoperative starvation but also has significant analgesic properties.

- Even if the most frequent indication for the awake caudal technique in neonates is inguinal hernia repair, this technique can also be very useful for lower limb venous cannulations (saphenous or femoral), and other lower limb procedures.

24.4.3 Anatomical Considerations

Anatomical differences between neonates and older children spine have already been highlighted in Fig. 24.1. The sacrum of infants is narrower, and flatter as compared to adult population. At birth, sacral vertebrae are not completely ossified and continue to fuse till child reaches 8 years of age. Incomplete fusion of lower sacral vertebrae forms sacral hiatus which serves as an entry point for caudal epidural injection. Epidural fat is less densely packed in children than in adults, and this facilitates spread of LA and unimpeded advancement of epidural catheter. Generally, the epidural space is found at a depth of 1 mm/kg body weight; however, there are considerable variations.

24.4.4 Technique and position for Caudal Block

The baby is usually placed in lateral position with knees drawn up to the chest or in prone position with a roll under the hips. After identifying the coccyx, continue to palpate in midline moving the finger in cephalad direction. The sacral hiatus is felt as a depression between two bony prominences of sacral cornua. Under full asepsis, short bevelled 22 G, styletted needle is inserted at around 45 degrees to the skin until a "pop" is felt as the sacrococcygeal ligament is punctured. At this point, the angle of needle is reduced to 20–30 degrees and needle is advanced for 2–4 mm into the caudal canal. Any further needle advancement is not recommended as risk of dural puncture increases significantly. Absence of subcutaneous bulging and lack of resistance upon injection of LA are additional signs of correct needle placement. While injecting the drug, aspiration-injection sequence must be followed, and all aspirations should be negative for blood and CSF.

The "whoosh" test, which involves injection of air in caudal space is not recommended as it can lead to patchy block or venous air embolism if needle is accidently placed in epidural vessel.

24.4.5 Local Anesthetics and Adjuvants

High concentrations of LA are hardly used in paediatric population. In children, body weight is a better correlate than age in predicting the spread of LA.

- Larger volumes of dilute concentrations are used such as 0.125%–0.25% L-bupivacaine or 0.2% ropivacaine.

- For continuous caudal epidural infusion, bupivacaine 0.2 mg/kg/h is recommended for neonates.
- Lidocaine is not often used due to its short duration of action.
- Always take into consideration the maximum allowable dose of LA to avoid overdosage and toxicity.
- Clonidine is the most common adjuvant used in dose of 0.5–2 mcg/kg to prolong the analgesic effect of caudal epidural.
- Epidural opioids prolong analgesia but have the potential of respiratory depression and unfavourable side effects as vomiting, itching, and urinary retention, necessitating bladder catheterization. Use of caudal epidural opioids should be restricted to special circumstances.

24.4.6 Complications

Major complications from single shot or continuous epidural blocks are rare if proper technique is used. Box 24.2 enumerates the list of possible complications, although rare.

Box 24.2 Complications

1.	Neurological injury
2.	Epidural hematoma
3.	Infection
4.	Dural puncture
5.	Total spinal
6.	LA toxicity

24.5 Some Technical Aspects of Epidural Block in Neonates

24.5.1 Site of Epidural Insertion

Insertion at the appropriate dermatomal level in relation to the surgical intervention is of paramount importance to achieve a well-functioning epidural block. This means that the tip of the epidural catheter is situated at an intraspinal level that corresponds to the dermatomal center of the surgical procedure. Thus, having the tip of the catheter at the lumbar level will not produce adequate analgesia if the patient is undergoing a thoracotomy. Rather, performing epidural at T8 for major upper laparotomy and at T4 or T5 for thoracotomy would ensure optimum pain relief. However, to make this technique reliable, it is important not to insert more than a few centimeters of the catheter into the epidural space.

Despite the low risk for major damage associated with thoracic epidural in children, the risk for traumatic spinal cord injury does exist. In order to avoid even the slightest risk for traumatic cord injury, and to reduce the risk of catheter dislodgment many paediatric anesthetists favor alternative methods for epidural catheter insertion, as Caudal approach. Blind caudal catheter technique as first described by Bosenberg is quite useful. Since neonates have not yet developed the adult pattern of spinal curvatures, it is possible to access the epidural space at the caudal hiatus, and then insert a predetermined length of the catheter to reach the desired spinal level. A very high success rate has been claimed with this blind approach, but some controversy exists regarding there confirmation radiographically. Although this approach is appealing due to its simplicity, the need for radiographic verification increases complexity. With use of high-performance USG machine, it is possible to see catheter tip at bed side.

Testing for proper placement of epidural catheters include LOR, Test dose, Epidural electrical stimulation test (Tsui test) and ultrasound guided placement.

24.5.2 Loss-of-resistance (LOR)

- Epidural block in neonates requires considerable experience and level of skill, unlike for caudal block.
- The distance to the epidural space is short in neonates. Changes in body habitus with increasing age are variable. These make it difficult to accurately predict the distance from the skin to the epidural space.
- Connective tissue is soft, thereby limiting the tactile feedback of loss of resistance (LOR) in identifying the epidural space.
- Besides, since regional block in children is usually performed under deep sedation or GA, subjective warning signs of neural injury during needle insertion cannot be detected.
- The use of air for loss-of-resistance (LOR) is not advocated because of risk of intravascular air embolism as well as permanent spinal cord injury. Only saline should be used for LOR, especially in neonates.

24.5.3 Test Dose

Due to the limited size of the equipment used in small children, inadvertent intravascular placement of the epidural catheter cannot be reliably identified solely from spontaneous backflow in the catheter or from an aspiration test. There is controversy over the use of adrenaline containing test dose. The occurrence of heart rate increase or T-wave changes on ECG following inadvertent intravascular injection of LA is influenced by the inhalational anaesthetic agents and anticholinergics used prior to the test dose. Since a negative result is not conclusive, many clinicians do not routinely use it in children.

24.5.4 Nerve Stimulation-guided Technique: 'Tsui-technique'

Tsui et al described this technique whereby the catheter with a stimulating tip is attached to a nerve stimulator. The catheter is inserted through the sacral hiatus or at thoracic level, and gradually the current is increased to 10 mA. The catheter is then slowly advanced in the cranial direction. The major advantage with this technique is that the operator is able to follow the muscular response as the tip of the catheter advances through the spinal canal **(this obviously requires that the patient be not paralyzed!).** The tip of the catheter is advanced until muscle contractions are visible or palpable at the appropriate level for the planned surgical procedure. An unexpected muscular response will alert the clinician that the catheter is not threading as expected and the catheter is slightly withdrawn and the patient position modified and the catheter re-advanced until the desired response and desired level is achieved.

24.5.5 Ultrasound Guided (USG) Caudal Epidural Catheter Placement

The application of US is particularly useful for regional epidural blocks in small babies since incomplete vertebral ossification facilitates the penetration of the US beam into the posterior vertebral column and makes identification of spinal structures easier.

The neonate is placed in a lateral position with the hips, maximally flexed. A high frequency linear probe is used to scan lumbo-sacral area. The US probe is placed transversely over the coccyx and scanning is performed in the cephalad direction till the two cornua of sacrum are seen as two humps (marked as stars) and hypoechoic space between them (frog eyes sign). Just beneath the hypoechoic space, hyperechoic line (sacrococcygeal ligament) is visualized (marked with arrow). The hypoechoic space between the "humps" and hyperechoic dorsum of the pelvic surface of the sacrum is the sacral hiatus (Fig. 24.2). Also, make a note of how superficial the sacral hiatus (0.5 cm).

If the probe is turned in longitudinal direction, sacral vertebrae (black arrow) and thick hyperechoic sacrococcygeal ligament (white arrow) covering the space from inferior S3 to the distal end of the sacrum can be seen. Anechoic caudal space (red

Fig. 24.2 Caudal sonoanatomy in transverse view

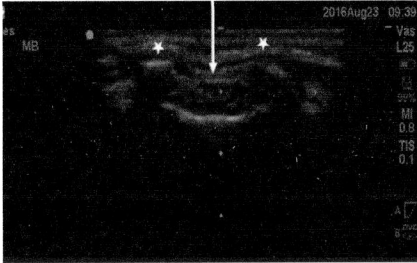

Fig. 24.3 Caudal sonoanatomy in longitudinal view

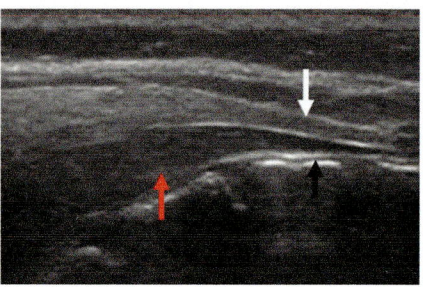

arrow) can also be observed (Fig. 24.3). Moving cephalad, the dural sac ends, cauda equina fibres, filum terminale, and conus medullaris can be visualized.

24.5.6 Technique of Caudal Placement Using USG

Under all aseptic precautions, the probe is first placed in transverse view, the needle tip is placed at the point of insertion, and then the probe is shifted to the longitudinal plane and the needle is advanced slowly till it reaches the caudal space. The LA solution is injected, and mass movement of the drug observed. The needle placement and success rate of USG caudal block are highly dependent on operator skill. However, USG caudal block increases the success rate of insertion at the first attempt and can reduce complications including vascular puncture and subcutaneous bulging. During caudal block, short bevelled and stylet needle should be used. Sharp needle can easily injure or even cut across the sacral base, causing damage to the pelvic or retroperitoneal organs.

24.6 Conclusion

Central neuraxial blocking technique is a boon to the neonatal anaesthesia practise. In specific surgical conditions, these can be used as sole anaesthesia techniques, and avoiding the use of GA, associated polypharmacy, and adverse consequences, chiefly, respiratory related. Specifically in premature and ex-premature neonates, procedures below the umbilicus can be performed under caudal or SAB, reducing the risk of postoperative apnea. While SAB has an end point, it is difficult to assess success of epidural puncture in neonates. Various tests have been described to confirm placement of epidural catheters or needle point for single shot technique, but Tsui test and Ultrasound have greatly improved the success rate and reduced the complication rates. However, proper knowledge of neuroanatomy, LA and additive drug dosages and their side-effects, availability of appropriate needles (spinal and Tuohy), monitoring facilities and readiness to manage any complications is of paramount importance for successful central neuraxial blocks in neonates.

Suggested Readings

Hadzic A. Textbook of regional anesthesia and acute pain management; 2016

Kil HK. Caudal and epidural blocks in infants and small children: historical perspective and ultrasound-guided approaches. Korean J Anesthesiol. 2018;71:430–9.

Tsui BC, Gupta S, Finucane B. Confirmation of epidural catheter placement using nerve stimulation. Can J Anaesth. 1998;45(7):640–4. https://doi.org/10.1213/01.ANE.0000080609.05942.38.

Tsui BC, Sze CK. An in vitro comparison of the electrical conducting properties of multi-port versus single-port epidural catheters for the epidural stimulation test. Anesth Analg. 2005;101(5):1528–30. https://doi.org/10.1213/01.ANE.0000181006.36917.3E.

Anaesthesia or Sedation for Procedures Outside the Operation Theatre

25

Sukanya Mitra, Kompal Jain, and Swati Jindal

25.1 Introduction

Key points to remember while giving sedation or anaesthesia to this age group are difficult airway, reduced functional residual capacity (FRC), reduced respiratory reserve, high oxygen consumption, rate dependent minute ventilation and cardiac output, dominant vagal tone, higher proneness to hypoglycaemia and hypothermia, and different pharmacokinetics and pharmacodynamics. They have increased sensitivity to anaesthetic drugs, leading to deeper level of sedation and loss of protective airway reflexes and impaired airway patency. It can further cause respiratory depression, apnea, laryngospasm, and cardiovascular instability. Immature liver and kidney prolong the action of drugs, demanding post sedation monitoring. Unfamiliar environment, lesser expert help, lack of immediate back up, and specific concerns related to procedures add to the challenges faced by anaesthesiologist in sedating and anaesthetising term and preterm newborns and neonates outside the operation theatre [1, 2].

25.2 The Context and the Challenges

The goal is to provide analgesia, relief from anxiety, amnesia, sedation, and most importantly prevent movements of the neonate, so that the diagnostic procedure can be done safely, to get meaningful results. The continuum of depth of sedation is classified as minimal, moderate, and deep sedation, and general anaesthesia, based on the responsiveness, airway, breathing and heart function.

S. Mitra (✉) · K. Jain · S. Jindal
Department of Anaesthesia & Intensive Care, Government Medical College & Hospital, Chandigarh, India

© The Author(s), under exclusive license to Springer Nature Singapore Pte Ltd. 2023
U. Saha (ed.), *Clinical Anesthesia for the Newborn and the Neonate*, https://doi.org/10.1007/978-981-19-5458-0_25

Human trials including GAS (General Anesthesia Spinal 2016) [3], Pediatric Anesthesia Neurodevelopment Assessment (PANDA 2016) [4], and Mayo Anesthesia Safety in Kids (MASK 2018) [5] concluded that no adverse neurodevelopmental outcome was observed in children after being exposed to general anaesthesia for short durations of less than 60 minutes.

Food and Drug Administration (FDA) issued warning against the use of general anaesthetic drugs, mainly medications acting on NMDA and GABA receptors, effect on the morphogenesis and synaptogenesis of the developing brain, triggering aponeurotic cell death and neurodegeneration, because of their effects in the neonatal period. However, this research studied neuro-inflammation induced by surgery and perioperative stress. Hence, the human trials are inconclusive regarding short- and long-term potential of anaesthetic drugs on neurodevelopment. Research also suggests that there might be increased risk of anaesthetic exposure in patients with specific genetic or epigenetic backgrounds and cognitive disabilities. A threefold increased incidence of desaturation had been noticed in paediatric age group with developmental disabilities as compared with normal children [6].

25.3   General Considerations

25.3.1 Infrastructure and Resources

This is required both for general and emergency management. A procedure might be performed in various settings: hospital, surgical centre, free standing imaging facility, dental facility, or private office. The major issue is the infrastructure, available resources in-situ, and immediate availability and accessibility of trained individuals competent in emergency resuscitation. Understandably, these are better in a hospital or similar setting rather stand-alone facilities. A dedicated area is required not only for the procedure but also for the recovery, with rescue drugs, equipment, and monitoring facilities [7, 8].

25.3.2 Clinicians' Skill and Training

Although non-anaesthesiologist practitioners can provide procedural sedation for neonates and infants, they must be adequately trained and have experience because skills are the most important asset for ensuring both safety and effectiveness of the procedures. Competency in airway management and handling emergency situations is a must. The clinician responsible for administering sedation must be prepared to manage emergency situations including aspiration, loss of airway, airway obstruction, laryngospasm, apnea, hypoventilation, hypoxemia, hypotension, bradycardia, arrhythmias, cardiac arrest, seizures, allergic reactions, and paradoxical reactions [9]. The practitioners must also be equipped with the right knowledge, skills, as well as attitude/affective component to deal with the neonates and their caregivers (all three medical educational domains-cognitive, psychomotor, and affective are tested during these procedures).

25.3.3 The '3-P's: Physical, Psychological, and Pharmacological

Pain and distress resulting from procedures can be mitigated by a combination of three general elements: physical, psychological, and pharmacological (the "3-P" approach) [10].

Physically comforting situation can be created by the environment (room, colours, lighting, sounds, music, and pictures on the wall), by various comforting positions when applicable (e.g., sitting upright rather than lying down, in the care-giver's lap, 'kangaroo' positioning), and by infant-focused tactics (breastfeeding, sucrose administration, sweetened pacifier, and 'swaddling') [11]. These can provide psychological comfort to the caretaker, along with various distraction techniques and psychological preparations. Finally, the pharmacological strategies are important, which are discussed below.

25.3.4 Selection and Screening

Patient selection and pre-sedation screening are vitally important, both to avoid pain arising out of less needed procedures (if other options are available) and to adequately prepare for the procedure, including for unexpected emergencies, in case it is selected. Pre-sedation screening is discussed below in details.

25.3.5 Specific Procedures

The sedation/analgesia protocols will vary according to specific procedures in question, because of differing pain-generating potentials, settings, duration, and parts of the body targeted by the procedures. Hence, knowledge and skills related to the specific procedures are required (discussed below).

25.4 Pre-sedation Screening

It is imperative that during screening multidisciplinary decision should be taken by anaesthesiologist, radiologist, and paediatrician regarding the importance weighing the benefits in comparison to risks, necessity, choice, and duration of the procedure. The procedure should only be undertaken if it provides meaningful information that will help in the neonatal care and outcome.

The procedures can be classified as painless and painful. Painless procedures include MRI, CT scan, radiotherapy, transthoracic ECHO, and electroencephalography (EEG). Painful procedures include cardiac angiography, interventional radiology, dental procedures, and cannulation for extracorporeal membrane oxygenation (ECMO). The requirements of the procedure including immobility, pain, amnesia and anxiolysis are assessed before the procedure along with the preanesthetic check-up including physical status evaluation, risk assessment of airway and respiration.

Emphasis should be on history of upper airway obstruction, gestational age (as prematurity can be associated with subglottic stenosis or apnea, behavioural problem, developmental delay, genetic disorders including Down's syndrome, trisomy, Pierre Robin syndrome), family history of malignant hyperthermia, pseudocholinesterase deficiency, muscular dystrophy, and allergies, history of previous sedation or hospitalisation and drug history. As per Scottish Intercollegiate Guidelines Network (SIGN), some of the contraindications of sedating the children include cardiac failure, liver failure, bowel obstruction, active respiratory tract disease, raised intracranial pressure, and known allergy to sedatives [12].

Prior to sedation, the WHO safety checklist should be followed for anaesthesia outside the operation theatre, regarding checklist for minimum staff, equipment and emergency checklist including resuscitation equipment, monitoring devices and drugs. Environment in which sedation or anaesthesia is to be given should include size-appropriate suction catheters and airway equipment, an adequate O_2 supply with functioning flowmeter, suction apparatus and monitors, special equipment like defibrillator, and basic and emergency drugs (acronym SOAPME; Panel 25.1) [13]. Monitors include pulse oximetry, blood pressure cuff, electrocardiogram, end tidal carbon dioxide and stethoscope. The team members should be assigned their roles, and communication should be clear and loud.

Minimum pre-sedation fasting time is 2 h for clear fluids, 4 h for breast milk. Baseline clinical observations include saturation, heart rate, temperature, respiratory rate, level of consciousness (using Paediatric Glasgow coma scale (PGCS)), sedation score, age, and weight in kilograms (kg) [14, 15].

Documentation includes informed consent, preanesthetic evaluation, baseline clinical observations, time-based record of the procedure including vitals every 5 min, drugs used and their doses, duration of the procedure, post-procedure vitals and instructions regarding start of feeding, and discharge criteria [2, 7].

Both pharmacological and nonpharmacological methods have been adopted for sedation and anaesthesia. Volatile anaesthetics, benzodiazepines, intravenous agents, opioids, sedative hypnotics, and others including xenon and dexmedetomidine have all been used. (Table 25.1) [16–18] Different routes of pharmacological sedation and anaesthesia include intraosseous (IO), intravenous (IV), intranasal, intramuscular (IM), per oral (PO) and inhalational via face mask, SGA/ LMA/ ETT. Nonpharmacological methods include good preparation, parental presence, parents lap or kangaroo care, facilitated tucking, distraction, feeding, non-nutritive sucking, and hypnosis. 'Feed and swaddle' or 'feed and wrap' or 'feed and sleep' technique includes feeding of the neonate 30–45 min prior to the procedure and induction of natural sleep followed by swaddling for immobilisation.

Factors contributing to failure of sedation in neonates include overstimulation, failed administration, length of procedure, procedural pain, timing, dosing, and adverse effects of drugs [8, 9].

Table 25.1 Various pharmacological drugs used for sedation

Drug group	Drug	Primary mechanism of action	Route	Dose	Precautions
Opioids	Fentanyl	Opioid receptor (especially mu) agonist	IV infusion IV single dose Intranasal	1–5 µg/kg/h 0.5–4 µg/kg 1.5–2 µg/kg	Slow administration Chest wall rigidity Respiration depression
Benzodiaz-epine	Midazolam	Gamma—Aminobu-tyric acid (GABA) receptor agonist	IV <32 week GA >32 week GA 6 mth–5 year IM Per rectal Sublingual Intranasal	0.03 mg/kg/h 0.06 mg/kg/h 0.05–0.1 mg/kg (max 6 mg) 0.1–0.15 mg/kg 1 mg/kg 0.5–0.75 mg/kg 0.2–0.3 mg/kg (max 10 mg/kg)	Rapid onset and short duration
Alpha 2 adrenergic receptor agonist	Dexme-detomidine	Alpha 2 adrenergic receptor agonist	Intranasal IV IM	0.2–2 µg/kg 1–2 µg/kg over 10 min, then 0.5–1.5 µg/kg/h 1–4 µg/kg	Preserves respiration Watch for hypotension, bradycardia
Dissociative anaesthetics	Ketamine	N methyl D aspartate receptor (NMDA) antagonist	IV Intranasal IM Oral	0.5–2 mg/kg 0.5–4 mg/kg 4–5 mg/kg 6–10 mg/kg	Increased secretions Hallucinations given with antisialogogue and benzodiaz-epine though can increase recovery time, vomiting
General anaesthetics	Propofol	GABA agonist	IV IV infusion	2.5–3.5 mg/kg 125–150 µg/kg/min	Watch for respiration, hypotension
	Ketofol	NMDA antagonist & GABA agonist	IV	0.5 mg/kg–1 mg/kg	Lower incidence of vomiting, adverse respiratory events
	Etomidate	GABA agonist	IV	0.1–0.3 mg/kg	Adrenocortical suppression

(continued)

Table 25.1 (continued)

Drug group	Drug	Primary mechanism of action	Route	Dose	Precautions
Hypnotics	Chloral hydrate	GABA agonist	Oral	25–75 mg/kg	Nausea, vomiting, postoperative agitation, moderately addictive
Barbitu-rates	Thiopental	GABA agonist	IV	2–4 mg/kg	Dose varies, limited usage
	Phenobar-bital	GABA agonist	IV IM	1–3 mg/kg 2–6 mg/kg	Nausea, vomiting

25.5 Cannulations

These are the commonest procedures in neonates that require sedation depending on the procedure, whether intravenous (IV) cannulation, arterial cannulation for sampling, monitoring or for ECMO.

Methods used in infants less than 3 month are ingestion of 24% sucrose and a pacifier, breast feeding during the procedure or intranasal midazolam 0.2 mg/kg. They can be made comfortable by distraction or placing the baby in the parental lap during cannulation (Topical EMLA cream (2.5% lidocaine and 2.5% prilocaine) application is recommended only after 3 months of age. Its benefit in neonates is not proven though a study did not find significant difference in meth Hb levels in groups with or without EMLA application) [19]. Topical 4% lidocaine, or 4% amethocaine cream, applied 30 min before, can be used.

The chances of difficult cannulations are very high especially premature and small for date babies. Difficulty can be predicted by DIVA score (Difficult IV assessment). It scores 3 points each for prematurity and younger than 1 year, 1 for 1–2 years of age, and 2 each for vein not palpable or not visible. Total score more than 4 predicts more than 50% failure of 1st attempt at cannulation [20].

Cannulation for ECMO requires standardized anaesthesia consisting of IV midazolam (0.2–0.5 mg/kg), fentanyl (1–3 mcg/kg), ketamine (1–2 mg/kg), infusion of midazolam or dexmedetomidine (0.24 μg/kg/h).

25.6 Radiological Procedures

Magnetic resonance imaging (MRI) is commonly performed for evaluation of the brain, spinal cord parenchyma, and other soft tissues in neonates. The main requirement of MRI is a motionless patient to prevent artefacts and compromised image quality; however, there are many MRI specific patient and anaesthesia concerns, including:

- Vulnerable patient with congenital disorders, medical, and surgical diseases
- Noisy and claustrophobic environment (not a problem in neonates)
- Limited access to the baby
- Ferromagnetic particles acting as projectiles
- Need for MRI safe and compatible monitoring and anaesthetic equipment
- Longer duration
- Heat generation

Earlier chloral hydrate 50–100 mg/kg orally was used for MRI in children, but FDA warning and nonavailability, limited its use. Nonsedating techniques like feed and wrap, parental presence, IV dextrose are successful in infants under 3 months. Sedation can be provided using airway maintaining spontaneous or controlled respiration, and O_2 given by the O_2 hood, LMA or ETT. Drugs that can be used are dexmedetomidine, midazolam, propofol, ketamine, fentanyl, and sevoflurane. Equipment such as head stabilisers, earmuffs and head coil are required to stabilize the baby.

Computed tomography (CT) - Since CT has radiation exposure, it is only done in selected cases where MRI cannot be done. It is useful in unstable babies, babies with ferrous objects, and to visualize bony structures (skull deformity or haemorrhage). It is of short duration (around 5 min) and requires calm and sleeping baby and can be performed under feed and wrap technique, and oral sucrose (0.1 mL/kg of 24% sucrose or 0.5 mL–1 mL of 25% glucose). If this fails, chloral hydrate syrup (50 mg/kg orally), IV midazolam (0.05-0.2 mg/kg) or IM phenobarbital (5 µg/kg) can be used. With Feed and wrap technique, most CT can be easily done without any sedation.

25.7   Cardiac Procedures

25.7.1 Echocardiogram (ECHO)

ECHO uses sound waves to study the structure and function of heart requiring around 15–20 min, with baby in supine position with slight tilt, or in parent's lap. The concerns include hypothermia as ECHO requires a bare chest up to the waist. Gel application, for better images, also calms the baby.

Preparation includes the following:

- Confirming fasting status
- Mild sedatives—oral chloral hydrate (50–100 mg/kg), or IV midazolam (0.05–0.2 mg/kg)
- Nonpharmacological techniques—distraction, feed and wrap technique and parental presence

Similar techniques can be used for **ultrasound also**.

25.7.2 Cardiac Catheterization

Babies requiring this investigation may have poor cardiac output and heart failure including poor growth, difficulty feeding and medication history of anticoagulants and angiotensin converting enzyme inhibitors (ACEI). It is usually accessed by the Femoral route in neonates. Inhalation technique using sevoflurane, or IV induction (propofol/ketamine) can be used. Maintenance with mixture of air and O_2 as high inspired O_2 (>30%) can lead to increase in left to right shunt fraction, ROP and BPD. At the time of insertion of femoral sheaths or oesophageal ECHO probes, a small dose of fentanyl may be required.

Insertion of Pacemaker or an implantable cardioverter-defibrillator (ICD) requires general anaesthesia with endotracheal intubation. There is a high risk of hypotension, and rate and rhythm disturbances. Multimodal approach includes local anaesthetic infiltration, IV paracetamol (10–15 mg/kg), and an opioid.

Cardiac angiography can be managed as for MRI and CT, using 'feed and wrap' regimen; however, GA is preferred.

25.8   Other miscellaneous procedures included are as follows:

- Interventional Radiology
- Minor Oncologic procedures
- Catheterization
- Repeated lumbar punctures
- Bone marrow aspirations
- Percutaneous biopsies of solid organ
  Central venous catheterisation

The nonpharmacological method with local anaesthesia is a reasonably successful technique. IV ketamine, midazolam, fentanyl, singly or in combination, can also be used for sedation. General anaesthesia rarely needs to be administered.

25.9   Radiotherapy, EEG, Evoked Potentials

Radiotherapy, EEG, and evoked potentials requires a sleeping baby as EEG and evoked potentials can be affected by movement and sedation. Melatonin at 2–10 mg orally, earlier sleep deprivation followed by induction of natural sleep (by feeding or pacifier) often works. Deep sedation or general anaesthesia can be provided to neonates undergoing brain evoked potentials and radiotherapy. The latter mostly lasts for 10–20 min.

25.10 Gastrointestinal Procedures: Insertion of Ryle's Tube, Esophago-Gastroscopy, and Colonoscopy

Ryle's tube can be inserted after minimal sedation by midazolam or non-pharmacological methods. For esophago-gastroscopy, general anaesthesia is preferred to abolish gag reflex, and to maintain airway patency as the endoscope itself can cause airway obstruction.

25.11 Specific Issues for Different Levels of Sedation

Sedation levels vary, and the issues are different depending on the levels, mild, moderate, and severe, and the risk and requirements for these levels [8].

Mild sedation is basically drug-induced anxiolysis when the subjects are awake but calm. They respond normally to verbal commands and don't require more than observation and intermittent assessment unless they develop deeper levels of sedation.

Moderate sedation is drug-induced depression of consciousness during which patients respond purposefully to verbal commands or after light tactile stimulation. No interventions are required to maintain the airway and respiration is spontaneous and adequate, with maintained hemodynamics. It is important to remember that there is no loss of consciousness.

Deep sedation is a drug-induced state of depression of consciousness during which patients cannot be easily aroused but respond purposefully after repeated verbal or painful stimulation. There may be partial or complete loss of protective airway reflexes and patients may require assistance in maintaining the airway. Spontaneous respiration may be inadequate, but CVS function is usually maintained. During this stage, patients may pass from a state of deep sedation to the state of general anaesthesia, which is a drug-induced loss of consciousness during which patients are not arousable even on painful stimulation. As patients can easily pass from one lower level to another higher level, this should be always done under proper monitoring and in the presence of a trained practitioner skilled in emergency airway management in the neonate in situations of apnea, laryngospasm, and airway obstruction. Basic monitoring includes for vital functions and peripheral O_2 saturation. Running O_2 supply, suction equipment, proper documentation, emergency checklists, rescue cart stocked with rescue drugs and age and size-appropriate equipment, and a dedicated recovery area are essential prerequisites. More intensive monitoring includes (ECG, $EtCO_2$), rescue resources (defibrillator), recording of monitoring (every 5 min for moderate sedation), personnel trained in providing advanced airway and tracheal intubation, will be required for deep sedation and general anaesthesia.

25.12 Scope of Regional Anesthesia/Analgesia

For deep sedation/anaesthesia, the commonest procedures employed are monitored anaesthesia care (MAC) by IV route and general anaesthesia. Regional anaesthesia, though rarely administered outside the paediatric OT, can be useful in certain circumstances [21, 22]. Indications for local or regional anaesthesia in neonates in NORA settings, include Cardiac catheterization, Lumbar punctures, Bone marrow aspiration, lung and rib biopsies, chest tube placement, biliary or subphrenic drainage procedures, and insertion of biliary stents.

- Intercostal nerve blocks are useful for lung and rib biopsies, chest tube placement, biliary or subphrenic drainage procedures, and insertion of biliary stents.
- Brachial plexus by axillary, interscalene, or supraclavicular routes can be given catheterization via brachial approach.
- Neuraxial block of the lower extremities for femoral catheterizations and percutaneous approaches to the kidney.
- Spinal anaesthesia has been used for repeat, painful radiotherapy on lower extremities, in conjunction with regional hyperthermia and limb exsanguinations.
- Caudal anaesthesia/analgesia and deep sedation provides prolonged perioperative pain of cardiac catheterization.
- Caudal anaesthesia is effective for sub-umbilical analgesia.

The choice of local anesthetic should prioritize long duration with weak motor blockade, making 0.25% bupivacaine an ideal choice [23].

25.13 Some Specific Complications of High Concern

Competency with emergency airway management procedure algorithms is fundamental for safe sedation practice and successful patient rescue, especially because babies can rapidly transit to a deeper level of sedation than intended. Four complications of very high concern and possible fatal outcome if not managed urgently, are as follows: [24–27]

1. Airway obstruction
2. Apnea
3. Laryngospasm
4. Local anesthetic systemic toxicity (LAST)

25.13.1 Airway Obstruction

The suggested step-by-step management algorithm for this condition is (move to the next action if the preceding one is not successful): reposition the airway → perform a jaw thrust → insert oral airway → call for help → insert nasal trumpet → insert supraglottic device (LMA or other) → tracheal intubation → surgical airway (needle cricothyrotomy or tracheostomy).

25.13.2 Apnea

The suggested step-by-step management algorithm for this condition is (move to the next action if the preceding one is not successful): bag/mask ventilation → reposition the airway → perform a jaw thrust → insert oral airway → call for help → insert nasal trumpet → insert supraglottic device (LMA or other) → tracheal intubation → surgical airway.

25.13.3 Laryngospasm

The suggested step-by-step management algorithm for this condition is (move to the next action if the preceding one is not successful): gentle positive pressure ventilation → deepen sedation (IV propofol) → call for help → give muscle relaxation (succinylcholine plus atropine) → tracheal intubation → surgical airway.

25.13.4 Local Anesthetic Systemic Toxicity (LAST)

Although the incidence of complications from LA administration in children is low (0.76 patients per 10,000 procedures), accidental systemic injection or inappropriate dosing can result in life-threatening neurological or cardiovascular complications. The suggested steps are as follows: [28]

1. **Get help:** Ventilate with 100% O_2. Alert nearest facility with cardiopulmonary bypass capability.
2. **Resuscitation**: Airway/ventilatory support, chest compression. Avoid vasopressin, calcium channel blockers, b-blockers, or additional LA. Reduce epinephrine dosages. Prolonged effort may be required.
3. **Seizure management**: Benzodiazepines preferred (IV midazolam 0.1–0.2 mg/kg), avoid propofol if cardiovascular instability.
4. **LA binding:** Administer 1.5 mL/kg 20% lipid emulsion over 1 min to trap unbound amide LA. Repeat once or twice or initiate infusion (0.25 mL/kg/minute) until circulation is restored. If BP remains low, double the infusion rate. Continue infusion for at least 10 min after attaining circulatory stability. Recommended upper limit is about 10 mL/kg.
5. **Fluid bolus** of 10–20 mL/kg balanced salt solution to correct hypovolemia.
6. **Phenylephrine infusion** (0.1 mg/kg/min) to correct peripheral vasodilation and maintain BP.

25.14 Conclusion

The scope of sedation or anaesthesia for neonates for procedures outside the operation theatre has been increasing. This is required for a wide range of procedures ranging from cannulations in various settings, radiological procedures including MRI and CT, several cardiac procedures and number of other special diagnostic and interventional procedures. The sedation in neonates is different from in children and adults. in neonates and small infants, the goal of sedation is to relieve pain, anxiety, modify behaviour, immobility, and allow safe completion of the procedure. The effective achievement of these goals depends on many factors other than the intervention itself: gestational and postnatal age, brain development, cognitive-emotional development, characteristics of the procedure (duration, pain arousing potential, anxiogenic paraphernalia, need for immobilization), and the environment including presence of caring figures and soothing and/or distracting elements.

Major concerns along with efficacy of the interventions are safety, especially because very young infants and preterm babies are vulnerable, as well as the fact that they may progress to a deeper level of sedation than initially intended. Hence, the general principles are extremely important: proper patient selection, adequate infrastructure, and resources, trained and experienced personnel, monitoring, rescue facilities, and documentation.

References

1. Shih G, Bailey PD Jr. Nonoperating room anesthesia for children. Curr Opin Anaesthesiol. 2020;33(4):584–8.
2. Setiawan CT, Landrigan-Ossar M. Practice horizons in pediatric nonoperating room anesthesia. Curr Opin Anaesthesiol. 2020;33(3):395–403.
3. McCann ME, de Graaff JC, Dorris L, Disma N, et al. GAS Consortium: Neurodevelopmental outcome at 5 years of age after general anaesthesia or awake-regional anaesthesia in infancy (GAS): An international, multicentre, randomised, controlled equivalence trial. Lancet. 2019;393:664–77.
4. Vutskits L, Culley DJ. GAS, PANDA, and MASK: no evidence of clinical anesthetic neurotoxicity! Anesthesiology. 2019;131:762–4. https://doi.org/10.1097/ALN.0000000000002863.
5. Warner DO, Zaccariello MJ, Katusic SK, Schroeder DR, et al. Neuropsychological and behavioral outcomes after exposure of young children to procedures requiring general anesthesia: The Mayo Anesthesia Safety in Kids (MASK) Study. Anesthesiology. 2018;129:89–105. https://doi.org/10.1097/ALN.0000000000002232.
6. Setiawan CT, Landrigan-Ossar M. Pediatric anesthesia outside the operating room: case management. Anesthesiol Clin. 2020;38(3):587–604.
7. Tobias JD, Cravero JP, editors. Procedural sedation for infants, children, and adolescents. Elk Grove Village, IL: American Academy of Pediatrics; 2016.
8. Coté CJ, Wilson S, American Academy of Pediatrics, American Academy of Pediatric Dentistry. Guidelines for monitoring and management of pediatric patients before, during, and after sedation for diagnostic and therapeutic procedures. Pediatrics. 2019;143(6):e20191000.
9. Krmpotic K, Rieder MJ, Rosen D. Canadian Paediatric Society. Recommendations for procedural sedation in infants, children, and adolescents. Paediatr Child Health. 2021;26(2):128. https://www.cps.ca/en/documents/position/recommendations-for-procedural-sedation-in-infants-children-and-adolescents

10. Doody O, Bailey ME. Interventions in pain management for persons with an intellectual disability. First Published May 17, 2017. doi: https://doi.org/10.1177/1744629517708679.

11. Trottier ED, Doré-Bergeron MJ, Chauvin-Kimoff L, et al. Managing pain and distress in children undergoing brief diagnostic and therapeutic procedures. Paediatr Child Health. 2019;24(8):509–35.

12. Petrie J. Scottish intercollegiate guidelines network. SIGN 50. A guideline developers' handbook. Edinburgh; February 2001.

13. Greenwood J. Back 2 Basiscs Series: your simple RSI checklist—SOAP ME. UMEM Educational Pearls. University of Maryland School of Medicine posted on April; 2014.

14. Jennett B, Teasdale GM. The child's Glasgow coma scale. Lancet. 1977:878–81.

15. Healey C, Osler TM, Rogers FB, et al. Improving the Glasgow Coma Scale score: motor score alone is a better predictor. J Trauma. 2003;54(4):671–8. https://doi.org/10.1097/01. TA.0000058130.30490.5D.

16. Maddirala S, Theagrajan A. Non-operating room anaesthesia in children. Indian J Anaesth. 2019;63:754–62.

17. Hu Y, Xu W, Cao F. A meta-analysis of randomized controlled trials: combination of ketamine and propofol versus ketamine alone for procedural sedation and analgesia in children. Intern Emerg Med. 2019;14:1159–65.

18. Krauss B, Green SM. Procedural sedation and analgesia in children. Lancet. 2006;367(9512):766–80.

19. Taddio A, Ohlsson A, Einarson TR, et al. A systematic review of lidocaine-prilocaine cream (EMLA) in the treatment of acute pain in neonates. Pediatrics. 1998;101(2):e1. https://doi. org/10.1542/peds.101.2.e1.

20. Riker MW, Kennedy C, Winfrey BS, et al. Validation and refinement of the difficult intravenous access score: a clinical prediction rule for identifying children with difficult intravenous access. Acad Emerg Med. 2011;18(11):1129–34. https://doi.org/10.1111/j.1553-2712.2011. 01205.x.

21. Faddoul A, Bonnet F. Is there a place for regional anesthesia in nonoperating room anesthesia? Curr Opin Anaesthesiol. 2020;33(4):561–5.

22. Mahmoud M, Holzman RS, Mason KP. Anesthesia and sedation outside the operating room. In: Andropoulos DB, Gregory GA, editors. Gregory's pediatric anaesthesia. New York: John Wiley and Sons; 2020. p. 1012–39.

23. Wong T, Georgiadis PL, Urman RD, Tsai MH. Non-operating room anesthesia: patient selection and special considerations. Local Reg Anesth. 2020;8(13):1–9.

24. Bellolio MF, Puls HA, Anderson JL, et al. Incidence of adverse events in paediatric procedural sedation in the emergency department: a systematic review and meta-analysis. BMJ Open. 2016;6(6):e011384.

25. Hartling L, Milne A, Foisy M, et al. What works and what's safe in pediatric emergency procedural sedation: an overview of reviews. Acad Emerg Med. 2016;23(5):519–30.

26. Heydinger G, Tobias J, Veneziano G. Fundamentals and innovations in regional anaesthesia for infants and children. Anaesthesia. 2021;76(Suppl 1):74–88.

27. American Academy of Pediatrics, American College of Emergency Physicians. Advanced pediatric life support. 5th ed. Boston, MA: Jones and Bartlett Publishers; 2012.

28. American Society of Regional Anesthesia (ASRA). Checklist for treatment of local anesthetic systemic toxicity. https://www.asra.com/guidelines-articles/guidelines/guideline-item/guide-lines/2020/11/01/checklist-for-treatment-of-local-anesthetic-systemic-toxicity (posted Nov 1, 2020; last accessed Jun 6, 2021).

Pain Management in Neonates

26

M. R. Vishnu Narayanan and Anju Gupta

26.1 Introduction

Pain perception is an inherent quality of life that appears early in development. Neonates are frequently exposed to painful diagnostic and therapeutic interventions. The need for these interventions is increased in premature neonates especially those <30 weeks' gestation, as they are more likely to undergo various procedures and interventions. Historically, treatment of pain in children was regarded as unnecessary. It was a widely held myth that the neonates do not perceive pain to noxious stimuli due to their immature nervous system [1].

Before 1970, there was no formal research looking at pain management in children. However, later evidence made it clear that neonates do experience pain but lack the adaptive mechanisms that modulate painful stimuli as manifested by older children [2]. A fetus at 20 weeks' gestation has a functional pain system and can mount a stress response. NMDA-mediated windup and central sensitization are in fact more pronounced in neonates [3]. Exposure to repeated pain-related stress early in life is known to have short- and long-term adverse sequelae including physiologic instability, altered neurodevelopment, specific learning deficits, poor adaptive behavior, and decreased pain threshold which can alter their response to future events of painful or nonpainful stimuli [4, 5]. Furthermore, high numbers of painful experiences in the neonatal period have been associated with poor quality of cognitive and motor development at 1 year of age [6]. Pain in the neonatal period is often under-recognized and undertreated. A large observational study in France reported that about 34% neonates received any kind of analgesia following painful procedures [7]. Neonates cannot verbally communicate their pain and discomfort but express their susceptibility to pain and stress through specific behavioral,

M. R. Vishnu Narayanan · A. Gupta (✉)
Department of Anaesthesiology, Pain Medicine and Critical Care, AIIMS, New Delhi, India

© The Author(s), under exclusive license to Springer Nature Singapore Pte Ltd. 2023
U. Saha (ed.), *Clinical Anesthesia for the Newborn and the Neonate*,
https://doi.org/10.1007/978-981-19-5458-0_26

physiological, and biochemical responses. Hence, the several pain assessment tools which have been developed for neonates rely on these surrogate markers of pain [8].

Pain is subjective. The International Association for the Study of Pain (IASP, 2003) defined pain as "an unpleasant sensory and emotional experience associated with actual or potential tissue damage or described in terms of that damage" [9]. For neonates and other preverbal children, the definition should be broadened to include behavioral and physiologic indicators.

Consequences of acute painful stimuli in neonates include increases in heart rate, blood pressure, intracranial pressure and decreases in oxygen saturations. The accompanying changes in cerebral blood flow may increase the risk of intraventricular hemorrhage (IVH) and periventricular leukomalacia [10].

It is therefore recommended that each healthcare facility that cares for neonates and young infants should establish a pain management program that includes routine pain detection and assessment, documentation and implementation of appropriate therapeutic interventions. Regular use of pain assessment tools has been strongly recommended by the American academy of pediatrics (AAP) [11]. Training of staff is mandatory to ensure its proper implementation. A previous multicentric study found that regular postoperative pain assessment and documentation substantially increased the odds of administration of pharmacologic analgesic agents, but their use did not correlate to surgical severity [12].

26.2 Pain Pathways in Neonates

1. **Peripheral Nervous System**

   The anatomic pathways of peripheral nervous system become functional by 20 weeks postconception with the nociceptor distribution being similar to that of adults by around 24 weeks. The nociceptors are connected to the developing spinal cord by A-delta and C fibers, with variably myelinated tracts [13]. Myelination takes 12 years of life to be completed, but lack of myelination does not imply lack of pain perception. Rather, the dense distribution of nociceptors makes the neonate more sensitive to pain than adults [14]. Moreover, the thick myelinated a beta fibers transmitting light touch and proprioception in adults also transmit noxious stimuli to pain processing areas of the spinal cord in the fetus and neonate. Also, recurrent painful stimuli in the early neonatal period leads to nociceptor recruitment and **primary hyperalgesia**. It also contributes to tissue damage and profound dendritic sprouting of local sensory nerve terminals leading to hyper innervation lasting into adulthood [2].

2. **Spinal Cord**

   The spinal cord plays an important role in perception of pain in neonates. The dorsal horn to which the peripheral pain pathways terminate develops by 20–24 weeks of gestation. Mechanoreceptors via the A-delta fibers synapse at Rexed's laminae I, II, and V. Mechano-, thermo-, and chemoreceptors via C fibers terminate at laminae II and III. The axons from the projection neurons carry sensory information to supraspinal area via spinothalamic, spinoreticular, and spinomesencephalic tracts. The fibers after synapsing in the dorsal horn spread signals to the anterior horn cells resulting in withdrawal reflex and muscle spasm. Signals are also transmitted to preganglionic sympathetic neurons, producing vasoconstriction of the skin [13]. On entering the dorsal horn, the A-delta and C fibers divide and make connections at the dermatomes above and below, increasing the excitability of surrounding neurons. This is experienced in preterm as a lower pain threshold, longer pain response and increased reactivity of the surrounding area. This is known as the **Windup phenomenon** [15].

3. **Supraspinal Area**

A-delta fiber impulses are carried via spinothalamic tract to the ventral posterolateral nucleus of the thalamus. C fiber impulses terminate in the thalamic nuclei via the spinoreticular tract, with connections to the limbic system. The pain impulses are then integrated and modified in the thalamus before transmitting to the cortex. The thalamus also regulates alertness and emotional aspects of pain which are revealed behaviorally in the preterm as well as term neonates. The fetal cortex begins to develop by 8 weeks of gestation, neurons develop by 20 weeks, and thalamocortical connections are established by 24 weeks. These tracts reach the somatosensory area of the parietal lobe, hippocampus, temporal lobe for memory and learning, and to the frontal lobe for associative function.

The periaqueductal gray matter plays an important role in pain modulation, interpretation, and response. It modulates the autonomic responses to pain (tachycardia, tachypnoea) by 22 weeks. Stimulation of this area is also responsible for facial expressions of pain which are evident by 25–26 weeks. Interconnections with the reticular activating system are responsible for the arousal effects of pain.

From the cortex and periaqueductal gray matter, descending inhibitory fibers arise which modulate pain, by inhibiting spinal processing of pain via release of inhibitory neurotransmitters. The release of inhibitory neurotransmitters starts only by 40–48 weeks postconception. The expression of inhibitory neurotransmitters in preterm spinal cord is significantly reduced [13, 16]. Hence, this modulation is lacking in preterm newborns.

26.3   Neonatal Pain Control Program

In 2006, the American Academy of Pediatrics [11] and the Canadian pediatric society [17] recommended that each health care facility treating newborns should establish a neonatal pain control program, that includes the following:-

- Routine neonatal pain assessment,
- Reduction of number of painful procedures,
- Prevention and treatment of acute pain during invasive procedures,
- Postoperative pain management, and
- Avoiding prolonged/repetitive pain or stress during NICU care.

26.4   Importance of Understanding Neonatal Pain

Neonates, especially those premature (<32 weeks' gestation), are exposed to numerous painful/stressful stimuli in early life. Failure to treat pain in neonates not only leads to short-term complications [3, 6], but also is responsible for variety of long-term physiological, behavioral, and cognitive sequelae, such as:

(i) Altered pain processing
(ii) Attention-deficit hyper-reactivity disorder (ADHD)
(iii) Impaired visual-motor integration
(iv) Poor executive function

Though NICU has increased the survival of preterm and low birthweight newborns, it is often accompanied with adverse outcomes related to pain and stress. Despite the knowledge of the vast multitude of pain management options available and the long-term adverse sequelae associated with untreated pain, there is still a stigma among practitioners in treating pain in the neonatal population. Leaving pain untreated is clinically indefensible, unethical, and illegal.

Some of the causes of inadequate management of pain in neonates are as follows:

(a) The diverse range of developmental and physiological changes during neonatal period that interfere in the interpretation,
(b) Difficulty in assessing pain in nonverbal patients,
(c) Fear of prescribing opioids in neonates because of overdosing and adverse effects,
(d) Pain is managed by pediatric physicians and surgeons in the wards who may be hesitant in prescribing appropriate doses,
(e) Limited knowledge of analgesic drug metabolism, dosing and side effects in neonates,
(f) Disinterest, lack of concern for the crying neonate, or habituation to crying neonates,
(g) Interobserver variability and subjectivity of pain assessment tools, and
(h) Time-consuming multidimensional assessment tools, which often lack consideration for the type of the noxious stimulus or body part involved.

26.5   Measuring Pain

26.5.1 Pain Assessment Tools

A multitude of pain assessment tools have been proposed for pediatric patients. It is important to make a correct selection of the pain assessment or scoring too, based on the subgroup of population (neonates) and type of pain to be assessed (acute, postoperative, or persistent) [2, 8, 11]. Pain assessment is challenging particularly in neonates, preterm, and nonverbal babies, as they rely on caregivers to interpret their behavior changes and other signs in response to pain. Neonatal pain assessment scales can be classified as **unidimensional** (single parameter) or **multidimensional composite pain scales** (based on physiological, behavioral, stress hormone levels) [8, 18, 19]. Multidimensional pain scales have been demonstrated to have more clinical utility with better validity and reliability as changes in physiological parameters and behavioral patterns are the most predictable clinical responses to pain in neonates [19]. Various physiological and behavioral

Table 26.1 Multidimensional pain assessment tools—Physiological /behavioral parameters in neonates

Physiologic parameters [3, 5]	Heart rate, blood pressure, heart rate variability, respiratory rate, breathing pattern, oxygen saturation, vagal tone, intracranial pressure, skin color, palmar sweating, pupillary size
Behavioral responses [5, 18, 19]	Sleep and crying patterns, facial expression, hand and body movement, behavioral state changes, muscle tone, consolability. Specific facial features such as eye squeeze, brow bulge, nasolabial furrow, and open mouth are associated with acute pain

Table 26.2 Commonly used pain assessment tools for neonates

Pain assessment tool	Variables included	Remarks
Wong-Baker FACES Pain Rating Scale	Wong-Baker FACES Pain Rating Scale 0 NO HURT — 2 HURTS LITTLE BIT — 4 HURTS LITTLE MORE — 6 HURTS EVEN MORE — 8 HURTS WHOLE LOT — 10 HURTS WORST From Wong D.L., Hockenberry-Eaton M., Wilson D., Winkelstein M.L., Schwartz P.: Wong's Essentials of Pediatric Nursing, ed. 6, St. Louis, 2001, p. 1301. Copyrighted by Mosby, Inc. Reprinted by permission.	
Premature Infant Pain Profile (PIPP)	Heart rate, saturation, facial expressions, gestational age	For acute and postoperative pain, reliable, valid, clinical utility established
FLACC scale	Facial expression, leg movement, activity, cry, consolability	Good inter-rater reliability and validity, quick, versatile, can be used in infants / older children / developmental disabilities
CRIES	Crying, require O_2 for SpO_2 95%, increased vital signs, facial expression, sleeplessness	Validated for postoperative pain Reliable
N-PASS (Neonatal Pain, Agitation and Sedation Scale)	Crying, irritability, facial expression, extremity tone, vitals	Reported for postoperative pain, includes sedation level, does not distinguish pain from agitation, reliable, validated against PIPP
COMFORT scale	Movement, calmness, facial tension, alertness, respiration rate, muscle tone, heart rate, blood pressure	Reported for postoperative pain. Reliable, validated against Numeric Rating Scale, clinical utility well established

(continued)

Table 26.2 (continued)

Pain assessment tool	Variables included	Remarks
NIPS (Neonatal Infant Pain Score)	Facial expression, crying, breathing patterns, arm and leg movements, arousal	Reliable, valid
NFCS (Neonatal Facial Coding System)	Facial expressions	Studied for postop pain (abdominal / thoracic surgery), reliable, valid, clinical useful, high degree of sensitivity to analgesia

Table 26.3 Indicators and scoring system for PIPP

Indicators/Scores	0	1	2	3
1. Gestational age	**>36 weeks**	**32–35 weeks**	**28–31 weeks**	**< 28 weeks**
2. Behavioral state	Active awake, eyes open, facial movements present	Quiet awake, eyes open, no facial movements	Active sleep, eyes closed, facial movements present	Quiet sleep, eyes closed, no facial movements
3. Maximum HR	0–4/min increase	5–14/min increase	15–24/min increase	> 25/min increase
4. Minimum SpO2	0–2.4% decrease	2.5–4.9% decrease	5.0–7.4% decrease	> 7.5% decrease
5. Brow bulge/ frown	None (0–9% of time)	Minimum (10–39% of time)	Moderate (40–69% of time)	Maximum (> 70% of time)
6. Eye squeeze	None (0–9% of time)	Minimum (10–39% of time)	Moderate (40–69% of time)	Maximum (> 70% of time)
7. Nasolabial furrow	None (0–9% of time)	Minimum (10–39% of time)	Moderate (40–69% of time)	Maximum (> 70% of time)

parameters of the multidimensional pain assessment tools are listed in Table 26.1 and commonly used pain assessment tools in Table 26.2 [3, 8, 11, 17, 20, 21].

Premature Infant Pain profile (PIPP) was developed and validated in 1996 for use in premature neonates (GA < 37 weeks), with limited validity in extremely premature babies (<28 weeks). It is a 7-item composite pain scoring system that includes 3 behavioral, 2 physiological, and 2 contextual parameters, each scored 0–3 [22–24] (Table 26.3).

26.5.2 Method and Interpretation

Step 1—Observe for 15 s before the painful event and note down the baseline parameters.

Step 2—Repeat scoring after the painful event, and 30 min and 1 h after administration of pain medication. Any change from baseline should be noted for 30 s.

Interpretation of Total Scores at Each Assessment—Total scores range from 0 to 21, i.e., nil to excruciating severe pain.

- </= 6—Minimal to no pain
- 7–12 —Mild pain
- >12—Moderate pain

26.5.3 Frequency of Pain Assessment

Frequency of pain assessment will depend on the clinical situation and can be increased or decreased in an individual context [11, 17, 21]. Following are the general guidelines for postoperative pain assessment:

i. Baseline postoperative pain scoring in all neonates.
ii. Hourly scoring until pain stabilizes and optimal analgesia is achieved.
iii. Thereafter, minimum 4 hourly assessment up to 48 h postoperatively.
iv. Reassessment 30 min after any rescue dose to establish its effectiveness.
v. Neonates on mechanical ventilation assessed 4 hourly.
vi. Pain scores documented in the progress notes every time it is completed.
vii. Patient background should also be documented at scoring (awake/asleep, sedated/paralyzed).
viii. Analgesic interventions and their efficacy should be recorded.
ix. Any special concerns should also be documented.
x. Handing over to the person in next shift to ensure continuity of care.

26.6   Neonatal Pain Management

Research is ongoing to add objectivity to pain assessment tools by using measurable end points to assess and quantify pain. Neuroimaging (functional magnetic resonance imaging [fMRI], near-infrared spectroscopy (NIRS)) and neurophysiologic techniques [amplitude-integrated EEG (aEEG), changes in skin conductance, and HR variability] are being used for research for acute or persistent pain but none has sufficient reliability or universal applicability to be considered as "the gold standard" [8, 18, 20].

26.6.1 Approach to Pain Management in Neonates

An individualized multimodal pain management approach should be adopted. American association of pediatrics (AAP) recommends [11] that all neonates should receive postoperative analgesia (Grade 1B evidence). Preemptive analgesia with systemic analgesics and continuous central neuraxial and peripheral nerve blocks instituted before surgical incision and continued perioperatively greatly reduce postoperative analgesic requirements. Treatment plan is dependent on the type of surgical procedure performed. This is generally accomplished with a combination of nonpharmacologic and pharmacologic techniques in a stepwise tiered approach with increasing intensity of analgesia as the degree of anticipated pain increases. The suggested pain management approach is only a guide to individual clinical judgment, with collaboration between multidisciplinary pain management teams.

26.6.2 Recommendations

The following are the general recommendations in the management of pain in neonates:

1.1. Analgesics should be titrated by following trends in pain scores.
1.2. A stepped approach as recommended by AAP (2016) [11] and Canadian Pediatric Society (CPS) [17] for prevention and treatment of neonatal pain and pain management:
    1.2.1. Nonpharmacologic nursing comfort measures should be provided at first step to complement systemic analgesia.
    1.2.2. Nonopioid analgesics for mild to moderate pain.
    1.2.3. Opioid analgesics in combination with nonopioid analgesics reserved for moderate to severe pain.

Nonpharmacologic Therapies (Step 1)

Step 1: Nonpharmacologic measures (breastfeeding, pacifier use, facilitated tucking, swaddling, skin-to-skin contact [kangaroo care], sensorial saturation), and oral sucrose. A combination of these measures may be most appropriate [25].

Pharmacologic Management (Steps 2–5)

Step 2: Topical Anesthetics
Step 3: Oral, intravenous (IV), or rectal acetaminophen.
Step 4: Subcutaneous infiltration of LA or specific nerve/neuraxial blocks.
Step 5: Deep sedation opiates (combination of opioids and other adjuvant drugs).

26.6.3 Step 1: Nonpharmacologic Interventions

Nonpharmacological approaches for pain management in neonates have been underutilized and unappreciated. Several studies have demonstrated the effectiveness of these methods in alleviating stress in newborns [26–28]. The following nonpharmacological/nursing control measures have been found to be effective in reducing pain scores in neonates: [29]

- Limit environmental stressors by reducing noise and light levels.
- Cluster nursing care and limited handling of the baby to allow undisturbed sleep.

- Kangaroo care.
- Facilitated touch/gentle massage.
- Oral sucrose and glucose.
- Breastfeeding when appropriate.
- Pacifiers/encouraging non-nutritive sucking.
- Swaddling and positioning with facilitated tucking.

Reduction of Painful Events: Reducing the number of procedures performed and episodes of patient handling without compromising care, use of noninvasive monitoring as much as possible, using devices that can perform multiple laboratory test analysis with single small blood sample, using peripheral arterial or central venous catheters in infants requiring multiple heel sticks per day.

Skin-to-Skin Care (SSC)-Kangaroo Care (KC): SSC with or without sucrose or glucose administration, has been shown to decrease some measures of pain in preterm and term infants. KC has shown to decrease crying time, improve pain scores, and decrease stress response in neonates. A meta-analysis of 19 studies of nonpharmacologic interventions used during minor invasive procedure (heel lance and IV catheter insertion) found that sucking-related and swaddling/facilitated-tucking interventions were beneficial for preterm neonates and that sucking-related and rocking/holding interventions were beneficial for term neonates [30]. The mechanism for SSC is unclear but proposed mechanisms include response to maternal heartbeat, decreased maternal stress, and enhanced self-regulation.

Non-nutritive Sucking, Sucrose, and Glucose: Non-nutritive sucking and sweeteners provide pain relief by releasing endogenous endorphins. Sweeteners, in addition, augment antinociceptive responses. Oral sucrose is commonly used to provide procedural analgesia during mild to moderately painful procedures. However, appropriate dosing, mechanism of action, soothing vs analgesic effects, and long-term consequences are not well known. Glucose is also effective in decreasing the response to brief painful procedures. Meta-analysis of studies has concluded that sucrose and glucose are safe and effective for reducing procedural pain from a single event [26, 31]. Breastfeeding, when accompanied by SSC, is also efficacious in reducing pain due to heel sticks. Literature is lacking on the role of these methods in postoperative analgesia.

Massage Therapy and Acupuncture: Massage therapy includes gentle hands-on and skin-skin manipulation like gentle stroking, compression, and nerve strokes. It is thought to modulate pain by enhancing vagal activity and reducing pain scores. In addition, it also releases insulin and insulin-like growth factor promoting weight gain in preterm neonates. Acupuncture and its role in pain relief have been inadequately studied in neonates [32].

26.6.4 Pharmacologic Treatment Strategies

26.6.4.1 Step 2: Topical Anesthetics

Though multiple topical anesthetic formulations are available for pediatric usage, EMLA is the only established and safe formulation available for use in neonatal population [33]. It is a eutectic creamy mixture of 2.5% lignocaine and 2.5%

prilocaine and is recommended in mild painful conditions like venous and arterial cannulation, lumbar puncture, and circumcision [34]. It is not recommended for heel sticks. It is applied over the intended area in a dose of 0.5–1g and with occlusive dressing for 45–60 min (max dose –1 g). Side effects include skin irritation and methemoglobinemia, though rare [35].

26.6.4.2 Step 3: Acetaminophen

Acetaminophen (paracetamol) has been used in the management of mild to moderate procedural (heel prick, circumcision) and postoperative pain (dressing changes, wound treatment). Alone, it is not effective enough to reduce acute severe pain and should be used as adjunctive analgesia (combined with topical LA or opioid therapy) to prevent or treat acute pain in neonates undergoing painful procedures [6, 36]. IV acetaminophen has a useful opioid-sparing action which is beneficial in reducing the dose and risk of adverse opioid effects [37]. Rectal acetaminophen has minimal opioid-sparing effect possibly due to inadequate rectal absorption or inadequate dosing, although it is commonly used as adjunctive analgesia in neonates who cannot receive oral therapy [38]. It can be given per oral (10 mg/kg every 6 hourly) and per rectal (15 mg/kg, 8 hourly) (Box 26.1).

IV preparation for neonates is also available. IV dose varies with the gestational age of the baby:

- 32–44 weeks GA—loading dose 20 mg/kg and then maintained at 10 mg/kg every 6 h.
- ≤31 weeks GA—dosing interval is lengthened to 12 h.

Total daily dose for neonates born between 37–42-week GA is 50–60 mg/kg/day, 31–36 weeks is 35–50 mg/kg/day, and 24–30 weeks is 20–30 mg/kg/day [39–41].

Side Effects: Unlike in older children and adults, acetaminophen rarely causes hepato-renal toxicity in neonates, but caution should be used in presence of malnutrition and hypoalbuminemia [42].

Box 26.1: Paracetamol in Neonates—Summarized
Decreased clearance
Hepatic metabolism and conjugation with glucuronic acid and sulfate
Renal excretion
Dose—Loading 20 mg/kg followed by 10 mg/kg 6 hourly (term /preterm)
Oral and per rectal dose—similar
Max daily doses
30-wk GA—25–30 mg/kg/24 h
34-wk GA—45 mg/kg/24 h
Term baby—60 mg/kg/24 h
In preterm newborns—high dose is used to induce PDA closure
Potential relationship of perinatal paracetamol to atopy in later age

Nonsteroidal Anti-Inflammatory Drugs (NSAID) are avoided in neonates and infants (<6 months age) because of concerns regarding gastrointestinal bleeding, renal insufficiency, platelet dysfunction, and development of pulmonary hypertension [6, 18]. However, IV ketorolac (0.5 mg/kg), an NSAID, has been documented for neonates and infants [18].

26.6.4.3 Step 4: LA Infiltration, Peripheral Nerve Blocks, Neuraxial Blocks

Local infiltration of lignocaine reduces pain in procedures like vascular access, lumbar puncture, and circumcision.

The use of peripheral regional anesthetic techniques including peripheral nerve blocks and neuraxial blocks is effective as components of multimodal analgesia management of postoperative pain [43].

Adjuvants like clonidine, fentanyl, and morphine are generally avoided in neonates because of potential side effects which must be weighed against any possible gains related to prolongation of analgesia. Use of continuous regional analgesic techniques should be considered when the need for analgesia is likely to exceed the duration of effect of a single injection.

Safe LA doses are lower for neonates and should be carefully maintained well within the recommended safe doses for single injection or continuous infusions, and infusions should be limited to less than 36 h. Ultrasound-guided blocks reduce complications and local anesthetic dose and are preferred whenever the equipment, skills, and expertise are available [43].

It is strongly recommended to vigilantly monitor neonates who receive central neuraxial analgesia, especially if additives are added

26.6.4.4 Step 5: Opioids and Adjuvant Drugs

The most effective therapy for moderate to severe pain relief is opioids. They provide both analgesia with ensuing sedation and calming effect, have a relatively wide therapeutic window, and also effectively attenuate physiologic stress responses. Morphine and fentanyl are most commonly used in neonates especially for intraoperative analgesia. Other more potent opioids are also available such as sufentanil, shorter-acting alfentanil and remifentanil, and mixed opioids codeine and tramadol and are used depending on the availability and local protocols.

Codeine and tramadol are gradually falling out of favor from pediatric practice because of reports of pharmacogenetic changes associated with their use [6, 18].

Morphine has been used as a continuous low-dose infusion or intermittent boluses in neonates following major surgeries. Both approaches are safe and effective. Parental or nurse-controlled analgesia is a useful modality to reduce opioid dosing compared with continuous opioid infusions [44, 45]. The dose is 0.05–0.1 mg/kg/dose IV. For a 2.5 kg baby, dose will be 0.125 mg–0.25 mg. (**Note:** Each 1 ml ampoule has 15 mg morphine, and dilutions need to be done appropriately. Insulin syringe should be used and loaded so that each one division has 0.125 mg or 0.25 mg so as to avoid large volumes, especially during neuraxial blocks).

Side Effects—The most dreaded side effect of morphine in the neonate is **respiratory depression,** which is an aid in babies on mechanical ventilation, or may necessitate postoperative ventilatory support in others. **Hypotension** is not common unless associated with high level of block, excess dose, or hypovolemia. **Prolonged duration** of effect is a cause of **delayed arousal** and **delay in start of feeds**. **Urinary retention** is a problem, especially with spinal administration, but often these neonates have bladder catheterization either for surgical procedure or for monitoring of urine output in the perioperative period; hence, there is no retention of urine or related problem. There are no reports of long-term adverse cognitive/behavioral outcomes after use of morphine in the neonatal period.

Fentanyl has been used for postoperative analgesia for all major surgeries and especially in patients with pulmonary hypertension, or congenital heart disease. The advantage of fentanyl is rapid onset of analgesia due to its lipophilicity, with minimal blood pressure fluctuations and lesser gastrointestinal dysmotility and urinary retention than morphine, but causes greater opioid tolerance and withdrawal [44]. Continuous infusion of fentanyl is not advocated in preterm neonates as per AAP and CPS guidelines because of lack of evidence for significant benefit over morphine and potential for adverse effects [17, 39]. Fentanyl and tramadol were found to be equally effective for postoperative analgesia in preterm neonates, with no differences regarding the duration of mechanical ventilation and the time to reach enteral feeds [46]. It is used intravenously in a dose of 0.5–1 μg/kg. Though IM route has been recommended, it has no advantage over IV administration. Other routes are transmucosal, aerosolized, and by inhalation. **Side effects** include bradycardia, respiratory depression, and chest wall rigidity. Slow administration of fentanyl over 3–5 min decreases the incidence of chest wall/skeletal rigidity [47].

Remifentanil, a shorter-acting fentanyl derivative, is an alternative for short procedures. It is twice potent as fentanyl with an ultra-short duration of action of 3–15 min and is administered as an IV infusion. It is metabolized by plasma esterase independent of liver and kidneys [44]. Its main advantage is lack of cumulation after prolonged infusion.

Sufentanil and alfentanil are also congeners of fentanyl with a short duration of action, but the efficacy and safety of these drugs in neonatal population are lacking.

26.7 Alternative/Adjuvant Medications

Methadone, ketamine, and dexmedetomidine have been proposed for pain management in neonates, but their use is limited because of lack of evidence of effectiveness, adverse effects, and potential for neurotoxicity [44, 48, 49].

Ketamine is a dissociative anesthetic widely used for procedural, operative, or postoperative analgesia and sedation in neonates and small infants [50]. In lower doses (IM/IV: 0.5–2 mg/kg/dose), it provides good analgesia, amnesia, and sedation, while maintaining respiratory drive and preserving hemodynamic status. Safety has not been established in neonates because of concerns regarding possible neurotoxicity [51]. Ketamine is an effective analgesic option for hemodynamically unstable neonates or in situations where opioids would not be suitable.

Dexmedetomidine has been used in preterm and term neonates and demonstrated effective analgesia while being devoid of respiratory depressant effect at usual doses [49]. However, because of the limited data on its safety and efficacy, its routine use is not recommended in neonates until larger randomized trials demonstrate that its beneficial and safety profile in newborns. Case reports of seizures or bradycardia have raised concern on use of dexmedetomidine in neonates [52].

26.8 Regional Anesthesia in Neonates

26.8.1 Caudal Block

This is the most widely useful central neuraxial blockade in children. Awake-caudal technique has been used as an alternative to general anesthesia in ex-premature neonates with BPD undergoing inguinal herniotomy [53, 54]. It has also been used for reduction of gastroschisis soon after birth [55]. However, most commonly, caudal block is used along with general anesthesia to provide surgical analgesia.

Indication include surgery below or up to umbilicus such as urologic, orthopedic, lower abdominal, and inguinal surgeries. An increased volume of LA can provide analgesia up to midthoracic region [43].

Technique of Caudal Block It is usually given after induction of general anesthesia in neonates, except where the technique is awake-caudal.

Landmark Guided—Sacral hiatus is formed by the failure of fusion of 5th sacral vertebral arch. It is found at the apex of an equilateral triangle whose base is formed by a line drawn between the 2 posterior superior iliac spines. The hiatus is palpable as a depression bound by the sacral cornua on each side.

Position—Lateral with knees flexed.

Technique—A 22-G needle is inserted into the sacral hiatus at 45° from the skin. As it enters the sacral canal, the sacrococcygeal membrane is pierced, felt as a "pop" after which the needle is brought to 30° and advanced 0.5 cm. LA is injected after aspiration is negative for CSF and blood [56, 57].

Ultrasound Guided—The sacral hiatus and bony landmarks can be identified by USG guidance. One can also see the spread of LA in the caudal-epidural space [57, 58].

LA Dosage—Modified Armitage formula
1. Urogenital/lower limb surgeries—0.5 ml/kg
2. Subumbilical abdominal surgeries—1 ml/kg
3. Mid-thoracic level surgeries—1.25 ml/kg

26.8.2 Epidural Analgesia

Epidural blockade has emerged as a standard intra- and postoperative pain management care in major abdominal and thoracic procedures in all population. In neonates, its advantage in reducing the need for postoperative ventilation especially following TEF repair is established [59]. It also attenuates the neuroendocrine stress response during major abdominal surgeries and shortens the period of postoperative ileus [60].

Technique

Position—Mostly performed under general anesthesia in lateral position with knees flexed.

Needle—Pediatric 20-G Tuohy needle (5 cm length) is used. This will take a 24-G epidural catheter.

Loss of Resistance—The epidural space is located by loss of resistance to air or saline. If air is used, the volume should be less than 1 ml to prevent air embolism. Use of saline is a safer option. Air is more sensitive than saline in neonates.

Depth of Epidural Space—1 mm/kg.

Catheter Placement—Tip of the catheter should be threaded so as to be in proximity with the dermatomal level of surgery.

Alternative Method—Catheter may be introduced via caudal space.

Ultrasound Guidance is used to locate the epidural space in case spine is deformed, and it is difficult to locate the midline. It also helps to see the location of catheter tip and also monitor the drug spread [61].

Dosing—For thoracic and high lumbar epidurals, volume is 0.25–0.5 ml/kg of 0.2% ropivacaine as an initial bolus, followed by infusion with 0.1% ropivacaine at a maximum rate of 0.2 mg/kg/hour. Adjuvants are not recommended [62, 63].

26.8.3 Spinal Anesthesia

Awake-spinal anesthesia has been described in ex-premature neonates and infants for infraumbilical surgeries especially inguinal hernia repair. Avoiding general anesthesia in this group of patients is useful as it decreases the risk of apnea, hypoxia, and bradycardia as well as the depressant effects of general anesthetics. However, the duration of spinal anesthesia is shorter due to large volume of CSF and increased drug uptake from spinal cord [64].

Performance—22-G needles are used in neonates. Position can be sitting or lateral decubitus. An assistant should firmly grasp the baby to provide head support and avoid unnecessary movements. As the spinal cord ends more caudal, a low approach (L4-5) is advocated.

Dosing—Higher dosing is required in neonates. Isobaric or hyperbaric 0.5% bupivacaine or ropivacaine, in a dose of 0.5–1 mg/kg is recommended. Adjuvants should not be used [14].

26.8.4 Peripheral Nerve Blocks

The indications of peripheral nerve blocks in neonates are limited. Most commonly used are as follows:

(a) Infra-orbital nerve block, for cleft lip surgery [65, 66].
(b) Suprazygomatic maxillary nerve block for cleft palate repair [67].

(c) Ilioinguinal/iliohypogastric nerve blocks for inguinal herniotomy and orchidopexy [68, 69].

(d) Dorsal penile nerve block for circumcision [70].

(e) TAP/Rectus sheath block for abdominal surgeries [71].

(f) Paravertebral block for thoracic surgeries [72, 73].

(g) Femoral nerve block for lower extremity surgeries [74].

(h) Brachial plexus block for upper extremity surgeries [74].

26.9 Family-Centered Care

Parents should be empowered to be involved in the care of their baby by educating them preoperatively for what to expect in the postoperative period, the basis for pain evaluation, and therapeutic interventions. They can be informed about the behavioral cues of pain and stress, and the information should be sought from them during pain assessment. They should be encouraged in giving support and consolation to their baby, which will boost their morale and help them feel involved in the care of their baby [75, 76].

26.10 Training

Formulation and implementation of a uniform neonatal postoperative pain management program can increase the awareness of the staff regarding its ubiquitous presence and the importance of its adequate control. The Joint Commission standards have necessitated pain assessments for all hospitalized patients. Many signs used in these assessment tools require the subjective evaluation by observers. Training of staff in accurate neonatal pain assessment and in uniform evaluation of behavioral responses to pain, so as to improve interobserver reliability, is crucial to determine whether neonates obtain adequate postoperative pain relief [77].

26.11 Conclusion

Neonatal pain is largely being neglected due to challenges in its assessment and management. Pediatric anesthesiologist should continuously strive to prevent, assess, and manage postoperative pain. A validated neonatal pain assessment tool should be regularly used perioperatively. Multimodal stepwise approach to postoperative pain with appropriate monitoring is the key to its successful management. Caution should be exerted when considering novel medications which are not yet approved for this age group or have limited data. Further research is needed in the field of regional anesthesia in neonatal age group.

References

1. Schechter NL, Berde CB, Yaster M. Pain in infants, children, and adolescents: an overview. In: Schechter NL, Berde CB, Yaster M, editors. Pain in infants, children, and adolescents. Baltimore, MD: Williams & Wilkins; 1993; pp. 3–9.
2. Anand KJ, Hickey PR. Pain and its effects in the human neonate and fetus. N Engl J Med. 1987;317:1321.
3. Craig KD, Whitfield MF, Grunau RV, et al. Pain in the preterm neonate: behavioral and physiological indices. Pain. 1993;52:287.
4. Shomaker K, Dutton S, Mark M. Pain prevalence and treatment patterns in a US children's hospital. Hosp Pediatr. 2015;5(7):363–70.
5. Guinsburg R, Kopelman BI, Anand KJ, et al. Physiological, hormonal, and behavioral responses to a single fentanyl dose in intubated and ventilated preterm neonates. J Pediatr. 1998;132:954.
6. World Health Organization. (2012). Persisting pain in children package: WHO guidelines on the pharmacological treatment of persisting pain in children with medical illnesses. http://apps.who.int/iris/bitstream/handle/10665/44540/9789241548120Guidelines.pdf?sequence=1.
7. Simons SHP, van Dijk M, Anand KS, et al. Do we still hurt newborn babies? A prospective study of procedural pain and analgesia in neonates. Arch Pediatr Adolesc Med. 2003;157:1058–64.
8. Giordano V, Edobor J, Deindl P, et al. Pain and sedation scales for neonatal and pediatric patients in a preverbal stage of development: A systematic review. Published online ahead of print, 2019 Oct 14. JAMA Pediatr. 2019. doi: https://doi.org/10.1001/jamapediatrics.2019.3351.
9. Warfield C, Bajwa Z, Wootton RJ. Principles and practice of pain medicine. 3rd ed. McGraw-Hill Education; 2016. p. 728–9.
10. Perlman JM. Neurobehavioral deficits in premature graduates of intensive care–potential medical and neonatal environmental risk factors. Pediatrics. 2001;108:1339–48.
11. American Academy of Pediatrics. Committee on Psychosocial Aspects of Child and Family Health, Task Force on Pain in Infants, Children, and Adolescents. The assessment and management of acute pain in infants, children, and adolescents. Pediatrics. 2001;108(3):793–7.
12. Australia and New Zealand College of Anaesthetics and Faculty of Pain Medicine (ANZCA). Acute pain management: Scientific evidence. 4th ed; 2015. p. 413–4.
13. Hall RW, Anand KJS. Physiology of pain and stress in the newborn. NeoReviews. 2005;6(2):e61–8.
14. Davis PJ, Cladis FP. Smith's Anesthesia for Infants and children. 9th ed. USA: Elsevier Health.
15. Hatfield LA. Neonatal pain: What's age got to do with it? [Internet]. [Cited 2021 Aug 30]. Available from: https://www.ncbi.nlm.nih.gov/pmc/articles/PMC4253046/
16. Evans JC. Physiology of acute pain in preterm infants. Newborn Infant Nurs Rev. 2001;1:75–84.
17. Canadian Paeditric Society Statement. Prevention and management of pain and stress in the neonate. Paediatric Child Health. 2000;5(1):31–8.
18. Shah P, Siu A. Considerations for neonatal and pediatric pain management. ASHP. 2019:1–10. https://doi.org/10.1093/ajhp/zxz166.
19. Burton J, MacKinnon R. Selection of a tool to assess postoperative pain on a neonatal surgical unit. Infant. 2007;3:188–96.
20. AAP Committee on Fetus and Newborn and Section on Anesthesiology and Pain Medicine, Policy Statement. Prevention and management of procedural pain in the neonate: an update. Pediatrics. 2016;137:e20154271.
21. Cong X, McGrath JM, Cusson RM, Zhang D. Pain assessment and measurement in neonates: an updated review. Adv Neonatal Care Off J Natl Assoc Neonatal Nurses. 2013;13(6):379–95.
22. Stevens B, Johnston C, Petryshen P, Taddio A. Premature infant pain profile: development and initial validation. Clin J Pain. 1996;12(1):13–22.

23. Stevens B, Johnston C, Taddio A, Gibbins S, Yamada J. The premature infant pain profile: evaluation 13 years after development. Clin J Pain. 2010;26(9):813–30.
24. Stevens BJ, Gibbins S, Yamada J, Dionne K, Lee G, Johnston C, et al. The premature infant pain profile-revised (PIPP-R): initial validation and feasibility. Clin J Pain. 2014;30(3):238–43.
25. Anand KJS, Stevens BJ, McGrath. Pain research and clinical management-pain in neonates and infants. 3rd ed. Elsevier; 2007. p. 19. 87–90
26. Gray L, Garza E, Zageris D, et al. Sucrose and warmth for analgesia in healthy newborns. Pediatrics. 2015;135:3.
27. Lopez O, Subramanian P, Rahmat N, et al. The effect of facilitated tucking on procedural pain control among premature babies. J Clin Nurs. 2014;24:183–91.
28. Landier WN, Tse A. Use of complementary and alternative medical interventions for the management of procedure-related pain, anxiety, and distress in pediatric oncology: an integrative review. J Pediatr Nurs. 2010;25:566–79.
29. Lago P, Garetti E, Pirelli A, Merazzi D, Bellieni CV, et al. Non-pharmacological intervention for neonatal pain control Ital J Pediatr 2014; 9 40(Suppl. 2): A52.
30. Johnston C, Campbell-Yeo M, Fernandes A, et al. Skin-to-skin care for procedural pain in neonates. Cochrane Database Syst Rev. 2014;23(1):CD008435.
31. Bueno M, Yamada J, Harrison D, et al. A systematic review and meta-analyses of nonsucrose sweet solutions for pain relief in neonates. Pain Res Manag. 2013;18(3):153–61.
32. Raith W, Urlesberger B, Schmölzer GM. Efficacy and safety of acupuncture in preterm and term infants. Evid-Based Complement Altern Med ECAM. 2013;2013:739414.
33. Lillieborg S, Otterbom I, Ahlen K, Long C. Topical anaesthesia in neonates, infants and children. BJA Br J Anaesth 2004 1; 92(3): 450–451.
34. Gourrier E, Karoubi P, el Hanache A, Merbouche S, et al. Use of EMLA cream in premature and full-term newborn infants. Study of efficacy and tolerance. Arch Pediatr Organe Off Soc Francaise Pediatr. 1995;2(11):1041–6.
35. Taddio A, Ohlsson A, Einarson TR, Stevens B, Koren G. A systematic review of lidocaine-prilocaine cream (EMLA) in the treatment of acute pain in neonates. Pediatrics. 1998;101(2):E1.
36. Witt N, Coynor S, Edwards C, Bradshaw H. A guide to pain assessment and management in the neonate. Curr Emerg Hosp Med Rep 2016 1; 4(1): 1–10.
37. Ceelie I, de Wildt SN, van Dijk M, van den Berg MMJ, et al. Effect of intravenous paracetamol on postoperative morphine requirements in neonates and infants undergoing major noncardiac surgery: a randomized controlled trial. JAMA. 2013;309(2):149–54.
38. van der Marel CD, Peters JWB, Bouwmeester NJ, et al. Rectal acetaminophen does not reduce morphine consumption after major surgery in young infants. Br J Anaesth. 2007;98(3):372–9.
39. American Society of Anesthesiologists Task Force on Acute Pain Management. Practice guidelines for acute pain management in the perioperative setting: an updated report by the American Society of Anesthesiologists Task Force on Acute Pain Management. Anesthesiology. 2012;116(2):248–73.
40. Bartocci M, Lundeberg S. Intravenous paracetamol: the "Stockholm protocol" for postoperative analgesia of term and preterm neonates. Paediatr Anaesth. 2007;17(11):1120–1.
41. Mian P, Knibbe CA, Tibboel D, Allegaert K. What is the dose of intravenous paracetamol for pain relief in neonates? Arch Dis Child. 2017;102(7):649–50.
42. Palmer GM, Atkins M, Anderson BJ, Smith KR, et al. I.V. acetaminophen pharmacokinetics in neonates after multiple doses. Br J Anaesth. 2008;101(4):523–30.
43. Lönnqvist P-A. Regional anaesthesia and analgesia in the neonate. Best Pract Res Clin Anaesthesiol. 2010;24(3):309–21.
44. Hall RW, Anand KJS. Pain management in newborns. Clin Perinatol. 2014;41(4):895–924.
45. Association of Paediatric Anaesthetists of Great Britain and Ireland. Good practice in postoperative and procedural pain management, 2nd ed. Paediatr Anaesth 2012; 22(Suppl. 1): 1–79.
46. Alencar AJC, Sanudo A, Sampaio VMR, Góis RP, et al. Efficacy of tramadol versus fentanyl for postoperative analgesia in neonates. Arch Dis Child Fetal Neonatal Ed. 2012;97(1):F24–9.
47. Eventov-Friedman S, Rozin I, Shinwell ES. Case of chest-wall rigidity in a preterm infant caused by prenatal fentanyl administration. J Perinatol. 2010;30(2):149–50.

48. Ranger M, Johnston CC, Anand KJS. Current controversies regarding pain assessment in neonates. Semin Perinatol. 2007;31(5):283–8.
49. Piastra M, Pizza A, Gaddi S, Luca E, Genovese O, et al. Dexmedetomidine is effective and safe during NIV in infants and young children with acute respiratory failure. BMC Pediatr 2018 25; 18(1); 282.
50. Analgesia for neonates I BJA Education I Oxford Academic [Internet]. [cited 2021 Aug 30]. Available from: https://academic.oup.com/bjaed/article/10/4/123/380855
51. Young C, Jevtovic-Todorovic V, Qin Y-Q, Tenkova T, et al. Potential of ketamine and midazolam, individually or in combination, to induce apoptotic neurodegeneration in the infant mouse brain. Br J Pharmacol. 2005;146(2):189–97.
52. Kubota T, Fukasawa T, Kitamura E, Magota M, Kato Y, et al. Epileptic seizures induced by dexmedetomidine in a neonate. Brain Dev. 2013;35(4):360–2.
53. Bouchut JC, Dubois R, Foussat C, Moussa M, Diot N, et al. Evaluation of caudal anaesthesia performed in conscious ex-premature infants for inguinal herniotomies. Paediatr Anaesth. 2001;11(1):55–8.
54. Daftary SR, Jagtap SR. Caudal epidural as a sole anaesthetic in preterm, former preterm and high risk infants. Indian J Anaesth. 2005;14(49):195–8.
55. Bianchi A, Dickson AP, Alizai NK. Elective delayed midgut reduction-No anesthesia for gastroschisis: Selection and conversion criteria. J Pediatr Surg. 2002;37(9):1334–6.
56. Caudal Anesthesia [Internet]. NYSORA. 2019 [cited 2021 Aug 30]. Available from: https://www.nysora.com/techniques/neuraxial-and-perineuraxial-techniques/caudal-anesthesia/
57. Wiegele M, Marhofer P, Lönnqvist P-A. Caudal epidural blocks in paediatric patients: a review and practical considerations. BJA Br J Anaesth. 2019;122(4):509–17.
58. Chen CPC, Tang SFT, Hsu T-C, Tsai W-C, Liu H-P, et al. Ultrasound guidance in caudal epidural needle placement. Anesthesiology. 2004;101(1):181–4.
59. Bösenberg AT, Hadley GP, Wiersma R. Oesophageal atresia: caudo-thoracic epidural anaesthesia reduces the need for post-operative ventilatory support. Pediatr Surg Int. 1992;7:289–91. https://doi.org/10.1007/BF00183983.
60. Wolf AR, Eyres RL, Laussen PC, Edwards J, et al. Effect of extradural analgesia on stress responses to abdominal surgery in infants. BJA. 1993;70(6):654–60. https://doi.org/10.1093/bja/70.6.654.
61. Tsui BCH, Suresh S. Ultrasound imaging for regional anesthesia in infants, children, and adolescents: a review of current literature and its application in the practice of neuraxial blocks. Anesthesiology. 2010;112(3):719–28.
62. Jöhr M. Regional anaesthesia in neonates, infants and children: an educational review. Eur J Anaesthesiol. 2015;32(5):289–97.
63. Suresh S, Ecoffey C, Bosenberg A, Lonnqvist P-A, et al. The European Society of Regional Anaesthesia and Pain Therapy/American Society of Regional Anaesthesia and Pain Medicine recommendations on local anesthetics and adjuvants dosage in pediatric regional anesthesia. Reg Anesth Pain Med. 2018;43(2):211–6.
64. Kachko L, Simhi E, Tzeitlin E, Efrat R, Tarabikin E, et al. Spinal anesthesia in neonates and infants - a single-center experience of 505 cases. Paediatr Anaesth. 2007;17(7):647–53.
65. Bösenberg AT, Kimble FW. Infraorbital nerve block in neonates for cleft lip repair: anatomical study and clinical application. Br J Anaesth. 1995;74(5):506–8.
66. Abdellatif AA, Elagamy AE, Elgazzar K. Ultrasound-guided infraorbital nerve block for cleft lip repair in pediatrics: a new technique for an old block. Ain-Shams J Anesthesiol. 2018;10(1):3.
67. Echaniz G, De Miguel M, Merritt G, Sierra P, Bora P, et al. Bilateral suprazygomatic maxillary nerve blocks vs. infraorbital and palatine nerve blocks in cleft lip and palate repair: a double-blind, randomised study. Eur J Anaesthesiol. 2019;36(1):40–7.
68. Schoor ANV, Boon JM, Bosenberg AT, et al. Anatomical considerations of the pediatric ilioinguinal/iliohypogastric nerve block. Pediatr Anesth. 2005;15(5):371–7.

69. Willschke H, Bösenberg A, Marhofer P, Johnston S, et al. Ultrasonographic-guided ilioingui-nal/iliohypogastric nerve block in pediatric anesthesia: what is the optimal volume? Anesth Analg. 2006;102(6):1680–4.
70. Spencer DM, Miller KA, O'Quin M, Tomsovic JP, et al. Dorsal penile nerve block in neonatal circumcision: chloroprocaine versus lidocaine. Am J Perinatol. 1992;9(3):214–8.
71. Hamill JK, Rahiri J-L, Liley A, Hill AG. Rectus sheath and transversus abdominis plane blocks in children: a systematic review and meta-analysis of randomized trials. Paediatr Anaesth. 2016;26(4):363–71.
72. Vecchione T, Zurakowski D, Boretsky K. Thoracic paravertebral nerve blocks in pediatric patients: Safety and clinical experience. Anesth Analg. 2016;123(6):1588–90.
73. Thompson ME, Haynes B. Ultrasound-guided thoracic paravertebral block catheter experience in 2 neonates. J Clin Anesth. 2015;27(6):514–6.
74. Bosenberg A, Flick RP. Regional anesthesia in neonates and infants. Clin Perinatol. 2013;40(3):525–38.
75. Marfurt-Russenberger K, Axelin A, Kesselring A, et al. The experiences of professionals regarding involvement of parents in neonatal pain management. J Obstet Gynecol Neonatal Nurs 2016 1; 45(5): 671–683.
76. Ramezani T, Hadian Shirazi Z, Sabet Sarvestani R, Moattari M. Family-centered care in neonatal intensive care unit: a concept analysis. Int J Community Based Nurs Midwifery. 2014;2(4):268–78.
77. Khoza S, Tjale A. Knowledge, attitudes and practices of neonatal staff concerning neonatal pain management. Curationis 2014 28; 37(2): E1–E9. doi:https://doi.org/10.4102/curationis.v37i2.1246.

Perioperative Complications and Critical Incidents During Anesthesia in a Surgical Neonate

Geeta Kamal

27.1 Introduction

There are several variable components of the system that can cause complications and critical incidents during anesthesia, with numerous cross connections and interactions, result of which cannot at times be predicted and averted. Besides, under anesthesia (especially GA), patient is unable to complain and the entire onus lies on the capability of the attending anesthesiologist to diagnose timely, take appropriate treatment measures, and avert adverse consequences or major harm to the patient. This becomes even more important in small nonverbal children like **newborns and neonates**.

Most literature reports CIs in adults and children, with only a small proportion of included patients being in the neonatal age group. The results of such studies become inconsequential regarding provision of any significant information on CIs unique to this age group.

Most of this topic is extrapolated from the available literature and authors knowledge and experience. In this chapter, we will discuss about perioperative complications and CIs in neonates, historical aspects of reporting and its significance, severity classification, risk factors, possible complications, and recommendations to avert them and improve patient outcome.

A summary of some reports is also included for the benefit of the reader interested in research.

G. Kamal (✉)
Chacha Nehru Bal Chikitsalya, Delhi, India

27.2 Special Concern in Neonates

- All children are at a risk of surgery and anesthesia. Newborns and neonates are more vulnerable. Preterm (<37 weeks GA) neonates, especially low birthweight (<1500 g), are at highest risk of developing CIs, often leading to mortality, as:
- The incidence of CIs is double in infants compared to adults.
- Mortality of pediatric anesthesia complications is quite high (nearly 10 times that in adults).
- Reported incidence of anesthesia-related cardiac arrest in infants is 0.19–0.24%, compared to in children (0.01–0.07%).
- Mortality following cardiac arrest in anesthetized neonates is very high (>70%).
- Though the 5-year outcomes for GA and conscious sedation in neonates are comparable.

27.2.1 What Makes Neonates at Greater Risk of Anesthesia Related Adverse Events (CIs)?

1. Poor tolerance to anesthetic drugs, interventions, and stress of surgery due to immaturity of various organ systems.
2. The transitional changes and adaptations from intra- to extra-uterine environment are still ongoing
3. The risk of reversion to fetal circulation even with minor insult is quite high.
4. Premature neonates have low surfactant concentration and lung volumes, poor alveolar compliance, intrapulmonary shunting, and ventilation /perfusion (V: Q) mismatch. These all are precursors for respiratory problems and high morbidity.
5. Low O_2 reserve, weak cough, and loss of protective airway reflexes under GA make them more prone to respiratory events.
6. They are extremely susceptibility to low O_2 concentration and hypoxia.
7. They are equally susceptible to high O_2 concentrations, O_2 toxicity.
8. High pressures and volumes during assisted/controlled ventilation increase the risk of pulmonary barotrauma.
9. Anesthesia, especially for minor procedures with short operating time (often few minutes) and minimal trauma and stimulation, poses a high risk for delayed recovery and perioperative respiratory events.
10. Most common CIs in neonates are respiratory and cardiac arrest.

27.2.2 Definition

Critical incidents are defined as -

- Any incident or occurrence which affected or could have affected safety of the patient under anesthetic care, including near misses, or

- An event under anesthesia care which had the potential to lead to an undesirable outcome if left to progress, or
- An occurrence that could have led (if not discovered or corrected in time) or did lead to an undesirable outcome.

Anesthesia-related CI may involve any organ system, but respiratory system is commonly affected. Literature lists common adverse events as follows:

 (i) **Respiratory**—difficult or failed intubation, airway trauma and edema, gum injury, endobronchial intubation, ET disconnection, bronchospasm, laryngospasm, stridor,
 (ii) **Drug errors**—wrong drug or wrong dose, adverse reactions (anaphylactoid reaction, thrombophlebitis, rash, nephrotoxicity, ototoxicity),
(iii) **Cardiac**—bradycardia, hypotension, arrhythmias, ventricular tachycardia, and fibrillation,
(iv) **Neurological,** and
 (v) **Others**—vascular (extravasation, occlusion of IV tubing), allergic (latex, rubber), or equipment related.

27.3   History and Development of CI Reporting

Critical incident technique was 1st described by Flanagan in 1954 to improve safety among military pilots and subsequently refined for nonmedical and medical use. Cooper et al. (1978) adapted this to anesthesia to uncover patterns of frequently occurring incidents. It was subsequently developed into a national plan in the Australian Incident Monitoring Study in 1988.

Presently, there are many CI monitoring programs including ASA Committee on Patient Safety and Risk Management, and National Patient Safety Agency in UK.

National Reporting and Learning System (NRLS) in England and Wales (UK National Patient Safety Agency) identifies and analyzes CIs in pediatric anesthesia.

27.3.1 Utility of CI Reporting in Anesthesia

- Discussion of CIs helps learning from problems and thereby improving patient safety,
- Is an appropriate tool for quality improvement and control in anesthesia,
- Helps improve patient safety by identifying potential risks by analyzing CIs,
- Helps uncover frequently occurring incidents under anesthesia,
- Captures "near misses" and tracks interventions in situations where no harm was done and enhances learning,
- CI analysis can help reach the root cause of the problem,
- Cost incurred in CI reporting at the level of the institute is very low, but benefits are huge.
- Last and not the least, *we can learn from mistakes of others*.

27.3.2 Limitations of CI Reporting

Learning from CI reporting has several limitations, chiefly because of **underreporting or underestimation of true numbers**

1. Underreporting may be from—complicated form design, time constraints, fear of blame or punitive action, lack of feedback, lack of clarity on what should be reported, or even what constitutes as CI. For example, anesthesiologists may only report major adverse events, and not minor events.
2. Different clinicians define CIs differently due to variations in perception and experience.
3. People do not want their name to be known, and so do not report. Making personal details optional in the form may allow more events to be reported (anonymity).
4. Reporting should be done by any staff who witnesses an adverse event, but one may miss important details, making analysis and reaching conclusions difficult and meaningless.
5. Often, if one already knows the outcome, it influences the judgment, evaluation, and reporting.
6. Each institution will have different categories and classification of CIs, and a particular event may not fit clearly into any one category, leading to errors in reporting, misses, and underreporting.
7. Incidence of adverse events varies with the operator's skill. This may lead either to under-reporting or to over-reporting.
8. Analysis of CIs must take the skill level into account when reaching conclusions and making recommendations.

27.4   Classification of Critical Incidents

CIs are classified by the severity of harm defined by the **National Patient Safety Agency (2005)** –

(i) No harm,
(ii) Low harm—Those that require extraobservation or minor treatment and caused minimal harm,
(iii) Moderate harm—Those that require moderate increase in treatment and which cause significant but not permanent harm,
(iv) Severe harm—Those that result in permanent harm, and
(v) Cardiac Arrest, Death, Loss of life.

27.5   Risk Factors for CIs

Various factors that increase the risk of anesthesia-related adverse or critical incidents can be classified as patient, surgery, and anesthesia related and can operate any time in the extended perioperative period. Risk factors can be mitigated by proper preoperative assessment, advance preparation, skilled assistance, open communication, knowledge and training, and experience of all personnel involved. Continuity in care from preoperative to intraoperative and into the postoperative period is one of the most important factors that can reduce the incidence of CIs, their consequences, and improved postoperative outcome.

These become highly significant in the term and preterm newborns and neonates, who are still undergoing adaptive changes and are in the process of growth and maturity.

(I) *Patient related*—gestational age at birth, birthweight, APGAR score, age at surgery, congenital anomalies or malformations, medical diseases, ASA, and nutritional status.

(II) *Surgery related*—surgical diagnosis, degree of hemodynamic, metabolic, acid base and electrolyte derangements, extent of dissection and duration of surgery, amount of 3rd space fluid shift, blood loss, and blood transfusion.

(III) *Anesthesia related*—preoperative workup and risk stratification, type of anesthetic technique, degree of monitoring, hypothermia, amount of blood transfusion, anesthetic drugs related adverse reactions, their diagnosis, and management.

(IV) *Human factors*—fatigue, anesthesiologist/ surgeon's/staff skill and experience, fatigue.

(V) *Equipment /Drug related*—failure to check the equipment, drug and dosage errors, wrong dilutions, allergic reactions.

(VI) *System or administrative related*—out of hours surgery, availability of equipment, staff.

27.6 Literature Search

1. In 2008, an audit report of pediatrics perioperative incidents in 10,000 anesthetics over a period of 2 years in Singapore (May 1997–April 1999) was published. Surgical procedures ranged from ambulatory to open heart surgeries, 80% patients being ASA I/II, and 73.3% elective surgeries. The incidence of CIs was 2.97%, 4 times more common in under 1 year age than older children, and no mortality. Most CIs occurred during the maintenance phase, commonest being respiratory events (laryngospasm), followed by cardiovascular (hypotension, hemorrhage, sepsis, dysrhythmias) events. Equipment and pharmacologically related events were low in this audit.

2. Procedural sedation is a common technique for investigative and short procedures in children outside the OT; they easily slip from sedation to anesthesia stage. Pediatric Sedation Research Consortium (2009) published a data of 49,836 Propofol sedation records (July 2004–August 2007) in 0-8 years ages (3.89% <6 months of age), from 37 centers. Procedures undertaken were airway/pulmonary, fracture reduction, cardiology, dental, FB removal, GI procedures, oncological, nerve conduction, eye, radiological, and minor surgeries. Patients had coexisting problems of the airway, cardiac and craniofacial anomalies, immune and hepato-renal-metabolic disorders, prematurity, and traumatic. Complications

or unplanned treatment during sedation were classified as none or present (agitation, delirium, airway related and unexpected airway management, cardiac events, hypothermia, inadequate anesthesia, IV related, delayed recovery, unplanned admission, need of reversal, allergic reactions, and gastrointestinal problems). The commonest CIs were pulmonary, followed by delayed recovery, and failed anesthesia or failed procedure.

3. In 2011, identification and analysis of CIs relating to pediatric anesthesia were reported from the UK National Reporting and Learning System in England and Wales. Data were obtained from the UK National Patient Safety Agency. Incidents were classified according to age, degree of harm sustained, and clinical category. 606 incidents were reported (including 6 deaths, 48 severe harm). CIs reported were medication issues (35.6%), airway/ventilation related (18.8%), equipment-related (failure or unavailability) (15.7%), communication and organizational problems (8.6%), and cardiovascular (5.9%). They recommended that anesthetists must be encouraged to take ownership and contribute high-quality descriptions of incidents to the national systems.

4. In 2016, a retrospective review of CI during anesthesia at a tertiary care hospital in Singapore, was published. Of 98502 anesthetics, 441 incidents were reported (0.44%). Age ranged up to 91 years. Neonates were 0.1%, with 0.2% CI component. They found that odds of having a CI increased with increasing ASA status, out-of-hours surgeries, under GA or combined epidural and GA and under MAC (monitored anesthesia care). Most common CIs were pulmonary, followed by drugs, infusion related, and surgery related. Less common were related to equipment, anesthesia, cardiac, and administrative. Cerebrovascular and transfusion-related CIs were few. 87% were drug errors, with human and system factors, staff shortage, poor communication, haste, and fatigue as contributory factors.

5. In 2018, retrospective CIs in pediatrics (up to 12 years age), over a period of 15 years, at a tertiary care hospital in Pakistan was published. 34% were infants. 451 CIs were recorded, 96% during elective, and 4% during emergency surgery, with poor outcome in 7%. Equipment-related, respiratory and drug-related CI occurred in similar frequency. Human factors contributed to 74% CIs, equipment failure in 10%, patient factors in 8%, and system errors in 5%. Most common human factors were failure to check equipment, drugs, or doses.

27.7 List of Possible Critical Incidents

Any organ system can be involved in adverse events or CIs. We have classified in order of commonest to less common CIs.

1. Pulmonary system related
2. Medication errors, anaphylaxis, systemic LA toxicity
3. Surgery related—operation on incorrect site, operation on incorrect patient
4. Transfusion reaction
5. Unplanned ICU admission

6. Vascular access related—vascular injury, pneumothorax
7. Neuraxial block related—infection, epidural hematoma, high spinal, postdural puncture headache
8. Regional anesthesia—peripheral neurologic deficit, infection
9. Delayed recovery
10. Hypothermia
11. Equipment related
12. Malignant hyperthermia
13. Cardiac arrest
14. Others—minor injuries and burns

27.7.1 Critical Incidents Related to the Pulmonary System are the Most Common

In neonatal anesthesia, such as difficult airway, reintubation, bronchospasm, laryngospasm, pulmonary edema, oropharyngeal injuries, aspiration, and subglottic stenosis.

(a) *Difficult airway*: For reporting of unrecognized difficult airway, we refer to the ASA's Practice Guidelines for Management of the Difficult Airway: The clinical situation in which a reasonably experienced anesthesiologist experiences difficulty with face mask ventilation, laryngoscopy, intubation, and/or ventilation.

Management

(i) Increase to FiO_2 to 1, maintain continuous O_2 flow during airway management
(ii) Call for expert help and difficult airway cart (laryngoscopes, different tubes, stylet, rigid bronchoscope, fiber-optic laryngoscope, and tracheostomy kit)
(iii) If unable to mask ventilate, ask for 2-handed assistance.
(iv) Insert oral airway (never try nasal airway or intubation), if unsuccessful,
(v) Insert supraglottic airway (e.g., LMA)
(vi) Decompress stomach with orogastric tube
(vii) Consider reversing neuromuscular blocker (if used)
(viii) Consider awakening the neonate if surgery not started
(ix) **Consider alternative approach for intubation**—different blade, reposition head, use intubating stylet /intubating LMA /different operator/videolaryngoscope /fiber-optic scope
(x) If still fail to achieve the airway, consider emergency surgical airway (cricothyrotomy or tracheostomy) or
(xi) Abandon the procedure, awaken the baby, postpone surgery, and plan tracheostomy electively before surgery when posted another time.
(xii) In neonates with macroglossia (Beckwith-Wiedemann, Pierre-Robin) or mediastinal mass— consider prone or lateral position

Care—NEVER Try Blind Oral or Nasal Approach in Newborns and Neonates

(b) *Reintubation*—Patient requires placement of tracheal tube or other airway devices for mechanical/assisted ventilation within 6 h after extubation because of severe respiratory distress, hypoxia, hypercapnia, or respiratory acidosis.

(c) *Bronchospasm*—Moderate-to-severe bronchospasm intraoperatively is accompanied by desaturation and dusky skin coloration. Most common cause is light planes of anesthesia, inadequate analgesia, overhydration, and silent aspiration. Management includes increase in FiO_2, bronchodilator and steroid nebulization or intravenously, assisted bag mask ventilation, subcutaneous adrenaline, and if still not relieved, management for pulmonary aspiration should be followed.

(d) *Laryngospasm*—usually occurs at induction of anesthesia when airway handling and instrumentation is done in light planes or awake neonate. Neonate becomes hypoxic, cyanotic, and desaturates. Management includes increase in FiO to 1 and gentle assisted ventilation with face mask and bag. If laryngospasm persists, deepening the plane of anesthesia usually resolves the issue. Nest attempt at intubation of trachea must be done with a smaller size tube.

- Laryngospasm may also occur at the time of extubation. Management is same as described above.
  Care at Extubation
- Either extubate in deeper plane of anesthesia and then use face mask and bag ventilation till spontaneous respiration and reflexes recover, or
- Extubate when the baby is fully awake

  Negative Pressure Pulmonary Edema can develop following severe unresolved laryngospasm at the time of induction or at extubation. Neonate becomes hypoxic, desaturates, develop noisy respiration, crepitations over the chest, and pink frothy sputum at the mouth. Management is by increase in FiO2 to 100%, tracheal intubation, diuretics, stop IV fluids, and controlled ventilation with PEEP.

(e) *Oropharyngeal Injuries*—These are common in neonates, especially premature and small babies, and often are due to improper handling, use of inappropriate instruments especially at induction and extubation, nasopharyngeal instrumentations. These are usually mild CIs, but in case of gums and tongue injuries, it can bleed profusely, risking the baby to pulmonary aspiration.

(f) *Aspiration*—Clinical diagnosis of aspiration during anesthesia and postoperatively consistent with radiologic findings should be reported. Risk factors for aspiration in surgical neonates are disease-related (intestinal obstruction, pyloric stenosis, TEF, CDH), patient-related (emergency surgery in a fed neonate, full stomach), and anesthesia-related (at the time of induction of anesthesia, laryngoscopy, and intubation). Management includes tracheal intubation and ventilation until chest condition improves and neonate recovers.

(g) *Subglottic Stenosis*—This is a late complication when healing of damaged tracheal mucosa occurs with fibrosis. This is usually due to attempts at intubation with a larger size ET (because at laryngoscopy, glottic opening seems bigger while the narrowest part is subglottic). If severe, baby may require tracheostomy below the level of stenosis and tracheal repair surgery later. All precautions must be taken to avoid this complication because of its severe adverse long-term consequences.

27.7.2 Medication-Related CIs Include Anaphylaxis, LA Toxicity, Wrong Drug, and Wrong Dose

(a) *Anaphylaxis* is broadly defined as a severe, systemic allergic reaction characterized by multisystem involvement including skin (rash, erythema), airway (bronchospasm), vascular system, and gastrointestinal tract, potentially resulting in hypoxemia, desaturation, cardiovascular collapse, shock, and death. This should be diagnosed immediately and managed because of its potential lethal implications. **Management**—increase in FiO_2 to 1, remove suspected triggers, if latex is suspected, thoroughly wash the area, ensure adequate ventilation/oxygenation, gas exchange and acid base balance, and if hypotensive, turn off anesthetic agents and use IV fluid boluses and sympathomimetic infusion (dopamine)

(b) *LA toxicity*—**This** is broadly defined by the ASRA recommendations on systemic toxicity of LA. The major systemic effects observed following injection of LA should be reported and should include features to allow reporters to report observed effects—seizures, somnolence, loss of consciousness, respiratory depression/apnea, bradycardia/asystole, or ventricular tachycardia/fibrillation.

(c) *Wrong drug, wrong dose*—These CIs occur due to lack of knowledge about drug dosages, similar packaging of different drugs, in hasty and tense situations, emergency, lack of adequate staff and help, wrong dilutions of drugs, and wrong infusion rates.

27.7.3 Surgery Related

(a) *Operation on incorrect site*: Surgery or anesthesia (including regional nerve block) on the wrong body part or wrong side of patient.

(b) *Operation on incorrect patient*: Surgery or procedure on the wrong patient.

Both these are Sentinel events and must be reported.

27.7.4 Transfusion Reactions

Most critical reactions to incompatible blood or blood products transfusion are hemolytic and anaphylactic reactions. Non-hemolytic reactions are usually benign and of mild severity. Any doubt or suspicion regarding incompatible transfusion must be managed as confirmed reaction until proved otherwise. This needs to be reported to the blood bank for rechecking and confirmation.

Management of suspected or definite transfusion reactions

(i) Stop transfusion immediately
(ii) Disconnect donor product and IV tubing from the IV cannula
(iii) Flush and infuse normal saline through a new IV tubing
(iv) Recheck and re-examine the blood product labeling and patient details
(v) Send the product, patients' blood, and urine sample to blood bank to confirm mismatch transfusion
(vi) Administer pheniramine maleate (Avil) or any antiallergic, hydrocortisone, and in case of hypotension and shock like state, start dopamine infusion

27.7.5 Unplanned ICU Admission

Unplanned admission to the NICU within 24 h of induction of anesthesia, due to any reason. This does not include those cases where either the neonate is brought from NICU or where preoperative decision is taken for postoperative NICU admission.

27.7.6 Vascular Access-Related CIs

Central venous line related, intra-arterial cannulation related vascular injury, and pneumothorax.

(a) *Complications of central venous (CV) cannulation* are well known. CIs are those injuries which are of sufficient severity, needing additional interventional therapy
  • Accidental intra-arterial placement of CV catheter
  • Pneumothorax
  • Thoracic duct injury, or
  • Other injuries requiring surgical or interventional radiologic management. They all need to be diagnosed, treated, and reported.
(b) *Pneumothorax*—occurs following difficult or failed vascular access or regional anesthesia. In neonates, these can occur with greater frequency because bony landmarks are not palpable and because the depth of insertion is very short, often in millimeters. Fall in heart rate, blood pressure, oxygen saturation should make the operator suspicious of this CI. The most critical incident is tension pneumothorax, diagnosed on clinical presentation (HR, BP and SpO2 changes, tracheal deviation, and mediastinal shift). Confirmation is by imaging studies (X-ray, CT, ultrasound). Imaging studies take time, and tension pneumothorax, if left undiagnosed, can be fatal in a neonate. Hence, treatment should be instituted immediately, on clinical findings:

- Stop N_2O
- Increase FiO_2 to 1
- Secure airway with endotracheal tube
- Assisted ventilation with low tidal volume and low pressure, no PEEP
- Administer vasopressors for circulatory collapse
- Needle decompression of the pneumothorax and once air exudes (confirmation), introduce a continuous underwater seal chest drain in ipsilateral 2nd intercostal space.
- Proceed with surgery if baby is stable.
- If neonate unstable hemodynamically, abandon surgery until neonate becomes stable.

27.7.7 Neuraxial Block Related

Infection, epidural hematoma, high spinal, postdural puncture headache
  (a) *Infection following epidural or spinal anesthesia*: Infectious complications associated with neuraxial anesthesia and analgesia are of great concern because of their potentially devastating sequelae including meningitis, paralysis, and death.
    - **Superficial soft tissue infection** along the course of an epidural/spinal needle or catheter placement track presents as local swelling, erythema, and tenderness in combination with any of the following:
      – Fever (>38.0 °C)
      – Drainage, positive culture from the area
      – Leukocytosis >12,000/deciliter or CRP >20 mg/L
    - *Epidural abscess*—Radiological evidence of a mass in the epidural space is consistent with an epidural abscess within 30 days following the neuraxial procedure in combination with any of the following—
      a. Fever (>38.0 °C)
      – Positive drainage culture from the local area
      – Leukocytosis >12,000/deciliter or CRP >20 mg/L
      – Local erythema, and tenderness
      – Focal back pain—may not be evident in a surgical neonate, and/or
      – Neurologic deficit
    - *Meningitis*—may be associated with central neuraxial block if symptoms appear within 72 h of neuraxial puncture, block or catheter insertion or removal, in combination with—
      – New onset of central neurologic symptoms
      – Headache (not evident in neonates)
      – Stiff neck
      – Fever >38.0 °C
      – Positive CSF culture
  (b) *Epidural hematoma following spinal or epidural block*—This can be confirmed by MRI and should be reported.

(c) *High spinal*: The unintentional high spinal as indicated by paralysis higher than T4, along with hypotension, bradycardia, respiratory insufficiency, necessitating intubation should be reported. This may be difficult to diagnose in a neonate, as neuraxial block is mostly used in conjunction with GA.

(d) *Dural puncture*—This occurs when accidentally dura is punctured when performing epidural block using a Tuohy needle. Often anesthesiologists perform epidural block in neonates using a hypodermic needle (sharp tipped and long bevel) or a spinal needle (sharp tipped short bevel) when appropriate needle for dural puncture in neonates is not available. If undetected and the drug meant for epidural block is injected, it will lead to high spinal or even total spinal, with its physiological consequences. Ignorance of the occurrence of these complications can lead to unnecessary multidrug interventions and high postoperative morbidity and mortality. In adults, it is easier to diagnose but in neonates, under concomitant GA, it is often missed. Hence, neonatal anesthesiologists should be aware of this potential lethal event and be vigilant and careful during epidural puncture and thereafter, monitoring for suspicious clinical signs. PDPH (postdural puncture headache) following this event is common but is obviously not a feature in neonates.

27.7.8 Regional Anesthesia Related

Peripheral neurologic deficit, infection

(a) *Peripheral neurologic deficit*—**is c**linically diagnosed when there is residual sensory and/or motor and/or autonomic block after 72 h after last injection of LA without other identifiable etiology. when no regional anesthetic/analgesia-related infection is present.

The diagnoses can be confirmed, where appropriate by:

   i. Paresthesia in affected nerve distribution area—neonate is unable to complain

  ii. New loss of deep tendon reflexes—can be detected on examination

 iii. New loss of vibration sensation—cannot be detected in neonates

 iv. Sensory/motor and/or autonomic deficit consistent with dermatomes or nerve distribution affected by the regional anesthetic technique—possible to detect in neonates

  v. Electrophysiological evidence of new nerve damage (MEP, SEP, nerve conduction study, EMG)—these studies are undertaken on patients complain of neurological symptoms but are not done as a routine in all patients following regional nerve blocks. Utility in neonates needs to be explored.

(b) *Infection*—Superficial and deep soft tissue infection within 30 days of block, with accompanying local swelling, erythema, and tenderness along the catheter or needle placement track in combination with any of the following:

   i. Fever (>38.0°C)

ii. Drainage or discharge

iii. Positive culture from the area

27.7.9 Delayed Recovery

This is quite common in neonates after GA and is often due to excessive or untimely (near the end of surgery) administration of anesthetic drugs, such as narcotics, muscle relaxants, or inhalational agents, or untimely reversal of neuromuscular block. This is a reason for need of prolonged postoperative care, ventilatory assistance, intense monitoring, and longer time to discharge from the hospital, higher cost incurred, and a matter of concern, especially following short minor procedures, done on daycare basis in a healthy neonate. Other factors that can cause delayed recovery after anesthesia are hypothermia, acid base and electrolyte imbalance, or any anesthetic or surgical complication. Knowledge, care, and vigilance can mitigate this complication.

27.7.10 Hypothermia

Hypothermia is quite common occurrence in neonates and is a cause of several complications in the perioperative period (discussed in a separate chapter) and is avoidable.

27.7.11 Equipment Related

Malfunction or failure of anesthesia machine or workstation, gas delivery system and pump, can lead to unanticipated, unavoidable CIs of varying severity. Regular maintenance care and check of equipment before anesthesia administration can avert this problem.

27.7.12 Malignant Hyperthermia

Malignant Hyperthermia is a rare, potentially fatal complication following exposure of a susceptible patient to certain triggering anesthetic drugs, halothane, and succinylcholine specifically. True incidence is not known but may range from 1:5000–15,000 to 1:50,000–100,000 anesthetic exposures. Incidence is higher in males, patients less than age of 50 and in children specifically with history of rheumatoid arthritis.

In neonates, it is difficult to predict their susceptibility to MH, and difficult to diagnose. Literature suggests that MH may be a cause in SIDS (sudden infant death syndrome), but no concrete evidence was found. Hence during preoperative evaluation, one must ask for family history suggestive of MHS (susceptibility to MH) so that precautions can be taken.

Malignant Hyperthermia Association of the United States (MHAUS) recommends that each OT or OPD, where anesthesia or sedation is given for surgery, must be equipped with a MH cart so as to prevent any delay in institution of treatment. If recognized, diagnosed, and treated timely, mortality is less than 10%; otherwise, it may be as high as 80%.

Treatment of MH
  i. Stop volatile anesthetic, succinylcholine.
 ii. High FGF with 100% O_2 @ 10 L/min
iii. Hyperventilation to reduce $EtCO_2$
 iv. Dantrolene 2.5 mg/kg IV through central vein, every 5 min until symptoms resolve. Usually, maximum dose needed is 10 mg/kg
  v. Sodium bicarbonate 1–2 mEq/kg IV for metabolic acidosis
 vi. Cool patient if temperature >39 °C—Apply ice externally to axilla, groin and around head, cold IV fluids, gastric lavage with cold water.

27.7.13 Cardiac Arrest

Anesthesia-related cardiac arrest is defined as cessation of mechanical activity of the heart, confirmed by absence of signs of circulation during anesthesia, surgery, or postoperatively, criteria being *"use of cardiac compressions and/or defibrillation within 24 hours of induction of anaesthesia."* Death within 24 h after induction of anesthesia is defined as *"anesthesia related death."* Death within 24 h of anesthetic induction should be tracked and reported within 24 h of surgery.

There are several causes of cardiac arrest which are reversible, and if detected timely, it can be treated. Table 27.1 lists the reversible causes of cardiac arrest.

Management
 – Give 100% O_2
 – Turn off all anesthetic gases
 – Check for Hs and Ts of cardiac arrest
 – Follow **NALS** (Neonatal Advanced Life Support) protocol.

Table 27.1 Reversible Causes of Cardiac arrest Hs and Ts

i. Hypovolemia	i. Tension Pneumothorax
ii. Hypoxemia	
iii. Hydrogen ion (acidosis)	ii. Tamponade (Cardiac)
iv. Hyperkalemia/Hypokalemia	iii. Thrombosis/Thromboembolism
v. Hypoglycemia	iv. Toxin (drugs, anesthetic, β-blocker)
vi. Hypothermia	v. Trauma

27.7.14 Others

Minor injuries are of common occurrence, e.g.

    a. *Cautery burns*—from improperly placed cautery plate, or improper earthing, or not following the instructions given by the company. Burns can be of varying severity.

    b. *Forced air warmer-related burns*—if it is placed too near the baby, especially an exposed limb and finger, leading to burn and gangrene, or if temperature is set high.

    c. *IV-line-related* phlebitis or extravasation.

    d. *Intra-arterial catheter-related* distal limb/finger ischemia, and possible gangrene.

27.8 Key Points and Recommendations for Prevention of CIs in Surgical Neonates (Table 27.2)

- Higher ASA status is the most important contributory factor for actual or potential harm.
- CIs are higher in the maintenance phase of anesthesia and more likely in out of hours surgeries, not necessarily emergency surgeries.
- Most events are related to human errors (slips, lapses).
- Most common are pulmonary and airway related.
- Anesthesia-related CIs and deaths should be reported within 24 h.
- Often CIs are underreported, e.g., by the anesthesiologists. Also, when the outcome is known, it influences the judgment and evaluation of the reporter regarding the significance of an incident.
- Care planning, efficient communication, and teamwork are critical to prevention of anesthesia-related CIs.
- Incident reportioning helps identify and mitigate risk factors and is a valuable part of learning and quality assurance.
- Anesthesiologists must assume greater responsibility and onus.
- A national critical incident reporting scheme should be developed in each country and hospital to track and analyze CIs and find safety solutions to improve outcome in surgical neonates.

To summarize, inhalational anesthesia in neonates enables precise breathing control with retained spontaneous respiration, avoids the need for muscle relaxants, and permits use of LMA for airway maintenance without invading the airway. These enhance the safety of GA in term and preterm neonates with multiple high-risk factors as even mild intraoperative incidence can be fatal. Sevoflurane is the most recommended inhalational agent because of its unique characteristics suitable for premature neonates, like quick onset and short-acting, no respiratory irritation, stable, with few postoperative complications.

Table 27.2 Recommendations to Prevent CIs and Complications in Neonates

1.	Preventive levels	Recommendations
2.	Teaching and Training	Quality improvement projects Training of residents and staff in managing airway-related problems in neonates
3.	Administrative	Invest in reporting of CIs, incident analysis, improvement plans to reduce risk and enhance patient safety Preventive strategies to decrease the future occurrence of CIs Medications and equipment areas need to be looked at more closely Mitigating factors—vigilance by staff involved and monitor alarms. Improving awareness of errors, establishing a safety culture, reducing system complexity.
4.	Anesthesiologists	Anesthesiologists must be familiar with all neonatal anesthesia techniques, choose most appropriate, ensure good effect, reduce complications. Anesthetists encouraged to take ownership and contribute high-quality descriptions of CIs to the national reporting systems. Postoperative follow-up system to capture major complications. Identifying and mitigating risk factors as listed above.
5.	Recording, Reporting, Analysis, and Auditing	Mandatory audit forms for all anesthetics. Mandatory recording of CIs and significant events and management. Incidents may not fit clearly in a category—forms should be simple. Improve the rate of reporting by encouraging feedback and creating a more conducive environment. Anonymity of the reporter encourages better reporting.
6.	Anesthesia Technique	Sevoflurane based GA and LMA ideal technique for short surgeries. Inhalational anesthesia retains spontaneous respiration. Avoids the need for muscle relaxants. Avoids the need for invasive airway (tracheal intubation).
7. 8.	Human Factors and Drug errors	Minimizing anesthesia out of hours. Managing human factors esp. fatigue. Standardizing packaging, presentation, and administration, Improving environment and workflow. Chart with common drugs, dosages, side effects, and management in OT.

Further Reading

Abbasi S, Khan FA, Khan S. Pediatric critical incidents reported over 15 years at a tertiary care teaching hospital of a developing country, 2018. J Anaesthesiol Clin Pharmacol. 2018;34(1):78–83. https://doi.org/10.4103/joacp.JOACP_240_16.

Butterworth JF, Mackey DC, Wasnick JD. Morgan and Mikhail's Clinical Anesthesiology. 5th ed. New York City, NY: McGraw-Hill Companies, Inc.; 2013.

Cravero JP, Beach ML, Blike GT, et al. The incidence and nature of adverse events during pediatric sedation/anesthesia with propofol for procedures outside the operating room: A report from the pediatric sedation research consortium. Anesthesia & Analgesia. 2009;108(3):795–804. https://doi.org/10.1213/ane.0b013e31818fc334.

Dewachter P, Mouton-Faivre C, Emala CW. Anaphylaxis and anesthesia: controversies and new insights. Anesthesiology. 2009;111:1141–50.

Flanagan JC. The critical incident technique. Psychological Bulletin. 1954;5:327–58. https://doi.org/10.1037/h0061470.

Galante D. Regional caudal blockade in a pediatric patient affected by the Joubert syndrome. Acta Anaesthesiol Scand. 2009;53:693–4.

Galante D. Ultrasound needle guidance in neonatal and infant caudal anesthesia. Pediatr Anesth. 2008;18:1233–4.

Kim DC. Malignant hyperthermia. Korean. Journal of Anesthesiology. 2012;63(5):391–401. Retrieved from 10.4097/kjae.2012.63.5.391

Andrew I MacLennan, Andrew F Smith. An analysis of critical incidents relevant to pediatric anesthesia reported to the UK National Reporting and Learning System, 2006–2008. 10.1111/j.1460-9592.2010.03421.x Pediatric Anesthesia, 2019 online – ISSN:1460-9592. 2011; 21(8): 841-847

Malignant Hyperthermia Association of the United States. Emergency treatment for an acute MH event. Retrieved from https://www.mhaus.org/healthcare-professionals/.

Naguib M, Brull SJ. Update on neuromuscular pharmacology. Curr Opin Anaesthesiol. 2009;22:483–90.

Rawicz M, Brandom B, Wolf A. The place of suxamethonium in pediatric anesthesia. Pediatr Anesth. 2009;19:561–70.

Spaeth JP, Kurth CD. The extremely premature infant (micropremie). In: Cote CJ, Lerman J, Todres ID, editors. 2009. A Practice of Anesthesia for Infants and Children. Philadelphia: Saunders.

Tay CLM, Tan GM, Ng SBA. Critical incidents in paediatric anaesthesia: an audit of 10,000 anesthetics in Singapore; 2008. https://doi.org/10.1046/j.1460-9592.2001.00767.x.

Zeng LA, Ng SY, Thong SY. Analysis of Critical Incidents during Anesthesia in a Tertiary Hospital. International Journal of Clinical Medicine. 2016;7:320–33. https://doi.org/10.4236/ijcm.2016.75034.

Part IV

Case-Based Anesthesia Management: Common Procedures

Tracheoesophageal Fistula in the Neonates

28

Radhika Agarwala and Rajeshwari Subramaniam

28.1 Introduction

TEF is a common congenital malformation with an incidence of 1:2500–4000 live births. Most common type is type C, which accounts for 80% of all TEFs [1, 2]. It is more common in males (M:F = 25:3) and in preterm babies (10–40%). It is a life-threatening condition if left undiagnosed and untreated, and requires urgent surgical intervention. Unlike many other anomalies, TEF does not lend itself to antenatal diagnosis. Polyhydramnios and small/absent stomach air bubble should make one suspect esophageal atresia (EA), but it is not a definitive sign.

EA with or without TEF is the most challenging condition for the anesthesiologist. The patients are usually in their first few days of life, might be premature, with low birthweight, associated anomalies, and immaturity, while undergoing adaptation from fetal to extra uterine life.

Duration of surgery usually ranges between 85 and 145 min. Increase in surgical time and prolonged duration of anesthesia exposes neonates to adverse effects of anesthetic agents (inhalational agents, narcotics, muscle relaxants), hemodynamic and ventilatory compromise, desaturation, increased fluid shifts, hypothermia, and need for blood transfusion, influencing the postoperative outcome in the form of delay in extubation, need for postoperative ventilation, prolonged hospital and NICU stay, infections, thereby contributing to high postoperative morbidity [2–4].

R. Agarwala (✉)
Department of Anesthesiology, Pain and Palliative Care, Lady Hardinge Medical College, Smt Sucheta Kriplani and Kalawati Saran Childrens Hospitals, New Delhi, India

R. Subramaniam
Department of Anesthesiology, Pain Medicine and Critical Care, AIIMS, New Delhi, India

This chapter will be dealing with the unique problems related to the classification of TEF and its clinical implications, risk stratification, preoperative care and optimization, and anesthesia requirements and management for surgical repair of TEF in the newborn and neonate.

28.2 Tracheoesophagea Fistula (TEF) [5–7]

28.2.1 History

TEF was described by Thomas Gibson in 1697 and by Thomas Hill in 1839. Surgery for EA was performed by Charles Steels in 1888. First surgical repair was performed by Cameron Haight in 1943 [8]. In the early 70s, postoperative mortality was more than 70% [9], but with improvement in anesthetic management, neonatal care, and surgical skills, the survival rate has increased tremendously, to more than 90% [10].

28.2.2 Development

Both esophagus and trachea develop from the primitive foregut. When the embryo is 4–6 weeks old, a ventral diverticulum forms at the caudal part of the foregut. This elongates and evolves into the trachea. The tracheoesophageal fold fuses to form the septum that divides the foregut into laryngotracheal tube (ventral) and esophagus (dorsal). As the septum develops, the respiratory and esophageal parts get completely separated. Incomplete fusion of the laryngotracheal septum fails to separate the esophagus from the laryngotracheal tube, resulting in TEF. It is often associated with esophageal atresia (EA). There are several anatomic variations of EA with or without a TEF, most common being blind proximal esophageal pouch and a distal TEF.

28.2.3 Etiology

There is no definite cause for occurrence of TEF. It may have a multifactorial etiology. Cases are sporadic and incidence of recurrence in siblings is 1% [11]. Its association with trisomy 18, 21, and 13 has been reported. Maternal use of decongestants containing imidazoline derivatives during first trimester increases the risk for TEF [12].

28.2.4 Pathophysiology

Severity of symptoms and signs may vary with the type of TEF, with or without EA, whether hospital or home delivery, oral feeds received, and age of the baby at presentation and diagnosis. The presence of pooled saliva in the blind upper pouch leads to pulmonary aspiration, pneumonitis, ventilation perfusion mismatch, and hypoxemia. The communication between the trachea and the lower pouch of the esophagus will also lead to pulmonary aspiration of gastric secretions, further aggravating the acid pneumonitis.

If the baby receives feed, e.g., home delivery, he is unable to swallow because of the blind upper esophageal pouch and the feed spills out through the nose, and into the trachea, with choking, gasping, and cyanosis (flow diagram). With no feeds and nutrition, they become dehydrated and hypoglycemic.

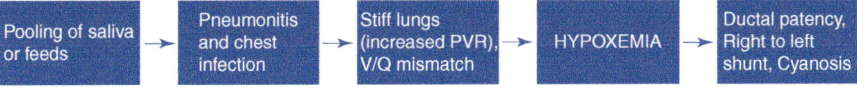

28.2.5 Classification

TEF is classically divided into five types, A to E (Gross classification) and into four types, II, III, IIIb, IIIa (Vogt classification) (Fig. 28.1). Gross and Vogt classifications are used interchangeably in different centers. Each type presents differently and carries different risks and morbidity rates.

These classes are described in the decreasing order of their incidence.

1. **Type C**—This is the commonest type, with an incidence of about 85%. The upper esophageal pouch is blind ended and the lower esophagus communicates with the trachea. When a feeding tube is passed, it coils up in the upper pouch. There is air in the stomach. The coiled feeding tube and gastric air bubble can be seen on X-ray chest.
2. **Type A**—This is the next common type with incidence of 8%. There is no fistulous connection between the esophagus and trachea. This is isolated EA without TEF. In this, secretions collect in the upper pouch and spill over into the trachea causing aspiration pneumonitis. There is no air in the stomach.
3. **Type E**—This is also known as H type TEF and has an incidence of 4%. There is no EA. The esophagus is patent throughout but there is a fistula between the

| Gross classification: | A | B | C | D | E |
| Vogt classification: | II | III | IIIb | IIIa | |

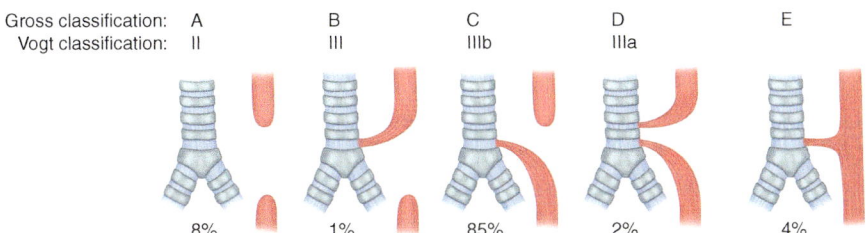

Fig. 28.1 Classification of subtypes of TEF and EA [13]

trachea and esophagus. Secretions and food reach the stomach, but some aspiration does occur through the fistula. This usually presents late (even beyond neonatal period), especially if the fistula is very narrow. Symptoms in the form of choking and respiratory difficulty occur on oral feeding, especially with liquids. There is no coiling of gastric tube and there is air in the stomach. The baby usually presents with history of recurrent chest infection in infancy.

4. **Type D**—There is EA with esophageal discontinuity and has an incidence of 2%. Both proximal and distal segments of esophagus communicate with trachea. There are two TEFs. Aspiration occurs as in type C, both of saliva and gastric acid. There is air in the stomach.

5. **Type B**—EA with proximal TEF is the rarest type, with an incidence of 1% or less. The upper pouch communicates with the trachea and the lower pouch is blind. Aspiration occurs directly through the fistula. The gastric tube does not coil, but will increase the respiratory distress from entry into the trachea via the fistula. There is no air in stomach. These babies present soon after birth with respiratory distress.

28.2.6 Associated Anomalies

The incidence of other congenital anomalies with TEF is 17–70%, including Down syndrome, and VACTERL anomaly [11, 14]. Components of VACTERL anomaly are:

1. **Vertebral (17%)—scoliosis,** hemivertebrae, vertebral defects
2. **Anal 12%**—imperforate anus, duodenal atresia, malrotation, Meckel diverticulum.
3. **Cardiac 20%**—VSD, PDA, TOF (tetralogy of Fallot), ASD, right-sided aortic arch.
4. **Tracheal, esophageal**—TEF, EA
5. **Renal** 16%—renal agenesis, horseshoe/polycystic kidney, hypospadias.
6. **Limb 10%**—radial anomalies, polydactyly/syndactyly, lower limb defects

There may be one or more components of this anomaly, which must be looked for in the preoperative evaluation. Presence of congenital anomalies, wide or pericarinal fistula, increase risk of the surgery and anesthesia, and intraoperative and postoperative complications.

28.3   Prognosis and Risk Stratification

Common complications associated with TEF are recurrent chest infections, pneumonia, acute lung injury, acute respiratory distress syndrome, lung abscess, poor nutrition, bronchiectasis, respiratory failure, and death.

Surgical and perioperative management of congenital TEFs has improved significantly. Average survival rates of more than 90% can be achieved in the surgical babies. In those with no associated congenital anomalies, survival of nearly 100% can be achieved, while in those with comorbidities or unfit for early repair, survival rate is around 80% [15]. Postoperative complication rate (62%) is reported after primary repair of type C TEF in presence of congenital heart disease [16].

Factors which increase the duration of anesthesia, such as patient factors (gestational age, birthweight, age at diagnosis and surgery, associated anomalies), anesthesia factors (hypothermia, difficult airway, hemodynamic instability, ventilation difficulties, desaturation, metabolic derangement), and surgical factors (type of TEF, surgical time, bleeding, surgical complications, duration of surgery), all increase the morbidity [3]. Schmidt et al. in 2017 found that in extremely and very low birthweight neonates undergoing primary repair for type C TEF, the surgical outcomes were similar irrespective of body weight, and so there was no indication of staged repair, unless babies are unstable [17]. Overall survival in type H TEF is 97%, with low complication rate (16%), main complications being postoperative leak (8%) and recurrent laryngeal nerve injury (22%) [18]. Waterston and Spitz classifications are the most widely used prognostic classifications for EA with or without TEF.

The Waterston classification (1997) correlates birthweight, chest condition, and presence of congenital anomalies for deciding the timing and the type of surgical repair, suited to the baby for improved survival. (Table 28.1). They used a cutoff birthweight of 2500 g as safe for surgery, 1800–2500 g with chest involvement or other congenital defects, to be optimized preoperatively, while babies with birthweight of less than 1800 g, severe pneumonia or congenital anomaly, to undergo staged repair.

Waterston stated that in babies with BW more than 2.5 kg and with no other comorbidity, survival was 95%, which reduced to 68% in the presence of one comorbidity and in babies with BW less than 2.5 kg without any comorbidity. The survival rate was 6% when BW was between 1.8 to 2.5 kg with comorbidity or BW less than 1.8 kg with no comorbidity (Table 28.2).

In **2007 Spitz L** used a cutoff of 1500 g birthweight and presence of major cardiac anomalies and heart failure to assess the survival, predicting 98% survival in babies weighing over 1500 g with no cardiac problem, presence of one risk factor reduced the survival to 82%, and in presence of both risk factors, survival was 50% [11] (Table 28.2).

Table 28.1 Waterston classification [14, 19]

Category	Weight/Comorbidities	Surgical Timing
Category A	>2500 grams	Can undergo surgery
Category B	1800–2500 grams or pneumonia or congenital anomaly	Short term delay, needs stabilizing treatment prior to surgery
Category C	<1800 grams or severe pneumonia or congenital anomaly	Requires staged repair

Table 28.2 Co-existing anomalies and survival in TEF [7]

Prognostic Scheme	Class	Birthweight kg	Anomaly	Survival rate (%)
Waterston 1997 [20]	A	≥2.5	Nil	95
	B	≥2.5	Lobar pneumonia mild–moderate anomaly (limb anomalies, cleft palate, ASD, PDA)	68
	C	1.8–2.5	Nil	6
		1.8–2.5	Severe pneumonia	
			Severe anomaly (transposition of great arteries, other bowel atresia, renal insufficiency), or combination of moderate anomalies	
Spitz 2007 [11]	I	≥1.5	Nil	98
	II	≥1.5	CHD	82
		≤1.5	Nil	50
		≤1.5	Major cardiac anomaly (CHD, treatment for heart failure)	
Okamoto 2009 [21]	I	≥2.0	Nil	100
	II	<2.0	Nil	81
	III	≥2.0	Major cardiac anomaly	72
	IV	<2.0	Major cardiac anomaly	27

Okamoto et al. revised Spitz classification in **2009** [21] (Table 28.2) using cardiac anomalies as a major predictor for survival, and cut off of 2000 g for birthweight, and grouped patients into 4 classes:

Class I (low-risk group)—no major cardiac anomaly, birthweight >2000 g;

Class II (moderate-risk group)—no major cardiac abnormality, birthweight <2000 g;

Class III (relatively high-risk group)—major cardiac anomaly, birthweight >2000 g; and

Class IV (high-risk group)—major cardiac anomaly, birthweight <2000 g.

28.4   Diagnosis

TEF and EA are reasons for the inability of the fetus to swallow amniotic fluid. During the antenatal period, maternal hydramnios may be the only feature which should alert the physician to the presence of TEF/EA. Prenatal ultrasound at 18 weeks' gestation showing a small or absent stomach bubble, along with hydramnios, is a pointer toward TEF/EA.

TEFs are often associated with life-threatening complications, so they are usually diagnosed early in the neonatal period. Immediately after birth, the inability to swallow salvia and presence of frothing at the mouth are noticeable signs. (Fig. 28.2a) In babies delivered at home or unsupervised, choking, cyanosis, and respiratory distress when attempts are made to feed the newborn, may be the first signs.

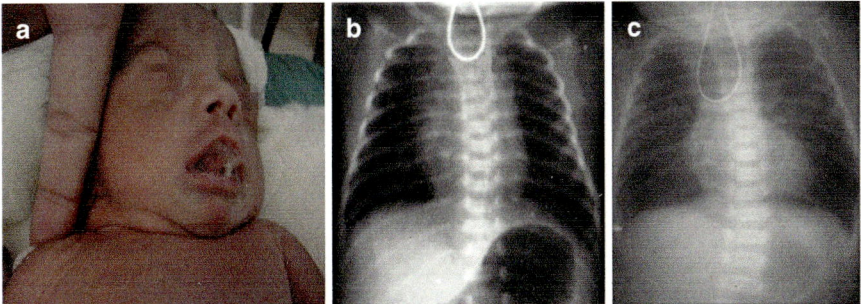

Fig. 28.2 (**a**) Frothy secretions. X-ray chest (**b**). TEF; (**c**). TEF with EA. (coiled gastric tube in upper pouch)

Diagnosis is confirmed by inability to pass an orogastric tube into the stomach (beyond 10 cm length). X-ray chest and abdomen will reveal a coiled feeding tube in the upper pouch and absent or small gastric air bubble (Fig. 28.2b, c). Complete absence of gastric air bubble is seen in pure EA (Type A).

28.5 Preoperative Care

Preoperatively these babies should be nursed in the head up position with continuous low pressures suction of the upper pouch by a Replogle tube. Replogle tubes however are not fail-safe and might get blocked with secretions, with a potential for pulmonary aspiration. It is a practice in many centers to use regular, frequent suction with a conventional naso-esophageal or oro-esophageal tube [13]. They are kept nil per oral and maintained on IV fluids; hence, definite surgery is required within the first few days of life.

28.6 Treatment

This is one congenital defect which can only be corrected by surgery. It is an emergency procedure, undertaken as early as possible after diagnosis, preferably before the baby receives feeds and aspirates, and only to be deferred if the neonate has a very poor general condition or if postponement will optimize or improve the chest condition. Approach can be open or thoracoscopic-aided surgery, at centers where facilities and expertise are available [22]. It can be done as:

1. **Primary repair**—done within 24–48 h of life.
2. **Staged repair**—3 stage procedure:
   a. 1st stage—Feeding gastrostomy +/- esophagostomy
   b. 2nd stage—TEF repair, i.e., ligation of the fistula and esophageal anastomosis
   c. 3rd stage—Closure of gastrostomy

Primary repair or one-stage repair is the first choice. Staged repair allows the sick neonate to recover better after each short procedure, along with allowing gastric intake and time for optimization. **Indications for staged repair are—**

   i. Poor general condition
  ii. Hemodynamic instability
 iii. Poor chest condition, severe hypoxemia
 iv. Long-gap EA
  v. High-risk babies (low or extremely low birthweight, major cardiac, or other congenital anomalies)

28.7 Anesthetic Management

28.7.1 Preoperative Evaluation

All neonates should undergo a detailed preoperative evaluation. Specific points to be noted are:

   i. **General condition**—Birthweight, gestational age at birth, age at diagnosis, home, or hospital delivery.
  ii. **Pulmonary status**—If the diagnosis has been made late, that is, after baby has received oral feeds, and most likely aspirated, there would already be involvement of the lungs and associated hypoxemia. Presence and severity of aspiration and pulmonary signs must be looked for.
 iii. **Congenital anomalies**—There is a 50% chance of associated congenital abnormalities, commonly in the form of components of VACTERL anomaly. These must be looked for and excluded. It is also important to identify congenital cardiac lesions as they will lead to a poorer prognosis. Renal abnormalities (especially single kidney) and vertebral defects could complicate the intraoperative and postoperative course.

     Note: If any one congenital anomaly is present in the baby, look for other associated or incidental anomalies. A complete workup should include an ECG and echocardiography for diagnosing the cardiac defect and its severity, as well as to delineate the aortic arch for proper planning of thoracotomy, especially for thoracoscopic surgery.

28.7.2 Investigations

Following investigations should be done prior to surgery.

  a. **Blood**—Complete blood counts, blood grouping and cross-matching, and serum electrolytes.
  b. **Chest X-ray**—Pneumonitis and lung changes.

c. **Echocardiography**—To diagnose the cardiac disease and its severity.

d. **Blood gas analysis**—Is indicated in sick neonates and on ventilatory support.

28.7.3 Optimization and Preoperative Preparation

Optimization and preoperative preparation (Box 28.1) are aimed at minimizing further aspiration, correcting fluid and electrolyte status, improving pulmonary status and oxygenation, and maintaining body temperature, preventing hypoglycemia, and informed consent.

Box 28.1: Preoperative Care and Optimization
1. **Minimize Aspiration**
   a. Withhold oral feeds
   b. Suction of upper pouch and oral secretions to prevent collection
   c. Nurse in an upright position (propped up) so oral secretions do not go into lungs, but collect in blind pouch and can be sucked out
2. **Correct fluid and electrolyte status**
   a. I/V access—Right upper extremity preferred because of intraoperative left lateral position and easy access
   b. IV fluids and nutrition
3. **Optimize pulmonary status by**
   a. Minimize aspiration
   b. Chest physiotherapy
   c. Tracheal toilet (suction)
   d. Antibiotics
4. **Improve oxygenation**
   a. Humidified oxygen inhalation
   b. CPAP
   c. Intubation and ventilatory support (if needed)
5. **Maintain body temperature and blood glucose**
6. **Informed consent**

28.7.4 An Informed Consent

An informed consent is vitally important keeping in mind the fact that the relative with the baby may not be the parent. So, a record of relatives' name and relationship to the baby must be made.

28.7.5 Monitoring

Monitoring includes HR, ECG, NIBP, SpO_2, $EtCO_2$, temperature, and fluid intake.

Precordial stethoscope is fixed in the left axilla. This will help in hearing the cardiac and respiratory sounds, and early detection of endobronchial intubation.

In the operation theater, oral suction is done to clear the oral cavity before induction of anesthesia. All monitors are attached. The ECG electrodes should be placed with care keeping the incision site clear (right lateral thoracotomy). IV is preferred in the right arm as this makes it easier for the anesthetist to reach, since the baby is in the left lateral position with the right arm stretched over the right side of the head. If the IV is on the left arm, it is more likely to get compressed and lead to inadequate fluid delivery.

28.7.6 Induction and Intubation

Anesthesia can be induced with either inhalational or intravenous agents, in a manner to preserve spontaneous ventilation by use of inhalational agents and small incremental doses of IV agents. Sevoflurane, in O_2 and air or N2O mixture, is a suitable technique.

A number of strategies have been proposed for tracheal intubation [7, 13]. Tracheal intubation may be performed at an optimal anesthetic depth, after spraying the laryngeal inlet with local anesthetic, or with the use of muscle relaxants. Direct laryngoscopy, using Millers straight blade or fiberoptic bronchoscopy, can either be used.

Special care is taken in proper placement of ETT. The tip of ETT should lie beyond the fistula opening to prevent gastric distension. The bevel of the ETT should face anteriorly as fistulae always are on the posterior wall of the trachea.

1. **Conventional laryngoscopy and intubation**—After laryngoscopy, the endotracheal tube is advanced till it meets with resistance (endobronchial intubation) and then gradually withdrawn till breath sounds are equally audible bilaterally, which indicates that the ETT is positioned beyond the fistula. In very small fistulae, ETT can be placed normally in mid-trachea.
2. **Check bronchoscopy**—To confirm the position of the ETT. This is fraught with the possibility of the ETT getting displaced into the fistula, leading to inability to ventilate and severe hypoxemia.
3. **Rigid bronchoscopy and Fogarty Catheterization** (Fig. 28.3)—This is done to visualize the exact size and number of fistulae and placement of 4/5Fr Fogarty catheter into the fistula under direct vision. The balloon is inflated to occlude a large pericarinal fistula. There is the danger of the Fogarty slipping back into the trachea and causing central airway obstruction. Hence, after the rigid bronchoscope is withdrawn, and a standard sized ETT is placed alongside the Fogarty at the same sitting. The stiff Fogarty catheter also serves to locate the fistula at

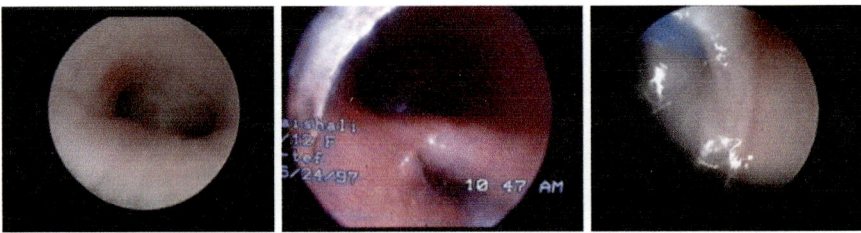

Fig. 28.3 Identification of fistula (arrow) while withdrawing rigid bronchoscope from carina. Fogarty catheter being introduced into fistula

thoracotomy and differentiates it from the bronchus. Ventilation during bronchoscopy is assisted from the side arm. Fogarty catheter is placed in case of repeated intubation of a large fistula.
4. Use of **flexible tracheoscopy** (2.0, 2.4, 2.8 mm) has been reported in neonates with TEF [7]. The tracheoscope is passed through the ETT. Fistulae are "opened" by applying PEEP. Tracheal transillumination aids in identification of multiple fistulae. Use of high airway pressures to identify fistulae has the potential of barotrauma.
5. **Fiber-optic-aided intubation**, under direct vision.

Air entry must be checked after positioning as the ETT could migrate into one of the bronchi. ETT should be fixed securely and note made of the measurement at the mouth level.

Awake induction is reserved for very sick neonates and for those with difficult airway.

28.7.7 Care During Ventilation

Although it is recommended to maintain spontaneous ventilation till the ligation of the fistula, in practice it is often difficult as these neonates desaturate in the lateral decubitus position and because of high metabolic rate and O_2 requirement, necessitating ventilatory assistance. Retaining of spontaneous ventilation till fistula ligation has been facilitated with continuous caudal epidural for analgesia [23, 24].

Special care must be taken when ventilating neonates with TEF. They are at risk of:

1. **Ineffective/inadequate ventilation** and hypoxemia (Box 28.2), and
2. **Gastric distension,** consequent respiratory compromise by the upward splinting of the diaphragm during spontaneous respiration, and danger of gastric reflux into the trachea (Fig. 28.4a).

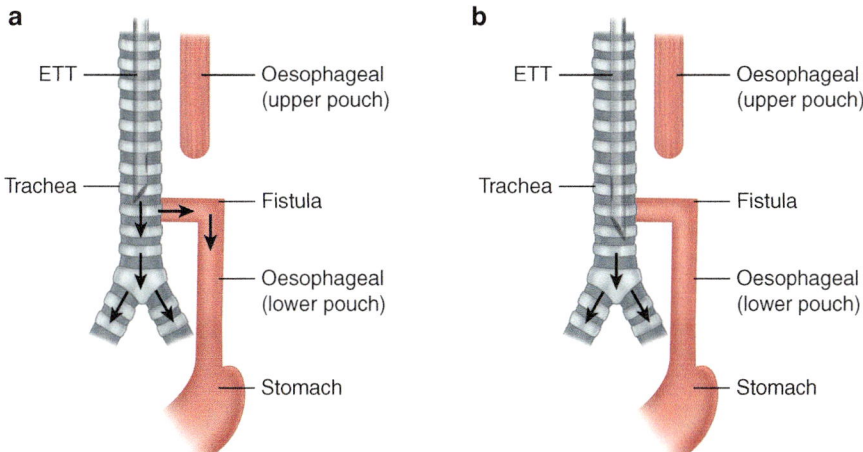

Fig. 28.4 Positioning of ETT in relation to the fistula (**a**) Tip of ETT above the level of Fistula - Incorrect positioning of ETT. (**b**) Tip of ETT below the level of fistula and bevel directed away - Correct positioning

Hence, following precautions must be taken:

   i. If a gastrostomy tube is in place, it must be left open to the atmosphere during induction, especially prior to intubation.

   ii. When ventilating with a face mask, it should be gentle, with low volume (3–5 ml/kg) and low pressures (<10 cm H_2O). At higher pressures and volume, the gases will preferentially get diverted through the fistula into the stomach, if the fistula is larger (>3 mm diameter) causing gastric distention.

   iii. Fistulae <3 mm diameter (less than the neonate's tracheal diameter) pose no problems with PPV.

   iv. Pericarinal fistulae or tracheal "trifurcation" is most problematic, because of their location near the carina, and also because they are usually wide. All gases will get diverted into the stomach both with face mask and ETT ventilation. Hence, these should be identified and blocked using Fogarty catheter.

   v. In patients with pure esophageal atresia (type A), ventilation is easier and more efficient, as there is no communication between the trachea and esophagus.

   vi. In neonates with stiff lungs as they require high ventilator pressures to overcome poor pulmonary compliance, e.g., HMD (hyaline membrane disease). (4) Tobias 2004

   vii. Majority of neonates tolerate neuromuscular blockade and gentle bag mask ventilation.

   viii. ETT should be placed with its tip below the level of fistula and bevel directed anteriorly (Fig. 28.4b).

Box 28.2: Causes of Inadequate Oxygenation and Ventilation During Surgery
   i. Leakage through fistula
   ii. ETT misplacement, compression, blockade, kinking
   iii. Lateral decubitus position
   iv. Retraction of nondependent lung
   v. Inadequate ventilation of dependent lung
     Management
     – high FiO_2
     – Intermittent inflation of the lungs,
     – Tracheal suction/adjustment

28.7.8 Maintenance of Anesthesia

Baby should be placed on a warm mattress and all exposed parts and head wrapped in cotton wool to retain heat. Heating devices, warm fluids, and warm humidified gases should be used to maintain body temperature of the baby as open chest increases the risk of hypothermia. Eyes should be padded and taped shut and ensure that there is no pressure on the dependent ear lobule and eye.

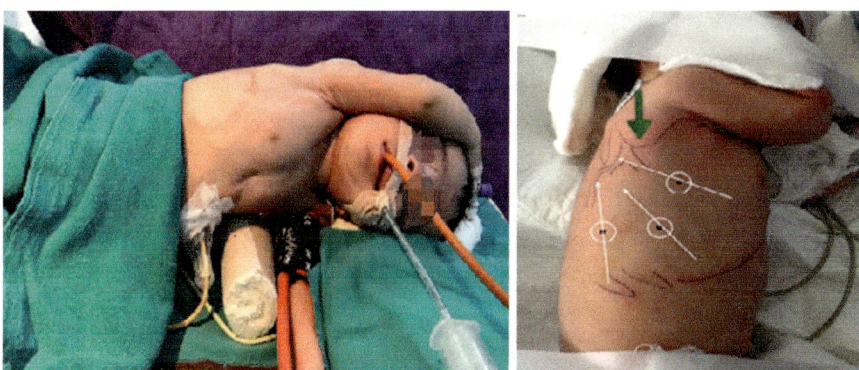

Fig. 28.5 Neonate positioned for open thoracotomy; port sites for thoracoscopic TEF Repair

Induction and intubation are performed in supine position. An oro-esophageal tube is placed in the upper pouch. A naso-esophageal tube is also inserted at the same time, as it is required after the esophageal anastomosis (becomes difficult to place intraoperatively), before positioning the baby for surgery.

The **surgical approach** is through a **lateral thoracotomy** from the side opposite to the aortic arch. Most neonates have a left aortic arch and are kept in the left lateral position for an open thoracotomy (Fig. 28.5). It is useful to have venous access on the right arm which is stretched above the head and strapped down.

Recent advances in **thoracoscopy** have shown comparable outcomes to thoracotomy [22]. The neonate may be made almost prone with elevation of right hemithorax (Cuschieri position) or kept in left lateral position (Fig. 28.5). Generally, left main bronchus intubation is preferred, with or without CO_2 insufflation for good surgical conditions. Problems with thoracoscopy in neonates include hypercarbia, respiratory acidosis, hypoxemia, and hypothermia consequent to lung collapse.

Always check air entry after positioning.

The anesthesiologist also aids the surgeon in locating the blind upper pouch by gently pushing or maneuvering the oro-esophageal tube in the upper pouch. After division of the fistula, manual ventilation may be requested to look for leaks and integrity of fistula ligation. Tracheal manipulation and pulling by the surgeon can initiate a vagal response and bradycardia. This subsides with cessation of stimulus.

Once both esophageal ends are located, the nasogastric tube is pushed down for the surgeon to thread into the lower esophagus and stomach, over which esophageal anastomosis is done. If the esophageal ends are too far apart (long-gap atresia) and preclude primary closure, a cervical esophagostomy and gastrostomy are done pending formal repair.

Before closure of chest, a chest drain is paced, and lungs are expanded with positive pressure. At this time, intercostal nerve block can be given for postoperative analgesia. Extrapleural approach does not need an intercostal drain.

After right thoracotomy, the ventilatory pattern should be altered to allow collapse and retraction of the upper nondependent lung. Ventilation usually becomes more effective after the fistula has been ligated.

Intermittent reinflation of nondependent lung with 100% O_2 may be done, to maintain oxygenation and alveolar integrity, at regular intervals. Anesthesia is continued with FiO_2 of 0.4–0.5, inhalational agent, air or N2O, nondepolarizing muscle relaxant, and short-acting narcotics. There is concern regarding use of N2O before ETT placement because of its potential to cause gastric distension, but clinically this does not pose a problem if induction time is kept short.

Blood loss is usually minimum. Blood transfusion is indicated in babies with preoperative low Hb, or major blood loss.

28.7.9 Recovery from Anesthesia

In babies at low risk and good lung condition, spontaneous respiratory activity is allowed to return, muscle relaxation reversed with neostigmine and glycopyrrolate. Trachea is extubated only when baby is awake, respiratory efforts and muscle tone are good, and saturation is maintained.

Box 28.3 highlights special care to be taken before extubation and Box 28.4 shows indications for elective postoperative ventilation.

Box 28.3: Special Care Before Extubation
   i. Intercostal nerve block by surgeon before closing the thorax
  ii. Complete expansion of right lung before chest closure
 iii. Slow, prolonged inspiration
  iv. Do not use large volumes or rigorous ventilation
   v. Ensure full lung expansion before extubation (air can drain via ICD)
  vi. Fix nasogastric tube firmly, should not get pulled out
 vii. No neck extension (esophageal anastomosis may give away)
viii. Reverse neuromuscular blockade only when respiratory effort is present
  ix. Extubate trachea only when -
       a. Baby is fully awake
       b. Tidal volume is adequate
       c. Baby is maintaining SpO_2
       Note: - Keep lungs expanded during extubation by gentle positive pressure

Box 28.4: Indications of Elective Postoperative Ventilation
1. Poor general condition, aspiration pneumonitis, RDS, CHD
2. Preop ventilatory support
3. Prolonged duration of surgery or surgical complications
4. Hypothermia
5. Inadequate respiratory efforts at the end of surgery

28.8   Postoperative Management

28.8.1 General Care

- No neck extension
- Fix NGT securely as it acts as a stent and also for feeding
- Maintain oxygenation, fluid balance, and temperature.
- Keep the baby warm and comfortable and hands tied in a fist to prevent accidental pulling of NG tube.

28.8.2 Pain Management

Provision of good analgesic is an important step to hasten extubation and reduce duration of postoperative ventilator support. Good perioperative analgesia facilitates early extubation and avoids mechanical ventilation and problems of tracheal suction-related trauma to the fistula site [6, 24]. Multimodal analgesia works the best while reducing the side effects of a single high-dose modality. Various modalities are:

- I/C block and local infiltration, given at the time of chest closure
- Rectal paracetamol at 8–12 hourly intervals
- IV fentanyl if baby is on ventilator support. No other drug is needed
- Epidural analgesia—lumbar epidural catheter threaded to thoracic level can be placed before surgery and used for both intraoperative and postoperative analgesia.

28.8.3 Nutrition

- Babies can be provided feeds via the NGT started 4–6 h postoperatively.
- Oral feeds are started on day 6 if there is no leak.

- Barium studies may be done to check for leaks, if in doubt. This is not done routinely.
- Parenteral nutrition is started in babies who cannot tolerate oral feeds or if feeding is delayed.
- If the gastrostomy tube is in situ, feeding can be done through it.

28.8.4 Postoperative Ventilation is Indicated

- Poor general condition, Aspiration pneumonitis, RDS, CHD
- Preop ventilatory support
- Prolonged duration of surgery or surgical complications
- Hypothermia
- Inadequate respiratory efforts at the end of surgery

28.9   Complications

28.9.1 Intraoperative Complications Include

(i)   Migration of ETT through the fistula leading to gastric distension,
(ii) Occlusion of ETT lumen with blood during ligation of the fistula,
(iii) Accidental ligation of the right main bronchus
(iv) Accidental extubation
(v)   Rarely, the IVC drains through the azygos vein which has to be ligated; a check on blood pressure should be made when the surgeon "check occludes" the azygos to prevent IVC obstruction.

28.9.2 Postoperative Complications

(i) Immediate complications, requiring attention, and requiring exploration is anastomotic leak.
(ii) Delayed and late complications include:
   a. GERD—Abnormal esophageal motility is always present with TEF because of abnormal innervation. Even after surgical repair, these babies are prone to developing gastroesophageal reflux disease later in life.
   b. Dysphagia
   c. Vocal cord paresis/paralysis occurs more often following thoracoscopic repair and may be due to the dissection of the esophagus high into the thoracic inlet [25].
   d. Tracheomalacia,
   e. Recurrent aspiration,
   f. Esophageal stricture—Placement of a transanastomotic tube is associated with higher rates of stricture, and interposition of prosthetic material with higher leak rates [16].

28.10 Conclusions

Anesthesia for TEF repair is very challenging. Surgery is imminent and cannot be delayed. Successful management requires careful preoperative evaluation with reference to associated anomalies, especially cardiac, precautions during face mask ventilation at induction, care in ETT placement, one lung ventilation and its consequences in the lateral position, intermittent expansion of both lungs, and potential for hypoxemia, hypothermia and vagal reflex stimulation, their prevention and management, and readiness for postoperative ventilation, in case needed. Results in babies more than 2500 g birthweight and with no associated anomalies are nearly 100%. This increases the anesthesiologists' responsibility much more so as not to create any iatrogenic problems. Provision of perioperative analgesia is very important. Thoracoscopic approach can reduce the duration of postoperative ventilation and hospital stay.

References

1. Rayyan M, Embrechts M, Van Veer H, Aerts R, et al. Neonatal factors predictive for respiratory and gastro-intestinal morbidity after esophageal atresia repair. Pediatr Neonatol. 2019;60(3):261–9.
2. Okata Y, Maeda K, Bitoh Y, Mishima Y, Tamaki A, et al. Evaluation of the intraoperative risk factors for esophageal anastomotic complications after primary repair of esophageal atresia with tracheoesophageal fistula. Pediatr Surg Int. 2016;32(9):869–73.
3. Yeung A, Butterworth SA. A comparison of surgical outcomes between in-hours and after-hours tracheoesophageal fistula repairs. J Pediatr Surg. 2015;50(5):805–8.
4. Puri A, Yadav PS, Saha U, Singh R, Chadha R, Choudhary SR. A case series study of therapeutic implications of type IIIb4: a rare variant of esophageal atresia and distal tracheoesophageal fistula. J Pediatr Surg. 2013;48(7):1463–9.
5. Tobias JD. Anesthesia for neonatal thoracic surgery. Best Pract Res Clin Anaesth. 2004;18:303–20.
6. Schalkwyk AS, Flaherty J, Hess D, Horvath B. Erector spinae catheter for post-thoracotomy pain control in a premature neonate. BMJ Case Rep. 2020;13:e234480. https://doi.org/10.1136/bcr-2020-234480.
7. Broemling N, Campbell F. Anesthetic management of congenital tracheoesophageal fistula. Pediatr Anesth. 2011;21:1092–9.
8. Nomura A, Yamoto M, Fukumoto K, Takahashi T, et al. Evaluation of developmental prognosis for esophageal atresia with tracheoesophageal fistula. Pediatr Surg Int. 2017;33(10):1091–5.
9. Alshehri A, Lo A, Baird R. An analysis of early non mortality outcome prediction in esophageal atresia. J Pediatr Surg. 2012;47(5):881–4.
10. Diaz LK, Akpek EA, Dinavahi R, Andropoulos DB. Tracheoesophageal fistula and associated congenital heart disease: implications for anesthetic management and survival. Paediatr Anaesth. 2005;15(10):862–9.
11. Spitz L. Oesophageal atresia. Orphanet J Rare Dis. 2007;2:24. https://doi.org/10.1186/1750-1172-2-24.
12. Yau WP, Mitchell AA, Lin KJ, Werler MM, Hernandez-Diaz S. Use of decongestants during pregnancy and the risk of birth defects. Am J Epidemiol. 2013;178(2):198–208. ISSN: 1476-6256
13. Knottenbelt G, Skinner A, Seefelder C. Tracheo-oesophageal fistula and oesophageal atresia. Best Pract Res Clin Anaesth. 2010;24:387–401.

14. Gayle JA, Gómez SL, Baluch A, Fox C, Lock S, Kaye A. Anesthetic considerations for the neonate with tracheoesophageal fistula. M.E.J. Anesth. 2008;19:1241–54.
15. Holder TM, Ashcraft KW, Sharp RJ, Amoury RA. Care of infants with esophageal atresia, tracheoesophageal fistula, and associated anomalies. J Thorac Cardiovasc Surg. 1987;94(6):828–35.
16. Lal DR, Gadepalli SK, Downard CD, et al. For the Midwest Pediatric Surgery Consortium. Challenging surgical dogma in the management of proximal esophageal atresia with distal tracheoesophageal fistula: Outcomes from the midwest pediatric surgery consortium. J Pediatr Surg. 2018;53(7):1267–72.
17. Schmidt A, Obermayr F, Lieber J, Gille C, Fideler F, Fuchs J. Outcome of primary repair in extremely and very-birth-weight infants with esophageal atresia/distal tracheoesophageal fistula. J Pediatr Surg. 2017;52(10):1567–70.
18. Fallon SC, Langer JC, St Peter SD, et al. Congenital H-type tracheoesophageal fistula: a multicenter review of outcomes in a rare disease. J Pediatr Surg. 2017;52(11):1711–4.
19. Gupta B, Agarwal M, Sinha SK. Recent advances in anesthetic management in repair of tracheoesophageal fistula. Indian Anaesth Forum. 2018;19:39–44.
20. Teich S, Barton DP, Ginn-Pease ME, King DR. Prognostic classification for esophageal atresia and tracheoesophageal fistula: Waterston versus Montreal. J Pediatr Surg. 1997;32(7):1075–9; discussion 1079–80. https://doi.org/10.1016/s0022-3468(97)90402-4. PMID: 9247237.
21. Okamoto T, Tatamizawa S, Arai H, et al. Esophageal atresia: prognostic classification revisited. Surgery. 2009;145(6):675–81. https://doi.org/10.1016/j.surg.2009.01.017.
22. Hiradfar M, Gharavifard M, Shojaeian R, Joodi M, et al. Thoracoscopic esophageal atresia with tracheoesophageal fistula repair: the first Iranian group report, passing the learning curve. J Neonatal Surg. 2016;5(3):29. https://doi.org/10.21699/jns.v5i3.344.
23. Hosking C, Motshabi-Chakane P. Thoracotomy in a spontaneously breathing neonate undergoing trachea-oesophageal repair. South Afr J Anaesth Analg. 2018;19:321–2.
24. Bosenberg AT, Hadley GP, Wiersma R. Oesophageal atresia: caudo-thoracic epidural anaesthesia reduces the need for post-operative ventilatory support. Paediatr Surg Int. 1992;7:289–91.
25. Woo S, Lau S, Yoo E, Shaul D, Sydorak R. Thoracoscopic versus open repair of tracheoesophageal fistulas and rates of vocal cord paresis. J Pediatr Surg. 2015;50(12):2016–8.

Further Reading

Barash P, Cullen B, Stoelting R, Cahalan M, Stock M, et al. Clinical anesthesia. 5th ed. p. 1198–9.
Ioannides A, Copp A. Embryology of oesophageal atresia. Semin Pediatr Surg. 2009;18(1):2–11.
Wylie W, Churchill-Davidson H. Wylie and Churchill-Davidson's a practice of anesthesia. 5th ed. London: Llyod-Luke Publication; 1984.
Wylie W, Churchill-Davidson H, et al. Wylie Churchill-Davidson's a practice of anesthesia, vol. 2. 7th ed. London: Hodder Education; 2003. p. 941–55.

Anesthesia for Congenital Diaphragmatic Hernia

29

Ranju Gandhi and Rajeshwari Subramaniam

29.1 Introduction

CDH is a rare entity, described by Bochdalek in 1848, with an incidence of 1:2000–1:5000 live births [1, 2]. Almost 50% cases have other congenital anomalies. Mortality rate is very high (20–50%) and is related to the degree of lung hypoplasia, pulmonary hypertension, right ventricular dysfunction, and coexisting cardiac defects.

There is a defect in the diaphragm leading to varying degrees of bowel herniation into the thorax with lung hypoplasia and pulmonary hypertension. Majority of hernias (75%) occur through the posterolateral defects (foramen of Bochdalek) with 80% left preponderance. Etiology is unclear. Patients usually present with respiratory distress at birth or soon after. However, 5–10% cases may present after the first month of life and sometimes well into adulthood [3, 4]. Only cure is early surgery, which can be life-saving.

Anesthetic management can be very challenging especially with large defects, with variable outcomes, because of pulmonary hypoplasia and gas exchange abnormalities, mediastinal shift, hemodynamic instability, pulmonary hypertension, persistent fetal circulation, and need for ventilatory support [1, 2, 5, 6].

R. Gandhi (✉)
VMMC and Safdarjung Hospital, New Delhi, India

R. Subramaniam
Department of Anesthesiology, Pain Medicine and Critical Care, AIIMS, New Delhi, India

© The Author(s), under exclusive license to Springer Nature Singapore Pte Ltd. 2023
U. Saha (ed.), *Clinical Anesthesia for the Newborn and the Neonate*,
https://doi.org/10.1007/978-981-19-5458-0_29

543

There is a wide variability in management and outcome of CDH in different centers. The European task force for CDH, in 2015 (CDH Euro Consortium) [7], proposed an updated protocol for standardized postnatal treatment, and in 2019, the Canadian CDH Collaborative developed an evidence-based guideline to standardize care practices across Canada. Advances in neonatal care have improved survival from 50 to 80% over the past three decades.

29.2   Classification of CDH

CDH is classified by the location of the defect, as **posterior**, **anterior** and **central**. (Fig. 29.1) A Bochdalek hernia is a defect in the posterior part of the diaphragm in 80% of the cases. A Morgagni hernia is a defect involving anterior part of the diaphragm in 20% of the cases. Other types, in the central region of the diaphragm, or where the diaphragm muscle is absent and there is a thin membrane instead, are extremely rare. Most common (80%) is the posterior left-sided defect.

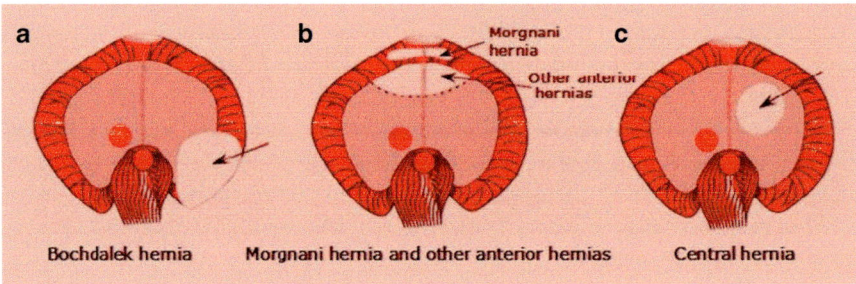

Fig. 29.1 Classification of CDH by location of defect (**a–c**)

29.3 Etiology

The exact etiology of CDH is unclear. There is some evidence that links its occurrence to the abnormalities in the retinoid signaling pathway in early gestation (vitamin A deficiency or abnormality), affecting the retinoid-regulated target genes that may be involved with development of the diaphragm [8]. Apart from coexistence of chromosomal abnormality and other congenital defects, no one antenatal factor can predict occurrence of CDH [9].

29.4 Embryology

In the fetus, diaphragm, lungs, and gastrointestinal tract develop synchronously, and to begin with, the pleuroperitoneal cavity is a single compartment. The membranous or the ventral part of the diaphragm is formed by 3rd or 4th week of gestation, and by the 8th week, it envelops the esophagus. Between the 5th–10th weeks, the gut is extruded into the extraembryonic coelom. The IVC and aorta fuse with the foregut mesentery to form the posterior and medial portions of the diaphragm. Lateral margins of the diaphragm are derived from the muscular part of body wall. By the 9th week, the pleuro-peritoneal canal closes, and all the membranous portions of the diaphragm fuse together, separating the thoracic and the abdominal cavities. The formation of the diaphragm is completed by the 10th week of gestation.

There are two **hypotheses** for the occurrence of CDH. **First hypothesis** is the failure of different parts of the diaphragm to fuse by the 10th week leads to patency of the pleuroperitoneal canal, encouraging bowel herniation or extrusion into the thorax, as normal rotation of mid-gut occurs before the 10th week (when the pleuroperitoneal canal is patent). **Second hypothesis ("dual hit")** states that the primary defect is lung hypoplasia which encourages diaphragm shift and bowel herniation (Fig. 29.2) [10].

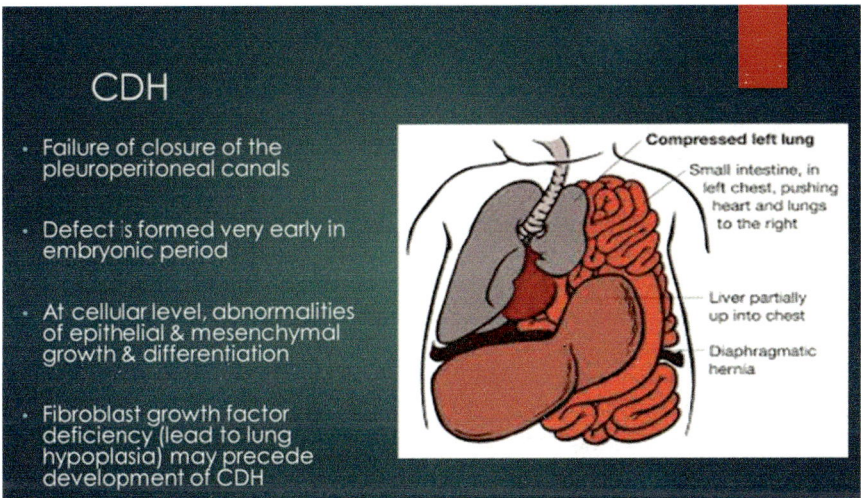

Fig. 29.2 Genesis of CDH

At cellular level, abnormalities of epithelial and mesenchymal growth and differentiation occur. It is proposed that fibroblast growth factor deficiency leads to lung hypoplasia which may precede development of CDH. Alterations at the molecular, cellular, and tissue levels contribute to the pathophysiologic pulmonary vasoreactivity and pulmonary hypertension PHT).

As the fetus grows, the abdominal organs also grow within the thorax. They occupy the space meant for the lungs and heart and cause growth impairment of the ipsilateral lung. The defect in the diaphragm can be isolated or associated with one or more other congenital abnormalities. 90% of CDH are through the left posterolateral defect, with no gender preference.

29.5 Associated Congenital Anomalies

Anomalies or defects involving other organ systems may occur in 50% of the newborns born with CDH. It may also be a part of several syndromes in 10–15% of affected neonates, caused by changes in single gene or by chromosomal abnormalities affecting several genes. Commonly associated anomalies are:

(a) **Central Nervous System** (28%): Spina bifida, hydrocephalus, acephalous
(b) **Cardiovascular System** (13–23%): ASD, VSD, Co Aorta, TOF
(c) **Gastrointestinal System** (20%): Malrotation, atresia
(d) **Genitourinary system** (15%): Hypospadias, and
(e) **Pentalogy of Cantrell** (omphalocele, anterior CDH, sternal cleft, ectopia cordis, VSD).

29.6 Pathophysiology

Abdominal viscera, most commonly bowel, herniate through the defect in the diaphragm into the thoracic cavity, effectively acting as a SOL (space-occupying lesion) (Fig. 29.2). Compression of the lung and heart by the herniated abdominal viscera during early fetal growth leads to following changes-

i. **Abnormal pulmonary development**—Ipsilateral pulmonary hypoplasia, immature lung with subsequent inadequate gas exchange,
ii. **Increased PVR** (pulmonary vascular resistance) with subsequent PHT (pulmonary hypertension),
iii. **Contralateral atelectasis**—collapse of part or whole opposite lung
iv. **Acidosis**—Respiratory acidosis due to hypercarbia and metabolic (lactic) acidosis due to hypoxia, and
v. **Persistent fetal circulation (PFC)** due to hypoxia, hypercarbia, acidosis, increased PVR

The pulmonary changes are characterized by reduction in the terminal branching of bronchioles and decreased number of bronchopulmonary segments and acinar hypoplasia. The consequent reduction in number of alveoli translates into less gas exchange surface area. This is further hampered by thickening of the alveolar walls and increase in interstitial tissue. There is thickening of arteriolar smooth muscle that involves alveolar capillaries as well. The cross-sectional area of the ipsilateral pulmonary vascular bed is markedly reduced. Because of the mediastinal shift to the opposite side, the contralateral lung is also similarly affected. The result is impaired pulmonary function, increased pulmonary artery pressure (PAP) and right-to-left shunting, and ultimately "**Fixed**" (or **irreversible**) and **persistent pulmonary hypertension (PPHN)** of the newborn (Fig. 29.3, Box 29.1).

The blood flow through the ductus venosus and IVC is naturally toward the right ventricle (RV). Left-sided CDH is associated with LV hypoplasia due to its underfilling and LV diastolic dysfunction, which is associated with failure of response to pulmonary vasodilator therapy [11]. The hypoplastic, underfilled LV, reduced pulmonary vascular bed area, coupled with PHT, affects the normal transition from fetal to neonatal circulation, and baby may be born with hypoxemia, hypercarbia, acidosis, and PFC (Box 29.1). Significant LV hypoplasia is associated with 100% mortality.

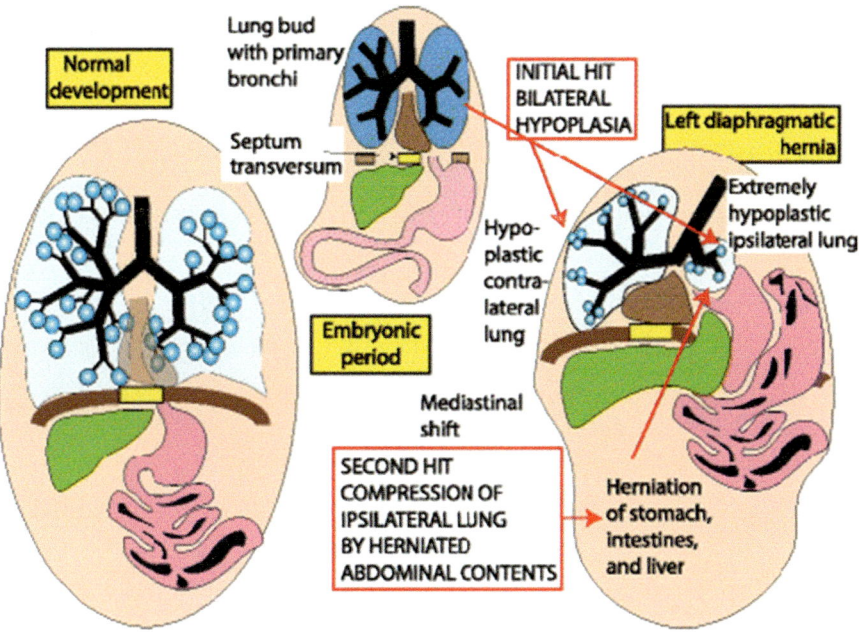

Fig. 29.3 Pathophysiology of CDH—compressed L lung, small intestine in the chest push heart/lungs to the right. Liver partially in the chest

Nearly 60% of CDH can be diagnosed on antenatal sonography and imaging studies, but liver herniation may be difficult to diagnose because of similar echogenicity of lung and liver, and is associated with high mortality.

At birth, newborn is noticeably tachypneic, with chest wall retractions, cyanosis, and tachycardia. Physical examination reveals full or "barrel-shaped" chest and a "scaphoid" abdomen. Breath sounds are absent on the ipsilateral side with mediastinal shift (displacement of the apex beat).

To pathophysiological changes are summarized in Box 29.1.

Box 29.1: Pathophysiological Changes in CDH (Fig. 29.3)
- Abdominal viscera, commonly bowel, herniate through the defect into the thorax, acting as SOL
- Abnormal ipsilateral pulmonary development and hypoplasia
- Mediastinal shift and contralateral pulmonary hypoplasia/ atelectasis
- Decrease in bronchopulmonary segments and alveolar surface area
- Thickening of arteriolar smooth muscle that extends to involve alveolar capillaries
- Impaired pulmonary vasculature, increased PVR, PHT, right-to-left shunt
- Acidosis: Respiratory acidosis due to hypercarbia and metabolic (lactic) acidosis due to hypoxia
- PFC due to hypoxia, hypercarbia, and acidosis

29.7   Clinical Presentation

The Classic Triad of clinical features in CDH is cyanosis, dyspnea, and displaced apex beat.

Physical examination confirms the pathophysiology of CDH:

- Scaphoid abdomen and barrel-shaped chest
- Decreased or absent breath sound on the ipsilateral side
- Bowel sounds in ipsilateral chest
- Mediastinum and apex beat shift to the opposite side

Chest X-ray confirms the findings for a left-sided CDH (Fig. 29.4): (a). bowel loops with air gas shadows in the left chest, (b). heart deviated to the right chest, (c). gastric tube for decompression, endotracheal tube (ETT) in a baby on assisted ventilation, and (e). mediastinum shift to right side. Morgagni type of CDH has more of GI symptoms than of respiratory compromise.

Fig. 29.4 X-ray
chest—Left CDH

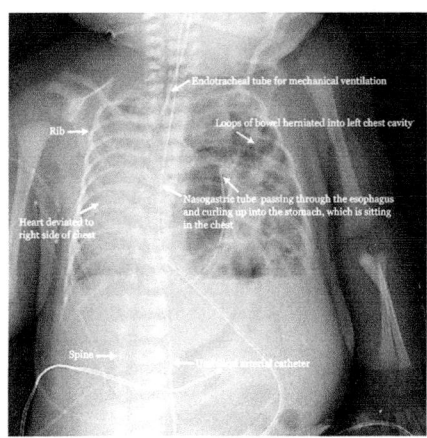

29.8 Diagnosis [12]

29.8.1 Antenatal Diagnosis

Antenatal imaging and sonography in the early 2nd trimester can identify CDH. Other important findings are:

 i. Exact location and size of the defect,
 ii. LHR, observed/expected lung to head (**O/E LHR**),
 iii. Amount of lung hypoplastic area,
 iv. Position of the liver (intra-abdominal or intrathoracic),
 v. Additional congenital anomalies or syndromes, and
 vi. Fetal MRI for lung volume and liver herniation.

29.8.2 Antenatal Management

Once antenatal diagnosis is made, appropriate measures can be taken, in the form of tracheal occlusion, to minimize pulmonary hypoplasia and PHT by the time of birth:

(a) **Open approach—Prenatal tracheal occlusion (TO)** prevents fluid egress from the lung and accelerates lung parenchymal growth, and even reverse the pulmonary arterial structural changes. Tracheal plug is placed through fetal neck dissection following laparotomy in the mother [13].

(b) **Fetoscopic endoluminal tracheal occlusion (FETO)** and reestablishment of fetal airways have now replaced the open approach. This is an endoscopic procedure, whereby FETO plug is deployed by trans-uterine fetal endoscopy at around 26–30 weeks of gestation. Two prerequisites for the procedure are maternal hemodynamic stability and fetal immobilization. The technique involves passage of the endoscope through the fetal mouth into the trachea and deployment of the balloon just above the carina. Postprocedural ultrasound surveillance is done every 2 weeks to ensure balloon's integrity and to measure fetal pulmonary response. At around 34 weeks, the balloon is deflated and removed. FETO is thought to improve outcome, decrease mortality, and allow better neonatal stabilization. Following delivery, neonates still require surgical repair [14–17]. The procedure can be done under general anesthesia, sedation and local infiltration, subarachnoid block, or epidural anesthesia.

29.9 Predictors of Survival in the Perinatal Period

Accurate prediction of survival of neonates with CDH is difficult. Babies with near absence of the diaphragm have a survival rate of 57% compared with 95% in those with defects small enough for primary repair. Several variables are used to predict morbidity/mortality [11, 18–22]:

1. Presence of polyhydramnios (amniotic fluid index >25 cm),
2. Right-sided CDH,
3. Intrathoracic liver/ solid organs,
4. ATR (abdomen to thorax ratio <0.777),
5. LHR ratio (for pulmonary hypoplasia) (O/E LHR <25%),
6. Fetal lung volume (<20 ml),
7. Predicted lung volume <15% (fMRI planimetry),
8. Presence of chromosomal abnormality,
9. Presence of major cardiac abnormality, and
10. LV hypoplasia (fetal ECHO)—fractional shortening of <1.2 indicates nonsurvival.

29.10 Intrapartum Management—In the Delivery Room

This includes prenatal diagnosis and transfer of the mother to a center experienced with management of neonates with CDH. Elective induction of labor is done at 38 weeks of gestation. Intubation is planned for immediately after delivery. During resuscitation, bag and mask ventilation must be avoided or minimized. If there is severe respiratory distress at birth, ETT must be performed (preferably while the baby is still on placental support) with the use of gentle or minimal ventilation. **The carina is higher than normal in CDH newborn, mandating care in placement of the ETT to prevent right mainstem intubation.** Synchronized or assist control ventilation is employed along with sedatives, and muscle relaxants are reserved for selected cases. After intubation, an orogastric tube is placed for stomach decompression by intermittent or continuous low suction. Preductal arterial access is desirable if neonate is critical and hemodynamically unstable. Baby is nursed in lateral position with ipsilateral side dependent. Management also involves that for PHT.

29.11 Ventilation Specifics

There has been a significant improvement in survival over the past 20 years. Conventional mechanical ventilation is the optimal initial strategy by the CDH EURO Consortium, American Heart Association/ American Thoracic Society and the American Pediatric Surgical Association (APSA) followed by lung protective ventilation. Recommendations are for use of **lung protective strategy**: [7, 23, 24]

a. Permissive hypercapnia—$PaCO_2$ 50–70 mmHg,
b. Avoid high inflation pressures—Peak inspiratory pressure < 25 cm H_2O, PEEP < 5 cm H_2O,
c. Accept relative hypoxemia—Preductal SpO_2 80–90% and postductal > 70%,
d. Use minimal FiO_2 (< 50%) to maintain preductal saturation,
e. Respiratory rate 40–60/min,
f. Monitor tidal volume and minute ventilation,
g. HFOV employed as rescue therapy if traditional ventilatory modes not adequate,
h. ECMO is indicated if HFOV fails to maintain oxygenation (see below).

29.12 Management of Pulmonary Hypertension (PHT)

Inhaled nitric oxide (iNO) is useful in neonates where ECHO demonstrates severe degree of right-to-left (R-L) shunting and preductal desaturation. It is a pulmonary vasodilator and helps in stabilizing and bridging the time to ECMO.

29.13 Predictors of Poor Postnatal Survival in Neonates with CDH

- Birthweight <1.5 kg,
- 5-min Apgar score <7,
- Decreased lung volume (measure bedside with Helium dilution computerized system),
- Pulmonary hypertension,
- Presence of chromosomal abnormality,
- Presence of major cardiac abnormality,
- High pre-ECMO $PaCO_2$ (>60 mmHg) [22]

29.14 Surgical Management

In 1940, Ladd and Gross advocated early surgery as the proper treatment for CDH in neonates. However, there is evidence in literature to the contrary. Open surgical repair should be delayed until physiologic stability has been achieved, usually takes about 5–15 days. Increased pulmonary vascular resistance (PVR) may require use of pulmonary vasodilators (prostaglandin E, IV infusion of milrinone, tolazoline, iNO) or in severe cases ECMO, allowing time for remodeling of pulmonary vasculature and also delays compliance changes associated with corrective surgery. Low-dose noradrenaline has been used to improve oxygenation in severe cases. Point of care ECHO can be used to guide cardiovascular support. Milrinone is preferred if there is both systolic and diastolic dysfunction. A reduction in PAP and improvement in RV dysfunction can improve outcome.

Preparation and planning involve discussion with the surgeon, with the team, with patient attendant, and make a clear strategy.

The goals of treatment

1. Avoid surgery in a hypoxic and acidotic baby if cardiorespiratory status is labile.
2. Medical management. Aim of medical treatment is:

   i. Increase pre-ductal saturation to > 90 mm Hg,
   ii. Correction of acidosis,
   iii. Decrease in R-L shunt
   iv. Improve in pulmonary perfusion (decrease PVR)

29.15 Preoperative Assessment of Prognosis

Factors which affect the prognosis in CDH are:

- Age at presentation
- Adequacy of preparation (hypothermia, hypoxia, acidosis)
- Adequacy of transitional adaptations, and presence of fetal circulation
- Associated congenital anomalies (especially cardiac)
- Hemodynamic instability and shock
- Pneumothorax

A. **Assess by the Degree Pulmonary Hypoplasia**—The difference between alveolar and arterial partial pressure of oxygen $(PAO_2–PaO_2)$ is calculated with the baby breathing 100% O_2 for 10 min [25, 26]. Results are analyzed as below:
   >500 mmHg—Predicts nonsurvival

   –500 mmHg—Survival uncertain
   <400 mmHg—Better prognosis.

B. **Bohn`s index** [27]—Uses ventilatory index VI (mean airway P x RR) and $PaCO_2$ to predict prognosis.

Neonate with $PaCO_2 < 40$ mmHg and VI<1000—always survive
$PaCO_2 > 50$ mmHg and VI<1000 or $PaCO_2 < 40$ mmHg and VI >1000—usually die.

Preoperative medical management salvages neonates too sick for surgery and reduces the need for ECMO.

29.15.1 Extracorporeal Membrane Oxygenation (ECMO) [11, 28–30]

ECMO is used in selective cases of severe lung hypoplasia and refractory PHT, in an attempt to reverse the respiratory pathology, in a baby with $PaO_2 < 50$ mm Hg @ FiO_2 of 1.0 despite optimal ventilatory strategy. ECMO allows for stabilization of the neonate while waiting for surgery. It is associated 50–60% survival rate. Approach may be veno-arterial (IJV and common carotid artery) or veno-venous.

29.15.2 Indications of ECMO

1. When LV function does not improve with milrinone and vasopressin therapy,
2. Refractory hypotension,
3. Preductal saturation < 80%, and refractory to ventilatory and medical therapy,
4. Oxygenation index (OI) > 40 (= $FiO_2 \times MAP$ (mean airway pressure)/PaO_2. OI is calculated before and after initiation of therapy (HFOV or iNO). Decreasing trend is a sensitive predictor of survival,
5. Severe air leak, and
6. Mixed acidosis (pH < 7.2).

29.15.3 Contraindications to ECMO

- Post conception age < 35 weeks
- Weight < 2 kg
- ICH
- Contraindication to use of heparin

29.16 Surgical Approach

Approaches for surgical repair of CDH are:

- **Invasive or open surgery**: Laparotomy/ thoracotomy,
- **Noninvasive surgery**: Laparoscopic repair/ thoracoscopic repair [31, 32]

29.16.1 Timing of Surgery

1. If **hemodynamic parameters are stable** and oxygenation is maintained without ECMO, surgical repair can be carried out in the presence of unresolved PHT. However, the incidence of acute postoperative decompensation is less if PAP is < 80% of systemic arterial pressure. Alternatively, ECHO evidence of L → R shunt across the PDA can be taken as an indication of reduction in PAP.
2. If the **neonate is on ECMO**, guidelines recommend surgery within 24–48 h if the neonate can be weaned and decannulated.

    Adequacy of Clinical Stabilization (CDH (EURO) consortium) (27) (Snoek et al. 2016):
    - Normal mean arterial blood pressure,
    - Preductal SpO_2 > 85% on < 0.5 FiO_2,
    - Lactate <3 mmol/L, and
    - Urine output >1 ml/kg/h
3. If neonate **cannot be weaned off ECMO** within two weeks, surgical decision is controversial. Surgery may be undertaken while the neonate is on ECMO, with the benefit of reduction of the mass effect within the thoracic cavity, support of CVS and renal dysfunction in the postoperative period, and reduced overall duration of ECMO support. Perioperative antifibrinolytic therapy can reduce the bleeding complications. Survivors of severe CDH with ECMO are at risk of long-term sequalae including neurodevelopmental delay.

29.17 Preanesthetic Assessment

History should include gestational age, birth history, current age and weight, and significant perinatal events such as low APGAR scores, symptoms soon after birth, respiratory distress requiring support, hypoglycemic episodes, NICU admission, evidence of sepsis or any antenatal concerns such as maternal illness. Polyhydramnios is a predictor of poor prognosis. Assess the associated anomalies.

Examination—The neonate should be examined carefully, particularly for signs of respiratory distress (RR, nasal flare, subcostal recession), and CVS compromise (HR, BP, peripheral perfusion, capillary refill). Check SpO_2. Chest auscultation may reveal apex beat on the right side, reduction of breath sounds, and presence of bowel sounds on the side of defect. The abdomen may be scaphoid. Examine for other congenital defects.

29.18 Preoperative Investigations

Relevant investigations are guided by the clinical findings and underlying condition of the neonate, with special emphasis on the degree of pulmonary and cardiac dysfunction. Investigations include complete blood count, serum electrolyte, blood sugar, liver and renal function tests, coagulation studies, blood grouping and cross-matching, ABG (capillary/arterial), and urine output. Other perinatal investigations such as sonography and MRI should also be evaluated. X-ray chest will confirm the CDH and lung condition (Fig. 29.4). ECG and ECHO are desirable to assess presence of PHT, R-L shunt, and cardiac anomalies.

Note: Frequent arterial blood gas (ABG) measurements are done during the course of management. The sampling site should be chosen well, because PPHN with R-L ductal shunt often complicates CDH, and preductal PaO_2 may be higher than post ductal (lower limb).

29.19 Consent Taking

The anesthetic plan including the risks should be discussed with the parent(s) or guardian, and informed consent taken for anesthesia including regional technique, if planned, for blood transfusion, as well as postoperative ventilatory support.

29.20 Preoperative Preparation

29.20.1 Preoperative Optimization

Preoperative optimization—check for adequacy of optimization by, i.e.,

- Normal mean arterial blood pressure,
- Preductal $SpO_2 \geq 85\%$ on < 0.5 FiO_2,
- Lactate < 3 mmol/L, and
- Urine output ≥ 1 ml/kg/h
- PAP less than systemic blood pressure
- If ABG shows acidosis, it should be corrected to $PaCO_2$ of 45–60 mm Hg and pH 7.25–7.4. An ongoing metabolic acidosis, requiring repeated large doses of base, should alert anesthesiologist to underlying risk factors such as myocardial ischemia, sepsis, or strangulated bowel.

IV access—usually these babies already have an IV line in situ in the NICU for drug and fluid administration. For anesthesia, there should be 2 patent and accessible IV lines, preferably one in the upper limb for easy access under the surgical drapes, using 22/24 G cannula.

Confirm the patency of the **orogastric tube** for gastric and bowel decompression. Babies are kept **NPO** and receive dextrose containing IV fluids.

Intramuscular Vit K must be administered as is advocated in all newborns, as single daily dose for three days.

Minimize sympathetic discharge by sedatives and narcotics in intubated and ventilated neonates, and maintaining thermoneutral environment and hypothermia.

29.20.2 Maintaining Systemic Blood Pressure

Signs of poor peripheral perfusion are capillary refill time >3 s, serum lactate > 3 mmol/l, urine output < 1ml/kg/hr, and mean arterial pressure less than normal for gestational age. Such babies should receive IV crystalloids @ 10–20 ml/kg. If poor perfusion continues, inotropes (dopamine, epinephrine, and/or norepinephrine) are started to maintain blood pressure within normal range. Neonates with CDH and PHT and refractory systemic hypotension may benefit from hydrocortisone.

29.20.3 Transport from NICU to Operation Theater

Baby is transported in a temperature-controlled incubator, and all infusions and ventilation must continue, as in the preoperative period. If the baby is on T-piece or mechanical ventilator, transport team must keep a careful watch on peak airway pressure and avoid inadvertent high pressure and overdistension of the lungs. During handing over and taking over in the OT, the infusion rates and ventilator settings must be checked and recorded.

29.21 Anesthesia Management

This will be discussed under following headings:

1. Monitoring
2. Premedication
3. Induction and maintenance
4. Positioning for surgery
5. Ventilation strategy
6. Laparoscopic approach
7. Fluid therapy
8. Pain management
9. Intraoperative complications
10. Extubation and postoperative care

29.21.1 Intraoperative Monitoring

Standard monitoring special monitoring for CDH repair is listed in Box 29.2. Usually, noninvasive monitoring is adequate for most cases. Invasive monitoring is reserved for babies with large defects, anticipated prolonged duration of surgery, major blood loss, and critically ill babies.

> **Box 29.2: Monitoring**
> - Precordial/ esophageal stethoscope
> - Pulse oximeter above and below the nipple for preductal and post ductal SpO_2
> - CVS—HR, ECG, NIBP, IBP (right radial artery for preductal BP and PaO_2)
> - Capnography
> - Airway pressures—PIP, MAP, PEEP
> - CVP—for volume status, right ventricular function, inotrope infusion
> - ABG
> - Temperature—esophageal/rectal
> - Urine output

29.21.2   Premedication

In an otherwise healthy neonate with isolated CDH, and no airway compromise, intranasal midazolam (0.3 mg/kg) or rectal/oral midazolam (0.5–0.75 mg/kg) can be given if there is no IV line, 15–20 min prior to induction. Prokinetics and H_2 antagonists can be given as these babies are at risk of regurgitation and aspiration. IV atropine (0.02 mg/kg)/glycopyrrolate (0.01 mg/kg) is administered for its vagolytic and antisialagogue action. Babies on ventilator may already be receiving sedatives.

29.21.3   Induction and Maintenance

After pre-oxygenation inhalation, induction is done with halothane/sevoflurane in 100% O_2. IV line can now be placed if already not in place, in the upper limb. Care at induction:

- **Avoid mask ventilation** before intubation to prevent overdistension of the intrathoracic stomach and respiratory compromise, and if essential, gentle assisted ventilation can be provided.
- **Avoid N2O** as it can cause bowel expansion and further respiratory compromise, and abdominal compartmental syndrome.
- **Endotracheal intubation** is done with uncuffed ETT after administering atracurium (0.5 mg/kg) or succinylcholine (1–2 mg/kg).
- **Awake intubation** is reserved for very low birthweight babies and those with severe respiratory or hemodynamic compromise.

Anesthesia is maintained with sevoflurane in 100% O_2 or in air O_2 mixture with high FiO_2. Atracurium is supplemented in 0.125 mg/kg dose during surgery and controlled ventilation, and analgesia is provided with Fentanyl (1–3 mic/kg).

29.21.4 Positioning for Surgery

Surgical correction of CDH is done by open approach or minimally invasive surgery by abdominal or thoracic approach.

- **Abdominal approach**—The neonate is placed in supine position (open/ laparoscopic).
- **Thoracic approach**—The neonate is placed in lateral position with ipsilateral side up (open/laparoscopic).

In abdominal open approach, a subcostal or a transverse incision is made and the herniated viscera is reduced into the abdomen. The diaphragmatic defect is closed primarily or with a prosthetic patch if defect is large.

29.21.5 Ventilatory Strategy-Intraoperative

Ventilation is controlled during surgery, always keeping the following objectives in mind:
- Peak inspiratory pressure (PIP) < 25 cm H_2O
- Prevent barotrauma to contralateral lung and pneumothorax
- Preductal saturation $\geq 90\%$
- Use least FiO_2 to maintain sufficient saturation and PaO_2.
    HFOV (High-Frequency Oscillating Ventilation) [33]
    Aims—To reduce barotrauma to contralateral lung associated with high airway pressures of controlled ventilation.
- The rate of ventilation is very high with a mean airway pressure of 18–20 cm H_2O.
- Gas exchange takes place through diffusion rather than bulk gas flow.
- The chief benefit of HFOV is recruitment of lung with minimal barotrauma.

29.21.6 Laparoscopic Approach

Minimal access surgical repair, a relatively recent addition, has benefits over conventional surgical repair [34, 35]. Thoracoscopic repair of CDH is common nowadays. However, the operative time is significantly longer than open procedure, with concomitant increase in the incidence of hypoxemia, hypercarbia, respiratory acidosis, and higher recurrence rate [31].

Repair can also be carried out in the NICU if the baby is unstable, with good results.

High-dose opioid anesthesia (fentanyl 10–30 μg/kg), with neuromuscular blockade, is normally used. Good venous access is necessary, and blood should be available. Care should be exercised in avoiding positive pressure ventilation with high pressures, which can result in contralateral pneumothorax, hypoxemia, and hemodynamic instability. Continued communication with the surgeons is necessary, especially if hypotension is observed or ventilation becomes difficult after returning the displaced organs into the abdomen.

(a) **General anesthesia without lung separation:** CO_2 insufflation into the operative hemithorax is particularly useful in smaller patients where lung isolation is not possible and there is inadequate separation of the two lungs with overflow ventilation into the operative side. Meticulous cardiopulmonary monitoring is mandatory as displacement of intrathoracic contents and creation of an excessive pneumothorax can lead to significant CVS compromise (decreased venous return to high LV afterload). The effects of artificial pneumothorax can be minimized by adopting slow CO_2 insufflation rate @ ≤ 1 L/min and limiting the inflating pressure to 4–6 mmHg. Direct insufflation of CO_2 into the lung parenchyma can cause sudden rise in $EtCO_2$, with subcutaneous emphysema and CO_2 embolism. Monitoring should include that for detection of gas embolism prior to the onset of CVS collapse. TEE (transesophageal Echo) is most sensitive and can even detect 0.1 ml of gas, while precordial doppler can detect 0.5 ml of gas, and end-tidal nitrogen monitoring. The combination of standard tracheal intubation with prone position and CO_2 insufflation may provide good exposure in some cases [23].

(b) **General anesthesia and one-lung ventilation:** During general anesthesia and positive pressure ventilation, intrathoracic visualization and surgical access can be impaired by lung movement. To overcome this, thoracoscopy is performed using techniques to isolate the lung and provide one-lung ventilation. This allows the lung on the operative side to be collapsed and motionless, facilitating exposure and surgical instrumentation, while gas exchange (oxygenation and CO_2 elimination) is maintained by ventilating the nonoperative dependent lung. **Techniques for one-lung ventilation in children include:**

   i. **Selective mainstem intubation** is used in babies whose small size precludes placement of a DLT or Univent tube. Bronchoscopy or fluoroscopy can aid correct placement.

   ii. **Bronchial blockers,** e.g., Fogarty embolectomy catheter, Swan-Ganz catheter, or Arndt bronchial blocker, can be placed in the mainstem bronchus of the operative side under direct vision via fiberoptic bronchoscope. With an inflated blocker balloon, the airway is completely sealed, providing more predictable lung collapse and better operating conditions than with an ETT in the bronchus. Blockers with a central suction channel allow for deflation of the operative lung and also for application of CPAP.

   iii. **Double lumen tubes**: The smallest available DLT is 26 Fr tube for placement in patients weighing 30 kg or age more than 8 years.

Once successful separation of the nonoperative and operative lung has been accomplished, anesthesia is maintained with a combination of IV and inhalational drugs. Isoflurane (MAC limited to 0.5–1.0 MAC) preserves HPV, while fentanyl, ketamine, benzodiazepines, and barbiturates have little or no effect. Standard anesthesia drugs can be safely used.

29.21.7 Fluid Therapy

Goals of fluid therapy:
- Correct preoperative deficit with maintenance fluid and replace intraoperative blood loss.
- Glucose should be given as neonate have decreased glycogen reserve.
- Maintenance fluid used is 5% dextrose in 1/4th–1/2 strength normal saline at 4 ml/kg/hr.
- Intraoperative and 3rd space losses are replaced by Ringer lactate or Saline 6–8 ml/kg/hr.
- Each milliliter of blood loss is replaced by 3 ml Ringer lactate or 1 ml of 5% albumin.

Note: refer to the chapter on fluid therapy

29.21.8 Complications

Anesthesiologist should watch for intraoperative complications like hypothermia, hypotension, pneumothorax, and PHT.
   i. **Hypothermia** may lead to cerebral and cardiac depression, increased O_2 demand, acidosis, hypoxia, and intracardiac shunt reversal. Measures to avoid hypothermia and maintain OT temperature must be strictly taken.
  ii. **Hypotension** can be caused by venous return impairment or hypovolemia. Treatment includes IV fluid bolus. If it does not improve, inotropic support is instituted.
 iii. **Pneumothorax** occurs on the contralateral side. It may manifest by sudden fall in lung compliance, sudden fall in blood pressure, and drop in SpO_2. Treatment is immediate placement of a chest tube.
  iv. **Pulmonary hypertension** causes ECG changes in the form of ST depression and t wave inversion in V1-4. PHT increases the R-L shunt (i.e., increased gap between preductal and postductal saturation). Identify causative factors such as hypoxia, acidosis, pain, stress, and hypothermia. Management consists of continued ventilation in NICU in the postoperative period, fentanyl to blunt autonomic cardiovascular response, hyperventilation with low VT and high RR (60–120/min) to improve the oxygenation and reduce $PaCO_2$, maintain pH 7.5–7.6 to induce pulmonary vasodilatation, restrict IV fluids (2–4 ml/kg/hr), administer pharmacological pulmonary vasodilators (morphine, prostaglandin E, tolazoline, inhaled nitric oxide), and minimize sympathetic discharge by opioids.

29.21.9 Extubation and Postoperative Care

Extubation should be done only if neonate is awake and opening eyes, breathing spontaneously with normal respiratory rate, maintaining SpO_2 of more than 95% on $FiO_2 < 50\%$, after administration of neostigmine and glycopyrrolate.

29.22 Postoperative Care

There already reduced pulmonary compliance decreases further after surgery; hence, continued ventilation should be planned in the postoperative period. FiO_2 is adjusted to maintain $PaO_2 > 150$ mmHg. If not extubated, continue gentle ventilation in NICU using fentanyl 1–3 µg/kg/h or morphine 0.1 mg IV 6–8 hourly, to blunt autonomic CVS responses. Hyperventilation with low tidal volume and high RR (60–120/min) improves oxygenation and reduces $PaCO_2$. Fluids are restricted (2–4 ml/kg/h). Pulmonary vasodilators (morphine, prostaglandin E, iNO, sildenafil, or bosentan) are used if PVR is elevated [36].

Neonate is slowly weaned off the ventilator to avoid vasoconstrictive rebound effect or **honeymoon phenomenon** (pulmonary vasoconstriction, lethal persistent pulmonary hypertension, hypercarbia, and acidosis) [37].

Noninvasive ventilation modalities may play a role during weaning from mechanical ventilation.

29.22.1 Postoperative Pain management

Multimodal approach is used to provide good pain relief. Thoracoscopic procedures offer the advantage of small incisions without either splitting of the serratus anterior or latissimus dorsi muscles or spreading of the ribs, two techniques which markedly contribute to postoperative pain. In order to minimize pain, patients breathe rapidly with small tidal volumes. This type of breathing promotes atelectasis, retention of secretions, decrease in functional residual capacity, and increase in V/Q mismatching all of which contribute to hypoxemia. Good pain relief by any method is mandatory:

1. **Oral**: Nonsteroidal anti-inflammatory drugs, paracetamol.
2. **Rectal** suppositories: Paracetamol/diclofenac provide long-lasting analgesia and reduce opioid requirements.
3. **Intravenous** route: Morphine or fentanyl or ketamine provide satisfactory analgesia
4. **Intercostal** nerve blocks / intrapleural installation of bupivacaine relieves pain from chest tubes or instrument insertion point.
5. **Epidural analgesia** by catheter placement can be used both for intraoperative and postoperative analgesia.

29.23 Long-Term Outcome in CDH

With advances in pediatric critical care, 70–90% of non-ECMO infants and up to 50% of infants needing ECMO may survive. Survivors of CDH may develop sequel in the long-term requiring multidisciplinary long-term follow-up:

- Chronic lung disease with impaired obstructive and restrictive lung function,
- Growth failure,

- Oral aversion,
- GERD,
- Neurocognitive delay and behavioral disorders,
- Chest wall deformities and scoliosis, and
- Recurrence.

29.24 Conclusion

CDH is a physiologic emergency and not a surgical emergency. The hallmarks are pulmonary hypoplasia and pulmonary hypertension. A thorough understanding of pathophysiology, meticulous preoperative preparation, perioperative care, one-lung ventilation, and continuous vigil leads to better outcomes. Surgical repair should be performed after clinical stabilization. Minimal access surgery does not mean minimally invasive anesthesia. Support of oxygenation, ventilation, hemodynamic stability, and lung protective ventilation, while minimizing ventilator-associated lung injury (VALI), barotrauma, and O_2 toxicity before and after surgery are the goals of management. Multidisciplinary approach between neonatologist, surgeon, anesthesiologist, and intensivist is vital for successful management of neonates with CDH. They should be managed in tertiary care centers with standard operating procedures.

References

1. Merin RG. Congenital diaphragmatic hernia from the anesthesiologist viewpoint. Anesth Analg. 1966;45:44–52.
2. Cullen MI, Klein MD, Philippart AI. Congenital diaphragmatic hernia. Surg Clin North Am. 1985;11:1115–38.
3. Berman L, Stringer D, Ein S, Shandling B. Childhood diaphragmatic hernias presenting after the neonatal period. Clin Radiol. 1988;39:237–44.
4. Reynolds VR, May RB. Delayed-onset Bochdalek hernia in a 3-year-old child. Am J Emerg Med. 1988;6:594–5.
5. Snoek KG, Reiss IKM, Greenough A, Capolupo I, et al. Standardized postnatal management of infants with congenital diaphragmatic hernia in Europe: The CDH EURO consortium consensus—2015 update. Neonatology. 2016;110:66–74.
6. Quinney M, Wellesley H. Anesthetic management of patients with a congenital diaphragmatic hernia. BJA Educ. 2018;18:95–101.
7. Snoek KG, Copolupo I, Van Rosmalen J, et al. CDH EURO consortium. Conventional ventilation versus high frequency oscillatory ventilation for congenital diaphragmatic hernia: a randomized clinical trial (the VICI trial). Ann Surg. 2016;263:867–74.
8. Greer J, Babiuk R, Thebaud B. Etiology of congenital diaphragmatic hernia: The retinoid hypothesis. Pediatr Res. 2003;53:726–30.
9. Sokol J, Bohn D, Lacro RV, Ryan G, et al. Fetal pulmonary artery diameters and their association with lung hypoplasia and postnatal outcome in congenital diaphragmatic hernia. Am J Obstet Gyynecol. 2002;186:1085–90.
10. Quinney M, Wellesley H. Anaesthetic management of patients with a congenital diaphragmatic hernia. BJA Educ. 2018;18:95–101.

11. Chatterjee D, Ing RJ, Gien J. Update on congenital diaphragmatic hernia. Anesth Analg. 2020;131:808–21.
12. Puligandla PS, Skarsgard ED, Offringa M, Adatia I, et al. Diagnosis and management of congenital diaphragmatic hernia: a clinical practice guideline. CMAJ. 2018;190:E103–12.
13. Kanai M, Kitano Y, von Allmen D, Davies P, et al. Fetal tracheal occlusion in the rat model of nitrofen-induced congenital diaphragmatic hernia: tracheal occlusion reverses the arterial structural abnormality. J Pediatr Surg. 2001;36(6):839–45. https://doi.org/10.1053/jpsu.2001.23950.
14. Al-Maary J, Eastwood MP, Russo FM, Deprest JA, Kejizer R. Fetal tracheal occlusion for severe pulmonary hypoplasia in isolated congenital diaphragmatic hernia: a systematic review and meta-analysis of survival. Ann Surg. 2016;264:929–33.
15. Van der Veeken L, Russo FM, De Catte L, et al. Fetoscopic endoluminal tracheal occlusion and reestablishment of fetal airways for congenital diaphragmatic hernia. Gynecol Surg. 2018;15:9. https://doi.org/10.1186/s10397-018-1041-9.
16. Ruano R, Ali RA, Patel P, Cass D, et al. Fetal endoscopic tracheal occlusion for congenital diaphragmatic hernia: indications, outcomes, and future directions. Obstet Gynecol Surv. 2014;69(3):147–58. https://doi.org/10.1097/OGX.0000000000000045.
17. Tsaoi KJ, Johnson A. Fetal tracheal occlusion for congenital diaphragmatic hernia. Semin Perinatol. 2020;44(1):151164. https://doi.org/10.1053/jsemperi2019.07.003.
18. Lee JY, Jun JK, Lee JH. Prenatal prediction of neonatal survival in cases diagnosed with congenital diaphragmatic hernia using abdomen-to-thorax ratio determined by ultrasonography. J. Obstet Gynaecol Res. 2014;40(9):2037–43. https://doi.org/10.1111/jog.12473.
19. Spaggiari E, Stirnemann J, Ville Y. Outcome in fetuses with isolated congenital diaphragmatic hernia with increased nuchal translucency thickness in first trimester. Prenat Diagn. 2012;32:268–71.
20. Ruano R, Takashi E, da Silva MM, Campos JA, et al. Prediction and probability of neonatal outcome in isolated congenital diaphragmatic hernia using multiple ultrasound parameters. Ultrasound Obstet Gynecol. 2012;39:42–9.
21. Mullassery D, Ba'ath ME, Jesudason EC, Losty PD. Value of liver herniation in prediction of outcome in fetal congenital diaphragmatic hernia: a systematic review and meta-analysis. Ultrasound Obstet Gynecol. 2010;35:609–14.
22. Hoffman S, Massaro A, Gingalewski C, et al. Predictors of survival in congenital diaphragmatic hernia patients requiring extracorporeal membrane oxygenation: CNMC 15-year experience. J Perinatol. 2010;30:546–52. https://doi.org/10.1038/jp.2009.193.
23. Boloker J, Bateman DA, Wung JT, et al. Congenital diaphragmatic hernia in 120 infants treated consecutively with permissive hypercapnia/spontaneous respiration/elective repair. I Pediatr Surg. 2002;37:357–66.
24. Morinini F, Capolupo I, Weteringen W. Ventilation modalities in infants with congenital diaphragmatic hernia. Semin Pediatr Surg. 2017;26:159–65.
25. Stranak Z, Zabrodsky V, Simak J. changes in alveolar-arterial oxygen difference and oxygenation index during low-dose nitric oxide inhalation in 15 newborns with severe respiratory insufficiency. Eur J Pediatr. 1996;155:907–10. https://doi.org/10.1007/BF02282844.
26. Gentili A, Giuntoli L, Bacchi L, Masciopinto F. Neonatal congenital diaphragmatic hernia: Respiratory and blood-gas derived indices in choosing surgical timing. Minerva Anestesiol. 2012;78(10):1117–25.
27. Bohn D, Tamura M, Perrin D, Barker G, Rabinovitch M. Ventilatory predictors of pulmonary hypoplasia in congenital diaphragmatic hernia, confirmed by morphologic assessment. J Pediatr. 1987;111(3):423–31. https://doi.org/10.1016/s0022-3476(87)80474-2.
28. Vaja R, Bakr A, Sharkey A, Joshi V, Faulkner G, et al. The use of extracorporeal membrane oxygenation in neonates with severe congenital diaphragmatic hernia: a 26-year experience from a tertiary center. Eur J Cardiothorac Surg 2017; 52:552–557.
29. Mc Honey M, Hammond P. Role of ECMO in congenital diaphragmatic hernia. Arch Dis Child Fetal Neonatal Ed. 2018;103:F178–81.

30. Grover TR, Rintoul NE, Hendick HL. Extracorporeal membrane oxygenation in infants with congenital diaphragmatic hernia. Semin Perinatol. 2018;42:96–103.
31. Schneider A, Becmeur F. Pediatric thoracoscopic repair of congenital diaphragmatic hernias. J Vis Surg. 2018;4:43.
32. Qin J, Ren Y, Ma D. A comparative study of thoracoscopic and open surgery of congenital diaphragmatic hernia in neonates. J Cardiothoracic Surg. 2019;14:118.
33. Edipoglu IS, Celik F, Ozdogan T, Comert S, Guvene BH. Anesthetic management of a neonate with congenital diaphragmatic hernia under high-frequency oscillatory ventilation. Clin Pract. 2018;8:1057.
34. Tobias JD. Anaesthetic implications of thoracoscopic surgery in children. Paediatric Anaesthesia. 1999;9:103–10.
35. Vijfhuije S, Deden AC, Costerus SA, Sloots CE, Wijnem RM. Minimal access surgery for repair of congenital diaphragmatic hernia: is it advantageous? An open review. Eur J Pediatr Surg. 2012;22:364–73.
36. Kinsella JP, Ivy DD, Abman SH. Pulmonary vasodilator therapy in congenital diaphragmatic hernia: acute, late, and chronic pulmonary hypertension. Semin Perinatol. 2005;29(2):123–8.
37. Da Costa KM, Fabro AT, Becari C, Figueira RL, et al. Honeymoon period in newborn rats with CDH is associated with changes in the VEGF signaling pathway. Front Pediatr. 2021; https://doi.org/10.3389/fped.2021.698217.

Anesthesia for Thoracic Surgery in Neonates

30

Rajeshwari Subramaniam

30.1 Introduction

Thoracic anesthesia for noncardiac surgery in neonates and infants is a very specialized and niche area. The neonate presenting for surgery may range from an otherwise healthy, term baby to a very sick neonate with severe cardiopulmonary illness on extracorporeal membrane oxygenation (ECMO) support. Surgical indications may be relatively elective (e.g., pulmonary sequestration) or an emergency, a large lung cyst with airway leak (Table 30.1). Anesthesia for thoracic procedures is challenging for many other reasons. Respiratory physiology is altered in the lateral decubitus position in neonates compared to older children and adults. The small airway size limits the availability of suitable equipment and demands high levels of expertise and skill. With the advent of thoracoscopy options for airway management for VATS are rapidly emerging and changing the anesthetic management scenario. Regardless of the neonates' condition, the anesthesiologist should meticulously plan out airway management with a back-up plan, ensure adequate vascular access, and last but not least, an effective analgesic technique. This chapter will cover the surgery for lung conditions in the neonate. TEF and CDH are discussed separately in other chapters.

Table 30.1 Indications for thoracotomy/VATS for noncardiac surgery in neonates

1.	Tracheoesophageal fistula (TEF)
2.	Congenital diaphragmatic hernia (CDH)
3.	Congenital cyst adenomatous malformation (CCAM)
4.	Congenital lobar emphysema (CLE)
5.	Broncho-biliary fistula (BBF)

R. Subramaniam (✉)
Department of Anaesthesiology, Pain Medicine and Critical Care, All India Institute of Medical Sciences, New Delhi, India

© The Author(s), under exclusive license to Springer Nature Singapore Pte Ltd. 2023
U. Saha (ed.), *Clinical Anesthesia for the Newborn and the Neonate*,
https://doi.org/10.1007/978-981-19-5458-0_30

30.2   Physiological Changes in the Lateral Decubitus Position [1–3]

Surgical neonates tend to have high airway resistance and airflow limitation as a result of poor lung compliance (due to prematurity or soiling), and intraoperative airway manipulation. The tendency toward lung collapse on the dependent side, with high O_2 consumption, sets the stage for respiratory compromise and complications. In the lateral decubitus position, the highly compliant cartilaginous rib cage on the dependent side gets deformed by the pressure of the operating table (Fig. 30.1).

Added to this is the weight of the mediastinum which compresses the dependent lung from above, and abdominal pressure transmitted through the diaphragm. As a result, the dependent lung gets little ventilation and FRC is close to residual volume. The hydrostatic pressure gradient is reduced from the nondependent to dependent lung owing to the small chest size. Thus, a significant amount of lung perfusion continues to stay in the upper, operated lung. When the operated lung is collapsed manually, by surgical sponges and retractors, it results in diversion of ventilation to the dependent lung. The hypoxic pulmonary vasoconstriction in the nondependent lung further diverts some blood to the dependent lung. Despite factors favoring V/Q mismatch and hypoxemia in the lateral decubitus position, majority of neonates tolerate DLV well, barring as in necrotizing pneumonia.

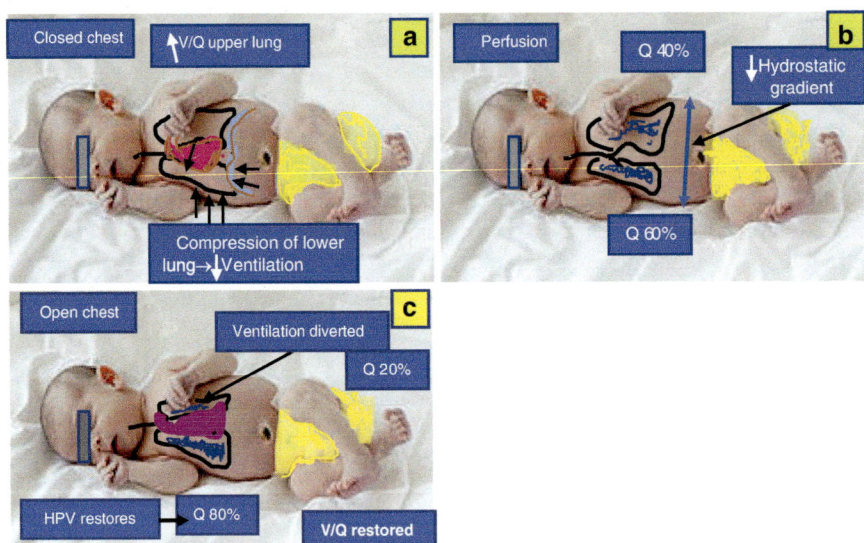

Fig. 30.1 V/Q changes in lateral decubitus position in a neonate: **a** and **b**, closed chest; **c**, open

30.3 Preoperative Evaluation [3, 4]

The goal of preoperative evaluation is (a) to identify potential anesthetic complications related to presence of comorbid conditions (cardiac /airway abnormalities), (b) to determine whether further diagnostic imaging/other laboratory investigations are required, and (c) to plan airway management. Many congenital malformations like TEF and CDH have significant association with congenital heart disease (CHD), with an odds ratio of 3.5 for 30-day mortality in presence of CHD. Conversely, babies with CHD have a high incidence of airway abnormalities. The neonate should be examined for facial features or dysmorphism suggestive of syndromes associated with difficult intubation. Respiratory symptoms (grunting, subcostal/suprasternal recession, alar flaring, sweating, inability to feed without interruption, sleeping in prone position) offer insight into severity of airway involvement and warrant planning of multiple management options. Other areas to be examined are status of hydration and suitability for vascular access.

If pertinent, history of prior airway management, venous access, and extubation should be obtained. Parental informed consent is very important, especially with reference to any additional risk, as in a neonate with anterior mediastinal mass.

Particular emphasis is on 4 aspects of anesthesia preparation:

1. **Induction of anesthesia**: routine, or with special preparations like rigid bronchoscopy?
2. **Airway management**: Does the procedure warrant lung isolation/OLV [equipment, skills]? Is the baby syndromic or having obstructive symptoms [difficult airway, video laryngoscopy]?
3. **Monitoring**: Will arterial blood gases (ABG) be necessary for management [arterial cannula placement]?
4. Is there likelihood of **major blood loss** [large bore vascular access]?
5. What would be the **analgesia plan**?

30.4 Fasting Guidelines and Premedication

Neonates can be breastfed 4 hours prior and administered clear fluids till 2 hours prior to the procedure. Premature babies and newborns within 48 hours of birth are prone to hypoglycemia and should receive 10% dextrose containing IV fluids.

Premedication generally includes airway nebulization /dexamethasone in neonates with hyperreactive airway, atropine/glycopyrrolate to dry secretions and prevent bradycardia (4).

30.4.1 Investigations

A preoperative echocardiogram and ECG should be carried out in all neonates with anomalies necessitating thoracotomy. A pediatric cardiac consultation is beneficial to plan hemodynamic goals in the perioperative period. CHD is associated with significant incidence of airway anomalies like subglottic stenosis and tracheal bronchus (bronchial variation arising from the trachea directed toward the upper lobe, usually arises within 2 cm of the carina, but can arise anywhere below the cricoid cartilage). An enlarged screening X-ray chest ("babygram") should be done and evaluated to confirm/exclude significant airway anomalies.

Hypoglycemia, hyponatremia, hypernatremia, hyperkalemia, hypocalcemia, and hypomagnesemia are all common in premature neonates and should be corrected. Anemic neonates may need preoperative blood transfusion. Low platelets and increased INR need prompt evaluation and correction. Packed RBCs and fresh-frozen plasma (FFP) should be arranged and available.

30.4.2 Blood Products and Vascular Access

In general, thoracic surgery in the neonate is not associated with significant blood loss. However, the proximity to large vascular structures and likelihood of inadvertent injury mandates blood to be crossmatched, as also for large masses with vascular supply. If the neonate does not have vascular access, blood can be drawn for cross-matching while placing the intravenous (IV) cannula after induction. The sites of possible vascular access should be examined. Plan should be made for a central line if venous access is poor or the neonate is likely to require prolonged postoperative fluid therapy and/or inotropes. Cannulation of the umbilical vein in the NICU is useful for perioperative IV fluid management. Vascular access sets should be kept ready.

30.4.3 Operation Room (OR) Preparation

Heat loss is a major concern in thoracotomies. The operation room should be warmed to 27°C before receiving the neonate. All exposed body parts should be covered with waterproof dressing ("cling wrap" or foil) or cotton wool. A warming mattress and forced air warming must be available. IV fluids and inspired gases should be humidified and warmed.

30.4.4 Induction of Anesthesia

In a neonate without hemodynamic instability or respiratory compromise, inhalational (sevoflurane, halothane) or intravenous (IV) induction with thiopentone/propofol can be safely performed. Helium can be added to the inhaled mixture in babies with obstructive lesions (tracheal stenosis, mediastinal mass), to improve gas flow past the obstruction [4]. After checking for mask ventilation, neuromuscular blockade can be done and airway secured as per plan.

30.5   Airway Management for Thoracotomy

30.5.1 Indications for Lung Isolation and One-Lung Ventilation (OLV)

Airway management for thoracotomy should ensure accurate placement of ETT and provision of lung isolation and OLV if indicated and/or feasible. Lung isolation is not necessary for all thoracotomies. The small size of the neonatal trachea is the main limiting factor, which necessitates specially designed equipment that may be available only in specialized centers.

There are very few absolute indications for lung isolation and OLV in neonates, both to improve the surgical field but also to reduce the risk of lung barotrauma and pneumothorax. The indications are:

1. **Absolute Indications** [1, 5]
    (i) Congenital lobar emphysema,
    (ii) giant unilateral lung cyst, and
    (iii) VATS.
2. **Less Common Indications** [5, 6]
    (i) To protect soiling of healthy dependent lung by secretions, blood, bile,
    (ii) To divert ventilation away from airway leak (bronchopleural fistula), and
    (iii) For lung lavage in pulmonary alveolar proteinosis.

Even for VATS, the highly compliant rib cage allows CO_2 insufflation at the expense of low pressures. Surgical retraction of the lung further improves exposure, and OLV is not "mandatory." However, OLV is instrumental in successful completion of surgery by VATS and reduces the incidence of conversion to thoracotomy.

30.5.2 Techniques of OLV

1. **Single lung ventilation**: Endobronchial intubation of the nonoperated side
    a. Blind or
    b. FOB/fluoroscopy guided.
2. **Extraluminal (parallel) bronchial blocker (BB) placement,** and
3. **Marraro pediatric bilumen tube.**

The techniques, advantages, and disadvantages of all the three will be discussed briefly. Fiber-optic guidance for correct placement is mandatory as margin of error is low. Because of the tendency to desaturaxte in lateral decubitus position, rapid access to both lungs should be available.

30.6   Single Lung Ventilation (SLV) by Endobronchial Intubation

Advantages
- Useful for very small children
- The right bronchus can be intubated blindly
- Useful in emergency situations, such as contralateral pneumothorax

Disadvantages [6]
- Blockade of ETT by blood/secretions,
- Inadequate seal of intubated lung,
- Inadequate collapse of the operated nondependent lung,
- Risk of soiling of healthy lung,
- Inability to provide CPAP and/or suction to operated lung, and
- Blockade of right upper lobe bronchus during right mainstem bronchus intubation.

When choosing SLV, it is preferable to intubate the left mainstem bronchus as the upper lobe bronchus on the right side arises <1 cm from the carina; the take-off of the upper lobe bronchus on the left side is 3 times that of the right upper lobe bronchus, increasing the margin of safety. The diameter of the left main bronchus is smaller than the trachea, and ETT, ½ size smaller must be selected. Uncuffed tubes have a Murphy eye. Intubation of right main bronchus with an appropriately placed Murphy eye may help to ventilate the upper lobe bronchus. The left main bronchus may be intubated "blind" by rotating the level of the ETT 180°, and turning the neonates' head to the right while advancing the tube down (1). Left bronchial intubation can be performed over a fiber-optic bronchoscope (FOB) or using fluoroscopy.

30.6.1 Bronchial Blockers

These are balloon-tipped narrow lumen catheters which have to be placed under fiber-optic guidance. They may be placed alongside the ETT (**parallel placement**) or down the lumen of the ETT (**co-axial placement**). The issues to be kept in mind are [5]:

(a) During co-axial placement, in order to permit **good ventilation**, the cross-sectional area of the bronchoscope (CSA_B) should be less than 50% of the cross-sectional area of the ETT lumen ($CSA_B/CSA_{ETT} <$ **0.5**).
(b) For a well-lubricated bronchoscope **to physically fit** inside the lumen of the ETT (and not get stuck due to friction), the outer diameter (OD) of the bronchoscope (OD_B) needs to be <90% of the internal diameter (ID) of the ETT (ID_{ETT}) [$OD_B/ID_{ETT} <$ **0.9**].

(c) The smallest FOB in general use (2 mm), which if placed inside a 2.5 mm ID tube, may give mobility (2/2.5 = 0.8), but is very unsatisfactory for ventilation.

(d) The blocker is placed in parallel outside the ETT. The combined OD of ETT + OD of blocker should be less than the tracheal diameter. The AP diameter of the neonatal trachea is 4.3 mm, and its lateral diameter 4.7 mm, which can tightly accommodate a 3.5 ID (4.8 mm OD) ETT with a 5 Fr BB (1.7 mm) (Fig. 30.2).

(e) The smallest ETT that can accommodate a 2.2 mm FOB and 5 Fr BB is 4.5 mm ID.

30.6.2 Varieties of Bronchial Blockers (Fig. 30.3)

1. **Vascular Catheters** - low volume, high inflation pressures (>700 cm H_2O with 2 ml air).
   a. Fogarty and
   b. Miller septostomy

Fig. 30.2 Parallel technique of blocker placement [5]

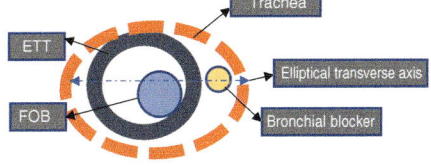

Fig. 30.3 Bronchial blockers: **a**. Fogarty 4 Fr; **b**. Arndt 5 Fr blocker with multiport adaptor

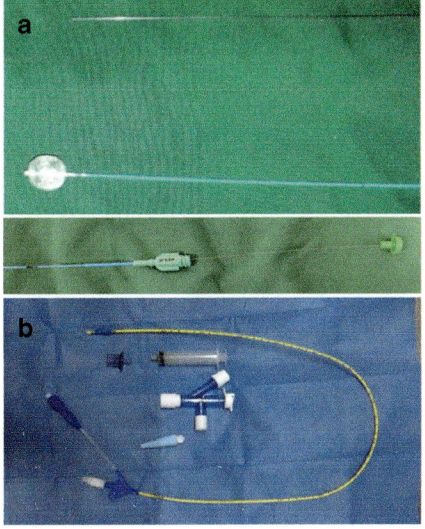

2. **High-Volume Low-Pressure Blocker**—(low pressure of 340–350 cm H_2O with 2 ml air).
   a. Arndt [7] and
   b. Fuji Uniblocker

Advantages
- Can transition from OLV to two-lung ventilation,
- Useful for very small children, and
- Useful in intubated/tracheostomized neonates.

Disadvantages
- High cuff pressure can cause bronchial mucosal damage,
- High chance of displacement with lung manipulation,
- Adequate lung isolation may not be achieved even with good blocker placement, and
- Significant hypercarbia common, even if oxygenation is maintained.

30.6.3 Technique of Placement of BB (Fig. 30.4)

1. Bronchial blockers may be placed extraluminally (parallel) through ETT guided into a mainstem bronchus, ETT removed, and another inserted into the trachea. This is the only available option for BB in children less than 2 years.
2. They may be classically placed using the loop approach as described for the Arndt blocker.
3. Templeton et al. [7] have described the bending of an Arndt blocker by 15°, introducing it into the trachea, then pass an ETT along it (using to advantage the larger transverse tracheal diameter), finally directing the blocker into position by FOB through the ETT.
4. Other innovative workers have done away with the multiport adaptor to give more flexibility to the apparatus [8].

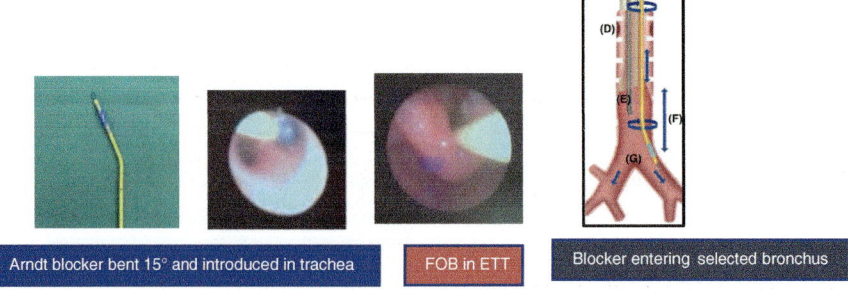

Arndt blocker bent 15° and introduced in trachea   FOB in ETT   Blocker entering selected bronchus

Fig. 30.4 Novel way of extraluminal blocker placement in a 9-day infant [7]

30.6.4 Marraro Bilumen Tube [9] (Fig. 30.5)

This tube was constructed from two uncuffed PVC tubes of different lengths attached laterally, with a radio-opaque line in 1994. The longer tube has a Murphy eye and is bent at 5° before the eye, which is useful for ventilating the right upper lobe when the longer tube is placed in the right main bronchus. Both tubes end in a lip shape facing outwards. There is no carinal hook. They can be connected to a single Y adaptor or to different circuits. Small sizes for newborns and neonates are available (Table 30.2).

It is placed under laryngoscopic view with both lumina antero-posteriorly oriented. After both cross the vocal cords, the tube is rotated 90° to the desired side. Confirmation is by clamping and auscultation or X-ray. The small lumen permits only 1.8 mm FOB.

Fig. 30.5 The Marraro Bilumen Tube [9] with Radio-Opaque Line (from Portex Brochure)

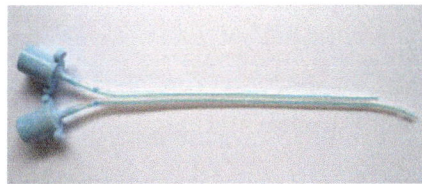

Table 30.2 Suggested sizes of Marraro Bilumen tubes [9]

Age	Caliber (mm)
Premature (1400–2500) g	2+2
Newborn (2500–4000) g	2.5+2 or 2.5+2.5
1 month	2.5+2.5
6 months	3+2.5
12 months	3.5+3

30.7   Pain Management for Thoracotomy

Neonates have immature neural development; pain pathways are poorly understood, and pain is generally unrecognized and untreated. Theoretically, adequate regional analgesia (RA) can avoid exposure to potential neurotoxic effects of general anesthetics and reduce surgical stress response. Inadequately treated pain may impact neurobehavioral impairment, emotional, behavioral, and learning disabilities [10].

Opioids as infusion or boluses (fentanyl 1 μg/kg/hr or 1 μg/kg bolus), or morphine 10 μg/kg/hr or 100 μg/kg bolus) are the mainstay of analgesia in neonates after thoracotomy. In neonates that have been extubated, caution must be exercised as they are at risk of respiratory depression. Paracetamol is an useful adjunct, and its dose should be limited to 7.5 mg/kg 6 hourly.

Epidural, paravertebral, and intercostal nerve blocks have all been used. Both neuraxial or fascial plane blocks (erector spinae plane) provide superior quality analgesia, reduce intraoperative inhalational anesthesia and opioid dose, and reduce or eliminate the need for postoperative ventilatory support [11–14].

30.7.1 Epidural Analgesia

Epidural analgesia in neonates is shown to be safe. It is associated with reduced need for both muscle relaxants and opioids and need for postoperative ventilatory support [11, 14].

Single bolus dose of bupivacaine has been described for neonates undergoing TEF surgery, which provided analgesia up to 8 h postoperatively. However, catheter-based techniques are more popular for providing extended postoperative analgesia.

A short skin-to-epidural space distance, soft ligamentum flavum, and narrow epidural space are characteristics of the neonatal epidural space. A minor leak of drug from the catheter insertion site may occur due to different calibers of the needle and catheter (19 G and 23 G), and the short skin-epidural distance. Higher technical challenge and sporadic reports of spinal cord damage and death warrant high levels of care and skill. Caudally introduced catheters are a better option for the novice anesthesiologist. A caudal block can produce adequate anesthesia up to the mid-thoracic region if an adequate volume and dose is given.

Thoracic catheters can be inserted through the caudal route in neonates owing to the nature of the epidural space. Although thought to be safer, it may be associated with more trauma, malposition and infection. Further, caudally threaded catheter migration occurs commonly in smallest and youngest patients, neonates, and infants, and postoperative imaging is crucial to confirm catheter tip location after its placement [15]. It is strongly recommended to use ultrasound guidance to track the catheter real-time during insertion, as a wide discrepancy between the actual length of catheter inside and the physical distance from the sacral hiatus to the desired vertebral level has been seen [16].

Bolus dosing and infusions have both been described, but risk of accumulation and resultant drug toxicity is higher with infusion, partly due to immature

Table 30.3 Doses of local anesthetics for neonates

Local anesthetic	Recommended dose	Issues
Bupivacaine	1 mg/kg	Commonly used for field blocks and wound infiltration
Ropivacaine	1.5 mg/kg	Less motor block less cardiotoxic Vasoconstrictor effect (avoid digital/penile blocks)
Lidocaine	2.5 mg/kg	Short acting
Prilocaine	Not recommended	Risk of methemoglobinemia
Chloroprocaine	7 mg/kg	No plasma accumulation due to short T 1/2
Eutectic mixture of LA (EMLA)	1g	Equal parts lidocaine and prilocaine Maximum skin contact—1 h Risk of methemoglobinemia

Table 30.4 Adjuncts for neuraxial block [13]

Drug/Route	Dose
Morphine—Caudal/epidural bolus	3–5 µg/kg
Fentanyl—Caudal/epidural bolus Epidural infusion	1.0–1.5 µg/kg 3–5 µg kg^1 24 h^1
Sufentanil—Epidural bolus Epidural infusion	0.6 µg/kg 2 µg kg^1 24 h^1
Clonidine—Caudal/epidural bolus Epidural infusion—limited data in < 12 mth age	1–2 µg/kg
Ketamine—Caudal bolus, racemic ketamine Caudal bolus, S (+) ketamine	0.25–0.5 mg/kg 0.5–1.0 mg/kg

metabolism and partly due to a more permeable blood-brain barrier (BBB). Ropivacaine 0.1–0.2% is the local anesthetic (LA) of choice with adjuncts (Tables 30.3 and 30.4). It is advisable not to run continuous epidural infusions of bupivacaine for more than 48 hours as there is a cumulative effect, resulting in local anesthetic systemic toxicity (LAST).

Intrathecal morphine—A dose of 3–5 µg/kg provides analgesia for 12–24 h.

30.7.2 Erector Spinae Plane Block (ESPB) [17, 18]

ESPB is performed under ultrasound guidance and has a good margin of safety because of its more superficial placement and greater distance from important structures (spinal cord, pleura). The catheter is placed congruent to the planned incision. In contrast to paravertebral or neuraxial blocks where coagulopathy is a contraindication, ESPB is safe and has been used in a preterm neonate undergoing TEF repair. The potential risk of a pneumothorax offsets its use for thoracotomy. However, it is effective and safe alternative to epidural and paravertebral catheters in neonates for thoracic procedures.

30.8   Special Surgical Conditions and Concerns

30.8.1   Congenital Cystic Adenomatoid Malformations (CCAM)
[17, 19–22]

CCAM is a rare congenital anomaly with an incidence of 1:25,000 to 1:35,000 live births. It is the second most common congenital lung lesion, with a male preponderance, postulated to occur as a result of embryologic insult before the 7th week of gestation, which eventually leads to maldevelopment of the terminal bronchiolar structures. CCAM is also known as Congenital Pulmonary Airway Malformation (CPAM). It is classified (Stocker classification) on the basis of the cyst size (Type I: 2–10 cm; Type II: 0.5–2 cm; Type III: microcystic). In CPAM, an entire lobe of lung is replaced by a cystic abnormal lung tissue, which is nonfunctional.

CCAM can be diagnosed on antenatal ultrasound. In the case of large cysts causing fetal hydrops, serial aspirations or ultrasound-guided placement of thoracic-amniotic shunts can be helpful. Untreated large masses causing airway compression can lead to severe ventilatory compromise at birth, warranting immediate tracheal intubation. For such cases, it would be prudent to plan an ex utero intrapartum (EXIT) procedure so that the airway is secured while the neonate is still on placental support.

Large malformations result in ipsilateral lung compression, pulmonary hypoplasia, and occasional mediastinal shift. At birth, the majority are asymptomatic. About 25% of CPAM may present as respiratory distress, cyanosis, tachypnoea, and intercostal retractions. On examination, hyper-resonance at percussion, diminished vesicular murmur, and an asymmetrical thorax may be found. Associated (renal, intestinal, bony, cardiac) anomalies and malignancies may be present in up to 25% patients which worsen prognosis [19].

Features of severe respiratory distress (tachypnoea, hypoxemia, increased work of breathing) respiratory failure requiring ventilatory support, mediastinal shift and hypotension, are indications for urgent emergency thoracotomy for curative excision of the affected lobe (lobectomy).

Investigations: Chest X-ray and CT scan are mandatory investigations to delineate anatomy and precise location of the cystic lobe. Chest X-ray may show marked hyperlucency if the lesion is aerated and may be mistaken for a pneumothorax. Lesion may also appear as air-filled cysts or a consolidation. Large lesions with mediastinal shift will show depression or inversion of the diaphragm [19] (Fig. 30.6). Apart from confirming radiological, CT may reveal mediastinal shift, downward displacement of the diaphragm, compression atelectasis of surrounding lung tissue, and occasionally herniation of involved lobe across the mediastinum. It may also detect a narrowed bronchus of the affected or collapsed lobe. The left upper lobe is most commonly involved. Bronchoscopy may be indicated to rule out a foreign body or mucus plug. The association of CPAM with CHD is in 15-20% babies, and a 2D echo is indicated in babies presenting with murmur or failure to thrive.

Coagulation parameters and ABG help to guide preoperative optimization.

Fig. 30.6 Chest X-ray in
CCAM (R)

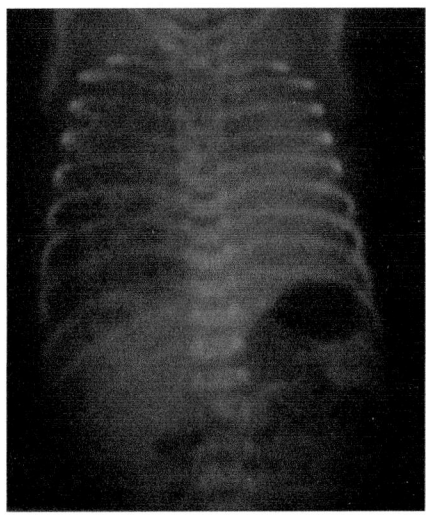

Inhalational induction is slowed due to lung pathology and intrapulmonary shunting. IV induction with thiopentone, propofol, or ketamine is preferred. In case of large CPAMs and risk of rupture with positive pressure ventilation (PPV), spontaneous ventilation is best preserved with sevoflurane and IV fentanyl till the chest is opened and the malformed lobe allowed to prolapse out of the chest. PPV and PEEP may lead to cyst expansion and rupture, or cause compression of lung and mediastinal shift with possibility of pneumothorax and/or severe hemodynamic compromise and hypotension. Hence, ventilation should be gentle in these patients. Nitrous oxide should be completely avoided.

Provision of OLV has problems due to the small size of the airways. Often surgeons manage with retracting the functional lung. Lung isolation can be done using techniques as described above, such as parallel placement of a 3Fr Fogarty into the left mainstem bronchus for left lung isolation [21], balloon-tipped BB (extraluminal) (Fogarty catheters (3, 4, 5 Fr G), Arndt endobronchial blocker (smallest 5 Fr G)], (7) and Marraro DLT (9). Selective mainstem endobronchial intubation with a single ETT is not preferred because of the inability to suction the operated lung. However, in case of nonaerated lung, OLV is not mandatory.

There is potential for many intraoperative issues:

- Airway problems include hypoxemia due to lateral decubitus position and retraction of functional lung tissue.
- Cardiovascular events include hypotension resulting from aortic/IVC compression/bleeding.
- Trauma to adjoining structures and bleeding.

Thoracic /caudal epidural catheters and ultrasound-guided paravertebral blocks have all been used for analgesia [20–22]. If instituted after induction, these blocks help limiting the inspired concentration of inhalational anesthetic and opioid dose. ESPB has also been used [17]. Short-acting opioids like fentanyl/remifentanil or paracetamol are used as a part of multimodal analgesia.

Pre- and post-ductal SpO2 monitoring is a must to detect cardiac shunting and desaturation. Invasive arterial monitoring is useful in large CPAM with risk of hemodynamic compromise and also for ABG monitoring. In addition to routine monitoring like temperature, ECG, and EtCO2, a precordial stethoscope is recommended for OLV.

Postoperative nasal CPAP/HFNC helps to maintain FRC and support gas exchange, thus reducing work of breathing. Effective postoperative analgesia is invaluable in facilitating breathing and early extubation [17].

30.8.2 Congenital Lobar Emphysema (CLE) [8, 23–29]

CLE or congenital lobar overinflation (CLO) is a rare condition with incidence of 1:20,000–1:30,000 births. The affected neonates may require lobectomy in early infancy. CLE accounts for 10% of all congenital lung malformations [24, 25] (Fig. 30.7). The association of CHD with CLE is significant (15–20%) [24]. Frequently, hypertensive or dilated pulmonary arteries with VSD or PDA are found in association with CLE. The most frequent site for emphysema is the left upper lobe followed by the right middle lobe. The bronchi of affected lobes are often compressed by dilated pulmonary vessels. Very often the neonate undergoes surgery for correction of the cardiac defect and CLE is discovered either during surgery or due to postoperative respiratory embarrassment. It is therefore important to evaluate the heart and airways thoroughly in the preoperative period, using whichever modality is relevant [contrast-enhanced computed tomography (CECT), MRI, or even cardiac catheterization in selected cases], to plan the operative procedure. CLE may improve with management of CHD, as in neonates who are symptomatic primarily because of enlarged pulmonary vessels, when symptoms of CLE may improve with

Fig. 30.7 Congenital lobar emphysema (L)

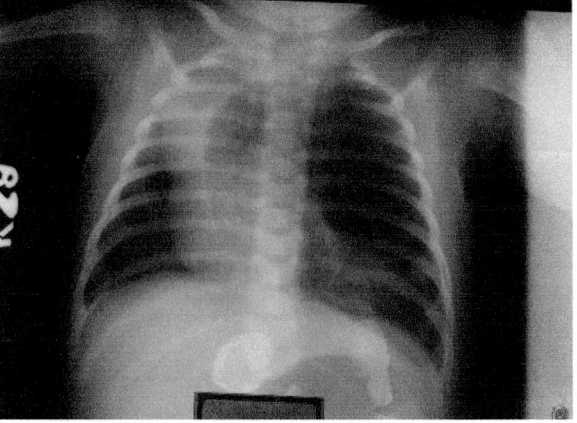

symptom control for CHD. Highly symptomatic neonates will benefit from early lobectomy.

Respiratory distress is the hallmark of CLE. It may have already been diagnosed antenatally. Symptoms worsen as the emphysematous lobe enlarges, with onset of cyanosis. It may be difficult to differentiate bronchopneumonia, cyanotic CHD, and other pulmonary abnormalities from CLE. Often, diagnosis of tension pneumothorax is made, with unfortunate insertion of chest tube, and worsening clinical condition [26].

Anesthetic management is on similar lines to CPAM. Anesthesia is induced with sevoflurane in 100% oxygen. Injudicious PPV during induction may result in expansion of the emphysematous lobe, with potentially disastrous consequences as compression of the surrounding normal lung, mediastinal shift, pneumothorax, and cardiac arrest. Occasional gentle assistance with minimum airway pressures is sometimes used. Nitrous oxide is avoided in all cases.

CLE is one of the few conditions mandating OLV, for preventing expansion of the cyst and consequent rupture and pneumothorax, but also to provide optimal conditions for VATS. OLV is generally established with an end-hole bronchial blocker like the Arndt blocker, to facilitate collapse of the operated lobe. Schmidt et. al. [8] have described co-axial placement of a 5 Fr Arndt blocker through a 4.0 mm ID ETT. Jacob et.al [27]. have described successful left endobronchial intubation with spontaneous ventilation using sevoflurane, passing a Fogarty down the ETT, then removing the ETT and intubating the right bronchus with another ETT.

Caudal epidural catheters have been used for analgesia in neonates with CLE, retaining spontaneous ventilation until thoracotomy to allow the cyst to extrude [24]. Thoracic epidural has been used for postoperative analgesia [28, 29].

30.8.3 Congenital Broncho-Biliary Fistula (CBBF) [30]

CBBF is a rare anomaly, characterized by very high mortality. It occurs consequent to an abnormal fistulous connection between the segmental bronchus (usually the right side) and the biliary tree. These neonates develop choking and respiratory distress with intermittent cyanosis soon after birth. Copious greenish secretions are vomited and also suctioned from the ETT. 3-D CT reveals the fistulous connection originating from the bronchus (usually right) and terminating in the biliary tract. Concomitant findings are air in the intrahepatic biliary tract and lower lobe pneumonia.

As part of preoperative preparation, these neonates are kept fasting, with gastric decompression and IV fluids. Antibiotics are administered as per protocol. Head-elevated position and CPAP reduce respiratory distress and promote secretions to localize in the dependent lobe. Parenteral nutrition and sedation are initiated depending on the duration of preoperative waiting.

Induction can be through inhalational or IV route. Since these fistulae are distal to the carina, there is no danger of distending the stomach, unlike in TEF, and neuromuscular blockade and mask ventilation can be carried out to facilitate atraumatic intubation.

Intraoperative issues relate mainly to poor lung compliance and hypoxemia. An arterial cannula is helpful to monitor ABG and guide ventilation. The fistula is localized and ligated through thoracoscopy if the infant is able to tolerate the CO_2 insufflation, or by thoracotomy.

As highlighted previously, good analgesia should be provided as described above. Recovery is usually good after a brief period of elective postoperative ventilation.

30.9 Conclusion

Thoracic anesthesia in neonates requires careful preoperative evaluation with reference to additional systemic disorders, airway evaluation and planning, and an effective analgesia plan. With advent of thoracoscopy, more neonates will be subjected to this technique, highlighting the concerns of OLV. All regular pediatric anesthesiologists should train themselves in at least one technique of lung isolation and be well versed with neonatal fiber-optic bronchoscopy. Advances in antenatal care and fetal surgery will also result in survival of more babies, where indicated. Anesthesiologists should be facile with a variety of regional anesthetic techniques which can immensely contribute to a good postoperative outcome.

Declaration I hereby declare that all clinical photographs and X-ray images are my personal ones and not copied from any site.

References for Further Reading

1. Templeton TW, Piccioni F, Chatterjee D. An update on one-lung ventilation in children. Anesth Analg. 2021;132:1389–99.
2. Fabila TS, Menghraj SJ. One lung ventilation strategies for infants and children undergoing video assisted thoracoscopic surgery. Indian J Anaesth. 2013;57:339–44.
3. Semmelmann A, Kaltofen H, Loop T. Anesthesia of thoracic surgery in children. Pediatr Anesth. 2018;28:326–31.
4. Tobias JD. Anesthesia for neonatal thoracic surgery. Best Pract Res Clin Anaesth. 2004;18:303–20.
5. Letal M, Theam M. Paediatric lung isolation. BJA Educ. 2017;17:57–62.
6. Tognon C, Meneghini L, Fascetti Leon F, Gamba PG. The different approaches of single lung ventilation in infants with pulmonary malformation. Int J Pediatr Res. 2018;4:030. https://doi.org/10.23937/2469-5769/1510030.
7. Templeton TW, Downard MG, Simpson CR, Zeller KA, et al. Bending the rules: a novel approach to placement and retrospective experience with the 5 French Arndt endobronchial blocker in children <2 years. Pediatr Anesth. 2016;26:512–20.
8. Schmidt C, Rellensman G, van Aken H, et al. Single-lung ventilation for pulmonary lobe resection in a newborn. Anesth Analg. 2005;101:362–4.

9. Marraro G. Selective endobronchial intubation in paediatrics: the Marraro paediatric bilumen tube. Pediatric Anesthesia. 1994;4:255–8. https://doi.org/10.1111/j.1460-9592.1994.tb00174.x.

10. Ponde V, Puri K, Nagdev T. Regional anaesthesia in neonates: a narrative review. S Afr J Anaesth Analg. 2020;26:S4–8.

11. Solanki NM, Engineer SR, Vecham P. Comparison of epidural versus systemic analgesia for major surgeries in neonates and infants. J Clin Neonatol. 2017;6:23–8.

12. Jayaram K, Durga P. Regional anesthesia for thoracotomy pain in newborns and infants- a systematic review. Trends Anaesth Crit Care. 2017;17:11–6.

13. Lonnqvist PA. Regional anaesthesia and analgesia in neonates. Best Pract Res Clin Anaesth. 2010;24:309–21.

14. Bosenberg AT. Epidural analgesia for major neonatal surgery. Paediatr Anaesth. 1998;8:479–83.

15. Simpao AF, Gálvez JA, Wartman EC, England WR, Wu L, et al. The migration of caudally threaded thoracic epidural catheters in neonates and infants. Anesth Analg. 2019;129:477–81.

16. Ponde VC, Bedekar VV, Desai AP, Puranik KA. Does ultrasound guidance add accuracy to continuous caudal-epidural catheter placements in neonates and infants? Paediatr Anaesth. 2017;27:1010–4.

17. Adler AC, Yim MM, Chandrakantan A. Erector spinae plane catheter for neonatal thoracotomy: a potentially safer alternative to a thoracic epidural. Can Anesth. 2019;66:607–8.

18. Schalkwyk AS, Flaherty J, Hess D, Horvath B. Erector spinae catheter for post-thoracotomy pain control in a premature neonate. BMJ Case Rep. 2020;13:e234480. https://doi.org/10.1136/bcr-2020-234480.

19. Gupta B, Chaudhary K, Hayaran N, Neogi S. Anesthetic considerations in patients with cystic pulmonary adenomatoid malformations. J Anaesthesiol Clin Pharmacol. 2021;37:146–52.

20. Rajgire V, Tandale SR, Kelkar K, Band R. Neonate with congenital cystic adenoid malformation of lung for lobectomy: Anesthesia concerns. J Anaesthesiol Clin Pharmacol. 2018;34:561–2.

21. Guruswamy V, Roberts S, Arnold P, Potter F. Anaesthetic management of a neonate with congenital cyst adenoid malformation. Br J Anaesth. 2005;95:240–2.

22. Cho AR, Kim KH, Shin SW, Hong JM, Kim HY. Anesthetic management of a neonate with giant bronchopulmonary sequestration. Anesth Pain Med. 2010;5:351–4.

23. Kanakis M, Petsios K, Bobos D, Sarafidis K, Nikopoulos S, et al. Left upper lobectomy for congenital lobar emphysema in a low birth weight infant. Case Rep Surg. 2016:4182741. https://doi.org/10.1155/2016/4182741.

24. Kylat RI. Managing congenital lobar overinflation associated with congenital heart disease. Children. 2020;7:113. https://doi.org/10.3390/children7090113.

25. Moideen I, Nair SG, Cherian A, Rao SG. Congenital lobar emphysema associated with congenital heart disease. J Cardiothorac Vasc Anesth. 2006;20:239–41.

26. Tempe DK, Virmani S, Javetkar S, Banerjee A, Puri SK, Datt V. Congenital lobar emphysema: pitfalls and management. Ann Card Anaesth. 2010;13:53–8.

27. Jacob M, Ramesh GS, Narmada LN. Anesthetic management of congenital lobar emphysema. Med J Armed Forces India. 2015;71(2015):S287–9.

28. Dogan R, Dogan OF, Yilmaz M, Demircin M, Pasaglou I, Kiper N, et al. Surgical managements of infants with congenital lobar emphysema and concomitant congenital heart disease. Heart Surg Forum. 2004;7:E644–9.

29. Raghavendran S, Diwan R, Shah T, Vas L. Continuous caudal epidural analgesia for congenital lobar emphysema: a report of three cases. Anesth Analg. 2001;93:348–50.

30. Yin H, Zhao G, Du Y, Zhao P. Anesthesia management in neonatal congenital bronchobiliary fistula: case report and literature review. BMC Anesthesiol. 2020;20:135.

Abdominal Wall Defects in Newborns and Neonates: Exomphalos and Gastrochisis

31

Geeta Kamal

31.1 Introduction

Neonates with Exomphalos (Omphalocele) and Gastroschisis have developmental defects in their anterior abdominal wall with external herniation and exposure of the abdominal contents. They may manifest with impaired blood supply to the herniated/exposed viscera, intestinal obstruction, and major intravascular fluid deficits. These are two distinct clinical entities present at birth. Majority of these anomalies are diagnosed antenatal, allowing planned delivery. Surgical closure of the defect under general anesthesia is the only solution, and in case of large defects, repeated surgeries and anesthesia become imminent. About 70% of neonates with exomphalos have an associated anomaly which further increases the risk to the life of the newborn. These neonates are highly susceptible to severe dehydration and hypothermia, often necessitating an initial surgery within hours of birth, when the newborn is still struggling to adapt to the extrauterine life and undergoing transitional changes. Delay in correction may affect the baby adversely with delayed or failure of closure of the cardiac shunts. Hence, meticulous post-delivery or preoperative care, maintenance of volume, electrolyte, acid base, urine output, and temperature can greatly aid the anesthesiologist in the intra- and postoperative management and better survival of such babies.

This chapter describes exomphalos and gastrochisis with the developmental differences, etiology, pathophysiological implications, preoperative evaluation and stabilization, anesthetic management and postoperative complications and management.

G. Kamal (✉)
Chacha Nehru Bal Chikitsalya, New Delhi, India

583

31.2 Exomphalos (Omphalocele) and Gastrochisis

31.2.1 Embryology

During the sixth week of development, the embryonic intestine develops rapidly and migrates through the umbilical ring into the umbilical cord. The intestine returns to the abdominal cavity within the following 4 weeks, i.e., by the tenth week of gestation. This return is associated with a 270° anti-clockwise rotation of the gut on its mesenteric base.

31.2.2 Etiopathology

Exomphalos occurs when the intestine fails to return to the abdominal cavity from the yolk sac. It is postulated that this is due to delayed closure of the lateral folds in association with a large umbilical ring. The viscera are covered with a membrane consisting of Wharton's jelly, peritoneum, and amnion. The liver, spleen, and ovaries are frequently present in the sac. These babies usually have associated non-rotation or malrotation of the intestines.

Gastroschisis is a smaller defect in the abdominal wall, periumbilical, commonly located to the right side of the anatomically normal umbilical cord. One theory suggests that a vascular incident involving the omphalo-mesenteric artery is responsible for the defect. Usually, it is the intestines that herniate. Testes, ovary, and liver are much less commonly involved. There is no membranous covering over the viscera; therefore, the herniated bowel is directly exposed to the amniotic fluid in the uterus and to the atmosphere after birth. As a result, the bowel wall develops an inflammatory peel, mesentery becomes thickened, and the exposed gut is inflamed, and edematous. There is a of fluid and heat loss from the exposed gut, as well as of compromise of circulation to the gut with ischemia and infarction.

Simply put, exomphalos is herniation while gastroschisis is exposure of abdominal contents.

31.2.3 Epidemiology

Abdominal wall defects are associated with low maternal age, low parity, low gestational age, low birth weight, maternal smoking, and use of nasal decongestants and aspirin. Gastroschisis has a greater association with younger maternal age (<20 years) as compared to Exomphalos. These defects are more common in males (M:F::3:2).

Exomphalos occurs in 1:3000 live births, whereas **Gastroschisis** is less common with incidence of 1:6000–10,000 live births, which has steadily increased over the last three decades because of better diagnostic facilities and awareness among public.

31.2.4 Associated Anomalies

Exomphalos is very frequently associated with congenital anomalies. Nearly 70% of neonates born with exomphalos have an associated anomaly, 20% being cardiac in origin, commonly tetralogy of Fallot and ASD. There is also an association of exomphalos with **various syndromes**, such as:

(a) **Chromosomal abnormalities** - Trisomy 13, 14, 15, 18, or 21.
(b) **Beckwith – Wiedemann syndrome** - macrosomia (large birth weight and length), hemihypertrophy/hemihyperplasia (overgrowth of one side or one part of the body), macroglossia (large tongue, that may interfere with breathing and feeding), gigantism, pancreatic islet cell hyperplasia, congenital heart disease, and exostrophy of bladder.
(c) **Pentalogy of Cantrell** consists of five defects - exomphalos, CDH, sternal defect, cardiac anomaly (VSD), and pericardial defect. This should be suspected when a baby with exomphalos has cyanosis also.
(d) **Lower Midline Syndrome** has all the midline defects, below the level of umbilicus – bladder and or cloacal exostrophy, imperforate anus, colonic atresia, vertebral anomalies, and meningomyelocele.

Gastroschisis is much less frequently associated with congenital anomalies, incidence being 10–15%, and most involving the gastrointestinal tract, chiefly as intestinal atresia. Meckel's diverticulum and intestinal duplication have also been reported.

31.3   Diagnosis

Abdominal wall defects are usually diagnosed antenatal, during routine sonographic screening in the first trimester, at about tenth week of gestation. Once an exomphalos is identified, further investigations (including amniocentesis and fetal echocardiography) should be carried out to exclude other associated anomalies. Antenatal diagnosis allows timing, location, and mode of delivery to be planned in advance, depending on the size of the defect and other anomalies.

In most cases, pregnancy is allowed till term (>36 weeks) and delivery planned at 37 weeks, to limit further bowel damage from exposure to amniotic fluid, while allowing full fetal maturity. This improves the chance of survival of the newborn.

Baby can be delivered vaginally if the defect and the size of herniated viscera is small, but large or major exomphalos and gastroschisis benefit from planned operative delivery at early term (37 weeks), to reduce the risk of trauma to the viscera or its coverings during vaginal delivery. Ideally, these babies should be delivered in a tertiary care center where both neonatal and surgical expertise is available.

31.4　Post-Delivery Management

These babies should be transferred to a special care unit/NICU soon after initial resuscitation at birth. Since the viscera is covered with a membrane and not directly exposed to the environment, babies with **Exomphalos** ideally should be optimized and stabilized, and surgery planned as elective. Babies with **Gastroschisis**, and those in whom the covering membrane of exomphalos is damaged, exposing the gut, need to be taken up for surgery as early as possible. This is a surgical emergency. Babies delivered at home are usually sicker, and have a poorer prognosis as compared to those born in the hospital settings.

The mainstays of the initial or early management are as follows:

1. Care of herniated bowel/viscera and their blood supply.
2. Bowel decompression using a nasogastric tube (NGT).
3. Temperature regulation.
4. Fluid resuscitation.

Inspection of the exposed or herniated viscera must be done to see the integrity of the covering membrane. If the sac covering the bowel in an exomphalos is intact, it should be covered with saline-soaked gauze. In case it is not intact or in **gastroschisis**, because of extreme susceptibility to significant fluid and heat loss from the gut exposure, the bowel is covered with a waterproof cellophane bowel bag (Fig. 31.1). All babies with abdominal wall defects should be nursed in the right lateral position with the bowel supported, and kept in an incubator to reduce heat loss. NGT is inserted for bowel decompression.

In addition to receiving maintenance fluid of 10% dextrose and 0.18% sodium chloride @ 80 mL/kg/day, they may require multiple fluid boluses to compensate for the excessive fluid losses. These are usually given as 4.5% human albumin solution in 10 mL/kg increments. Fluid requirement is determined by clinical parameters: pulse, arterial pressure, and capillary refill.

IV antibiotics are started to prevent infection.

Fig. 31.1 Waterproof cellophane bowel bag

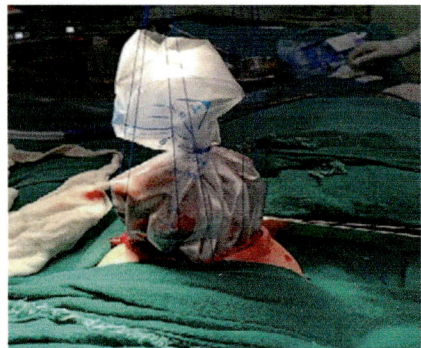

Initial basic investigations include complete blood counts (CBC), capillary blood gases, and radiographs of the abdominal and chest.

Because of greater association of exomphalos with other anomalies, Echocardiogram, Renal ultrasound, Chromosome studies and CT scan of head, become mandatory investigations. Cross-matched blood should be available for transfusion, if required.

Management in NICU is the continuation of the initial care after birth (Box 31.1).

Box 31.1 Abdominal Wall Defects—Initial Management

1. Fluid resuscitation and maintenance,
2. Care of exposed/herniated bowel/viscera and their blood supply,
3. Bowel decompression using an NGT,
4. Temperature regulation and prevention of hypothermia,
5. Baby nursed in right lateral position with bowel supported.

31.5   Preoperative Management

Since surgery for exomphalos is mostly an elective procedure, it is expected that neonate will be stable in terms of fluid, electrolyte, oxygenation and temperature status and well resuscitated. In case of ruptured sac of an exomphalos or in gastroschisis, which are taken up for surgery as an emergency, anaesthesiologist must ensure and assess the adequacy of optimization, at preoperative evaluation:

1. **Volume status** should be assessed for the degree of dehydration and hypovolemia. Signs of severe hypovolemia/dehydration/circulatory insufficiency such as tachypnoea, tachycardia, cold peripheries, poor skin perfusion (skin is pale or mottled), and delayed capillary refill, must be made a note of. Hypotension is a late sign. These babies will require fluid boluses, preferably before surgery, so as to avoid circulatory collapse at the time of induction of anaesthesia, as described above, or PRBC in case of severe anaemia, along with maintenance fluids.
2. **CBC, electrolytes, acid base and blood gas analysis** can be done using capillary blood sample, and any abnormality detected can be corrected preoperative and paid heed to during anaesthetic management.
3. **Other investigations** Abdominal and Chest x-rays, and Echo. Look for features of pulmonary hypoplasia, aspiration, infection, intrapulmonary shunting; note NGT and ETT position if in place.
4. **Blood grouping and availability of cross-matched** blood must be confirmed. In case of major defects, it may be prudent to have one pediatric unit of PRBC in hand at the time of induction.

31.6   Surgical Management

Surgery can be urgent, semi-urgent or elective, single stage or staged reduction of the bowel and closure of the abdominal wall defect.

Exomphalos: Surgery with intact sac is elective or semi-urgent, but it should be undertaken once the baby is adequately hydrated and resuscitated. In case of sac is rupture, the defect must be repaired within a few hours of birth.

A small defect may be repaired in a **single stage**, whereas larger defects may require the formation of a **silastic pouch and gradual reduction** over the next several days at 24–48 h intervals (Fig. 31.2). The initial reductions may need to be done under general anesthesia. In case of exomphalos major, the contents will not accommodate in the abdominal cavity even after creation of a surgical pouch. Hence, the sac is left intact and allowed to epithelialize. A ventral hernia results which is repaired at a much later date.

Conservative management: Antiseptic desiccating agents (silver sulfadiazine ointment or povidone iodine spray) are applied to the sac, which gradually contracts in size. The abdominal closure is done as the defect becomes smaller, but if the sac ruptures any time, urgent surgery is required.

Gastroschisis: Surgery is usually performed within a few hours of birth, but in case the bowel perfusion is compromised, it is taken up without further delay, as an emergency.

There are a number of surgical options for the repair of **gastroschisis**. If possible, the exposed bowel is returned to the abdominal cavity in its entirety and a **primary closure** performed. However, some centers have moved towards a **staged reduction** in routine practice.

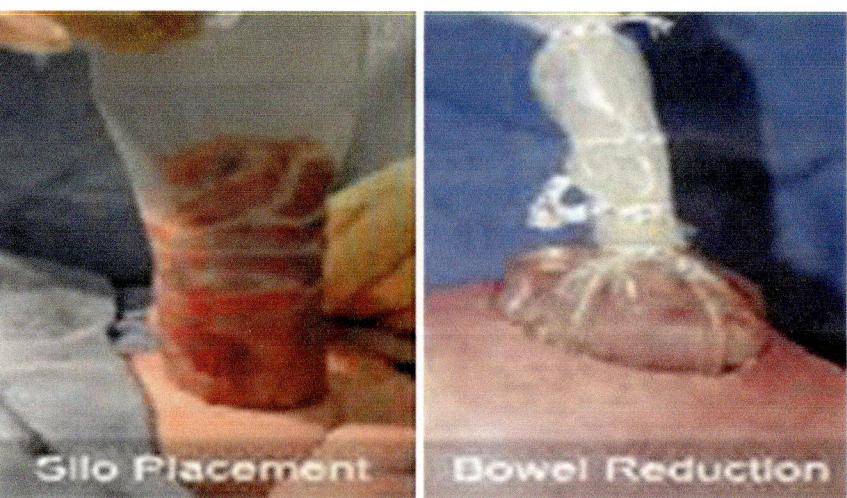

Fig. 31.2 Silastic pouch and gradual reduction

Staged surgery requires 'silo' to cover the hernial contents, which is sutured to the edge of the fascial defect. A sterile plastic sheeting is kept between the intestines and the silastic covering. IV fluid bags and urinary bags have also been used as covers. The silo is suspended above the baby. The bowel gets reduced under gravity over 4–7 days and the silo is intermittently reduced (Fig. 31.2). The silo is applied under general anaesthesia and once the contents are reduced significantly, abdominal closure is done at a second surgery under anaesthesia.

Spring loaded, self-retaining silastic pouch has been developed which can be inserted in the NICU without anesthesia. G- More recently, a preformed, silastic spring loaded silo has been developed for the management of gastroschisis. The device is inserted and serial reductions are performed on the NICU without any sedation or analgesia and a delayed surgical closure is achieved when the bowel is adequately reduced. This technique prevents the neonate from being exposed to multiple anaesthetics and does not require the baby to be ventilated in NICU. The use of a preformed silo followed by delayed fascial closure in infants with gastroschisis is associated with improved fascial closure rates, fewer ventilator days, more rapid return of bowel function, and fewer complications compared with attempts at initial early repair. It would seem to be a technique ideally suited to use for management of gastroschisis in the developing world.

EDMR-No GA (elective delayed midgut resection – no general anaesthesia) is a novel technique, by Bianchi et al. in 2002, for neonates with poor general condition, significant vital organ anomaly, bowel-to-abdomen disproportion and "at risk" bowel circulation. But the development of distress and progressive metabolic acidosis during and after EDMR-No GA limit its utility and is an indication for urgent conversion to open surgery, to avoid serious bowel injury.

Table 31.1 summarizes the important features of Exomphalos and Gastroschisis.

The goal of surgery is to return the bowel to the abdomen and close the fascia in single surgery. Before repositing the bowel inside the abdomen, it must be inspected for any atretic segments or rotation abnormalities and accordingly managed with resection of atretic or unhealthy segment and anastomosed. Once confirmed that remaining intestine is healthy, the bowel is returned to the abdominal cavity and closure attempted, but this may be associated with increase in intra-abdominal pressure and respiratory compromise (Fig. 31.3).

Table 31.1 Exomphalos (Omphalocele) and Gastroschisis

	Exomphalos (Omphalocele)	Gastroschisis
Incidence	1:3000, M:F::3:2	1:6000–10,000, M:F::3:2, maternal age <20 year
Etiology	Failure of gut to migrate from yolk sac into the abdomen. Herniation within the umbilical cord.	Defect in abdominal wall (usually right side). Umbilical cord normal
Location of the defect and status of viscera	Central defect. Viscera covered with membrane, bowel in condition good, may contain liver. Small abdominal and thoracic cavities, greater pulmonary hypoplasia.	Periumbilical commonly on the right. Exposed gut inflamed, edematous, shortening. May involve stomach, bladder, uterus, liver (rare). Less pulmonary hypoplasia
Associated lesions	Common (70%) - malrotation, intestinal atresia/stenosis, prematurity, cardiac(20%)	Uncommon (15%) - Malrotation, volvulus, poor gut motility, intestinal atresia/stenosis
Association with syndromes	Chromosomal anomalies, Beckwith–Wiedemann syndrome, pentalogy of cantrell, lower midline syndrome	GI atresia (15%) Meckel's diverticulum Intestinal duplication
Management	Elective/semi-urgent surgery unless sac ruptures	Urgency - cover bowel with cellophane, IV fluids, NGT, antibiotics, urgent surgery
Surgery	Single stage for small defect. Staged reduction for large exomphalos	Single stage for small defect. Staged reduction. EDMR No-GA

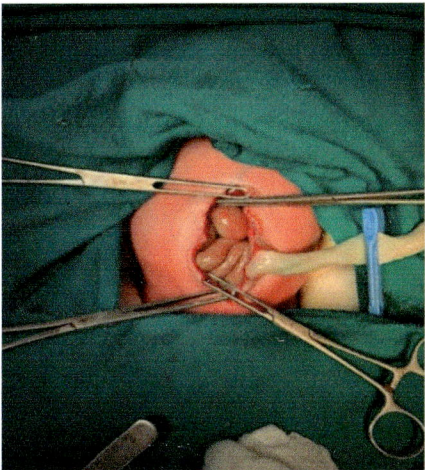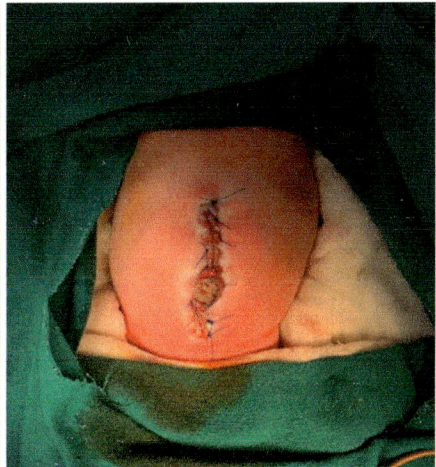

Fig. 31.3 Gastroschisis - abdominal closure

31.7 Anaesthetic Management - Gastroschisis/Exomphalos

31.7.1 Preoperative Assessment

Baby should undergo a detailed preoperative evaluation, as for any procedure in this age group. Besides, assessment should include that pertaining to the abdominal wall defect and surgery:

1. **History** – Gestational age, Birth weight, APGAR, apnea and apneic spell, Vit k and Surfactant administration, present age and weight. Assess for adequacy of transition from intra- to extrauterine life.
2. **Airway** assessment is important because of associated anomalies and syndromes, e.g., macroglossia in Beckwith – Wiedemann syndrome. Some babies may already be intubated. In such a case, check for the ETT size and positioning.
3. **Pulmonary assessment** – in exomphalos major, the abdomen is scaphoid. Respiratory assessment is important as after repositioning of contents and abdominal closure, there is a risk of respiratory compromise. If the baby is already in distress (tachycardia, tachypnoea, retraction, nasal faring, and low sPO$_2$), they will need to be on mechanical ventilation after surgery. Intraoperative care must be taken to adjust the ventilation to maintain normoxia and normocarbia. Make a note of the FiO$_2$, ventilator settings if baby already ventilated and SpO$_2$, so that same may be continued in the OT.
4. **Cardiovascular assessment -** Look for signs of volume deficit (look above). Check HR, pulse volume, capillary refill, and NIBP. If there are signs of hypovolemia or circulatory shock, baby must receive 10 ml/kg fluid boluses, intubated and mechanically ventilated.

5. **Cardiac evaluation** - Look for intracardiac shunts, cardiac defects, and adequacy of transitional changes. An absent femoral pulse may lead to suspicion of coarctation of aorta. Echocardiography and cardiology opinion should be taken.
6. **Associated anomalies** and syndromic findings must be looked for and noted.
7. **Check records** of drug/fluids/feeds/output/daily GC and temperature charting.

31.7.2 Investigations

- CBC, blood grouping, and crossmatch of one paediatric unit of blood.
- Capillary blood gas and acid base status to assess the adequacy of resuscitation and ventilation.
- Chest X-ray.
- Echocardiogram.
- Renal ultrasound, in syndromic neonates.
- Head ultrasound scan to exclude ICH in premature babies.

31.7.3 Readiness for Anesthesia and Surgery

Surgery should be carried out in a OT specialized for neonates, regarding temperature, equipment, drugs, and staff.

- **OT preparation** - Ensure OT temperature is 28–30 °C, warming mattress on the table, availability of heated (36 °C) and humidified inhaled gases and fluids, overhead warming device, cotton wrapped in gauze for covering the head and exposed parts of the baby.
- **Fasting status** – usually these babies are on parenteral nutrition and not allowed oral feeds. But confirm that baby is fasting for 4 h.
- **Premedication** – no sedative premedication is needed. IV atropine can be given at induction. If the baby is already on ventilator and narcotics, they may be supplemented if need be.
- **Plan the anesthesia technique** – general anesthesia with muscle relaxants, tracheal intubation, narcotics and assisted/controlled ventilation is the most suitable technique. Single shot caudal epidural or continuous (via a catheter) is a good option to reduce the dose of relaxants and narcotics, and may improve extubation outcome.
- **Check for consent**, which should include for general anesthesia and baby's condition, blood transfusion, postoperative ventilation, and high risk because of associated anomalies and surgical complications.
- **Trained anaesthesia team** with assistants, technicians, and nurses.
- **Equipment** -check the functioning status of all equipment, syringe infusion pumps, appropriate sizes of laryngoscope and ETT, suction catheters and gastric tubes, and drugs.

- **Monitoring equipment** - Pulse oximetry, ECG, NIBP, $EtCO_2$, esophageal/rectal temperature probes are basic monitoring. Invasive arterial monitoring may be done especially if repeated arterial sampling is indicated. CVP monitoring can be done as often these babies are on TPN via a central line placed in NICU, which can also be used for TPN in the postoperative period. Intra-abdominal pressure monitoring may be needed especially in case of primary closure. This can be done by monitoring intragastric or urinary bladder pressures using a manometer.
- **NGT** aspiration and bowel decompression before induction. It can be removed for induction and reinserted after tracheal intubation.
- Check for **IV access** – an IV line will already be in place in most babies which can be used for induction of anaesthesia. Another IV line (peripheral/central) can be placed appropriately after induction.

31.7.4 Induction on Anesthesia

All **emergency drugs** should be loaded and kept ready in appropriate dilutions, for emergency use, especially atropine, adrenaline, calcium, and saline. Care should be taken to minimize exposure of the baby to cold temperature during shifting from an incubator to the OT table. Attach all monitors (SpO_2, ECG, NIBP, and temperature) while preoxygenating. Before induction, nasogastric tube is aspirated to ensure bowel decompression. Invasive monitoring is not usually required.

In case neonate is already intubated, check for the ETT size and positioning and refix securely, and continue with relaxants narcotic and controlled ventilation.

Modified RSI technique can be used for induction in major exomphalos and gastroschisis repair, using IV (thiopentone 3–4 mg/kg) or inhalational induction(sevoflurane/halothane). Suxamethonium (2 mg/kg) or atracurium (0.5 mg/kg) or rocuronium (0.8–1.2 mg/kg) can be used to facilitate tracheal intubation, with an appropriately sized tracheal tube (usually 3.0–3.5 mm ID). A slight leak should be apparent with airway pressures of 20–25 cmH_2O in order to prevent compression damage to the tracheal mucosa. Correct tracheal tube placement should be confirmed by auscultation of the chest and $EtCO_2$ measurement.

A single shot **caudal epidural** block may be performed to provide analgesia in a volume of 0.75–1 mL/kg of 0.25% L-bupivacaine (keeping the toxic dose in mind). An epidural or caudal catheter requires an experienced anaesthetist but provides very good intra- and post-operative analgesia and has the added benefit of abdominal wall relaxation. Hepatic clearance of local anaesthetics may be reduced if there is any abdominal compression, as well as the epidural spread may be higher.

Anesthesia is **maintained** with O_2, air, and a low concentration of sevoflurane (1–2%). Nitrous oxide should be avoided in order to prevent further bowel distension. Muscle relaxation is maintained with atracurium 0.5 mg/kg. Intraoperative analgesia may be provided by fentanyl 1–2 µg/kg or morphine 20–50 µg/kg if postoperative ventilation is anticipated.

Maintenance **fluid** therapy with isotonic 10% dextrose and 0.18% sodium chloride or RL/ 4.5% albumen/colloid/blood should be continued intraoperatively. third space losses may be significant and require replacement with 10–20 mL/kg boluses of crystalloids or colloids (4.5% albumen). 30–60 mL bolus may be given in case of sudden loss intraoperatively, maintaining hemodynamic parameters. Gastric losses are replaced with normal saline in equal volume. TPN from postoperative day two, TPN should be started until return of gut motility. Assessment for volume status is a continuous process.

Intraoperative **blood glucose** should be maintained within normal range and levels below 3 mmol/L (54 mg%) merit addition of dextrose to IV infusion.

Calculate **allowable blood loss** even before induction of anesthesia. In an anemic neonate, there may be no allowable blood loss. Blood loss must be monitored throughout surgery and PRBC transfused to maintain Hb 10–12 g% (4 mL PRBC > Hb by 1 g%). Generally, blood loss of more than 10% of blood volume (term 80 mL/kg, preterm 90 mL/kg), should be replaced, unlike in adults who have a wider margin. Platelets and FFP are given in aliquots of 10 mL/kg especially if platelet count or coagulation screen is abnormal, and cryoprecipitate (5 mL/kg) if fibrinogen levels are low.

Extubation: Babies with extremely small defects may be extubated successfully at the end of surgery, and reversal of residual neuromuscular blockade must be ensured by administering neostigmine 50 µg/kg and Glycopyrrolate 10 µg/kg after some return of neuromuscular transmission. Extubation should be done only in an awake, active neonate with adequate respiration and stable hemodynamics and saturation.

31.8 Postoperative Care

The great majority of babies who have undergone surgical repair of an abdominal wall defect and having multiple risk factors, such as low birth weight and gestational age, multiple congenital anomalies, and on preoperative respiratory or hemodynamic support, will be returned to NICU intubated and ventilated. **Sedation** is usually provided with morphine 10–20 mg/kg, low dose atracurium/cisatracurium infusion (0.5–1.0 mg/kg/h or 3 mg/kg/min). The duration of **respiratory support** is governed by the return of the bowel to the abdominal cavity which may take up to 10 days. Classically, the contents of the silastic pouch are reduced manually every 12–24 h, in the NICU. In case of preformed, spring-loaded pouches, the bowel is allowed to passively re-enter the abdominal cavity under gravity.

During this period the neonate requires vigilant monitoring for signs of excessive intraabdominal pressure or hemodynamic compromise. Besides this may also cause hypoperfusion of liver, kidneys, intestines, and lower limbs, heralding 'abdominal compartment syndrome.' This necessitates reduction in intra-abdominal pressure. If a primary repair has been performed, the abdomen is re-opened and a silastic pouch formed, and in case this happens after reduction of the pouch contents, then the tension on the pouch must be reduced and portion of bowel allowed to re-herniate.

After complete return of the bowel to the abdomen, the neonate is taken to the OT for surgical closure of the abdominal wall.

Antibiotics should be continued until the silastic pouch is removed.

Feeding - The first enteral feed is commenced once the volume of gastric aspirate has reduced and is non-bilious. Full enteral feeding following gastroschisis repair often takes several weeks until bowel has recovered from damage by exposure to amniotic fluid. Hence, TPN is continued until then.

Fluid management – In the immediate postoperative period, fluids should be restricted to 60% of maintenance, to reduce the cardiac load with increase in abdominal pressure. Only isotonic fluids should be used (10% dextrose or 4% dextrose 0.18% saline). GI losses are replaced with normal saline. Colloids (albumin preferred) are used to replace third space losses. Fluid balance, urine output, and electrolytes must be frequently checked. Daily maintenance fluids are started at 60 mL/kg/day on day 1, and increased by 30 mL/kg/day to reach 150 mL/kg/day by day five.

Blood sugar - Babies within 48 h of birth, especially premature, small for gestational age and those born to diabetic mothers are prone to hypoglycaemia. It is important to measure blood glucose levels regularly and to treat hypoglycaemia with 1–2 mL/kg of 10% glucose, as boluses or as a continuous infusion.

Temperature regulation - Measures to prevent hypothermia must be taken in the postoperative period. Babies should be nursed in a warmed incubator, in lateral position, with the silo/ intestines supported.

Analgesia - Babies on ventilatory support are on fentanyl or morphine therapy. For remaining neonate multimodal analgesia regimen should be adopted, including small doses of IV fentanyl (0.5 µg/kg), and or caudal epidural analgesia using bupivacaine and fentanyl, and paracetamol (10 mg/kg) 6 hourly IV/PR.

31.9 Complications

These can be classified as gastrointestinal or non-gastrointestinal (Table 31.2).

Table 31.2 Complications of exomphalos repair

A. GI complications	Delayed establishment of enteral feeding, NEC, Adhesive intestinal obstruction, TPN-related metabolic derangements, cholestasis GE reflux, Short gut syndrome, Pylorospasm, Abdominal compartment syndrome.
B. non-GI complications	Sepsis, Wound infections, VAP, UTI, IVC compression.

GI complications include prolonged ileus because of gut handling and motility dysfunction, persistent hypotension (low dose dopamine infusion may be needed), necrotising enterocolitis, gastroesophageal reflux and cholestasis. **Non-GI complications** include renal insufficiency, pneumonia, patent ductus arteriosus, and cellulitis or necrosis of the abdominal wall.

"**Abdominal compartment syndrome**" may occur if the abdominal contents are reduced under pressure, particularly in exomphalos major if the abdominal cavity is small. There is splinting and upward shift in the diaphragm interfering with ventilation, decrease in venous return and abdominal organ perfusion. Reduction in renal perfusion can result in oliguria or even anuria, reduced mesenteric blood flow can result in gut necrosis and reduction in liver perfusion. Forceful closure of the abdominal wall will also cause significant tension of the skin resulting in a high incidence of skin necrosis with secondary infection. It is associated with high morbidity and mortality. This is why many centres prefer staged repair especially if high intragastric pressure (>20 mmHg) or high inspiratory pressure (>30 cmH$_2$O) are anticipated after closure.

31.10 Prognosis

Increased morbidity in neonates born out of hospital settings may be related to factors uncontrolled, such as hypothermia, lack of proper care of exposed viscera, dehydration, and injury to the prolapsed gut during transportation. The mortality has decreased dramatically over recent two to three decades due to advances in surgical, neonatal and anesthesia care. In the 1960s, up to 70% of these neonates failed to survive. With improved resuscitative measures, the outcome is now excellent, nearly 90% survival, and vast majority of neonates without associated cardiac or respiratory abnormalities now survive to lead normal adult lives.

31.11 Conclusion

Early antenatal diagnosis and planned delivery improves the chances of survival of babies with large abdominal defects. Preoperative assessment, understanding of the pathophysiological consequences of corrective surgery, basic care during anesthesia and surgery, limiting the duration and extent of surgery, and preferred use of staged approach in case of large defects, can markedly improve postoperative outcome. Fluid management and maintenance of temperature, oxygenation, hemodynamics and nutrition, are of paramount importance in the peri-surgical period until the return of normal bowel movements.

Good communication between the surgeon and the anesthetist is vital during the management of these defects. Overenthusiastic attempts by surgeons to close the defect inevitably can lead to abdominal compartment syndrome, an avoidable life-threatening postoperative complication. Readiness for postoperative ventilation and specialized NICU care is vital in the immediate postoperative period.

Over the past two to three decades, as there has been an increase in these cases because of better diagnostic techniques, so has prognosis has markedly improved, and now parents can be assured of a normal baby who can grow into anormal adult, after surgical repair.

Further Readings

1. Berg S. Paediatric and neonatal anaesthesia. In: Allman K, Wilson I, editors. Oxford handbook of Anaesthesia. 2nd ed. Oxford University Press; 2006. p. 757–93.
2. Bianchi A, Dickson AP, Alizai NK. Elective delayed midgut reduction-no anesthesia for gastroschisis: selection and conversion criteria. J Pediatr Surg. 2002;37(9):1334–6. https://doi.org/10.1053/jpsu.2002.35003; PMID: 12194127.
3. Continuing education in anesthesia, critical care & pain a (Indian ed). 2009; 2:2.
4. Cote C, Lerman J, Todres ID. Practice of anesthesia for infants and children. 4th ed. Philadelphia: Saunders, Elsevier; 2008, ISBN-13: 978-1-4160-3134-5.
5. Gormky SMC, Crean PM. Basic principles of anaesthesia for neonates and infants. BJA CEPD Rev. 2001;1:130–3. https://doi.org/10.1093/bjacepd/1.5.130.
6. Kitchanan S, Patole SK, Muller R, Whitehall JS. Neonatal outcome of gastroschisis and exomphalos: a 10-year review. Published online 30 sept 2008. https://doi.org/10.1046/j.1440-1754.00551.x.
7. Motoyama E. Smith's Anesthesia for infants and children. 8th ed. In: Davis Peter J, Cladis Franklyn P, editors; 2010; eBook ISBN: 9780323081696. Hardcover ISBN: 9780323066129.
8. Pai VK, Dhar M, Singh AP, Kumar AA. Neonate with omphalocele and dextrocardia: anesthetic goals and challenges. J Med sci. 2016;36:81.
9. Wouters K, Walker I. Neonatal anaesthesia 2: anaesthesia for neonates with abdominal wall defects. September 2007. isabeau@isabeau.demon.co.uk.

Anesthesia for Gastrointestinal Surgical Conditions in Neonates

32

Poonam Motiani and Zainab Ahmad

32.1 Introduction

GI-related problems are quite frequent in the newborn baby and neonates suggestive of features of structural malformations, motility disorders, obstruction, and or GI bleeding, as major causes of morbidity, frequently requiring surgical intervention under general anesthesia.

Most common presentation is obstruction. Intestinal Obstruction may be **Mechanical** (IHPS, malrotation, volvulus), **Functional** (meconium ileus, HD) or **Congenital** (web, atresia, stenosis, duplication, annular pancreas, ARM). The classical presentation is vomiting, abdominal distention, poor feeding, and failure to pass meconium within first day of life.

IHPS is gastric outflow tract obstruction due to pyloric smooth muscle hypertrophy forcing food back into the esophagus and vomiting. Most babies present during infancy, but nearly 30% present in the first month of life. **HD** is due to a defect in the development of neural crest resulting in severe constipation and sometimes bowel obstruction. **ARM** has a strong association with other congenital anomalies, especially VACTERL and CHARGE. **Bowel Atresia/Stenosis** can affect any part of the intestine, more common is jejunoileal. **Malrotation** is caused by an aberrant embryological rotation of the midgut with abnormal and narrow fixation and is a common entity. **Volvulus** is caused by twisting of the small bowel around the narrow mesenteric base causing closed loop obstruction and intestinal ischemia. **Anal atresia** involves lack of or incomplete development of the anus often an aberrant or absent anal opening.

P. Motiani (✉)
Pediatric Anesthesia, Super Specialty Pediatric Hospital and Postgraduate Teaching Institute, Noida, Uttar Pradesh, India

Z. Ahmad
Anesthesia and Critical Care, AIIMS, Bhopal, Madhya Pradesh, India

Of all the GI surgical conditions, most common neonatal GI emergency is **NEC**. It is associated with highest mortality and morbidity, particularly in very low birth weight preterm neonates (BW <1500 g, gestational age <32 weeks), with survivors suffering from long-term consequences including poor growth and neurodevelopmental abnormalities. Early recognition and aggressive treatment can improve the outcome.

This chapter will cover the effects on various systems of the GI dysfunction in the neonates and their anesthetic implications, preoperative optimization, and management followed by the anesthetic management of each individual surgical condition.

32.2   Common Congenital GI Abnormalities

Table 32.1 is the listing of the common GI surgical conditions encountered by the anesthesiologist in the newborns and neonates. Their incidences (adjusted to per 1000 live births for easy comparison) in ascending order, are also shown along with gender preference. As can be noticed biliary atresia has the lowest incidence and malrotation, volvulus and IHPS have maximum incidence. Most diseases are more common in males.

Table 32.1 Common congenital GI conditions in neonates

GI abnormality	Incidence (calculated as per 1000 live births)
1. Biliary atresia*	0.01–0.2 (1:5000–1:20,000) F:M 1.25:1
2. Gastroschisis*	0.1–0.2 (1:6000–1:10,000) M: F 3:2
3. Ano rectal malformations (ARM)	0.1–0.2 (1:3000–5000) M>F
4. Hirschsprung's disease (HD)	0.2(1:5000) M:F-5:1(1:100 in Down syndrome)
5. Atresia/stenosis	0.2 (1:5000) M=F
6. Congenital diaphragmatic hernia (CDH)*	0.2–0.5 (1:2000-1:5000) more in males
7. Necrotizing enterocolitis (NEC)	0.3–2.4
8. Exomphalos/Omphalocele*	0.3–0.4 (1:3000) M:F 3:2
9. EA-Tracheo esophageal fistula (TEF)*	0.3–0.4 (1:3000) M:F 25:3
10. Intestinal obstruction	0.6–0.7 (1:1500)
11. Volvulus/malrotation	2
12. Idiopathic hypertrophic pyloric stenosis (IHPS)	2–5

Note: *Biliary atresia, gastroschisis, CDH, omphalocele, EA/TEF- are discussed in separate chapters

32.3   Anesthesia Considerations in Major GI Surgery (Table 32.2)

Table 32.2 Physiological concerns in relation to anesthesia for abdominal surgery

I. Respiratory control and respiratory mechanics

A. Newborns have higher O_2 consumption (5–8 mL/kg/min), low TV (4–6 mL/kg); high RR (40–60/min).

B. Low pulmonary compliance and increased chest wall compliance.

C. At risk of reduction in lung volumes, FRC and development of atelectasis; can be counteracted by low PEEP.

D. Increased risk of airway obstruction and thoracoabdominal asynchrony.

E. Diaphragm: susceptible to fatigue, due to lesser oxidative type I fibers.

F. Hypercarbia stimulates respiration but to a lesser extent than in adults.

G. Hypoxia leads to transient tachypnea, followed by sustained respiratory depression.

H. Neonates including ex-premature infants: at increased risk of postoperative apnea (until 60 wk PCA).

II. Cardiovascular considerations

1. Myocardium
   - Relatively noncompliant.
   - More resistant to hypoxia and ischemia.
   - More dependent on extracellular calcium.
   - Very sensitive to afterload increase.
2. Limited functional reserve, especially early in the neonatal period.
3. Autonomic nervous system - parasympathetic predominates.
4. Changes in preload significantly affect SV and CO.
5. Less response to inotropes.

III. Temperature regulation

1. Unfavorable body surface-to- body weight ratio - increased heat loss.
2. Incapable of shivering thermogenesis.
3. Unique capacity for nonshivering thermogenesis and brown fat metabolism (interscapular area).

Note: All volatile anesthetics inhibit nonshivering thermogenesis, increasing the risk of hypothermia.

IV. Blood volume and fluid balance

1. Higher total body water (neonates: adults: 75%:60%), mainly due to larger ECF (40% vs. 20% in adults).
2. Blood volume larger (85–90 mL/kg) compared to adults (65 mL/kg).
3. Plasma volume fairly constant (50 mL/kg); hematocrit varies due to placenta-to-neonate transfusion at birth.
4. Hugh caloric requirement: 100–150 kcal/kg/24 h.
5. Daily electrolyte requirements: sodium 2.5 mmol/kg, potassium 2.0 mmol/kg, calcium 0.5 mmol/kg.

V. Nociceptive system and stress response

1. Neonates, incl. preterm, have fully operational nociceptive system.
2. Nociceptive stimulation causes negative long-term behavioral changes to subsequent painful stimulation.
3. Undeveloped descending pain inhibitory pathways: neonate more vulnerable to pain stimulation.
4. Lack of proper anesthesia and postoperative analgesia: detrimental neuroendocrine surgical stress response.

I. Respiratory System

Neonates are prone to hypoxemia because of increased O_2 requirement (5–8 mL/kg/min vs. 2–3 mL/kg/min in adults) and reduced reserves (low FRC). Abdominal distention, surgical retraction or replacement of bowel into the abdominal cavity (gastroschisis, omphalocele, CDH), may further reduce lung volumes and reserves. Additionally, preterm neonates may have RDS, surfactant deficiency, and atelectasis.

Apnea is cessation of respiration, may be Central (due to immaturity or depressed respiratory drive), Obstructive (due to loss of airway patency) or Mixed (most common). Due to small size of the airways, the work of breathing in a neonate is comparatively higher which is further increased by the use of an ETT. Preterm neonates are susceptible to apnea (Central), anemia, sepsis, hypothermia, hypoglycemia, and hypocalcemia, but major GI abnormality may make even the term neonates susceptible. There is an increased risk of postoperative apnea, especially in those with postconceptual age (PCA) < 44 wk, which persists up to PCA of 60 wk. The risk is inversely proportional to gestational age, PCA, and hemoglobin concentration. Apnea may also be a result of prolonged action of anesthetics, severe electrolyte and acid base derangement, and respiratory muscle fatigue. Preoperatively, the degree and type of respiratory support, FiO_2, and SpO_2 (pre- and postductal) should be noted.

Safe anesthesia delivery requires optimal ventilation (i.e., without increase in work of breathing), using assisted/controlled ventilation, via an ETT, with adequate inflation pressures, using a circle absorber system, and a judicious plan of extubation/postoperative ventilation.

II. Cardiovascular System (CVS)

The gas exchange during intrauterine life is a function of the placenta. At birth, the lungs expand, PVR (Pulmonary Vascular Resistance) falls, and SVR (Systemic vascular resistance) rises, causing closure of ductus arteriosus and foramen ovale, with establishment of and neonatal circulation. Conditions that increase PVR (stress, pain, hypothermia, hypoxemia, hypercarbia, acidosis, high inflating airway pressures) may cause reversal of these shunts and persistent fetal circulation (PFC), leading to severe hypoxemia in the perioperative period.

Maintenance of blood pressure (BP) in a neonate, requires maintenance of cardiac output (CO) via heart rate (HR) as they have a fixed stroke volume (SV), due to a poorly compliant myocardium. The myocardium is more resistant to hypoxia and ischemia; however, its response to inotropes is poor, and any increase in afterload is not well tolerated. Further, large arteries, due to incomplete sympathetic innervation, are unable to fully contract in response to hypovolemia. Hence, knowledge of the CVS condition at birth is as important as the history of the current status, including degree of CVS decompensation, fluid resuscitation, use of inotropes, and choice of sites for invasive monitoring. The cardiovascular system should be examined thoroughly particularly focusing on volume status by noting HR, BP, capillary refill, core/peripheral temperature, and urine output. Presence of metabolic acidosis indicates continued poor perfusion and also dead or critically ischemic gut.

Sepsis-induced decompensation may also cause derangement of coagulation and necessitate transfusion of packed cells, clotting factors, or platelets.

Babies who do not respond to fluid resuscitation should undergo echocardiography for evaluation of the cardiac status. Some neonatal GI units recommend inotropes at mean arterial pressure (MAP) <30 mm Hg, while others recommend when there are signs of poor perfusion regardless of MAP. Choice of inotrope depends on the clinical condition. There should be no hesitation in starting inotropes preoperatively, especially if the CVS decompensation is anticipated, as it is easier to increase the rate of an infusion of an already in progress than to commence one after the onset of a critical event.

For surgeries involving major fluid shifts and in hemodynamically unstable neonates, intra-arterial catheters should be placed for invasive BP monitoring, arterial blood gases, and metabolic status. Adequate venous access, in the form of two peripheral cannulae, preferably sited in the upper limbs and well secured, should be ensured preoperatively. Peripherally inserted central catheters (PICC lines) are usually used for large fluid boluses in extenuating circumstances. Decompensated neonates may merit transfer to a unit with neonatal cardiological expertize.

III. Temperature Regulation

Neonates are extremely susceptible to hypothermia due to large body surface area to weight ratio, thin skin, decreased body fat, and inability to shiver. The nonshivering thermogenesis that generates heat, is hampered by anesthetics. The consequences of hypothermia include pulmonary hypertension, delayed drug metabolism, hypoxemia, and apnea. Use of warm humidified inspired gases, warm antiseptic solutions, warm irrigating fluids, warm blood and IV fluids, heated mattress, radiant warmer, convective air warmers, all assist in maintaining normal body temperature. Care should be taken during transport.

IV. Fluid and Electrolyte Management

In neonates, increased insensible fluid losses may occur in the OT. In conditions such as gastroschisis and omphalocele, due to exposure of large mucosal surfaces, insensible losses are markedly increased. Anesthetic drugs mask subtle CVS responses secondary to hypovolemia. Renal immaturity, effect of neuroendocrine surgical stress response, and variable body fluid composition, make accurate administration of fluids to maintain circulating volume a challenging task. Conversely, overzealous fluid administration can lead to overloading and worsen third spacing.

Glycogen stores do not develop in the fetus till late gestation, hence preterm, small for gestational age (SGA), excessive fasting duration, babies of diabetic mothers, and those on TPN, are prone to hypoglycemia. Glucose infusion @ 8–10 mg/kg/min in preterms and 5–8 mg/kg/min in term neonates prevents hypoglycemia during the nil per oral period. Blood glucose should be maintained between 3 and 11 mmol/L (54–198 mg/dL).

Maintenance fluid rate: Hypotonic glucose solution (D10 in water or 0.2% NS) @ 4 mL/kg/h.

Replacement fluids (for insensible (third space)/small volume blood loss): Isotonic fluid @ 3–10 mL/kg/h.

Critically ill neonates are particularly susceptible to hypocalcemia due to parathormone (PTH) deficiency, parathyroid resistance, and inadequate calcium supplementation. Serum Ca+ <1 mmol/L (4 mg/dL) in term and <0.75 mmol/L (3 mg/dL) in preterm neonates is defined as Neonatal hypocalcemia. Symptomatic hypocalcemia is treated with slow IV Calcium Gluconate @ 100 mg/kg, followed by 100–200 mg/kg/day for maintenance (1 mg/dL = 0.25 mmol/L or 0.5 mEq/L).

V. Neurologic Development

Immaturity of the brain and its blood vessels, especially in the preterm, increases the risk of intraventricular hemorrhage (IVH) in the neonatal period. BP fluctuations, hypoxia, hypercarbia, and pain increase this risk. "Awake laryngoscopy and intubation" raise the same concerns. Repeated or prolonged use of general anesthetics (isoflurane, N2O), and sedatives (ketamine, midazolam), may be associated with negative effects on the developing brain. Hyperoxia is associated with ROP. Though optimal SpO_2 is not defined, a preductal saturation of 91–95% is considered appropriate.

32.4   Anesthestic Management

32.4.1 Preoperative Assessment

A detailed evaluation including history and examination, focusing on identifying risk-associated conditions which would forewarn the anesthetist and/or allow for optimization of the neonate should be done. Also, airway difficulties should be ruled out as many congenital conditions may have an associated difficult airway. Other details regarding pregnancy, delivery, birth weight, Apgar scores, PCA, and gestational age should be obtained.

Investigations: A preoperative Hb, Hct, blood typing, and compatibility screening, should be performed in all neonates scheduled for major GI surgery. Repeat laparotomies can be notoriously bloody due to adhesions compounded by coagulopathy. Keeping a close watch on blood loss and ensuring availability of packed cells, platelets, and fresh-frozen plasma (FFP) are paramount.

- **Hemoglobin (Hb):** Neonates have higher Hb values (17–24 g/dL) compared to adults, and baseline value decides when to commence blood preoperative transfusion. Goal should be to maintain the Hb within normal range, and for this reason, in an already anemic neonate the criterion used in adults may not be appropriate and even 10–15% blood loss may need to be replaced. However, because of the risks associated with blood transfusion, many neonatal anesthesiologists follow restricted blood transfusion policy.

- **Coagulation**: In term neonates, platelet counts are similar to adults (250–300 × 109/L), while in preterm babies, levels are lower (50–150 × 109/L). Platelet function is usually preserved despite low counts, except in sepsis. Vitamin K administration should be ensured.
- **Cross-match**: Packed red cells (PRBC), FFP, and platelets—Ensure availability as per need.
- **Electrolytes and Blood Gas**: A formal laboratory analysis is preferable for electrolytes; Arterial blood gases help to assess respiratory function and shunt; Capillary blood gases can assess pH, bicarbonate, base excess, and glucose. If possible, all deviations should be corrected preoperatively.
- **ECHO and Chest X-ray**: On a case-to-case basis.

32.4.2 Perioperative Management

General principles and recommendations for conduct during the perioperative period, for GI surgeries in the newborn and neonate, are outlined in Box 32.1.

Box 32.1: Recommendations for Conduct of Anesthesia for GI Surgery in a Neonate

- Preoperative evaluation; Concerned Specialist consultation, if required.
- Consider Anticholinergic; Sedative premedication +/-
- Discuss the plan of anesthesia with surgeons and parents, including postoperative ventilation, if anticipated.
- Written, informed consent.
- Ensure presence of a trained anesthesia assistant and technical and nursing staff.
- Prepare appropriate equipment including airway equipment (e.g., 3–3.5 ETT for a term neonate, 2.5 ETT for preterm; Straight Blade Laryngoscope#1, Infant face mask and Oral airway, breathing circuit, etc).
- Ensure availability of Anesthesia delivery system, blood and fluid administration, fluid and patient warming devices.
- Ensure availability of all drugs, including emergency drugs and fluids, in appropriate doses.
- Ensure availability of blood and blood products.
- Prevent hypothermia.
- Ensure minimum monitoring: ECG, NIBP, Saturation, EtCO$_2$, temperature monitoring.
- Invasive monitoring—Consider intra-arterial, CVP monitoring in select cases.
- Check adequacy of IV access. Place a second line after induction, if required.
- Ensure access to a peripheral pulse and a body part (to test capillary refill).
- Meticulous assessment of blood loss during surgery.
- Provide good intraoperative analgesia and Plan for postoperative pain relief.

Infrequently, if the neonate is too unstable to transfer to the OT or is ECMO-dependent, a decision to operate in the NICU may be taken. This requires meticulous preparation by a flexible and experienced multidisciplinary team to deal with issues such as inadequate space, lighting, equipment, and technique modification.

Preoxygenation: Standard preoxygenation though difficult to perform, is still recommended in neonates. The median time to achieve an end-tidal oxygen concentration of 90% using a tight-fitting mask @ 6 L/min O_2 flow is 40 s. Preoxygenation for 60 s is recommended in neonates and children under 5 years of age. However, desaturation (SpO_2 <90%) may still occur, following prolonged periods of apnea (80–90 s) in neonates, even after 2 min of preoxygenation with 100% O_2, following anesthesia induction and muscle relaxation.

32.4.3 Induction of Anesthesia

Most neonates planned for a laparotomy have a nasogastric tube (NGT) in situ, and decompression before induction is recommended along with the use of a modified RSI, with intravenous induction and neuromuscular blockade followed by gentle mask ventilation before the initial intubation attempt. IV or inhalation induction, or a combination, can be used safely.

32.4.4 Airway Management

Maintaining and securing the airway is very important in babies undergoing GI surgeries, especially if there is risk of regurgitation of the gastric or GI contents, during manipulation, as in obstructive diseases. Tracheal intubation is the safest and effective method for securing the airway, using either a nondepolarizing (e.g., atracurium) or depolarizing neuromuscular blocking agent, succinylcholine. Neonates, though more sensitive to the effects of nondepolarizing muscle relaxants, due to a higher volume of distribution, have a dosing similar to adults.

32.4.5 Ventilation Strategy

Controlled ventilation can be challenging in neonates undergoing laparotomy, especially as the anesthesia ventilators lack the sophistication of NICU ventilators. Moreover, use of surgical retractors, limited access and visibility of the baby's chest intraoperatively, and detrimental effects of anesthesia on pulmonary vascular mechanics, compound the problem. Ideally, ventilation should maintain an adequate and consistent tidal volume at low airway pressures, ensure oxygenation, and minimize the risk of barotrauma and intracerebral bleeds. PCV (pressure-controlled ventilation) with adequate paralysis and at high frequency reduces the risk of ventilator asynchrony, reducing the risk of barotrauma. Low PEEP helps to prevent collapse of smaller airways and atelectasis. The adequacy of ventilation in neonates is difficult to measure as $EtCO_2$ does not produce a clear square trace, mirroring alveolar CO_2, as in adults, because of relatively large dead space. Arterial or even capillary gases may help guide the anesthetist to optimize ventilation. The desired SpO_2 should be in the mid-90s. Hyperoxia should be avoided to reduce the risk of ROP and BPD in preterm neonates.

32.4.6 Cardiovascular Stability and Fluid Therapy

Most neonates presenting for a laparotomy are already on maintenance IV fluids, and continuing the same regime is recommended along with periodic blood capillary glucose measurements.

Ongoing losses can be divided into insensible loss and blood loss. It is quite feasible for a neonate undergoing laparotomy to lose 8–10 mL kg^{-1} h^{-1} through evaporation and this should be replaced using warmed lactated Ringer solution. Constant vigilance of cardiovascular status (HR, BP, capillary refill, core temperature) is required to guide the fluid administration. Decision-making for PRBC administration is more difficult, as there is no consensus on appropriate transfusion triggers and volume to be transfused. Total blood volume should be estimated before surgery (Table 32.2). Initial Hb, Hct, gestational age, and co-morbidities are important factors in blood transfusion decision-making. Weighing swabs and measuring suction loss may be used to estimate blood loss. In sick neonates, many anesthesiologists consider transfusion at 10% of total blood loss depending on initial Hb, comorbidities, and the surgical procedure. In the smallest babies, this may be 15 mL or less. In very small neonates, it is safer to use syringe infusion pumps rather than IV infusion sets to accurately transfuse fluids and blood, and avoid volume overload.

32.5 Postoperative Care

A multimodal approach to postoperative analgesia is required. Regional analgesia in the form of a caudal or lumbar epidural provides excellent intra- and postoperative analgesia, but may not be appropriate in the presence of intra-abdominal sepsis; IV / rectal paracetamol may be used. The total dose of local anesthetics, opioids, and paracetamol, should be titrated carefully, as neonates lack mature liver enzymes for the efficient metabolism of drugs.

32.6 Anesthetic Consideration for Individual Surgical Conditions – NEC, IHPS, Hirschsprung's Disease, ARM, Intestinal Obstruction. *Biliary Atresia, Gastroschisis, CDH, Omphalocele, EA/TEF- are Discussed in Separate Chapters*

32.6.1 Necrotizing Enterocolitis (NEC)

One of the commonest neonatal gastrointestinal emergencies, NEC, is associated with a high mortality and morbidity, particularly in very low birth weight (VLBW)

Fig. 32.1 Distended abdomen in a neonate with necrotizing enterocolitis

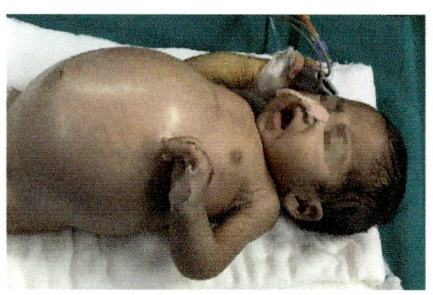

preterm infants (BW <1500 g and gestational age [GA] <32 weeks). The incidence is 0.3–2.4/1000 live births (USA). It is called "**the disease of survivors**" as it characteristically affects preterm neonates, who are also dealing with other life-threatening complications such as RDS, IVH, ROP, and congenital cardiac anomalies. It is characterized by ischemic necrosis of the intestinal mucosa, invasion of enteric gas-forming organisms, and dissection of gas into the intestinal wall and portal venous system. Early recognition and aggressive treatment may improve outcome.

32.6.1.1 Clinical Presentation

Affected neonates usually present with poor feeding, lethargy, vomiting, bloody diarrhea, respiratory distress, shock, and body temperature instability, usually within 3–10 days of birth, usually preterm. Examination may reveal a distended, tender abdomen (Fig. 32.1). Typically, NEC develops after the first enteral feed when the intestinal lumen becomes colonized with bacteria. With fulminant disease, it rapidly progresses to septic shock with hemodynamic instability.

Predisposing Factors: These include prematurity, gut ischemia, immature immune system, infection, and hyperosmotic enteral feeds.

32.6.1.2 Pathophysiology

The pathophysiology of NEC is poorly understood. Predisposing risk factors for ischemic bowel injury in NEC are perinatal asphyxia, umbilical artery cannulation, polycythemia, exchange blood transfusion, RDS, and cyanotic congenital heart disease. Indomethacin, commonly used for pharmacological closure of PDA, has also been implicated. Intraluminal fermentation of undigested lactose from milk feeds, by the normal or pathogenic gut flora, leads to gas production (raising intra-abdominal pressure), decreased gut perfusion, and subsequently intestinal intracellular acidosis. Gas in the intestinal wall (pneumatosis intestinalis) (Fig. 32.2), hepatobiliary tract or portal venous system, on radiography, is pathognomonic of NEC. If bowel perforation occurs, free gas under diaphragm is seen.

Radiological and laboratory tests aid in the diagnosis of NEC:

Fig. 32.2 Pneumatosis
intestinalis on chest x-ray
in a neonate with NEC

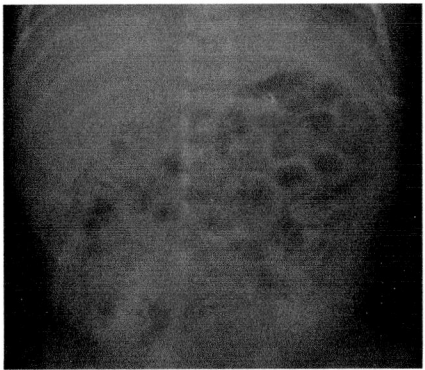

(i) Plain X-rays in supine may determine free intraperitoneal air, dilated bowel
loops, ascites, along with pneumatosis intestinalis.

(ii) Ultrasound with Doppler (demonstrating the absence of mesenteric blood flow)
confirms the presence of necrotic bowel and portal venous gas.

Laboratory findings, of sepsis, thrombocytopenia, neutropenia, metabolic acidosis, and coagulopathy, though not diagnostic on their own, help to support the diagnosis of NEC.

Differential diagnosis includes Congenital bowel strictures/perforation, malrotation, intussusception, pseudomembranous colitis, meconium ileus, and hemorrhagic disease of the newborn.

32.6.1.3 Management

On the basis of the severity of illness, signs and symptoms, laboratory and radiological investigations, NEC is classified using modified Bell staging criteria (1978),
into three stages, which though not distinct, help to define various management
strategies.

I. **Stage I**: Mild disease; Nonspecific symptoms (vomiting, apnea, bradycardia /
tachycardia, and guaiac-positive stools); No definitive radiologic evidence.
Management: Supportive.

II. **Stage II:** Definitive NEC; clinical symptoms as in Stage I; definitive radiological evidence present. Radiographs document pneumatosis intestinalis or portal
venous air. **Management**: Supportive; Those who fail to respond may need
surgical intervention.

III. **Stage III:** Advanced disease, with evidence of intestinal necrosis/ perforation,
signs of hemodynamic, respiratory, and hematologic instability. **Management:**
Surgical intervention.

Walsh and Kleigman (1986) expanded the classification, but the primary framework of suspected, definite, and advanced disease persists.

Medical management includes supportive care and discontinuation of enteral feeding, gastric decompression with intermittent NGT Suction, TPN, judicious fluid replacement, PRBC, FFP, Platelet concentrate to correct anemia and coagulation abnormalities, cardiovascular and respiratory support (as required), and empiric antibiotic therapy (to be initiated after obtaining blood/stool cultures). If pneumoperitoneum occurs, adequate anaerobic antibiotic cover should also be ensured. Serial examinations, laboratory and radiologic monitoring are done to monitor the course of the disease. If disease progresses, surgical intervention is required, in 20–40% babies.

Surgical Management

Surgical intervention is indicated by the presence of bowel perforation, gangrenous bowel, and pneumoperitoneum (Absolute Indications) and also by laboratory findings of severe, persistent hematological derangements and the radiological signs of generalized intestinal distension (Relative Indications) (Table 32.3).

The main surgical procedures performed are:

I. **Primary Peritoneal Drainage**: Usually done bedside, under local anesthesia, to provide pressure relief by evacuation of some air and stool contaminated ascites. This also allows some bowel to recover before resection of nonviable bowel. This is a preferred procedure in sick and extremely low birth weight neonates.

II. **Laparotomy**: Involves resection of the affected bowel segment and exteriorization of a proximal enterostomy (usually ileostomy). Re-anastomosis, is usually required, 4–6 weeks later. If a short segment of bowel is affected, limited resection and primary anastomosis is done to avoid ileostomy and its associated complications. Ileostomy-related problems include fluid and electrolyte abnormalities, delayed resumption of oral feeding, poor growth, enterostomy site stenosis, and a second surgical procedure for re-anastomosis.

Table 32.3 Indications for surgery in NEC

Absolute indications	Relative indications
1. Pneumoperitoneum	1. Clinical deterioration
2. Intestinal gangrene	2. Metabolic acidosis
	3. Ventilatory failure
	4. Hypovolemia, oliguria
	5. Thrombocytopenia, leukopenia, leucocytosis
	6. Portal vein gas
	7. Generalized intestinal distention (radiography)
	8. Erythema of abdominal wall
	9. Fixed abdominal mass

The cardinal principle of surgery is to excise all necrotic bowel while preserving maximum healthy bowel length. This may require multiple segmental resections and second-look operation to reassess bowel viability. A few patients may tolerate resection and primary re-anastomosis. Enterostomies are closed 4 weeks to 6 months after the initial surgery.

32.6.1.4 Anesthetic Management of NEC

All neonates with NEC should be optimized before surgery; however, a critically ill neonate may require life-saving surgery while resuscitation is in progress, in the NICU itself. This option, however, should only be considered in extreme circumstances. A very unstable patient with NEC, for example, requiring high-frequency jet ventilation might necessitate the urgent surgical intervention, such as insertion of an abdominal drain, in the NICU itself. This option, however, should only be considered in extreme circumstances, as sterility of the surgical field may be compromised. Subsequent operative procedures can be carried out in the operating theater, after stabilization of the baby.

(i). Preoperative Evaluation

A detailed history and physical examination should include gestational age, significant events at birth (asphyxia, meconium aspiration, Apgar score), ventilatory support, evaluation of metabolic and hydration status, and co-existing diseases. Anemia, thrombocytopenia, and coagulopathy are quite common. Judicious colloid and crystalloid therapy is needed in hypovolemic babies with massive third space losses, bleeding, and DIC. Exaggerated electrolyte disturbances and acidosis may occur due to acute renal failure (ARF), secondary to shock or abdominal compartment syndrome. As abdominal distention and/or metabolic and respiratory acidosis worsen, respiratory support needs to be increased. Preoperative assessment focuses on evaluating and correcting the respiratory, circulatory, metabolic, and hematological disturbances. Preoperative preparation includes a discussion with parents regarding the plan of conduct of anesthesia, informed risk consent, pain relief, postoperative monitoring, blood transfusion, invasive monitoring, and admission to intensive care unit (ICU).

(ii). Intraoperative Management

Intraoperative monitoring includes in addition to minimum monitoring, invasive blood pressure (IBP), and central venous pressure (CVP) monitoring. Invasive monitoring is not done routinely and is reserved for critically ill and unstable neonates.

Optimal intraoperative monitoring includes pulse oximetry (SpO_2), capnography ($EtCO_2$), noninvasive blood pressure monitoring (NIBP), electrocardiography (ECG), and temperature monitoring (esophageal/rectal probe). A 5Fr feeding tube is used for bladder catheterization and monitoring of urine output. In the critically ill (hypotension, shock, on vasopressors, coagulopathy), an arterial cannula is placed for IBP monitoring and to facilitate samples for arterial blood gas and metabolic analysis. A peripheral and a central catheter is placed for fluid, PRBC, FFP, and platelet transfusion. Commonly 22/24 G are the largest IV catheters that can be inserted peripherally.

Neonates are extremely susceptible to hypothermia. The consequences of hypothermia include pulmonary hypertension, delayed drug metabolism, hypoxia, and apnea. Use of warm humidified inspired gases, warm antiseptic solution, warm irrigating fluids, warm blood and intravenous (IV) fluids, heated mattress, radiant warmer, convective air warmers, all help in maintaining normal body temperature. Care should also be taken to transport them in a heated module.

(iii). Intraoperative Fluid and Electrolyte Management

- **Maintenance fluid** consists of Hypotonic glucose solution (D_{10} in water or 0.2% NS) @ 4 mL/kg/h.
- **Replacement fluid** (for insensible (third space) and small volume blood loss): Isotonic fluid is usually administered at 3–10 mL/kg/h.
- Vigorous fluid therapy to compensate for losses from necrotic bowel during open laparotomy.
- Inotropes to maintain hemodynamic parameters and to avoid massive IV fluid therapy.

Response to fluid therapy is monitored by variations in HR, BP, CVP, and urine output.

Large fluid requirements secondary to exposed bowel/peritoneal cavity during open abdominal surgery, may lead to hypothermia, complicating intraoperative care.

Blood glucose should be monitored at regular hourly intervals, intraoperatively. Hypoglycemia is defined as blood glucose less than 45 mg/dL in the first 3 days of life and below 75 mg/dL thereafter. Further, glucose intolerance may accompany sepsis.

FiO_2 should be adjusted to produce an SpO_2 of 90% - 95%. N2O is avoided in the presence of air in the intestines and portal venous system.

An IV anesthetic, narcotic, and nondepolarizing muscle relaxant-based anesthesia via an infusion pump is preferred to inhalational induction in sick neonates.

32.6.1.5 Postoperative Management

Postoperatively, mechanical ventilation and cardiovascular support are universally required in these babies. Parenteral nutrition is essential after sepsis control and metabolic stabilization The perioperative anesthetic management is summarized in Table 32.4.

32.6.1.6 Outcome

The mortality from NEC has decreased from 80% to 20% over the last three decades due to early recognition and diagnosis and better intensive care. But morbidity is still high (10–30%) related to post-NEC complications, particularly intestinal stricture 10–40%, and short gut syndrome (if more than 70% of small bowel is resected). The preservations of the terminal ileum and ileocecal valve are important surgical considerations for survival.

Table 32.4 Summary of anesthetic management for NEC

Preoperative	Intraoperative	Postoperative
1. Optimize hemodynamic and coagulation status	1. Standard monitoring, IBP, CVP	1. Mechanical ventilation
2. Blood product availability ensured	2. Maintain hemodynamic stability	2. Sedation
3. ETT, if required	3. Consider inotropes—dopamine/epinephrine	3. Analgesia
4. Know acceptable hemodynamic parameters (BP, FiO_2)	4. Prefer opioids to inhaled anesthetics	4. TPN
5. Adequate venous access	5. Neuromuscular paralysis	
	6. Check glucose levels and electrolytes	
	7. Fluid resuscitation	
	8. Blood products—PRBC, FFP, cryoprecipitate	
	9. Temperature homeostasis	

Prevention - Feeding exclusively with human milk and conservative enteral feeding practices, especially in high-risk infants, can reduce the incidence of NEC; however, antenatal steroids, IgA and arginine supplementation, erythropoietin, oral antibiotics, and probiotics have been used to prevent the disease, with questionable efficacy though.

32.6.2 Congenital/Infantile Hypertrophic Pyloric Stenosis (IHPS)

IHPS is an outflow tract obstruction of the gastric antrum. Pylorus in Greek means gatekeeper. IHPS occurs due to smooth muscle hypertrophy and hyperplasia of the gastric pylorus, thus causing obstruction to the forward motion of the peristaltic wave. It is the most common surgical cause of vomiting and the most common cause of gastric outlet obstruction in small babies.

32.6.2.1 Epidemiology and Etiology
It manifests in the first year of life. About 30% patients present in the first month itself. Usual presentation is between 3 and 12 weeks of age.

Etiology: Exact etiology is unknown. Both genetic and environmental factors are implicated which indicates multifactorial etiology. There is a male preponderance with M:F::4–6:1. Annual incidence is approximately 2–5 per 1000 live births. Risk factors include maternal (Caucasian origin, young age, history of smoking, first order birth) and patient (macrolide antibiotics, bottle feeding, hypertonic feeds, prematurity, operative delivery).

32.6.2.2 Pathophysiology
There is hypertrophy and hyperplasia of both the circular and longitudinal smooth muscle of the pylorus, causing luminal narrowing and elongation of the pylorus. Peristalsis fails to get conducted beyond the pylorus. This results in gastric outlet obstruction along with gross distention and retrograde peristalsis (Fig. 32.3).

Fig. 32.3 IHPS—anatomy

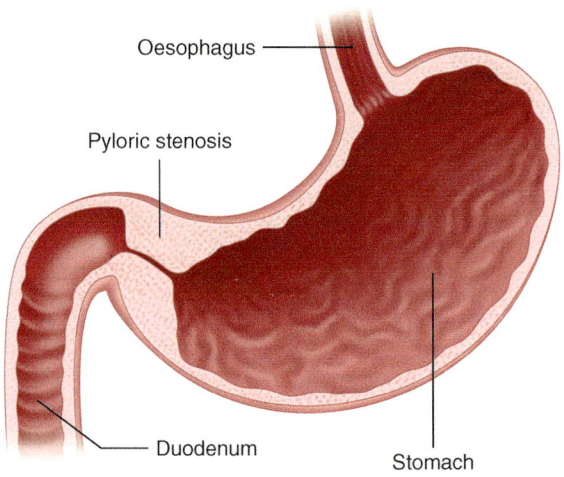

32.6.2.3 Presentation

Usual presentation is of a previously healthy baby presenting with projectile/forceful, nonbilious, nonbloody vomiting, typically after feeds. Baby is immediately hungry (**Hungry Vomiter**). Baby may present with dehydration, electrolyte, and acid-base imbalance as well as weight loss particularly if diagnosis or presentation is delayed. On abdominal examination, a firm and nontender "**olive**" (**palpable thickened pylorus**) may be present in the epigastric region. Visible peristaltic waves may be present. Most common acid base abnormality is a hypochloremic hypokalemic metabolic alkalosis caused by excessive loss of gastric hydrochloric acid in the vomitus (**Contraction alkalosis**). There is net increase in HCO_3^- which overwhelms the absorptive capacity of the renal tubules. Initially the kidneys try to compensate and preserve H^+ ions by alkalinizing the urine by exchanging H^+ ions inside the renal tubule with Na^+ and K^+ to maintain serum pH. Persistent vomiting causes contraction of extracellular volume. The kidneys are forced to preserve ECF volume (by preserving Na^+) in preference to pH due to aldosterone secretion. This causes excretion of acidic urine despite severe metabolic alkalosis termed as paradoxical aciduria. Cl^- reabsorption in exchange of HCO_3^- does not occur with nonresolving alkalosis because of Cl^- depletion. Hypernatremia may be present in patients with long duration of symptoms (3 weeks). Dehydration may be severe enough to cause hypovolemic shock and prerenal AKI. Metabolic acidosis may be paradoxically present. Babies nowadays present with less classic symptoms and signs due to early presentation and diagnosis.

   Diagnosis in neonates is based on clinical presentation, imaging, and sonography. History and clinical examination are diagnostic. It can be confirmed on **Ultrasound**, which is reliable, highly sensitive, and specific. Pyloric wall thickness >3 mm or pyloric channel length >15 mm along with gastric distention confirm the diagnosis. Other investigations as X-Ray abdomen and Barium swallow are reserved for older infants. Unconjugated hyperbilirubinemia may be present (nutritional/dehydration) which is known as **icteropyloric syndrome,** and if associated with elevated conjugated bilirubin, ALT, or AST, underlying liver disease may be present. Other investigations required are CBC, KFT, serum electrolytes, and ABG.

Differential Diagnosis: Pylorospasm, gastroesophageal reflux, and intestinal obstruction should be considered in babies presenting with bilious vomiting, abdominal distention or bloody stools.

32.6.2.4 Management

(i). Medical Management:
It is not a surgical emergency but is a medical emergency. Preoperative management centers toward assessment and optimization of hydration, electrolyte, and acid base status which may take 24–48 h for stabilization. Mucus membranes, tearing, skin turgor, capillary refill time, and fontanelles must be examined for the degree of dehydration.

A NGT is inserted to relieve gastric distention and the baby is kept NPO. IV hydration with Cl containing fluids is started. Goals of resuscitation and fluid therapy in neonates with mild, moderate and severe dehydration are outlined in the Table 32.5. Strict Input/Output charting should be maintained. Serial blood sugar, electrolytes, and ABG should be monitored.

(ii). Surgical Management:
Surgery is undertaken only after optimization. Corrective surgery performed is **Ramstedt pyloromyotomy** (Fig. 32.4), by open or laparoscopic approach. The

Table 32.5 Resuscitation in IHPS

Goals of resuscitation—pH 7.35–7.45, Base excess >3.5, Bicarbonate 28–30 mmol/L, Sodium > 132 mmol/L, Potassium > 3.5 mmol/L, Chloride > 100 mmol/L, glucose > 40 mg/dL	
No/mild dehydration (Deficit <5% body weight)	**Moderate/severe dehydration (>10% deficit)**
D5 with 0.45% NaCl @ 1.5 times maintenance rate KCl 1–2 meq/100 mL IVF once urination established. Gastric drainage replaced with NS 1:1	NS bolus 20 mL/kg over 30 min Same regimen as for mild dehydration **BUT** @ 1.5–2 times the maintenance rate Extra NS bolus as required per degree of dehydration

Fig. 32.4 Ramstedt pyloromyotomy

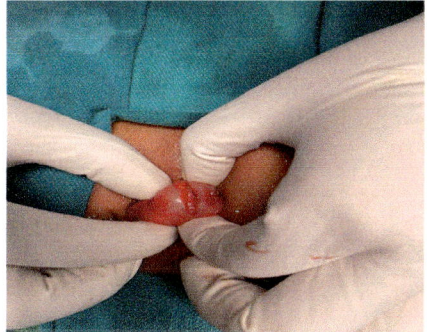

muscle of the pylorus is incised longitudinally to the submucosa, which relieves the obstruction and allows the normal conduction of peristalsis. Laparoscopic approach has the advantage of early recovery, less pain, and faster bowel recovery. However, there is a risk of incomplete incision (pyloromyotomy) with this approach.

32.6.2.5 Anesthetic Management
(i). Perioperative Considerations
1. Usual neonatal anesthesia considerations especially temperature, cardiovascular, and respiratory considerations.
2. Fluid and electrolyte imbalance must be corrected prior to surgery.
3. Full stomach and attendant risk of aspiration due to gastric outlet obstruction.
4. Persistent CSF alkalosis even if ABG picture improves, increases the risk of postoperative apnea.

(ii). Perioperative Management
After adequate resuscitation, baby is taken up for surgery. A wide bore (at least 10F) NGT is inserted if not already present. Thorough gastric suction in the right and left lateral, supine and prone positions is recommended to thoroughly empty the stomach. The NGT should be removed and reinserted after intubation to reduce difficulty in mask ventilation at induction.

A modified RSI is recommended. Very good airway skills are required, as tolerance of loss of mask ventilation or time for adjustment of mask or apnea is poor. Many anesthesiologists use an inhalational induction too, which offers the advantage of slow controlled induction and better airway maintenance. Intubation in awake or under sedation is preferred by some but has the risk of trauma, breath holding, bronchospasm, laryngospasm, regurgitation, and aspiration. IV Atropine is administered just prior to induction of anesthesia. After preoxygenation, mRSI with IV Propofol (2–3 mg/kg) or Etomidate (0.2–0.3 mg/kg) followed by succinylcholine (2 mg/kg) is done. Often after intubation with succinylcholine followed by nondepolarizing relaxant during maintenance, causes delayed recovery from anesthesia, as surgery is short lasting. Rocuronium in a low dose (0.3 mg/kg) may be used as an alternative for intubation and maintenance. Cricoid pressure is controversial as it can cause difficulty during intubation by distorting the larynx and is unproven to prevent aspiration. Gentle manual ventilation with low peak inspiratory pressure is continued due to risk of fast desaturation. Intubation is carried out only when the baby is completely paralyzed because attempts in a struggling baby may cause aspiration.

Maintenance of anesthesia is with volatile agents. Sevoflurane or Desflurane are preferred for faster wake up times and reduced risk of postoperative apnea. N_2O can be used. Opioids and hypocarbia are avoided. Standard noninvasive monitoring and maintenance fluids suffice in adequately resuscitated babies.

It is important to check for mucosal integrity after making the incision in the pyloric mucosa and before closure of abdomen. This is done by injecting air through the NGT.

Local infiltration, IV (7.5 mg/kg maximum 60 mg/kg in 24 h) or rectal (30–40 mg/kg) paracetamol, Rectus sheath block are the common options for postoperative pain relief.

Extubation is carried out in the lateral position when the baby is fully awake and active (Box 32.2).

Postoperatively, they are watched for apnea and hypoglycemia. Otherwise, the recovery and prognosis are generally good.

Box 32.2: IHPS—Summary of Perioperative Management
1. Standard neonatal care, focus on temperature, glucose homeostasis, hemodynamics, and oxygenation.
2. Preoperative optimization.
3. No premedication, only IV atropine.
4. 4 quadrant NGT suction immediately before induction of anesthesia.
5. Standard noninvasive monitoring.
6. Preoxygenation, mRSI, intubation.
7. Maintenance with Sevoflurane/Desflurane, N_2O, O–. Avoid opioids.
8. Pain management—IV or rectal paracetamol, local infiltration, rectus sheath block.
9. Extubation when fully awake and vigorous.

32.6.3 Congenital Aganglionic Colon (Hirschsprung's Disease) (HD)

This is classified as a neurocristopathy, that is a defect in the development of neural crest. The most accepted etiology is failure of migration of neuroblasts (which later develop into ganglion cells) to the colon in the embryological period. This condition shows a male to female preponderance of 4–5:1. Affected babies may also have other gastrointestinal, neurological, cardiovascular, or urological anomalies. Trisomy 21 is a known association of this condition.

32.6.3.1 Etiopathogenesis
Absence of ganglion cells in the intramuscular and submucosal mesenteric nerve supply (Auerbachs's and Meissner's plexus) extends from the anal sphincter to varying length of the colon, and results in failure of coordinated intestinal motility, and spasm of the affected portion with proximal dilatation. In 80% cases, it is limited to the sigmoid colon and rectum. Small intestine may be involved in 5% cases.

32.6.3.2 Presentation
It presents as poor feeding, bilious vomiting, progressive abdominal distention, and difficult bowel movement or obstruction. Only a small proportion of neonates

present as failure to pass meconium in the first day of life. About 80% neonates are diagnosed in the neonatal period. In older children, it presents as constipation and obstipation, failure to thrive, irritability, distention, fecal impaction, and diarrhea due to enterocolitis.

Diagnosis: CBC, KFT with electrolytes, ABG, CXR are ordered. They may reveal electrolyte or Hb disturbances, depending on the clinical condition. X-ray abdomen, Barium enema, and rectal biopsy can confirm diagnosis in older children. Intestinal obstruction being an emergency, colostomy is undertaken following clinical and radiological evaluation, in neonates.

32.6.3.3 Surgical Management
A primary colostomy is performed, followed by pull through surgery later (Duhamel's, Swenson's, Soave) which involves resection of the aganglionic segment and anastomosis of ganglionic segment with anus, followed by colostomy closure at a third sitting. A combined abdominoperineal or laparoscopic approach may be used. A single-stage pull through surgery is also one of the surgical options.

The anesthetic management for the colostomy depends on the associated anomalies and the degree of the abdominal distention. Perioperative management is similar as for intestinal obstruction.

32.6.3.4 Perioperative Considerations
1. Extensive bowel preparation is done.
2. Fluid and electrolyte imbalance must be corrected.
3. Consider as full stomach with risk of aspiration.
4. Supine followed by lithotomy position.
5. Intraoperative frozen section may be planned to verify the transition of aganglionic segment with normal.
6. Anesthesia as for other GI surgeries.
7. Usually not associated with significant blood loss. Major surgery is associated with prolonged duration, third space fluid shifts, and hypothermia.
8. Surgeon may use perineal muscle stimulation intraoperatively.
9. IV analgesics or continuous epidural analgesia can be used for intra- and postoperative analgesia.

32.6.4 Anorectal Malformations (ARM)

ARMs include a group of congenital anomalies of the anorectum and the genitourinary tract (often erroneously referred to as imperforate anus), and may range in severity from simple imperforate anus to a complex genitourinary syndrome associated with other congenital anomalies.

32.6.4.1 Epidemiology
Incidence is 1:3000 to 1:5000 live births, with a slight male preponderance. About 50% of patients have associated anomalies. Severe ARMs have a stronger

Table 32.6 Wingspread classification of ARM

Anomaly level	Female	Male
High	Anorectal agenesis (with rectovaginal fistula or without fistula); rectal atresia	Anorectal agenesis (with recto prostatic-urethral fistula or without fistula); rectal atresia
Intermediate	Recto vestibular/Rectovaginal fistula, anal agenesis without fistula	Rectobulbar-urethral fistula, anal agenesis without fistula
Low	Anovestibular/Anocutaneous (perineal) fistula, anal stenosis	Anocutaneous (perineal) fistula, anal stenosis
Rare	Persistent cloacal abnormality, rare malformations	Rare malformations

association with congenital anomalies (90%). The common associations are VACTERL (Vertebral, anal, cardiac, tracheoesophageal, and limb) and CHARGE (choanal atresia/coloboma, anal, renal, GI, and ear).

32.6.4.2 Etiopathogenesis
Both genetic and environmental factors have been associated with ARM. A chromosomal anomaly is found in 10% of cases including Trisomy 21 (especially in anal stenosis without fistula) and DiGeorge Syndrome. Trisomy 13 and 18 are also associated with ARM.

32.6.4.3 Presentation
The classical types of ARM were described as high, intermediate, and low depending on the relation of the rectal termination in relation to the levator plate, the Wingspread Classification (Table 32.6). The babies with higher anomalies have less well-developed anorectal muscle complexes and sacral anomalies are common. The usual presentation is of an abnormal or no anal opening with failure to pass meconium in the first day of life. Depending on the level of ARM, varying degrees of vomiting and bowel distention may be present.

32.6.4.4 Anesthetic Management
(i). Investigations/Workup
In high ARM, renal USG, ECHO, X-ray Chest, spinal column radiography, spinal USG to rule out tethered cord, and sacral vertebral anomalies are indicated. Other workup is similar to intestinal obstruction.

(ii). Surgery
Ranges from simple primary anoplasty/repair for mild/low ARMs to major three-stage procedure. Severe/high ARMs require a colostomy on the first day of life followed by definitive corrective repair the extent of which is variable and depends on the extent of the anomaly 2 weeks later, and colostomy closure thereafter. Most surgeons use a posterior sagittal approach (PSARP—posterior sagittal anorectoplasty). Other approaches are anterior sagittal, abdominoperineal, and laparoscopic (Box 32.3).

(iii). The anesthetic

Management for the colostomy depends on the associated anomalies, and degree of abdominal distention. Perioperative management is similar to intestinal obstruction. Baby will have a NGT in situ and will be NPO. Assessment of dehydration, fluid and electrolyte status, degree of abdominal distention, and consequent respiratory distress due to reduced FRC must be evaluated. Signs of sepsis, acidosis, peritonitis, obstructive uropathy should also be evaluated.

Box 32.3: Hirschsprung's Disease and ARM—Summary of Perioperative Management

Anesthesia management similar to intestinal obstruction. Plan should be adapted based on clinical condition, prematurity, anomalies, and plan of surgery.

1. Posture – supine or prone with elevated pelvis or lithotomy. Laparoscopic assisted approach may be used.
2. Ensure fluid resuscitation, acid base, and electrolyte imbalance have been corrected.
3. NGT suction immediately before induction of anesthesia.
4. Standard noninvasive monitoring. Invasive monitoring if indicated. Urine output should be monitored.
5. IV access in upper limb.
6. IV Atropine followed by preoxygenation.
7. mRSI with or without cricoid pressure. Inhalational induction if no significant abdominal distention.
8. Maintenance of anesthesia with inhalational agent and opioids. Avoid N_2O to prevent bowel distention. Relaxant may have to be avoided if perineal muscle or anal sphincter stimulation is planned.
9. Maintenance fluids and third space losses must be administered depending on the extent of the surgery. Blood loss in colostomy is expected to be minimal.
10. Pain management—IV or rectal paracetamol, local infiltration, TAP block (Transverse abdomens plane block) are the usual options. Epidural anesthesia using a lumbar or caudal approach may be used if no sacral/vertebral anomalies are present.
11. Extubation when fully awake and vigorous.

32.6.5 Intestinal Obstruction

Neonatal bowel obstruction may be **mechanical** (malrotation, volvulus), **functional** (meconium ileus, Hirschsprung's disease) or **congenital** (web, atresia, stenosis, duplication affecting any part of the small or large intestine, annular pancreas,

ARM). The classical presentation is vomiting, abdominal distention, poor feeding, and failure to pass meconium within hours of birth.

32.6.5.1 Bowel Atresia

Atresia/ Stenosis can affect any part of the intestine, though the jejunoileal is more common. Incidence is about 1:5000 live births with equal gender predilection. Atresia accounts for 95% cases of obstruction. Affected neonates are frequently premature and low birth weight. Duodenal atresia or stenosis occurs usually due to failure of recanalization during embryological development. It is commonly associated with other GI anomalies (malrotation, biliary atresia, annular pancreas) and congenital anomalies like renal/cardiac or vertebral. Subglottic stenosis may also be present. Trisomy 21 is also a known association of duodenal atresia with its attendant risk of atlantoaxial instability and congenital heart disease. Jejunal-ileal and colonic atresia are associated with conditions predisposing to maternal thrombosis and compromised vascular supply. Colonic atresia/stenosis are associated with Hirschsprung's disease, GI, and VACTERL anomalies.

(i). Presentation:

A baby born to a mother with polyhydramnios presenting with bilious vomiting (if obstruction is below the ampulla of Vater), abdominal distension, and failure of passage of meconium in the first day of life. If a high obstruction scaphoid abdomen and nonbilious vomiting are present, diagnosis is confirmed by X- ray abdomen which shows air-fluid levels. The classic double bubble appearance is seen in duodenal atresia which shows two bubbles (gastric and duodenal along with no other air-fluid levels beyond the duodenum). Investigations required are CBC, KFT with electrolytes, ABG, Coagulation, CXR, and ECHO (especially in duodenal anomalies) as clinically indicated.

(ii). Management:

Treatment is by resection and anastomosis of the stenotic/atretic segment. Outcome is determined to a large extent by the nature of congenital anomalies and the degree of prematurity.

32.6.5.2 Malrotation/Volvulus

Malrotation is a common entity with an incidence of 1:500 live births, caused by aberrant embryological rotation of the midgut around the superior mesenteric artery, i.e., twisting of the small bowel around the narrow mesenteric bases causing a closed loop obstruction and intestinal ischemia. There are many subtypes depending on the degree and direction of rotation. It may be associated with congenital heart disease, other GI anomalies (atresia, stenosis, Hirschsprung disease, intussusception), asplenia or polysplenia, omphalocele, gastroschisis, and CDH.

(i). Presentation:

There are signs of obstruction and strangulation within the first 2 months of life with 60% presenting within the first month. Volvulus is a true surgical emergency. Usual symptoms include bilious emesis, abdominal distension, diarrhea or constipation. Signs of peritonitis may be present. A tense tender abdomen, with vomiting, bloody stools, and shock may indicate strangulation of the bowel. A closed loop obstruction will rapidly cause ischemia of the entire bowel and the neonate may decompensate rapidly. Diagnosis is clinicoradiological. X-Ray abdomen, Upper GI series or CT scan may be required to confirm the diagnosis. Urgent biochemical investigations CBC, KFT with electrolytes, LFT, ABG, blood sugar, Chest X-Ray, Coagulation profile are required. Delay in investigations does not preclude proceeding with surgery in a sick neonate.

(ii). Perioperative Considerations and Management (Box 32.4)

1. Full stomach, gastric distention, risk of aspiration.
2. Respiratory distress and hypoxemia due to reduced FRC, acidosis, aspiration, pneumonia.
3. Hypovolemia and electrolyte abnormalities (hyponatremia/hypokalemia) are expected. Hypoglycemia is also common.
4. Fever increases O_2 consumption. Increase in maintenance fluid requirement by 10%/°C rise.
5. Hypothermia is common due to requirement of large volume resuscitation, and sepsis.
6. Sepsis with coagulopathy, neutropenia, anemia, thrombocytopenia.
7. Metabolic acidosis, sign of gut ischemia, is ominous.
8. Reperfusion of ischemic bowel can precipitate acute decompensation and cardiac arrest.

(iii). Management:

Delay in anesthesia for correction of metabolic derangements resuscitation should be weighed against the emergency nature of the surgery. Neonates with bowel ischemia are urgently taken to the OT along with ongoing resuscitation. LADD procedure is carried out which involves derotation of the bowel, gut repositioning of the small bowel on the right side and the large bowel on left side, adhesiolysis of the thick LADD bands and appendicectomy. Resection and anastomosis of the gangrenous bowel or resection with stoma formation may be needed. A Second look laparotomy may be carried out after 24–48 h if bowel viability is doubtful.

Box 32.4: Intestinal Obstruction: Summary of Perioperative Management

1. OT prepared with warming, drugs (epinephrine, bicarbonate, calcium, dextrose, insulin, glucose, dopamine).
2. Ongoing resuscitation and treatment of electrolyte abnormalities.
3. Aggressive warming measures; sterile cling film may be used to wrap the neonate.

4. Aspiration by large bore NGT in supine, left and right lateral positions.
5. Two venous access—one in upper limb as IVC may be compressed, and other may be a central line.
6. Standard noninvasive monitoring; Invasive arterial access depending on patient condition, extent of surgery. Blood sugar and urine output monitoring also indicated.
7. Preoxygenation as tolerated; Induction with mRSI with Propofol (2–3 mg/kg)/Etomidate 0.2–0.3 mg/kg) followed by Succinylcholine 2 mg/kg or Rocuronium 1–1.2 mg/kg.
8. Awake intubation in severely compromised babies in antiaspiration position (reverse Trendelenburg).
9. Maintenance—Low concentration of Sevoflurane/Isoflurane (poorly tolerated in shock) with O_2 and air. Small doses of Atracurium or Cisatracurium; ventilation controlled; Avoid N2O; Low dose opioids.
10. Administer fluid accurately through syringe pump; Aggressive loss replacement by RL @ 10 mL/kg/h; 5% Albumin/Plasma in case of high crystalloid requirement, PRBC if loss >10% estimated blood volume. 10% Dextrose at maintenance rate.
11. Cardiac arrest due to reperfusion injury may require large volumes of IV fluids, albumin, plasma/blood.
12. Inotropes (Dopamine is preferred) may be required.
13. Postoperative elective ventilation.
14. If extubation planned, extubate in lateral position when neonate fully awake and vigorous.
15. Postoperative analgesia - IV PCM, local infiltration, TAP block, low dose IV opioid infusion.
16. Lumbar or caudal epidural analgesia may be used intra- and postoperatively. The catheter is threaded up the epidural space congruent to the dermatome of incision. Local anesthetic drugs in low doses can be infused through the catheter.

32.7 Conclusion

Surgical and anesthetic care for neonates requiring laparotomy is best delivered in units which have the multidisciplinary support for these challenging patients and where these operations are performed regularly. A logical approach to preoperative optimization, meticulous attention to perioperative anesthetic concerns, and postoperative nursing in an NICU, PICU, or in a highly skilled pediatric surgical ward will achieve the best results.

Further Reading

Bell MJ, Ternberg JL, Feigin RD, et al. Neonatal necrotizing enterocolitis: therapeutic decisions based upon clinical staging. Ann Surg. 1978;187:1–7.

Chandrashekhar S, Davis L. Anesthesia for neonatal emergency laparotomy. BJA Educ. 2015;15(4):194–8.

Choi YY. Necrotizing enterocolitis in newborns: update in pathophysiology and newly emerging therapeutic strategies. Korean J Pediatr. 2014;57:505–13.

Christensen RD, Gordon PV, Besner GE. Can we cut the incidence of necrotizing enterocolitis in half—today? Fetal Pediatr Pathol. 2010;29(4):185–98. https://doi.org/10.3109/1551381 5.2010.483874.

Craig R. Anesthesia for pyloromyotomy. BJA Educ. 2018;18(6):173–7.

Dhayagude S, Dave N. Principles and practice of pediatric anesthesia. 1st ed. Jaypee; 2017.

Gregory GA, Andropoulod DB. Gregory's pediatric anesthesia. 6th ed. Wiley Blackwell; 2020.

Holzman R, Mancuso T, Polaner D. A practical approach to pediatric anesthesia. 2nd ed. Lippincott Williams & Wilkins; 2016.

Houck P, Hache M, Sun L. NEC. Handbook of pediatric anesthesia. Lange; 2015.

Lerman J. Neonatal anesthesia. 1st ed. New York: Springer-Verlag; 2015.

Neu J, Walker WA. Necrotizing enterocolitis. N Engl J Med. 2011;364:255–64.

Shah TA, Meinzen-Derr J, Gratton T, et al. Hospital and neurodevelopmental outcomes of extremely low-birth-weight infants with necrotizing enterocolitis and spontaneous intestinal perforation. J Perinatol. 2012;32(552):558.

Sims C, Weber D, Johnson C. A guide to pediatric anesthesia. 2nd ed. Springer; 2020.

Walsh MC, Kliegman RM. Necrotizing enterocolitis: treatment based on staging criteria. Pediatr Clin North Am. 1986;33:179–201.

Anesthesia for Genitourinary Surgery in the Neonate

Nitin Hayaran and Preeti Varshney

33.1 Introduction

Of all abdominal masses nearly two-thirds are of renal origin, and 15% can be detected in the antenatal period. Congenital renal tumors are rare (7% of all neonatal tumors), and are usually benign. Cystic masses are more common than solid, such as Hydronephrosis, Multicystic Dysplastic Kidney (MCDK), and Hereditary Polycystic Kidney Disease (PKD). Of the solid tumors, malignant Wilms tumor (WT) is most common, that presents in the first year of life, followed by Congenital Mesoblastic Nephroma (CMN), Rhabdoid Tumor of The Kidney (RTK), and Clear Cell Sarcoma of the Kidney (CCSK). Two-thirds of solid tumors in the neonates are CMN, followed by WT and RTK, and CCSK (rare) [1–3].

Congenital Anomalies of Kidney and Urinary Tract (CAKUT) have an incidence of 3–7/1000 livebirths, varying from mild (small PUV) to severe (renal agenesis) abnormality. All these may not be correctable by surgery, or may require more than one surgery, with renal transplantation at a later stage [4].

Urogenital anomalies may also be associated with other congenital anomalies usually as a part of a syndrome. A thorough understanding of the pathology as well as evaluation of the baby is important for the anesthetist to plan and provide the best perioperative care.

This chapter reviews the general anesthetic considerations for urological surgeries and the brief description of common anomalies requiring attention in the neonatal period.

N. Hayaran (✉) · P. Varshney
Lady Hardinge Medical College, SSK and Associated Hospitals, New Delhi, India

U. Saha (ed.), *Clinical Anesthesia for the Newborn and the Neonate*,
https://doi.org/10.1007/978-981-19-5458-0_33

33.2   Embryology

Urogenital system has two different systems: (1) **Urinary or excretory and (2) Genital or reproductive systems**. They are generally discussed together as they have common embryology and both grow simultaneously, interconnected with each other. Both develop from a common mesodermal ridge along the posterior wall of the abdominal cavity, and the excretory ducts of both the systems enter a common cloacal cavity [5, 6].

33.2.1 Excretory System

Development of the excretory system begins in the third week from the intraembryonic mesoderm along the posterior wall of the abdominal cavity. In the intrauterine life, there are three different renal systems, the pronephros, mesonephros, and metanephros. **Pronephros** is the earliest, in the cervical region, disappears by the end of fourth week, and is replaced by the intermediate system, **Mesonephros,** extending from lower cervical to upper lumbar segments. This disappear by the end of second month and is replaced by **Metanephros**, the permanent kidney which arises in the lower lumbar and sacral regions. It continues to grow and differentiate into Bowman's capsule, renal pelvis, calyces, collecting tubules and collecting duct, the excretory units of the urinary system, and becomes functional by the end of pregnancy. In the fourth to seventh week, cloaca subdivides into a posterior (anorectal canal), and anterior (primitive urogenital sinus) portions.

Abnormalities at any stage give rise to developmental anomalies in the urinary system. Failure of proliferation of the metanephric tissue cap results in **renal agenesis** (unilateral or bilateral). Uterus and major portion of the vagina are also absent. These babies die soon after birth.

During early development, kidneys are pelvic organs (lower lumbar) and ascend to upper lumbar area as the fetus elongates, failure of which rise to **Pelvic kidney,** unilateral or bilateral. Sometimes, during ascent, both kidneys are pushed close together resulting in **Horseshoe** kidney [5].

33.2.2 Genital System and Gonads

Sex of the embryo is determined at the time of fertilization, but gonads only acquire sexual characteristics by the seventh week. A large ovoid organ (developing gonad) is formed on each side of midline at 4- 6 weeks of gestation, projecting into the coelomic cavity, attached to the posterior abdominal wall by a mesentery and with a urogenital ridge in between. In the sixth week, germ cells invade the genital ridges (failure leads to **gonadal agenesis**). The gonads have two pairs of genital ducts – **Wolffian** (mesonephric) and **Mullerian** (paramesonephric), and depending on the sex of the embryo, either duct develops; in male embryo, the Wolffian duct forms the main genital duct (ductus deferens) and Mullerian disappears, while in female embryo the Mullerian duct develops to form oviducts, uterus, and vagina, and

Wolffian duct disappears. By the eighth week, either duct has disappeared. Testis are formed at 6–8 weeks and continue to differentiate up to the fourth month of life. The testis cords are composed of primitive germ and epithelial cells and remain solid until puberty. When sexual maturity is reached, they acquire a lumen, forming the seminiferous tubules. The External genitalia is formed in the third to fourth months. In males, genital (scrotal) swellings are in the inguinal region, they move caudally, each swelling making up half of the scrotum, separated by the scrotal septum. The pelvic portion of the urogenital sinus develops into the urethra (prostatic, membranous, and penile parts). In females, genital tubercle forms the clitoris, unfused urethral folds form labia minora, genital swellings enlarge to form labia majora, and urogenital sinus forms the urethra and the vestibule [5].

Etiology of Gonadal Abnormalities - Development of the genital system is dependent on sex chromosomes, fetal differential development, and hormonal sensitivity, making it prone to several abnormalities [7]:

(a) Deletion of **Protein Transcription Factors (FOX a1 and a2)** results in persistent cloaca, incomplete separation of urinary, genital, and anorectal tracts, hypospadias and urethral fistula [8].
(b) **Bone Morphogenetic Protein (Bmp4),** an essential growth factor for initiating genital tubercle outgrowth, regulates formation of distal urethral epithelium [9, 10].
(c) **Differences of Sex Development (DSD)** are congenital conditions with atypical gonads and anatomical sex, of heterogenous etiology [11, 12].

33.3   General Considerations

Congenital anomalies account for majority of urological surgeries in the pediatric age group; however, most surgeries are not performed in the neonatal period, unless they are not urgent, because of high neonatal morbidity and mortality. Common congenital urogenital anomalies encountered in the neonatal age are summarized in Table 33.1.

Disorders of the Genitourinary System include disorders with minimal or major manifestations, such as Hypospadias, Epispadias, duplications, and atresia. Isolated hypospadias is seen in 0.8% of newborns and isolated cryptorchidism in 5% term and 15% preterm newborns. These are usually not associated with endocrine abnormality. Severe hypospadias or nonpalpable testes are associated with DSD, and cryptorchidism with hypospadias may have 25% incidence of DSD. Micropenis is secondary to insufficient testosterone secretion in the third trimester. Other disorders include complete or partial gonadal dysgenesis, sex reversal, Ovo testicular disorder, Congenital adrenal hyperplasia, Chromosomal aberrations, Aromatase deficiency associated with midline congenital anomalies, Congenital anorchia (vanishing testis – teratogenic, idiopathic, Congenital midline defects, Inadequate masculinization of males), and rare and sporadic partial or complete gonadal agenesis (associated with cardiac defects, WT, osteoporosis, sensorineural hearing loss, congenital adrenal hyperplasia, androgen insensitivity syndrome).

Table 33.1 Congenital urogenital anomalies in the neonatal age [6, 13–17]

	Malformation	Incidence	Diagnosis/associations
Urological anomalies			
1.	Posterior urethral valve (PUV)	1:5000 male births	Antenatal/postnatal
2.	Bladder exstrophy/ Ectopia vesicae	1:10,000–50,000 live births (2–3 times more in males affected)	Antenatal USG or at birth
3.	Renal agenesis	Bilateral 1:4000 live births, unilateral 1:500–1300 live births M > F:2.5:1 [13]	Bilateral not compatible with life
4.	Double /Ectopic ureter	Up to 6%, R > L F > M [14]	One ureter may open in uterus/vagina/ urethra
5.	Urachal cyst and fistula	Very rare	Presents in childhood
6.	Ureterocele	1:4000 more in females	Antenatal USG or later in life
7.	Vesicoureteral reflux (VUR)	1:100, more in males	Antenatal USG or later in life
8.	Pelviureteric junction (PUJ) obstruction	1:500, more in males, L > R	Antenatal USG
9.	Congenital cystic dysplasia of the kidneys	Unilateral 1:4300 live births, L > R,	Antenatal/postnatal/childhood,
10.	Pelvic/Horseshoe/ Ectopic kidney	1:500 people, M:F:2:1	Presents in childhood/adolescence
11.	Prune belly syndrome	1:30,000–40,000 births, in males	Antenatal/postnatal/infancy. Often stillbirth
12.	Wilms tumor or nephroblastoma (WT)	Rare <0.16% incidence	Presents in childhood (3–5 years)
Genital anomalies			
1.	Congenital inguinal hernia	Term—3–5% Preterm—up to 30% Males > females	At birth or in infancy
2.	Duplication/atresia of uterovaginal canal	Rare, in females, Turner syndrome	At birth
3.	Hypospadias	1:250–350 male births (0.8% in newborns)	At birth or during circumcision or later
4.	Epispadias	1:1,00,000 male births	At birth
5.	Cryptorchidism	1:100 male births (1/ third bilateral) Term −5%, preterm 15%	At birth (pelvic/intra-abdominal testis)
6.	Partial or complete gonadal dysgenesis	Rare, sporadic	At birth, at puberty in females, associated with cardiac defects, WT, osteoporosis, sensorineural hearing loss, congenital adrenal hyperplasia, androgen insensitivity syndrome

Surgical Approach in a Neonate For Urogenital Surgeries: Traditional approach to these procedures is open surgery. Development of smaller devices and expertize in pediatric laparoscopy has encouraged its use in neonates also. However, drawbacks that may limit minimally invasive surgeries in neonates, including Robotics, are lack of knowledge of extent of hemodynamic and respiratory alterations occurring during these procedures and their management, and its effects on growth and development [18].

33.4 Preanesthetic Evaluation

It is thus important to thoroughly evaluate the neonate before taking up for surgical correction, irrespective of the procedure and anesthesia technique planned.

33.4.1 Preanesthetic Evaluation

Preanesthetic evaluation should include:

i. Age and maturity of the neonate and problems associated with prematurity.
ii. Identification of clinically apparent other congenital anomalies.
iii. Assessment of each organ system by blood investigations or radiological scan, especially in a syndromic neonate (Common anomalies in the neonatal period are listed in Table 33.2).
iv. Hematological and biochemical investigations to rule out anemia, electrolyte imbalance, and metabolic derangements. In most neonates, hemoglobin, blood urea, and urinalysis (routine and microscopic) are sufficient.
v. Spinal abnormalities should be ruled out in a baby with cloacal defects and bladder exstrophy before planning for central neuraxial block.

Table 33.2 Congenital syndromes associated with urological malformations in neonates

	Syndrome	Gene defect	Characteristic malformations
1	Branchio-oto-renal syndrome	EYA1, SIX1	Branchial cysts, ear malformations, preauricular pits, renal agenesis, or dysplasia
2	CHARGE syndrome	CHD7	Coloboma, heart defects, choanal atresia, growth retardation, genital and urinary abnormalities, ear and hearing defects
3	DiGeorge syndrome	22q11	Cardiac defects, abnormal facies, thymic hypoplasia, immunodeficiency, cleft lip/palate, hypocalcemia, renal agenesis/Vesicoureteric reflux (VUR)
4	Renal coloboma syndrome	PAX2	Renal hypoplasia, VUR, optic nerve malformation, retinal coloboma
5	Townes- Brocks syndrome	SALL1	Imperforate anus, ear and hearing defects, renal dysplasia, hypoplasia or VUR, thumb malformations

(continued)

Table 33.2 (continued)

	Syndrome	Gene defect	Characteristic malformations
6	VACTERL association	Multiple genetic and environmental factors	Vertebral defects, anal atresia, cardiac defects, TEF, renal anomalies, limb abnormalities
7	Complete androgen insensitivity syndrome (CAIS)	one X and one Y chromosome	Abnormal sexual development—genetically male but do not respond to androgens, prevents the masculinization of male genitalia, not much impairment in females
8	Denys-Drash syndrome (DDS)	Genetic disorder. Wilms tumor suppressor gene (WT1) mutation	Affects kidneys and genitalia—congenital nephropathy, early renal failure, Wilms tumor in 90%, DSD in males, normal genitalia in females
9	Turner syndrome (TS)	Rare, Monosomy X (45X or 45X0) - one X chromosome than XX =	Affects females—short stature, webbed neck, low-set ears, low hairline at the nape, swollen hands and feet at birth. Most can lead normal life with regular medical care
10	Perrault syndrome	Rare, 46XX karyotype	XX gonadal dysgenesis + early sensorineural hearing loss delayed growth, neurological (frequent falls, lack of coordination). Females—Ovarian dysfunction and primary ovarian insufficiency (POI), late puberty, early menopause

33.4.2 Preoperative Investigations

Many of the congenital and developmental renal abnormalities can be diagnosed at routine antenatal ultrasound done in the first and second trimester, and parents advised on the postnatal prognosis and care of the baby. Postnatal confirmation of the genitourinary defects is done by renal ultrasound, voiding cystourethrogram (VCUG), intravenous pyelography (IVP), and blood biochemistry. Hemoglobin, serum electrolytes, urea, and creatinine are done for the purpose of preoperative evaluation.

33.5 Anesthetic Management

33.5.1 General Anesthesia

General anesthesia with controlled ventilation is the preferred mode technique of anesthesia for urogenital procedures in the newborn and neonate. Airway can be secured either by LMA or endotracheal tube, and depending on the duration of surgery, can be either with neonate maintaining spontaneous, assisted, or controlled respiration, with use of muscle relaxants and reversal at the end. Intraoperative analgesia can be provided using fentanyl [18].

33.5.2 Epidural Anesthesia

Epidural anesthesia, caudal block or regional nerve blocks can be supplemented with general anesthesia for intraoperative as well as postoperative pain relief [19]. If regional anesthesia is planned, it is important to block the correct nerve distribution for the surgical area [20, 21]. The important nerve supplies relevant to urogenital procedures are:

- Kidney-T10 to L1.
- Procedures on ureters and bladder require blockade up to T10 level.
- Pelvic parasympathetic supply from S2, S3, and S4 via the pelvic splanchnic plexus.
- Pelvic sympathetic supply from T11 and T12 from the hypogastric plexus.
- Pudendal nerve carries motor and sensory fibers from S2 to 4. It is blocked for surgeries on perineum and external genitalia.
- Penile nerve block by blocking dorsal nerve of penis (branch of pudendal nerve) which supplies the distal 2/third of penis. It is mainly used for circumcision.
- Ilioinguinal/iliohypogastric nerve (L1) block for inguinal surgeries.

33.5.3 Spinal Anesthesia

Spinal anesthesia has been successfully used in neonates for various surgical procedures, chiefly, cystoscopy for PUV, ureterocele, and in neonatal emergency surgery for torsion testis [19, 22].

33.5.4 Intraoperative Positioning

Urinary outflow tract procedures are performed in lithotomy position, and surgeries on kidneys in lateral, semi lateral or prone position. Procedures related to gonads and genitalia are performed in supine position. Lithotomy positioning requires proper preparation as even pediatric operation tables are too wide for a neonate, and excessive abduction and lateral rotation of the hip joint must be avoided. Proper padding of pressure points is mandatory to avoid nerve injuries associated with lithotomy position.

Latex free gloves should be used for urogenital surgery in neonates, as they are repeatedly exposed through multiple surgical procedures especially in the first year of life; using latex gloves make them prone to develop latex allergy. The allergic reaction may manifest as bronchospasm and cardiovascular collapse as late as 30–60 min after induction, and watery eyes, sneezing and coughing after 6–48 h of exposure as delayed type IV hypersensitivity reaction. Latex free gloves should be used to prevent severe anaphylactic reactions.

33.6 Anesthesia Management of Individual Surgeries

33.6.1 Circumcision

Circumcision is the procedure of removing foreskin to expose the glans of penis. Although it is not performed for congenital anomaly, but it is the most common surgical procedure around the world. In neonates, circumcision is performed for cultural reasons and rarely for some absolute indication [23]. Newborn circumcisions are commonly performed in the ward by using a Gomco clamp, Mogen clamp or Plastic bell device. Baby may be premedicated with oral paracetamol drops (15 mg /kg). Lignocaine infiltration or EMLA cream is used to provide local anesthesia. When performed in the OR, it is done under general anesthesia with tracheal intubation or LMA and controlled ventilation. Analgesia can be provided by caudal route, dorsal penile nerve block or subcutaneous penile ring block. Care must be taken to not to add adrenaline to the LA drug as the end arteries may constrict leading to ischemia and necrosis of distal penile skin. Circumcision should be avoided in a preterm newborns, within 12 h of birth, presence of hypospadias, ambiguous genitalia, or bleeding disorders [24–26].

33.6.2 Posterior Urethral Valves (PUV)

PUV is the most common cause of bladder outlet obstruction in a male newborn accounting for renal failure and need for renal transplantation in later childhood. It is a disease of male lower urinary tract in which mucosal folds are present anywhere in the prostatic urethra to the external urinary sphincter causing obstruction to urinary outflow. The severity of obstruction may be variable leading to renal changes ranging from mild hydronephrosis to severe renal dysplasia. The diagnosis may be possible in antenatal USG if there is obvious obstructive uropathy. In severe obstruction, neonate may present with anuria and palpable bladder. However, the diagnosis may be delayed in cases of mild obstruction having poor urinary stream and is confirmed by voiding cystourethrography (VCUG). Moreover, there can be bladder wall hypertrophy to overcome partial obstruction by generating high voiding pressures. VCUG has characteristic findings of dilated proximal urethra with a thickened bladder neck, valve leaflets in urethra and Vesicoureteric reflux (VUR) in 50% cases. Thus, persistent PUV will eventually lead to bilateral hydronephrosis either due to VUR or because of elevated bladder pressures. Oligohydramnios is a clue to obstructive uropathy. The neonatal survival may be doubtful in cases of severe obstruction associated with oligohydramnios and renal dysplasia. Since amniotic fluid is important for the development of bronchial tree and alveoli, these babies also have pulmonary hypoplasia [27].

The management ranges from early bladder catheterization with a small size feeding tube (8 FG) to vesicostomy for bladder and kidney decompression in severe cases. Cystoscopic resection of PU valve leaflets can be performed as corrective surgery, and avoid vesicostomy, if done timely, before development of renal dysfunction. Preoperative evaluation must include assessment of hydration status and renal function to rule out electrolyte imbalance (hyperkalemia, hyponatremia, acidosis) as well as renal failure in severe cases.

If endoscopic resection or primary ablation of valve leaflets is attempted, depth of anesthesia should be maintained to avoid any movement, coughing, or straining during the procedure to prevent inadvertent urethral damage with the baby in lithotomy position. Temperature monitoring is important as hypothermia is a concern both due to anesthesia and use of irrigation fluid in endoscopic procedure.

In neonates with PUV, most often, vesicostomy is performed either because of severe renal disease, failure to catheterize or due to lack of small size cystoscope for the neonatal urethra. Intravenous or inhalational anesthesia with endotracheal tube is preferred, with controlled ventilation. High peak pressures and permissive hypercapnia may be required in neonates with associated pulmonary hypoplasia. Transurethral valve ablation followed by vesicostomy closure may be undertaken later in infancy, after improvement in general condition and renal functions. Spinal anesthesia is a safer option in neonates, that avoids the adverse neurological effects of general anesthetics [19, 28]. Postoperative analgesia can be provided with local infiltration of LA agent, intravenous paracetamol, or caudal block.

33.6.3 Hypospadias/Epispadias

Hypospadias is a common congenital defect characterized by abnormal ventral opening of urethral meatus. In 70–80% of cases, it is distal, i.e., meatus is located on the glans or distal shaft, which may be discovered during neonatal circumcision or later in life. In some cases, the meatus is in the middle shaft associated with downward curvature of penis known as **chordee**. Rarely, the urethral opening is located in the scrotum or perineum making surgery more complex, requiring staged procedure for correction. The repair is never an emergency and is usually performed after 3 months of age. There is no renal dysfunction or urinary obstruction, but there may be associated inguinal hernia, cryptorchidism, or low birth weight. The combination of proximal hypospadias and ambiguous genitalia or the impalpable testis should raise the suspicion of intersex condition and the genetic and endocrine investigations should be performed [29]. **Epispadias** is the condition when the urinary meatus is present on dorsum of penis, and is mostly associated with other anomalies such as anterior abdominal wall defects and bladder exstrophy. General, spinal caudal anesthesia have all been found suitable for surgical repair of hypospadias in children; however, in neonates light general anesthesia in combination with regional technique, would be most appropriate [30].

33.6.4 Ureterocele

Ureterocele is a sac-like pouch of distal ureter causing varying degree of obstruction at the uretero-vesical junction. It is more common in girls and may be associated with duplication of ureters. The baby may be asymptomatic at birth; however, the diagnosis may already be made in antenatal ultrasonography. Ectopic or large ureterocele may cause bladder outlet obstruction. A voiding cystourethrogram may be required to see the degree and level of obstruction, and renal and bladder USG to see the extent of hydronephrosis.

Surgery for ureterocele repair is not an emergency. But in cases of urinary obstruction urine retention, neonates may need surgery urgently. With severe obstruction, it is mandatory to drain the ureterocele early, within the first few days of life. Minimal intervention in the form of endoscopic drainage and placement of a ureteric stent is preferred. The more definitive repair is carried out later in infancy.

Open surgery is performed under GA, with baby in supine position. Spinal anesthesia has also been used [19]. Prophylactic antibiotics should always be administered to prevent the perioperative urinary infection.

33.6.5 Prune Belly Syndrome

This is a rare syndrome with incidence of 1:30000–40,000 births. Also known as Eagle-Barrett syndrome, or triad syndrome, involving three organs in the body, the abdominal wall, gonads, and urinary tract. Specifically, it consists of abdominal wall muscular hypoplasia or weakness, bilateral cryptorchidism or undescended testes, and abnormal distended hypotonic bladder, and problems related to the upper urinary tract (kidney, ureters, bladder). There may also be other birth defects, involving the skeletal system, intestines, and cardiac. Some babies may be still born or die within a few months.

The diagnosis can be made on clinical examination, and distinct lax, thin "prune" like appearance of the abdomen wall. Weak or ineffective cough due to abdominal wall deficiency, causes retention of secretions. Investigations include renal USG (to assess renal parenchyma, extent of dilation, and renal blood flow), VCUG (for reverse flow of urine), IVP (intravenous pyelogram) (for rate and path of urinary flow), and blood tests (for renal function and electrolyte and metabolic status, and hemoglobin level).

The neonate may present for vesicostomy to relieve urinary obstruction or for other anomalies, such as colostomy for imperforate anus. Surgery for undescended testes is usually delayed for post neonatal age. These neonates are at high risk of perioperative urinary infection and must receive prophylactic antibiotics. The more definitive procedure in the form of surgical remodeling of the abdominal wall and urinary tract are undertaken at a later age. Despite surgical interventions, these patients are at risk of developing extensive renal failure [31–33].

33.6.6 Cryptorchidism

Cryptorchidism represents unilateral or bilateral nondescent of testes from abdomen to the scrotum during fetal development. The testes normally descend into the scrotum during the seventh month of gestation. Overall incidence is 1:100 male births (1/third being bilateral) and is seen in 5% term and in up to 15% preterm babies. Unilateral undescended testis is present in 3% term male newborns, right side more common. In about 80% of such cases, the testis spontaneously descends by 3–6 months of age. Cryptorchidism may occur as an isolated anomaly or may be associated with other congenital anomalies. It is usually associated with inguinal hernia of the same side.

Management aims to locate the testis and perform an orchidopexy. Most of the time, testicular descent is arrested during its passage through the inguinal canal, the most common site of undescended testes. It can be relocated into the scrotum by a single surgery along with herniotomy. If the testis is abdominal with short spermatic vessels, two staged surgical procedure may be required. The unattended cryptorchidism can progress to infertility, torsion, or germ cell tumor [33–36]. The optimal time of surgery is 6–18 months age [37]. In a neonate, the only indication for testicular surgery is torsion of testis. Most common procedure is EUA (examination under anesthesia) [38].

33.6.7 Testicular Torsion

Torsion of testis leading to its vascular compromise is a surgical emergency. Anatomically, the testes along with the spermatic cord are covered with tunica vaginalis, which fixes the testes posteriorly to the scrotal wall. If there is defect in these attachments, there are likely chances of testicular torsion. Also, torsion is more common in the neonatal age as the recently descended testis lies relatively free in the scrotum.

Clinically, the baby may be excessively crying because of acute severe pain. On examination, the affected testes are edematous and the ipsilateral hemiscrotum is enlarged, hardened, tender with bluish to red discoloration of the overlying skin. The testicle is difficult to palpate. Diagnosis is confirmed either by colored doppler to see the vascular compromise or by conventional USG of the scrotum showing heterogenous, hypoechoic testes with a brightly echogenic rim.

Immediate intervention is surgical detorsion and orchidopexy. Salvage rates are higher if the surgery is performed within 6 h of onset of pain. Even if in doubt, the decision for surgery is taken up with high index of clinical suspicion, instead of waiting for diagnostic imaging tests or to achieve recommended fasting status. Orchidectomy is required if the testicular infarction has already occurred. Orchidopexy of the contralateral testis is almost always performed along with primary surgical procedure [39, 40].

The baby may be dehydrated. Fluid resuscitation should be done preoperatively and continued intraoperatively. General anesthesia with endotracheal intubation remains the preferred technique. Baby is always considered as full stomach as the pain delays gastric emptying. Caudal block is commonly supplemented for reducing intraoperative anesthesia requirements as well as for managing postoperative pain. It also reduces chances of intraoperative bradycardia which may be caused by vagal response during manipulation of testes. Atropine and glycopyrrolate should be available and kept ready. Postoperative nausea and vomiting associated with testicular surgery is not frequently observed in neonates [41].

There are reports of prenatal testicular torsion (torsion occurring before birth). The scrotal examination findings remain the same, except that the testis is nontender. Imaging studies are required to confirm the diagnosis. By the time diagnosis is made, testes are unsalvageable in most cases. Surgical exploration is required for orchidectomy as well as to perform contralateral orchidopexy to prevent the torsion of the other testes and anorchia. Since, the testes are already beyond salvage and nontender, surgery and anesthesia can be planned as an elective procedure. Bilateral torsion of testes has also been reported and requires immediate surgical exploration.

33.6.8 Hydrocele

Hydrocele is the nontender enlargement of scrotum, characterized by accumulation of serous fluid around the testes in tunica vaginalis. It is clinically confirmed by transillumination of scrotum. Scrotal ultrasound may be required to confirm the diagnosis. Surgery is rarely required as spontaneous resorption of fluid takes place within first year of life. Decrease in size of scrotum by compressing it, indicates communication with the abdomen and a patent processus vaginalis. In such patients, hernia may also be present. Surgical correction is required as there is possibility of incarceration of bowel. However, the neonate can be placed under close observation.

33.6.9 Renal Masses

Majority of congenital renal masses are benign, and cystic masses being more common than solid, common being hydronephrosis, MCDK, and hereditary polycystic kidney disease (PKD). Common solid renal tumors in pediatric age are Wilms tumor or Nephroblastoma (WT), Rhabdoid tumor of the kidney (RTK), and clear cell sarcoma of the kidney (CCSK). Tumors rarely develop in utero but have been reported in neonatal period, though they are extremely rare. However, two-thirds of all solid renal tumors in the neonates are Congenital Mesoblastic Nephroma (CMN), followed by WT, RTK, and CCSK (Rarest). CMN presents with an abdominal mass and requires imaging studies and biopsy for confirmation [17, 42].

33.6.9.1   Cystic Masses

These can be classified as Benign (hydronephrosis, multicystic dysplastic kidney, polycystic renal disease) or Malignant (multilocular cystic nephroma, cystic partially differentiated nephroblastoma, cystic Wilms tumor). Three cystic masses of the kidney seen in neonatal age are:

(i) *Hydronephrosis*: 40% of all neonatal abdominal masses are due to hydronephrosis and renal cystic disease. Depending on the severity of hydronephrosis in the newborn and onset of symptoms in the neonate, baby undergoes radiological and sonographic investigations, early. The causes of hydronephrosis are obstruction to urinary out flow tract, e.g., ureteropelvic junction (UPJ) obstruction, ureterovesical junction obstruction, vesicoureteral reflux (VUR), primary megaureter, neurogenic bladder, PUV, and Prune-Belly syndrome.

(ii) *Multicystic Dysplastic Kidney (MCDK)*: Unilateral MCDK has an incidence of 1:4300 live births, more common on left side, and most common cystic renal disease of the newborn. It thought to be because of ureteral obstruction from atresia or developmental insults during the eighth week of gestation. MCDK results in a nonfunctioning mass, that looks like a bag of grapes, composed of primitive tubules and immature glomeruli. It can be differentiated from hydronephrosis in the newborn by renal sonography.

(iii) *Polycystic Kidney Disease (PKD) (Recessive Type and Dominant Type)*: In neonates, PKD is predominantly of recessive type, though dominant type can also be seen. Its severity varies with age of onset and if it presents in the neonatal age, it is likely to very severe. The kidney is nondysplastic (differentiate from MCDK) and contains normal nephrons. Sonographic findings are suggestive of very large, homogeneously hyperechogenic kidneys with loss of corticomedullary differentiation. Oligohydramnios is often present.

33.6.9.2 Solid Renal Masses

These are classified as Benign (Renal vein thrombosis, ectopic or horse shoe kidney), or Malignant (CMN, Wilms tumor, Rhabdoid tumor of kidney).

(i) **Wilms Tumor** (nephroblastoma) (WT) is most common childhood renal malignancy, with peak incidence (80%) at 3–4 years of age. It is rarely seen in neonates. It accounts for 87% of pediatric renal masses and has an incidence of 1:10,000 persons. It is **very rare** in neonates (incidence less than 0.16%). WT can be distinguished from other masses because of the vascular invasion and displacement of adjacent structures. In 10% neonates it is bilateral. Surgical procedure is early nephrectomy [43].

(ii) **Renal Vein Thrombosis** (RVT) is associated with serious morbidity in the newborn of hypertension and chronic renal disease. Two-thirds of all cases occur within the first 3 days of life. In utero detection rate is low (7%). It is the most common noncatheter-related thrombotic event in the neonatal period, and nearly 80% of cases present in the first postnatal month. Risk factors for RVT are fetal or birth asphyxia, diabetic mother, severe hypovolemia, and coagulation abnormalities. Factors that can initiate thrombus formation include vascular injury, reduced blood flow, increased blood viscosity, hyperosmolality, and underlying thrombophilia. Classic triad of signs of RVT is gross hematuria, flank mass (unilateral/bilateral), and thrombocytopenia. Blood **investigations** can confirm hematuria and proteinuria, and reveal polycythemia, hemolytic anemia, and thrombocytopenia. Renal sonography reveals a large kidney diffusely echogenic, with loss of corticomedullary junction and few calcifications. Thrombus, extending from the renal vein into the inferior vena cava can be seen in 50% cases if extra renal vessels are involved. In 1/third cases, it is bilateral, which has a poor prognosis. **Management** is conservative with heparinization, thrombolytic therapy, or conventional anticoagulant to decrease the risk of thrombus progression and embolism. Simultaneously, hypertension and renal failure must be managed. Surgical thrombectomy is usually not done as thrombus may extend into intrarenal branches rather being restricted to the main renal vein. Surgery is indicated only in case of bilateral or IVC involvement [44, 45].

(iii) **Horseshoe Kidney** (HSK) is the most common renal fusion anomaly occurring in 1:400–666 people, twice as common in males. There are two distinct renal units fused at their inferior poles by a fibrous isthmus crossing the midline, at the level of L3–L4 level. In less than 5% cases, fusion occurs at the upper poles. This takes place in the 4th -sixth week of gestation. A slight alteration in the orientation of the fetal kidneys allows them to fuse during their ascent. Due to incomplete ascent, there may be aberrant or duplication or even triplication of the renal vessels, and ureters inserting higher on the renal pelvis than in normal kidneys, that may cause obstruction of the upper Pelviureteric junction. **Diagnosis** of HSK can be done at antenatal sonography, or postnatally on visualizing low-lying kidneys bilaterally, malrotated, and poorly defined inferior poles. In 80% cases, isthmus visualization is confirmatory. Further confirmation can be done by CT scan, MRI or renal scintigraphy. Radionucleotide scans with technetium 99 m dimercaptosuccinic acid (DMSA) can visualize the isthmus in 100% cases. A newborn with HSK is frequently associated with one or more other **congenital anomalies** that may affect neonatal survival, and stillbirths. These fatal anomalies primarily involve the gastrointestinal, skeletal, cardiovascular, central nervous systems, and chromosomal aberrations (Trisomy 18, Turner syndrome). Nonfatal anomalies are gonadal, e.g., hypospadias, undescended testes, bicornuate uterus and septate vagina, ureteral duplication, UPJO, and vesicoureteral reflux. These neonates may need to undergo surgery for other anomalies and defects. In an otherwise healthy neonate, no treatment is required. However, associated congenital anomalies necessitate supportive therapy. HSK is prone to UPJ obstruction, renal stones, UTI, and malignancy, later in life [2].

(iv) **Congenital Mesoblastic Nephroma** (CMN) is the most common solid renal tumor of the newborn, accounting for 66% of tumors identified during the first 2 months of life with slight male predilection (M:F: 1.5:1). In relation to other congenital tumors, the incidence of CMN decreases with age from 54% in the first month to 16% in the third month of life. CMN has some favorable characteristics: almost-exclusive occurrence in the first year of life, nonaggressive, nonmalignant, and mesenchymal origin. Histologically, there are three varieties of CMN: classic (49%), cellular (30%), and mixed (21%). The classic CMN is diagnosed at a median age of 17 days, while other two present later. Though nonmalignant, they recur locally if resection is incomplete. **Diagnosis** is by presence of abdominal lump on antenatal ultrasound or postnatal examination, unilateral or bilateral, and hematuria (microscopic and macroscopic). Antenatal diagnosis is associated with polyhydramnios, preterm labor, labor complications, and high perinatal morbidity and mortality. Acute fetal distress, anemia, and respiratory distress at birth have been described. Hence, these babies should be delivered at pediatric tertiary care center, for mechanical ventilation or immediate surgery. Associations with CMN include paraneoplastic syndromes, hypercalcemia secondary parathyroid hormone-like peptide secretion, though uncommon (10% incidence), may warrant intense medical therapy prior to surgical resection in case it is severe, hypertension (22 incidence) secondary to elevated plasma renin activity needing ACEI therapy. Often, surgical resection of the tumor normalizes hypertension and hypocalcemia. CMN should be differentiated from other extrarenal retroperitoneal masses (WT and adrenal hemorrhagic cyst). Investigations are as described for other renal masses. Preoperative investigations include complete blood count with differential counts liver function tests, electrolytes, serum creatinine, serum calcium, and urinalysis. Coagulation profile must be done especially for Acquired von Willebrand (incidence 4–8%) prothrombin time, partial thromboplastin time, and von Willebrand factor antigen. Prior to surgical resection. Confirm the origin of the mass and establish its spread to regional lymph nodes or IVC (inferior vena cava), and for presence of normal functioning contralateral kidney, and other urological anomalies. Histopathological staging grades CMN into five stages from a confined resectable tumor to bilateral CMN with metastasis to liver, bone, and brain. In neonates, most CMN are of stage I/II (resectable with no metastasis, and good prognosis). Tumor extension into the renal vein though rare but can increase surgical complications and bleeding [2, 46–48].

Management of neonatal renal tumors requires multidisciplinary approach in which **complete excision of the mass** is paramount. For unilateral solid renal mass, preferred treatment is radical nephrectomy with lymph node biopsy via laparotomy. Surgeon must take precautions to prevent its spread because of the potential of malignant pathology of all solid tumors. Retroperitoneal lymph node dissection is associated with high morbidity and is not advocated in neonates. Partial nephrectomy is associated with risk of recurrence and malignant spread and is not advocated [2].

Anesthesia technique of choice is general anesthesia with tracheal intubation and controlled ventilation. For intraoperative and postoperative analgesia, a caudal epidural catheter can be placed for continuous analgesia, to supplement IV fentanyl intraoperative. Cross-matched blood should be available for anemic neonates and surgeries with high anticipated blood loss. Intraoperative hypothermia should be avoided. Monitoring includes noninvasive HR, ECG, NIBP, SpO2, rectal or esophageal temperature, blood loss, volume status, and urine output. Anesthetist must be vigilant intraoperatively, because of the potential for hypertensive crisis and cardiac arrest. All emergency medications must be kept ready for administration in an emergency.

Postoperative complications are common and include hemorrhage, small-bowel obstruction, chylous ascites, intussusception, recurrence, and spread from incomplete or partial excision. Extensive and long duration surgery may result in major blood loss and fluid shifts, hypothermia, and postoperative ventilatory support. Postoperative pain management is mandatory [2].

Prognosis and outcome after resection of unilateral CMN is good with no need of adjuvant therapy and there is no current role for adjuvant therapy with complete excision of the mass, and if performed early, within the first week of life.

33.6.10   Anesthesia for Urological Disorders of the Urinary Tract

(i) **Vesicoureteral Reflux (VUR)**

Anatomically, the distal ureter travels through the submucosal layers of the bladder wall in a tunnel like path to make a flap valve mechanism which prevents reflux of urine from the bladder back into the ureter. Defects in insertion of ureter into bladder lead to vesicoureteral reflux (VUR) and subsequent reflux nephropathy. This is also known as Primary VUR and is more common in boys. The diagnosis is made later in life when the child develops urinary tract infection (UTI). Rarely the VUR may be severe enough to cause ureteral dilatation with gross hydronephrosis, which may be diagnosed in antenatal USG. VCUG is required to confirm the diagnosis and to know the severity of reflux. Secondary VUR results from urinary blockage after repeated UTI especially in girls. It may also be associated with other urological abnormalities like ureterocele and posterior urethral valve. Medical management includes antibiotics to prevent UTI, pyelonephritis, and renal scarring. Ureteric reimplantation will always be required later in life. In cases of VUR associated with other anomalies, surgical correction of the primary defect is always desired. Surgery is performed on elective basis in the childhood age or infancy if severe, though the defect is since birth [49].

(ii) **Pelvi-Ureteric Junction (PUJ) Obstruction**

Congenital stenotic defect at the PUJ causes obstructive uropathy and hydronephrosis. It is mostly diagnosed on antenatal sonography as hydronephrosis without ureteral dilatation. Renal function may be impaired due to pressure atrophy. Of the renal cortex, early intervention in the form of pyeloplasty is favored to prevent further damage to renal parenchyma, yet surgery is deferred beyond the neonatal period to prevent the risks associated with surgery and anesthesia. The indications for surgery in the neonatal age are ipsilateral PUJ obstruction with <40% functioning kidney or with bilateral severe PUJ obstruction with renal parenchymal atrophy.

Preoperative renal function and serum electrolyte levels should be assessed. Open surgical approach is conventionally used. General anesthesia with endotracheal intubation and controlled ventilation is preferred. Caudal block provides good pain relief. Analgesia can also be provided by Transverse abdominis plane block or by infiltration of local anesthetic at the surgical incision site and intravenous paracetamol. The patient is placed in semi lateral position with the lateral tilt of 15–20^0 and a wedge is placed at the level of anterior superior iliac crest to improve the surgical access to kidney. Care should be taken to prevent the extreme wedging as it may compromise the venous return. Liberal fluid therapy is desired to maintain perioperative urine output.

Laparoscopic pyeloplasty is also commonly performed these days with the improved surgical expertize. With CO_2 insufflation, as the diaphragm moves cephalad, the position of ETT should be reconfirmed to exclude endobronchial displacement. The insufflation pressure should be limited to 8–10 mmHg. Higher pressures may cause a rise in peak inspiratory pressures, $EtCO_2$, and hypotension. Hypothermia is to be prevented by using warm fluids and warming blanket. Since laparoscopic procedures are less painful, IV paracetamol and local infiltration at port insertion sites are sufficient for postoperative analgesia.

33.6.11 Gonadal Masses [50]

(i) **Neonatal Testicular Tumors** like teratomas and Para testicular neuroblastomas may present as prenatal testicular torsion. The diagnosis of torsion is excluded by ultrasonography and color doppler. If tumor is suspected, a biopsy by inguinal approach is taken before planning for major surgical procedure.

(ii) **Vaginal Rhabdomyosarcoma** (botryoid sarcoma) appears as a cluster of grayish masses like bunch of grapes prolapsing through the introitus. The baby may present with vaginal bleeding. Surgical intervention is done after thorough evaluation and assessment of the patient.

33.7 Conclusion

Congenital abnormalities of the genitourinary system are very common at birth, but only a few need surgical intervention during the neonatal age, except when it compromises the renal function or causes urinary obstruction. A few conditions that need attention in early age after birth are PUV, upper PUJ obstruction, bilateral renal disease or solid renal masses, inguinal testes with hernia causing GI obstruction, torsion testes, and CMN, which if operated early has a good prognosis. Often they are associated with anomalies of other systems, namely, cardiac and GIT. All surgeries are performed under general anesthesia, with intubation or LMA, spontaneous or controlled ventilation, vigilant monitoring of temperature, blood loss, and fluid shifts. Preanesthetic evaluation of the GU anomaly and its biochemical and physiological effects, presence of other anomalies, anemia, prematurity, must be done and care provided as for any other surgery in this age. GU surgeries are limited to the lower abdominal and pelvis, and pain management can be done with IV analgesics supplemented by caudal anesthesia or analgesia. Pulmonary hypoplasia, an association with birth defects must be taken heed of during controlled ventilation. Postoperative ventilatory support may be needed in neonates after prolonged surgery, major fluid shifts and blood loss, hypothermia and preoperative anemia, and coagulation abnormalities. However, in general, outcome and prognosis, in neonates undergoing GU surgeries, is extremely favorable.

References

1. Weinberg AE, Kennedy WA II. Renal masses and urinary ascites December 28, 2016. Obgyn Key https://obgynkey.com/renal-masses-and-urinary-ascites.
2. Payne RP and Kennedy WA II. Congenital renal masses. Dec 28, 2016. In Pediatrics.
3. Weitzman S, Finkelstein Y, Arceci RJ. Neonatal Oncol. 2017;
4. Capone VP, Morello W, Taroni F, Montini G. Genetics of congenital anomalies of the kidney and urinary tract: the current state of play. Int J Mol Sci. 2017;18(4) pii: E796 https://doi.org/10.3390/ijms18040796. Review
5. Langman J. Special embryology: urogenital system. Chapter 11. pp. 148–182. Medical embryology—human development-normal and abnormal. Langman. 2nd Asian edition 1973 reprint. The Williams & Wilkins Company, Igaku Shoin Ltd.
6. DeUgarte CM. Chapter 2. Embryology of the urogenital system & congenital anomalies of the genital tract. In: DeCherney AH, Nathan L, Laufer N, Roman AS, editors. Current diagnosis & treatment: obstetrics & gynecology. 11th ed. McGraw Hill; 2013. https://accessmedicine.mhmedical.com/content.aspx?bookid=498 & sectionid=41008590.
7. Hill MA. Embryology developmental signals—Fox. 26 October 2021; https://embryology.med.unsw.edu.au/embryology/index.php/DevelopmentalSignals_-_Fox.
8. Kerschner JL, Gosalia N, Leir SH, Harris A. Chromatin remodeling mediated by the FOXA1/A2 transcription factors activates CFTR expression in intestinal epithelial cells. Epigenetics. 2014;9(4):557–65. https://doi.org/10.4161/epi.27696.
9. Weber S. Genetic aspects of human congenital anomalies of the kidney and urinary tract. In: Kidney development, disease, repair and regeneration, 2016.
10. McCabe MJ, Dattani MT. Bone morphogenetic protein 4 and the sonic hedgehog pathway. In: Clinical neuroendocrinology 2014.
11. Moore KL, Persaud TVN. The developing human: clinically oriented embryology. 6th ed. Saunders; 1998.; Ch 13. p. 303–46.
12. Schoenwolf GC. Larson S. Human embryology. 2nd ed. Nov 2014; Chapter 10, pp. 261–306. Churchill Livingstone. ISBN 10: 1455706841.
13. Bronshtein M, Amit A, Achiron R, etal. The early prenatal sonographic diagnosis of renal agenesis: techniques and possible pitfalls. Prenat Diagn 1994; 14:291.
14. Arumugam S, Subbiah NK, Senthiappan AM. Double ureter: incidence, types, and its applied significance—a cadaveric study. Cureus. 2020;12(4):e7760. https://doi.org/10.7759/cureus.7760.
15. Dwyer PL, Rosamilia A. Congenital urogenital anomalies that are associated with the persistence of Gartner's duct: a review. Am J Obst Gynecol. 2006;195(2):354–9. https://doi.org/10.1016/j.ajog.2005.10.815.
16. Jana M, Gupta AK, Prasad KR, Goel S, etal. Pictorial essay: congenital anomalies of male urethra in children. Indian J Radiol Imaging 2011;21(1):38–45. https://doi.org/10.4103/0971-3026.76053.
17. Densmore JC and Oldham KT. Chapter on abdominal masses. In Nelson pediatric symptom-based diagnosis. 2018, pp. 283–301. e2 SCOPUS ID: 2-s2.0-85054348886 01/01/2018; https://doi.org/10.1016/b978-0-323-39956-2.00017-0.
18. Bellon M, Skhiri A, Julien-Marsollier F, etal. Paediatric minimally invasive abdominal and urological surgeries: Current trends and perioperative management. Anaesthesia Crit Care Pain Med 2017; 37(5) https://doi.org/10.1016/j.accpm.2017.11.013.
19. Ebert KM, Jayanthi VR, Alpert SA, Ching CB, et al. Benefits of spinal anesthesia for urologic surgery in the youngest patients. J Pediatr Urol. 2019;15(1):49.e1–5. https://doi.org/10.1016/j.jpurol.2018.08.011. PUV-Ureterocele
20. Zeigler LN, Modes KB, Deshpande JK. Anaesthesia for pediatric urologic procedures. Ch 32, Gregory's Pediatric Anesthesia, 2020, pp. 813–833.
21. Williams RK, Lauro HV, Davis PJ. Anesthesia for general abdominal and urologic surgery. In: Davis PJ, Cladis FP, editors. Smith's anesthesia for infants and children. 9th ed. Philadelphia, Pennsylvania: Elsevier; 2017.

22. O'Neill DB, Ramji F, et al. Neonatal urologic emergencies. Ch 54. Pediatric Urol. 2010;

23. Simpson E, Carstensen J, Murphy P. Neonatal circumcision: new recommendations & implications for practice. Mo Med. 2014;111(3):222–30.

24. Maxwell LG, Yaster M, Wetzel RC, Niebyl JR. Penile nerve block for newborn circumcision. Obstet Gynecol. 1987;70(3 Pt 1):415–9.

25. Williamson PS, Williamson ML. Physiologic stress reduction by a local anesthetic during newborn circumcision. Pediatrics. 1983;71(1):36–40.

26. Fontaine P, Toffler WL. Dorsal penile nerve block for newborn circumcision. Am Fam Physician. 1991;43(4):1327–33.

27. Sharma S, Joshi M, Gupta DK, Abraham M, et al. Consensus on the management of posterior urethral valves from antenatal period to puberty. J Indian Assoc Pediatr Surg. 2019;24(1):4–14. https://doi.org/10.4103/jiaps.JIAPS_148_18.

28. Daisy TM, Rangam MT, Matthews L. Anaesthesia in extremely low birth weight and preterm neonate—a case report. Chettinad Health City Med J. 2020;9(3):202–4. https://doi.org/10.36503/chcmj9(3)-10.

29. Stokowski LA. Hypospadias in the neonate. Adv Neonatal Care. 2004;4(4):206–15. https://doi.org/10.1016/j.adnc.2004.05.003.

30. Splinter WM, Kim J, Kim AM, Harrison MA. Effect of anesthesia for hypospadias repair on perioperative complications. Paediatr Anaesth. 2019 Jul;29(7):760–7. https://doi.org/10.1111/pan.13657.

31. Henderson AM, Vallis CJ, Sumner E. Anaesthesia in the prune-belly syndrome—a review of 36 cases. Anaesthesia. 1987;42:54–60.

32. Goyal S, Gupta SK, Kothari N, et al. Prune-belly syndrome: anesthetic implications and management. Indian Anaesthetists Forum. 2019;20(1):47. https://doi.org/10.4103/TheIAForum.TheIAForum_2_19. LicenseCC BY-NC-SA

33. Arlen AM, Nawaf CM, Kirsch AJ. Prune belly syndrome: current perspectives. Pediatric Health Med Ther. 2019;10:75–81. https://doi.org/10.2147/PHMT.S188014.

34. Khatwa UA, Menon PS. Management of undescended testis. Indian J Pediatr. 2000;67(6):449–54.

35. Shin J, Jeon GW. Comparison of diagnostic and treatment guidelines for undescended testis. Clin Exp Pediatr. 2020;63(11):415–21.

36. Hadziselimovic F. On the descent of the epididymo-testicular unit, cryptorchidism, and prevention of infertility. Basic Clin Androl. 2017;27:21.

37. Rodprasert W, Virtanen HE, Mäkelä JA, Toppari J. Hypogonadism and cryptorchidism. Front Endocrinol (Lausanne). 2019;10:906.

38. Zakaria OM, Hokkam E, Kadi EI, etal. Examination under anesthesia for management of impalpable undescended testis: a traditional technique revisited. World J Surg 2013; 37(5):1125-1129. https://doi.org/10.1007/s00268-013-1973-1.

39. Kaye JD, Levitt SB, Friedman SC, Franco I, Gitlin J, Palmer LS. Neonatal torsion: a 14-year experience and proposed algorithm for management. J Urol. 2008;179(6):2377–83. https://doi.org/10.1016/j.juro.2008.01.148.

40. Riaz-Ul-haq M, Mahdi DEA, Elhassan EU. Neonatal testicular torsion: a review article. Iran J Pediatr. 22(3):281–9.

41. Fernandez N, Santander J, Ceballos C. Regional anesthesia. An alternative to general anesthesia in the management of neonatal testicular torsion. Urology. 2020;146:219–21. https://doi.org/10.1016/j.urology.2020.06.037.

42. Pinto E, Guignard JP. Renal masses in the neonate. Biol Neonate. 1995;68(3):175–84. https://doi.org/10.1159/000244235.

43. Lowe LH, Isuani BH, Heller RM, et al. Pediatric renal masses: Wilms tumor and beyond. Radiographics. 2000;20(6):1585–603. https://doi.org/10.1148/radiographics.20.6.g00nv051585.

44. Beaufils F, Schlegel N, Brun P, Loirat C. Traitement des thromboses veineuses rénales du nouveau-né [Treatment of renal vein thromboses in the newborn]. Ann Pediatr (Paris). 1993;40(2):57–60.

45. Moudgil A. Renal venous thrombosis in neonates. Curr Pediatr Rev. 2014;10(2):101–6. https://doi.org/10.2174/1573396310021405113101845.
46. Khashu M, Osiovich H, Sargent M. Congenital mesoblastic nephroma presenting with neonatal hypertension. J Perinatol. 2005;25:433–5. https://doi.org/10.1038/sj.jp.7211304.
47. Traore F, Maiga B, Diabate K, Coulibaly Y, et al. Treatment of congenital mesoblastic nephroma at pediatric oncology unit of Gabriel Toure teaching hospital. J Pediatr Pediatric. 2018;
48. Pachl M, Arul GS, Jester I, Bowen C, etal. Congenital mesoblastic nephroma: a single-centre series. Ann R Coll Surg Engl 2020;102(1):67-70. https://doi.org/10.1308/rcsann.2019.0111.
49. Gandhi M, Vashisht R. Anaesthesia for paediatric urology. Contin Educ Anaesthesia Crit Care Pain. 2010;10(5):152–7. https://doi.org/10.1093/bjaceaccp/mkq025.
50. Basta AM, Courtier J, Phelps A, Copp HL, Mackenzie JD. Scrotal swelling in the neonate. J Ultrasound Med. 2015;34(3):495–505. https://doi.org/10.7863/ultra.34.3.495.

Anesthesia for Ophthalmic Procedures in the Newborn, Neonate, and Premature

34

Renu Sinha

34.1 Introduction

Congenital anomalies involving craniofacial development, genetic abnormalities, and syndromes, may lead to ocular abnormalities with ocular manifestations. Ophthalmic involvement may not be evident in the neonatal period as it progresses gradually; however, some ophthalmic diseases do manifest in the neonatal age and require urgent medical or surgical intervention. Neonates cannot cooperate for ophthalmic examination so anesthesia is required for evaluation of the disease before a surgery. They often need multiple anesthesia exposures for diagnosis, further evaluation to plan the management, and for surgery [1–4].

Some of the conditions that require urgent attention and surgery in the neonatal age group, include congenital cataract, congenital glaucoma, lid coloboma, keratitis, corneal ulcers, nasolacrimal duct (NLD) blockage, retinoblastoma, retinopathy of prematurity, ocular trauma, evisceration, and enucleation.

(a) **Congenital glaucoma** does not respond optimally to medical management and needs urgent surgical intervention to control the intraocular pressure (IOP).
(b) **Nasolacrimal duct (NLD) obstruction** requires urgent syringing and probing if it does not respond to manual milking.
(c) **Evisceration,** removal of the contents of the globe leaving the sclera behind, is a shorter and less painful procedure than enucleation.

R. Sinha (✉)
Department of Anesthesiology, All India Institute of Medical Sciences, New Delhi, India

(d) **Enucleation,** removal of the whole eyeball as for Retinoblastoma, is a prolonged, painful and traumatic procedure.
(e) **Vitreoretinal surgeries** are painful and require strong analgesics.
(f) **Retinopathy of prematurity (ROP)** is associated with high risk of retinal detachment (RD) and vision loss if treatment is delayed. It needs anesthetic intervention for diagnostic purposes, repeated eye examinations (EUA) to evaluate progression of the disease, and for therapeutic reasons **(laser photocoagulation of retina, intravitreal injection, vitreoretinal and other surgeries)** [5].

Timing of Anesthesia – All eye pathologies in neonates do not require surgery and can be often managed conservatively but will still require examination under anesthesia (EUA). Often the ophthalmic condition is associated with congenital defects and systemic involvement of one or more systems, most common being cardiac and central neural system (CNS). Delaying eye surgery until correction of the systemic defect may not be feasible, as valuable time will be lost and return of optimal vision will be hampered. Hence, such neonates need to be taken up for ophthalmic procedures under general anesthesia, early, to save vision. However, babies with craniofacial involvement may also have airway-related difficulties, which must be kept in mind.

Even after a minor procedure, under general anesthesia, it is prudent to keep the neonate in NICU for a few hours for observation, especially preterm babies, with comorbidities or congenital defects. First episode of apnea usually occurs within the first 4 h of anesthesia exposure. Monitoring for 6 h is adequate for 46–60 weeks postconceptual age (PCA), but longer for under 46 weeks PCA.

Parents should be counseled by ophthalmologist, neonatologist, pediatric genetic experts, and anesthesiologist regarding the need for urgent intervention (investigation or surgery), visual prognosis, and possibility of postoperative NICU stay. Informed consent must be obtained preferably from both parents and caretaker.

Anesthesiologist must understand ocular physiology and its responses, as well as the interaction of ophthalmic drugs and anesthetic agents to prevent complications, some of which may be life or vision threatening.

34.2   Physiology of IOP (Intraocular Pressure) and Factors Affecting

The knowledge of physiology of IOP, effects of anesthesia techniques and drugs, systemic effects of the ophthalmic drugs and drug interactions, effects of surgical manipulation, and mechanism of ocular cardiac reflex (OCR), is important for conduct of safe anesthesia in neonates for ophthalmic procedures.

34.3   Aqueous Humor [6, 7]

Eye is a relatively avascular structure and is lubricated by watery Aqueous humor (AH), secreted by the ciliary epithelium. It circulates over the lens into the anterior chamber through the pupil from the posterior chamber. It is a protein poor ultra-filtrate of plasma, provides nutrition to the eye, removes metabolic waste, keeps the globe of the eye tense by maintaining IOP. Aqueous gets absorbed by the trabecular meshwork and drains into the Canal of Schlemm. AH is produced at a rate of 2 μL/min. In adults, the volume of AH is 0.25 mL (anterior chamber) and 0.06 mL (posterior chamber), with IOP of 10–20 mmHg.

Ciliary muscles have both α and β adrenergic receptors. β_2 stimulation (epinephrine) increases production of AH whereas α_2 (norepinephrine) stimulation reduces AH production (both mediated via cAMP). Increased chloride secretion increases the volume of AH and is regulated by the bicarb production and carbonic anhydrase enzyme.

Contraction of the ciliary muscles and sphincter pupillae causes miosis, increasing AH outflow. Muscarinic antagonists or sympathetic α_1 agonists (cause mydriasis) obstruct the outflow.

Parasympathetic stimulation decreases drainage, but this has a minor effect.

Prostaglandins ($PGF_{2\alpha}$) cause ciliary muscle relaxation, reabsorption of AH, and drainage by the uveoscleral outflow.

Obstruction to free drainage of AH causes increase in IOP. Carbonic anhydrase inhibitors decrease production of the aqueous and reduce IOP.

At birth, IOP is about 9.5 mmHg with diurnal variation of 3–6 mmHg. Various factors affect IOP (Table 34.1). It increases by 5 mmHg during blinking, and by

Table 34.1 Factors affecting IOP

S. no.	Factors increasing IOP	Factors lowering IOP	Fluctuation/variation
1	Obstruction to AH outflow	↓AH secretion–carbonic anhydrase inhibitor (acetazolamide)	Diurnal variation
2	↑CVP (coughing, bucking, vomiting, sneezing, Valsalva maneuver)	↓Venous pressure (head up)	Cardiac cycle
3	↑Choroidal blood volume (respiratory acidosis, hypoxia)	↓Vitreous volume (mannitol induced)	Respiration
4	Hypercarbia, hypertension	Hypotension, hypocarbia	Posture
5	External pressure on the eye, large volume of LA injected	Open globe	

26 mmHg during sneezing and Valsalva maneuver, and fluctuates with cardiac cycle (1–2 mmHg) and respiration (3–5 mmHg). It is affected by changes in choroidal blood volume, central venous pressure (CVP), and extraocular muscle tone. IOP becomes equal to atmospheric pressure in open globe injury and perforation. Elevated IOP decreases intraocular volume by increasing drainage of AH or vitreal extrusion (Figs. 34.1 and 34.2).

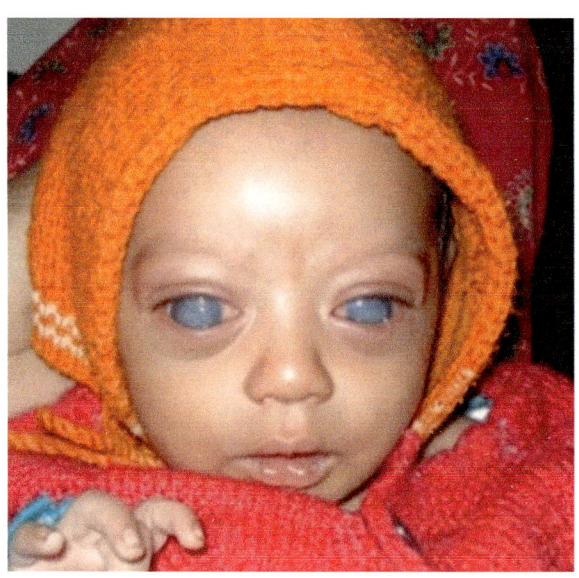

Fig. 34.1 5-days age, bilateral corneal opacity due to primary congenital glaucoma

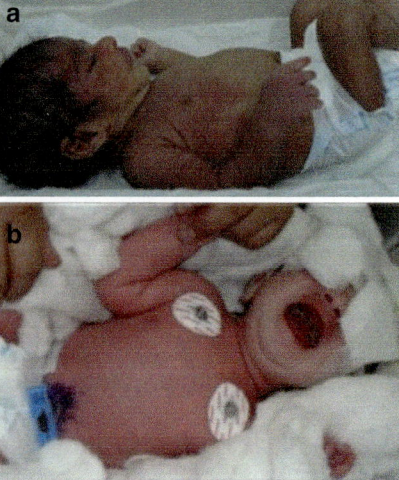

Fig. 34.2 (**a**) Sturge-weber syndrome with glaucoma, (**b**) 1-day age, postglaucoma surgery

34.4 Anesthetic Implications of Drugs Used in Ophthalmology

Topical ophthalmic drugs trickle through the punctum in the medial canthus, into the NLD, absorbed by the nasal mucosa into the systemic circulation. Neonates are more susceptible for the drug-related side effects due to lack of availability of lower concentration of ophthalmic eye drops, e.g., risk with use of higher concentration of phenylephrine is pulmonary edema [8]. Measures to reduce systemic effects include –

- Use of micro dropper.
- Instillation of small amounts (1–2 drops).
- Lower concentration of drugs.
- Occlusion of medial punctum during instillation.
- Increase in viscosity of drug, and.
- Use of alternative drugs.

Various ophthalmic drugs, their concentrations, route of administration, and side effects, in neonates, are given in Table 34.2.

34.4.1 Oculocardiac Reflex (OCR)

OCR occurs during ocular procedures especially strabismus surgery, enucleation, scleral banding, vitreoretinal surgery, and orbital blocks, due to traction on the extraocular muscles (especially medial rectus) or pressure on the globe. Strabismus surgery is not done in the neonatal age, but other ophthalmic procedures can precipitate OCR. Afferents travel through the long and short ciliary nerves to the ciliary ganglion, and via the ophthalmic branch of the Trigeminal nerve to the Gasserian ganglion and sensory nucleus of the Trigeminal nerve. Efferent pathway is via the motor nucleus of vagus (tenth cranial) nerve to the SA node, resulting in dysrhythmias (bradycardia, ventricular ectopics, ventricular fibrillation, and sinus arrest). Postoperative nausea and vomiting is common in children who develop intraoperative OCR [9–12]. Neonates have parasympathetic predominance and so this reflex is more common in them. Hypercapnia increases its sensitivity. It is usually self-limiting once the stimulus is withdrawn. Atropine premedication (20 µg/kg) can prevent this reflex.

Bradycardia response is more with Propofol induction. Sevoflurane is safer with less risk of OCR. Rocuronium and hyperventilation can attenuate OCR but can induce bradycardia because of hypocarbia. Atracurium is a greater risk than Pancuronium but is preferred because of shorter duration of action and nonhepatic metabolism. OCR can be managed by temporary cessation of the surgical stimulus until heart rate increases, simultaneous hyperventilation, maintenance of oxygenation, and increasing depth of anesthesia. If it persists or recurs, atropine (7–10 mcg/kg) or glycopyrrolate (10 mcg/kg) must be administered intravenously. Infiltration of the rectus muscle with local anesthetic (LA) and/or sub-Tenon block is also helpful [12].

Table 34.2 Topical and systemic ophthalmic drugs

Action	Class		Drug	Route	Concentration	Side effects
Mydriasis	Anticholinergic		Atropine	Topical drop/ointment	0.5%, 1%	Tachycardia, fever, anticholinergic effects
			Tropicamide	Drops	0.5%	Dry mouth, drowsiness, tachycardia
	α agonist		Phenylephrine	Drops	2.5%	Transient hypertension, bradycardia, pulmonary edema, cardiac arrest
	Catecholamine		Adrenaline	Topical (Infusion bottle)	0.1 mg in 500 ml RL	Tachycardia, hypertension, tachyarrhythmias
Reduces IOP	β blocker	Nonselective	Timolol	Drops, gel	0.25%, 0.5%	Bradycardia, hypotension. CHF, exacerbation of asthma
		Cardio-selective	Betaxolol	Drops	0.25%	Bradycardia, Sinus arrest
	Parasympathomimetic		Pilocarpine	Drops	1%	Bronchospasm, bradycardia, increase mucous secretion
	Osmotic diuretic		Mannitol	Intravenous	20% - 0.5 g/kg	Hypervolemia, electrolyte imbalance, CHF
	Carbonic anhydrase inhibitor		Acetazolamide	Tablet	8–30 mg/kg/day	Metabolic acidosis, hypokalemia, dehydration
			Dorzalamide	Topical	2%	Headache, strange taste in mouth, dizziness

34.5   Anesthesia Considerations

Most eye surgeries in the neonates are performed in an apparently healthy baby, generally fit to tolerate anesthesia, and may be done on day-case basis. But with increase in survival of preterm and LBW babies, who have several developmental and congenital anomalies and syndromes, many of which have ophthalmic manifestations, now present for treatment. Eye is the most sensitive organ and examination requires a still baby, to prevent injury to the eye during instrumentation at examination. This requires some form of anesthesia or sedation.

Essential considerations in neonates for procedures on the eye are same as for any other surgery in this age group, irrespective of the choice of anesthesia technique, but the goals and anesthetic requirements differ in some ways

34.5.1 Goals of Anesthesia for Ophthalmic Surgery

1. Complete ocular akinesia.
2. Smooth induction and prevention of increase in IOP.
3. Prevention of OCR.
4. Prophylaxis and treatment of PONV – not a problem in neonates.
5. Maintenance of IOP, SpO2, and EtCO2 (avoid aggravation of ROP).
6. Prevention of drug interactions of ophthalmic and anesthetic drugs.
7. Prevention and management of side effects of ophthalmic medications that are continued till the day of surgery.
8. Prevention of pressure on the eye during induction by face mask or hand.
9. Complete asepsis.
10. Care at extubation – cough, strain, airway obstruction, laryngo / bronchospasm.
11. Adequate pain relief using multimodal analgesia.

34.5.2 Preoperative Evaluation (PAE)

A detailed PAE must be done irrespective of the type and duration of the procedure. Few important basic points for neonates planned for anesthesia for eye surgery, are (preferably):

(a) Preferably admit and do as in-patient with adequate postoperative monitoring.
(b) Should be done early in the list so that proper postoperative monitoring can be done.
(c) Informed consent including possible need for NICU stay postoperatively.
(d) Record keeping.

34.5.3 Special Attention Must Be Paid to

1. These babies often require repeated anesthesia for diagnostic purposes (EUA, IOP measurement, USG, CT scan or MRI, etc.). They are under specialist care and expected to have undergone thorough evaluation by the neonatology and ophthalmic teams. Check for the past anesthesia records and note details especially relating to the airway and complications, so that requisite care can be taken in the next anesthesia exposure.
2. However, if the baby is presenting for the first time, a detailed evaluation is a must. Most data can be obtained from the neonatology and ophthalmic records. Of special significance for the anesthesiologist are Birth history (birth weight, gestational age at birth, APGAR score, need for special care (NICU), O2 or ventilatory support).
3. Many eye disorders are associated with **chromosomal or metabolic disorders** (mucopolysaccharidosis, Marfan's Syndrome) with anesthetic implications and must be evaluated and recorded. Common cues are abnormal facies and airway-related symptoms.
4. Accompanying global **developmental delay or mental health** issues require appropriate approach and empathy.
5. **Congenital syndromes** and Ophthalmic manifestations (usually as cataract or glaucoma) –.
     (i) **Hallerman–Strieff syndrome (HSS)** characterized by craniofacial malformations (bird like facies), eye and dental defects, skin atrophic changes, and psychiatric anomalies.
    (ii) **Stickler's syndrome** with Retinal detachment and with glaucoma.
   (iii) **Pierre Robin syndrome** with small lower jaw (problems at laryngoscopy and intubation), tendency of tongue to fall back (risk of airway obstruction at induction with face mask).
   (iv) Syndromes such as **Down's, Marfan, Crouzon's, Fraser, Apert, Sturge Weber, and Pfeiffer.**
    (v) **Craniofacial malformations** such as **Craniosynostosis, Goldenhar, and Treacher–Collins syndrome** [13–15].

34.5.4 Laboratory Investigations

Laboratory investigations required will depend on the preoperative status of the neonate. Usually Hb, Hct, SpO2, and blood sugar suffice. Other investigations include, serum bilirubin, electrolytes, and ABG status, if indicated and for major surgery. Serum calcium should be done as preterm babies are at risk of hypocalcemia and delayed recovery. Surgery or EUA may be urgent as visual prognosis might be compromised due to delay, hence only relevant necessary investigations depending on comorbidities should be advised.

34.5.5 Preoperative Fasting

Preoperative Fasting Instructions - Preterm babies may be on orogastric feeds due to poor sucking reflex. Obtain feeding history and intervals between feeds, so that appropriate nil per oral (NPO) instructions can be given. Fasting guidelines with dextrose containing IV fluids should be followed. About 2–3 h of preoperative nil per oral (NPO) is sufficient in neonates, and 2 h in a newborn baby (within 24 h of birth).

34.6   Anesthesia Techniques

Babies will require anesthesia either for Examination or for Surgery.

Examination Under Anesthesia (EUA) is usually performed bilaterally, and involves IOP assessment, biometry for intraocular power calculation, fundoscopy, and retinoscopy. The duration may range from 15 to 45 min and at times longer, especially if EUA is combined with a short surgical procedure. It must be noted that while all babies will undergo EUA, may be more than once, all babies may not need surgery. Hence EUA is the commonest procedure performed in the neonatal age group.

Surgery may also vary from being a short procedure or of long duration and a major one. Ideal technique is tracheal intubation and balanced anesthesia with assisted or controlled ventilation. Usually only one eye is operated in one sitting because of risk of infection.

General Anesthesia can be administered in many ways, depending on the available facilities, skill of the anesthetist, and ophthalmological requirements.

1. **Face Mask and Bag with a Spontaneous Ventilation** has the advantage of quick induction and recovery, avoidance of airway invasion, laryngoscopy and its adverse effects, and necessary polypharmacy, but has certain limitations needing attention and care:
   (i) **Patient selection** - all neonates are not suited to mask-based anesthesia. Those with airway difficulty are the ones where one would like to avoid airway invasion (ETI/SGD) and are also at-risk during facemask anesthesia. Careful planning and discussion with the surgical team and keeping EUA short, mask-based technique might be a safer option. In babies with major craniofacial anomalies, airway must be secured even for EUA. For surgery, it is always better to secure the airway with ETI /SGD and assisted or controlled ventilation.
   (ii) This requires **skill in mask holding** without airway obstruction, especially in newborns, LBW, premature, and very small neonates, for the duration of 30–60 min.
   (iii) Appropriate **well-fitting face mask** and neonatal fit breathing circuit.
   (iv) Requires **constant hand adjustments** of the anesthetist in holding the mask - with left hand for right eye examination and with the right hand for left eye examination to allow the ophthalmologist to perform the EUA on both eyes,

(v) An **assistant** must be available, as both hands of the anesthetists are busy.

(vi) **Crowding at the head end** of the little baby under EUA, with the anesthetist, ophthalmologist, and one assistant, etc.

(vii) Constant hand adjustments and associated head and neck movements expose the baby to **airway-related problems** like obstruction, laryngospasm, aspiration of secretions, hypoxemia, CO_2 retention, bradycardia, and apnea.

2. **SGD/LMA**: This is a more convenient technique as the anesthetist can stay out of the eye examination field, allowing a clear wide field for the ophthalmologist to perform unhindered procedure. This avoids tracheal intubation and its risks. Besides, anesthetists' hands are free for monitoring and drug administration. Additional advantage is in case of unanticipated prolongation in the procedure when ventilation can be assisted or controlled [16–19]. Limitations with this technique are:

(i) Need for appropriate size small LMA.

(ii) Anesthetist skill in placing the LMA, especially in babies with orofacial anomalies.

(iii) Risk of displacement of the LMA and loss of airway in case of head movements or light anesthesia.

(iv) Alternative airway devices must be always at hand (ET and laryngoscope).

3. **Tracheal Intubation**—is the only definitive airway option, but has several risks associated with it, such as:

(i) Need for adequately deep anesthesia for ET toleration.

(ii) Need for poly pharmacy—muscle relaxants, narcotics, and reversal agents.

(iii) Risk of bradycardia at laryngoscopy and intubation.

(iv) Risk of laryngeal edema and damage to tracheal mucosa.

(v) Problems at extubation.

(vi) Delay in extubation and recovery.

(vii) High risk of postoperative apnea.

4. **Regional Blocks** are useful adjuncts to general anesthesia in neonates also. Their usefulness lies in the fact that they reduce the requirement of anesthetic agents and narcotics, especially in sick babies and those with airway difficulty, lower the risk for postoperative apnea, and thereby better recovery from anesthesia. Limitations of Eye blocks are:

(i) Since blocks are performed under GA, risk of complications is higher.

(ii) Risk of needle stick injury to the eye structure.

(iii) Risk of LA overdose and toxicity.

(iv) Increase in IOP.

(v) Eye hemorrhage.

(vi) Requires skill.

(vii) Contraindicated in conditions such as Retinoblastoma and other eye tumors, anatomical deformation of the orbit and globe, and microphthalmos.

34.7 Examination Under Anesthesia (EUA)

34.7.1 General Principles

General anesthesia is required for ocular disease evaluation, staging, refraction, IOP measurement, ultrasonography, fundus examination, suture removal, corneal tattooing, etc. Any sort of examination in neonates requires general anesthesia.

34.7.2 Special Care During EUA and IOP Measurement

- Duration of EUA may be short, a few minutes or longer, lasting up to 30–45 min. Anesthetist must discuss with the ophthalmologist regarding what all that will be done during the examination, and accordingly plan for anesthesia.
- Risk of stimulation of OCR and severe bradycardia, e.g., when too much pressure or traction is exerted on the eyeball. Due precautions must be taken to prevent this and anesthetist be ready to manage it.
- Eye examination (EUA)is usually performed as a day care procedure, but preterm neonates and those with medical diseases and congenital abnormalities and syndromic babies, should be admitted.
- Most anesthetic agents reduce IOP. Injudicious anesthesia may reduce the IOP to an extent as to mask the higher IOP, affecting management.
- No premedication.
- IOP reading should be taken at the beginning of induction as higher concentrations of Sevoflurane and prolonged exposure may result in underestimation of IOP.

34.7.3 Anesthesia Considerations

- Intravenous and inhalation induction is suitable depending on the anesthesiologist choice.
- Can be performed using Face mask, SGD or tracheal intubation depending. Be prepared to intubate in case of failure of SGD placement.
- Proper seal of face mask without pressure on eyeball to facilitate eye examination needs expertize.
- An intravenous cannula can be inserted before or after induction of anesthesia.
- Spontaneous or assisted ventilation with O_2, N_2O/air, and inhalational agent is preferred.
- Sometimes eye examination is done under topical anesthesia alone with oral sucrose or dextrose. This technique is used for neonates who need only short examination without any intervention.
- IOP should not be checked if neonate is crying as it can give spurious high reading.
- Ketamine is preferable despite a slight increase in IOP following its administration. But this is preferable to the fall in IOP by other anesthetic agents, especially when measuring IOP.

- Sevoflurane also does not cause a fall in IOP except when used in higher concentrations (>5%).
- Succinyl choline does not produce muscle fasciculations in neonates but does increase IOP.

Nondepolarizing muscle relaxants (NDMR) per se have no effect on IOP. But apnea and hypercarbia will increase IOP and hyperventilation and hypocapnia will reduce IOP.

34.8   Anesthesia for Surgical Procedures

34.8.1   General Principles

- Both inhalational and intravenous (IV) induction can be adopted. Thiopentone and Sevoflurane are agents of choice for induction.
- Preterm neonates may have an IV cannula in situ for preoperative fluid administration, or can be secured preoperatively, and titrated dose of IV agent can be administered for induction.
- Intravenous induction is preferred with big orbital mass due to chances of compression of the mass with face mask during inhalational induction.
- Caution to avoid eye injury and pressure during mask ventilation.
- IV cannula is preferred in lower limb as neonate will be far away from the anesthesiologist during ophthalmic surgery. Dextrose containing IV fluid should be used.
- Drugs should be used with caution because of the effect on IOP. Drugs and procedures that can affect IOP are listed in Table 34.3.

Table 34.3 Drugs and procedures that can affect IOP

Drugs/procedure	Effect on IOP
Thiopentone, propofol, inhalational agents	↓
Ketamine	↑
Succinylcholine	↑
NDMR	↓ or no effect
Laryngoscopy, intubation, extubation	↑
SGD insertion	May have no effect
Spontaneous ventilation	↑ If $EtCO_2$ rises
Controlled ventilation	↓ If ↓ in $EtCO_2$
Coughing, bucking, airway obstruction	↑
Pressure on eyeball	↑

34.8.2 Airway Management

Endotracheal intubation (ETI) and supraglottic devices (SGD) have been used for ophthalmic surgeries. Face mask can be used for short EUA. Avoid ocular pressure with face mask. SGD is preferable for EUA and short surgery in neonates weighing more than 3 kg, as rescue device in case of difficult ventilation and conduit for fiberoptic-guided intubation. Smaller size ET should be available as neonates may have history of previous intubation. Video laryngoscopy is helpful for simple as well as difficult intubation. ET position should be carefully confirmed by auscultation and properly secured.

34.8.3 Neuromuscular Block (NMB)

For short EUA, muscle relaxants are not required. NLD, Oculoplastic and vitreoretinal, and ROP surgeries should be done under balanced anesthesia technique using NMB, ETI, and controlled ventilation.

In neonates with difficult airway, succinylcholine can be used for intubation. In other cases, use of succinylcholine for intubation depends on anesthesiologist choice. Succinylcholine is useful in case laryngospasm occurs. Among NDMR, atracurium and cisatracurium are the relaxants of choice for neonates. Before administering a muscle relaxant, always check for feasibility of unobstructed mask ventilation.

Anesthesia is usually maintained with O_2 in nitrous oxide (N_2O) or air, sevoflurane/ isoflurane/ desflurane depending on availability. N_2O should be avoided in vitreoretinal surgery if injection of gas is planned.

These babies are prone to and may need calcium supplement at the time of extubation.

34.8.4 Pain Relief

- Long-acting opioids can cause postoperative apnea, more in up to 46 weeks PCA.
- Short-acting opioids (Fentanyl, Remifentanil) are preferred, in titrated doses and with arrangement for postoperative respiratory support.
- Regional blocks like peribulbar block, sub-Tenon block, and topical anesthesia may be helpful in reducing opioid requirement.
- IV or rectal acetaminophen can be used intraoperative and postoperative analgesia, in a dose of acetaminophen is 7.5 mg/kg 8 hourly (<32 weeks gestation), 6 hourly (33–36 weeks), and 10–15 mg/kg 6 hourly (>36 weeks gestation), intravenously.
- During procedures under topical anesthesia, allowing sweetened pacifier for baby to suck on has a calming and probably some analgesic effect [20].

34.9   Regional Anesthesia Techniques

Topical and regional blocks are used as adjuncts to general anesthesia in neonates. Though useful, they are associated with complications like LA overdose, vascular injury, injury to eyeball structures, increase in IOP, chemosis, subconjunctival hemorrhage, and infection [21].

1. **Topical Ophthalmic Anesthesia** can be administered using eye drops and gel preparations. This is low cost and avoids complications of needle block. Commonly used drugs are Proparacaine 0.5%, Lignocaine drops 4%, Lignocaine gel 2%, and Tetracaine drops 1%. Combination of topical and intracameral anesthesia gives good results.
2. **Regional Block**: Lignocaine 2%, Bupivacaine 0.5%, and Ropivacaine 0.5% are suitable for regional blocks in neonates. These drug concentrations are the same as those used in adults, so care must be taken not to exceed the safe dose limit.
    (i) **Peribulbar block** is administered after general anesthesia. This helps to reduce opioid requirement and incidence of OCR. Either the anesthetist or ophthalmologist can administer the block. Do not exceed the safe volume and dose limit, to avoid increase in IOP and complications.
    (ii) **Sub-Tenon block** has been used in neonates for various ophthalmic surgeries. It requires less volume of LA. Subconjunctival hemorrhage and chemosis are the main side effects [11].

34.10 Monitoring

Standard monitoring including ECG, heart rate (HR), arterial oxygen saturation (SpO$_2$), noninvasive blood pressure (NIBP), EtCO$_2$ is routinely applied for ophthalmic surgery. In case of SGD, cuff pressure monitoring can be used.

Temperature monitoring and blood glucose monitoring are done in preterm infants. Radiant warmer, second pulse oximeter are also used in neonates.

Monitoring is difficult in ophthalmic surgery as airway is away from the anesthetist and head end is crowded with two ophthalmologist, microscope, and surgical trolleys. Displacement of SGD or circuit disconnection can be detected early with inspired and expired tidal volume and EtCO$_2$. One should avoid movement of the operating table as it can disturb microscopic vision.

34.11 Extubation

Extubation or removal of SGD should be smooth, without coughing and straining, to prevent increase in IOP and bleeding from the surgical site. Deep extubation in neonates needs expertize. Incidence of reintubation is high as compared to older children because of apnea and delated recovery. Preparation of reintubation should always be done before extubation. Care should be taken to avoid pressure on eyeball and face mask after extubation. Proper seal of face mask is difficult due to the eye bandage. Baby should be kept lateral with operative side up to prevent pressure on the eye.

34.12 Postoperative Care

Postoperative breath holding, apnea, and episodic bradycardia are potentially serious complications for premature and ex-premature neonates due to fragile cardiorespiratory system. Perioperative risk of apnea depends on the PCA and gestational age. Apnea at emergence from anesthesia, periodic breathing in the recovery room, and history of anemia confers moderate additional risk for delayed breath holding.

Any intervention or intercurrent illness can aggravate cardiorespiratory instability. Neonate should be kept in incubator for temperature control and oxygenation.

Postoperative monitoring should include SpO_2, ECG, and respiration in PACU/NICU. O_2 supplementation should continue. High-risk neonates should be shifted to NICU as mechanical ventilation may be required.

Breast-feeding or formula feed needs to be initiated once the neonate is fully awake. Until then maintenance intravenous fluids should be continued.

Postoperative analgesia should be provided with intravenous or rectal acetaminophen.

34.13 Complications

- Intraoperative arrhythmias, bradycardia, and even asystole are not uncommon during eye surgery.
- Bradycardia, hypertension, and pulmonary edema can occur after phenylephrine eye drops which may need NICU admission.
- Postoperative apnea and bradycardia are common in preterm neonates.

34.14 Common Ophthalmic Surgeries in Neonates

Specific requirements with each procedure will be discussed here.

(i) *Congenital Cataract*: This is seen as a white reflex observed by parents or pediatrician, is usually bilateral and commonly associated with systemic disease and syndromes (Down syndrome, Peter's anomaly, congenital rubella syndrome). [22] Surgery is performed early to avoid amblyopia [23]. Good mydriasis is needed for surgery and is achieved by topical mydriatic drugs (atropine, tropicamide, phenylephrine) applied preoperatively. Intraoperative mydriasis is maintained with adrenaline in balanced salt solution as irrigant.

Intracameral adrenaline can also be used to maintain intraoperative mydriasis. Mydriatics cause tachycardia, which may not be due to pain or light anesthesia.

In neonates, lens aspiration is done along with posterior central curvilinear capsularhexis (PCCC) and anterior vitrectomy. Intraocular lens (IOL) implantation is usually done after 2 yr age, as the lens capsule is too small to accommodate commercially available IOL. Anesthesia should provide complete akinesia and meticulous control of IOP with controlled ventilation. In neonates, topical anesthesia and paracetamol provide adequate analgesia. Postoperative pain after cataract surgery is minimal and can be managed with paracetamol.

(ii) *Corneal Surface Disorders*: Keratoplasty may be required for corneal diseases. Vit A deficiency may lead to corneal melting and perforation. Lid coloboma leads to corneal opacity and if not treated can lead to secondary infection and perforation. In Peter's anomaly, corneal opacity is usually present. Optical iridectomy provides some vision till keratoplasty is done at a later stage. Depending on the thickness of corneal opacity, lamellar keratoplasty may be required after shaving of opacity. There are many types of keratoplasties including optical, therapeutic, tectonic, and lamellar. Corneal dermoid needs excision especially if it is obstructing pupillary area. General anesthesia is required for these surgeries, regional block should be administered with caution as it can increase IOP.

(iii) *Glaucoma*: Primary congenital glaucoma (PCG) is a rare genetic disorder. It may be associated with congenital abnormalities (craniofacial dysostosis, chromosomal trisomies, Sturge weber and Crouzon syndromes) [24]. It has the classic triad of tearing, photophobia, and blepharospasm. Corneal "clouding" and buphthalmos may be clinically evident at the time of birth. Its incidence is 1:2000–1:10,000 births, is bilateral in 75% cases, and more common in males (65%).

The treatment is early surgery under general anesthesia. Combined trabeculotomy with mitomycin C (MMC 0.2–0.4 mg/mL) is the preferred procedure. Surgery is moderately painful due to incision of conjunctiva and sclera. Preoperatively, raised IOP is managed by oral acetazolamide (15 mg/kg/day) and topical medications like dorzolamide (carbonic anhydrase inhibitor), timolol and betaxolol (beta blockers), or pilocarpine (alpha-2 agonist). Topical drugs also have several side effects (bradycardia, hypotension, bronchospasm, respiratory obstruction, and decreases myocardial contractility) due to systemic absorption. Side effects of antiglaucoma drugs should be ruled out during preanesthetic evaluation.

The aim of anesthetic management is to maintain IOP within normal range and prevent its increase during anesthetic procedures (laryngoscopy, intubation, extubation). Both intubation and extubation increase IOP especially during coughing and straining on ET which may lead to visual damage [16]. SGD provides definitive advantage as it does not increase IOP during inser-

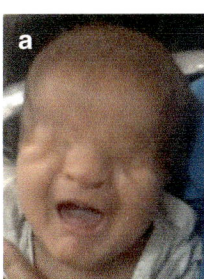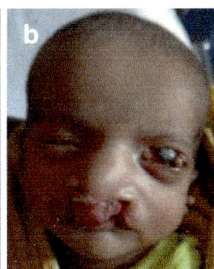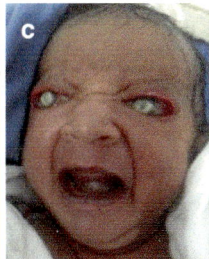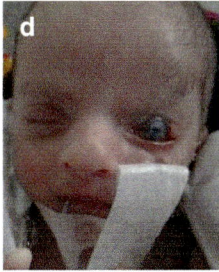

Fig. 34.3 Oculoplastic disorders: (**a**) 28-days crypophthalmos, (**b**) 19-days Goldenhar syndrome, (**c**) 20-days microblepharon and corneal melting, (**d**) 12-day lid coloboma and corneal opacity

tion and removal. Subconjunctival LA injection at the start of surgery and in the sub-Tenon's space at the end of surgery provides analgesia. Short-acting opioid and paracetamol may be used for multimodal analgesia. Mannitol is administered at a dose of 0.5 g/kg within 15 min before the start of surgery. There is no recommendation for use of mannitol and its dosage in preterm babies due to increased risk of intraventricular hemorrhage. Postoperative pain can be managed with NSAIDs.

(iv) *Oculoplastic Disorders*: Surgery is required in neonatal period for anophthalmos, microphthalmos, cryptophthalmos, buphthalmos, lid coloboma, microblepharon, NLD obstruction, dermoid, burns, etc. (Fig. 34.3). These anomalies may be a part of syndrome. Common procedures are syringing and probing (for NLD blockage), lid reconstruction with or without skin grafting (for lid coloboma and microphthalmos), skin grafting for burn, dermoid excision, and tarsorrhaphy (for exposure keratopathy).

Eye protection should be done during mask ventilation to prevent injury especially in case of lid coloboma and orbital swelling. Face mask should be soft with proper fitting as poor fitting mask will lead to pressure on the eye. Author prefers Rendell-Baker mask due to its round shape as it hugs the bridge of the nose and tapers away from the eyes.

Sino-orbital massage is the initial treatment for NLD blockade in neonates, and if it fails, then syringing and probing is done. Methylene blue or betadine mix saline is injected through either of punctum after probing to check patency of the NLD. If colored saline is aspirated from ipsilateral nostril, then procedure is successful. It is usually done on day care basis. ETI or SGD can be used with continuous suction through ipsilateral nasal cavity or pharynx. Proper size neck role is kept under the shoulders to divert irrigation fluid away from the larynx. Chances of respiratory complications are more during this procedure [17–19]. Lid reconstruction is usually done by local flap raising or transplanting skin from posterior surface of ear on ipsilateral side. Tarsorrhaphy is done after lid reconstruction. Many a times amniotic membrane grafting is done to protect cornea along with lid reconstruction.

(v) *Neonatal Retinoblastoma*: Retinoblastoma (RB) is responsible for 4–29% of solid neonatal cancers that make up 1–3% of childhood malignancy. Up to 7–10% RB is diagnosed in neonatal period. Prenatal genetic testing can diagnose it before birth. If prenatal genetic test is positive, screening is done by USG or MRI during third trimester. Diagnosis of RB in preterm infants has been increased due to ROP screening. Neonatal RB is characterized by definitive familial history, unilateral at the time of diagnosis but with higher rate of becoming bilateral, usually of higher grade with macular involvement. Screening of term neonate of parents with familial history of RB is done within 2 weeks of birth and then every 2 weeks. RB can be treated successfully if diagnosed early. However, if left untreated it leads to significant morbidity and mortality due to metastases.

Common presenting features are leucocoria (60%), strabismus (20%), red painful eye (5%), poor vision, orbital cellulitis, unilateral mydriasis, heterochromia iridis, and hyphema. Ultrasound, CT, MRI, bone scan, bone marrow aspiration, lumbar puncture, and genetic analysis are done for tumor classification, extent of tumor and treatment planning. MRI is superior to CT scan for optic nerve evaluation and detection of extraocular extension; however, it cannot detect calcification [25–27].

Current treatment of RB includes eye-preserving therapy with photo or cryo coagulation, transpupillary thermotherapy, external radiation brachytherapy, and chemotherapy (cisplatin, carboplatin, vincristine, cyclophosphamide, etoposide, topotecan, and doxorubicin, given IV, periocular in sub-Tenon space, in ophthalmic artery and intravitreal). In advance cases, enucleation is done. Side effects should be considered at PAE. IV access may be difficult.

Standard chemotherapy is not very effective due to lack of significant vascular supply in the neonatal period. Transpupillary thermotherapy is also not very effective as neonatal fundus is lightly pigmented which does not absorb enough heat to kill small focus. Ophthalmic artery chemosurgery and radioactive plaque may be more effective. Vitreous seedlings occur early leading to increase chances of vitreous relapse. Incidence of enucleation is minimal as diagnosis is sometimes delayed and other treatment options are considered.

General anesthesia is required for EUA, laser photocoagulation, transpupillary thermotherapy, and intravitreal injection. GA with ETI and balanced anesthesia is preferred for therapeutic procedures. During enucleation, OCR can occur at the time of indentation of sclera or at dissection of extraocular muscles and when eye is stretched to cut the optic nerve. Adrenaline-soaked bandage pack is used after enucleation to decrease bleeding. Blood should be arranged according to the preoperative hemoglobin. An implant is inserted in the empty orbit for normal growth. Enucleation is a painful surgery so multimodal analgesia including fentanyl, paracetamol, and sub-Tenon block should be considered.

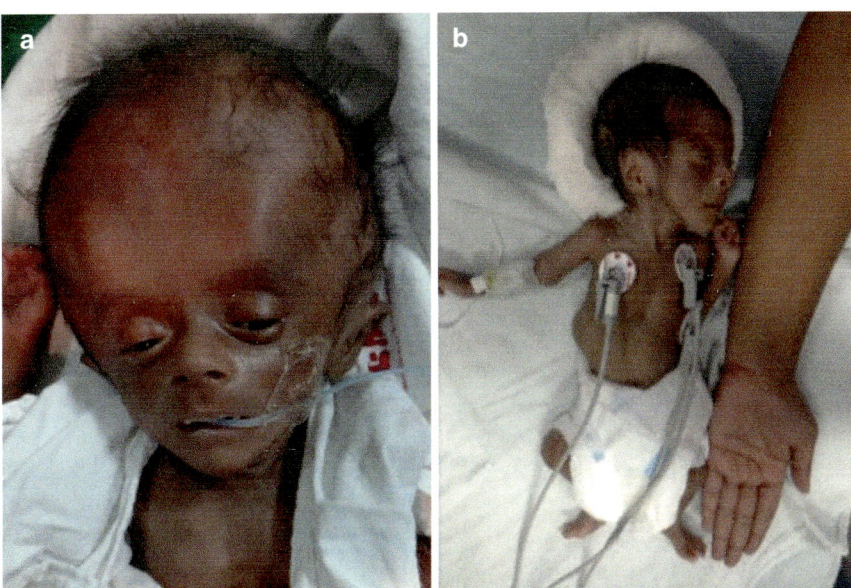

Fig. 34.4 Preterm with ROP. (**a**) 35-weeks PCA hydrocephalus, (**b**) 32-weeks PCA 1.0 kg for intravitreal injection

(vi) ***Retinopathy of Prematurity***: ROP is a vaso proliferative disorder due to arrest of normal retinal neurovascular development followed by compensatory aberrant vascularization in preterm (BW < 1250 g/<31 week GA) neonates (Fig. 34.4). It is a leading cause of preventable blindness. In utero, retinal vascularization occurs in the second and third trimesters and peaks prebirth (36–40 weeks). This gets disrupted in preterm births and retina becomes ischemic and hypoxic. Hypoxia stimulates growth factors like VEGF (vascular endothelia growth factor) leading to neovascularization. Subsequently, retina undergoes cicatricial changes, folds on itself, and leads to RD. International classification for ROP (ICROP) is according to location of retinal involvement, severity of ROP (stage 1–5), plus disease, preplus disease, and aggressive posterior ROP [28–30]. **Treatment Options:** Early intervention is needed for good visual outcome. Treatment guidelines are based on the Early Treatment for Retinopathy of Prematurity (ETROP) trial. Laser photocoagulation is done in ROP Stage III [5]. Scleral buckling and lens sparing vitrectomy are performed in ROP Stage IV while vitrectomy is performed in ROP Stage V. Serial examinations are advised for type 2 ROP which include absence of plus disease in stage 1/2 ROP in Zone I and stage 3 ROP in Zone II. Intravitreal injection of antivascular endothelial growth factor (anti-VEGF), peripheral ablation of avascular retina and retinal surgery are done to treat type 1 ROP. Type 1 ROP includes: Zone I any stage ROP with plus disease, Zone I, stage 3 ROP with or without plus disease and Zone II, stage 2 or 3 ROP with plus disease [31–44].

Examination of Eye: Eye examination is done via Retcam under topical anesthesia. Retinal images are saved for future reference for staging, evaluating progression of disease, effect of treatment and for teaching.

Anesthesia/Sedation for Laser Therapy for ROP: Laser ablation for ROP can be done either in the OT or in NICU while keeping baby in incubator. Spontaneous head or eye movements can lead to inadvertent laser application of the adjoining unaffected parts of the retina. Pupillary dilatation is done 10 min before the laser with 1–2 micro drops of 2.5% phenylephrine. Laser therapy is a painful, especially if beam strikes on iris or reaches till sclera at the path of long and short ciliary nerves. It requires scleral indentation to reach periphery of retina. Duration of laser is 60–90 min to hit more than 1000 spots in retina. The procedure results in significant stress response and may result in cardiorespiratory changes due to scleral indentation, deep retinal/pupil margin burns, and globe manipulation. Protective goggles should be used by the anesthesiologists, neonatologist, and staff according to the type of laser light.

Anesthesia and sedation protocols for laser therapy are variable at different centers. These include topical anesthesia with oral sucrose, topical anesthesia combined with oral or rectal sedation (chloral hydrate and/or paracetamol), topical anesthesia with IV ketamine, general anesthesia (ETI/SGD, controlled ventilation), remifentanil/ morphine/ fentanyl infusion and sub-tenon's block. Topical anesthesia alone results in more frequent adverse cardiorespiratory events in comparison to other techniques. Topical proparacaine 0.5% significantly reduces pain scores in preterm neonates during eye speculum insertion. The baby should be wrapped inside the drapes to keep warm and to prevent limb movements during the procedure. The assistant should support both head and chin to reduce head and neck movement. Sweetened Pacifier may reduce the baby's distress and cry [20]. Monitoring SpO_2, ECG, and respiration helps early diagnosis of bradycardia, apnea, and desaturation.

Sub-tenon's anesthesia with oral/rectal sedation can be performed in NICU in incubator, that reduces the delay in treatment along with risks of IV sedation, intubation, and complications during transportation. Performing sub-tenon's block in very small eye is challenging. However, a careful pre-procedural assessment is essential to select the most suitable anesthesia technique for each baby based on history of duration of mechanical ventilation, requirement of CPAP or higher FiO_2, and recent episodes of desaturation or bradycardia [11].

Intravitreal Injection: Injection of anti-VEGF [bevacizumab (0.063–0.25 mg) or ranibizumab (0.1–0.2 mg)] has been used for ROP treatment. Recent studies showed better effect of intravitreal injection with fewer complications in comparison to laser therapy. It can be administered in NICU, OPD or OT settings. Sterility should not be compromised as there is risk of intraocular infection. Anti-VEGF can lead to potential local and systemic developmental effects and frequent follow-ups are required. Variable anesthesia techniques have been practiced including topical anesthesia with oral sucrose, sub-Tenon's block with oral sucrose, and anesthesia with sevoflurane. Preterm neonates should be monitored in NICU as they are between 30 and 38 weeks PCA. An IV cannula should always be inserted to treat bradycardia and for fluid administration during fasting period.

(vii) **Vitreoretinal Surgery**: Many ophthalmic centers are stand-alone or far away from NICU facility. Preterm infant should be transferred to the OT and back to NICU in incubator with proper monitoring along with neonatologist or anesthesiologist. Bilateral VR surgery or laser of one eye and VR surgery of the other eye may be planned in single sitting. 25 G and 27 G scleral ports are made which do not require suturing. Duration of surgery varies from 45 to 120 min.

Inhalational or IV induction with ETI/SGD can be used. Author prefers ETI as there are more chances of intraoperative displacement of SGD in preterms and intraoperative repositioning of airway device can lead to eye injury and infection. N2O should be avoided. As fluctuation between hypoxia and hyperoxia produces greater neovascularization, SpO2 should be maintained within a restricted, tight range (87–92% or NICU prescribed limits) to prevent further neovascularization and progression of ROP. Since concentration, duration, timing, and fluctuations of O_2 levels have a role in ROP progression, optimal intraoperative SpO_2 has yet to be clearly elucidated. In chronic lung disease, higher FiO_2 during surgery reduces the likelihood of severe hypoxemia, lowers pulmonary arterial pressure, and decreases airway resistance. Adequate depth of anesthesia prevents OCR. Dextrose containing IV fluid should be administered by infusion pump, especially in LBW babies or those requiring TPN preoperatively. Blood glucose should be monitored to avoid hypoglycemia. Ex-preterm neonates (<44 weeks gestation) are at high risk of apnea and need postoperative monitoring for 12–24 h. Multimodal regimen consisting of minimal/low dose opioids (fentanyl /remifentanil) combined with regional blocks (sub-Tenon's/ peribulbar), topical anesthesia, and acetaminophen can be used [45, 46].

(viii) **Emergency Eye Surgery**: Traumatic or chemical burn eye injury, endophthalmitis, foreign body should be treated urgently to prevent visual loss. It may be associated with head injury or injuries of other organs. Corneal and or scleral perforation repair, globe repair, lid repair are performed as early as possible depending on the extent of injury. Decision to delay in surgery should be taken with the ophthalmologist after establishing the degree of urgency and need for optimization of systemic disease to gain maximum visual prognosis. Penetrating injuries need urgent attention due to the risk of infection, endophthalmitis, vitreous loss, and RD. Proper preoperative evaluation should be done to rule out any other medical or surgical disease and other injuries. Rapid sequence induction technique is preferred in neonate with full stomach. There is always a caution for the use of succinylcholine with open globe due to increase in IOP. SGD with gastric drain or ETI can be used depending on the anesthesiologist choice. Short-acting opioid, regional anesthesia and paracetamol should be administered. In case of open eye injury, peribulbar block should not be administered as it may lead to increase in IOP.

References

1. Gayer S, Tutiven J. Anaesthesia for pediatric ocular surgery. Opthalmol Clin N Am. 2006;19(2):269–78.
2. Bret CM, Zwass MS. Eyes, ears, nose, throat and dental surgery. In: George A. Gregory, editor. Pediatric anaesthesia, 4th ed. London: Churchill Livingstone, 2003. pp. 663–706.
3. Hauser MW, Valley R, Bailey AG. Anesthesia for pediatric ophthalmic surgery. Smith's Anesthesia for infants and children. 7th ed. Elsevier; 2006. p. 770–86.
4. Feldman MA, Patel A. Anesthesia for eye, ear, nose, and throat surgery. In: Miller's anesthesia, 7th ed. Elsevier, 2010, pp. 3423–3472.
5. Early Treatment for Retinopathy of Prematurity Cooperative Group. Revised indications for the treatment of retinopathy of prematurity: results of the early treatment for retinopathy of prematurity randomized trial. Arch Ophthalmol. 2003;121:1684–94.
6. Krupin T, Wax M, Moolchandani J. Aqueous production. Trans Ophthalmol Soc U K. 1986;105(Pt 2):156–61.
7. To CH, Kong CW, Chan CV, et al. The mechanism of aqueous humor formation. Clin Exp Optom. 2002;85(6):335–49.
8. Renu S. Topical phenylephrine induced pulmonary odema: few suggestions. Paediatr Anaesth. 2009;19(5):553.
9. Sauerbrei A, Wutzler P. Herpes simplex and varicella-zoster virus infections during pregnancy: current concepts of prevention, diagnosis and therapy. Part 2: Varicella-zoster virus infections. Med MicrobiolImmunol. 2007;196(2):95–102.
10. Braun U, Feise J, Mühlendyck H. Is there a cholinergic and an adrenergic phase of the oculocardiac reflex during strabismus surgery? Acta Anaesthesiol Scand. 1993;37(4):390–5.
11. Steib A, Karcenty A, Calache E, Franckhauser J, et al. Effects of subtenon anesthesia combined with general anesthesia on perioperative analgesic requirements in pediatric strabismus surgery. Reg Anesth Pain Med. 2005;30(5):478–83.
12. Misurya VK, Singh SP, Kulshrestha VK. Prevention of oculocardiac reflex (O.C.R) during extraocular muscle surgery. Indian J Ophthalmol. 1990;38(2):85–7.
13. Sinha R, Maitra S. The effect of peribulbar block with general anesthesia for vitreoretinal surgery in preterm and Ex-Premature infants with retinopathy of prematurity. Anesth Analg Case Rep. 2016;6(2):25–7.
14. Jean YK, Kam D, Gayer S, Palte HD, Stein ALS. Regional anesthesia for pediatric ophthalmic surgery: a review of the literature. Anesth Analg. 2020;130(5):1351–63.
15. James I. Anaesthesia for paediatric eye surgery. Continuing Educ Anaesth Crit Care Pain. 2008;8:5–10.
16. Madan R, Tamilselvan P, Sadhasivam S, Shende D, et al. Intra-ocular pressure and haemodynamic changes after tracheal intubation and extubation: a comparative study in glaucomatous and nonglaucomatous children. Anaesthesia. 2000;55:380–4.
17. Gulati M, Mohta M, Ahuja S, Gupta VP. Comparison of laryngeal mask airway with tracheal tube for ophthalmic surgery in paediatric patients. Anaesth Intensive Care. 2004;32:383–9.

18. Langenstein H, Möller F, Krause R, Kluge R, Vogelsang H. Safe handling of the laryngeal mask airway in eye surgery. Anaesthesist. 1997;46:389–97.
19. Sunder RA, Joshi C. A technique to improve the safety of laryngeal mask airway when used in lacrimal duct surgery. Paediatr Anaesth. 2006;16:130–3.
20. Stevens B, Yamada J, Lee GY, Ohlsson A. Sucrose for analgesia in newborn infants undergoing painful procedures. Cochrane Database Syst Rev. 2013;1:CD001069.
21. Sinha R, Patel N, Kumar KR. Local anaesthetic systemic toxicity in paediatric patient: tips to prevent. Saudi J Anaesth. 2020;14:561–2.
22. Givens KT, Lee DA, Jones T, Ilstrup DM. Congenital rubella syndrome: ophthalmic manifestations and associated systemic disorders. Br J Ophthalmol. 1993;77:358–63.
23. Zetterstrom C. Cataract surgery in the pediatric eye. In: Buratto L, Osher RH, Masket S. editors. Cataract surgery in complicated cases. Thorofare: SLACK Inc.; 2000. pp.1–4.
24. Sinha R, Sharma A, Singh A, Patel N, et al. Anesthetic management of a preterm infant with Crouzon's syndrome. Acta Anaesthesiol Belgica. 2017;68:147–9.
25. Abramson DH. Retinoblastoma: diagnosis and management. CA Cancer J Clin. 1982;32:130–40.
26. Herrema I, Clarke M. Anaesthesia for retinoblastoma screening—a dilemma. Anaesthesia. 2001;56:486–7.
27. Kivela TT, Hadjistilianou T. Neonatal retinoblastoma. Asia Pac J Oncol Nurs. 2017;4:197–204.
28. Chawla D, Agarwal R, Deorari A, Paul VK, et al. Retinopathy of prematurity. Indian J Pediatr. 2012;79:501–9.
29. Maheshwari R, Kumar H, Paul VK, Singh M, et al. Incidence and risk factors of retinopathy of prematurity in a tertiary care newborn unit in New Delhi. Natl Med J India. 1996;9:211–4.
30. International Committee for the Classification of Retinopathy of Prematurity. The International Classification of Retinopathy of Prematurity revisited. Arch Ophthalmol. 2005;123:991–9.
31. Dempsey E, McCreery K. Local anaesthetic eye drops for prevention of pain in preterm infants undergoing screening for retinopathy of prematurity. Cochrane Database Syst Rev. 2011;(9):CD007645.
32. Chen SD, Sundaram V, Wilkinson A, Patel CK. Variation in anaesthesia for the laser treatment of retinopathy of prematurity—a survey of ophthalmologists in the UK. Eye (Lond). 2007;21:1033–6.
33. Haigh PM, Chiswick ML, O'Donoghue EP. Retinopathy of prematurity: systemic complications associated with different anaesthetic techniques at treatment. Br J Ophthalmol. 1997;81:283–7.
34. Eipe N, Kim J, Ramsey G, et al. Anesthesia for laser treatment for retinopathy of prematurity—all clear now? Pediatr Anesth. 2008;18:1103–5.
35. Sammartino M, Bocci MG, Ferro G, Mercurio G, et al. Efficacy and safety of continuous infusion of remifentanil in preterm infants undergoing laser therapy in retinopathy of prematurity: clinical experience. Pediatr Anaesth. 2003;13:596–602.
36. Woodhead DD, Lambert DK, Molloy DA. Avoiding endotracheal intubation of neonates undergoing laser surgery for retinopathy of prematurity. J Perinatol. 2007;27:209–13.
37. Gunenc F, Kuvaki B, Iyilikci L, Gokmen N, et al. Use of laryngeal mask airway in anesthesia for treatment of retinopathy of prematurity. Saudi Med J. 2011;32:1127–32.
38. Sekeroglu MA, Hekimoglu E, Sekeroglu HT. Topical anesthesia for laser treatment of retinopathy of prematurity. Pediatr Anaesth. 2012;22:1224–5.
39. Sinha R, Ray BR. Laser treatment for retinopathy of prematurity under topical anesthesia—prospective from our experience. Pediatr Anaesth. 2013;23:376.
40. Dogra MR, Vinekar A, Viswanathan K, Sangtam T, et al. Laser treatment for retinopathy of prematurity through the incubator wall. Ophthalmic Surg Lasers Imaging. 2008;39:350–2.
41. Misra A, Kersey JP, Astbury NJ, Allen LE. Laser treatment in infants with retinopathy of prematurity using sub-Tenon's lidocaine anaesthesia and sedation with chloral hydrate. Anaesthesia. 2007;62(1):103.

42. Stahl A, Lepore D, Fielder A, Fleck B, et al. Ranibizumab versus laser therapy for the treatment of very low birthweight infants with retinopathy of prematurity (RAINBOW): an open-label randomised controlled trial. Lancet. 2019;394(10208):1551–9.

43. Tokgöz O, Sahin A, Tüfek A, Çınar Y, et al. Inhalation anesthesia with sevoflurane during intravitreal bevacizumab injection in infants with retinopathy of prematurity. Biomed Res Int. 2013;2013:435387.

44. Aoyama K, Kondou Y, Suzuki Y, Sakai H, et al. Anesthesia protocols for early vitrectomy in former preterm infants diagnosed with aggressive posterior retinopathy of prematurity. J Anesth. 2010;24:633–8.

45. Sinha R, Talwar P, Ramachandran R, Azad R, et al. Perioperative management and postoperative course in preterm infants undergoing vitreo-retinal surgery for retinopathy of prematurity: a retrospective study. J Anaesthesiol Clin Pharmacol. 2014;30(2):258–62.

46. Sinha R, Maitra S. The effect of peribulbar block with general anesthesia for vitreoretinal surgery in preterm and ex-premature infants with retinopathy of prematurity. Anesth Analg Case Rep. 2016;6(2):25–7.

Neural Tube Development and Defects: Meningocele, Encephalocele, Hydrocephalus

Indu Mohini Sen and Kiran Jangra

35.1 Introduction

The neural tube is a primordial structure extending along the entire length of the embryo. It gives rise to the brain and the spinal cord [1]. Neural tube defects (NTD) occur due to defect in the midline fusion of neural tube resulting in cranial or spinal dysraphism, and may involve nerve roots, spinal cord, or bony vertebrae [2]. These are serious birth defects as they may result in paralysis or death, affecting 300,000 births each year, worldwide. The Incidence of this defect is highest in South-East Asia. As per hospital records from major cities in India, reported incidence was 3.9–8.8 per 1000 births (live and dead), and from rural areas was 6.57–8.21 per 1000 live births [3, 4].

Neural Tube Defects are of two types (Table 35.1, Fig. 35.1):

1. **Open (Aperta)** - there is no overlying skin, neuroepithelium protrudes externally and there is cerebrospinal fluid (CSF) leak. These defects have poor neurological outcome especially when they are associated with other CNS abnormalities.
2. **Closed (Occulta)** - skin covering the lesion is intact [1], and the spinous process and part of the lamina is absent. Other CNS malformations are usually absent, and prognosis is better than open NTD.

According to the anatomical location in the vertebral column, it can be classified as follows:

1. **Cranial.**
2. **Spinal.**

I. M. Sen (✉) · K. Jangra
Department of Anaesthesia & Intensive Care, PGIMER, Chandigarh, India

Table 35.1 Types of neural tube defects

Type		Presentation
Open cranial dysraphism (Aperta) *Incompatible with life*	Anencephaly	Partial or complete absence of skull bones with no overlying tissues. Rudimentary malformed brain tissues
	Iniencephaly	Characterised by defect in occipital bone, cervical spina bifida with extreme retroflexion of head on cervical spine. Death in inevitable
	Craniorachischism	Rare, severe NTD. Complete failure of neural tube formation due of non-closure of cranial and caudal ends. Combination of rachischism & anencephaly with exposed brain & spinal cord. Incompatible with life
Closed cranial dysraphism	Meningocele	Characterised by herniation of meninges and CSF through skull defects
	Encephalocele	Protrusion of intracranial tissue (meninges, brain) through skull defect
Spina bifida aperta	Myelo meningocele	Herniation of spinal cord, nerves, meninges, CSF through spinal defects
	Myelocele	Herniation of spinal cord tissue through defect in the vertebral column
	Hemi myelocele/ meningocele	Spinal cord is split in two and one of the hemicords has a small meningocele or myelomeningocele
Spina bifida occulta	Split cord malformations	Longitudinal division of the spinal cord into two hemi-cords by bony spur/ fibrocartilaginous ridge
	Dorsal dermal sinus	Epithelium-lined tract from skin to Spinal Canal
	Meningocele	Herniation of meninges and CSF leakage through the defect
	Lipomyelo meningocele	Focal disjunction of cutaneous and neuroectoderm that allows the mesenchyme to enter the neural tube
	Spinal lipoma	Focal premature disjunction of neurocutaneous ectoderm
	Others	Terminal syringo-hydromyelocele, abnormal filum terminale, caudal agenesis

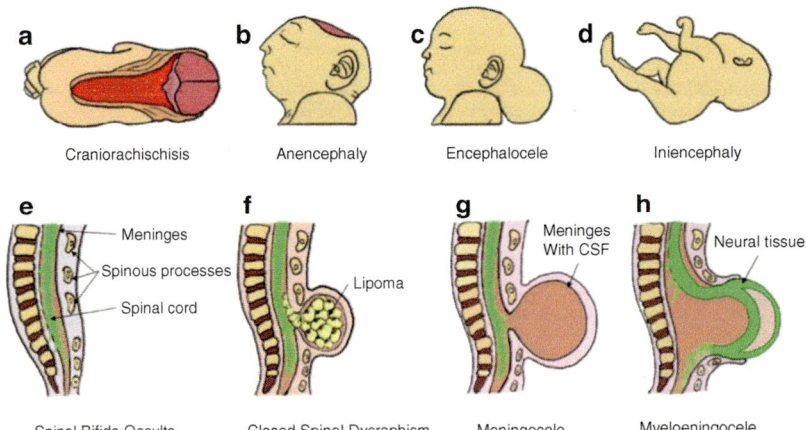

Fig. 35.1 Diagrammatic representation of various NDT; (**a**) Craniorachischisis, completely open brain and spinal cord; (**b**) Anencephaly, Open brain and absent skull vault; (**c**) Encephalocele, herniation of meninges and brain; (**d**) Iniencephaly, Occipital Skull and spine defect and Extreme retroflexion of head; (**e**) Spinal Bifida Occulta, Vertebral arches not completely fused, overlying skin intact; (**f**) Closed Spinal Dysraphism, Deficiency of vertebral arches with overlying lipoma; (**g**) Meningocele, Protrusion of meninges filled with CSF; (**h**) Myelomeningocele, Open NDT with meningeal cyst

35.2   Neuro-Embryology

The development of CNS starts at third week post-conception by primary neurulation as a thickening in the ectoderm, the neural plate (Fig. 35.2). The process of development of the CNS is known as Neurulation.

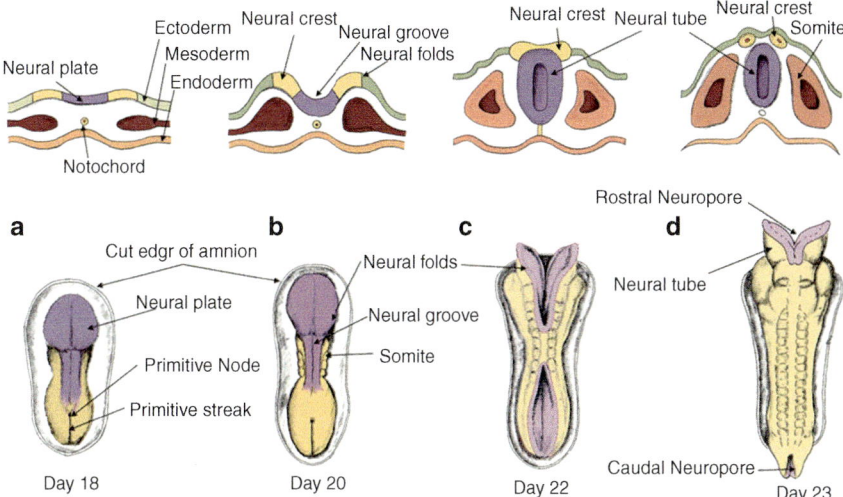

Fig. 35.2 Transverse sections (upper row) and dorsal view (lower row) at various stages of development of an embryo; (**a**) Day 18 - Late presomite embryo, the amnion has been removed, and neural plate is visible; (**b**) Day 20 - the somites and the neural groove and neural folds; (**c**) Day 22 - seven distinct somites visible on each side of the neural tube; (**d**) Day 23, the nervous system is in connection with the amniotic cavity through the cranial and caudal neuropores

35.2.1 Primary Neurulation

The lateral edges of neural plates elevate to form neural folds, which fuse in midline to form the neural tube [5, 6]. Fusion begins in the cervical region and proceeds in both cranial and caudal directions. The cranial part forms the brain, while the caudal part forms the spinal cord. The end openings of the neural tube are known as neuropores.

There are two neuropores:

- Cranial or anterior neuropore, and
- Caudal or posterior neuropore.

The fusion and closure of the cranial neuropore occurs by 25th day, and of the caudal neuropore by the 30th day of gestation, and closure of both neuropores is usually complete by the end of fourth week of gestation.

Abnormalities or failure of fusion of neuropores at any level of the neural tube during primary neurulation leads to NTDs:

1. **Anencephaly** - Failure of closure of anterior neuropore.
2. **Spinal Bifida** - Failure of closure of caudal neuropore.
3. **Rachischisis** - Failure of closure of the entire length of the neural tubes (Fig. 35.1).

35.2.2 Secondary Neurulation

At 5–6 weeks of gestation, the neural tube hollows, medullary cord, and its cavities appear, and formation of sacral and coccygeal spinal cord segments occurs. Abnormalities or interruption in the secondary neurulation leads **Closed Dysraphism,** as these defects are sub-ectodermal and have overlying skin [7].

Rarely, same neonate may have two or more NTD. This has been explained on the basis of "multiple site closure model". Accordingly, closure of neural tube is initiated at five sites, and failure in closure can cause multiple defects [8, 9].

35.3 Etiopathogenesis

There is a wide variation in prevalence of NTD, ranging from 0.3–199.4 per 10,000 births. Almost 300,000 babies born each year worldwide, have NTD. Spina bifida being the commonest followed by anencephaly and encephalocele [10, 11].

In India, the birth prevalence, live birth, and stillbirth prevalence is 4.1, 1.3 and 1.7 per 1000 births, respectively. An incidence of NTD, reported from major cities in India, in 2005, was 3.3–8.8 per 1000 births, and from rural India as 6.57–8.21 per 1000 live births [3, 4]. Anencephaly is the most prevalent (2.1 per 1000 births) followed by spina bifida (1.9 per 1000 births) [5]. The incidence of NTD has declined over the past 20 years due to folic acid supplementation to the expectant mothers.

NTD have a multifactorial etiopathogenesis, genetic, environmental, and nutritional factors.

1. **Genetic Factors** -There is an association with complex genetic disorders with a strong epigenetics (extrinsic influences) that makes identification of genetic risk factors difficult. Even though siblings, monozygotic twins and offspring from consanguineous marriages are affected more, majority of cases are sporadic. Various genes that increase the risk of NDT include methionine synthase (MTR), 5-methionine synthase reductase (MTRR), 10-methylene tetrahydrofolate reductase (MTHFR), and cystathionine synthase [12, 13]. NTD is associated with various chromosomal disorders and syndromes, such as:

   Trisomy 13 and 18,

   Partial aneuploidy or triploidy.

   PHAVER (Pterygia, Heart anomalies, Autosomal recessive inheritance, Vertebral defects, Ear anomalies, and Radial defects), and one of the sibs also has MMC,

   VATER (Vertebral anomalies, Anal atresia, Tracheal anomalies, Esophageal abnormalities, Renal or Radial abnormalities) syndrome,

   Meckel–Gruber syndrome, and

   X-linked disorders.

2. **Environmental factors** include:
   (a) **Use of medications** - anti-epileptic drugs (Valproic acid, Carbamazepine), hypervitaminosis A, nitrates, cytochalasin.
   (b) **Antenatal factors** - maternal diabetes, obesity, advanced age, alcoholism, exposure to lead, febrile illness, and.
   (c) History of NDT in the sibling or previous offspring.

3. **Nutritional Factors – Micronutrient deficiencies** - zinc, vitamin B12 and folic acid. There is prevalence of vitamin B12, iron, folic acid deficiency in Indian women [14, 15]. Vitamin B12 and folate are methyl donors in one-carbon metabolism which influences DNA synthesis and epigenetic regulation, and thereby cell growth and differentiation. A strong causative association has been found between maternal vitamin B12 deficiency, hyperhomocysteinemia, and low birth weight and incidence of NTD. WHO recommends pre-emptive (before conception) folic acid (400 mcg/day) to all women of childbearing age and early pregnancy, and higher dose (4 mg/day) in high-risk women, along with Vit B 12 [16]. However, folate deficiency leading to NTD is a controversial and its deficiency poses a risk only in the presence of other predisposing factors [8, 17, 18].

35.4 Spinal Dysraphism

35.4.1 Meningomyelocele

Meningomyelocele (MMC) or spina bifida cystica is the most common type of NTD with defect in the vertebral arches leading to protrusion of membranous sac that may contain CSF, meninges, and or neural tissue. If this sac contains only CSF, then it is known as meningocele [7].

The commonest site of MMC is the lumbosacral (>85%), followed by thoracic (10%) and cervical (5%) regions. Involvement of high spinal levels carries a poorer prognosis compared to lower levels, [6, 19–21]

35.4.1.1 Pathophysiology

The neuronal damage due to NTD is described as two-hit theory.

- The first hit is the defect in neurulation.
- The second hit is the exposure of the neuroepithelium to the amniotic fluid in-utero (as in the open type NTD) [13, 22]

This results in neuronal tissue damage and degeneration. The CSF leak through the defect hampers the distension of neurocranium and results in the formation of small posterior fossa and maldevelopment of the CNS [20, 23].

35.4.1.2 Clinical Presentation

The baby usually presents with a swelling over the back since birth. The lesion is usually cystic and is covered with intact skin or membrane. If these coverings are disrupted, there will be CSF leak and risk of meningitis. There may be variable degrees of neurological deficits depending on the site of the lesion and age. Presenting features are as follows:

- Swelling over the back.
- Neurological deficits - Motor and sensory deficits.
- Bowel/bladder involvement.

Paralysis may be partial or complete along with loss of sensation below the level of the lesion. Bowel and bladder dysfunction is commonly seen due to the loss of autonomic control. Several other neurological pathologies may be associated with MMC, e.g.,

- Hydrocephalus.
- Arnold-Chiari malformation (ACM) II.
- Corpus Callosal Agenesis.
- Microgyria.
- Arachnoi/Porencephalic cysts.
- Tethered spinal cord.
- Syringomyelia 23.

Hydrocephalus occurs due to the blockage in the CSF pathway. There may be congenital stenosis of cerebral aqueduct obstructing the CSF flow from third to fourth ventricle or tonsillar herniation secondary to ACM obstructing flow from fourth ventricle to the foramen of Magendie and Luschka [24]. Often signs of hydrocephalus are not present due to the CSF diversion into the MMC Cyst or leak through the breach in the covering. Symptoms of raised intracranial pressure (ICP) usually appear by second week of birth or after the surgical closure of MMC. If hydrocephalus is not treated prior to MMC repair, it may lead to severely high ICP with CSF leak through the surgical wound.

In ACM II, there is herniation of cerebellar vermis, tonsils, fourth ventricle, and medulla into the spinal canal below the level of C 2, leading to compression of the brainstem and lower cranial nerves, and brainstem dysfunction, in the form of difficulty in breathing, feeding and swallowing, apnea, stridor and or visual disturbances. CM is unique to MMC, that means it invariably presents along with MMC unless proven otherwise. Symptomatic ACM is usually fatal, hence early recognition and timely treatment is warranted.

Systemic involvements include renal, cardiac, and gastro-intestinal tract malformations, and lower extremity deformities (club foot). Common cardiac defects include ASD, VSD, TOF, bicuspid aortic valve, coarctation of aorta, and total anomalous pulmonary venous drainage (TAPVD). Presence of autonomic cardiovascular disturbances due to paraplegia and associated mobility disorders should be evaluated preoperatively.

35.4.1.3 Diagnosis Prenatal Diagnosis A

MMC can be diagnosed in-utero and timely intervention can improve fetal outcome and better preservation of neurological functions.

The two main diagnostic modalities are in-utero USG, and amniocentesis (α fetoprotein (α AFP), levels and acetyl cholinesterase).

1. (i) Availability of USG avoids the need for invasive amniocentesis for diagnosis. USG is done in two stages.
   (a) 1st for screening during the second trimester, and
   (b) 2nd (level II USG) for evaluation of brain and spinal cord.

USG also helps recognising the type and severity of NTD, and presence of other anomalies.

Three sonographic signs of MMC are Banana sign, Lemon sign, Ventriculomegaly, and spinal sign.

1. **The Banana sign** indicates downward shift of the posterior fossa structure (ACM II) and represents distorted cerebellum.
2. **Lemon sign** is the shape of skull bone in transverse view and occurs due to the concavity of parietal bones.
3. **Ventriculomegaly** indicates the onset of hydrocephalus.
4. **Spinal sign** is the cystic lesion with splaying of posterior elements.

(ii) Amniocentesis
(a) AFP is checked during the second trimester between 15 and 22 weeks. An abnormally high AFP level indicates the open NTD [25–27].
(b) Acetylcholine esterase, highly specific marker for neural tissue, is usually absent from the amniotic fluid, and its presence indicates NTD.

B. Postnatal Diagnosis
Bony abnormalities of the brain, spinal cord, hydrocephalus, and vertebral column are delineated on X-ray and CT scan. MRI of head assesses brain parenchymal abnormalities (ACM II), posterior fossa and spinal cord defects. MRI of spinal cord delineates the sac contents and other abnormalities (split cord malformations) [28].

35.4.1.4   Management
Multidisciplinary approach is needed for spinal dysmorphism as the neonate may require repeated surgeries for MMC and other anomalies [29]. Open NDT may be repaired antenatally (in-utero) or postnatally [30].

(i) Antenatal Management
The exposure of neural tissue to amniotic fluid damages the neural tissues and worsens neurologic outcome [31]. Early in-utero repair may be necessary to halt the neuronal damage, reduce the incidence of hydrocephalus, need for shunt surgery, improve neurological and motor outcome, and reversal of ACM. Despite promising results of antenatal surgery, there are associated maternal and fetal risks, preterm delivery and uterine dehiscence. Presence of ventriculomegaly is contraindication to antenatal repair [30–34].

(ii) Perinatal Management
The most important concern is the mode of delivery, vaginal or operative, depending on the size of the head and the swelling and obstetric condition. The goal is to prevent any trauma or compression of the swelling and its neural contents [35–37].

(iii) Postnatal Management
- The newborn with NTD should be nursed in prone or lateral position to avoid pressure on the sac and its rupture [38].
- The timing of surgery depends on the general condition of the neonate, pressure in the cyst, and associated anomalies.
- If condition permits, proper evaluation of the baby should be done and best possible optimization, preoperatively.
- In case of ruptured sac, antibiotics should be started, and surgery undertaken on urgent basis [39, 40].

35.4.1.5   Perioperative Considerations

Associated abnormalities, especially ACM make these neonates vulnerable to postoperative respiratory problems, impaired swallowing, and gag reflexes, mandating careful decisions regarding postoperative airway management and ventilatory support. It is prudent to avoid use of latex products in case of possible latex allergy [41].

Lesion must be protected at induction and positioning for surgery. Custom-made cotton pads and rings, or commercial gel rings can be used to prevent harm to the fragile sac [42].

35.4.1.6   Preanesthetic Preparation

A thorough detailed preoperative evaluation is a must:

1. To rule out or confirm presence of any anomalies, Assess the degree of physiological impact, and pathophysiological disturbances secondary to the primary condition (MMC),
2. A complete history including ANC (antenatal) history for risk factors, birth history (mode of delivery/perinatal problems) and presenting complaints.
3. Clinical examination should focus on the developmental abnormalities of the CNS and other organ systems [43], and history and signs of the brain stem or lower cranial nerve involvement. Neurological involvement below the affected segment may result in weakness of respiratory and abdominal muscles, and weak and ineffective cough, necessitating decision for postoperative mechanical ventilation ([6, 24, 30, 44–46].
4. Investigations should include a complete hemogram, serum electrolytes, renal and liver function tests, blood grouping and cross matching, and basic coagulation profile. Chest x-ray to assess the airway and length of trachea (may have short trachea or TEF), lung parenchyma (for signs of aspiration), and cardiac silhouette (for cardiac anomalies).
5. Specific investigations to rule out associated illnesses must be done. ECG may show rate and rhythm disturbances, abnormalities in conduction, and ectopics, mandating Echocardiography for a detailed evaluation for congenital cardiac defects and degree of shunt.
6. USG is useful to diagnose and assess difficult airway, tracheal length, and to mark the trachea if invasive airway is required.
7. Fetal MRI report should be checked to rule out or establish other anomalies [47, 48].
8. **Premedication** - Usually no premedication is required. Sedatives and narcotics should be avoided in a closed NTD with possible raised ICP, until the opening of the sac.

35.4.1.7   Surgical Procedure

- Surgery is usually performed in prone position. Semi-prone position has also been used. It is imperative that care is taken to avoid undue pressure on the abdomen and IVC.
- Abdominal compression creates difficulty in ventilation and obstructs venous drainage.
- IVC compression reduces venous return resulting in hypotension, or increased oozing at the surgical site due to engorgement of vertebral venous plexus.
- All pressure points should be padded, and eyes covered and protected to avoid damage from external compression.
- Head should be placed in neutral position or turned to one side, avoiding excessive traction or twisting of the neck.
- Large MMC tends to bleed. Sac is opened to release the pressure, redundant tissue removed, and surrounding skin flaps are raised so as to cover the defect. This can lead to massive blood loss. Therefore, meticulous assessment of blood loss must be done intraoperatively, with replacement if needed. So, adequate volume of blood and blood products should be cross matched and kept available.
- Duration of surgery may be prolonged, and neonate should be cared for to prevent complications, such as hypothermia, fluid loss and hypovolemia, electrolyte disturbances and coagulation defects.

35.4.1.8   Anaesthetic Management

The operation room (OR) should be prepared to manage neonates and strict aseptic precautions should be followed. A special emphasis should be on:

- Maintaining warm ambient temperature (around 27 °C),
- Body and fluid warming devices,
- Appropriate positioning aids,
- Adequate size and type of airway equipment.
- Avoid use of latex-containing equipment (surgical gloves, face masks, reservoir bags, ECG leads, stethoscope, BP cuff, IV tubing, and injection ports) [48, 49]

35.4.1.9   Monitoring

The standard intraoperative monitoring includes the following:

- SpO_2 (pulse oximetry),
- ECG,
- NIBP (non-invasive blood pressure),
- Temperature,
- Capnography, [50] and
- Intake output.

If available, non-invasive multiwavelength pulse oximetry with plethysmographic variability index and perfusion index is a better choice [51, 52]

35.4.1.10 Positioning

The most important concern is the positioning of the baby so that there is no external compression on the protruding sac. This can be achieved by placing a doughnut-shaped ring underneath the swelling and maintaining the child in supine position. Placing the baby in lateral position is also suitable but makes airway management challenging. Hence, to avoid chaos at the time of unsuccessful intubation, child should be comfortably positioned supine, with anaesthesiologist sitting comfortably.

Either inhalational or intravenous induction may be chosen depending upon the availability of intravenous access [53, 54].

Excessive neck movements and rotation must be avoided to prevent brainstem compression. Appropriate endotracheal tube (ET) size should be chosen, preferably uncuffed. Before fixing the ET, check for bilateral equal air entry as a short trachea may promote endobronchial intubation if ET is fixed based on a pre-calculated formula. A 5-point auscultation helps in identifying esophageal intubation. Lung sliding is a useful sign to confirm bilateral air entry [55].

35.4.1.11 Allergic Reactions

The severity of allergic reaction may vary from minor skin rash or urticaria to severe anaphylactic reaction. These babies are at risk of latex allergy due to prolonged catheterizations and insertion of latex implants. Repeated surgical exposures may lead to severe anaphylactic reaction, especially after mucosal exposure. The latex-containing equipment should be avoided. Various commonly used equipment should be latex-free including surgical gloves face masks, reservoir bags, ECG leads, stethoscope, blood pressure cuff and tubing, and intravenous injection ports [21].

35.4.1.12 Maintenance of Anaesthesia

- Both intravenous and inhalational anaesthetic agents may be used for maintenance. Sevoflurane has a better recovery profile than isoflurane but may be associated with emergence delirium [56].
- Shorter acting non depolarizing muscle relaxants (atracurium, cisatracurium) and opioids (fentanyl, remifentanil) should be used.
- Dexmedetomidine has an opioid-sparing effect. It maintains hemodynamics and reduces postoperative pain and emergence agitation when used with sevoflurane [57, 58]. however this is of not much concern in neonates.

35.4.1.13 Intraoperative Concerns

- High insensible losses,
- Massive blood loss,
- Hemodynamic derangement from blood loss,
- Bradycardia or asystole due to brain stem manipulation during cervical MMC,

- Hypothermia,
- Autonomic disturbances due to cord manipulation,
- Venous air embolism, and
- Other complications related to prone positioning include pressure injury, and vision loss.

35.4.1.14 Emergence from Anaesthesia

The emergence and extubation should be planned based on the preoperative neurological status of the neonate, hemodynamic stability, temperature, blood loss, metabolic derangements, airway edema and duration of surgery.

If decision to extubate the trachea is taken, then anaesthesia should be planned such that the baby is fully awake at the end of surgery, respiration is regular and adequate, and airway reflexes (esp. in cervical MMC) are intact.

35.4.1.15 Postoperative Care

The neonate should be nursed in the lateral or semi prone position, and closely monitored in the NICU [59, 60].

  i. **Early Postoperative Complications** should be looked for, such as:
     - Neurological deficits.
     - Apnea.
     - Stridor.
     - Autonomic disturbances.
 ii. **Delayed complications** to be watched for are as follows:
     - CSF leak.
     - Raised ICP due to aggravation of hydrocephalus.
     - Wound infection.
     - Meningitis.

These babies may require future surgeries for spinal column deformity, urological problems, anal sphincter dysfunction and limb deformities, etc.

35.4.2 Occult Spinal Dysraphism

There is a bony defect in the spinal column with overlying skin cover and no CSF leak. The defect is not visible externally. Only clue may be a cutaneous manifestation such as nevus, hypopigmentation, large dimple, tuft of hair, lipoma, hemangioma, true or pseudo tails, telangiectasias, dermal sinus, skin tags, and cystic or sinus tract lesions. As dura is intact and neural contents are not exposed to amniotic fluid, the AFP levels are not raised. These patients usually remain asymptomatic for years, and diagnosis is often incidental on imaging studies conducted for some other pathologies. Various occult spinal dysraphisms are enumerated in Table 35.1. MRI helps to differentiate spinal dysraphisms. The neurological prognosis of these defects is better than the open NTD.

(i) Lipomatous Malformations

Lipomas are the most common closed spinal NTD, commonest site being lower lumbar region and usually occurs with spina bifida. The sac containing only lipomatous tissue is known as lipomyelocele, and if a part of neural tissue is also present, it is called as lipomyelomeningocele. This presents as a mass of lipomatous tissue at filumterminale, conusmedullaris, within or attached to the spinal cord and subcutaneous fat and herniates through the bony defect. Thus, causing tethering of the cord. There may be compression of the cord. Tethering and compression are responsible for neurological manifestations. Management is surgical untethering and removal of the lipomatous tissue.

(ii) Meningocele

When the herniating sac through spinal column defects contains fluid-filled meningeal tissue without neural components and is covered by intact skin or membrane, it is known as meningocele. There is no deformation of the spinal contents. Hence, neurologic deficits and brain malformations are usually absent. The lumbar and sacral meningoceles are the closed types of NTD, the cervical meningoceles may be either open or closed. Surgical correction involves resection of herniated meninges and closure of the gap.

(iii) Congenital Dermal Sinus

In this condition, there is an epithelial lined sinus tract close to midline extending from the skin to near the conus medullaris. As this tract communicates with the spinal column, if infected, it can lead to meningitis. It may cause mass tethering of cord and mass effect if a dermoid cyst is present in the tract. Surgical excision of the tract and dermoid cyst is warranted.

(iv) Split Cord Malformations (SCM)

In this condition, the spinal cord is split into two cords. It is of two types: type-1 and type-2.

1. **Type-I SCM** – The hemi cords are in two separate spinal canals, each with its own meninges and set of dorsal and ventral nerve roots and is also known as Diastematomyelia. There is an-osteo-cartilagenous bony septum separating the two cords (Fig. 35.3). It is usually associated with overlying cutaneous manifestations. Neurological symptoms occur due to tethering of the cord. Motor weakness, limb atrophy, sensory deficit, and bladder dysfunction are frequent occurrences. Surgical detethering of the cord, removal of the septum, and reconstitution of dura into a single tube is needed. The anaesthetic concerns are as for surgery for MMC. An important concern during removal of the bony septum is the risk of bleeding, venous air embolism, and significant hypotension [61].

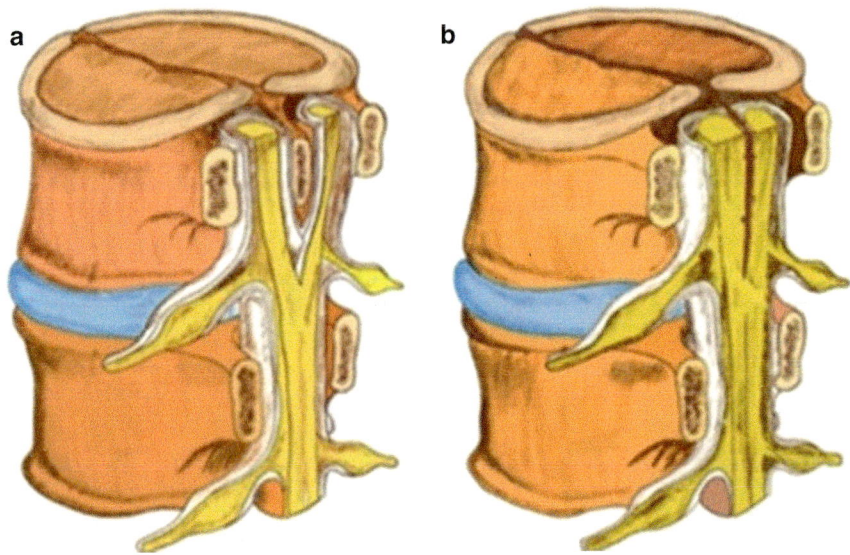

Fig. 35.3 Split cord malformations (SCM) as depicted by sketch; (**a**) Type-I SCM, characterized by two hemicords, each has its own dural sleeve and are separated by bony spur; (**b**) Type-II SCM, characterized by two hemicords within a single dural sleeve that are separated and tethered by a fibrous septum

2. **Type 2 SCM** -The two hemi cords along with four sets of dorsal and ventral nerve roots are enclosed within a single dural canal. They are separated by the **fibrous** septum, also known as diplomyelia. The fibrous band may result in tethering of cord. Surgical excision of the band and detethering of the cord is done to relieve the symptoms. Even though the risk of bleeding is there during excision of the fibrous band, it is much less than in type 1.

(v) Tethered Cord Syndrome

Tethered cord syndrome (TCS) is the constellation of signs and symptoms arising due to abnormal strain on the spinal cord. [27] With the growth of spinal cord, stretching of neural tissue occurs due to abnormal adherence resulting in restricted growth and ischemic changes. Any pathology that causes abnormal adherence of the spinal cord to adjacent structures, results in the restriction of spinal cord movement, such as thickened filum, congenital malformations of the spinal cord, spinal dysraphism, postoperative case of tumour or MMC excision, infection, and scarring.

The neurological manifestations may be subtle and progress gradually with age. The symptoms and signs vary from leg and back pain to the varied neurological deficits, scoliosis along with bowel and bladder involvements. A detailed neurological examination and MRI helps in making a diagnosis and identifying the level of tethering, and exact pathology.

The surgical technique involves release of abnormal attachment of the cord in prone position. The anaesthesia concerns are the same as for MMC excision. Intraoperative neurophysiological monitoring may be used to identify the motor roots. Accordingly, anaesthesia techniques should be modified. Total intravenous anaesthesia (TIVA) does not interfere with motor evoked potentials (MEP). Halogenated agents may be used in less than 0.5 MAC, and muscle relaxants should be omitted.

Transcortical MEP stimulation is used, and recording electrodes are placed on limb muscles and external anal sphincter.

The tibial or pudendal nerve may be used for somatosensory evoked potentials (SSEP), and response is recorded from epidural or cortex electrodes.

Electromyography (EMG) responses can be recorded from external anal sphincter muscles. Postoperatively, children should be nursed in the supine position to minimise CSF pressure on the surgical repair site.

Postoperative complications include CSF leak and wound infection [62].

35.4.3 Cranial Dysraphism - Encephalocele

As in spinal dysraphism, defects in development of brain or closure of skull result in various cranial dysraphisms (Fig. 35.1). The salient features are listed in Table 35.2. Encephalocele is discussed in detail here.

The intracranial tissue (meninges and brain parenchyma) herniates through a skull defect and forms a sac-like structure known as encephalocele. It may herniate through various locations, such as anterior or sincipital/frontoethmoidal (nasofrontal, nasoethmoidal, and naso-orbital), posterior or occipital, cranial vault (parietal,

Table 35.2 Presentation of encephalocele based on the location

Type	Defect for herniation	Presentation
Giant encephalocele	Larger that the head size	Difficulty in nursing
Frontonasal encephalocele	Herniation of intracranial contents through the foramen caecum and comes out at junction of nasal and frontal bones	Present as a nasal mass Difficulty in breathing
Transsphenoidal encephaloceles	Vertical midline skull base defect, with a diameter usually <1.5 mm Extends from the sellar floor to the nasopharynx	Involvement and dysfunction of pituitary gland, hypothalamus, and optic pathway CSF rhinorrhoea, visual defect (in older children), nasal and epipharyngeal mass causing respiratory obstruction, features of pituitary-hypothalamic insufficiency
Orbital encephaloceles	Herniation of intracranial tissue into orbit through basal defect	Proptosis
Occipital encephaloceles	Through a defect in occipital bone	Brainstem dysfunction Involvement of vital centres, respiratory distress Involvement of lower cranial nerves

temporal, or through anterior or posterior fontanelle), or basal (trans sphenoidal, transethmoidal, sphenoorbital, or sphenoethmoidal) [8, 2, 63].

There is regional variation in the location of encephalocele. In Europe and the United states occipital encephaloceles, while in Asia and Africa, frontoethmoidal encephaloceles are more common.

35.4.3.1 Pathogenesis

The pathogenesis is the same as that of spinal dysraphism, i.e., defect during neurulation where neural folds fail to fuse. Etiopathogenesis is diverse as the exact cause is unknown, and both genetic and epigenetics may be responsible. Approximately 15–20% of all NTD are encephaloceles. The estimated incidence of encephalocele is 1 in 10,000 livebirths worldwide [10, 11, 24].

Various congenital cranial and extracranial anomalies are associated with cranial dysraphism:
- Hydrocephalus.
- Craniosynostosis.
- Porencephaly, microcephaly.
- Arnold-Chiari II malformation.
- Agenesis of the corpus callosum.
- Cortical atrophy.
- Dandy-Walker malformation.

Various systemic anomalies include:
- Facial anomalies (cleft lip/palate or micrognathia).
- Polydactyly.
- Vertebral defects (spina bifida).
- Renal agenesis.
- Pulmonary hypoplasia.
- Cardiac anomalies (PDA, ASD, VSD, dextrocardia).

Presenting features:
- Developmental delay.
- Vision problems.
- Seizures.
- Mental and growth retardation.

Encephalocele is also recognized as a part of some other syndromes: [64]
- Knobloch syndrome.
- Meckel syndrome.
- Von Voss syndrome.
- Walker-Warburg syndrome.
- Aberrant tissue band syndrome

Most of these anomalies can be detected by fetal USG during ANC ([65, 46]

As these defects are closed NTD, the serum level of AFP is not raised. After birth, CT scan helps in detecting the bony defects and hydrocephalus, while MRI delineates the contents of the sac, and details other anomalies (corpus callosum agenesis, ACM, aqueductal stenosis).

Surgery should be done as early as possible, but if the sac ruptures or overlying skin is excoriated the surgery should be done on urgent basis to avoid the risk of meningitis. Closure of herniated MMC and encephaloceles can aggravate hydrocephalus [66, 67].

A comprehensive preanesthetic evaluation is warranted to rule out associated anomalies and to evaluate the risks associated with anaesthesia [68, 69].

Laboratory investigations including hemogram, serum electrolytes, renal function tests, chest X-ray. More advanced investigations such as ECG or echocardiography should be done if indicated. With the increasing use of USG in the perioperative setting, optical detection of intracranial pressure and perfusion changes is also useful.

Adequate amount of blood and blood products must be arranged preoperatively.

35.4.3.2 Perioperative Management

Technical difficulties during anaesthesia vary depending upon the site and size of encephalocele (Table 35.2) [24, 68, 69]. Care-providers should be explained in an understandable language about the possible benefits as well as risks of procedure. Antisialogogue (IV glycopyrrolate 10 mcg/kg) if airway difficulty is anticipated, is indicated. Preemptive analgesia in the form of intravenous paracetamol (15 mg/kg) can be given. Preoperative sedation should be avoided and only given under strict monitoring (Table 35.2).

35.4.3.3 Conduct of Anaesthesia

Warming the operating room to 80–85 °F (27–29 °C), using heating pads, HME (heat and moisture exchange) filters in the inspiratory limb of the breathing circuit and warm intravenous and irrigation fluids help maintain the neonate's temperature.

Difficult intubation cart should be available with appropriate size gadgets before induction of anaesthesia.

The cervical and occipital encephaloceles interfere with the head movement leading to difficulties in airway management.

Mask holding and positioning for intubation can also cause undue pressure on frontonasal sac or occipital sac, resulting in compression of the vital structures, increase in ICP and rupture of the sac.

Various techniques described in the literature. The goal is to avoid the pressure on the sac during mask holding for induction and intubation such as use of lateral decubitus position, or supine position with sac resting on the doughnut [24, 43, 49].

In patients with giant encephalocele, CSF may be drained to decompress the sac before anaesthesia induction to minimize morbidity [69].

Sevoflurane induction is advantageous as it allows rapid smooth induction and enough relaxation to permit check laryngoscopy in anticipated difficult airway. Wherever available videolaryngoscope guided endotracheal intubation with appropriate size endotracheal tube with stylet should be done. This improves first pass success without undue pressure on the sac. Short-acting anaesthetic agents should be preferred for maintenance to allow early awakening.

35.4.3.4 Major Complications are Related to Location of Encephalocele

(a) During resection of occipital encephalocele, rapid drainage of CSF or compression on brainstem can cause hemodynamic derangements such as bradycardia, hypertension, or hypotension, and even asystole. Tachycardia and hypothermia may also be seen. The surgeon should be notified and surgical stimulus should be removed instantaneously. In most of the cases, hemodynamic changes revert after removal of stimulus, if not, appropriate management should be started depending upon the presentation. Therefore, slow controlled drainage of CSF is advocated.

(b) Transsphenoidal encephalocele can cause refractory hypotension due to pituitary-hypothalamic or adrenal insufficiency, and hypothyroidism.

(c) Other anticipated intraoperative complications include blood loss, hypothermia, venous air embolism, and complications due to prone position such as dislodgement of endotracheal tube, intravenous and arterial cannula, catheters and raised abdominal pressure.

Postoperatively, before extubation, baby should be normothermic, fully awake, respiration and muscle power below the level of surgery must be adequate. After excision of occipital encephalocele, gag and cough reflexes should be specifically checked. Mechanical ventilation may be needed if there are major intraoperative complications and persistent metabolic derangements.

Postoperative apnea may occur in premature babies and in cases with high cervical and occipital encephalocele. These babies must be observed in NICU. They should be provided with good analgesia, preferably non opioid based drugs, especially in an extubated baby [70]. Late postoperative complications include hydrocephalus, CSF leak, and meningitis.

35.5 Hydrocephalus

Hydrocephalus, also known as **"water in the brain"** is characterized by increase in the amount of CSF. It can be caused by congenital anomalies or secondary to closure of NTD.

Hydrocephalus is of two types:

1. **Obstructive/non-communicating,** where flow of CSF is not present around the spinal cord, and.
2. **Non-obstructive/communicating**, where CSF can flow normally around the spinal cord.

Hydrocephalus is the most common neurosurgical condition requiring intervention [24, 70, 71]. In preterm neonates, post hemorrhagic hydrocephalus is grievous condition, needing immediate management [72].

35.5.1 Presentation

The most common symptoms are a rapid increase in head circumference, downward deviation of the eyes, irritability, sleepiness, poor feeding, vomiting, and breathing difficulty.

35.5.2 Etiology

1. Aqueduct stenosis,
2. NTD, and
3. Posterior fossa malformations (vein of Galen malformation obstructing flow at the aqueduct).

35.5.3 Treatment

The treatment is diversion of CSF out of the ventricular system. Various options include:

1. External ventricular drain,
2. Ventriculoperitoneal (VP) shunt (open and laparoscopic assisted) [73]
3. Ventriculo-pleural shunt,
4. Ventriculo-atrial shunt (VA), and
5. Internalized ventricular shunt,
6. Endoscopic third ventriculostomy.

VP shunt and ETV are commonly performed procedures. There is a one- way valve within the shunt that prevents CSF from flowing back into the ventricles. The invention of cost-effective Indian shunts has revolutionized the management of hydrocephalus in our country [74, 75]. Complications of surgery include:

- Failures or malfunction [76]
- Infections, and
- Disconnections.

35.5.4 Anaesthetic Management for VP Shunt Surgery

a. The main goal of anaesthetic management of hydrocephalus is to decrease ICP and prevent further rise. Factors that increase ICP must be avoided, such as:
- Hypoventilation.
- Hypoxia.
- Hypertension.

b. Premedication
Sedative premedication may lead to hypoventilation and causes rise in ICP. If at all, oral or intravenous midazolam may be given under supervision and strict monitoring. No narcotic premedication should be used.

c. Conduct of Anesthesia
1. If there are no signs and symptoms of raised ICP, any induction and maintenance technique may be adopted (inhalation or intravenous).
2. If there are features of raised ICP, induction with intravenous induction (propofol/thiopentone) is preferred, if venous line is in place. If not, then inhalational induction (sevoflurane) may be used with slow titration, and ventilation should be controlled to avoid hypercapnia, increased cerebral blood flow, and rise in ICP.
3. Rapid sequence induction (RSI) is used in patients with severely raised ICP and actively vomiting, using succinylcholine or rocuronium for muscle paralysis.
4. Shorter acting opioids should be used such as fentanyl or remifentanil.
5. Intubation may be challenging in these patients with large head. Rolled sheets should be used below the shoulders to appropriately align the oral, pharyngeal, and laryngeal axis (ear lobule and ipsilateral shoulder in one plane).
6. Standard monitoring is used. Advanced monitoring is indicated depending upon the co-morbidities present.
7. There is no consensus for the best maintenance anaesthetic agent. Complete immobility is warranted to avoid intraoperative complications.
8. Intraoperatively, normovolemia should be maintained using iso-osmolar crystalloids.
9. Dextrose containing solutions should be avoided except for babies who are high risk for hypoglycaemia such as premature neonates, babies of diabetic mothers, or critically ill babies. Blood sugar should be monitored. Both hypoglycaemia and hyperglycaemia must be prevented.

d. Special Concerns
Major intraoperative events can occur at various stages of surgery.

1. As the head and abdomen of the child is exposed during surgery, there is high risk of **hypothermia**, and adequate measures should be adapted to prevent that.
2. During ventricular tapping, sudden loss of CSF can lead to **reverse herniation** resulting in bradycardia, arrhythmias or even asystole. To prevent this complica-

tion, CSF should be gradually drained by intermittent clamping of the cranial cannula. If still haemodynamic instability occurs, titrated boluses of normal saline should be pushed inside the lateral ventricles through the same cannula.

3. Deeper plane of anaesthesia or opioid supplementation may be needed during subcutaneous tunnelling.

4. It is important to maintain hemodynamic stability all throughout, as cerebrovascular oxygenation correlates well with mean arterial pressure in neonates, including sick and preterm babies [77].

35.6   Special Concerns during Endoscopic Third Ventriculostomy (ETV)

In ETV, an endoscopic device is placed in lateral ventricle, and then passed into the third ventricle through foramen of Monroe. Multiple fenestrae are created in the floor of the ventricle to divert the CSF to the basal cisterns. Patient may develop arrhythmias, hypotension, or hypertension due to manipulation of vital structures (hypothalamus, brain stem) during the fenestration step. These changes are short-lasting and usually resolve after the removal of stimulus. Irrigation fluid used during ETV may lead to major hemodynamic disturbances. Rapid irrigation with slow return of fluid can cause sudden rise in ICP resulting in bradycardia and hypertension [78]. Management is prompt stoppage of irrigation fluid, and drainage of CSF. One dreaded complication is bleeding, ranging from mild intraventricular haemorrhage to major vascular injury to the venous network or basilar artery. Venous oozing is more frequent but manageable, whereas injury to arterial blood vessels can be catastrophic, warranting urgent craniotomy. A large volume of irrigation fluid may lead to electrolyte disturbances cerebral oedema, and delayed awakening.

35.7   Conclusion

NTD's are one of the most common congenital anomalies. They can be detected on antenatal ultrasound, and surgical repair of open NTD can be done in -utero. Various genetic, maternal and environmental factors have been implicated in its occurrence. The location of the defect, presence of hydrocephalus, Arnold-Chiari malformations and other co-existing congenital anomalies, pose tremendous perioperative challenges. However, better understanding of neonatal physiology, advancement in diagnostic modalities, availability of NICU care, better preoperative optimization, can help reduce perioperative morbidity and mortality. Anesthetic management demands for meticulous planning and good team dynamics. The anesthesiologist should take special care to protect the out-growth from trauma or rupture, by proper positioning in the preoperative period, and at the time of induction of anesthesia. It is imperative that optimum hemodynamic stability be maintained during anesthesia and surgery, as cerebral oxygenation correlates well with the systemic blood pressure. All care to maintain OT temperature, prevent hypothermia, maintain adequate depth of anesthesia and analgesia, fluid management, intense monitoring, must be taken, and anesthesiologist must be ready to tackle any adverse events, in the intra-operative period. often these babies require multiple surgeries (redo or for other anomalies) and hence, a multispecialty team approach must be adopted to improve the quality of life.

Cervical MMC with hydrocephalus for VP Shunt

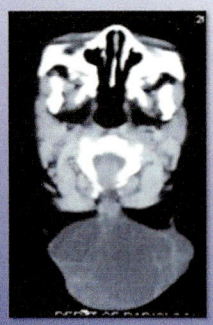 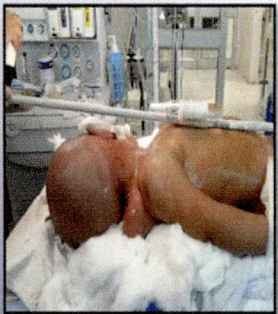 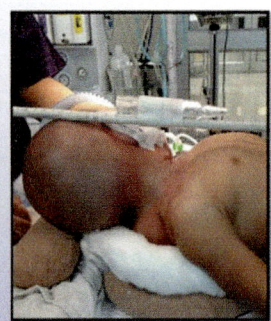

Airway Management

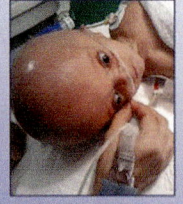 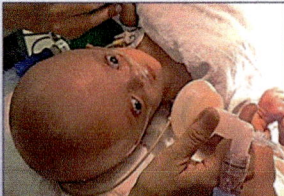 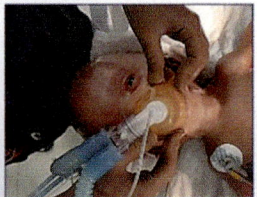

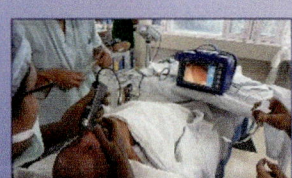 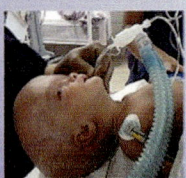 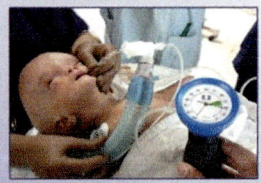

Spina Bifida- Cyst on baby's lower back area
Repair of Lumbar Meningomyelocele &
Healed Scar on the back

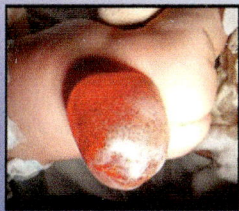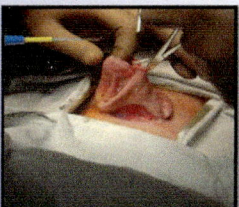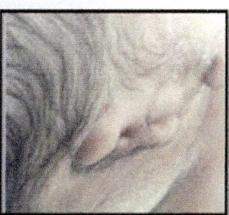

References

1. Copp AJ, Brook FA, Estibeiro JP, et al. The embryonic development of mammalian neural tube defects. Prog Neurobiol. 1990;35(5):363–403.
2. Greene ND, Copp AJ. Neural tube defects. Annu Rev Neurosci. 2014;37:221–42.
3. Cherian A, Seena S, Bullock RK, Antony AC. Incidence of neural tube defects in the leastdeveloped area of India: a population-based study. Research Letters. 2005;366(9489):930–1. https://doi.org/10.1016/S0140-6736(05)67319-9.
4. Flores AL, Vellozzi C, Valencia D, Sniezek J. Global Burden of Neural Tube Defects, Risk Factors, and Prevention. Indian J Community Health. 2014;26(Suppl 1):3–5. PMID: 26120254; PMCID: PMC4480200.
5. Darnell D, Gilbert SF. Neuroembryology. Wiley Interdiscip Rev Dev Biol. 2017;6:1. https://doi.org/10.1002/wdev.215.
6. Eagles ME, Gupta N. Embryology of spinal dysraphism and its relationship to surgical treatment. Can J Neurol Sci. 2020;47(6):736–46.
7. Acharya UV, Pendharkar H, Varma DR, Pruthi N, Varadarajan S. Spinal dysraphism illustrated; Embroyology revisited. Indian J Radiol Imaging. 2017;27(4):417–26.
8. Van Allen MI, Kalousek DK, Chernoff GF, Juriloff D, et al. Evidence for multi-site closure of the neural tube in humans. Am J Med Genet. 1993;47:723–43.
9. Mahalik SK, Vaze D, Kanojia RP, Narasimhan KL, Rao KL. Multiple neural tube defects may not be very rare. Childs Nerv Syst. 2013;29(4):609–19.
10. Allagh KP, Shamanna BR, Murthy GV, Ness AR, et al. Birth prevalence of neural tube defects and orofacial clefts in India: a systematic review and meta-analysis. PLoS One. 2015;10:e0118961.

11. Zaganjor I, Sekkarie A, Tsang BL, et al. Describing the prevalence of neural tube defects worldwide: a systematic literature review. PLoS One. 2016;11(4):e0151586.
12. Greene ND, Stanier P, Copp AJ. Genetics of human neural tube defects. Hum Mol Genet. 2009;18(R2):R113–29.
13. Mishra PR, Barik M, Mahapatra AK. Molecular genetics involved in neural tube defects: recent advances and future prospective for molecular medicine. Neurol India. 2020t;68(5):1144–50.
14. Yadav U, Kumar P, Rai V. Maternal biomarkers for early prediction of the neural tube defects pregnancies. Birth Defects Res. 2021;113(7):589–600.
15. Behere RV, Deshmukh AS, Otiv S, Gupte MD, Yajnik CS. Maternal vitamin B12 status during pregnancy and its association with outcomes of pregnancy and health of the offspring: a systematic review and implications for policy in India. Front Endocrinol (Lausanne). 2021;12:619176.
16. Central Technical Co-Ordinating Unit and ICMR Central Technical Coordinating Unit, ICMR. Multicentric study of efficacy of periconceptional folic acid containing vitamin supplementation in prevention of open neural tube defects from India. Indian J Med Res. 2000;112:206–11.
17. Copp AJ, Stanier P, Greene ND. Neural tube defects: recent advances, unsolved questions, and controversies. Lancet Neurol. 2013;12(8):799–810.
18. Liu HY, Liu SM, Zhang YZ. Maternal folic acid supplementation mediates offspring health via DNA methylation. Reprod Sci. 2020;27(4):963–76.
19. John HM, Harvey BS, Laura FS. Malformations of the central nervous system. In: John HM, editor. Child neurology. Lippincott: Williams Wilkins; 2006. p. 285–366.
20. McComb JG. A practical clinical classification of spinal neural tube defects. Childs Nerv Syst. 2015;31(10):1641–57.
21. Jacobs RA. Myelodysplasia. In: Wolraich ML, editor. Disorders of development and learning. 2nd ed. St. louis: Mosby; 1996. p. 213–61.
22. Stiefel D, Copp AJ, Meuli M. Fetal spina bifida: loss of neural function in utero. J Neurosurg. 2007;106:213–21.
23. McLone DG, Knepper PA. The cause of Chiari II malformation: a unified theory. Pediatr Neurosci. 1989;15:1–12.
24. Carling N, Brady KM, Bissonnette B, Easley RB. Anesthesia for neurosurgical procedures. In: Andropoulos DB, George A, editors. Gregory's pediatric anesthesia. 6th ed; 2020. p. 571–602.
25. Bradley LA, Palomaki GE, McDowell GA, ONTD Working Group; ACMG Laboratory Quality Assurance Committee. Technical standards and guidelines: prenatal screening for open neural tube defects. Genet Med. 2005;7(5):355–69.
26. Gandy K, Castillo H, Rocque BG, Bradko V, et al. Neurosurgical training and global health education: systematic review of challenges and benefits of in-country programs in the care of neural tube defects. Neurosurg Focus. 2020;48:E14.
27. Chen Y, Wang X, Li L, Lu S, Zhang Z. New cut-off values for screening of trisomy 21, 18 and open neural tube defects (ONTD) during the second trimester in pregnant women with advanced maternal age. BMC Pregnancy Childbirth. 2020;20(1):776.
28. Zugazaga Cortazar A, Martín Martinez C, et al. Magnetic resonance imaging in the prenatal diagnosis of neural tube defects. Insights Imaging. 2013;4(2):225–37.
29. Eibach S, Moes G, Hou YJ, Zovickian J, Pang D. New surgical paradigm for open neural tube defects. Childs Nerv Syst. 2021;37(2):529–38.
30. Grivell RM, Andersen C, Dodd JM. Prenatal versus postnatal repair procedures for spina bifida for improving infant and maternal outcomes. Cochrane Database Syst Rev. 2014;2014(10):CD008825.
31. Meuli M, Meuli-Simmen C, Hutchins GM, Yingling CD, et al. In utero surgery rescues neurological function at birth in sheep with spina bifida. Nat Med. 1995;1:342–7.
32. Horzelska EI, Zamlynski M, Horzelski T, Zamlynski J, et al. Open fetal surgery for myelomeningocele - is there the learning curve at reduction mother and fetal morbidity? Ginekol Pol. 2020;91(3):123–31.

33. Tulipan N, Wellons JC 3rd, Thom EA, Gupta N, et al. Prenatal surgery for myelomeningocele and the need for cerebrospinal fluid shunt placement. J Neurosurg Pediatr. 2015;16:613–20.
34. Adzick NS, Thom EA, Spong CY, Brock JW 3rd, et al. A randomised trial of prenatal versus postnatal repair of myelomeningocele. N Engl J Med. 2011;364:993–1004.
35. McCurdy CM Jr, Seeds JW. Route of delivery of infants with congenital anomalies. Clin Perinatol. 1993;20(1):81–106.
36. Tolcher MC, Shazly SA, Shamshirsaz AA, Whitehead WE, et al. Neurological outcomes by mode of delivery for fetuses with open neural tube defects: a systematic review and meta-analysis. BJOG. 2019;126(3):322–7.
37. Waters JFR, O'Neal MA, Pilato M, Waters SH. Management of anesthesia and delivery in women with Chiari I malformations. Obstet Gynecol. 2018;132(5):1180–4.
38. Demirci J, Caplan E, Brozanski B, Bogen D. Winging it: maternal perspectives and experiences of breastfeeding newborns with complex congenital surgical anomalies. J Perinatol. 2018;38(6):708–17.
39. Kuo BJ, Vissoci JR, Egger JR, et al. Perioperative outcomes for pediatric neurosurgical procedures: analysis of the National Surgical Quality Improvement Program-Pediatrics. J Neurosurg. 2017;19:361–71.
40. Campbell E, Beez T, Todd L. Prospective review of 30-day morbidity and mortality in a paediatric neurosurgical unit. Childs Nerv Syst. 2017;33:483–9.
41. Bohle B, Wagner B, Vollmann U, Niggemann B, et al. Characterisation of T cell responses to Hev b 3, an allergen associated with latex allergy in spina bifida. J Immunol. 2000;164:4393–8.
42. Soriano SG, McManus ML. Pediatric neuroanesthesia and critical care. In: Cottrell JE, Patel P, editors. Cottrell and Patel's neuroanesthesia. 6th ed. Amstradam: Elsevier; 2017. p. 337–50.
43. Hamid R, Newfield P. Pediatric neuroanesthesia neural tube defects. Anesthesiol Clin North Am. 2001;19:219–28.
44. Deora H, Srinivas D, Shukla D, Devi BI, et al. Multiple-site neural tube defects: embryogenesis with complete review of existing literature. Neurosurg Focus. 2019;47(4):E18.
45. Singh D, Rath GP, Dash HH, Bithal PK. Anesthetic concerns and perioperative complications in repair of myelomeningocele: a retrospective review of 135 cases. J Neurosurg Anesthesiol. 2010;22:11–5.
46. Vavilala MS, Soriano SG, Krane EJ. Anesthesia for neurosurgery. In: Davis PJ, Cladis FP, editors. Smith's anesthesia for infants and children. 9th ed; 2017. p. 744–72.
47. Linh LT, Duc NM, Nhung NH, My TT, et al. Detecting fetal central nervous system anomalies using magnetic resonance imaging and ultrasound. Med Arch. 2021;75(1):45–9.
48. Aoki H, Miyazaki O, Irahara S, Okamoto R, Tsutsumi Y, et al. Value of parametric indexes to identify tracheal atresia with or without fistula on fetal magnetic resonance imaging. Pediatr Radiol. 2021;51:2027. https://doi.org/10.1007/s00247-021-05092-x.
49. Birmingham PK, Dsida RM, Grayhack JJ, et al. Do latex precautions in children with myelodysplasia reduce intraoperative allergic reactions? J Pediatr Orthop. 1996;16(6):799–802.
50. Humphreys S, Schibler A, von Ungern-Sternberg BS. Carbon dioxide monitoring in children - a narrative review of physiology, value and pitfalls in clinical practice. Paediatr Anaesth. 2021;31:839. https://doi.org/10.1111/pan.14208. Epub ahead of print.
51. Unal S, Ergenekon E, Aktas S, Beken S, Altuntas N, et al. Perfusion index assessment during transition period of newborns: an observational study. BMC Pediatr. 2016;16(1):164.
52. Goldman JM, Petterson MT, Kopotic RJ, Barker SJ. Masimo signal extraction pulse oximetry. J Clin Monit Comput. 2000;16(7):475–83.
53. Vanderhaegen J, Naulaers G, Van Huffel S, et al. Cerebral and systemic hemodynamic effects of intravenous bolus administration of propofol in neonates. Neonatology. 2010;98:57–63.
54. Matchett GA, Allard MW, Martin RD, et al. Neuroprotective effect of volatile anesthetic agents: molecular mechanisms. Neurol Res. 2009;31:128–34.
55. Sever F, Özmert S. Evaluation of the relationship between airway measurements with ultrasonography and laryngoscopy in newborns and infants. Paediatr Anaesth. 2020;30(11):1233–9.

56. Gupta P, Rath GP, Prabhakar H, Bithal PK. Comparison between sevoflurane and desflurane on emergence and recovery characteristics of children undergoing surgery for spinal dysraphism. Indian J Anaesth. 2015;59:482–7.

57. Gupta N, Rath GP, Prabhakar H, Dash HH. Effect of intraoperative dexmedetomidine on postoperative recovery profile of children undergoing surgery for spinal dysraphism. J Neurosurg Anesthesiol. 2013;25:271–8.

58. Squillaro A, Mahdi EM, Tran N, Lakshmanan A, et al. Managing procedural pain in the neonate using an opioid-sparing approach. Clin Ther. 2019;41(9):1701–13. https://doi.org/10.1016/j.clinthera.2019.07.014. PMCID: PMC6790974. Epub 2019 Aug 17. PMID: 31431300.

59. Wade C, Frazer JS, Qian E, Davidson LM, Dash S, et al. Development of locally relevant clinical guidelines for procedure-related neonatal analgesic practice in Kenya: a systematic review and meta-analysis. Lancet Child Adolesc Health. 2020;4(10):750–60.

60. Hoarau K, Payet ML, Zamidio L, Bonsante F, Iacobelli S. "Holding-cuddling" and sucrose for pain relief during venepuncture in newborn infants: a randomized, controlled trial (CÂSA). Front Pediatr. 2021;14(8):607900.

61. Kaloria N, Bhagat H, Singla N. Venous air embolism during removal of bony spur in a child of split cord malformation. J Neurosci Rural Pract. 2017;8(3):483–4.

62. Lew SM, Kothbauer KF. Tethered cord syndrome: an updated review. Pediatr Neurosurg. 2007;43:236–48.

63. Bhagwat SN, Mahapatra AK, et al. Encephalocoele and anomalies of the scalp. Pediatr Neurosurg. 1999 London Churchill Livingstone: 101–120.

64. Cohen MM, Lemire RJ. Syndromes with cephaloceles. Teratology. 1982;25:161–72.

65. Marinho M, Lourenço C, Nogueira R, Valente F. Prenatal diagnosis of frontal encephalocele. J Clin Ultrasound. 2020;48(9):557–9. https://doi.org/10.1002/jcu.22848. Epub 2020 Apr 24

66. Lo BW, Kulkarni AV, Rutka JT, Jea A, Drake JM, et al. Clinical predictors of developmental outcome in patients with cephaloceles. J Neurosurg Pediatr. 2008;2(4):254–7.

67. Flanders TM, Heuer GG, Madsen PJ, Buch VP, et al. Detailed analysis of hydrocephalus and hindbrain herniation after prenatal and postnatal myelomeningocele closure: report from a single institution. Neurosurgery. 2020;86(5):637–45. https://doi.org/10.1093/neuros/nyz302.

68. Mahapatra AK. Anterior encephalocele - AIIMS experience a series of 133 patients. J Pediatr Neurosci. 2011;6(Suppl 1):S27–30. https://doi.org/10.4103/1817-1745.85706.

69. Mahajan C, Rath GP. Anaesthetic management in a child with frontonasal encephalocele. J Anaesthesiol Clin Pharmacol. 2010;26:570–1.

70. Kahle KT, Kulkarni AV, Limbrick DD Jr, Warf BC. Hydrocephalus in children. Lancet. 2016;387:788–99.

71. Bawa M, Dash V, Mahalik S, Rao KLN. Outcome analysis of patients of congenital hydrocephalus with ventriculoperitoneal shunt at a tertiary care hospital in North India. Pediatr Neurosurg. 2019;54(4):233–6. https://doi.org/10.1159/000501018. Epub 2019 Jul 10.

72. Flanders TM, Kimmel AC, Lang SS, Bellah R, et al. Standardizing treatment of preterm infants with post-hemorrhagic hydrocephalus at a single institution with a multidisciplinary team. Childs Nerv Syst. 2020;36(8):1737–44.

73. Heye P, Su YS, Flanders TM, Reisen B, et al. Laparoscopy assisted ventriculoperitoneal shunt placement in children. J Pediatr Surg. 2020;55(2):296–9.

74. Lim J, Tang AR, Liles C, et al. The cost of hydrocephalus: a cost-effectiveness model for evaluating surgical techniques. J Neurosurg Pediatr. 2018;23:109–18.

75. Chhabra DK. The saga of the 'Chhabra' shunt. Neurol India. 2019;67:635–8.

76. Riva-Cambrin J, Kestle JR, Holubkov R, Butler J, et al. Risk factors for shunt malfunction in pediatric hydrocephalus: a multicenter prospective cohort study. J Neurosurg Pediatr. 2016;17(4):382–90.

77. Tsuji M, Saul JP, du Plessis A, et al. Cerebral intravascular oxygenation correlates with mean arterial pressure in critically ill premature infants. Pediatrics. 2000;106:625.

78. Yadav Y R, Jaiswal S, Adam N, Basoor A, Jain G. Endoscopic third ventriculostomy in infants. Neurol India [serial online] 2006;54:161–3. Available from: https://www.neurologyindia.com/text.asp?2006/54/2/161/25960

Anesthesia for Short Procedures

36

Shilpa Agarwal

36.1 Introduction

Newborns undergoing surgery present several challenges for the anesthesiologist, whether minor or major procedures. Concerns are more for short and minor procedures because the anesthesia requirement and risk remain the same, but with greater need for exercising care so that the baby recovers well after the procedure.

A multispecialty approach works the best as anesthesiologist is involved in the neonatal care only at the time of surgery. Communication and cooperation between the entire health care team (surgeon, anesthesiologist, neonatologist, nursing, and technical staff) is essential preoperative requirement for the best outcome. The anticipation, prevention, and efficient and prompt management of complications may be lifesaving.

Any surgery undertaken in a newborn or a neonate is critical. Many of these are minor procedures, and short in duration, and though usually elective, many are often done on emergency basis. Many of these minor or short procedures, if undertaken in the neonatal period, are done on emergency basis and are frequently associated with other multisystem abnormalities including congenital heart disease and RDS, and carry the same anesthesia risk as for any other major procedure. On top of that, since these are short minor procedures, they usually last for less than 60 min, and more often 30–45 min. The goal of anesthetic management is that the neonate recovers soon after surgery without need for postoperative ventilatory support or NICU care [1].

Anesthetic concerns and requirements, OT preparation, are the same as in any newborn or neonate, undergoing major surgery. All precautions to prevent hypothermia must be taken.

S. Agarwal (✉)
Department of Anesthesiology, Chacha Nehru Bal Chikitsalya, New Delhi, India

U. Saha (ed.), *Clinical Anesthesia for the Newborn and the Neonate*, https://doi.org/10.1007/978-981-19-5458-0_36

All care must be taken as described in the chapter on anesthetic considerations in the newborn, neonate, and premature.

Common short procedures that a newborn baby or a neonate may have to undergo, are follows:

1. **Lower Abdominal and Perineal Procedures -** Umbilical hernia, Inguinal hernia, Undescended testis, Hydrocele, Torsion testis, Circumcision, Cystoscopy, and PUV fulguration,
2. **Gastro Abdominal procedures -** Gastrostomy, Colostomy, Intraperitoneal drain placement,
3. **Tracheostomy,**
4. **Infective (drainage, debridement) -** Necrotizing Fasciitis (NF), septic arthritis,
5. **Birth injuries (BI), Neonatal care injuries (NCI),** and
6. **Ventriculoperitoneal (VP) shunt** placement.

36.2   Anesthetic Concerns for Short Procedures in Neonates

Anesthetic management and choice of anesthetic drugs largely depend upon the condition of the neonate, gestational age at birth, weight, birth weight, associated medical or other abnormality, and type of surgical emergency or procedure. Careful titration of drug dosage is important to reduce the risk of anesthesia, while achieving the desired effect. Factors to be kept in mind when planning anesthesia for such babies are as follows:

1. How well the baby has adapted to postnatal environment.
2. Immature organ systems, which are still growing and maturing. Immature hepatorenal system and effect of drug metabolism and excretion. Immature autonomic nervous system and poor hemodynamic adjustments and sympathetic responses. Immaturity of neuromuscular junction and sensitivity to muscle relaxants.
3. Presence of congenital abnormalities such as congenital cardiac defects, RDS, cleft lip or palate, and other anomalies. They may suffer from various medical conditions, which are undiagnosed and untreated and increase the surgical and anesthesia risk.
4. Brain and Blood Brain Barrier immaturity and sensitivity to anesthetic drugs (induction agents, narcotics, and sedatives).
5. Hematological and coagulation abnormalities, risk of hypothermia, hypoxemia, electrolyte changes, and dehydration and hypoglycemia with prolonged fasting.
6. Preoperative investigations may not be available and blood not arranged for transfusion.
7. On top of that, since these are short minor procedures, it is expected that both induction and recovery should be quick and rapid, with no residual effects, and monitoring takes a back step, and invasive monitoring is usually not considered.
8. There should be no need for postoperative ventilatory support, but need postoperative observation for a few hours at least, best for 12 h.

36.3 Anesthetic management – General Considerations

Patient and OT preparation: A detailed preoperative evaluation and risk stratification must be done, informed consent taken and documented, just as for any other surgery. Usually these procedures are short, not more than 60 min duration. OT preparation suitable for a neonate, prevention of hypothermia, and equipped with appropriate equipment. Anesthesiologist and other OR staff must be well-trained in caring for neonates.

Anesthesia induction and maintenance: GA is the usual technique of choice. Both inhalational and intravenous inductions are suitable depending on the availability of a peripheral IV line. Airway can be managed using SGD /LMA or ET tube. Wherever possible, SGD is preferred, avoiding need of muscle relaxant and endotracheal intubation. Most procedures, except abdominal, can be performed with baby retaining spontaneous respiration, assisted at intervals. Avoid or minimize the use of muscle relaxants and narcotics.

Analgesia: Any surgical intervention is painful. Multimodal analgesia is safer technique for both intra and postoperative pain, and babies should not be deprived of this, however short the procedure. Short-acting drugs, with predicted duration of action and effect, are preferred. Careful titration of drug dosages is advocated to get the desired effect, without adverse effects. Avoid unnecessary administration of drugs and undue polypharmacy.

Monitoring: Minimal basic monitoring includes heart rate, blood pressure (NIBP), respiratory rate, and saturation (SpO_2). Invasive monitoring is usually not mandated.

Preoperative fasting and Fluid therapy - Fluid loss and third space shifts are minimal. Careful calculation of fluid deficits, intraoperative losses, and replacement must be done, avoiding overloading and under transfusion. Blood loss is minimal and blood transfusion is not required, but always get blood grouping and keep cross-matched blood available. Main concern during short surgeries is inability to replace fasting deficits (which traditionally are calculated and given over 3-h period). This makes neonate at risk of hypovolemia even when there is hardly any intraoperative fluid or blood loss. Rapid fluid infusion puts the neonate at risk of fluid overload. To avoid this, keep NPO period to minimum (2 h for clear fluids). If longer preoperative NPO status is deemed necessary because of the type of surgery, start dextrose containing IV fluids to avoid dehydration and hypoglycemia.

Recovery from anesthesia: Anesthesia for short procedures in a newborn or neonate is a skillful task. Babies are at risk of delayed recovery from overdose of anesthetic drugs, inadequate recovery of neuromuscular block, opioids, hypothermia, fluid and electrolyte imbalance and hypoglycemia, etc. Increased proneness to pulmonary aspiration adds further to delayed recovery. Hence, these babies require monitored postoperative care.

36.4 Specific Short Procedures

Perioperative concerns, care, precautions, dos and don'ts, and anesthesia technique, specific to the procedure, will be discussed.

36.4.1 Lower Abdominal and Perineal Procedures

These are the most common short procedures undertaken in the neonatal period. Umbilical hernia, Inguinal hernia, Hydrocele, Undescended testis, Torsion testis, Circumcision, Cystoscopy, PUV fulguration, and Colostomy [2].

36.4.1.1 Umbilical Hernias
Umbilical Hernias are common in newborns, especially in premature and low birth weight babies. The incidence is as high as 84% in newborns weighing 1000–1500 g, and 20% in those weighing 2000–2500 g. After separation of the umbilical cord, the umbilical ring undergoes spontaneous closure through the growth of the rectus muscles and fusion of the fascial layers. Delay or incomplete closure leads to herniation of the intra-abdominal contents through the open ring. Umbilical hernias are quite common in healthy neonates, but may be associated with some specific conditions, like autosomal trisomies (Trisomy 21 and 18), metabolic disorders (hypothyroidism, mucopolysaccharidoses), and dysmorphic syndromes (Beckwith-Wiedemann and Marfan syndromes). It is important to identify isolated umbilical hernia from that associated with syndromes with features like macroglossia or hypotonia, as a clue warranting further evaluation. Surgical repair of umbilical hernia in neonates is usually delayed due to its low complication rate and also because majority of umbilical defects close spontaneously within 2 years. Surgery is indicated for large defects (>1.5 cm) and in case of complications such as incarceration, strangulation, or rupture. Surgery is performed under general anesthesia.

36.4.1.2 Inguinal Hernia and Hydrocele Repair: Herniorrhaphy
Testicles are enclosed in a peritoneal covering, the processus vaginalis, which is usually closed at birth. Failure of closure leads to development of hernia and hydrocele. Obliteration of processus vaginalis occurs late in gestation, and so incidence of inguinal hernia is high in premature (10–11%) and extremely low birth weight (ELBW) (40%) newborns. Incidence in term newborns is less than 5%. Ten percent hernias in term and up to 50% in premature and ELBW babies are bilateral.

Hydrocele is a fluid collection that may occur anywhere along the path of testicular decent and may be communicating or noncommunicating. Parents usually bring the baby with a history of a painless **intermittent swelling** in the groin, which appears only on straining, e.g., during crying. Often, the hernia is **reducible**. At times, it cannot be reduced by manipulation and is termed as **incarcerated hernia**. Bowel within the hernia can become erythematous and trapped within the hernia sac and progress on to **bowel obstruction.** In females the sac may also contain an ovary.

The progressive swelling and edema of the entrapped contents of the hernia cause vascular compromise of the entrapped bowel, which becomes ischemic and progresses onto the stage of **strangulation.**

Unlike in adults, inguinal hernias are surgically corrected soon after diagnosis to prevent the risk of incarceration, strangulation, bowel obstruction, or gonadal damage. Management of hydrocele is more conservative and usually resolves within 1–2 years of life. Surgical correction is required if hydrocele persists beyond 1 year.

The definitive treatment for hernia is manual reduction followed by surgical repair. Major surgical issue with unilateral inguinal hernia is whether to explore the contralateral side or not, with the risk of damage to the vas deferens and spermatic cord. So, each neonate must be examined thoroughly for the presence of bilateral hernia, preoperatively.

Asymptomatic hernias can be electively scheduled at a later convenient date and time, but they remain at risk of incarceration, progressing onto intestinal obstruction, strangulation, and gangrene. Therefore, even asymptomatic hernias must be repaired at the earliest [3, 4].

Anesthesia

Unilateral inguinal hernia repair is a short procedure of about 30–45 min, while a bilateral repair may last up to 90 min. The goal of anesthetic management is rapid induction, rapid recovery, and good analgesia. Surgery is at the inguinal region, so muscle relaxation is not an issue, but adequate depth of anesthesia is a necessity for the hernial contents to be reposited into the abdomen. Either general or regional anesthesia can be used for inguinal herniorrhaphy. GA carries the usual risks of a newborn and neonate. Shorter-acting agents such as Sevoflurane with caudal or ilioinguinal/iliohypogastric nerve block or Fentanyl or Remifentanyl for pain relief are acceptable techniques, with face mask, or LMA, baby breathing spontaneously or assisted. Fluid and blood loss is minimal. In premature neonates, GA carries the usual risk of postoperative apnea and delayed recovery. Subarachnoid block (SAB) is advocated to avoid complications of GA. Baby movements can be controlled by gentle strapping or light anesthesia with O2 and Sevoflurane with a face mask [4].

Anesthesia for incarcerated or obstructed hernia: These neonates may be sick because of incarceration, obstruction, or gangrene of intestines. They may be hypovolemic, dehydrated, anemic, acidotic, hypoxemic, febrile, and oliguric. Surgery is prolonged and is associated with fluid shifts because of handling of intestines, chances of intestinal perforation or tear because of edema, and hemodynamic disturbances (hypotension and bradycardia). Blood transfusion may be needed in anemic babies and if there is blood loss. They are at risk of delayed recovery from anesthesia because of hypothermia, acid base, and electrolyte disturbances and may need postoperative ventilatory support. General anesthesia is the technique of choice, with muscle relaxation, tracheal intubation / LMA, and controlled ventilation, followed by reversal with neostigmine and glycopyrrolate at the end. Glycopyrrolate premedication reduces the risk of bradycardia at induction, laryngoscopy, intubation, and handling of the intestines. Intraoperative care includes monitoring for vitals, meticulous fluid therapy, maintenance of acid base and electrolyte balance and calcium supplementation, and care to prevent reopening of intracardiac shunts. Postoperatively, babies must be under observation in the NICU, for at least 24–48 h, before shifting back to the ward., and discharge from hospital is usually delayed to 5–7 days depending on the intestinal handling.

In case of **gangrenous hernia**, after separation, intestines may need to be resected with colostomy usually done. Baby presents another time after 4–6 weeks for colostomy closure under anesthesia. General anesthesia with tracheal intubation and controlled ventilation is instituted, with facilities for postoperative ventilatory support and blood transfusion.

36.4.1.3   Undescended Testis: Orchidopexy

Orchiopexy is done for cryptorchidism in which there is a failure of normal testicular decent from abdomen into the scrotum. The undescended testicle may lie anywhere along its route of descent, within the abdomen, inguinal canal, or external ring. The incidence is 33% in preterm and 3% in full term males and reduces to 1% by 3 months of age. It is usually associated with a hernia. The chance for developing a malignancy is ten fold higher than in normal descended testes. It is not operated in the neonatal period, because of the risks involved in this age group, unless there is an emergency or there are indications for hernia surgery (see above).

Preoperative evaluation is important as there is high association of prematurity with undescended testes. One should look for various syndromes and cardiac defects and anatomical and physiological impact on anesthesia management, e.g., Noonan syndrome (congenital heart disease, bleeding problems, skeletal malformations, short neck, and small jaw), Prader Willi syndrome (muscle weakness, slow development, and usually not much problem in neonatal period), and cloacal exstrophy (OEIS syndrome – omphalocele, extrophy bladder, imperforate anus, and spinal defects).

The surgical procedure depends on the position of the testes. In babies requiring inguinal exploration, general anesthesia alone or in combination with a regional anesthesia can be used (Fig. 36.1). Anesthesia management is same as for inguinal

Fig. 36.1 Incision for undescended testis

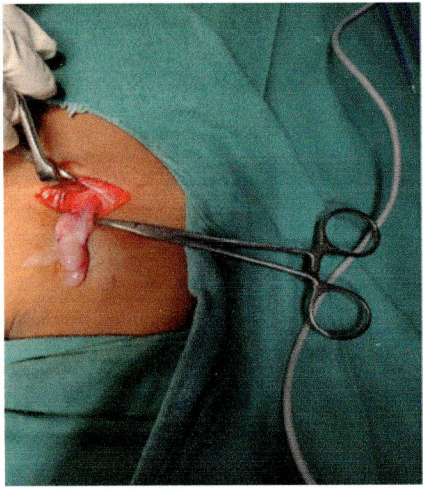

herniotomy. Unlike hernia surgery, here tissue dissection may be more, which is painful. Multimodal analgesia including acetaminophen, NSAIDS, short-acting opioids, and regional techniques can be used. Regional analgesia can be provided by caudal route, or ilioinguinal or iliohypogastric nerve block. Ensure adequate depth of anesthesia especially when surgeon puts traction on the spermatic cord, foreskin, or testis, as this may trigger laryngospasm. A small IV bolus of propofol or increasing the inspired concentration of volatile anesthetic can prevent triggering of laryngospasm [5].

36.4.1.4 Torsion Testis

Testicular torsion is a true surgical emergency. Testicular torsion is either intrauterine or postnatal. The presentation of both is different, but sequels are same [6]. Prenatal torsion is generally associated with minimal or no findings, and if of long duration, it shows calcification and a hyper vascular ring of tunica with a hypodense center, while a short duration torsion shows mixed echogenicity. Antenatal sonography does not detect testicular torsion. Diagnosis is made at routine postnatal examination. Postnatal torsion is an acute manifestation with considerable swelling and tenderness of a previously normal testicle. Testicular infarction can occur within few hours of torsion; in addition, unilateral torsion can lead to bilateral testicular damage and infertility. Testicular torsion is best managed by early exploration, detorsion, and fixation. Testis should be salvaged as far as possible, and orchidectomy is done only if it is unsalvageable. Atrophic testis is a precursor of testicular carcinoma. Surgery is usually done under GA with RSI with caudal analgesia or under spinal anesthesia.

36.4.1.5 Circumcision

There are very few absolute indications for circumcision in neonates, but in a newborn with hydronephrosis, circumcision reduces the risk of urinary tract infections. Indications for circumcision are for (a) Religious and sociocultural reasons, and (b) Medical indications (true phimosis, balanitis xerotica, recurrent balanoposthitis, and urinary outlet obstruction). Neonatal circumcision is generally inexpensive, has low complication rate, and usually performed in the nursery under local anesthesia, like:

- Topically applied lidocaine-prilocaine cream,
- Subcutaneous ring block, or/and
- Dorsal penile block.

In case GA is required, it is same as described for other short procedures in this chapter. It is painful. Intraoperative analgesia can be provided with short-acting Fentanyl or dorsal penile block. Postoperative analgesia can be provided with acetaminophen, NSAIDs, and opioids coupled with regional anesthesia (penile block, pudendal nerve block, or caudal analgesia).

Note - LA without adrenalin should be used to avoid risk of ischemia and necrosis of glans penis.

Complications of circumcision include Infection, bleeding, meatal stenosis, and residual redundant skin.

36.4.1.6   Cystoscopy and Fulguration for PUV (Posterior Urethral Valves)

PUV is the most common cause of obstructive uropathy in children, incidence being 1/5000. The severity of renal changes from back pressure depends on the degree of obstruction and age of onset [5, 7]. Prenatal diagnosis can be made by fetal ultrasound, along with associated abnormalities, like bilateral hydronephrosis, oligohydramnios, and distended thick walled urinary bladder. A diagnosis in the second trimester is associated with poorer prognosis than those detected postnatal. Newborns with severe PUV may present with palpable bladder and anuria at birth. Postnatal diagnosis is established by voiding cysto-urethrogram (VCUG or MCU). Priority in all patients with PUV is early stabilization, and once the bladder is catheterized, it is no longer a surgical emergency.

Preoperative evaluation includes assessment of renal functions, urinary tract anatomy, extent of urinary retention and fluid overload, and evidence of renal failure. As far as possible, hypertension, azotemia, hyperkalemia, and hyponatremia should be optimized preoperatively. Azotemia affects branching of the bronchial tree and alveoli, and these babies may have respiratory compromise, evidenced with small chest and poor breathing movements, ascites, and limb deformities. Fetal urine forms the amniotic fluid. Underdeveloped kidneys and oliguria lead to oligohydramnios **(Potters Syndrome).** Fetus is not well cushioned from the uterine wall and assumes a typical facial appearance, the **Potter Facies.**

1. If **serum creatinine returns to normal after birth**, transurethral ablation of the valve leaflets under GA is undertaken.
2. If urethra is too small for the endoscope, then suprapubic vesicostomy and bladder exteriorization or catheterization are the only options, with ablation of valves at a later stage.

Inhalational or IV induction can be used. Procedure is performed in lithotomy position at the foot end of the OT table. The small baby is placed at the end opposite to the anesthesiologist and covered with drapes. This places the baby far away from the anesthetist. Hence, proper securing of airway is a must, either with an endotracheal tube or LMA. Use of short-acting relaxants and analgesics allows early recovery after the short procedure. A penile nerve block or caudal block can be given for intraoperative and postoperative analgesia. Judicious use of fluids and anesthetic agents is warranted in case of hydronephrosis and renal failure. Neonates with pulmonary hypoplasia may need postoperative ventilation.

36.4.2 Gastro Abdominal Procedures: Gastrostomy, Colostomy, Intraperitoneal Drain Placement

36.4.2.1   Gastrostomy

Gastrostomy (draining or feeding) is usually done in case of congenital deformities of the esophagus and small bowel (atresia), complicated TEF, exomphalos and CDH, for the purpose of gastric decompression, where definitive surgery cannot be undertaken for various reasons. This has several benefits: improved ventilation, early enteral feeding, and patient comfort and better growth, allowing time for optimization before major surgery later, with better outcome. This is a short procedure, of 10–15 min duration, and can be performed under LA, with or without sedation, in the NICU itself.

36.4.2.2 Colostomy

Creation of colostomy is another common procedure in the newborn, often performed within 24–48 h of birth, on urgent basis in NEC, anorectal malformations, Hirschsprung's disease, and imperforate anus.

1. **Imperforate anus** can present as a simple membranous defect to more complex involving urogenital anomalies. The newborn will present with non-passage of stools in the first 24 h, abdominal distention, or passage of stools near the penis, scrotum, or vagina from a fistulous connection.
2. **Anorectal malformations:** The incidence of anorectal malformations is 1 in 5000 newborns and may be associated with other congenital abnormalities such as VACTERL (Vertebral, Anal, Cardiac, Tracheal Esophageal, Renal, and Limb) and REAR (Renal, Ear, Anal, and Radial) syndromes. Preoperatively, babies should be screened for these anomalies, and due care taken during surgery and anesthesia.
3. **NEC** is a common surgical diagnosis in very sick neonates. Definitive surgery includes exploratory laparotomy, gut resection, and anastomosis or exteriorization. These babies are very sick and the surgery carries a high mortality. Hence, colostomy is often undertaken to allow time for the baby to optimize and reduce the risk of surgery, in very sick and premature newborns. Extensive abdominoperineal repair (APR) is undertaken later when the baby is about 3 months old, and when risk of anesthesia and surgery is considerably low.

Anesthesia Technique
Surgical management may be a simple perineal anoplasty (cut in the covering membrane) or a loop or divided colostomy (Fig. 36.2). Usually when the baby presents

Fig. 36.2 Colostomy – the two exteriorized ends of the descending colon

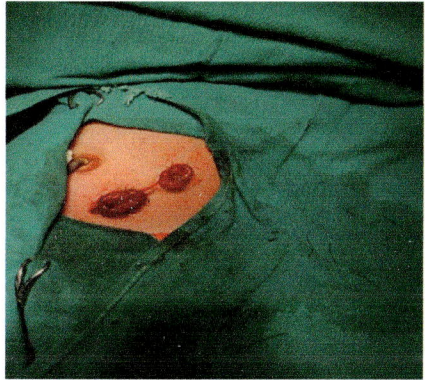

for anesthesia, an orogastric tube for stomach decompression is already in place. Before induction of anesthesia, its patency and proper placement must be checked and if any doubt it should be replaced, and stomach contents aspirated with a low pressure suction, or a syringe. GA with modified RSI, tracheal intubation with controlled ventilation, is the preferred technique. Nitrous oxide should be avoided at induction, to prevent further bowel distention and hemodynamic decompensation. For intraoperative analgesia, short-acting IV narcotics or caudal epidural can be used. A continuous caudal technique allows for postoperative analgesia too. Rectal suppositories cannot be used in these cases, but IV paracetamol can used to supplement postoperative analgesia. There may be large insensible and third space fluid losses associated with bowel handling and manipulation, so hydration and intravascular volume should be maintained. Blood loss is usually not significant to warrant transfusion. Babies can be extubated on the table and kept under observation in the NICU.

36.4.2.3   Intraperitoneal Drain (PD) Placement

Peritoneal drain is generally used as the initial management of intestinal perforation in premature neonates. Placement of an intra-abdominal PD relieves the acute respiratory and circulatory physiological effects of tension pneumoperitoneum, thus giving time for optimization of patient for definitive repair. It is generally done as a bedside procedure in the NICU under local anesthesia.

36.4.3 Tracheostomy

Tracheostomy is done for the maintenance of airway in neonates with neurologic impairment, pulmonary insufficiency, and acute airway obstruction, needing to be on prolonged ventilatory support [8, 9]. Common specific conditions are:

1. **Respiratory distress syndrome (RDS)**, very common in premature newborns, necessitating ventilatory support right from the time of birth. Duration of ventilatory support or assistance depends on the degree of lung maturity.
2. **Upper airway obstruction** is an absolute indication for tracheostomy. Proximal lesions such as Pierre Robin Syndrome and craniofacial abnormalities cause obstruction at the level of nasal and oral cavities, whereas subglottic stenosis, laryngomalacia, vocal cord paralysis, cysts, lymphangiomas, and hemangiomas cause obstruction at the level of larynx. Damage to the airway from trauma or infection may also need short-term tracheostomy.

Tracheostomy in newborn is a complex procedure due to anatomical and technical factors. Neonatal tracheostomy tubes (TT) are shorter than the pediatric TT and are usually uncuffed, but cuffed tubes are occasionally used in neonates requiring high ventilation pressures, as in RDS.

Technical issues in neonates: Trachea is small, pliable, and difficult to palpate in the short neck, more so in preterm and ELBW newborns. Pleura extends into the

Fig. 36.3 Transverse
tracheostomy

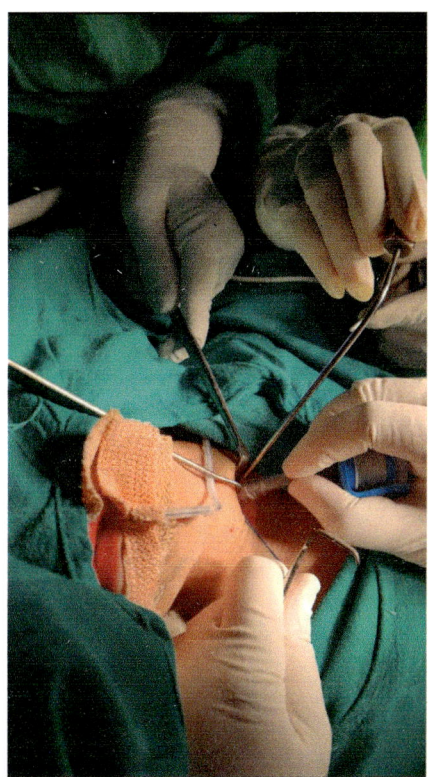

neck which poses the risk of pleural damage. Unlike in children, a vertical tracheostomy is preferred in neonates to avoid the risk of subglottic stenosis associated with a transverse tracheostomy (Fig. 36.3), but it poses a difficulty at the time of change of blocked or dislodged TT, until stoma maturation is complete.

The procedure is undertaken in the operation theatre. Most babies already have an endotracheal tube (ETT) in situ. Often an emergency tracheostomy is performed when such babies present for other surgeries with no apparent respiratory difficulty. Problems are encountered at the time of induction of GA, laryngoscopy, and intubation, when anesthetist fails to pass in even the smallest size ETT or causes injury to the upper airway with repeated attempts at intubation.

Preoperative assessment must include history of difficult mask ventilation, difficulty in securing the airway, and last feed time. At least 3 h should elapse from the last feed to avoid risk of regurgitation, vomiting, and pulmonary aspiration. Those with history of difficult laryngoscopy and intubation should have a backup plan at the completion of tracheostomy, like leaving an airway exchange catheter in the trachea during withdrawal of ETT, with the care that the tip is between the vocal cords so that ETT can be reinserted easily if need arises (as in failure of introducing TT).

Anesthesia Technique

In neonates with ETT in situ, tracheostomy can be done as an elective procedure, after initial stabilization. Anesthesia considerations and technique is as for any other airway surgery.

Babies who present for tracheostomy without ETT pose a greater challenge. It is important to maintain oxygenation and hemoglobin saturation within the normal range, using a face mask. Attempt should be made to secure the airway by intubation. In case of difficulty or failure to intubate, procedure can also be performed under LMA. Short-acting muscle relaxants and analgesics are preferred to allow early recovery without respiratory depression or compromise. It can also be performed with the baby breathing spontaneously, a mixture of O_2, air/N_2O, and sevoflurane, while surgeon instils LA at the incision site.

Postoperatively, babies must be cared for in NICU for postoperative ventilatory support, with maintenance of temperature, respiration and gas exchange, and analgesia. Feeding can be started after 3 h if there are no complications and bleeding.

36.4.4 Infective (Drainage, Debridement): Necrotizing Fasciitis (NF), Septic Arthritis

36.4.4.1 Necrotizing Fasciitis (NF)

NF is a rare life-threatening infection of the soft tissue, with fatal sequel. Bacterial invasion of the subcutaneous tissue releases endotoxins and exotoxins causing tissue ischemia and liquefactive necrosis. Accompanying systemic inflammation increases the morbidity. Mortality can be as high as 57% [10]. Cause of death is septic shock, DIC, and/or multiorgan failure [10]. Risk factors for NF in neonates include immunodeficiency, malnutrition, omphalitis, mammitis, balanitis, septicemia, NEC, fetal scalp monitoring, bullous impetigo, postoperative, diaper rash, burns, insect bites, hematologic malignancies, or nephrotic syndrome [10–12]. In as many cases no underlying diseases or triggering factor may be found. Even a small wound of capillary sampling site may provide entry point for the bacteria and can occur anywhere in the body (Fig. 36.4).

Fig. 36.4 NF on inner thigh in a neonate

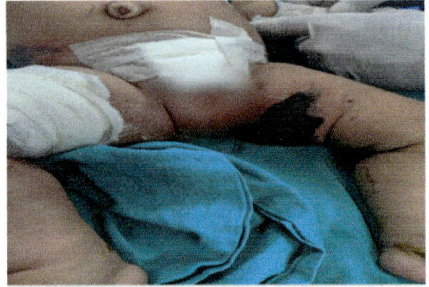

Presenting Features

Initial symptoms are nonspecific like fever, tenderness, erythema, pain, and edema, which may extend beyond the erythematous border since underlying tissue damage is much more extensive. If untreated, fulminant progression can occur within hours, with erythema progressing to violaceous necrotic lesions, vesicles, and bullae. **Primary NF** is monomicrobial and common in the lumbar area, while **secondary NF** is polymicrobial and common over the abdominal wall [10].

"Pain out of proportion" a typical sign in adult NF, but is not obvious in the neonate. Typical surgical findings are loose nonadherent fascia that gives away to blunt dissection and local edema (dishwater fluid) due to subcutaneous tissue necrosis which is gray non-bleeding. Once suspected, microbiological sampling is done and antibiotics started. Management is usually supportive. Surgical debridement of all necrotic tissue and drainage of affected fascial plane by fasciotomy improve the chances of survival.

Preoperative evaluation includes CBC, blood sugar, and coagulation profile. Neonates are anemic, with leukocytosis, abnormal coagulation profile, and hyper or hypoglycemic. Hemodynamic parameters must be optimized prior to surgery. All IM or SC injections must be avoided. Wound debridement is done under GA with controlled ventilation and good analgesia as it is very painful. There can be massive fluid and blood loss. Aggressive fluid therapy and fresh blood transfusion are needed. Blood sugar must be monitored and maintained in normal range. Urine output must be maintained at least 0.5–1 mL/kg/h, to preempt renal dysfunction.

36.4.4.2 Septic Arthritis

Septic arthritis is difficult to diagnose, particularly of deeper joints. The risk factors include umbilical catheterization, breech presentation, prematurity, sepsis, perinatal asphyxia, TPN (total parenteral nutrition), femoral venipuncture, and birth trauma [13, 14]. Delay in diagnosis can have potentially devastating sequelae: -

1. Pathologic joint instability,
2. Avascular necrosis,
3. Epiphyseal separation, or Premature epiphyseal closure,
4. Growth disturbance leading to limb length inequality, and.
5. Premature arthritis from joint destruction.

Neonates may be afebrile and have normal laboratory values, as TLC, ESR, and C-reactive proteins due to inappropriate immune response. Diagnosis is often delayed, increasing the risk of a poor outcome. The common presenting features are irritability, poor feeding, tenderness, limited range of motion, local swelling, difference in resting position of the affected extremity, erythema, warmth, and instability of the joint. Various imaging modalities can aid in the diagnosis of septic arthritis such as X Rays, USG, and MRI. USG is particularly useful as it can confirm joint effusion and identify periosteal separation or sub-periosteal collection, and cortical erosion. Treatment options include IV antibiotics with serial aspirations or surgical incision and drainage (I & D) as bedside procedure. Most important is to maintain asepsis and is best done in the OT under GA or regional anesthesia. Needle aspiration is a short procedure and can be done under LA and sedation and O_2, N_2O, sevoflurane inhalation by face mask. I & D procedure requires a still baby and is a slightly prolonged painful procedure. Usually, GA/IV induction and SGD/LMA suffice with baby breathing spontaneously, along with IV or caudal analgesia.

36.4.5 Birth Injuries (BI) and Neonatal Care Injuries (NCI)

Bi and NCI are causes of concern because of their contribution to neonatal morbidity and mortality. They contribute to nearly 2% mortality of all neonatal deaths.

36.4.5.1 Birth Injuries (BI)

Babies usually present within first 24–72 h of life. Earlier incidence of 2–7% of all deliveries (vaginal and operative) is on the decline with improvement in obstetric care [15, 16]. Many injuries can be managed conservatively such as **caput succedaneum, cephalic hematoma, minor intracerebral bleeds, fractures (clavicle, humerus, femur, slipped humerus epiphysis), shoulder or hip dislocation, and rib fracture** (following aggressive resuscitation) by splinting, bandaging, or POP, unless thoracic viscera is injured and bleeds. **Splenic rupture** is a serious condition. It occurs at during delivery, in babies with splenomegaly with associated coagulation disorders, vascular malformations, or hemangiomas. This is a surgical emergency. Baby becomes symptomatic and hemodynamically unstable within 24 h due to intra-abdominal bleeding, needing aggressive fluid and blood resuscitation, vasoactive drug infusion, and intubation and respiratory support for maintenance of oxygenation. The perioperative risk is high because of splenomegaly related abnormalities, hypothermia, need for large volume fluid and blood transfusion, and adverse outcomes. GA with ETT and controlled ventilation is adopted. Adequate analgesia must be provided. All care, monitoring, and precautions must be taken as in any newborn undergoing major emergency surgery. Postoperative ventilatory support for 12–24 h or till the baby becomes hemodynamically stable improves the outcome.

36.4.5.2 Neonatal Care Injuries (NCI)

These injuries occur during neonatal care, and usually present by 1–2 weeks, more commonly in premature babies in NICU than in home care [15]. Minor injuries, like **bruises or puncture marks, caustic burns from chemicals** used on the skin, and **fractures,** are managed conservatively. A common NCI is **finger-tip necrosis** following a tight SpO_2 monitor clip, leading to finger pulp amputation. **Cautery burns** usually heal with minor scarring. **Gastric perforation,** spontaneous, or due to prematurity, nasal ventilation at high pressures, sepsis, and steroid therapy, though rare, is usually fatal. Once diagnosed, it is a surgical emergency. GA is administered with standard care and precautions. Hyponatremia is a medical emergency. **Vascular life threatening conditions, like thrombosis, thromboembolism, vasospasm, vessel**

tear, and bleeding, need urgent management and are secondary to multiple attempts at IV or arterial cannulations. **Thrombosis** is managed conservatively by removal of catheter and anticoagulant and antifibrinolytic therapy. Surgical thrombectomy is not attempted because of high risk of GA and small size of the vessels.

36.4.6 Ventriculoperitoneal (VP) Shunt Placement

Hydrocephalus, accumulation of CSF in the skull, occurs because of obstruction to flow of CSF or due to excessive CSF production [17, 18]. Conditions associated with hydrocephalus are:

- **Inborn or Congenital** - Arnold-Chiari malformation, Dandy Walker syndrome,
- **Acquired** - brain tumors, intraventricular hemorrhage (IVH), infection, trauma.

36.4.6.1   Neuroanatomy and Physiology

The duramater is covered by the calvaria consisting of ossified plates connected by fibrous structures and fontanelle at the joints. This makes the skull of a newborn more compliant, so that with increase in CSF volume, though the skull /head will expand, there will be no increase in ICP. Presenting features are vague such as irritability, poor feeding, and lethargy. Parents notice disproportionate increase in head circumference, expanding sutures, bulging fontanels, "sundowning" of the eyes, and lower motor neuron deficit (weakness in the lower limbs).

Neonatal neurophysiological differences affect the management of intracranial hypertension. Normally, ICP in the neonate is low (2–4 mmHg) compared to that in adults (8–15 mmHg). The cerebral autoregulation limit is significantly lower with a MAP of 20–60 mmHg. This is inefficient in premature babies and in the presence of a pathological process. The global cerebral blood flow (CBF) is lower than that in children and adults. Large acute fluctuations in systemic blood pressure are poorly tolerated as systemic hypertension may cause IVH, while low mean arterial pressure may result in cerebral ischemia. The response to hyperventilation is exaggerated and ischemia may ensue at low $PaCO_2$ levels (<20 mmHg) due to intense cerebral arterial vasoconstriction. Untreated hydrocephalus is a cause of poor neurologic outcome due to ventriculomegaly, ischemia, and irreversible cellular damage.

Surgery aims at increasing CSF drainage, by making an alternative CSF flow path from the ventricular system to the **peritoneum (VP), pleural cavity, or right atrium.** A definitive procedure, removal of obstruction, is a major procedure, which is undertaken when the baby is mature enough to tolerate the cranial surgery.

Among the drainage procedures, **VP shunt** is the most common in neonates, with least risk. Complications include repeated blockage, infections, leaks, and over drainage from the valve failure, requiring frequent revision surgeries, on semi-emergency basis. In a near-term and full-term newborn with post-hemorrhagic hydrocephalus where surgical shunt is contraindicated, a ventricular assist device can be placed under LA at the bedside [19].

Anesthetic Considerations

Anesthetic management presents several challenges due to associated anomalies, prematurity, and associated comorbidities (Low birth weight, Anemia, Coagulopathy, Jaundice, RDS, and PFC), and distortion of airway anatomy by macrocephaly.

Preoperatively, baby should be assessed for coexisting diseases, medications, IV volume status, previous anesthetic history, evidence of raised ICP, vomiting and electrolyte imbalance, hormonal alterations, and seizures and anticonvulsant therapy (which need to be continued). Altered mental status or underlying pulmonary pathology may require preoperative blood gas analysis and postoperative airway and ventilatory support.

Preoperative sedatives should be used cautiously as indiscrete use can cause respiratory depression, altered sensorium, and further increase in ICP. Midazolam may be given orally. Ketamine is contraindicated as it increases CBF, ICP, cerebral metabolic rate, and O_2 consumption and lowers seizure threshold. GA with ETT and controlled ventilation is the technique of choice. IV induction with thiopentone (5–7 mg/kg) is preferred. Inhalational induction with sevoflurane is one if there is no IV access. Volatile anesthetics cause cerebral vasodilation and increase in ICP. Sevoflurane and Isoflurane have minimal effect on CBF, ICP, and cerebrovascular reactivity to CO_2 at low MAC (0.5–1.5).

Positioning at induction is challenging as macrocephaly distorts the normal skull anatomy and makes airway difficulty. The large occiput places the neck in extreme flexion, and large forehead obscures the line of sight during laryngoscopy or increase ICP due to jugular vein occlusion impeding venous drainage. A roll of towel placed under the shoulders can ease the airway difficulty, laryngoscopy, and intubation. A modified RSI is indicated as these babies are at risk for aspiration. The eyes should be adequately padded to protect from drying and injury (Fig. 36.5).

A short-acting opioid (fentanyl, remifentanil) will provide adequate intraoperative analgesia, allowing for rapid emergence and permitting timely postoperative neurologic assessment.

Because of the large head and its exposure during shunt placement, these neonates are prone to heat loss, **hypothermia,** and related sequel as peripheral vasospasm, increased O_2 consumption, metabolic acidosis due to increased lactate production, shift of the ODC to Left, decreased hepatic drug metabolism, delayed emergence from anesthesia, coagulopathy, immunodeficiency, hypoglycemia, and arrhythmias. Intraoperative temperature monitoring is crucial.

0.9% saline (NS) is commonly used as IV fluid for VP shunt surgery. It has slight hyperosmolarity (308 mOsm) which may attenuate cerebral edema. Neonates are at higher risk for hypoglycemia and must receive dextrose containing IV fluids (N/5). Hyperglycemia should be avoided as it can lead to cerebral ischemia and brain injury.

Nonsurgical measures (pharmacotherapy) to reduce raised ICP include:

1. Furosemide (loop diuretic),
2. Mannitol (osmotic diuretic), and
3. Hypertonic saline (3%).

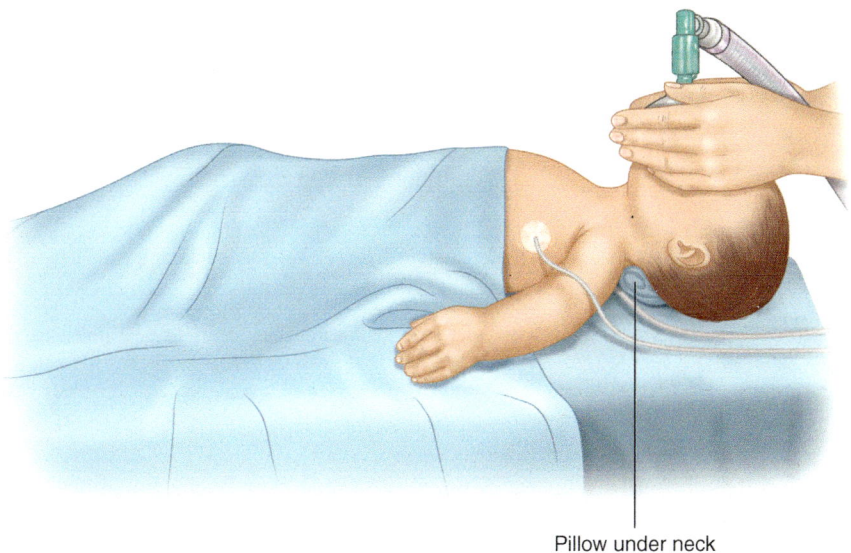

Pillow under neck

Fig. 36.5 Position at induction for VP shunt

These babies are at risk of delayed recovery and apnea, hence need postoperative monitoring.

36.5   Conclusion

Even for short minor procedures, the principles of anesthetic management and perioperative care remain same as for any major procedure including temperature control, glucose management, positioning, blood loss, meticulous fluid administration, maintenance of volume status, and vigilant monitoring. Difference in airway, respiratory, and cardiovascular anatomy, physiology, pharmacology, drug metabolism and excretion, and immature hepatorenal function are important considerations during anesthetic management.

The management of neonates with severe illness or major anomalies is challenging. Equally, or rather more challenging is when these babies undergo minor short procedures, because the anesthetic considerations, risks, and complications are same as in any other neonate, but with demand of quick induction and rapid recovery, without need for postoperative ventilatory support or other complications.

GA with IV or inhalational induction, LMA for airway control, and spontaneous respiration is most often appropriate. Endotracheal intubation is done only if indicated because of the risks associated with it. Preoperative evaluation should be as detailed, and with proper planning, and adequate knowledge of newborn and neonatal physiology, one can achieve good outcome after anesthesia. Basic care includes noninvasive vital monitoring, thermo neutral environment, meticulous fluid replacement (risk of overhydration), and readiness for management of any complication or critical event. Anesthesiologist and other OT staff must be well-trained in caring for neonates. If detected and managed early, morbidity and mortality related to short procedures under GA in the neonates can be minimized.

References

1. Pani N, Panda CK. Anaesthetic consideration for neonatal surgical emergencies. Indian J Anaesth. 2012;56(5):463–9. https://doi.org/10.4103/0019-5049.103962.
2. Wiliams RK, Lauro HV, Davis PJ. Ch 30: Anesthesia for feneral abdominal and urologic surgery. In: Davis PJ, Cladis FP, editors. Smith's anesthesia for infants and children. 9th ed. Amsterdam: Elsevier Inc; 2017. p. 789–816.
3. Wang KS. Assessment and management of inguinal hernia in infants. Pediatrics. 2012;130:768–73.
4. Ahmad N, Greenaway S. Anaesthesia for inguinal hernia repair in the newborn. BJA Edu. 2018;18(7):211–7.
5. Landsman IS, Zeigler LN, Deshpande JK. Ch 29: Anesthesia for pediatric Urological procedures. In: Gregory GA, Andropoulos DB, editors. Gregory's pediatric anesthesia. 5th ed. Hoboken: Wiley Blackwell; 2011. p. 744–7.
6. Riaz-Ul-Haq M, Mahdi DE, Elhassan EU. Neonatal testicular torsion; a review article. Iran J Pediatr. 2012;22(3):281–9.
7. Gharpure V. Posterior urethral valves in neonate. J Neonatal Surg. 2013;2(3):37.
8. Fiadjoe JE, Stricker PA, Litman RS. Ch 14: Pediatric airway management. In: Gregory GA, Andropoulos DB, editors. Gregory's pediatric Anesthesia. 5th ed. Hoboken: Wiley Blackwell; 2011. p. 317–8.
9. Doherty C, Neal R, English C, Cooke J, Atkinson D, et al. Multidisciplinary guidelines for the management of pediatric tracheostomy emergencies. Anesthesia. 2018;73(11):1309–12.
10. Hsieh WS, Yang PH, Fu RH, et al. Neonatal necrotizing fasciitis. Pediatr Res 1999; 45, 269. https://doi.org/10.1203/00006450-199904020-01602.
11. Hsieh WS, Yang PH, Chao HC, Lai JY. Neonatal necrotizing fasciitis: a report of three cases and review of the literature. Pediatrics. 1999;103(4):e53.
12. Zundel S, Lemaréchal A, Kaiser P, Szavay P. Diagnosis and treatment of pediatric necrotizing fasciitis: a systematic review of the literature. Eur J Pediatr Surg. 2016;27:127. https://doi.org/10.1055/s-0036-1584531.
13. Devi RU, Bharathi SM, Anitha M. Neonatal septic arthritis: clinical profile and predictors of outcome. Indian J Child Health. 2017;4(1):10–4. https://doi.org/10.32677/IJCH.2017.v04.i01.004.
14. Rai A, Chakladar D, Bhowmik S, etal. Neonatal septic arthritis: Indian perspective. Eur J Rheumatol 2020;7(1):S72-S77. https://doi.org/10.5152/eurjrheum.2019.19052.
15. Fette A. Birth and neonatal care injuries: a special aspect of newborn surgery. Pediat Therapeut. 2012;2:132. https://doi.org/10.4172/2161-0665.10001322.
16. Rijal L, Ansari T, Trikha V, Yadhav CS. Irth injuries in caesarian sections: cases of fracture femur and humerus following caesarian section. Nepal Med Coll J. 2009;11:207–8.
17. Vuksanaj D, Desphande JK. Anaesthesia for neurosurgery in infants and children. ASA. 2008;36:215–26.
18. Malinzak EB, Taicher BM. Anesthetic considerations for congenital hydrocephalus. Pediatric Anesthesia Crit Care J 2015; 3(1):10-14doi:https://doi.org/10.14587/paccj.2015.2.
19. Van Lindert EJ, Liem KD, Geerlings M, etal. Bedside placement of ventricular access devices under local anaesthesia in neonates with post haemorrhagic hydrocephalus: preliminary experience. Childs Nerv Syst 2019,35:2307–2312. https://doi.org/10.1007/s00381-019-04361-3.

Anesthetic Consideration in a Neonate with Congenital Heart Disease for Noncardiac Surgery

37

Samhati Mondal, Allison Ulrich, and Usha Saha

37.1 Introduction

CHD is estimated to affect between 3–5% of all newborns and is the most common birth defect [1]. Nearly 30% of all birth defects are CHDs, affecting approximately 40,000 births per year in the US with a reported incidence of 7–10/1000 live births [2]. The prevalence of CHD is on the rise because of better antenatal diagnosis and postnatal management, the most common being VSD [3]. Prevalence in India is 19.4/1000 live births (33% VSD, 19% ASD, 16% TOF, and others) [4–6]. About 25% babies with CHD have critical defects and need corrective or palliative surgery within 1 year of age. CHDs are a leading cause of birth defect-associated deaths, contributing to nearly 4.2% to the neonatal deaths and infant mortality rate of 10% in uncorrected CHD [4–7]. Prognosis depends on the type and size of the defect, time of diagnosis and treatment met, and associated genetic conditions (15%) [8, 9] Extra-cardiac malformations are observed in 7–50% of patients with CHD [1]. Incidence of syndromic anomalies associated with CHD is 53% for Down, 9% for Edward, 10% for Turner, 8% for Patau, and 4% for Noonan syndromes. Of the non-syndromic noncardiac anomalies, 30% are genitourinary, 17% respiratory, 16% gastrointestinal (GI), 10% craniofacial, 11% musculoskeletal, 9% neurologic, and 7% others [10].

S. Mondal (✉)
Cardiothoracic Division, Department of Anesthesiology, University of Maryland School of Medicine, Baltimore, MD, USA

A. Ulrich
Department of Anesthesiology, University of Maryland School of Medicine, Baltimore, MD, USA

U. Saha
Department of Anesthesia, Critical Care, Pain and Palliative Care, Lady Hardinge Medical College, SSK and KSC Hospitals, New Delhi, India

More than 30% patients with CHD undergo noncardiac surgeries within the first year of life for conditions such as tracheoesophageal fistula (TEF), esophageal atresia (EA), anorectal anomalies, cleft lip/palate, renal, skeletal pathologies, and inguinal herniorrhaphy. Of these, surgery for TEF, congenital diaphragmatic hernia (CDH), gut exteriorization for anorectal anomalies, wide cleft lip repair, inguinal herniorrhaphy, pyloromyotomy are often undertaken within the neonatal age. The risk of short-term and 30-day mortality is doubled in neonates, especially preterm, both after minor and major noncardiac surgeries [11].

Administration of anesthesia to such neonates is very challenging as they present for non-corrective noncardiac surgeries of varied range, from short minor procedures to major longer surgeries, accompanied by major fluid and electrolyte shifts, blood loss, ventilatory, and gas exchange difficulties. But, under experienced hands, anesthesia can still be conducted with manageable complications, by the anesthesiologist with knowledge of issues related to newborns and neonates, about the cardiac defects and their pathophysiology, their anesthetic implications, possible complications, and their prevention and management.

This chapter will cover a summary of fetal circulation and adaptive changes at birth, common cardiac defects, their classification, hemodynamic consequences, different types of shunts and their anesthetic implications, anesthetic considerations and management, and prevention and management of complications, especially TET or anoxic spell, when these patients present for noncardiac surgeries within 28 days of life.

37.2   Fetal Circulation and Changes at Birth

It is imperative that the anesthesiologist is well-versed with fetal circulation and changes that occur at birth. This is covered in detail in the chapter on Transitional changes at birth. In short, Foramen ovale closes immediately after birth, with the baby's first cry, Ductus venosus closes by 7–8 days, and Ductus arteriosus closes by within few hours of birth. The importance to the anesthesiologist of these changes lies in the fact that these three closures at birth are functional, meaning they can reopen any time when adverse conditions arise, as in the intrauterine life. This risk persists until anatomic closure occurs, which is 3–4 weeks for ductus arteriosus, and 3 months – 1 year for foramen ovale. Hence, the neonatal period (within 28 days of birth) is extremely critical. Acidosis, hypoxia, hypercarbia, alkalosis, and hypothermia can increase PVR (pulmonary vascular resistance) and Pulmonary arterial hypertension (PAH) with Persistence of fetal circulation (PFC). Preterm neonates are especially at risk. Pressures in different chambers of the heart at birth, compared to adults, and PaO_2 and O_2 saturation (fetus at birth) are listed in Tables 37.1 and 37.2.

Table 37.1 Pressure in chambers of heart (mm Hg)

	At birth	Adult
RA	10	0–6
LA	10	6–10
RV	60/10	25/0–6
LV	60/10	120/0–10
PA	60–40	25/10
Aorta	60–40	120/80

Table 37.2 Pressures and O2 saturation (fetus at birth)

	PaO$_2$ mm Hg	Saturation %
Umbilical V	32–35	80
IVC		70
SVC	12–14	40
PA	16–18	50–55
LV	26–28	65
Descending aorta	20–22	55–60

37.3 Etiology of CHD

Etiology of CHD is not clear but several factors may contribute to occurrence of CHD. Besides, it is associated with other anomalies and syndromes and with many other congenital defects (Box 37.1).

Box 37.1 Etiology and Associated Anomalies

1. Gender - equal incidence, right-sided common in females and left-sided in males
2. Heredity
3. Environmental factors- e.g., PDA, ASD more common at high altitude
4. Maternal factors – Diabetes (PDA, ASD, VSD, HCM, PFO), smoking, obesity, rubella in first trimester (PDA), drugs thalidomide, alcohol, lithium (TOF), phenylketonuria.
5. Genetic and chromosomal aberrations -trisomy 21/13/18, turner syndrome, Marfan syndrome, Ehler-Danlos syndrome, hurler syndrome, CATCH-22 syndrome (cardiac defects, abnormal facies, thymic hypoplasia, cleft palate, hypocalcemia, and microdeletion of band 22q11), diabetes (PDA, ASD, VSD, HCM, PFO), rubella syndrome (PS, PDA), phenylketonuria (TOF, Coarctation aorta).

Associated defects and anomalies with common CHDs
1. VSD - absent radius and ulna, syndactyly, polydactyly, trisomy 13–15, trisomy 17–18
2. ASD- arachnodactyly, Ellis-van-Crevald syndrome, Holt-Oram syndrome, down syndrome (endocardial cushion type of defect)
3. Coarctation of aorta - turner syndrome (with associated pulmonary and aortic stenosis)

Association of other birth defects and CHD
1. TEF - ASD (15%), VSD (7.5%), aortic anomalies (8%), TOF (2%).
2. CDH (15% incidence of CHD) – Critical CHD in 42% with poor survival in 32% [12].
3. MMC (3.8–17.5% incidence of CHD), multiple CHD more likely [13].
4. Abdominal wall defects (15% with gastroschisis, 45% with omphalocele) - PAH, VSD, ASD, Ectopia cordis, Coarctation of aorta [14].
5. Congenital lobar emphysema -14% incidence of CHD [15].
6. VACTERL association - vertebral and cardiac defects, anorectal, renal and limb anomalies, TEF /EA. [1]
7. NEC + CHD high mortality [11].
8. Syndromes with difficult airway–downs, Pierre Robin, Noonan, Goldenhar, Beckwith-Wiedemann

---

Table 37.3 Classification and incidence

1. According to the presence of cyanosis or not	
Acyanotic (L-R) volume overload	**Cyanotic (R-L) pressure overload**
VSD 35%	TOF 5%
ASD 9%	TGA 4%
PDA 8%	Eisenmenger's syndrome
PS 8%	Ebstein's anomaly
AS 6%	Truncus arteriosus
Coarctation 6%	Tricuspid atresia
Aorto-pulm fenestrations	Partially anomalous pulmonary venous connection

2. Physiological classification
1. **Shunt**: L → R (VSD, ASD, PDA = volume overload), or R → L (TOF, Eisenmenger = pressure overload)
2. **Mixing lesion**: TGA, single ventricle, anomalous venous return
3. **Obstructive lesion**: Coarctation aorta, (pulmonary, aortic or mitral stenosis) PS, AS, MS.
4. **Regurgitant lesion**: Epstein anomaly

37.4 CHDs are Classified

CHDs are classified according to the chief symptom (cyanosis) and the physiology. (Table 37.3).

37.5 Understanding of Hemodynamics in CHD

(a) Hemodynamic physiology follows Hagen Poiseuille law of laminar flow ($R \propto 1/r^4$), i.e., resistance to flow is inversely proportional to fourth power of the radius, such that if radius is decreased by 50%, resistance to flow increases 16 folds. Hence, when blood flows into a constriction (narrow diameter), its speed will be more and pressure will be lower than in a wider diameter (Bernoulli's equation) and blood viscosity (unlike water) causing additional pressure drop along the way, drop being proportional to the distance travelled. Hence, lower pressure and lower flow beyond the constriction or narrowing [16]. This is important in understanding the hemodynamics of stenotic lesions, in the manipulation of variables like systemic and pulmonary vascular resistance (SVR and PVR) by various drugs with dramatic changes in pulmonary and systemic hemodynamics, as well as the effect of anesthetic drugs.

(b) **Qp/Qs (shunt fraction), i.e.,** pulmonary: systemic blood flow, quantifies the intracardiac shunt and is normally 1:1 (no intracardiac shunt). Qp/Qs > 1 signifies higher pulmonary flow (from L → R shunt), < 1 signifies lower pulmonary blood flow (from R → L shunt), and Qp: Qs 2:1 indicates L → R shunt.

(c) **Pulmonary Hypertension (PAH)** - Mean pulmonary arterial pressure (PAP) is 25 mmHg at rest, with 35 mmHg during exertion. PAH occurs when baseline PAP is >25 mmHg or >50% of systemic pressure. Initially, the pulmonary vasculature is responsive to stress, pain, acidosis, hypercapnia, hypoxia, and high intrathoracic pressure, but as the disease progresses, PAH becomes fixed and nonresponsive [17].

(d) **Ductal dependence** refers to critical CHD that is dependent on PDA to maintain pulmonary or systemic circulation. Lesions that are **ductal-dependent for pulmonary circulation** (i.e., flow from aorta to PA) are right-sided obstructive lesions and include TOF, critical pulmonary atresia, pulmonary valve stenosis, and Ebstein's anomaly (R → L shunt lesions). Lesions that are **ductal-dependent for systemic circulation** (flow from PA to aorta) are left-sided obstructive lesions and include hypoplastic left heart syndrome, severe aortic valve stenosis, and aortic coarctation (L → R shunt lesions).

(e) **Diagnosis of CHD** – neonates cannot complain and have no symptoms, except distress crying, and one has to rely on the clinical acquity, hence detailed examination is extremely important. Signs depend on the type and severity of the defect. Milder defects may be asymptomatic, while larger ones may cause cyanosis, tachypnoea, tachycardia, fatiguability (on feeding), sleepiness, poor weight gain, murmur on auscultation, or signs of CHF. Early diagnosis is by antenatal Echocardiography; however, minor defects may remain undetected until after birth or later in life. **NADA's Criteria** consist of **Major** (Systolic murmur grade 3 or more, Diastolic murmur, Cyanosis, Congestive cardiac failure), and **Minor** (Systolic murmur < grade 3, Abnormal second heart sound, Abnormal ECG, Abnormal X-ray, Abnormal BP) criteria and presence of one major and two minor criteria should raise suspicion of a cardiac defect [18].

37.6   Individual CHD

37.6.1 Patent Foramen Ovale (PFO)/Atrial Septal Defect (ASD) (L → R Shunt)

In the process of transition, functional closure of the foramen ovale occurs soon after birth or within 24–48 h. Anatomic closure occurs by 3 months–1 year, hence, many neonates may have a patent foramen ovale (PFO) [19].

ASD is an abnormal connection between the two atria, with 6–10% incidence. It is more common in females and is of four types: Ostium primum (located inferior to fossa ovalis), Ostium secundum >75% (located in upper interatrial septum), sinus venosus, and coronary sinus. Nearly 40% ASD close spontaneously by 4 years of age. Spontaneous closure rate is 100% for defects smaller than 3–4 mm by 3 years. Bulk of the ASD < 8 mm close spontaneously by 5 years. Eighty percent for defects 3–8 mm, and 0% for larger than 8–10 mm [20, 21]. PAH develops by the age of 20–30 years if left untreated, followed by right heart failure. PAH is rare under 2 years of age. ASD makes the patient prone to paradoxical embolism [22].

Hemodynamic changes - The hemodynamic effects depend on the size of the defect. Functional closure of foramen ovale allows no shunting of the blood. If the defect is small (<3–5 mm), the pressure gradient is very low and shunting is minimal, with no hemodynamic changes and no murmur on auscultation. But if the size is larger, there will be increased blood flow from left atrium to right atrium, right ventricle (RV) overload and enlargement, increase in blood flow from RV to PA, and ejection systolic murmur will be heard. There will be increase in pulmonary blood flow. When pulmonary blood flow is <1.5 times the systemic blood flow, patient remains asymptomatic.

Hence, **presentation** will vary from no symptoms and signs to mild effort intolerance (fatigue on feeding) and frequent chest infection. Right heart failure is usually not seen in neonates. However, a large ASD may present with features of CCF by 2–3 weeks (tachycardia, tachypnea, hepatomegaly, and poor feeding). **Examination** may reveal ejection systolic murmur and left systolic thrill, delayed diastolic murmur at left second ICS, with split second heart sound. **X ray chest** may show mild-moderate cardiomegaly, RA and RV enlargement, and pulmonary plethora. **ECG** may show right axis deviation (RAD) and right ventricular hypertrophy (RVH). Diagnosis is confirmed by 2-D Echocardiography.

37.6.2 Ventricular Septal Defect (VSD) (L → R Shunt)

This is the most common congenital cardiac lesion (50% of all CHD), with a communication between the two ventricles [3]. VSD is pathological. VSD <3 mm diameter close spontaneously. Up to 40% VSDs close spontaneously within first 6 months of life, and 50% by 2–5 years of age [19, 23]. VSD can be isolated (20%) or part of complex syndromes with other types of CHD, e.g., ASD, TOF, Eisenmenger's syndrome, Tricuspid atresia, and TGA. As per their location, 70% are membranous or infracristal, 20% muscular (located in mid or apical portion of septum), 5% infra-aortic, and 5% located between aortic and mitral valves. Depending on the size of the defect, small VSD (diameter 1/3rd the size of aortic orifice, with large pressure difference between the two ventricles) may go undetected. Large defects become symptomatic early, often with CCF in early infancy:

i. Moderate c-diameter 1/2 of aortic orifice,
ii. Moderate to large
iii. Raised RV pressure, and
iv. Large diameter equal to aortic orifice, with equalization of pressures in the two ventricles.

Hemodynamic changes – During systole, blood from LV is directed both into the aorta and through the VSD into the RV, (pansystolic murmur at lower left sternal border). Increased pulmonary arterial blood flow results in ejection of systolic murmur, and consequent increased flow from LA into LV results in delayed diastolic murmur. Exposure of pulmonary vascular bed to high pressure and flow ultimately leads to PAH, and when pulmonary arterial pressure exceeds aortic pressure, shunt reversal occurs, i.e., Eisenmenger syndrome, and hypoxemia and cyanosis ensue [22].

Presentation depends on the size of the defect and PVR. Small defects and normal PVR generally remain asymptomatic, while large defects cause CCF by 6–8 weeks, and pulmonary vascular disease by 6–12 months of age. A high PVR: SVR (>0.7) is high risk for surgical closure and also for noncardiac surgeries in the neonatal period. Large VSD have features of pulmonary congestion, such as easy fatigue (while feeding), apathy, restlessness, poor weight gain, diaphoresis, tachypnoea, weak cry, facial/pedal edema, and hepatomegaly. **Examination** may reveal hyperkinetic precordium, systolic thrill, pansystolic murmur at lower left sternal border, widely split S2, loud P2, S3 over apex, and delayed diastolic murmur in mitral area. **ECG** may be normal or show LVH and RVH, if pulmonary hypertension is present (usually after 6 weeks age). **2-D Echo** is confirmatory and will show the size and location of the defect and magnitude and direction of the shunt. **Xray chest** may be normal or show cardiomegaly, LA and LV enlargement, and pulmonary plethora. Management includes O_2 therapy to maintain saturation and other measures for pulmonary congestion (raised position, diuretics, decreased IV fluids), antibiotics, and correction of anemia.

37.6.3 Patent Ductus Arteriosus (PDA) (L → R Shunt)

In fetal life ductus arteriosus is a normal connection between the pulmonary artery (PA) and descending aorta. It is muscular and goes into spasm soon after birth. Anatomic closure occurs by 2–3 weeks, latest by 8 weeks of age. PDA occurs because of failure of closure due to abnormal transition at birth. Various factors contribute to its **Etiology**, chiefly prematurity (<37 weeks), genetic (trisomy 21, carpenter's syndrome), Rubella syndrome, uncontrolled maternal diabetes, and drugs (Teratogens, amphetamine, phenytoin), and high altitude. The degree of shunt depends on the size of the duct as well as SVR: PVR. Anomalies associated with PDA include cardiac (PS/Atresia, Tricuspid atresia, noncardiac (CTEV, scoliosis, deafness, mental retardation), and syndromes (CHARGE, Goldenhar, VATER).

Hemodynamic changes – PDA is often diagnosed incidentally. It allows continuous blood flow from aorta to the PA, along the pressure gradient. Pulmonary to systemic blood flow ratio depends on the size of the defect, pressure gradient from aorta to PA, and PVR: SVR. Because of higher pressure in the aorta than PA, the flow through the PDA is L → R (acyanotic) all through the cardiac cycle (machinery murmur), with both systolic and diastolic overloading of PA, high pulmonary blood flow, and increased flow into LA (LA enlargement) and LV (accentuated S1, delayed diastolic murmur). The duration of LV systole is prolonged (delayed closer of aortic valve and dilatation of ascending aorta). However, soon after birth, it can reopen in conditions that increase PVR such as hypoxia, hypercarbia, acidosis, IPPV, and PEEP, allowing reversal of flow from PA to aorta (R → L shunt). Presence of PAH at birth is an ominous sign and these babies may develop CCF in the first week itself with poor prognosis. If diagnosis is made within 2 weeks of life, three doses of IV Indomethacin (0.1 mg/kg/dose) 12 h apart can close the ductus within 24 h. Alternately, single oral dose of Ibuprofen (10 mg/kg) is also useful. Increase in PA pressure to more than SBP causes shunt reversal (cyanotic) [24].

Presentation ranges from asymptomatic to symptoms of pulmonary congestion. Prominent finding is differential cyanosis (cyanosis only in lower limbs). Cardiac impulse is hyperkinetic, pulse is bounding, SBP is high, and DBP is low (due to flow diversion into PA). A delayed diastolic murmur, continuous machinery murmur (Gibson murmur), aortic ejection click, and ejection systolic murmur (PAH) may be heard. **ECG** axis is normal with LVH, Deep Q waves, and tall T waves in left chest leads due to volume overload of LV. **Chest x ray** may show cardiomegaly, prominent aortic knuckle, dilated PA, and pulmonary plethora. **2-D Echo** is diagnostic. **Doppler** can demonstrate the type and degree of shunt. **Preductal vs post-ductal PaO2** >20 mmHg is diagnostic. **Management** is symptomatic, for CCF and pulmonary congestion. Indomethacin, a nonselective NSAID, if administered within 72 h of life, can help close the PDA. Definitive surgery is undertaken after 1 month of age, and in case of refractory CCF, percutaneous closure with Duct Occluder can be done.

Eisenmenger's Syndrome describes severe PAH resulting in reversal of L → R shunt (acyanotic) to R → L shunt (cyanotic) at the atrial, ventricular, or pulmonary arterial level (ASD, VSD, PDA), while **Eisenmenger's Complex** is used only for VSD with severe PAH and R → L shunt (cyanotic). PAH is due to pulmonary vascular obstructive disease. If a communication is present at the PA (PDA) or ventricular level (VSD), RV pressure cannot exceed systemic pressure and R → L shunt decompresses the RV, which undergoes concentric hypertrophy without increase in size and mild parasternal impulse. Shunt reversal in PDA causes differential cyanosis, while at atrial or ventricular level, cyanosis is uniform. In patients without PDA/VSD, RV hypertrophies and dilates, with a parasternal heave. **Presentation** is similar as in cyanotic syndrome (TOF). **Management** is nonsurgical, i.e., avoid increase in PVR and decrease in SVR (Table 37.4), antibiotics for chest infections, phlebotomy with isovolumic replacement for hyperviscosity, anemia management, and Epoprostenol for reducing PVR.

Table 37.4 Management of TET spell

S no.	Measure	Dose/route	Mechanism of action
1.	Oxygen humidified	FiO_2 100% via O_2 tent/ mask/ CPAP	Prevent HPV & ↑PVR, improve PaO_2
2.	Morphine	0.1–0.2 mg/kg IV	Calming, ↓hyperpnea, central depression, ↓PVR
3.	IV crystalloids	15–20 mL/kg IV NS	Improve ventricular filling, ↓RVOT obstruction
4.	Epinephrine/Isoprin	0.1 μ/kg/min	↑SVR, ↓R → L shunt, ↑pulmonary blood flow
5.	Phenylephrine	5-10 μ/kg bolus or 2–5 μ/kg/min	↑SVR, ↓R → L shunt, ↑pulmonary blood flow
6.	Norepinephrine	0.05 mg/kg/min to 0.1 mg/kg/min	↑SVR, ↓R → L shunt, ↑pulmonary blood flow
7.	Methoxamine	0.1–0.2 mg/kg/dose IV	↑SVR, ↓R → L shunt, ↑pulmonary blood flow
8.	Dopamine	2–16 μ/kg/min, max 50 μ/kg/min	↑SVR, ↓R → L shunt, ↑pulmonary blood flow

Table 37.4 (continued)

S no.	Measure	Dose/route	Mechanism of action
9.	B blockers-Esmolol, propranolol, metoprolol	Esmolol (0.5 mg/kg → 50–300 µ/kg/min propranolol (0.01–0.1 mg/kg) metoprolol 0.1 mg/kg over 5 min → 1–2 mcg/kg/min.	↓infundibular spasm, ↓heart rate, ↑diastolic ventricular filling, ↓RVOT obstruction
10.	NTG	0.4 µ/kg/min	Pulmonary vasodilatation, ↓PVR
11.	SNP	0.5–0.8 µ/kg/min, discard after 4 h	Pulmonary vasodilatation, ↓PVR
12.	Calcium chloride	20–30 mg/kg slow IV	Vasoconstriction
13.	Calcium gluconate	3–4 mg/kg IV bolus	Vasoconstriction
14.	HCO3	1–2 mEq/kg IV	For metabolic acidosis-can be given without ABG
15.	Dexmedetomidine	0.2 mcg/kg/min	Central sympatholysis
16.	Knee chest position	Baby held up, knees flexed	↑SVR, ↓R → L shunt, ↑pulmonary blood flow
17.	Diazepam/midazolam	0.1–0.2 mg/kg IV	For treatment of convulsions

Note: **Mechanism of action - Morphine** relieves pain, ↓HR, RR, PVR, catecholamine release, causes pulmonary vasodilatation, ↓venous return, ↓infundibular spasm. Can be given IV, IM, S/c. **Midazolam, dexmedetomidine, and fentanyl** have also been used. **IV fluids** help correct hypovolemia and ↑CO, ↑mixed venous O_2 saturation, ↓risk of drug-induced hypotension. However, excessive fluids can lead to cerebral and pulmonary edema and dilute polycythaemia with aggravation of hypoxemia and must be avoided. **Systemic vasoconstrictors** (Phenylephrine, Norepinephrine, methoxamine) ↑SVR, reduce R → L shunt and ↑pulmonary blood flow. B blockers ↓HR and venous return, ↑cardiac filling, preload and may ↑SVR. Sodium bicarbonate for correction of acidosis. Knee chest position compresses femoral vessels, ↑afterload
If unresponsive to pharmacological therapy, mechanical ventilation and sedation may be required, to reduce the work of breathing and O_2 consumption

37.6.4 Tetralogy of Fallot (TOF) (R → L Shunt)

TOF is the commonest cyanotic CHD and is associated with various syndromes, specifically CATCH-22, VATER, and CHARGE. It has four anatomical components - large VSD, pulmonary stenosis (PS), Overriding of aorta, and RVH [25]. TOF has several variants:

1. **TOF with pulmonary atresia** – most severe variant of TOF and requires palliative PDA or prostaglandins to maintain ductal patency for decompression of the pulmonary trunk.
2. **TOF with absent pulmonary valve syndrome** – the pulmonary valve is dysplastic and pulmonary arteries are dilated that compress on the bronchi causing breathing difficulty.
3. **Pentalogy of Fallot** - TOF with ASD is the least common variant.
4. **Trilogy of Fallot** consists of PS, RVH, and ASD, incidence being 1.2% of all CHD.

Hemodynamic changes - TOF is associated with severe hemodynamic consequences. PS creates a fixed obstruction to the RV outflow tract (RVOT), decrease in pulmonary blood flow and LA filling, decreased LV filling, and decrease in CO, systemic hypoxia, and cyanosis. Large VSD results in equalization of pressures in the RV and LV, mixing of deoxygenated and oxygenated blood, hypoxemia, and cyanosis. Combined PS and VSD leads to RV pressure overload, RVH, RV dysfunction, and RV failure. Overriding of aorta allows venous (desaturated) blood from RV to enter the aorta during systole, compounding hypoxemia and cyanosis. Persistent hypoxemia and cyanosis results in compensatory polycythemia, increased blood viscosity, and hypercoagulability. Squatting, a feature of TOF, is a compensatory mechanism whereby there is increase in systemic vascular resistance with decrease in R $\rightarrow$ L shunt and symptomatic relief. But this feature is seen in older children and is absent in neonates.

Once RV and LV pressures equalize, there is little or no shunt and VSD is silent. Flow from RV into the stenosed PA results in ejection systolic murmur in the pulmonary area. Since RV gets decompressed by VSD, CCF does not occur, except if associated with anaemia, systemic hypertension, myocarditis, infective endocarditis, and aortic or pulmonary regurgitation. Anteriorly placed aorta (overriding) results in loud A2 and enlarged ascending aorta makes an aortic ejection click.

Changes in SVR affect the degree of shunt:

- Decrease in SVR increases the R $\rightarrow$ L shunting and severity of hypoxia,
- Increase in SVR reduces R $\rightarrow$ L shunt and increases pulmonary blood flow, which is beneficial.

Presentation – Symptoms develop soon after birth with central cyanosis (cf. from acrocyanosis), anoxic spells (TET spells), easy fatiguability, and dyspnea on exertion (feeding). Physical examination will confirm cyanosis, prominent jugular veins, large 'a' wave in CVP, mild parasternal impulse, and systolic thrill. Squatting and clubbing are not seen in neonates. On auscultation, S1 is normal, S2 is single, and an ejection systolic murmur of PS can be heard (intensity inversely proportional to severity of PS) in the pulmonary area. **Diagnosis** can be confirmed by cardiac investigations. ECG will have features of RAD, RBBB, and RVH. Echocardiography (for level and severity of RV outflow tract (RVOT) obstruction, and size of pulmonary artery, number and location of VSD) and Color Doppler for the type and degree of shunt and RVOT obstruction are confirmatory. Additionally, CT and MRI can also be done. **Laboratory investigations** will establish polycythaemia, hypofibrinogenemia, and decreased platelet aggregation. $PaO_2 < 50$ mmHg even with 100% FiO_2 is indicative of severe degree of RVOT obstruction and R $\rightarrow$ L shunt. X ray chest may show typical Boot-shaped heart (uplifted apex) (COR-EN-SABOT), decreased pulmonary vascularity (pulmonary oligemia), and concave main PA segment (PS).

Typical feature of TOF is TET or Anoxic spells (Hyper cyanotic spells), characterized by sudden desaturation, worsening cyanosis, tachypnea, loss of consciousness, seizures, cerebrovascular attacks (CVA), and even death. Mechanism postulated is that sympathetic stimulation from crying causes infundibular spasm, further narrowing of PA, increase in RVOT obstruction, and increased R $\rightarrow$ L shunt. In neonates, excessive crying, sudden fright, agitation, and distress can easily precipitate a TET spell and should be prevented. It can also be precipitated at induction of general anesthesia if it is associated with acute decrease in SVR, consequent decreased pulmonary blood flow, and increased R → L shunt. **Management -** The chief objectives are to decrease catecholamine production (remove the cause), increase blood oxygenation (100% O2 inhalation), increase SVR (α1 agonist), reduce RVOT obstruction and infundibular spasm (β blockers), and increase pulmonary blood flow [26] (Table 37.4).

Pink TET spell is a condition of anoxic spell, but without cyanosis. This may occur in two TOF variants:

(a) **TOF with minimal valvular or subvalvular stenosis** - Pulmonary blood flow is sufficient to keep deoxyHb content <5 gm%, hence no cyanosis, and.
(b) **TOF with pulmonary atresia or severe PS** – they have major aorto-pulmonary collateral arteries, and patient is asymptomatic or show signs of CCF due to L → R shunt through a PDA or collaterals.

Management of TOF – principal of management is similar as for TET spells and includes measures to prevent infundibular spasm, reduce PVR, increase SVR, and adequate hydration with a goal to prevent TET spells and worsening hypoxemia (Table 37.4). These babies should be kept in an O_2 tent, inhaling high FiO_2 (>50%), receive IV morphine, hold baby in knee chest position, and small IV fluid boluses. Early surgical management is palliative, with the goal to increase pulmonary blood flow (by creating a shunt), improve oxygenation, and promote pulmonary vascular growth:

(i) **Pott's shunt** (descending aorta to pulmonary artery),
(ii) **Blalock-Taussig (BT) shunt** (subclavian artery to pulmonary artery) most common procedure, or.
(iii) **Waterston's shunt** (ascending aorta to pulmonary artery), or.
(iv) **Modified BT shunt** (a conduit between subclavian artery and pulmonary artery).

Definitive Surgery (VSD closure, release of RVOT obstruction) is undertaken after 3–4 months age.

37.7 Complications of CHD

All neonates with CHD are at risk of several complications (Box 37.2), during the normal course, except for small ASD, the only lesion which can go undetected and patient is able to lead a full life.

Box 37.2 Complications of Untreated CHD

1. Failure to thrive
2. Infective endocarditis (IE)
3. Cardiac dysrhythmias, complete heart block
4. Hypertension (systemic/pulmonary), RVH, RVF
5. Erythrocytosis (polycythemia), coagulopathy
6. Thromboembolism, CVA, brain abscess
7. Sudden death

37.7.1 PLSVC (Persistent Left Superior Vena Cava)

PLSVC (Persistent left superior vena cava) is the result of persistent patency of the left anterior cardinal vein. The majority of PLSVC drain into the coronary sinus and are associated with no clinical symptoms. However, in some instances it drains directly into the LA and produce R → L shunt. When they present for surgery, considerations are as for cyanotic heart disease and TOF.

37.7.2 TAPVC (Total Anomalous Pulmonary Venous Connection)

TAPVC (Total Anomalous Pulmonary Venous Connection) occurs when the pulmonary veins do not return to LA, instead open into the RA or a systemic vein (SVC, IVC, azygos veins, coronary sinus), resulting in total mixing of pulmonary and systemic venous blood in RA. Patients present with dyspnea, heart failure, and cyanosis (>50% anomalous pulmonary venous drainage). **Angiography** demonstrates normal chamber pressures with increased right heart O_2 saturation. Life with TAPVC is not possible unless associated with R → L shunt (ASD, VSD). R → L shunt is required for survival as a palliative procedure. PPV (positive pressure ventilation) decreases pulmonary venous drainage into the RA by increasing right heart pressure. Even during corrective cardiac surgery, these patients may develop hemodynamic disturbances and arrythmias [27]. Such neonates will not present for noncardiac surgery.

37.7.3 Infective Endocarditis (IE)

Reported incidence of IE in neonates is 7.3%. This high incidence is because of increasing use of invasive techniques, long dwelling CVP/arterial/PICC lines, that are more often placed in babies with complex cardiac and noncardiac lesions. These lines provide entry portal for the bacteria. IE is more common in CHD, especially cyanotic lesions, with higher (31%) mortality in premature neonates. The most common infecting organisms are *S aureus*, coagulase-negative staphylococci, Gram-negative bacteria, and Candida [28]. Septic IE emboli create extra cardiac infective foci, e.g., osteomyelitis, meningitis, and pneumonia, and neonates often present with feeding difficulties, respiratory distress, tachycardia, hypotension, neurological signs (seizures, hemiparesis, apnea), and changing murmur pattern. **American heart association (AHA)** modified its original recommendations for IE prophylaxis in 2007, recommending restrictive antibiotic prophylaxis (AP). Most risk factors are not applicable to neonates with CHD undergoing noncardiac surgeries, e.g., dental procedures. On the positive note, AHA does not recommend AP for patients with valvular heart disease (who are at high risk of IE) for nondental procedures such as TEE, esophagogastroduodenoscopy, colonoscopy, cystoscopy, or minor surgeries, in absence of active infection. AHA Guidelines for AP that may be applicable to neonates are:

(a) Invasive Bronchoscopy procedures (excluding intubation),
(b) Invasive gastrointestinal / gynecological procedure,
(c) Incision and drainage,

(d) Unrepaired CHD, excluding uncomplicated ASD,

(e) Indwelling prosthesis following palliative or corrective surgery, and

(f) Hypertrophic cardiomyopathy and Mitral valve prolapse with regurgitation.

Additional high-risk factors enumerated by Rushani et al. (2013) in children with CHD, eligible for AP, include: [29]

(g) Lesions associated with cyanosis at birth (highest incidence of IE),

(h) Post-definitive repair of Dextro-transposition of great arteries and TOF,

(i) Left-sided lesions or endocardial cushion defects (L → R shunt),

(j) PDA frequent underlying condition in infants and neonates,

(k) Highest risk in under 3 years age.

ASD, VSD, and right-sided lesions are at least risk of IE.

There are no antibiotic prophylaxis guidelines specifically pertaining to neonates with CHD undergoing noncardiac surgeries within the neonatal period, and the concerned medical personnel should consult and discuss with a specialist.

37.8   Conduct of Anesthesia in Neonates with CHD for Noncardiac Surgery

37.8.1 Anesthetic Challenges

Anesthetic challenges in the management of these neonates arise from the age of the patient (<28 days age), type and complexity of the cardiac defect, type and degree of shunt, surgical indication and its bio-pathophysiological effects, associated anomalies and syndromes, airway difficulty, and emergency nature of surgery. Common cardiac defects include VSD, ASD, PDA, and TOF. Anesthesiologists' chief concern is to avoid factors that may reverse cardiac shunts and fetal circulation as these patients are still in the transition phase when closure of cardiac shunts is just functional and prevent worsening hypoxemia and precipitation of TET spells.

Generally, neonates with CHD presenting for noncardiac surgeries will either have an uncorrected cardiac defect or have undergone palliation by minimally invasive cardiac catheterization or by surgical creation of BT shunt in a baby with TOF (Total correction is done after 3 months of age).

37.8.2 Preoperative Evaluation Should Include

(a) **Detailed information relating to the cardiac lesion** - degree of altered physiology, its adverse effects, information about the palliative procedure and patients' clinical improvement, change in hemodynamic physiology, type and severity of shunt, presence and severity of pulmonary HT, extent of decrease or increase in pulmonary blood flow, degree of hypoxemia, polycythemia, coagulation abnormalities, hypercoagulability, thrombosis, and other complications (Box 37.2).

(b) **Detailed information relating to the surgical pathology** and its effects on the blood biochemistry, associated pathophysiological finding, and effect on other organ systems (renal and hepatic), and proposed surgery and its implications and feasibility,

(c) **Clinical status** of the neonate - level of consciousness and mental state, easy fatiguability, feeding history, cyanosis, pulse rate-rhythm-volume, body temperature, manifestations of heart failure (tachypnea, poor weight gain, HR >200/min, murmur, cyanosis), PAH, volume status, anemia, and urinary output.

(d) One must look for **noncardiac anomalies** because of their effects during anesthesia, e.g., neuromuscular drugs in musculoskeletal diseases, anesthetic drugs and narcotics in neurological diseases, fluid and electrolyte imbalance in GI and genitourinary diseases, and airway-related issues in down's syndrome (atlanto-occipital subluxation requires extra care during airway management), cleft lip and palate, neonates with a week cry, and suprasternal retraction.

(e) **Examination** should include palpation of all four peripheral pulses, NIBP, SpO_2 (pre and post-ductal), signs of CCF, murmurs, syndromes, airway, peripheral and central veins and arteries (for cannulation), and body temperature.

(f) **Risk assessment -** Faraoni et al. (2016) developed and validated a Risk Stratification Score for Children with CHD undergoing noncardiac surgery by using preoperative predictors which were scored: Emergency surgery (1), Severe CHD (1), single ventricle physiology (1), surgery within 30 days of birth (1), inotropic support (1), preoperative CPR (2), renal injury (3), and need for mechanical ventilation (4). Total score was sum of individual scores and was graded as – low risk (<3) (mortality 0.78–3.4%), medium risk (4–6 (mortality 4–6%), and high risk (>7) (mortality 15.06–32.59%) [30].

37.8.3 Investigations

Neonates coming for noncardiac procedures are already diagnosed and investigated for the cardiac defects. The array of investigations required for the purpose of anesthesia must be tailored to the surgical procedure being undertaken. Aim of these investigations is to confirm the cardiac findings, any change from the last status, for need of preoperative optimization, and in coordination with the surgeon, to decide on the extent of surgery safely tolerated by the neonate, plan the anesthetic technique, drugs to be used, and need for postoperative ventilatory support, so as to achieve a good postoperative outcome.

Basic minimal includes hemoglobin, WBC, blood sugar, coagulation profile (Prothrombin time (PT), partial thromboplastin time (PTT), platelet count, and function. For major prolonged and GI surgeries, serum electrolytes, KFT (urea, creatinine), and LFT (serum bilirubin, serum proteins, esp. albumin) are essential investigations. ECG and Echo are usually available as these neonates are already under pediatric cardiology care; however, a fresh ECG to confirm and assess changes in earlier pattern (LVH, strain, rhythm changes) and X-ray chest (for cardiac size, position, lung changes, vascular markings, position of diaphragm) can be asked for (Box 37.3).

Box 37.3 Investigation in CHD

- Raised Hb and polycythemia - ↑blood viscosity – cerebral/renal/pulmonary thrombosis and infarction
- Coagulation abnormalities - due to low fibrinogen, thrombocytopenia, platelet dysfunction, hyperviscosity
- Platelet count, PT, PTT
- Preoperative phlebotomy - for symptomatic hyperviscosity (Hct > 65%)
- Electrolyte changes (diuretic therapy and on TPN)
- ECG – LV strain or hypertrophy
- Echocardiography
- X-ray for heart position, size, atelectasis, respiratory infection,
- Pulmonary vascular markings – oligemia/hyperemia
- CT-MRI - neurological assessment

37.8.4 Preoperative Optimization

Preoperative optimization of the altered hemodynamic physiology, relative PVR to SVR ratio, effect of shunt, and oxygenation, can significantly improve anesthetic course and postoperative outcome. Drugs and infusions already started must continue (glucose, digoxin, β blockers, prostaglandins, vasomimetics). Diuretics put neonates at risk of hypochloremic hypokalemic metabolic alkalosis, necessitating ABG and electrolyte testing and correction. Epoprostenol is mildly effective in decreasing PVR and can be administered if available.

37.8.5 Preoperative Fasting

Preoperative fasting – neonates are extremely prone to dehydration and hypoglycemia with prolonged duration of fasting, added on by the pathological losses. Recommended NPO times are 2 h for clear liquids (water, apple juice, Pedialyte) and 4 h for breast milk. In case babies are NPO for surgical reasons or for long duration, they must receive IV fluids and dextrose to maintain intravascular volume and prevent hypoglycemia.

37.8.6 Premedication

Premedication—consists of **anticholinergics** (glycopyrrolate or atropine) (can be given orally) to prevent bradycardia during laryngoscopy and intubation, as well to achieve antisialagogue function in case ketamine induction is planned. Anxiety is not common in this age group; however, **oral midazolam** can quieten a crying baby and aid in placement of an IV cannula, in case not already in place. Continue β blocker till the day of surgery if patient is started on.

Preoperative phlebotomy with isovolumic replacement is indicated in cases of symptomatic hyperviscosity (Hct > 65%) despite correction of dehydration.

37.9 Cardiac Shunt and Anesthesia

1. In neonates with **L → R shunt,** pulmonary blood flow is increased with pulmonary hyperemia. This is the most common type of CHD (>50%) and includes ASD, VSD, PDA, and BT Shunt. There is minimal effect on SVR or PVR at IV (propofol, barbiturates, etomidate) and inhalational induction @ 1–1.5 MAC (Isoflurane, Halothane, Sevoflurane), and IPPV is well tolerated with no effect on shunt ratio. Isolated VSD or ASD with small defects are particularly safe, except for iatrogenic pulmonary vasodilatation, pulmonary congestion, and hypoxemia secondary to use of 100% O_2 and hyperventilation. Ketamine is proven to be standard induction agent for most CHDs, because of vasoconstriction and increase in SVR with reduction in R → L shunt, alone or along with other IV agents. For longer procedures, opioid-based induction is advised with similar benefits. However, pulmonary congestion itself can cause desaturation and must be avoided by preventing acute severe increase in SVR, severe decrease in PVR, volume overload, and negative intrathoracic pressure.

2. In neonates with **R → L shunt (Cyanotic CHD),** as may be seen in those with abnormal transition at birth, high PVR, pulmonary blood flow is reduced. This results in delayed inhalational induction, but faster IV induction because of R → L and reduced arm to brain circulation time. R → L shunt in ASD/VSD/PDA indicates severe PAH. Clinically, in R → L shunt at the level of PDA, there will be differential cyanosis, whereas at atrial or ventricular level, there will be uniform cyanosis. R → L shunt has serious implications in the form of risk of septic locus embolism in IE and paradoxical embolism in ASD, leading to cerebral ischemia and permanent brain injury. Hence, extreme caution is required in de-airing of syringes and IV lines and IE prophylaxis in indicated cases. Anoxic or TET spells usually respond to volume administration, systemic vasoconstriction with alpha agonists, and release of infundibular spasm with β blockers (Table 37.4). **Shunt Reversal (Eisenmenger syndrome) -** L → R shunt can reverse to R → L any time there is decrease in SVR or increase in PVR and should always be prevented.

3. **Factors that increase PVR** include low FiO_2, high $PaCO_2$, hypoventilation, acidosis, high airway pressure, PEEP, atelectasis, hypothermia, vasopressors, polycythemia, light anesthesia, and pain. **Factors that decrease PVR** include high FiO_2, low $PaCO_2$, hyperventilation, alkalosis, nitric oxide, and vasodilators (NTG, PGE1).

37.9.1 Goals of Anesthetic Management

- Prevent increase in PVR and PAH and decrease in SVR and myocardial function.
- Avoid stress, pain, acidosis, hypercapnia, hypoxia, and high intrathoracic pressure.
- Maintain HR and blood saturation to target SpO_2 of 92–94%.
- **Salient points that must be kept in mind:**
  - SpO_2 overestimates SaO_2 as SaO_2 decreases,
  - $EtCO_2$ underestimates $PaCO_2$, and
  - Discrepancy worsens with hypoxemia, and
  - If in doubt, get an ABG done.

PAH crisis intervention - Goal of management is to increase pulmonary blood flow and oxygenation, and maintain cardiac output. Management includes high FiO_2 (up to 100% O_2), administration of pulmonary vasodilators (iNO, phosphodiesterase inhibitors, prostacyclin analogues), and peripheral vasoconstrictors (inotropes). All emergency drugs must be kept ready. Incidence of PAH increases with tracheal intubation, and hence, many anesthetists prefer less-invasive airway management (supraglottic devices, or IV or spinal block-based anesthesia, while maintaining respiration and oxygenation via a face mask).

Ideal technique is general anesthesia, securing the airway with tracheal intubation or LMA, and controlled or assisted ventilation.

37.9.2 Care in Preoperative Period

(a) Maintaining hydration and volume status, specifically avoiding dehydration and hypoglycemia.
(b) **NPO can reduce preload** – adequate fluid resuscitation as soon as possible should be initiated.
(c) Avoiding intramuscular injections and excessive crying (crying increases PVR).
(d) Patients are usually on β blockers which should be continued till the day of surgery.
(e) Antibiotic cover to reduce the risk of IE.
(f) Avoidance of hypoxia, hypercarbia hypothermia, acidosis, and pain, all of which increase PVR.
(g) Transporting to OT and back to postoperative room or NICU should be done in a comfortable thermos-regulated incubator, with O_2-enriched air.
(h) All drugs as described in management of TET spell must be kept ready (Table 37.2).

37.9.3 Monitoring

Monitoring – of all available facilities, monitoring also needs to be tailored according to the clinical condition of the neonate, pathophysiological effects of the cardiac defect and the surgical pathology, the type and degree of cardiac shunt, and surgery planned. Basic monitoring includes continuous 5 lead ECG for HR and Rhythm, NIBP, SpO_2, $EtCO_2$, temperature, blood loss, and fluid administered. Usually, noninvasive monitoring suffices for noncardiac surgeries, except bladder catheterization for urine output and CVP, in select cases. (ref chapter on monitoring).

$EtCO_2$ monitoring is very important in this case since gradient between end-tidal and arterial CO_2 will indicate forward flow through pulmonary circulation. Increase in PVR will decrease forward pulmonary flow and thereby will increase the gradient between $PaCO_2$ and $EtCO_2$. This could be an early indicator of alteration of Qp: Qs, right to left shunt and hypoxemia.

37.9.4 Preoxygenation

Preoxygenation with 100% O_2 must be done in all neonates with CHD, for at least 3 min, and note made of the SpO_2 before and after. Care must be taken to never allow SpO_2 to fall below that achieved after oxygenation. This also give a clue as to the degree of shunt, and whether high FiO_2 should be continued all throughout surgery or not. As has been repeatedly advised, **use minimal FiO_2 to achieve target SpO_2 principal** that must be followed because of the danger of ROP and BPD with high FiO_2, especially in the premature neonate.

37.9.5 Induction

Induction - If an IV line is in place, IV induction is ideal. Ketamine is a preferred agent because it maintains SVR; theoretical risk of ketamine-induced pulmonary vasoconstriction is minimal here and it is widely used for induction in TOF patients. It can be combined with low-dose thiopentone or propofol, to achieve better anesthetic depth for intubation. In case there is no IV-line, inhalational induction can be done but with caution, as most volatile agents reduce SVR and myocardial contractility. A better option is to lightly induce with volatile agent, and then place an IV line for IV-based induction. Opioid induction using morphine has the benefit of maintaining hemodynamic stability, as well as has reducing PVR, but because of its prolonged duration of action and central respiratory depressant effect, its use is restricted for major surgeries, in neonates with critical CHD, on inotropic support, or in those who may need postoperative ventilation, and in those already on ventilatory support. A combination of opioids and IV agents can be safely used for induction (Table 37.5).

It must be remembered that onset of action of IV drugs will be rapid in the presence of R → L shunt, because of bypassing pulmonary circulation, and hence, less drug dose and slower rate of injection. On the contrary, inhalational induction is slower because of decreased pulmonary blood flow. However, sevoflurane, with low blood gas solubility, can overcome this drawback with faster induction. Laryngoscopy

Table 37.5 Anesthetic drugs and dosage

Drug	SVR	PVR	Dose/route
Inhalational agent	↓	↓	0.5–1 MAC
N2O	–	↑	≤ 50%
Fentanyl	↓	–	1–2 μ/kg or 0.5–2 μ/kg/h
Morphine	↓	↓	0.05–0.2 mg/kg or 0.02–0.2 mg/kg/h
Ketamine	↑	–	3–4 mg/kg PO, 1–2 mg/kg IV,
Propofol	↓	–	2–3 mg/kg. 100–300 μ/kg/min
Midazolam	–	–	0.5 mg/kg PO /0.1 mg/kg IV/ 0.2–0.3 mg/kg/h
Dexmedetomidine	↑	↓↓	1 μ/kg over 10 min, 0.2–1 μ/kg/h

and intubation can be facilitated by depolarizing or nondepolarizing muscle relaxant of choice, tube placement checked and well secured. To prevent adverse effects of laryngoscopy and intubation on PVR, adequate depth of anesthesia must be achieved and done under adequate relaxation.

37.9.6 Airway Management

Airway management – various options are available, depending on duration and extent of surgery, and clinical status of the neonate, and both tracheal intubation and supraglottic airway are acceptable, under direct laryngoscopy, or video laryngoscopy, or intubating LMA. Bronchoscopic intubation is restricted for babies with severe airway deformity. Appropriate size ETT or LMA are used and secured after placement is confirmed using 5-point auscultation. Uncuffed ETT are advisable because of the risk of the adverse effects of inadvertent high cuff pressure. Microcuff ETT are now available for use in neonates.

37.9.7 Maintenance of Anesthesia

Maintenance of anesthesia – neonates should not be left on spontaneous respiration because of the risk of early fatigue and hypoxia, especially under the effect of anesthetic drugs. Hence, ventilation should be always assisted or controlled, preferably using muscle relaxants, and FiO_2 of 0.5, or higher to maintain SpO_2. In some surgeries, especial repair of TEF/EA by thoracic route, expanding the lungs with 100% O_2, may be required at frequent intervals, to maintain saturation. Carrier gas for O_2 can be air or N_2O, as per the availability, and low-dose sevoflurane or desflurane. N_2O may affect PVR, but this action is not significant enough to warrant its disuse, especially with high FiO_2. More important effect of N_2O is its effect on increasing the size of air bubble in case of air embolism. Many neonatal anesthesiologists prefer to avoid N2O—ventilate with low tidal volume and low inflatory pressures; avoid hyperventilation.

Muscle relaxant - non-histamine releasing relaxants are preferred. Pancuronium (Pavulon), because of its sympathomimetic action, was preferred, but its chief drawback was prolonged action and delayed recovery. With the advent of newer short-acting relaxants Rocuronium and Atracurium, Pavulon went into disrepute. Rocuronium can be used for intubation and continued during surgery.

Analgesia – as has been stressed that pain and stress of surgery can itself increase PVR, it is important that pain is adequately managed during surgery in neonates, both term and preterm. Opioids are preferred agents for surgical analgesia. For short procedures, Fentanyl is preferred and Morphine for major prolonged surgeries (as described above). Regional anesthesia in the form of spinal and epidural analgesia is especially suitable as it helps reduce the requirement of inhaled anesthetics and muscle relaxants, with better hemodynamic stability and recovery. Single shot or continuous catheter-based caudal or lumbar epidural analgesia can be used. Surgeries have been performed under SAB (subarachnoid block) as sole technique, with O_2 inhalation by mask, in premature neonates undergoing inguinal herniotomy, with good results. 0.2% Ropivacaine or 0.25% Bupivacaine with opioid as additive may be used.

37.9.8 Intraoperative Concerns

1. De-airing of syringes and IV lines must be done so as to reduce the risk pf paradoxical air embolism.
2. Maintenance of SVR with phenylephrine is beneficial, with minimal N_2O and high FiO_2.
3. Avoid rate and rhythm disturbances, myocardial depression, and hypotension.
4. Gas flow should contain just enough FiO_2 to maintain target SpO_2 (92–94%). Avoid use of 100% O_2 and for long duration.
5. Slowing of HR improves myocardial contractility and reduces RVOT obstruction with improved pulmonary blood flow. IV Esmolol or Metoprolol as bolus can be used. But care must be taken to prevent bradycardia and decrease in CO and peripheral perfusion. Tachycardia reduces diastolic filling time and CO and must be also avoided.
6. Inhaled anesthetics are potent vasodilators and can increase R $\rightarrow$ L shunt. Small doses of ketamine can be used intermittently to maintain SVR. Phenylephrine (α agonists) must always be kept available and ready for use.
7. If the baby has BT shunt in situ, arterial line should not be placed on the same side, as it will give erroneous PaO_2 values.
8. Patients with TOF have compensatory polycythemia, hence hypovolemia and further decrease in peripheral blood flow must be avoided. Crystalloid-based IV fluids are preferred (ref chapter on IV fluids), with restricted blood replacement (to maintain hematocrit 45–50 and Hb > 14–16 g%).
9. Neonates with acyanotic CHD may also be coagulopathic from hypofibrinogenemia and platelet dysfunction, enhanced fibrinolysis, impaired coagulation

factors production, and contracted serum volume. Preoperative hemodilution or FFP (20 mL/kg) infusion can reduce the risk.

10. During controlled ventilation, avoid using large tidal volumes and inflation pressures, so as not to increase PVR. PEEP should be avoided or used minimally (2–3 cmH$_2$O) for the same reason. Avoid hypoxia and hypocarbia, rather mild hypercarbia is beneficial. Avoid hyperventilation.

37.9.9 Extubation

Goal is early extubation to reduce the risk of IPPV. Most neonates can be extubated at the end of surgery; however, NICU bed with ventilator facility must be available. The muscle relaxant effect must be reversed with and patient extubated after complete recovery. In case postoperative ventilation is deemed necessary, there is no need to reverse the relaxant effect; additional morphine dose is given for reflex suppression during transfer to NICU.

37.9.10   Complications After GA

Risk is highest in neonates and infants:

(a) **Airway events -** bronchospasm, laryngospasm, aspiration, apnea.
(b) **CVS events -** hypotension, arrest, arrhythmias, thromboembolic events.
(c) **Postop events** (nausea, vomiting, emergence agitation, apnea, hypoxia).
(d) Postoperative croup or respiratory distress is a serious complication that manifests after tracheal extubation. It occurs due to laryngeal edema and airway obstruction. Management includes humidified 100% O$_2$, IV steroids (Decadron 0.5–1 mg/kg), racemic epinephrine nebulization (2.25%, 0.05 mL/kg diluted in 5 mL), hydration, light sedation, and reintubation with a smaller size ETT, if needed.
(e) **Risk of CVA, Cardiac Arrest**, and **Postoperative period.**

All neonates should be transferred to the NICU under pediatric cardiology care, as their cardiac defect is still present along with the effects of surgery and anesthesia. Care provided during surgery and monitoring should continue in the postoperative period, specially:

1. Maintaining of hydration and volume status,
2. Adequate pain relief (morphine ideal choice for those on ventilatory support, or fentanyl infusion),
3. Maintaining hemoglobin and O$_2$ saturation, avoiding hypercarbia,
4. Prevention of hypothermia, shivering, acidosis, increase in metabolic O$_2$ demand,
5. Care in Ventilator settings to prevent increase in PVR, as discussed above.

6. Be vigilant for occurrence of complications – croup,
7. Early extubation and continue on noninvasive ventilation or continuous positive pressure ventilation (NIV/CPAP).

37.9.11 Role of Regional Anesthesia

Subarachnoid blockade (SAB) is indicated in premature with CHD for hernia, orchidopexy PUV, cystoscopy, with 0.5% Bupivacaine (1 mg/kg) and will provide analgesia for nearly 100 min [31]. The only contraindication is patients with bleeding tendency or on anticoagulant. (ref chapters on regional anesthesia and pain management).

37.10 Special Situations

1. **Cardiac catheterization** is indicated for therapeutic interventions, often under IV sedation by the cardiologist, and has a high complication rate [6, 32] - cardiac arrest (0.96%), hypoxia, acidosis, arrhythmias (bradycardia, SVT, VT, VF, AV blocks, junctional rhythm), vascular (thrombosis, arterial/venous tears, and perforations), bleeding (catheter site/retroperitoneal hematoma), catheter manipulation-related (cardiac perforation, tamponade, air embolism, wire break, knot), device-related (device embolization, balloon rupture), and others (drug interactions, infection).
2. **Laparoscopic surgery** is safe in neonates with CHD [33], and successful thoracoscopic repair of EA with TEF in newborn baby with single ventricle physiology [34] and of D type TEF in complex CHD [35] have been reported. Concerns in laparoscopic/video-assisted surgery are related to CO_2 insufflation, positioning (head down, lateral, prone), invasive monitoring (BP, CVP, ABG), and chiefly, failure of closed procedure and conversion to open surgery, with compounding risk.

37.11 To Summarize

Congenital heart defects (CHD) are the most common types of birth defects, accounting for nearly 30% of all birth defects, with a high mortality and morbidity, due to late presentation and delay in diagnosis, management, especially in critical defects. **ASD** is the mildest form of CHD, not directly affected by changes in PVR and SVR. However, goal is to prevent further fall in PVR (increasing L → R shunt) as well as in SVR (promoting R → L flow). Special care is for de-airing of injections and infusion lines because of risk of paradoxical embolism. In the neonatal period, PFO may be present deserving similar care. **VSD** is most common CHD, always pathological, and most common lesion complicated by IE. Factors that increase the risk of anesthesia are CCF, PAH, aortic regurgitation, IE, and potential increase in myocardial contractility that may increase RVOT resistance such as hypovolemia, vasodilatation, and PAH, which may cause shunt reversal. Most anesthetics and IPPV are well-tolerated; De-airing of injections and infusion lines because of risk of paradoxical embolism. **PDA** – ductus may remain patent in neonates especially with increase in PVR and PAH and decrease in SVR. Inhalational induction decreases L → R flow and improves systemic blood flow. Anesthetics and IPPV are well-tolerated. However, decrease in PVR and increase in SVR can increase the magnitude of L → R shunt, while increase in PVR and PAH will cause shunt reversal. Goal of management is to maintain PVR, slightly low SVR, and avoid hypovolemia. **TOF** –resistance to flow across the RVOT is fixed, hence drug-induced changes in SVR will significantly affect the magnitude of shunt. Decrease in SVR and increase in PVR are very detrimental in this CHD by increasing the R → L shunt and precipitate TET spell. Goal is to maintain high SVR, preventing increase in PVR and reducing infundibular spasm and early extubation. Ketamine induction is preferred. These neonates cannot tolerate IPPV, PEEP, and hypovolemia and fall in hematocrit. They may require vasopressor infusion throughout. Laparoscopic procedures increase the risk in all cardiac defects because of CO_2 insufflation (hypercarbia, acidosis, hypotension, and arrhythmias). General anesthesia with tracheal intubation is the ideal technique.

37.12　Conclusion

Neonates with cardiac defects, presenting for noncardiac surgery, pose a great challenge to the anesthesiologist. Many complex factors are involved – hemodynamic effects of the cardiac pathology, compounded by the biochemical effects of the surgical emergency, effect of surgery and its stress, and effect of anesthetics. Anesthetic management relies on the experience and knowledge of the anesthesiologist. Preoperative evaluation, thorough study of the medical records, understanding the hemodynamics of the cardiac lesion, type and degree of shunt, whether isolated or part of a syndrome, airway difficulty, are important for planning of the anesthetic technique and management. Preoperative optimization of saturation and hydration, intraoperative ventilation care, managing SVR and PVR as per the demand, adequate anesthetic depth and pain management, with the goal of early extubation, while readiness for prevention of and management of complications, coordinating with the surgical team, are important for a favorable outcome.

Needless to say, these neonates should be operated in a tertiary care center that can cater to the needs of these highly vulnerable population. Appropriate equipment, knowledge, expertise, technical skill to manage these vulnerable patients with variety of diagnosis and pathophysiology, and self-updating with latest advances will fortify anesthetic management.

References

1. Cunningham BK, Hadley DW, Hannoush H, Meltzer AC. Etal. Analysis of cardiac anomalies in VACTERL association. Birth Defects Res A Clin Mol Teratol. 2013;97(12):792–7. https://doi.org/10.1002/bdra.23211.
2. Reller MD, Strickland MJ, Riehle-Colarusso T, et al. Prevalence of congenital heart defects in Atlanta 1998-2005. J Pediatr. 2008;153:807–13.
3. Bjornard K, Riehle-Colarusso T, Gilboa SM, Correa A. Patterns in the prevalence of congenital heart defects, metropolitan Atlanta, 1978 to 2005. Birth Defects Res Part A Clin Mol Teratol. 2013;97(2):87–94.
4. Saxena A, Relan J, Agarwal R, Awasthy N, et al. Indian guidelines for indications and timing of intervention for common congenital heart diseases: revised and updated consensus statement of the working group on management of congenital heart diseases. Ann Pediatr Card. 2019;12:254–86.
5. Bhardwaj R, Rai SK, Yadav AK, et al. Epidemiology of congenital heart disease in India. Cong Heart Dis. 2015;10:437–46.
6. Junghare SW, Desurkar V. Congenital heart diseases and anaesthesia. Indian J Anaesth. 2017;61(9):744–52. https://doi.org/10.4103/ija.IJA_415_17.
7. Lee JY. Clinical presentations of critical cardiac defects in the newborn: decision making and initial management. Korean J Pediatr. 2010;53(6):669–79. https://doi.org/10.3345/kjp.2010.53.6.669. Epub 2010 Jun 23. PMID: 21189937; PMCID: PMC2994134.
8. Hartman RJ, Rasmussen SA, Botto LD, Riehle-Colarusso T, et al. The contribution of chromosomal abnormalities to congenital heart defects: a population-based study. Pediatr Cardiol. 2011;32:1147–57. https://doi.org/10.1007/s00246-011-0034-5.
9. CDC Data and Statistics on Congenital Heart Defects. 2014. https://www.cdc.gov/ncbddd/heartdefects/data.html
10. Egbe A, Lee S, Ho D, Uppu S, Srivastava S. Prevalence of congenital anomalies in newborns with congenital heart disease diagnosis. Ann Pediatr Card. 2014;7:86–91. https://www.annalspc.com/text.asp?2014/7/2/86/132474
11. Walker A, Stokes M, Moriarty A. Anesthesia for major general surgery in neonates with complex cardiac defects. Paediatr Anaesth. 2009;19(2):119–25.
12. Montalva L, Lauriti G, Zani A. Congenital heart disease associated with congenital diaphragmatic hernia: a systematic review on incidence, prenatal diagnosis, management, and outcome. J Peadiatr Surg. 2019;54:909–19.
13. Wilkes JK, Morris SA. Incidence of congenital heart disease among patients with myelomeningocele and associated increased mortality and length of stay; a database study. Pediatrics. 2020; 146(1_MeetingAbstract):604–605. https://doi.org/10.1542/peds.146.1MA7.604.
14. Gibbin C, Touch S, Broth RE, Berghella V. Abdominal wall defects and congenital heart disease. Ultrasound in Obst Gynec. 2003;21:334–7. https://doi.org/10.1002/uog.93.
15. Moideen I, Nair SG, Cherian A, Rao SG. Congenital lobar emphysema associated with congenital heart disease. J Cardiothorac Vasc Anesth. 2006;20(2):239–41. [PubMed: 16616669].
16. Sutera SP, Skalak R. The history of Poiseuille's Law. Ann Rev Fluid Mech. 1993;25:1–19. https://doi.org/10.1146/annurev.fl.25.010193.000245. Bibcode:1993AnRFM..25....1S.
17. Carmosino MJ, Friesen RH, Doran A, et al. Perioperative complications in children with pulmonary hypertension undergoing noncardiac surgery or cardiac catheterization. Anesth Analg. 2007;104:521–7.
18. Nadas AS, Robinson SJ, and Taussig HB. Nadas criteria. 2017. https://telegraph.ph/Nadas-criteria-pdf-11-21
19. Demir T, Oztunc F, Eroglu AG, Saltik L, Ahunbay G, et al. Outcome for patients with isolated atrial septal defects in the oval fossa diagnosed in infancy. Cardiol Young. Congenit Heart Dis. 2010;5(1):32–7. https://doi.org/10.1111/j.1747-0803.2009.00358.x.
20. Helgason H, Jonsdottir G. Spontaneous closure of atrial septal defects. Pediatr Cardiol. 1999;20(3):195–9. https://doi.org/10.1007/s002469900439.

21. Hanslik A, Pospisil U, Salzer-Muhar U, et al. Predictors of spontaneous closure of isolated secundum atrial septal defect in children: a longitudinal study. Pediatrics. 2006;118(4):1560–5.
22. Yen P. ASD and VSD flow dynamics and anesthetic management. Anesth Prog. 2015;62(3):125–30. https://doi.org/10.2344/0003-3006-62.3.125. PMID: 26398131; PMCID: PMC4581019.
23. Mostefa-Kara M, Houyel L, Bonnet D. Anatomy of the ventricular septal defect in congenital heart defects: a random association? Orphanet J Rare Dis. 2018;13:118.
24. Schneider DJ, Moore JW. Patent ductus arteriosus. Circulation. 2006;114(17):1873–82. https://doi.org/10.1161/CIRCULATIONAHA.105.592063.
25. Apitz C, Webb GD, Redington AN. Tetralogy of Fallot. Lancet. 2009;374(9699):1462–71. https://doi.org/10.1016/S0140-6736(09)60657-7. Epub 2009; Aug 14. PMID:19683809.
26. Gawalkar AA, Shrimanth YS, Batta A, Rohit MK. Management of tet spell –an updated review. Curr Res Emerg Med. 2021;1(1):1002–3.
27. Files MD, Morray B. Total anomalous pulmonary venous connection: preoperative anatomy, physiology, imaging, and interventional Management of Postoperative Pulmonary Venous Obstruction. Semin Cardiothorac Vasc Anesth. 2017;21(2):123–31.
28. Baltimore RS, Gewitz M, Baddour LM, Beerman LB, et al. Infective endocarditis in childhood: 2015 update. A scientific statement from the American Heart Association. Circulation. 2015;132(15):1487–515. https://doi.org/10.1161/CIR.0000000000000298.
29. Rushani D, Kaufman JS, Ionescu-Ittu, Mackie AS, et al. Infective endocarditis in children with congenital heart disease. Circulation. 2013;128:1412–9. https://doi.org/10.1161/CIRCULATIONAHA.113.001827.
30. Faraoni D, Vo D, Nasr VG, DiNardo J. Development and validation of a risk stratification score for children with congenital heart disease undergoing noncardiac surgery. Anesth Analg. 2016;123:824–30. https://doi.org/10.1213/ANE.0000000000001500.
31. Shenkman Z, Johnson VM, Zurakowski D, Arnon S, Sethna NF. Hemodynamic changes during spinal anesthesia in premature infants with congenital heart disease undergoing inguinal hernia correction. Paediatr Anaesth. 2012;22(9):865–70. https://doi.org/10.1111/j.1460-9592.2012.03873.x. Epub 2012 May 15.
32. Odegard KC, Bergersen L, Thiagarajan R, Clark L, Shukla A, Wypij D, et al. The frequency of cardiac arrests in patients with congenital heart disease undergoing cardiac catheterization. Anesth Analg. 2014;118:175–82.
33. Kim J, Sun Z, Englum BR, Allori AC, et al. Laparoscopy is safe in infants and neonates with congenital heart disease: a National Study of 3684 patients. J Laparoendosc Adv Surg Tech A. 2016;26(10):836–9. https://doi.org/10.1089/lap.2016.0232.
34. Mariano ER, Chu LF, Albanese CT, Ramamoorthy C. Successful thoracoscopic repair of esophageal atresia with tracheoesophageal fistula in a newborn with single ventricle physiology. Anesth Analg. 2005;101(4):1000–2. https://doi.org/10.1213/01.ANE.0000175778.96374.4F.
35. Rice-Townsend S, Ramamoorthy C, Dutta S. Thoracoscopic repair of a type D esophageal atresia in a newborn with complex congenital heart disease. J Pediatr Surg. 2007;42:1616–9.

Further Readings

Bland JW Jr, Williams WH. Anesthesia for treatment of Congenital Heart Defects. in Kaplan's cardiac anesthesia. Cardiac and noncardiac surgery. 7th ed.; 2016. pp. 281–346. ISBN: 9780323393782. eBook ISBN: 9780323463010. https://www.readbookpage.com/pdf/kaplans-cardiac-anesthesia.
Gravlee PG, Shaw AD, Bartels K. Hensley's practical approach to cardiothoracic anesthesia. Gravelee PG, editor, 6th ed.; 2018.
Hines RL and Marschall KE. Stoelting's anesthesia and co-existing diseases. 7th ed.; 2018. ISBN 978-0-323-40137-1.

Kaplan JA. Kaplan's cardiac anesthesia, 6th ed.; 2011. ISBN: 0323393780. https://www.readbook-page.com/pdf/kaplans-cardiac-anesthesia.

Yao SF, Malhotra V, Fontes ML. Yao and Artusio's anesthesiology: problem-oriented patient management. 6th ed. Philadelphia: Lippincott Williams & Wilkins, 2007. ISBN-10: 0781765102; ISBN-13: 978–0781765107.

Thoracic surgery. Yao & Artusio's anesthesiology problem-oriented patient management, 8th ed; 2016.

Part V

Anesthesia for Advanced Procedures and Uncommon Surgeries

Anaesthesia for Laparoscopic Surgery in Neonates

38

Sandhya Yaddanapudi

38.1 Introduction

Although laparoscopy has become a standard surgical technique in children as in adults, its practice in neonates remains less frequent. Presently, it is limited to a few paediatric centres. However, its use is increasing and therefore it is essential for all neonatal anaesthesiologists to be familiar with the technique and the effects of pneumoperitoneum, so that anaesthesia and perioperative care can be conducted in a safe manner [1–3].

38.2 Laparoscopic Surgery in Neonates

Pyloromyotomy was the first surgery performed laparoscopically in 1991, laparoscopic-assisted anorectal pull-through was reported by Georgeson in 1999 [4], followed by laparoscopic duodenal atresia repair by Bax in 2001 [5], and Rothenberg in 2002 [6]. Since then, a variety of surgical procedures have been successfully undertaken in neonates laparoscopically [7–9].

Neonatal laparoscopy has become possible because of the advances in technology and availability of appropriately sized instruments. Better understanding of the effects of pneumoperitoneum on the neonatal physiology and improvement in perioperative care have contributed to better outcomes and led to the acceptance of the technique for this age group [10–12].

There is a growing volume of literature on laparoscopy in neonates, but most of it includes retrospective studies and case series. There is no definite evidence regarding benefits or harms of laparoscopy over laparotomy due to very few prospective randomised studies comparing the outcomes after the two surgical techniques in

S. Yaddanapudi (✉)
Department of Anaesthesia and Intensive Care, PGIMER, Chandigarh, India

neonates. The purported benefits and the known limitations of laparoscopy are presented here. Future studies are required to address this issue.

38.2.1 Benefits of Laparoscopy

The advantages of laparoscopy in neonates are similar to those in adults and older children. Surgical incision-related outcomes such as tissue trauma, inflammation, pain, scarring, infection, dehiscence and herniation are proportional to the wound size and closing tension, which is determined by the square of the length of the incision. As the combined wound tension of the multiple small incisions of laparoscopy (3–5 mm size) is much less than that of one large laparotomy incision, these morbidities are expected to be less after laparoscopy, with better cosmesis [3].

The bowel is not exteriorized during laparoscopy which minimizes evaporative losses from the intestinal surfaces. Decreased handling of the bowel and less exposure of the tissues to talc, rubber, and polyisoprene from surgical gloves reduce the tendency for formation of adhesions after laparoscopic surgery. Therefore, laparoscopy is specifically beneficial in neonates as they have a high incidence of adhesive intestinal obstruction after laparotomy. Less tissue trauma, decreased ileus, and early return to oral feeds translate into faster recovery and early discharge from the hospital [3].

The surgeon has the advantages of a better view and easier access to the surgical field. The high-definition digital camera and monitor system provide a closer and magnified view of the field. Some of the structures which are difficult to access during open surgery, such as the lower esophageal sphincter complex, can be easily visualized and reached using angled telescopes. Better visualization can enhance greater surgical precision. The mechanical result after laparoscopy is similar or even better than the open procedure. Besides, laparoscopy allows exploration without an extra incision when there is clinical uncertainty, e.g., in malrotation or contralateral inguinal hernia [3].

38.2.2 Limitations and Harmful Effects of Laparoscopy

Laparoscopy in neonates is technically difficult. The vertical working space during laparoscopy in a 3-kg neonate is about 3 cm, which requires very fine and precise movement of the instruments for good outcomes. The degrees of freedom of movement are also limited. Besides, the surgeon cannot palpate and feel the structures which guide some surgical decisions during open surgery. Poor ergonomics and prolonged laparoscopy can lead to fatigue in the surgeon, imprecise surgical technique, and adverse outcomes. The use of electrocautery or ultrasound during laparoscopy can easily damage adjoining structures due to small volumes. Thus, paediatric surgeons require adequate training, proficiency as well as experience in neonatal laparoscopic surgery. It takes much longer for a surgeon to gain expertise in neonatal laparoscopy than in older children. The rate of conversion to open procedure is also high in neonates.

Neonatal laparoscopy requires specialized equipment which is not available at all paediatric centres. Laparoscopic procedures also incur higher operating costs due to the expensive equipment and the use of disposables. The nursing and technical staff also require training in the use and maintenance of the equipment. The high costs may be compensated to some extent by the savings due to faster recovery and shorter hospital stay.

Laparoscopic procedures usually take much longer than open procedures, more so during the initial learning phase of the surgeon. Setting up the equipment and creating pneumoperitoneum require additional time which adds to the overall operating time. A skilled and experienced surgeon may however perform some of the laparoscopic procedures as fast as open surgery.

38.3   Surgical Equipment and Techniques

Laparoscopy is used in neonates for both diagnostic and therapeutic purposes. Table 38.1 lists the common neonatal conditions for which laparoscopic surgery is performed.

Table 38.1 Common laparoscopic procedures undertaken in neonates

Surgical diagnosis	Laparoscopic procedure/technique	Perioperative implications/outcomes
Atresia - duodenal, jejunal, ileal, colon	Resection of atretic segment and anastomosis. Anastomosis is technically difficult, sometimes done extracorporeally by delivering the bowel out of umbilical incision. Multiple atretic segments may be present.	Anastomosis is time consuming. Bowel checked for patency of using saline infusion through gastric tube. Early oral feeding and discharge.
Gut malrotation, volvulus	Ladds procedure.	Urgent surgery due to the risk of vascular compromise. Early oral feeding and discharge.
Infantile hypertrophic pyloric stenosis (IHPS)	Pyloromyotomy. Microlaparoscopic pyloromyotomy with 2-mm instruments and small scope.	Preop correction of electrolyte/acid-base disturbance/hydration required. Early discharge.
Inguinal hernia	Herniotomy. Contralateral side can be evaluated for patent process vaginalis and undiagnosed inguinal hernia. 2-5 mm laparoscope through umbilicus and two small 2–3 mm 'needlescopic' ports on either side.	GA required for lap surgery, while open surgery can be done under regional anaesthesia. Risk of postoperative apnea in preterm neonates.
Ovarian cyst	Resection of large (>4 cm)/torsion cyst.	Early feeds and early discharge.

(continued)

Table 38.1 (continued)

Surgical diagnosis	Laparoscopic procedure/technique	Perioperative implications/ outcomes
Esophageal atresia, gastrostomies	Laparoscopic-assisted gastrostomy.	Gastrostomy site selected under vision, avoiding injury to viscera vs percutaneous endoscopic gastrostomy.
CDH	Reduction of hernia contents and repair of diaphragm.	Pulmonary hypoplasia, pulmonary hypertension. Postoperative ventilation. Risk of injury to viscera minimized examination of abdominal viscera possible for malformations.
GE reflux	Nissen fundoplication.	Better access and visualization
Hirschsprung's disease, high ARM	Colostomy/anorectal pull-through.	Less surgery time, better precision
Intestinal duplication	Excision.	Smaller incision
Acute abdomen	Diagnostic laparoscopy	Laparotomy avoided in case no surgical intervention required. If surgery required - proceed laparoscopically.
Prolonged jaundice	Diagnostic laparoscopy to differentiate between extrahepatic biliary atresia and neonatal hepatitis. Evaluation of liver, in conjunction with cholangiography if the gall bladder is present.	Laparotomy avoided in case no surgical intervention is required. If required Kasai procedure can be performed laparoscopically.

Insufflation of gas into the peritoneum is required during laparoscopy to allow visualization of the abdominal contents and conduct of surgery. The properties of an ideal gas for this purpose are similar to those in adults and should have limited absorption from the peritoneum, minimal physiological effects if absorbed, high solubility in blood so that intravascular embolization causes minimal adverse effects, and should not support combustion. Carbon dioxide (CO_2), though not ideal, is commonly used for this purpose. It is highly soluble, cheap, and non-combustible. However, it is readily absorbed from the peritoneum leading to hypercarbia and adverse cardiorespiratory effects (Table 38.2). Gas-less laparoscopy, in which devices are used to tent the abdominal wall, would be beneficial in neonates.

Table 38.2 Properties of carbon dioxide as insufflating gas for pneumoperitoneum

Properties of an ideal agent	Properties of carbon dioxide
Minimal absorption from peritoneum	Easily absorbed from peritoneum
Minimum physiological effects if absorbed	Major physiological effects
Rapid excretion if absorbed	Rapid excretion
Does not support combustion	Does not support combustion
High solubility in blood so that venous embolization causes minimal adverse effects	High solubility in blood
Low cost	Low cost

Laparoscopy can be performed at a much lower intra-abdominal pressure (IAP) in children than in adults, as their abdominal wall is less rigid. As cardiorespiratory adverse effects directly correlate with the intra-abdominal pressure, the lowest IAP that allows the procedure should be used. Commonly used IAP in neonates are of 5–12 mmHg, but lower pressures of 5–6 mmHg are recommended.

Gas insufflation should be carried out at low flow rates to prevent sudden increase in IAP. Most insufflators have a minimum flow rate of 1 LPM, while some may allow 0.5 LPM. If the device cannot provide low flows, insufflation should be done in stages and the required IAP be achieved in 1 min or longer. Nowadays, neonatal insufflators which release puffs of gas for only 1.7 s are available. Anaesthetists should monitor the IAP and gas flow rate throughout the period of pneumoperitoneum.

A Veress needle inserted blindly for creation of pneumoperitoneum can inadvertently puncture a patent umbilical vein and lead to air embolism. Therefore, an open technique with insertion of a blunt trocar through an umbilical incision is preferred in neonates.

The equipment used for neonatal laparoscopy includes a telescope with 0- or 30-degree vision, introduced through a 3–5 mm trans-umbilical camera port, 2–4 operative ports each 2–5 mm in size, and short length instruments (15 cm) and corresponding diameter. Self-retaining valved ports are advantageous as they do not get dislodged, can be pulled out to increase the abdominal space with minimum gas insufflation, and prevent gas leakage during change of instruments (Figs. 38.1 and 38.2). Mini-laparoscopy, micro-laparoscopy, or needle-scopy are the terms used when small diameter (<3 mm) trocars, telescopes, and instruments are used. These small incisions can be glued together and need not be sutured, providing good cosmesis. Better energy sources are now available which allow cuts with more precision and with less lateral thermal tissue damage. Tissue sealing devices which seal the vessels and tissue by liquefying and reforming the collagen and elastin are of great advantage over suturing or clipping in a small space. A miniature stapler (<6 mm) is useful in performing watertight anastomosis of the intestines.

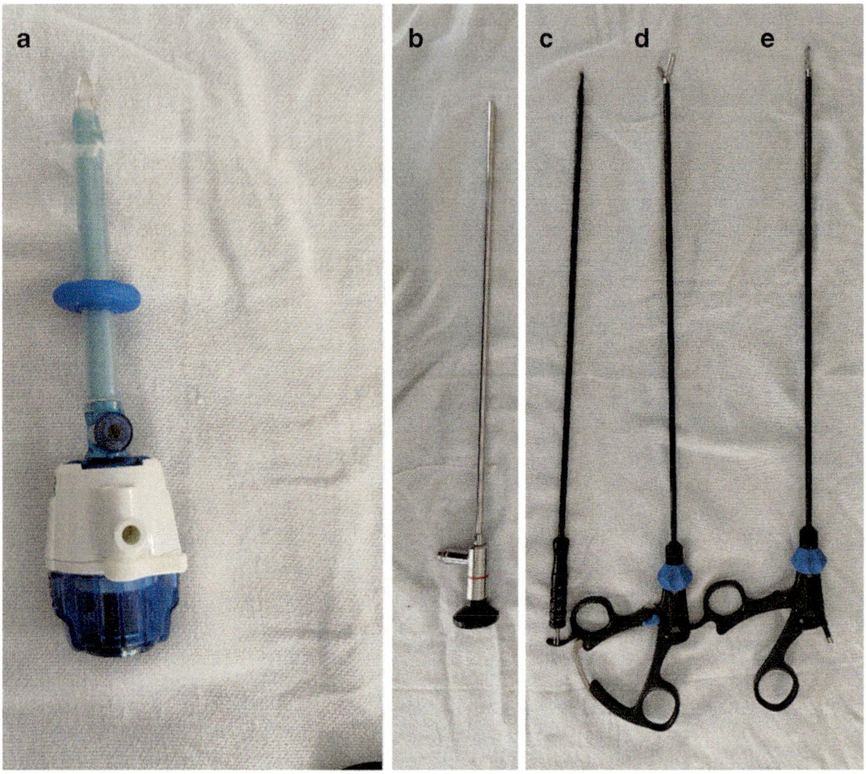

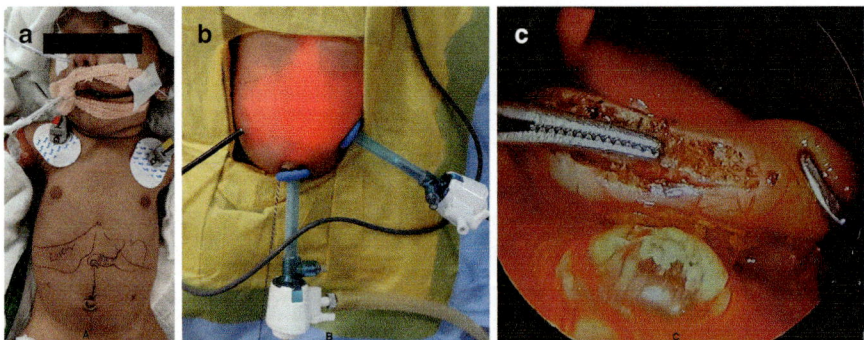

Fig. 38.1 Laparoscopic instruments. (**a**) 5 mm self-retaining valved port, (**b**) Telescope, (**c**) Electrocautery, (**d**) Bowel grasper, and (**e**) Scissors

Fig. 38.2 Laparoscopic pyloromyotomy in a 4-weeks old neonate with pyloric stenosis. (**a**) After induction of anaesthesia, (**b**) Laparoscopic ports and instruments in situ, and (**c**) Pyloromyotomy

38.4   Effects of Laparoscopy on Neonatal Physiology

The immature respiratory and cardiovascular systems of a neonate are very sensitive to the adverse effects of pneumoperitoneum. Pneumoperitoneum affects physiological functions mainly due to

1. Mechanical effects of increased IAP,
2. Systemic absorption of the insufflated CO_2 and
3. Other contributory factors such as position of the baby during the procedure, intravascular volume status, baseline cardiorespiratory status, anaesthetic drugs, and ventilatory technique.

These effects have been described mostly in infants and small children with a few studies in neonates.

38.4.1 Cardiovascular System

Cardiovascular effects of pneumoperitoneum have been studied using non-invasive methods such as esophageal aortic blood flow echo doppler, trans-esophageal echocardiography (TEE), and thoracic electrical bioimpedance. IAP of 5–6 mmHg is not associated with any haemodynamic changes, and the stroke volume and cardiac output remain in the normal range. On the other hand, IAP in the range of 10–12 mmHg results in decrease in stroke volume, cardiac output, and aortic blood flow, and increase in blood pressure, systemic vascular resistance (SVR), and left ventricular end-diastolic and end-systolic volumes. Septal hypokinesia has been observed at high IAP. Heart rate response is usually tachycardia, like in children, but bradycardia and asystole can also occur in neonates due to their parasympathetic overactivity. These cardiovascular changes are usually well-tolerated in healthy infants and are completely reversed on deflation of the pneumoperitoneum [13].

38.4.1.1 Mechanism
As pneumoperitoneum is created (especially when IAP is less than right atrial pressure (RAP)), blood from the splanchnic circulation is displaced, increasing the venous return to the heart. But, once IAP exceeds RAP, the inferior vena cava collapses, venous return declines, and cardiac output decreases significantly. Increase in afterload due to IAP-induced increase in SVR compounds the decrease in the cardiac output.

Hypercarbia due to CO_2 absorption stimulates the sympathoadrenal system leading to the release of vasoactive substances and resultant tachycardia, hypertension, increase in SVR, myocardial depression, and arrhythmias. The cardiovascular system in neonates is more sensitive to CO_2 than in older children. Neonatal cardiac output can only increase by increasing the heart rate, as myocardial contractility-induced increase in stroke volume cannot occur due to the immaturity of the myocardial fibres.

Reverse Trendelenburg position, anaesthesia-induced vasodilatation, and low intravascular volume worsen the reduction in the venous return and cardiac output, while Trendelenburg position improves the cardiac output. In neonates with congenital heart disease, the cardiorespiratory changes due to pneumoperitoneum can result in the reopening of intracardiac shunts, increasing the chances of paradoxical gas embolism in case of vascular injury during trocar insertion and gas insufflation, and cardiac failure.

38.4.2 Respiratory System

The insufflation pressures during pneumoperitoneum correlate with the changes in peak inspiratory pressure, end-tidal carbon dioxide ($EtCO_2$), tidal volume, and dynamic compliance in small babies, with almost no changes at 5 mmHg and significant changes at 10–15 mmHg IAP. A decrease in oxygen saturation (SpO_2) is reported in 40–60% and an increase in $EtCO_2$ in nearly 90% of babies during laparoscopy even after ventilatory adjustments [8, 14].

38.4.2.1 Mechanism

Increased IAP displaces the diaphragm cranially and restricts its movement, leading to a decrease in functional residual capacity (FRC), basal alveolar atelectasis, and increased intrapulmonary shunting. Pulmonary compliance decreases and airway resistance increases, resulting in high inspiratory pressure, hypoxaemia, and hypercarbia. These effects are exaggerated in neonates as they have low FRC to start with. Besides the IAP, the insufflating gas flow rate also influences the respiratory effects, with higher flows amplifying the changes.

The insufflated CO_2 gets absorbed rapidly into the systemic circulation, increasing the total body CO_2 content, augmenting hypercarbia. The amount of CO_2 absorption is directly proportional to IAP, gas flow rate, and duration of insufflation. It occurs more rapidly in neonates compared to older children, because of a thin and highly permeable peritoneum, larger peritoneal surface area to weight ratio, and lack of CO_2 absorbing peritoneal fat buffer. Neonates also decompensate quickly due to high metabolic rate and oxygen consumption.

The respiratory effects of pneumoperitoneum are accentuated in Trendelenburg position as the diaphragm is displaced further cephalad. Reverse Trendelenburg position improves oxygenation, ventilation, and compliance. Bronchospasm and increased airway secretions may occur during pneumoperitoneum.

Pneumoperitoneum and Trendelenburg position result in decrease in the length of trachea and shift the carina cephalad, reducing the distance between the tip of the endotracheal tube and the carina in adults. Similar changes are expected in neonates, with increased likelihood of endobronchial intubation.

38.4.3 Central Nervous System (CNS)

Effects of pneumoperitoneum on the CNS have not been well-studied in neonates. Laparoscopy in neonates and infants has been observed to have minimal effect on cerebral tissue oxygenation measured using NIRS (near infra-red spectroscopy). In an animal study, decreased venous return and hypercarbia during laparoscopy have been observed to increase the intracranial pressure, which along with low cardiac output results in a decreased cerebral perfusion pressure. These changes are likely to be more harmful in neonates who already have impaired cerebral autoregulation [15].

38.4.4 Renal System

The incidence of transient oliguria and anuria during laparoscopic surgery is higher in neonates and infants than in older children. It is completely reversible in children with normal renal functions and is followed by an increase in postoperative urine output. Increased excretion of N-acetyl-beta-D-glycosaminidase (marker of renal injury) has been observed following laparoscopy. However, other investigators found that renal tissue oxygenation and fractional tissue oxygen extraction did not decrease during laparoscopy of short duration in neonates. Serum creatinine, urine creatinine, and cystatin C also did not change after pneumoperitoneum. The possible causes of oliguria include low cardiac output, sympathoadrenal stimulation, release of vasoactive mediators (endothelin, vasopressin), and direct compression of renal vessels and parenchyma by the high IAP. Effect of different levels of IAP on renal functions has not been studied in neonates [15].

38.4.5 Other Systems

Effects of pneumoperitoneum and hypercarbia on perfusion of other abdominal organs have not been studied.

Laparoscopy of short duration produces minimal changes in buccal and sublingual microcirculation in neonates and small infants. The metabolic and endocrine response to surgical stress as evaluated by blood insulin, cortisol, prolactin, adrenaline, lactate, and blood glucose is similar in children after laparoscopic and open surgeries. However, interleukin-6, another measure of stress response, was lower in neonates undergoing laparoscopic surgery compared to age-matched controls undergoing the same procedure by open surgery.

38.5   Selection of Patients

Laparoscopy is a high-risk procedure in neonates. The advantages must be weighed against the risks and limitations specific to neonates. The neonate should be carefully evaluated preoperatively for the presence of conditions which increase the risks of laparoscopic technique and carry high risk of decompensation during pneumoperitoneum such as

- Neonates with haemodynamic instability,
- Uncorrected hypovolemia,
- Raised intracranial pressure and
- Alveolar distension.
- High risk of decompensation during pneumoperitoneum.

Such babies are not suitable candidates for laparoscopy.

There is a controversy regarding laparoscopy in neonates with prematurity or congenital heart disease.

38.5.1 Preterm Neonates

Preterm neonates have immature organs, less functional reserve, and tend to have other co-morbid conditions. Burgmeier and Schier [16] observed a higher incidence of postoperative cardiorespiratory complications requiring tracheal re-intubation and prolonged ventilation following laparoscopy in preterm than in term neonates (20.4% vs. 5.5%). In addition, the procedure was technically more difficult and took much longer in preterm neonates. However, thoracoscopic repair of congenital diaphragmatic hernia has been reported in a preterm baby weighing 1 kg [17]. Delaying a non-urgent surgery till the baby attains the body weight of about 2.5 kg is suggested as a safe alternative.

38.5.2 Congenital Heart Disease

The cardiorespiratory effects of pneumoperitoneum are exaggerated in children with congenital heart disease (CHD). The high IAP and hypercarbia during laparoscopy increase the pulmonary vascular resistance, resulting in a right to left shunt, hypoxemia, and decrease in cardiac output in children with intracardiac shunt lesions. Also, the cardiorespiratory changes which are completely reversed after deflation of pneumoperitoneum in healthy neonates persist into the postoperative period in those with CHD. Analysis of the data from the National Surgical Quality Improvement Program-Paediatric (2013–2014), which included a large number of infants and neonates, confirmed higher postoperative morbidity and mortality after laparoscopic surgery in children with CHD compared to matched controls without

CHD. A direct correlation was also observed between the severity of the CHD and postoperative morbidity and mortality [18–20].

On the other hand, the literature has many reports of safe conduct of laparoscopic surgery in neonates with CHD (cyanotic and acyanotic) of varying severity, with minimal or no cardiovascular complications. However, these publications being mostly case reports or retrospective studies are limited by selection and publication bias, with only the successful cases being reported and published. In addition, these reports are mostly published in surgical journals and provide minimal intraoperative haemodynamic and respiratory details of significance to the anaesthesiologist [18, 20].

Thus, the decision to undertake laparoscopic surgery in a neonate with prematurity or CHD should be made by a multidisciplinary team consisting of a paediatric surgeon, a paediatric anaesthetist, and a neonatal cardiologist, considering the risks and benefits on case-to-case basis. If laparoscopy is decided, it should be carried out by a skilled surgeon, and anaesthesia provided by an anaesthetist well-experienced in neonatal anaesthesia as well as familiar with the pathophysiology of the CHD. In case of any deterioration, an early decision to deflate the abdomen and convert to open procedure is required. Intensive monitoring and care are required in the entire intraoperative and postoperative periods.

38.6 Preoperative Assessment and Preparation

The neonate should be assessed for the presence of congenital anomalies, which may not only require further evaluation and preparation, but also affect the decision to use the laparoscopic technique. Hydration, electrolyte and metabolic status, and cardiovascular and respiratory functions should be optimized preoperatively, and adequate blood and blood products arranged as per the requirement of the surgery. Risks, benefits and outcomes of anaesthesia, and the procedure, including those due to the laparoscopic technique, should be communicated to the parents and a written informed consent obtained.

The operation theatre is prepared for the neonate with special attention to patient warming devices and the ambient temperature appropriate for the gestational age. Anaesthesia equipment and drugs are readied according to the age and body weight prior to transfer of the baby to the operation theatre. No premedication is indicated; however, prophylactic atropine may be used to prevent bradycardia secondary to CO_2 pneumoperitoneum, but may not always be effective and can cause undue tachycardia and arrhythmias.

38.7 Monitoring

The monitoring to be initiated prior to anaesthesia includes 5-lead ECG, pre- and post-ductal SpO_2 using two pulse oximeters, and non-invasive blood pressure (NIBP) using an appropriate-sized cuff. After induction of anaesthesia, $EtCO_2$ and core temperature (nasopharyngeal, esophageal, or rectal) probes are applied. Bladder catheterization and urine output monitoring is indicated for prolonged procedures.

A precordial or an esophageal stethoscope is used to monitor the quality, intensity, rate, and rhythm of the heart sounds. A precordial stethoscope also monitors breath sounds on the left side of the chest and is useful in detecting endobronchial intubation. It is essential to keep a constant watch on the respiratory parameters as frequent adjustments and changes are required during surgery, e.g., in peak and mean airway pressures, inspired and expired tidal volume, respiratory rate, and PEEP.

A 24 or 26 G arterial cannula is useful for continuous blood pressure monitoring and sampling for blood gas analysis. $EtCO_2$ does not accurately reflect $PaCO_2$ and adequacy of ventilation due to increased dead space during laparoscopy [8]. It is also not reliable in low cardiac output states. Capillary blood can be used for blood gas analysis in the absence of arterial cannulation, but it is difficult to obtain the sample due to restricted access to the patient. Alternatively, transcutaneous CO_2 monitoring may be useful during prolonged procedures [21].

38.8   Conduct of Anaesthesia

Clear communication between the anaesthetist and the surgeon is essential to titrate the IAP to a level which allows a good surgical access as well as satisfactory respiratory and hemodynamic parameters. Use of minimum IAP is encouraged as blood pressure in the normal range does not rule out low cardiac output. An orogastric tube is placed to deflate the stomach and allow better visibility. It is preferable to place the IV cannula in the upper limb, as increased IAP can delay the drug from lower limb from reaching the central circulation. Once the surgical procedure starts, access to the baby gets restricted (Fig. 38.3). Therefore, all monitoring probes, breathing circuits, and IV lines should be well-secured and within reach. An extension is required for the venous line.

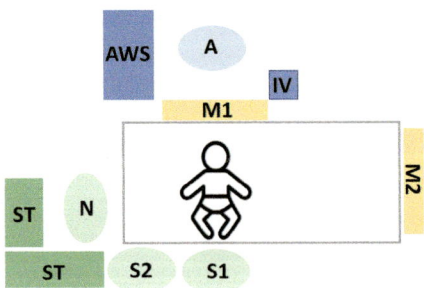

Fig. 38.3 Arrangement of OT personnel and equipment during laparoscopic pyloromyotomy. *A* Anaesthetist, *AWS* anaesthesia workstation, *IV* intravenous infusion and infusion pump, *M1* laparoscopic monitor, *M2* laparoscopic rack and monitor, *N* nurse, *S1* chief surgeon, *S2* surgical assistant, and *ST* surgical instruments' trolley

38.8.1 Induction and Maintenance of Anaesthesia

The choice of anaesthetic agents depends on the neonate's underlying condition and the anaesthetist's preference. Nitrous oxide is not preferred as it can diffuse into the intestines causing distension and interference with surgery, and into the peritoneal space where it can support combustion, when using electrocautery. Therefore, air is the favoured carrier gas. Multimodal analgesia is provided with titrated doses of fentanyl, intravenous paracetamol, and local anaesthetic (ropivacaine) infiltration at trocar insertion sites. Caudal block is suitable for lower abdominal procedures (inguinal hernia repair) [22].

Laparoscopic procedures are conventionally performed under general anaesthesia (GA). However, due to the concern of neurotoxic effects of anaesthetic agents on the developing brain of the neonate, feasibility of laparoscopy under regional anaesthesia has been explored. Laparoscopic pyloromyotomy has been performed under subarachnoid block with 1 mg/kg of hyperbaric bupivacaine in neonates with pyloric stenosis. However, conversion to GA was required in 25% of the cases. Laparoscopic hernia repair has also been reported under caudal block and intravenous anaesthesia consisting of dexmedetomidine and propofol with or without remifentanil, without any airway instrumentation [22].

38.8.2 Airway and Ventilatory Management

A non-depolarizing neuromuscular blocking agent is used to facilitate endotracheal intubation and the surgical procedure. In babies with risk of pulmonary aspiration (e.g., pyloric stenosis, intestinal obstruction, etc.), succinyl choline may be used for intubation in a modified rapid sequence induction technique. A cuffed endotracheal tube is preferred as it allows better ventilation and respiratory monitoring, with cuff pressure maintained below 10 cm of H_2O. It is essential to reconfirm the position of the endotracheal tube after abdominal insufflation as well as after any change in position [10].

Pressure controlled ventilation is the usual mode of ventilation in neonates, with inspiratory pressure adjusted to achieve a tidal volume of 8–10 mL/kg, PEEP of 4–5 cm H_2O, and respiratory rate of 30–40/min to achieve normocarbia. Mild to moderate hypercapnia (45–50 mmHg) is acceptable after pneumoperitoneum as it causes sympathetic stimulation and counteracts the low cardiac output effects of IAP, and increases O_2 delivery to the tissues due to Bohr effect. Also, the changes in ventilation required to maintain normocarbia may lead to pulmonary barotrauma, volutrauma, and increase in intrathoracic pressure impeding the venous return. Increase in respiratory rate shortens the expiratory phase and may result in air trapping [1, 10].

Increase in minute ventilation (by increasing peak inspiratory pressure and respiratory rate) by up to 40% and in PEEP may be required to maintain mild hypercarbia after CO_2 insufflation. The pressure limit and alarms are adjusted accordingly.

Increase in inspired O_2 concentration may also be required to maintain acceptable SpO_2 appropriate for the gestational age.

$EtCO_2$ and SpO_2 usually return to normal values after desufflation. The ventilatory settings should be adjusted accordingly. In some neonates, $EtCO_2$ may increase for a while after deflation, probably due to increase in cardiac output.

38.8.3 Hemodynamic Management

Hemodynamic parameters are stringently monitored during pneumoperitoneum. The intravascular volume is optimized before creation of pneumoperitoneum to prevent decrease in cardiac output. Fluid loss is minimal during laparoscopic surgery. Balanced isotonic electrolyte solution containing 1–2.5% dextrose is administered at a rate of 10 mL/kg/h. Additional fluid boluses of 10 mL/kg can be given if there is decreased perfusion, hypotension, or blood loss. Neonates are more prone to bradycardia on insufflation due to peritoneal stretch, and slow inflation is recommended. Moderate to severe hypothermia can also result in bradycardia.

38.8.4 Emergence

$EtCO_2$ and SpO_2 return to the baseline within 15 min of desufflation in most neonates. Trachea can be extubated in these babies once they are awake and have regained adequate muscle tone and respiration. In case ventilatory derangement or hemodynamic instability persists, postoperative ventilation is required. Reasons for delayed extubation include

- Prolonged surgery (>100 min of insufflation),
- Hypothermia,
- Major intraoperative incident,
- Metabolic derangement such as acidosis or alkalosis,
- Prematurity and
- Pre-existing condition such as CHD.

38.9   Intraoperative Adverse Events

38.9.1   Respiratory and Cardiovascular Events

Intraoperative anaesthetic incidents were reported in 10% (20/204) neonates undergoing laparoscopy in a large multicentric retrospective study by Kalfa et al. [19] These included O_2 desaturation, hypotension, hypercapnia, hypothermia, bradycardia and metabolic acidosis. The risk factors for these incidents were younger age, high insufflation pressure and flow, long duration of surgery, and inadequate preoperative resuscitation.

If hypotension persists despite fluid resuscitation, $EtCO_2$ increases despite appropriate changes in ventilation and/or SpO_2 remains low (<80%) despite 100% oxygen, the IAP and gas flow need to be reduced, or the insufflation can be stopped temporarily. If the changes do not revert to acceptable levels even after these measures, the abdomen should be deflated, laparoscopy abandoned, and surgery converted to open procedure.

38.9.2   Hypo- and Hyperthermia

Though there is less heat loss during laparoscopy compared to open surgery, a newborn baby can easily become hypothermic under anaesthesia, and external heat sources are required to keep the baby warm. The decrease in temperature is directly proportional to the duration of insufflation. Cold CO_2 contributes to hypothermia. CO_2 is also dry which leads to evaporation from the peritoneal surfaces, cooling the baby further and creating volume deficit. Use of warm gas and meticulous care in preventing leaks from the ports, so that lower flow of gas is required, are helpful in maintaining normothermia.

Hyperthermia has been also observed in neonates and infants during laparoscopy, often iatrogenic, due to patient warming devices, heated and humidified CO_2 for insufflation, and heat generated by laparoscopic light.

38.9.3 Gas Embolism

The incidence of major embolism during laparoscopy in neonates is not known. There are four reports of cardiac arrest in neonates due to gas embolism during laparoscopy as of this writing. The gas entrainment in these cases occurred at the start of pneumoperitoneum due to injury to a patent umbilical vein during insertion of Veress needle. The clinical effects of embolism depend upon the solubility, volume, and the rate of gas entrainment. CO_2, being soluble, is less likely than air to cause cardiovascular effects, unless a large bolus is rapidly entrained.

The risk of paradoxical embolism is high in neonates, as foramen Ovale and ductus arteriosus are only functionally closed in the first few weeks of life, and not anatomically. They can reopen due to changes in pressure gradients, allowing the embolus to move across the shunt to the systemic circulation (paradoxical embolism). A similar risk is present in children with cardiac shunts (VSD, ASD) [18, 20].

If gas embolism is suspected, the surgeon is immediately informed, gas insufflation stopped, and pneumoperitoneum deflated. Anaesthetic agents are stopped, 100% oxygen and fluid boluses are administered, and resuscitation initiated as per the clinical condition.

38.9.4 Other Complications

The incidence of major bleeding in neonates undergoing laparoscopy is not known but is known to occur in about 0.5% of adult laparoscopies. Immediate detection and rapid fluid resuscitation are required in such cases. At least two IV lines should be established before the start of the procedure in neonates. If the bleeding is not controlled, an early decision of conversion to open procedure should be made.

The insufflated CO_2 can diffuse into the subcutaneous tissues leading to subcutaneous emphysema from improper insertion of the Verres needle. Rarely, the gas may traverse into the fascial planes causing pneumomediastinum or pneumothorax, requiring urgent intervention.

Conversion to an open procedure occurs more often in neonates than in older children, common reasons being hemodynamic or respiratory compromise, surgical difficulty, bleeding, and long duration.

38.10 Postoperative Management

All neonates undergoing laparoscopic surgery require close monitoring and management in NICU. Respiratory events such as desaturation, hypoventilation, and apnea can occur requiring reintubation and ventilation. Reasons for reintubation are

- Continued high CO_2 excretion,
- Depression of the central respiratory drive,
- Apnea due to uncorrected alkalosis (e.g., IHPS),
- Prematurity,
- Pre-existing diseases such as Arnold Chiari syndrome, patent foramen ovale, or
- History of postnatal respiratory distress.

As in children, less postoperative pain is expected following laparoscopy in neonates compared to open surgery. In infants and neonates with pyloric stenosis randomized to undergo laparoscopic or open pyloromyotomy, postoperative pain scores and analgesic requirement were significantly lower after laparoscopy than open surgery. Intravenous paracetamol (30 mg/kg/day) in 3–4 divided doses usually suffices for postoperative analgesia. IV fentanyl can be also given in titrated doses.

Oral feeding is started as soon as possible and is much earlier following laparoscopy than after open procedures. This translates into shorter hospital stay and earlier discharge after procedures such as pyloromyotomy and inguinal hernia repair. The effect of laparoscopy on postoperative emesis is not certain, and both higher and lower incidences of vomiting have been reported.

The incidence of surgical complications after minimally invasive compared to the open procedures in neonates is not known. However, incomplete procedure, bowel injury, and perforation have been reported requiring re-exploration.

38.11 Conclusions

As the use of laparoscopic surgery in neonates is increasing, paediatric anaesthetists need to be prepared for the challenges by familiarizing themselves with the pathophysiology of pneumoperitoneum on the immature neonatal organs [23]. Neonates require careful selection for laparoscopic surgery in order to have a good outcome. Anaesthetists play a big role in titration of the IAP to maintain an acceptable physiological state, and in the decision to abandon the procedure in favour of open surgery. The intensive monitoring is continued postoperatively with many babies requiring postoperative ventilation.

References

1. Tobias JD. Anaesthesia for minimally invasive surgery in children. Best Pract Res Clin Anaesthesiol. 2002;16:115–30.
2. Ahmed A. Laparoscopic surgery in children - anaesthetic considerations. J Pak Med Assoc. 2006;56:75–9.
3. Blinman T, Ponsky T. Pediatric minimally invasive surgery: laparoscopy and thoracoscopy in infants and children. Pediatrics. 2012;130:539–49.
4. Georgeson K. Minmally invasive surgery in neonates. Semin Neonatol. 2003;8:243–8.
5. Bax NM, Ure BM, van der Zee DC, van Tuijl I. Laparoscopic duodenoduodenostomy for duodenal atresia. Surg Endosc. 2001;15:217.
6. Rothenberg SS. Laparoscopic duodenoduodenostomy for duodenal obstruction in infants and children. Pediatr Surg. 2002;37:1088–9.
7. Lee KH, Yeung CK. Laparoscopic surgery in newborns and infants: an update. J Paediatr. 2003;8:327–35.
8. Sanders JC, Gerstein N. Arterial to endtidal carbon dioxide gradient during pediatric laparoscopic fundoplication. Pediatr Anesth. 2008;18:1096–101.
9. Numanoglu A, Alexander A. Neonatal laparoscopy. S Afr J Surg. 2011;49:28–9.
10. Tobias JD. Anesthetic considerations for laparoscopy in children. Semin Laparosc Surg. 1998;5:60–6.
11. Fujimoto T, Segawa O, Lane GJ, Esaki S, Miyano T. Laparoscopic surgery in newborn infants. Surg Endosc. 1999;13:773–7.
12. Kalfa N, Allal H, Raux O, Lopez M, Forgues D, Guibal MP, et al. Tolerance of laparoscopy and thoracoscopy in neonates. Pediatrics. 2005;116:e785–90.
13. De Waal EEC, Kalkman CJ. Haemodynamic changes during low-pressure carbon dioxide pneumoperitoneum in young children. Paediatr Anaesth. 2003;13:18–25.
14. Bannister CF, Brosius KK, Wulkan M. The effect of insufflation pressure on pulmonary mechanics in infants during laparoscopic surgical procedures. Paediatr Anaesth. 2003;13:785–9.
15. Kamata M, Hakim M, Walia H, Tumin D, Tobias JD. Changes in cerebral and renal oxygenation during laparoscopic pyloromyotomy. J Clin Monit Comput. 2020;34:699–703.
16. Burgmeier C, Schier F. Cardiorespiratory complications after laparoscopic hernia repair in term and preterm babies. J Pediatr Surg. 2013;48:1972–6.
17. Choudhry M, Rusu S, Brooks P, Ogundipe E, Chuang S-L. Thoracoscopic repair of congenital diaphragmatic hernia in preterm neonate at 1 kilogram. J Pediatr Surg Rep. 2021;9:e13–6.
18. Burgmeier C, Schier F. Are cardiac anomalies and persistent fetal circulation a risk factor for cardiovascular events during minimally invasive surgery in neonates? J Laparoendosc Adv Surg Tech. 2019;29:694–7.

19. Kalfa N, Allal H, Raux O, Lardy H, Varlet F, Reinberg O. Multicentric assessment of the safety of neonatal videosurgery. Surg Endosc. 2007;21:303–8.
20. Chu DI, Tan JM, Mattei P, Costarino AT, Rossano JW, Tasian GE. Mortality and morbidity after laparoscopic surgery in children with and without congenital heart disease. J Pediatr. 2017;185:88–93.
21. Truchon R. Anaesthetic considerations for laparoscopic surgery in neonates and infants: a practical review. Best Pract Res Clin Anaesthesiol. 2004;18:343–55.
22. Krishnan P, Whyte SD, Baird R, Malherbe S. Caudal and intravenous anesthesia without airway instrumentation for laparoscopic inguinal hernia repair in infants: a case series. A&A Pract. 2020;14:e01251.
23. Chou C-M, Yeh C-M, Huang S-Y, Chen H-C. Perioperative parameter analysis of neonates and infants receiving laparoscopic surgery. J Chin Med Assoc. 2016;79:554–64.

Anesthesia for Bronchoscopy in Neonates

39

Rakhee Goyal

39.1 Introduction

Respiratory disorders are the commonest indication of admission in the NICU and are responsible for increased morbidity and mortality in the neonate. Bronchoscopy is an useful adjunct to diagnose and treat many respiratory and airway-related illnesses and pathologies.

In earlier times, until the introduction of the fiberoptic technology, rigid bronchoscopy was performed by the surgeons in small babies. Because of the wall thickness of the rigid scope the internal diameter was much smaller compared to the FOB, making clear detailed visualization a problem. It not only required smaller bronchoscope, but also general anesthesia with muscle relaxants, thereby making it more invasive and high risk in the neonates. It is now replaced by FOB, except in centers where appropriate size fiberoptic bronchoscope or expertise is not available.

Fiberoptic bronchoscopy (FOB) has been in clinical practice in adults since 1967. Robert Wood pioneered FOB in children in 1978, but it was in 1990s that it was first performed in neonates, but with limited use restricted mainly to the quaternary NICU setups. Technological advancement and better understanding of the neonatal anatomy and physiology have opened new doors in neonatal anesthesia and intensive care. The neonatal fiberoptic bronchoscopes are gradually being made available to many centers now, and the anesthesiologists are beginning to gain expertise and experience in the procedure.

R. Goyal (✉)
Madhukar Rainbow Children's hospital, New Delhi, India

39.2 Fiberoptic Bronchoscopy in Neonates

It was only in the last two decades that neonatal FOB has been truly possible, and in India mostly in the last 5 years. Limitations to its routine use are nonavailability of appropriately sized scopes, and/or the patient (neonate) was deemed to be too sick to undergo airway-related non-therapeutic procedure. It was mostly performed by either the otorhinolaryngologist, pulmonologist, or the neonatologist. Many of these centers have an airway team including all the above, and a pediatric surgeon, who would take a combined decision regarding the indication, best person, and place (NICU or operation theater) to perform the procedure. Anesthesiologists were usually not a part of the team. It is only in the last decade that anesthesiologists have gained expertise in performing FOB in children as well as neonates. Pediatric anesthesiologists have an edge over other members of the airway team, by virtue of their training in sedation in sick children as well as advance airway management.

39.3 Indications for Neonatal FOB

In the neonates, indications are both diagnostic and therapeutic (Table 39.1). The diagnostic indications are more common than the therapeutic usefulness [7, 8]. Sachdeva et al. found it particularly useful in diagnosis of persistent or unexplained airway and lung abnormalities and obstruction [9]. Failure or difficult to wean from mechanical ventilation is quite common in NICU patients, often due to ventilator-associated pneumonias (VAP) or ventilator-related lung disease. Bronchoalveolar lavage (BAL) through the bronchoscope provides sampling, considered as the best marker of lung infection. The in-house NICU bugs are known to be the commonest cause of nosocomial infection. BAL helps in making the right choice of antibiotics, and negative results save the babies from unnecessary medications. Better ventilator strategies can be planned to prevent lung injury [10]. Atelectasis due to airway blockade by the tracheal or bronchial secretions is another reason for weaning troubles. Bronchoscopy can be very useful for airway toilet without disrupting the ventilation

Table 39.1 Indications of FOB in neonates

Diagnostic indication	Therapeutic
Laryngomalacia, Tracheobronchomalacia, vocal cord paralysis, tracheal stenosis	Airway toilet in pulmonary atelectasis
Respiratory distress Stridor [1] Persistent or unexplained wheeze Persistent atelectasis Persistent radiological abnormalities	Endotracheal intubation in difficult airway (unanticipated or planned)
Difficult to wean from controlled ventilation [1]	Bronchoscopy-assisted neonatal tracheostomy (BANT) [2]
Preoperative assessment for TEF [3]or esophageal atresia [1, 4]	Necrotizing tracheobronchitis [5]
BAL	Tracheoscopy-assisted repair of TEF (TARTEF) [6]

in sick babies [11]. Vijayasekaran et al. observed that of 84 neonates in whom FOB was performed, in 57% neonates it helped in the modification of diagnosis [7].

Rigid bronchoscopy is still in use for all the above-mentioned indications in the neonates in centers where FOB is not available. However, its role over FOB is more in infants and children mainly for foreign body removal, massive hemoptysis, large tumor, etc.

39.4   Technique of FOB

FOB can be performed through an endotracheal tube (ET) or without directly through the mouth or nose. For evaluation of the airway dynamics, basic requirement is retention of spontaneous respiration, as in an awake or mildly sedated neonate. It is easier to diagnose upper airway anomalies such as airway malacias, edema, stenosis, vocal cord palsy, or paralysis when FOB is performed without the ET. Supraglottic airway (e.g., LMA, i-gel) also provides a good conduit for the bronchoscope. Preoxygenation and supplemental O_2 during the procedure are beneficial. Neonates usually do not tolerate longer duration of hypoventilation, and desaturate fast, therefore the procedure must be done quickly. Essential intraprocedural monitoring includes SpO_2, ECG, NIBP, and $EtCO_2$.

39.5   Fiberoptic Bronchoscope

Neonates require smaller diameter bronchoscopes, appropriate for their airway anatomy. Most neonates would need a 2.8 mm (outer diameter) bronchoscope, which can be maneuvered through a 3.5 mm (internal diameter) ET, with assisted ventilation, and 4.0 mm ET for FOB with spontaneous breathing. It has a 1.2 mm suction channel for airway secretions and BAL sampling. The distal tip has a maneuverability range of 180° and slight rotation of the shaft of the scope can help in moving the tip in and out of this range. The smallest size is 2.2 mm. It can just pass through a 2.5 mm ET. It has no suction channel and can be used only for diagnostic purpose. It is useful in premature neonates. However, this size may not be available in every center. Table 39.2 shows the details of available bronchoscopes and gives a guide to choose the right device.

Table 39.2 Bronchoscope size chart

Outer diameter (mm)	Working channel	Working length (mm)	Tip deflection	Field of vision	ET Size for assisted ventilation (id)	ET Size for spontaneous breathing (id)
2.2	Not present	550	Up 160° down 90°	75°	3.0 mm	3.5
2.8	1.2 mm	550	Up 180° down 130°	95°	3.5	4.0
3.5	1.2 mm	600	Up 180° down 130°	95°	5.0	5.5

The bronchoscope must be lubricated before insertion into the ET. The internal diameter of the ET should be at least 1 mm more than the outer diameter of the scope for easy maneuverability and prevention of ET blockage and inadvertent PEEP.

'Spray as you go' technique with lignocaine can be used, and care being taken not to exceed safe dose.

After its use, the bronchoscope should be cleaned and disinfected as per manufacturers' recommendations. It is best stored in a hanging position in a designated cabinet and transported in its prescribed container. It is a delicate and expensive equipment and should be handled with care to prevent breakage of internal fiberoptic fibers.

For diagnostic purposes, FOB is better performed without an ET and with spontaneous breathing. However, in neonates, on mechanical ventilation, only brief period of apnea may be tolerated.

Fiberoptic bronchoscopes do not have any O_2port and oxygen should be given separately by other suitable methods. The suction port of the elbow-shaped connector is commonly used with anesthesia circuit and support of ventilation.

39.6 Contraindications

There is no absolute contraindication for FOB, as most often it is indicated in sick neonates, suffering from respiratory, cardiovascular, or neurological illnesses. Therefore, the procedure should be done with due diligence and care to maintain oxygenation during and after FOB.

39.7 Limitation and Complications

FOB in neonates has some limitations.

- The smallest bronchoscope 2.2 mm does not have a suction channel; this difficulty in visualization is due to presence of secretions.
- BAL cannot be done without a channel.
- Even larger scopes do not allow forceps for biopsy or foreign body retrieval (though usually not required in neonates).
- The use of FOB for difficult intubation is limited by lack of expertise and shorter procedure time (neonates do not tolerate apnea or long periods of compromised ventilation).
- The scope needs to be withdrawn if SpO2 falls, and reintroduced, when optimized.
- Arrythmias, laryngospasm, and bronchospasm are known during or after the procedure.
- There are reports of pneumothorax, bleeding, or other mechanical trauma also [11].

Carefully planned and systematically performed bronchoscopy can be safely done in neonates [1, 7].

39.8   FOB and the Role of the Anesthetist

FOB can be performed in an awake neonate, as practiced by many caregivers in the NICU. However, as an anesthetist my personal experience entails safe and smooth procedure with mild to moderate sedation with retention and maintenance of spontaneous breathing.

39.8.1 Pre-Procedure Assessment

It is important to do a thorough assessment of the neonate before scheduling a bronchoscopy. The important concerns include

- Prematurity and low birth weight or both,
- Challenging or difficult airway,
- Frequent apneic episodes (poor respiratory reserve or on controlled ventilation - note the peak/plateau pressures, FiO_2, ABG if any),
- Hemodynamic instability (baby on inotropic support),
- Cardiac anomalies if any, and
- Sepsis.

Neonatal respiratory reserves are poor, have reduced functional residual capacity, are obligate nose breathers, and may not breathe well if the bronchoscope occludes one of the nostrils. Oral route may be used whenever nasal route is difficult.

39.8.2 Pre-Procedure Instructions

- It is mandatory to have an adequately fasted baby for the procedure.
- It is better to have an orogastric tube placed (to avoid gastric inflation during O_2 insufflation).
- Written informed consent from parents separately for sedation and bronchoscopy.

39.8.3 Pre-Procedure Preparations

- It is wise to perform FOB in a neonate in a safe and familiar environment.
- Unless the baby is too sick to be shifted from the NICU, it would be preferred to do the procedure in the operating room, with monitor settings suitable for a neonate.
- FOB should only be performed by someone experienced in FOB and well-versed with neonatal anatomy.
- There should be a separate anesthetist to administer sedation.
- A technical assistant, familiar with the equipment and briefed about the procedure, is vital.

39.8.4 Before Use, Bronchoscope Should be Checked for the Following

- **Sterility** - bronchoscopes are soaked in enzymatic detergent for 15–20 min, cleaned with 2% glutaraldehyde, and then wiped with 70% alcohol from the outside.
- **Integrity** – there should be no external damage.
- **Function** - the scope should be checked for adequate vision (white balance must be done) and maneuverability. The range of movement of the tip and the direction of rotation should be checked prior to insertion. The suction channel if present must also be checked.

39.8.5 Other Important Preparations

- The airway cart with appropriately sized devices such as nasal probes, mask, circuit, oral/nasal/pharyngeal airway, LMA (size 1), ET, laryngoscope, etc. should be ready.
- The anesthesia machine should be checked and set on neonatal mode. All standard monitoring including appropriate size SpO_2 probe, NIBP cuff, ECG leads, $EtCO_2$, and temperature probe should be ready.
- A good intravenous access should be ensured. Intravenous fluids with or without glucose, warmed adequately, may be given when required.
- Drugs for sedation and resuscitation must be loaded in dilution as per weight of the baby (midazolam, propofol, ketamine, glycopyrrolate, atropine, adrenaline, hydrocortisone, and any other if indicated).
- Diluted pediatric nasal decongestant drops can be instilled in the nostrils 5 min before the procedure if nasal route is being used.

39.8.6 FOB under Sedation

- After placing all monitors, checking patency of IV access, preoxygenation must be done using face mask or nasal prongs.
- Mild to moderate sedation can be given slowly over 5–10 min using midazolam, propofol, and/or ketamine in carefully titrated doses. Overzealous sedation may lead to apnea and therefore should be avoided. The dose to be used will depend upon the age, weight, post-conceptual maturity, and general condition of the baby.
- Strict monitoring should be done all through the procedure. The $EtCO_2$ sampling line can be manually held next to the nostrils to get a trace on the monitor (in intubated baby it would be part of the circuit). It may not show an ideal trace, but can give a fair estimate to guide the level of sedation (a visual chest rise is always reassuring).
- Supplemental O_2 can be given via a feeding tube through the other nostril (or both nostrils if bronchoscope is inserted orally). A rapidly falling SpO_2 may progress to hypoxic bradycardia, and therefore should be immediately conveyed

to the person performing FOB, who may then decide to withdraw the scope and reinsert once the baby stabilizes.

- Anticholinergic premedication (glycopyrrolate) can be given to reduce the secretions.
- The baby may move a little during the procedure, but excessive movements or struggle should not be allowed (prevent trauma).
- The sedation can be given as small boluses, although it is better to run a low dose continuous infusion. Ketamine can be used as a rescue drug during the procedure.
- 0.5% lignocaine should be loaded in a syringe for instillation through the suction channel of the scope (total not more than the 3 mg/kg).

Some clinicians do the bronchoscopy in awake babies. It helps in assessment of airway dynamics, but can be traumatic and unethical (excessive physical restraint).

39.8.7 The Procedure

The neck and shoulder of the baby can be supported and raised by a roll kept underneath for better extension (head being larger in neonates). Most studies show FOB in neonates via nasal route, but the risk of trauma and bleeding is more unless an ultrathin scope is used. If the size of the bronchoscope is relatively bigger for the nostril, then oral route is preferred (mouth guard can be used though not mandatory).

In my personal experience, I have done most bronchoscopies through the mouth, slightly more difficult to maneuver but easier to insufflate O_2 nasally, and without trauma. The bronchoscope can be inserted through an ET/LMA/tracheostomy tube, but this restricts movement of the scope and does not allow visualization of the larynx and trachea. Besides, their placement requires deeper sedation which in turn may lead to loss of spontaneous breathing (and airway dynamics as in laryngo / tracheomalacia). It is best to perform FOB without the ET, provided sedation is administered safely. If baby is already intubated, ET can be removed for the procedure and replaced afterwards.

The scope should be well-lubricated (special lubricant spray available for the bronchoscope or common jelly available in the OT-apply and gently wipe off) and advanced gently under direct vision on the external video monitor. No force should be applied to push it in any direction. Reinsert the scope when not able to progress or any resistance is felt.

The vocal cords are visualized, and the movement of the cords observed. The baby may move when the scope crosses the glottis, and therefore additional bolus of sedation or spraying of lignocaine is desirable at this step.

39.8.8 Pathologies Visualized

- **Laryngomalacia** is seen as a curled-up epiglottis.
- **Tracheomalacia** as collapsing of the tracheal wall.
- **Laryngeal web** as a cover of mucosa between the vocal cords.

- **Laryngeal perforation.**
- **Congenital laryngeal stenosis.**
- **Tracheal and bronchial granulomas.**
- **TEF** is seen as an opening in the tracheal wall.
- **Complete laryngotracheoesophageal cleft.**
- **Tracheobronchitis.**
- **Subglottic stenosis** is seen as a narrowed opening often not allowing the scope to advance further (these may be an indication for elective tracheostomy).
- The **mucus plugs** can be easily seen and sucked out (with saline irrigation) to relieve any blockage of bronchi.

In case of difficult airway, an ET may be mounted over the bronchoscope and advanced through the glottis. The scope should be withdrawn slowly while seeing all the structures again on the way out. The baby should be oxygenated well, monitored, and observed for any complications after the procedure in the recovery room. High pressures should never be used for suctioning in neonates.

39.9   Practical Trouble-Shooters

- The availability of appropriate sized bronchoscope is very important. Do not pass bigger scopes through the nose or trachea or the tracheal tube.
- Deep sedation can often lead to hypoventilation or complete apnea. It is very important to maintain a good balance between level of sedation and maintenance of adequate spontaneous breathing.
- The scope should be withdrawn, and ventilation assisted as soon as the baby begins to desaturate.
- Post-procedure nebulization may be required in sick babies using saline, steroids, or adrenaline.
- Neonatal FOB should never be done without proper planning and expertise. An extra hand is always useful.
- The presence of secretions can be troublesome in some cases. Increase the depth of sedation, use anticholinergic premedication and/or do a continuous oral suction/suction through the bronchoscope (the button has to be pressed in a sustained manner for effective suction).

39.10   Rigid Bronchoscopy in Neonates

Rigid bronchoscope has been used in the past for diagnostic purposes in the neonates. It involves a different set of equipment in smaller size for the neonates, preterms, and small for age babies. It is best done under deep sedation/general anesthesia with good muscle relaxation. The ET needs to be removed to give way to the rigid bronchoscope. These small rigid bronchoscopes do not have side port for O_2 and ventilation. This means that bronchoscopy is done in the apnea time, and therefore a limiting factor in sick neonates. Additionally, O_2 can only be insufflated through nasal prongs/feeding tube/any other device. Once the bronchoscope is removed, the ET is replaced until recovery and when extubation is possible. Standard monitoring is mandatory during the procedure. Rigid bronchoscopy is gradually fading because the FOB method is better, faster, less invasive, with minimal morbidity. Moreover, the rigid scope cannot be pushed beyond the carina as opposed to fiberoptic that can be manoeuvred into the bronchioles.

39.11 Conclusion

In the last few years, fiberoptic bronchoscopy has been successfully performed, for diagnostic and therapeutic indications, largely replacing rigid bronchoscopy in neonates. This has been possible because of the availability of smaller sized bronchoscopes and better monitoring and ventilating facility. It has helped in diagnosing dynamic airway abnormalities and lung pathologies. Its role is vital in determining the cause in difficult to wean neonates in intensive care units. It is found to be a safe when performed systematically in experienced hands. Thorough knowledge of neonatal anatomy, physiology, pharmacology, and experience in handling pediatric bronchoscopes is vital. Good planning, expertise, and assistance are the key to success. However, it should only be performed in centers where there is facility to undertake urgent thoracotomy and lung surgery in the neonate, in case required.

References

1. Lindahl H, Rintala R, Malinen L, Leijala M, Sairanen H. Bronchoscopy during the first month of life. J Pediatr Surg. 1992;27(5):548–50.
2. Pereira KD, Weinstock YE. Bronchoscopy assisted neonatal tracheostomy (BANT): a new technique. Int J Pediatr Otorhinolaryngol. 2007;71:211–5.
3. Atzori P, Iacobelli BD, Bottero S, et al. Preoperative tracheobronchoscopy in newborns with esophageal atresia: does it matter? J Pediatr Surg. 2006;41:1054–7.
4. Parolini F, Boroni G, Stefini S, Agapiti C, Bazzana T, et al. Role of preoperative tracheobronchoscopy in newborns with esophageal atresia: a review. World J Gastrointest Endosc. 2014;6:482–7.
5. Pietsch JB, Nagaraj HS, Groff DB, Yacoub UA, Roberts JL. Necrotizing tracheobronchitis: a new indication for emergency bronchoscopy in the neonate. J Pediatr Surg. 1985;20:391–3.
6. Deanovic D, Gerber AC, Dodge-Khatami A, Dillier CM, Meuli M, Weiss M. Tracheoscopy assisted repair of tracheo-esophageal fistula (TARTEF): a 10-year experience. Paediatr Anaesth. 2007;17:557–62.
7. Vijayasekaran D, Kalpana S, Ramachandran P, Nedunchelian K. Indications and outcome of flexible bronchoscopy in neonates. Indian J Pediatr. 2012;79(9):1181–4.
8. Soni A, Badatya S, Modi M, Saluja S. Neonatal bronchoscopy—a review. Curr Med Res Pract. 2016;6:192–201.
9. Sachdeva A, Chhawchharia R, Gupta D, Gupta N. Flexible fiberopic bronchoscopy directed interventions in neonatal intensive care unit. Indian Pediatr. 2019;56:563–6.
10. Mackanjee HR, Naidoo L, Ramkaran P, Sartorius B, et al. Neonatal bronchoscopy: role in respiratory disease of the newborn—a 7-year experience. Pediatr Pulmonol. 2019;415–20
11. Kohelet D, Arbel E, Shinwell ES. Flexible fibreoptic bronchoscopy – a bedside technique for neonatologist. J Matern Fetal Neonat Med. 2011;24:531–5.

Anaesthesia for Neurosurgical Procedures in Neonates

40

Pragati Ganjoo and Deepti Saigal

40.1 Introduction

A newborn can present with several conditions affecting the central nervous system (CNS) and involving the brain and spinal cord. Common neurological conditions are seizures, birth asphyxia, encephalopathy, hypotonia, intracranial hemorrhage (ICH), hydrocephalus, cerebrovascular (CV) malformations, congenital brain tumours, neural tube defects (NTDs), and Arnold Chiari malformations (ACMs). Some of these such as hydrocephalus, ICH, NTDs, ACMs, CV malformations, and tumours are amenable to surgical treatment.

Undertaking neurosurgery in neonates presents a set of major challenges to the neurosurgeon, anaesthesiologist, and the neonatologist providing pre- and post-surgical care. The surgeries are mostly high-end and the neonatal population precarious and delicate. Neonates have unique multi-system anatomical and physiological attributes and concomitant congenital anomalies. The neonatal CNS is particularly vulnerable to perioperative injury due to a still-developing brain and spinal cord, and a very different and evolving neurophysiology that is responsible for the variable and unpredictable responses to surgery and anaesthesia. The variety of neurosurgical lesions, each with a distinct pathophysiology, clinical manifestations, and management techniques, add to the challenges. Considerations of the interrelated pathophysiologic processes in neonates are thus important to fully understand the nature of the neurological abnormality and its effective treatment which would enable a successful interdisciplinary management of neurosurgery in neonates.

P. Ganjoo (✉)
Neuroanaesthesia Unit, Department of Anaesthesiology and Intensive Care, GB Pant Institute of Postgraduate Medical Education and Research (GIPMER), New Delhi, India

D. Saigal
Department of Anaesthesiology and Intensive Care, VMMC and Safdarjang Hospital, New Delhi, India

769

40.2   Neonatal Neurology

40.2.1   Cerebral Blood Flow and Perfusion Pressure

A very different cerebrovascular physiology and cranial bone development distinguishes neonates from older children and adults. An adequate cerebral perfusion pressure (CPP) is vital for delivery of oxygen, glucose, and other vital nutrients to the brain. Any perturbation in the cerebral blood flow (CBF) can lead to hypoxic brain injury and ICH. CBF in neonates is tightly coupled with cerebral metabolic oxygen ($CMRO_2$) requirements, and both increase proportionally immediately after birth. Based on the principle of flow-metabolism coupling, neonates have a lower $CMRO_2$ (2.3 mL/100 g/min) compared to adults (3.5 mL/100 g/min) and consequently a lower CBF (40–42 mL/100 g/min) than in adults (55 mL/100 g/min). Due to the fewer synaptic connections and a lower neuronal activity in the neonatal brain, neonates have a lower oxygen (O_2) requirement and a relative tolerance to hypoxemia. $CMRO_2$ increases to above adult values in infancy and older children to 5.2 mL/100 g/min with consequent increase in CBF to 90 mL/100 g/min at age of 6 months–3 years, and 100 mL/100 g/min between 3 and 12 years of age [1, 2].

The cerebral vascular response to $PaCO_2$ is poorly developed in neonates. Hypercapnia is a potent cerebral vasodilator in adults with linear increase in CBF between $PaCO_2$ of 20 and 80 mmHg, and hypocapnia, potent cerebral vasoconstrictor. The neonatal cerebral vasculature response to $PaCO_2$ is poorly developed. There is significant increase in total CBF in response to hypercarbia, but neonates are relatively immune to hypocapnia. They respond with lesser cerebral vasoconstriction to moderate hypocapnia ($PaCO_2 > 15$ mmHg) with maintenance of CBF. But, severe hypocapnia ($PaCO_2 < 15$ mmHg) results in decrease in CBF and increase in heart rate.

Contrarily, the response to PaO_2 is more pronounced in neonates compared to adults. The CBF in neonates increases even with a small decrease in PaO_2, while in adults it increases only when the PaO_2 falls below 50–60 mmHg. This heightened response in neonates can be attributed to their relative hypoxic state (normal PaO_2 is 65–70 mmHg in neonates vs 95–100 mmHg in adults) and increased affinity of O_2 to fetal haemoglobin (fHb) [2, 3].

40.2.2   Cerebral Autoregulation

Cerebral autoregulation is a vital protective mechanism controlling cerebral circulation with changes in mean arterial pressure (MAP) and extends from MAP of 50 to 150 mmHg in adults. The cerebral autoregulation limits in neonate vary with lower cerebrovascular reserve and are difficult to ascertain, but the lower limit of MAP of 40 mmHg is considered the critical CPP in neonates. While cerebral autoregulation may be intact in healthy term neonates, premature with low birth weight have a linear correlation between CBF. Extreme rise of blood pressure in absence of cerebrovascular autoregulation and fragile vasculature predisposes neonates to intraventricular hemorrhage (IVH), more so in a preterm neonate. Hence, there is a need of a tight blood pressure control during anaesthetic management to minimize both cerebral ischemia and risk of IVH [2, 4–6].

The percentage of cardiac output (CO) directed to the brain differs in neonates; CBF is 10–20% of CO during the first 6 months. The head of the neonate accounts for a large percentage of the body surface area and blood volume which places the neonate at risk for significant haemodynamic instability during neurosurgical procedures [7, 8].

40.2.3 Intracranial Pressure (ICP)

ICP also depends on age. It is 0–6 mmHg in infants, 6–11 mmHg in toddlers, and 13–15 mmHg in adolescents and adults. The newborn experiences physiological salt and water loss and consequent weight loss in the first 10 days after birth. There is a parallel decrease in cerebral volume and hence fall in ICP that can reach sub-atmospheric values along with overriding of membranous bones of the skull. Therefore, normal ICP values in neonates are not only lower than in adults, but also differ in the same neonate through the first month. The decrease in ICP during first 10 days can also lead to compensatory ventricular enlargement in accordance with Monroe Kelly Doctrine and lead to what is known as a physiological hydrocephalus that is usually mild. Drop in ICP and development of physiological hydrocephalus can mask diagnosis of a developing pathological hydrocephalus. Hence, hydrocephalus in neonates can be present even with ICP that is seemingly normal if adult standards are used; this is known as **normal pressure infantile hydrocephalus**. However, ICP is high if age-appropriate standards are used. Knowledge of age-appropriate ICP physiology and range allows for early detection and management of hydrocephalus in neonates [9].

The skull is a closed cavity with three compartments; the brain, blood, and cerebrospinal fluid (CSF) (Monroe-Kellie doctrine). An increase in volume of either of these three compartments causes increase in ICP unless compensated by reduction in other two, in adult brain. However, the neonatal cranial vault is in a state of flux. Open fontanels and cranial sutures result in a compliant intracranial space. Skull has open sutures and fontanelle, which not only provide locus for ICP monitoring and trans fontanelle ultrasound (USG), but also for slow increases in intracerebral volume. The mass effect of a slow-growing tumour or insidious haemorrhage is often masked by a compensatory distended fontanel and widening of the cranial sutures, increase in skull volume with minimal increase in ICP. However, acute increases in cranial volume due to massive IVH or an obstructed ventricular system cannot be attenuated by expansion of the immature cranial vault and often result in life-threatening intracranial hypertension. The closure of posterior fontanelle occurs by 6 months, of anterior fontanelle by 12–18 months, and of final cranial sutures by 10 years of age [2, 10].

40.2.4   Blood-Brain Barrier

Blood-brain barrier in neonate is immature and weak, permitting easy permeability of anaesthetic drugs, and thus increased sensitivity. Presence of increased amount of CSF coupled with immature myelination can shorten and decrease the potency of local anaesthetics in the CSF.

40.2.5   Spinal Cord

Spinal cord in neonates extends till L3, two segments below the adult level (L1) and the dural sac ends at S4 (S2 in adults).

Development of CNS is incomplete at birth and continues up to the age of 1 year and poses challenges to the anaesthesiologist for maintaining cerebral oxygenation and perfusion and preventing cerebral injury during neurosurgery [11]. The unique pathophysiologic mechanisms in neonates greatly impact the conduct and outcome of neurosurgical interventions. The biomechanical nature of their brain tissue, distensible skull, and widening sutures results in an abnormal head growth and resultant craniocephalic disproportions that lead to considerable neurosurgical difficulty. Congenital anomalies like open NTDs, despite timely intervention, may still result in neurological deficits due to presence of concurrent microscopic abnormalities like widespread synaptic miswirings which are not correctable by surgery. The unique plasticity of the neonatal CNS tissue determines its vulnerability to neurosurgical injury and its ability to its functional recovery, and hence, estimating prognosis after neurosurgery becomes extremely difficult in this age [12, 13].

40.3   Neurosurgical Conditions in the Neonate

A newborn can present with several neurological conditions attributable to congenital defects or premature or difficult delivery. Disorders like neonatal seizures, newborn stroke, encephalopathy, birth asphyxia, CNS infections, and congenital neuromuscular diseases including myasthenia and muscular dystrophies are mostly managed by medical treatment. Pathological conditions in neonates amenable to surgical treatment include hydrocephalus; NTD [meningomyelocele (MMC), encephalocele, spina bifida, syringomyelia, and tethered cord]; congenital brain and spine malformations like ACMs and arachnoid cysts; brain and spinal cord tumours; CV conditions (Vein of Galen malformation); traumatic brain and spinal cord injuries; craniosynostosis, craniofacial syndromes; and craniopagus conjunctions.

However, neurosurgery in neonates is generally avoided considering their frailty and increased perioperative morbidity and mortality due to a higher risk of developing cardiac and respiratory complications [14]. Hence, non-emergent surgical conditions are often deferred until after 3 months of age when surgical intervention is medically safer.

Neurosurgeries that may need to be undertaken in neonates, often as urgent interventions, include:

- Drainage or diversion of cerebrospinal fluid (CSF) and intracranial cysts.
- Closure of NTDs like MMCs and encephaloceles.
- Removal of neoplasms, anomalous masses, and haematomas secondary to brain and spinal cord trauma.
- Decompression of type-2 ACMs.
- Opening of bony fusions in craniosynostoses.

Sometimes, two or more of these surgeries may be necessary [12, 15].

Congenital CNS tumours include teratomas, astrocytomas, choroid plexus papillomas, glioblastomas, gangliogliomas, primary neuroblastomas, craniopharyngiomas, and embryonal, ependymal, and meningeal tumours. In view of their large size, mass effect, vascularity, and in context of a patient with low total blood volume, these tumours present formidable surgical and anaesthetic challenges. Malignant brain tumours are the second commonest cancers in children and most occur in the posterior fossa. Surgical resection is the primary treatment modality [16, 17]. Other rare neurosurgical conditions in a neonate are craniosynostosis, arterivenous (AV) malformations, and craniopagus twins. However, these conditions are seldom operated in the neonatal period. Preoperative embolization of choroid plexus tumours helps reduce intraoperative blood loss and protects the vulnerable neonate from haemodynamic instability [18, 19].

Neonatal head trauma may occur due to the birth process resulting in epidural, subdural, subarachnoid, and parenchymal hemorrhages that may require percutaneous aspiration of blood. A high head to torso ratio predisposes neonates to acceleration-deceleration injuries, more diffuse brain and upper cervical spine injuries, acute subdural hematomas, and air embolism [20]. The anaesthesiologist plays a vital role beginning from anaesthesia for diagnostic imaging such as CT scan, MRI, PET scan, preoperative assessment and optimization, and intraoperative management and the role extends further into postoperative neurocritical care.

40.4 Neuroembryology and Pathogenesis of Diseases of the CNS

The knowledge of embryology of the neural tube in fetal life is the foundation for understanding the genesis, clinical features, need for urgent neonatal surgical correction and the challenges encountered by the anaesthesiologist in the perioperative management of one of the most commonly encountered groups of neurosurgical conditions which comprise of **Neural Tube Defects, Arnold Chiari Malformations, and Hydrocephalus.**

40.4.1 Embryology and Pathogenesis of Neural Tube Defects (NTDs)

The development of CNS begins in the third week of gestation, around day 13–14 of embryonic life. The ectodermal cells rostral to the primitive node give rise to the neural plate. Bending of neural plate to form a pair of neural folds starts by 17–18 days post-fertilization. As the folds grow, they approach each other towards the midline, enabling fusion to occur, leading to formation of the neural tube (NT). Fusion of neural folds is a discontinuous process which starts at multiple but discrete points, starting at the junction of future hind brain and cervical spinal cord at day 22, extending bidirectionally, cranial and caudal. Another point of fusion is initiated at the rostral end of forebrain, from where it extends cranially and meets the upward closure wave from the hindbrain. Areas between the points that are initially not fused are known as neuropores. As the fusion progresses, neuropores shrink and close completely, ultimately leading to the formation of a closed neural tube in the fourth week. Cranial closure of rostral neuropore occurs earlier, by day 24, whereas closure of the posterior neuropore gets completed later, at day 26. This phase of formation of a completely closed neural tube is called **primary neurulation**. The neural tube gives rise to future brain and spinal cord till its upper lumbar level. Incomplete closure of neuropores during primary neurulation results in open NTDs. This phase of primary neurulation is followed by **secondary neurulation** which forms the neural tube in sacral and coccygeal regions. The caudal eminence of mesenchymal cells in tail end of embryo reorganizes to form longitudinal cell condensations. The dorsal portions of these cells (neural precursors) undergo canalization to form the secondary neural tube which is completed by the sixth week of gestation and gives rise to spinal cord at lower lumbar levels and extends till S2. Hence, secondary neurulation does not have a closure component. Most NTDs in this phase result from indistinct separation of neural and mesodermal tissues and are closed NTDs. The prevalence of NTDs is 1:1000 births, with regional variations [21–24].

40.4.1.1 Types of Neural Tube Defects
Spinal dysraphism ("Raphe" is a Greek word meaning line of union of two contiguous bilaterally symmetric structures) is a general term used for defects arising from incomplete fusion of neural tube and vertebral arches and is often used interchangeably with **Spina bifida**. It can be classified into:

Classification I
(a) **Spina bifida Cystica**: meningocele (outpouching of meninges) or myelomeningocele (outpouching of spinal neural tissue and meninges).
(b) **Spina bifida Aperta**: myeloschisis (absent or ruptured cyst).
(c) **Spina bifida Occulta**: external cutaneous lesion with defective fusion of vertebral arches. Neural tissue and meninges stay within the spinal canal.

In this classification, it is not possible to associate each class of spina bifida consistently with the neurological deficit. For instance, in spina bifida cystica, the neurological deficit may be either markedly present as in myelomeningocele, or limited to absent as in meningocele. The only class of spina bifida that is associated with CNS deficit is spina bifida Aperta. Because of the non-clarity of kind of neurological deficit in the above classification, a more useful classification was proposed. The above defects resulted from defective fusion of neural tube and were hence termed collectively as NTDs

Classification II

1. **Open neural tube defect:** These defects occur due to faulty closure of neural tube during the neurulation phase, leading to exposure of neural tube tissue. Chronic exposure of neural tissue to amniotic fluid in utero has toxic effect causing neuronal tissue degeneration, interrupted axonal connections, and neuronal cell death leading to loss of neurological function and disability. Therefore, fetal surgical attempts to cover the open neural tube lesion during fetal life have been encouraged, so as to arrest or prevent neurodegeneration when complete neural tube closure has failed. These defects are associated with CSF leakage and ACM.

   (a) **Myelomeningocele**: The dysplastic meninges along with the spinal cord protrude out through a defect in the posterior vertebral arches and extend beyond the spinal canal.

   (b) **Myeloschisis**: the neural placode gets plastered with the ventral part of spinal canal. There is no cystic formation.

   (c) **Hemi myelomeningocele**: Split cord malformation with part of the cord closed, the other part is open causing protrusion of neural elements along with meninges. Defects in pre-neurulation as well as neurulation lead to this anomaly.

   (d) **Craniorachischisis**: Severe open NTD in which there is failure of initiation of closure of the neural tube at day 22.

   (e) **Anencephaly**: Failed closure of cranial rostral neuropore.

2. **Closed neural tube defect:** The neural tube is closed. Hence, it is not associated with CSF leakage or marked CNS defects or ACM.

Defects in Secondary Neurulation Phase (a)

1. **Posterior lumbar, sacral, and thoracic meningocele**: Abnormality in spine leads to outpouching of meninges. Occasionally, there can be neural elements such as aberrant nerve roots, ganglion cells, or glial tissue adhered to the inner surface of the dome of meningocele.

2. **Anterior sacral meningocele**: There is anterior herniation of the dura mater beyond the spinal canal leading to the development of the anterior meningocele. These are occult lesions without visible abnormalities. The cysts are small to start with, and slowly enlarge over decades, displacing the rectum, bladder, and ureters, giving rise to difficulty with bladder and bowel function and dystocia in females.

3. **Lipomatous malformation:** Most common form of closed NTDs charecterized by presence of excessive lipomatous tissue.

4. **Abnormal filum terminale:** Presence of an abnormal filum that is shorter, thicker and contains increased amount of connective and adipose tissues. It often

co-exists with lipomatous malformations and presents as Conus Medullaris syndrome.

5. **Congenital dermal sinus:** Occurs due to abnormal separation of neural ecto-derm and cutaneous ectoderm. It is a tract lined by stratified squamous epithe-lium extending below the skin to subcutaneous tissue or deeper and often coexists with other cutaneous markers.

6. **Association with caudal regression:** Partial to complete absence of coccygeal, sacral, lumbar and lower thoracic vertebrae.

Defects in Primary Neurulation Phase (b)

1. **Posterior cervical meningocele and limited dorsal myeloschisis**: An abnor-mal midline endo mesenchymal tract grows that bisects the notochord and neural plate during the primary neurulation phase. Hence, there is a stalk with or with-out dysplastic glial elements extending to the dome or side of the meningo-cele sac.

2. **Myelo-cystocele**: This is an extension or a diverticulum from the central canal of spinal cord containing CSF that protrudes through a defect in the posterior vertebral arches to extend beyond the spinal canal; however, the spinal cord remains within the spinal canal. Common sites are posterior cervical and lumbosacral.

3. **Neureneteric (NE) cyst**: or enterogenous endodermal cysts, arising from more extensive disruption of the notochord and neural plate. However, they are rare, benign, with no neurological deficit.

4. **Split cord malformation**: Presence of two hemicords, each having a single set of laterally located dorsal and ventral nerve roots contained within two distinct dural sheaths [25].

40.4.2   Embryology and Pathogenesis of Arnold Chiari Malformation (ACM)

During the development of CNS, there is a temporary phase of spinal central canal occlusion for 2–8 days that occurs just prior to NT closure, hence CSF stays in the cranial compartment, under pressure, leading to distension of developing ven-tricles. This distension provides inductive stimulus for growth of cranial neuroecto-derm and surrounding mesenchyme. End of this occlusion phase is preceded by complete fusion of the NT. Therefore, the required distending pressure for develop-ment of cranial structures, after the occlusion phase is over, is maintained by closure of NT once the occlusion reverses. Failed closure of NT causes failure to sustain this adequate distending pressure leading to miscoding of volume determination and consequently a small posterior fossa, impaired supratentorial neuronal development with malformed cerebrum, and dysgenesis of corpus callosum as well as mesenchy-mal defects. The ventricular fluid also drains via the open NT, leading to defective development of ventricles, consequent ventricular atresia and hypoplasia. Since the posterior fossa is not well-developed and is small, it is unable to accommodate the developing cerebellum and brainstem. The hindbrain herniates cranially through the incisura compressing the aqueduct and breaking the collicular plate. Caudal displacement of the hind brain occurs through the foramen magnum into the cervical canal. The impaired development of ventricles along with impaired flow of CSF due to kinked aqueduct contributes to development of hydrocephalus. ACM is thus a precursor of hydrocephalus and 80% cases of ACM develop hydrocephalus, which can further exaggerate symptoms of hind brain compression. Overt hydrocephalus due to aqueductal stenosis is present in 15% neonates with MMC at birth. Closure of MMC defect will stop CSF drainage, thereby leading to progressive ventriculomegaly and precipitate hydrocephalus. The clinical manifestations of ACM are of hindbrain compression, brainstem dysgenesis, cranial nerve nuclei hypoplasia, and basal pontine nuclear hypoplasia, exaggerated by hydrocephalus. Presence of manifestations such as stridor, cyanosis, high pitched cry, abnormal breathing patterns, and feeding problems (nasal feed aspiration, choking while feeding, gastroesophageal reflux, and aspiration pneumonitis) are linked to poor outcomes.

The management of symptoms related to ACM II, central apnea, stridor, and vocal cord palsy involves CSF diversion as the first step and then consider decompression, if the neonate is normal at birth but develops acute symptoms despite effective CSF diversion [26, 27]. Closure of NTD promotes upward movement of herniated hindbrain. Treatment of hydrocephalus with shunting is crucial to prevent and reduce symptoms of hindbrain compression before undertaking decompression procedures. Anatomical malformations can lead to isolated lateral ventricles, leading to unilateral functioning of the shunt. Despite surgery, complete resolution of symptoms may not be possible since certain causative factors such as brain stem dysgenesis are not reversible and only hind brain herniation is amenable to surgical correction [28–32].

40.4.3 Embryology and Pathogenesis of Congenital Hydrocephalus

CSF maintains the internal environment of the brain and shields the brain from homeostatic disturbances, such as acute concentrations of serum electrolytes. CSF is produced by choroid plexus and secreted into the lateral ventricles at a rate of 0.3–0.4 mL/min across all age groups, except for being slightly lower in preterm neonates. Since the ventricular size is smaller in children than adults, turnover of CSF is also faster, and presence of non-communicating hydrocephalus leads to an acute rise in ICP in them. From lateral ventricles, CSF flows from the foramen of Monroe into the third ventricle, and then through the aqueduct of Sylvius into the fourth ventricle, from where CSF flows out via foramen of Mangendie medially and foramen of Luschka laterally, into the basal cisterns [33, 34].

Congenital hydrocephalus At can result from open NTD, Dandy-Walker syndrome, X-linked hydrocephalus, mucopolysaccharidosis, in utero IVH), and Maroteaux-Lamy syndrome. **Acquired hydrocephalus** can result from IVH, trauma, space occupying lesions (SOL) and infections. Preterm and LBW neonates have high incidence (30–50%) of IVH that causes post-hemorrhagic ventricular dilation (PHVD) and Progressive post-hemorrhagic hydrocephalus (PHH) [35, 36].

Management options include, medical treatment with diuretics (most commonly used), and surgical or endoscopic shunt placement. Invasive options for hydrocephalus include:

(a) **Surgical Ventriculostomy or Ventricular shunt: Ventriculo-peritoneal (VP) or Ventriculo-atrial (VA) shunt.**
(b) **Endoscopic third Ventriculostomy (ETV).**
(c) **External ventricular drain (EVD).**
(d) **Neuro endoscopic ventricular lavage** [37, 38].
(e) **Ventriculo-subgaleal shunts.**

All these procedures are conventionally performed in the operation theatre (OT) under general anaesthesia (GA). **A Ventricular access device** placement can be done outside the OT, by the bedside, under local anesthesia (LA), at low risk, especially in preterm neonates, as it avoids the need of GA and intubation [39].

40.5 Preoperative Assessment as per the Neurosurgical Condition

40.5.1 Hydrocephalus

Assessment begins with detailed history from parents, which reveals excessive increase in head circumference, anterior fontanelle fullness especially in upright position, episodic apnea, bradycardia, general lethargy, and abnormalities of ocular movement (restricted up gaze). Symptoms suggestive of **chronic hydrocephalus** are increasing head size, irritability, poor feeding, vomiting, altered behaviour, and developmental delays. These symptoms are non-specific and combination of vomiting and decreased feeding can mimic gastroenteritis. The rise in head circumference can be severe enough to increase difficulty in handling the airway. The normal rise in head circumference in first month of life is 2 cm [40]. **Acute hydrocephalus** can manifest as vomiting, dehydration, sluggishness, and altered sensorium, and if left untreated, may result in cerebral and brainstem herniation, cardiorespiratory arrest, and even death. The commonest form of hydrocephalus seen in neonates is due to abnormal resorption of CSF, mostly associated with IVH. VP shunting should be done judiciously in hemorrhagic hydrocephalus due to its several disadvantages and complications. Non-hemorrhagic hydrocephalus due to aqueductal stenosis, posterior fossa cysts, holoprosencephaly, or hydranencephaly can be shunted within 1–2 days of birth, to prevent subsequent massive head enlargement.

40.5.2 Intracranial Cystic Spaces

Interhemispheric, temporal fossa, posterior fossa, and other arachnoid cysts may be found incidentally or may present with macrocephaly or hydrocephalus in neonates. Those causing symptomatic mass effect or accelerated head growth may be fenestrated, endoscopically or by open microsurgical technique, into the basal cisterns or ventricle. fourth ventricular cysts and placement of shunts to drain them can elicit dangerous brainstem responses like apnea and bradycardia.

40.5.3 Neural Tube Defects

Abnormal developmental folding of the NT and anterior neuropore can vary from benign (spina bifida occulta with no neurologic sequelae) to the most severe presentation (anencephaly, craniospinal rachischisis, complete absence of NT closure). Open defects, such as MMC, or defects that leak CSF or interfere with airway patency (large nasofrontal encephalocele, open occipital encephaloceles, those with impending rupture) require urgent repair within a few days of birth. Surgeries for tethered cord syndrome, spinal lipomas, and other closed malformations are typically delayed until the patient is at least 3 months age [41, 42].

Neonates with NTDs present with swelling anywhere along the spine region. History of fever and discharge indicates rupture or infection of MMC. Assessment of motor function can be done by asking if the movement of all limbs is equal or not. Lower cranial nerve dysfunction, indication of ACM, can be assessed by eliciting history of weak or poor cry, inability to swallow feeds and nasal regurgitation of feeds, stridor, and cyanosis (cyanosis could also indicate co-existent cardiac anomaly). MMC may be associated with other systemic anomalies. (Table 40.1) [43–47].

The location of MMC is relevant for predicting difficult mask ventilation (frontonasal encephalocele), difficult laryngoscopy and intubation (occipital encephalocele), and risk of postoperative respiratory palsy (cervicothoracic MMC). Neurological deficit is expected to be present below the level of MMC, with interruption of the spinal cord at the site of the MMC, and paralysis of the legs, incontinence of urine and feaces, anaesthesia of the skin, and abnormalities of the hips, knees, and feet [24]. Only 1% of newborns with open NTD are free of handicap. Incidence of seizures is 15–25% and is most likely related to cerebral anomalies (cortical heterotopias, polymicrogyria), which are associated with ACM II [28].

History should include birth history (gestational age, birth weight, APGAR), exposure to risk factors for occurrence of NTD (antenatal exposure to drugs (anticonvulsants) or radiation, folic acid supplementation, similar defects in sibling / family members), maternal diabetes, and obesity [23]. Milestones achieved in the first month of life should be documented. Lastly, it is important to take history of vaccinations received as per the national guidelines. A detailed **general and systemic examination** of neonate should be done. Ascertain the size and location of MMC to predict the magnitude of intraoperative fluid shifts and blood loss. MMC

Table 40.1 Anomalies associated with MMC

Trisomy 18	**Common (>75%):** Cardiac (septal defects, PDA, poly valvular disease) **Frequent (25–75%):** Genitourinary (horse shoe kidney) **Less frequent (< 25%):** Gastrointestinal (omphalocele, TEF, pyloric stenosis, Meckel's diverticulum), CNS (cerebellar hypoplasia, corpus callosum agenesis, spina bifida, polymicrogyria), craniofacial (orofacial clefts), ocular (microphthalmia, coloboma, corneal opacities, cataract), limb (radial aplasia/ hypoplasia)
Trisomy 13	**Face:** Sloping forehead, small malformed ears, anophthalmia or microphthalmia, micrognathia, pre-auricular tags **CNS:** Midline anomalies, alobar holoprosencephaly **Limbs:** Postaxial polydactyly, congenital talipes equinovarus **CVS:** Septal defects, tetralogy of Fallot (TOF), double outlet right ventricle **Others:** Cryptorchidism, hypospadias, labia minora hypoplasia, bicornuate uterus, omphalocele, incomplete rotation of the colon, Meckel's diverticulum, polycystic kidney, hydronephrosis, horseshoe kidney
Meckel Gruber syndrome	Occipital encephalocele, bilateral large multicystic kidneys, fibrotic changes of liver, Polydactyly
HARD syndrome	Hydrocephalus, Agyria, retinal dysplasia
VACTERL group	Vertebral defect, anal atresia, cardiac defect, TracheoEsophageal fistula, renal anomalies, and limb abnormalities
OEIS complex	Omphalocele, Exstrophy, imperforate anus, and spinal anomalies
Jarcho-Levin syndrome	NTD, vertebral body/rib malformation, kyphosis, scoliosis, short stature short necks, limited neck movement, difficulty breathing, small malformed chest (crab-like appearance), defects – CNS, cardiac, genitalia, syndactyly, camptodactyly, typical facial features
Roberts (pseudothalidomide) Syndrome	Malformation of the bones in the skull, face, arms, and legs – Tetraphocomelia, growth retardation, hypoplasia, oligo -syn -clinodactyly, cleft lip-palate, elbow-knee contractures, micrognathia, exophthalmos, encephalocele, ear malformations, intellectual disability

and meningoceles are usually pedunculated and have positive transillumination test. Ruptured MMC with fever and pus discharge makes the neonate more susceptible to intraoperative hemodynamic disturbances. Raised ICP features may be present. CNS evaluation includes level of consciousness, measurement of head circumference, and cranial nerve functions. CVS examination is done to rule out cardiac defects. Look for abnormal facial features (may further increase airway difficulty), polydactyly, and gross anomalies of extremities. **Preoperative investigations** should include haematological (Hb to calculate maximal allowable blood loss and total leukocyte count to rule out infection), Biochemical (blood sugar, liver enzymes, serum bilirubin, blood urea, serum creatinine, electrolytes, calcium), Blood grouping and crossmatching, and others (USG abdomen, ABG, Echo) [48], radiological

(X-ray head and chest, CT, MRI, PET scans of brain and spine), and Transcranial doppler (to predict cerebral perfusion in babies with raised ICP). Altered flow signals in anterior cerebral artery upon compression of anterior fontanelle, at transcranial doppler study, suggest changes in ICP warranting shunt placement [49].

40.5.4 Craniosynostosis

Premature intrauterine fusion of one or more cranial sutures with abnormal skull growth causes craniosynostosis. Surgical management includes **strip (open) craniectomy** which should be carried out at the age of 3–6 months. Anaesthetic concerns include difficult airway, sudden and massive blood loss, and venous air embolism (VAE) during surgery, and facial oedema, need for sedation and pain management, total parentral nutrition or Ryles tube feeds, and ventilatory support in the postoperative period.

Multiple suture craniosynostosis may be associated with craniofacial abnormalities such as Apert's, Crouzen's, and Pfeiffer syndromes. Surgical correction of the syndromic categories is usually deferred for several months beyond the neonatal period. The **kleeblattschädel syndrome** (cloverleaf skull), when all sutures are prematurely closed, is the only craniosynostotic syndrome requiring treatment in the neonatal period. Currently, endoscopic procedures for single suture involvement are being carried out to prevent morbidities of open suturectomy. **Endoscopic strip craniectomy** is minimally invasive, used recently for surgical correction of craniosynostosis that offers advantages of decreased magnitude of blood loss and improved wound healing. This procedure has been carried out successfully in infants with age as low as 4–5 weeks [50, 51]. The advancement in minimally invasive surgical techniques, monitoring techniques, and neurocritical care, in conjunction with a multidisciplinary approach comprising of neonatologist, pediatric neurosurgeon, and pediatric neuroanaesthesiologist, can pave way for correction of craniosynostosis in the neonatal period in the coming future.

40.5.5 Large Cerebral Arteriovenous Shunts

The most frequent cerebrovascular anomaly in neonates is the **vein of Galen aneurysmal malformation (VGAM)**. Arteriovenous malformations (AVMs), AV fistulas (Dural and pial), and cavernous malformations have also been described. In neonates, VGAM often presents with high output cardiac failure requiring inotropes, pulmonary hypertension, and myocardial ischemia. Initial treatment of a high-flow fistula involves **endovascular embolization** by trans arterial or transvenous route in the radiology suite. Surgical resection of these vascular lesions is associated with massive blood loss, sudden postoperative hypertension, and hyperemic cerebral oedema, necessitating vasodilator therapy for the hypertensive crisis [52, 53].

40.6 Anesthetic Concerns in a Neonate Undergoing Neurosurgery

Neonates have an increased perioperative risk due to;

1. Emergency conditions of surgery.
2. Presence of undiagnosed congenital anomalies.
3. Persistence of transitional circulation in premature neonates.
4. Intracardiac shunting through patent ductus arteriosus or unclosed foramen ovale.
5. Possible congestive heart failure (CHF) associated with large cerebral arteriovenous (AV) malformations.
6. Airway difficulty - Management of neonatal respiratory system may be difficult because of the small-sized airway, craniofacial anomalies, laryngotracheal lesions, acute respiratory disease due to hyaline membrane disease or retained amniotic fluid, or chronic respiratory disease like bronchopulmonary dysplasia.
7. The immature neonatal organ systems, especially the myocardium which is highly sensitive to anaesthetic drugs and surgical stress.
8. Not-fully developed hepatic and renal systems.

Craniotomy for total or partial resection of brain tumours is a major, prolonged surgery with risk of hypothermia, hypoglycemia, fluid shifts, and massive blood loss. Neonatal brain tumours are usually infratentorial that mandate use of prone position. Poor intracranial compliance necessitates reduction in ICP and a relaxed brain that can be achieved by maintaining adequate depth of anaesthesia, hyperventilation and moderate hypocarbia, use of diuretics (Mannitol (0.5–2 g/kg), and/or Furosemide (0.5 mg/kg)), and head elevation. Preoperative embolization of choroid plexus tumours also helps reduce intraoperative blood loss and protect the vulnerable neonate from hemodynamic instability [18, 19].

The anaesthetic management for neurosurgery in neonates is impacted by:

(a) **Patient Factors** - Concerns related to the neonatal age, unique multi-system anatomical and physiologic variations, particularly of the CNS, and possible co-existing anomalies,
(b) **Disease Factors** - Concerns due to the underlying neurosurgical disease and its pathology, and.
(c) **Surgical Factors** - Concerns imposed by the neurosurgical procedure itself, craniotomy and open surgery, or endoscopic procedure.

40.6.1 Anesthetic Concerns Due to Neonatal Age

The neonate is not merely a miniature adult. There are several anatomical and physiological differences in all systems of the body when compared with adult which can have several anaesthetic implications. Although these have been discussed in detail in previous chapters, these general concerns have many unique implications when a neonate has to undergo a neurosurgery. Specific implications pertinent to neurosurgery are listed in Box 40.1.

Box 40.1 List Specific Implications Pertinent to Neurosurgery in a Neonate

- Presence of craniofacial abnormalities.
- Difficult airway.
- Prematurity and low birth weight – Immature CNS, liver, kidney, etc., postop apnoea.
- Associated congenital heart disease - hypoxemia, paradoxical air embolism, arterial air embolism.
- Hemodynamic disturbances - arrhythmias, hypotension, venous air emboli.
- Gastrointestinal reflux - aspiration pneumonia.
- Upper respiratory tract infection causing laryngospasm, bronchospasm, hypoxia, pneumonia.

40.6.1.1 Airway and Respiratory System

(a) Difficult airway: The airway in neonates is already an anticipated difficult airway, difficult mask ventilation, difficult laryngoscopy, and difficult intubation. Presence of hydrocephalus, occipital encephaloceles, and cervical MMC may further impede neck movements. Frontonasal encephaloceles result in difficult mask holding and difficult mask ventilation. Presence of syndromes with abnormal facial features can also impair airway handling. Hence, the already difficult airway of neonate can become even more difficult to handle. The difficult airway, coupled with a combination of low FRC (25 mL/kg, adults 35 mL/kg) and high metabolic O_2 demand, results in reduction of the safe apnea time, defined as time duration between last breath until SpO_2 falls below 90%, and consequently early desaturation. Safe apnea time of 25 s is reported in preterm neonates [54]. Thus, the importance of a meticulously performed preoxygenation with 100% O_2, which can prolong safe apnea time, cannot be overemphasized. However, attaining effective preoxygenation ($FeO_2 > 0.9$) itself is challenging because of non-compliant age group. Judicious use of sedation titrated so as to just facilitate preoxygenation can be tried to achieve target FeO_2.

(b) Due to higher alveolar ventilation (VA) to FRC ratio (**VA:FRC**), preoxygenation occurs faster in neonate; however, total O_2 reserves created are lower. Therefore, despite achieving target FeO_2, neonates remain at risk of **early desaturation**. Employment of apneic oxygenation methods from an auxiliary O_2 source during the entire apneic period (while laryngoscopy and intubation are being performed) can further prolong the safe apnea time.

(c) Apart from the risk of early desaturation, airway handling especially laryngoscopy and intubation can result in **hemodynamic instability** [55]. Laryngoscopy and intubation performed by an experienced anaesthesiologist trained in neonatal intubations and use of muscle relaxation can reduce the incidence of intubation-related adverse events [56].

(d) Impairment of lower cranial nerves in neonates with ACM and slow gastric emptying in presence of raised ICP can potentially increase the **risk of aspiration** in unprotected airway.

(e) Lungs are immature with **reduced compliance** and **increased work of breathing**. Mainstay of ventilatory strategy is thus use of lower tidal volumes, lower inspiratory pressures, use of low PEEP to avoid atelectasis, and higher respiratory rates, with acceptance for mild hypercapnia ($PaCO_2$ 45–55 mmHg) [57]. Application of **PEEP** and use of hypercapnia may not be tolerated by neonates with raised ICP. It is recommended to avoid hypocapnia ($PaCO_2 < 39$ mmHg), hypercapnia ($PaCO_2 > 60$ mmHg), as well as sudden fluctuations in $PaCO_2$ values during first 4 days of after birth, especially in preterm neonates who are more prone to develop IVH. Oxygen must be used judiciously because excessive O_2 predisposes to injury of the developing brain, although there are no conclusive outcome studies demonstrating poor neurodevelopmental outcomes in neonates receiving liberal O_2 (target SpO_2 91–95%) compared with neonates receiving restricted O_2 (target SpO_2 85–89%). There are no definite guidelines regarding the target SpO_2 for neonates. Most acceptable safe limits range from 87–88% up to 94%.

(f) **Length of trachea** is short, around 5 cm. Shorter tracheal length narrows the margin of safety for proper ETT positioning and predisposes both to endobronchial intubation with neck flexion and accidental extubation with neck extension. Either of these manoeuvres is usually required to obtain ideal surgical position during neurosurgery. Thus, presence of bilateral equal air entry by chest auscultation must be reconfirmed after final head positioning.

(g) The central control of respiratory rhythm and central and peripheral chemoreceptors are immature making the neonate susceptible to **postoperative apnea**. Preterm neonates experience apneic episodes up to 60 weeks postconceptional age. Breathing hypoxic mixture leads to a short period of hyperpnea followed by prolonged bradypnea and apnea. Ventilatory response to hypercapnia is present in term and is weak in preterm neonates.

(h) These factors along with brainstem pathologies and depressant effects of anaesthesia on respiratory system make the preterm and term neonate even more susceptible to **apnea and respiratory depression in the postoperative period**.

(i) **Delayed tracheal extubation** is expected in ACM and brainstem surgery due to intermittent postoperative apnea, vocal cord paralysis, respiratory irregularities, significant airway oedema, and pre-existing bronchopulmonary dysplasia [58].

40.6.1.2 Cardiovascular System (CVS)

(a) **Hemodynamic changes in neonates:** Cardiac output, which is a product of stroke volume and heart rate, is rate-dependent in neonates, therefore maintaining normal sinus rate and rhythm is crucial to maintain cardiac output and thus CPP. MAP and SBP increase by 8 mmHg in first 72 h of life in term as well as preterm infants. Also, hypotension even in non-anaesthetized neonates is not well-defined. **Physiological hypotension** is defined as MAP below which cerebrovascular autoregulation is lost leading to neonatal cerebral ischemia. Most widely used definition of hypotension is MAP below 5–10 percentile of MAP at a particular gestational or postnatal age. MAP above 30 mmHg is maintained in premature (born at 26–30 weeks) neonates to reduce occurrence of IVH. A rough guide to target MAP is the gestational age in weeks, and goal is to maintain MAP above the target value. Brainstem manipulations are accompanied by severe cardiac manifestations in the form of bradycardia, arrythmias, and sudden cardiac arrests.

(b) Neurosurgery can be associated with **major fluid shifts**. Estimation of fluid loss and adequate replacement of losses are important since baroreceptor responses to circulating blood volume are immature. Thus, hypovolemia does not lead to compensatory tachycardia to maintain cardiac output, and hypotension ensues with decrease in CPP. Over-correction with fluids can predispose to congestive heart failure (CHF) since left ventricle (LV) is less compliant and cannot tolerate overload.

(c) Hemodynamic monitoring concerns: Measurement of BP in neonate is technically challenging. The value of NIBP will be affected by the limb used and type of instrument. The bladder cuff width in oscillometer NIBP measurement technique should be half of mid arm circumference. 20 mmHg lower MAP in legs (than arms) in 8% of neonates and different readings between the two upper arms in 16% neonates have been reported with non-invasive methods [59, 60]. The gold standard method is MAP measurement, using invasive intra-arterial catheter. It is recommended in all critically ill neonates and if MAP recordings with oscillometer are less than 30 mmHg [61]. Hence, in neonates with neurosurgeries where major fluid shifts are expected such as large MMC, use of IABP in place of NIBP would be useful. For anaesthetized neonates, hypotension is defined as MAP less than 20% of baseline. Absolute target range for minimum SBP in neonates is 45.5–49.6 mmHg [62, 63].

(d) Perioperative hypoxia, hypercarbia, acidosis, hypothermia, and hypoglycemia can lead to **transition to fetal circulation** and **pulmonary hypertension**, which worsen perioperative outcome.

40.6.1.3 Hepatorenal System

Liver and Kidney are immature, and mature by the age of 2 years. GFR in term neonates is 35% of adults, with prolongation in drug clearance times of most drugs with prolonged duration of action. This can interfere with recovery and on-table extubation that is important after neurosurgery to assess the neurological outcome by a focussed post-extubation neurological evaluation of the neonate.

40.6.1.4 Thermoregulation

High surface area to volume ratio, less subcutaneous fat, lack of shivering, all make the neonate vulnerable to **hypothermia** especially during prolonged surgeries, and most neurosurgical procedures fall in this category. Hypothermia further delays anesthetic drug elimination, delays recovery, and interferes with early extubation post-neurosurgery. It also increases blood viscosity and shifts

ODC (oxygen dissociation curve) to left, with impaired cerebral O_2 delivery, transition to fetal circulation, and potential to increase ICP further. Opening up of functionally closed intracardiac shunts also predisposes them to systemic arterial embolism after paradoxical venous air embolism, cerebral embolism, and cerebral hypoxemia. All measures to prevent hypothermia are integral to neuroanaesthesia.

40.6.2 Anesthetic Concerns Due to Neurological Pathology

The neurological lesions induce multi-system abnormalities that need to be addressed in the perioperative period, e.g. lower cranial nerve involvement (altered sensorium, aspiration pneumonitis), brainstem lesions (respiratory insufficiency, cardiovascular abnormalities), pituitary lesions (diabetes insipidus, hypothyroidism, adrenal insufficiency), ACM (stridor, apnea), AV malformations (congestive cardiac failure), excessive vomiting (electrolyte imbalance), and seizures.

1. **Maintaining cerebral blood flow (CBF):** CBF is determined by CPP and cerebrovascular resistance (CVR). Preventing rise in ICP is crucial for maintaining CPP. In absence of an IV access, inhalational induction can be done to avoid rise in ICP due to crying of neonate at IV-line placement. Inhalational induction, laryngoscopy, intubation, and incision are times when increase in ICP can occur. Drugs and anaesthetic techniques can be deployed to maintain adequate plane of anaesthesia and prevent rise in ICP at these time points. Increase airway pressures (intraoperative bronchospasm) and application of PEEP increase intrathoracic pressures, thereby increasing CVP and decreasing CPP. Hence, maintaining target MAP at all times, during induction and in the intraoperative period, is essential to maintain CPP.
2. **Brainstem dysfunction-** Neonates with ACM have brainstem dysgenesis and dysfunction that predispose to perioperative hemodynamic instability and postoperative stridor and apneic episodes.
3. **Implications of drugs** - Antiepileptics can induce hepatic enzymes and increase the requirements of anaesthetic drugs, diuretics such as acetazolamide, lasix and mannitol can lead to dyselectrolytemia, and steroids can be associated with metabolic disturbances.
4. **Maintaining cerebral O_2 delivery** to prevent cerebral hypoxia - $CMRO_2$ or cerebral O_2 consumption can be reduced by maintaining adequate depth of anaesthesia, and use of antiepileptics, if indicated. Cerebral O_2 delivery can be ensured by maintaining O_2 flux and cerebral blood flow. Hb concentration, PaO_2, and cardiac output are the major global determinants of cerebral blood flow and O_2 concentration. Prompt replacement of lost blood is needed.
5. **Cerebral autoregulation** is impaired by inhalational agents, hypercapnia, and vasodilators [64].

40.6.3 Anesthetic Concerns Due to Neurosurgical Intervention

Neurosurgery in the neonate generates several perioperative concerns depending on the approach used, craniotomy vs endoscopic, from prolonged duration of surgery, sharing of the airway field, intraoperative position-related, excessive blood loss, haemodynamic disturbances, raised ICP, venous air embolism (VAE), hypothermia, delayed awakening, and seizures due to pneumocephalus. The most commonly encountered conditions requiring neurosurgical treatment in a neonate are excision of MMC, decompression of ACM-II, and shunt insertion of congenital hydrocephalus. Early postnatal repair of MMC should ideally be performed within first 48 h of neonatal life to minimize further neurological damage, risk of infection, and rupture of MMC [23, 24, 65, 66].

ACM is characterized by caudal displacement of cerebellum, fourth ventricle, and medulla into the cervical spine, and it co-exists in almost all neonates (>90%) with MMC; however, clinical manifestations are present in 15–35% neonates with MMC. Presence of symptoms of MMC, especially stridor, worsens the prognosis even after decompression surgery. Kyphosis is the commonest spine anomaly associated with MMC and kyphectomy may need to be performed simultaneously with MMC repair in the neonate [67]. The common concerns during neurosurgery are as follows:

1. Neurosurgeries are usually procedures with **long time duration** with consequent risk of perioperative hypothermia, blood loss, and drug accumulation; all contributing to delayed awakening after surgery.
2. There is an unavoidable **sharing of the airway field** with the surgeon with ETT malpositioning and kinking, and accidental extubation due to manipulation of the head during surgery. Proper communication between neurosurgeon and neuroanaesthesiologist before head movements, gentle head movements when required, and close monitoring of respiratory parameters (EtCO$_2$, airway pressures, ventilator waveforms) aid in prevention and early detection of these mishaps. Special ETT such as flexometallic and south pole RAE tubes can be considered as these can be directed away from patient's head and operative field and are kink-resistant. Use of cuffed ETT has several advantages such as better optimization of ventilation, accurate EtCO$_2$ monitoring, minimal air leak, continuous lung recruitment, and prevention of aspiration; however, their use is associated with development of subglottic stenosis in 0.3–11% neonatal population. Special cuffed ETT with low-pressure, high-volume cuffs (microcuff tubes) have reduced the incidence of cuff pressure-related complications and subglottic stenosis.
3. **Blood loss**: Except for ventriculoperitoneal (VP) shunt insertion, most are major procedures, associated with significant blood loss, hypovolemia, decreased cardiac output, and CPP. Also, reduction in Hb leads to fall in O$_2$ content of blood, decreasing cerebral O$_2$ delivery. Blood grouping and cross matching are a must during preoperative preparation.

4. **Surgical positioning:** This is a huge problem in neonates due to their diminutive size, increased risk of fractures, and epidural hemorrhage due to thin skull. **Prone position** is deployed for operating on posterior fossa surgery and NTD. It increases the risk of accidental extubation, ETT kinking, pressure neuropathies, and ocular sequalae. Therefore, proper eye padding, securing of ETT with its connectors, and padding of various pressure points are prerequisites. Careful placement of proper sized bolsters should be done to avoid abdominal compression that can raise the epidural venous pressures and increase in surgical site bleeding. Inadvertent pressure on the chest from a large bolster can impede ventilation and should be avoided. Neurosurgeries in head region often require change in head positions from flexion to extension and lateral rotation. In adults, neck flexion is permitted till the point where at least two fingers can be insinuated between the chin and chest, but there is no such definite end point for neonatal population. Excessive flexion can cause endobronchial intubation, ETT kinking, and obstruct cranial venous drainage leading to decrease in CPP. **Lateral rotation** of neck is permissible up to 45° in adults. Further rotation can cause obstruction to ipsilateral vertebral vessels. Excessive flexion and extension can lead to brainstem compression and aggravate hemodynamic instability. VP shunt insertion is performed in **supine position** with neck extension. Care should be taken to avoid accidental extubation.
5. **Haemodynamic disturbances** like arrythmias or sudden cardiac arrests.
6. **Raised intracranial pressure during surgery**.
7. **Venous air embolism** (VAE); more likely in surgeries using head elevated position.
8. The neonate is a **small individual** who can get hidden under surgical drapes. It is imperative that the anaesthesiologist should have unrestricted access to ETT, ventilatory circuits, and IV lines. Before handing over the neonate to the surgeon, check that all connections are tight and well-secured.
9. **Hypothermia,**
10. **Delayed awakening,**
11. Seizures due to **pneumocephalus**.

40.7 Effects of Anaesthetic Agents on Cerebral Perfusion

40.7.1 Intravenous Agents

Barbiturates decrease CBF by decreasing $CMRO_2$ and direct cerebral vasoconstriction, decreasing cerebral blood volume (CBV), and thus decreasing ICP in accordance with Monroe Kelly Doctrine. Caution must be exercised to avoid fall in CPP secondary to fall in MAP. Autoregulation and cerebrovascular reactivity to CO_2 are maintained.

    Thiopentone has neuroprotective properties by virtue of attenuation of ischemia-induced glutamate release, inhibition of cortical intracellular calcium increase, and free radical scavenging activity. **Propofol** also decreases $CMRO_2$, CBF, CBV, and thereby decreases ICP. Fall in SVR and cardiac output cause fall in MAP and consequent fall in CPP. Cerebral autoregulation and cerebrovascular reactivity are preserved. Neonates are vulnerable to propofol-induced hypotension that may be severe and persistent and must be avoided [68].

Etomidate reduces $CMRO_2$, CBF, CBV, and ICP. It causes lesser cardiovascular instability than propofol and thiopentone, with no decrease in MAP and CPP. However, it causes severe cerebral vasoconstriction that can lead to cerebral ischemia and also causes adrenocortical suppression. These properties warrant cautious use of etomidate in neonates during neurosurgery.

Ketamine increases $CMRO_2$, CBF, CBV, and ICP and should be avoided in cases with raised ICP.

40.7.2 Volatile Anaesthetic Agents

Nitrous oxide- N_2O increases $CMRO_2$ and causes cerebral vasodilation, preferentially in the supratentorial grey matter and consequent increase in regional blood flow. This is mediated via sympathoadrenal stimulation and mitochondrial activation. Increased CBF can lead to rise in ICP. N_2O impairs cerebral autoregulation and can also impair CO_2 reactivity of cerebral vasculature, especially in conjunction with other volatile halogenated agents.

Halogenated agents: Like most of the anaesthetic agents, volatile anaesthetic agents (VAA) cause decrease in $CMRO_2$ that is expected to decrease CBF. However, these agents cause direct cerebral vasodilation and increase in cerebral perfusion, which in excess of metabolic O_2 needs is known as **luxury perfusion**. The magnitude of increased CBF by an inhalational agent is determined by the balance between direct vasodilation and potential of the agent to decrease $CMRO_2$. **Halothane** has greatest propensity to increase CBF. In children, this increase is known to persist even after halothane concentration has been reduced, leading to **cerebrovascular hysteresis. Isoflurane, desflurane,** and **sevoflurane** decrease $CMRO_2$ more than halothane and thus lead to lesser increase in CBF than halothane. However, children are more sensitive to the vasodilatory effects of volatile agents on brain. Cerebrovascular autoregulation is also impaired by volatile agents. Sevoflurane has the minimum increase in CBF, maintains cerebral autoregulation at lower concentrations (<1.0 MAC), and has better preservation of cerebral vasculature CO_2 reactivity and is therefore the preferred agent for inhalational induction. Sevoflurane and isoflurane are the preferred agents for maintenance of anaesthesia [33].

40.7.3 Opioids and Sedatives

Cause minimal changes in $CMRO_2$, CBF, CBV, and ICP. They blunt catecholamine release and rise in ICP following laryngoscopy and intubation. Premedication with opioids can cause respiratory depression and hypercapnia, leading to cerebral vasodilation and rise in ICP. Hence, it should be used under supervision and monitoring. **Morphine** causes stimulation of Edinger Westphal nucleus and interferes with pupillary assessment. Pethidine metabolite, norpethidine, has proconvulsant action and is excreted via kidneys. Renal immaturity predisposes to accumulation of proconvulsant metabolite. **Fentanyl**, **remifentanil**, **alfentanil**, and **Sufentanyl** are the preferred opioids for their shorter duration of action. Remifentanil has a very short half-life and short context-sensitive half time. It can be given as an infusion and effect wears off within minutes of cessation. Fentanyl achieves peak brain concentration 4 min after its administration with effect lasting 15 min.

Benzodiazepines cause decrease in $CMRO_2$, CBF, CBV, and ICP. They are useful for sedation for diagnostic procedures and in babies on ventilator.

40.7.4 Muscle Relaxants

Succinylcholine raises ICP which can be offset by opioid premedication, additional incremental doses of thiopentone or propofol, and mild hyperventilation. It is useful in situations of difficult airway.

Non-depolarizing muscle relaxants that cause sympathetic stimulation can potentially lead to increase in ICP. Pancuronium increases the heart rate, Vecuronium causes bradycardia, while Rocuronium has minimal effect on heart rate and rhythm. All these drugs are metabolized in the liver and excreted by the kidneys. Atracurium and Cisatracurium do not rely on hepatorenal excretion and are preferred, as they will have minimal effect on recovery after surgery, allowing better neurological assessment of the neonate.

40.8 Anesthesia Technique: Basic Principles

40.8.1 Preoperative Fasting

Neonate should be kept fasting using 6-4-2 rule that means at least 6 h for formula milk, 4 h for breast milk, and 2 h for clear liquids [69]. Neonates with ACM and lower cranial nerve dysfunction are prone to aspiration. Gastric emptying can also be slowed by raised ICP. Such neonates may be considered as full stomach and candidates for rapid sequence induction, in the modified (mRSI) or controlled RSI (cRSI) form [70].

40.8.2 Premedication

Premedication is seldom administered in neonates; first, because of absence of separation anxiety, and second, unsupervised administration can cause sedation leading to respiratory depression, hypercapnia, and rise in ICP. Premedication just prior to induction of general anaesthesia under monitoring in the OR can be administered to blunt responses to laryngoscopy and intubation.

40.8.3   OT Preparation

Apart from routine check of OR, preparation for neonate undergoing neurosurgery includes control of ambient OT temperature, warming instruments and techniques, and readiness with age-appropriate difficult airway aids that includes appropriately sized cuffed and uncuffed endotracheal tubes, stylets, video laryngoscope with blades for neonatal age group, and flexible fibreoptic bronchoscope. Above all, presence of experienced anaesthesiologists and OT personnel cannot be undermined.

40.8.4   Induction of Anesthesia

The prime goal at induction of anaesthesia in neonates undergoing cranial surgeries is to maintain CPP and prevent increases in ICP, and these can be achieved by correct choice of drugs, avoidance of fall in MAP, maintaining eucapnia, avoidance of high pressure during bag mask ventilation (BMV), maintaining adequate depth of anaesthesia, and reflex suppression with adequate muscle relaxation and good analgesia.

40.8.5   Inhalational induction

Inhalational induction is preferred in neonates who do not have IV line in place. Neonates have high alveolar ventilation to FRC ratio, making inhalational induction faster, and also avoid ICP rise from neonatal crying. However, inhalational agents are known to cause increase in CBF secondary to cerebral vasodilatory effect, despite decrease in $CMRO_2$, and increase in ICP. Halothane has the highest potency to increase CBF, followed by isoflurane, desflurane, and lowest with sevoflurane. Hence, Sevoflurane is the preferred induction agent with its favourable cerebral effect profile and lower MAC.

Induction can be done with 1% sevoflurane to start with, and 1% increment every 4–6 breaths until neonate is induced, or alternatively, with 8% sevoflurane for rapid induction. Simultaneously, ECG, NIBP cuff, and pulse oximeter should be attached, along with establishing an IV access, preferably in lower limbs, for easy access. IV fentanyl (2–4µg/kg) along with muscle relaxant (vecuronium bromide or atracurium besylate) to facilitate tracheal intubation should be administered, followed by reduction in sevoflurane concentration. If cRSI is being opted for, rocuronium 1 mg/kg can be used to achieve intubating conditions at 1 min. Succinylcholine (1–2 mg/kg) can be used in neonates with anticipated difficult airway along with additional dose of IV thiopentone or propofol, and mild hyperventilation, to offset the rise in ICP.

Intravenous induction is preferred if an IV access is already in situ, beginning with fentanyl 2–4µg/kg, as premedicants, 5 min prior to induction, to achieve its peak effect, followed by thiopentone (5–7 mg/kg) or propofol (1–2 mg/kg). After confirming successful BMV, muscle relaxant of choice is administered.

40.8.6 Bag-mask Ventilation

Bag-mask ventilation precautions include:

- Avoiding pressure over the eyes and soft tissues of neck as this can impede venous drainage from head and increase CVP, reducing CPP.
  Hyperventilation can lead to hypocapnia and decreased CBF and must be avoided.

40.8.7 Laryngoscopy and Intubation

After ensuring adequate relaxation using a neuromuscular monitor if available, gentle and swift direct laryngoscopy and intubation should be performed by an experienced anaesthesiologist using an adequately sized cuffed ETT (micro cuff) and correct position confirmed by five-point auscultation before it is secured safely. ETT position is again confirmed after final positioning, before the baby is draped. Avoid placing an oral airway to secure the ETT, as it can lead to tongue edema and macroglossia by the end of surgery, which may cause airway obstruction after extubation. A soft bite block may be inserted if neonate is being placed in prone position.

40.8.8 Anesthesia Maintenance

Controlled ventilation using pressure control or volume control mode with O_2 air mixture and FiO_2 to target SpO_2 of 87–94% can be used. N_2O has the potential to raise ICP and worsens the effect of VAE, hence is avoided. However, there are no outcome studies negating the use of N_2O in neurosurgery. Spontaneous ventilation comes with the risk of raised ICP from coughing or bucking, increased chances of VAE due to generation of negative intrathoracic pressures during inspiration, decreased CPP and MAP as an effect of increase in inhalational anaesthetic drug requirement due to more myocardial depression in a neonate who is already sensitive to the cardio-depressant effects of volatile agents, and increase in ICP due to cerebral vasodilatation. Moreover, neonates generate auto-PEEP by various mechanisms when awake to maintain their FRC and prevent atelectasis, and this is abolished in spontaneously breathing neonates under general anaesthesia. Therefore, spontaneous ventilation is not recommended during neurosurgery.

Volatile agents for maintenance can be used for anaesthesia maintenance at concentrations up to 1.0 MAC that do not increase ICP. Isoflurane, desflurane, or sevoflurane can be used.

TIVA for maintenance leads to better control of ICP and CPP, especially in neonates where intracranial compliance is reduced. Propofol, fentanyl, and remifentanil are the agents for TIVA. Dexmedetomidine is approved by FDA for use in neonates and is neuroprotective. But there is not much evidence on its use as an agent for TIVA in neonates for long surgeries.

There is no evidence suggesting preference of TIVA over inhalational maintenance in neonates.

Neonate is then positioned for the surgical procedure, pressure points and eyes padded and protected, and ETT and circuit connections secured tightly, avoiding any drag on the ETT. Check that all monitoring equipment is well-placed and secured. Also confirm that IV, arterial, central venous lines, and urinary catheters are also well-secured and without kink or drag on them after positioning.

40.8.9 Prevention of Hypothermia

Prevention of hypothermia must be done using warmed mattress, fluid warmers, warm humidified breathing gases, warm fluids for surgical irrigation, body warmers, overhead radiant heaters, covering of all exposed parts of the neonate body, etc.

40.8.10 Analgesia

Analgesia can be provided with IV paracetamol, hourly supplements of short-acting opioids (fentanyl or remifentanil), local infiltration at the site prior to incision, and repeated at closure, depending on surgical duration. Epinephrine (1:200,000) when added to LA solution provides vasoconstriction, helps reduce bleeding, and prolongs its duration of action. Specific nerve blocks can be employed too; supraorbital and supratrochlear nerve blocks provide analgesia from frontal area to midcoronal portion of the occiput, and greater occipital nerve block provides analgesia from posterior of the occiput to the midcoronal area of the occiput, though multimodal analgesia is the modern pain management technique advocated and used. However, in neonates with low body weights and low gestational age, the safe dose limit of LA drugs should not be exceeded to prevent toxicity, remembering the potentiation of effect by other concomitantly administered analgesics, and that there should be no effect on recovery and postoperative neurological assessment.

40.8.11 Intraoperative Monitoring

Intraoperative monitoring must consist of non-invasive ECG, $EtCO_2$, SpO_2, temperature, NIBP, and urine output if indicated, and agent monitoring to keep MAC below 1.0. Monitoring of $EtO2$ should be done during preoxygenation and it is deemed adequate when EtO_2 of 85–90% is achieved. In event of VAE, EtN_2 falls earlier than $EtCO_2$. Hence, EtN_2 monitoring too is indicated for early detection of VAE. FiO_2 should be monitored throughout the surgery to avoid delivery of hypoxic mixtures and of very high FiO_2 for long periods because of the risk of ROP and BPD. In most cases, non-invasive monitoring suffices.

(a) **Invasive hemodynamic monitoring**: Neurosurgeries can be prolonged procedures with large volume shifts and hemodynamic changes, and neonates with brainstem dysfunction can be even more hemodynamically vulnerable. Since NIBP measurements may be technically challenging and not always accurate, arterial blood pressure monitoring can provide accurate beat to beat reading of MAP. Intra-arterial line is also useful for repeated blood sampling for blood gases, electrolytes, and haematocrit. Central venous line can be inserted for major neurosurgeries such as large NTD and can also be used for therapeutic aspiration of air from right heart in event of VAE.

(b) **Continuous monitoring of EtCO$_2$, EtN$_2$ and hemodynamic, precordial doppler** is advocated for early detection of VAE.

(c) **Neuromuscular monitoring** can aid in correct dosing of NMBs so as to maintain optimum intraoperative relaxation, prevent overdosing, and to help in on-table extubation.

(d) **Neuromonitoring** helps prevent inadvertent neurological damage in surgeries on spine and spinal cord and is an established monitoring technique in adult patients. Although incomplete myelination makes interpretation of intraoperative neuromonitoring (IONM) challenging in neonates, yet motor-evoked potentials, somatosensory-evoked potentials, and bulbocavernous reflex monitoring have been reported in neonates and require close communication and cooperation between the neurosurgeon and neuroanaesthesiologist, as at the time of monitoring, anaesthesiologist will need to adjust and titrate the anaesthetic technique and accordingly use short-acting agents and time the dose of muscle relaxant [71–74].

(e) **Monitoring of blood sugar, blood loss, fluid loss, and urine output** (0.5–2 mL/kg/h) should be done. The goals of fluid therapy are to maintain normovolemia, euosmolarity, euglycemia, and prevention of dyselectrolytemia. As discussed above, hypovolemia and hypervolemia are both poorly tolerated by neonates, leading to decreased cardiac output by decreasing preload and precipitating congestive heart failure, respectively. This reduces CBF and cerebral oxygenation and potentiates brain injury. Normal saline (NS) is slightly hyperosmolar and hence the preferred crystalloid during neurosurgery. However, neonates have renal immaturity and cannot handle high sodium loads and also prolonged use of NS leads to hyperchloremic metabolic acidosis. Ringer lactate (RL) is hypo-osmolar and its solitary use can precipitate cerebral edema. Moreover, neonates, especially preterm, are susceptible to hypoglycemia and require glucose supplement. All these factors have to be borne in mind to guide the fluid therapy. Glucose infusion should be given at 5–6 g/min to maintain normoglycemia and RL is used for maintenance and losses.

Craniotomies can cause significant blood loss; prior estimation of the patient's blood volume is essential in determining the amount of allowable blood loss and the time to transfuse blood. Brainstem manipulations can cause cardiorespiratory disturbances that should be immediately communicated to the neurosurgeon.

40.8.12 Lowering ICP

Raised ICP due to brain edema can be managed by:

- Increasing the depth of anaesthesia.
- Ensuring adequate muscle relaxation.
- Slight head elevation.
- Hyperventilation (moderate hypocapnia).
  Diuretics - Osmotic diuretic mannitol in a dose of 0.25–1.0 g/kg IV (it raises serum osmolality by 10–20 mOsm/kg), or Furosemide 0.1 mg/kg.

40.8.13 Prevention of VAE

Neonates are more vulnerable to the hemodynamic impact of VAE because the same amount of air enters a relatively lower circulatory volume than adults. Posterior fossa tumours are operated in prone positions and carry the risk of VAE. Although TEE and precordial doppler are most sensitive for diagnosis of VAE, $EtCO_2$ and EtN_2 are usually used for intraoperative diagnosis. Neonatal miniaturized TEE probes are available, but intraoperative use has not been documented in neurosurgery, though it was found successful in a neonate undergoing laparoscopic repair of duodenal atresia [75].

40.8.14 Extubation

Presence of normothermia and hemodynamic stability are prerequisites before considering extubation. On-table extubation followed by a focussed neurological examination has advantages of less sympathetic response related to retained ETT and lower ETT-related complications. Extubation should be smooth, avoiding coughing and bucking, without fluctuations in hemodynamic parameters, and maintaining normocapnia. Lignocaine 1.5 mg/kg can be used to block response to extubation. Residual NM blockade is reversed using glycopyrrolate and neostigmine (50μg/kg). Once the neonate is conscious and responsive, moving all limbs which are not neurologically involved and NM recovery has been ascertained, on-table extubation can be performed. Neonates who have hemodynamic instability, hypothermia, and metabolic disturbances should be electively ventilated until these disturbances are corrected. Neonates with poor preoperative level of consciousness are also difficult candidates for early extubation. A close communication with neurosurgeon to know the status of brain compliance, cerebral oedema, and brainstem handling is important before deciding for extubation. Neonates with brainstem dysfunction can undergo elective ventilation till the brainstem and lower cranial nerve functions improve.

40.8.15 Delayed Awakening

Delayed awakening in neonates could be because of metabolic factors such as hypoglycemia, hypothermia, hypocalcemia, dyselectrolytemia, or residual effect of anaesthetic drugs. Once the metabolic factors have been ruled out and neonate has still not regained consciousness even after prolonged interval from last anaesthetic drug dosage, neurological cause must be determined by using NCCT of brain.

40.8.16 Postoperative Management

Neonate should be nursed in HDU with ambient temperature maintained. O2 supplementation should be provided. Meticulous monitoring of cardiorespiratory parameters should be continued and with special vigil for occurrence of apnea in extubated neonates. Irregular respiration, apneic spells, and sleep apnea are more common in neonates with ACM and brainstem involvement. Neurogenic stridor can aggravate in postoperative period in neonates with lower cranial nerve dysfunction, necessitating re-intubation. Incomplete resolution of lower cranial nerve dysfunction, despite surgical correction, can also occur and these neonates usually require tracheostomy and have poor prognosis. Postoperative analgesia can be provided using paracetamol and short-acting opioids. Antiepileptics should be continued to prevent seizure activity. Drugs that may be used for control of seizures are phenobarbitone or phenytoin (20 mg/kg loading followed by 5 mg/kg/day) or levetiracetam (50 mg/kg loading followed by 40 mg/kg/day) [76].

40.9 Some Special Concerns in Particular Neurosurgical Procedures

40.9.1 Ventriculoperitoneal (VP) Shunt Insertion

Apart from the general concerns imposed by neonatal age, neuropathology and neurosurgery as discussed above, challenges during shunt insertion are prevention of further increase in ICP and maintenance of CPP. Due to the raised ICP, neonates who have vomited may be dehydrated and require rehydration. Raised ICP also slows gastric emptying and increased risk of aspiration, and cRSI should be considered. A large head poses problems during laryngoscopy and intubation and mandates preparedness with difficult airway cart and rescue plans. Also, surgical position requires head extension and lateral rotation that can cause accidental extubation, kinking, and signs of brainstem compression. Tunnelling of the shunt is a noxious stimulus; adequate depth of anaesthesia and adequate analgesia should be maintained at this point. Exposure of head and abdomen can lead to heat loss and hypothermia; measures for dealing with the same must be taken. Rapid drainage of

CSF from the shunt should be avoided to prevent arrythmias and hemodynamic disturbances. The complications of shunt insertion are listed in Box 40.2 [77].

Box 40.2 Complications of Shunt Insertion

- Allergic reaction to shunt material
- Hematoma formation
- Infection
- Migration into pleural cavity or heart
- Shunt fracture
- Shunt occlusion
- Valve malfunction
- Disconnection
- Over-drainage
- Outgrown shunt
- Bleeding - into subdural space/ventricles/brain parenchyma
- Injury – bowel, abdominal viscera

Neonates are particularly at high risk of complications of VP shunt, especially infection and malfunction, because of relatively thin skin, nutritional difficulties, delayed wound healing, and more proteinaceous CSF and to injury to bowel or other abdominal viscera due to the fragility of these tissues. Migration of the catheter can result in penetration into the pleural cavity or heart. Rapid decompression of large ventricles can cause bleeding into the subdural space, ventricles, or brain parenchyma. Thus, only moderate amounts of CSF are removed at the time of surgery, and patients are nursed flat immediately postoperative. Use of higher-pressure valves and programmable valves is useful [78–80].

40.9.2 Neonatal Brain Tumour Resection

Craniotomy for total or partial resection of neonatal brain tumour is a major surgery with prolonged duration in neonate. The risks include hypothermia, hypoglycemia, fluid shifts, and massive blood loss. Neonatal brain tumours are usually infratentorial that mandate use of prone position. Intracranial compliance is poor and measures to relax the brain by decreasing ICP need to be implemented. Adequate depth of anaesthesia, hyperventilation, mannitol (0.5–2 g/kg), and furosemide (0.5 mg/kg) are the strategies used for reducing ICP. TIVA is preferred over inhalational agents for maintenance of anaesthesia. Antiepileptics should be continued in the perioperative period. Posterior fossa tumours are operated in prone positions and carry the risk of VAE. Continuous monitoring of $EtCO_2$, ETN_2, haemodynamic parameters, and if available, precordial doppler aids in early diagnosis of this lethal condition. Brainstem manipulations can cause cardiorespiratory disturbances that should be immediately communicated to the neurosurgeon. Craniopharyngiomas occur in the sellar region and may be associated with endocrine disturbances, requiring steroid supplementation. They may develop diabetes insipidus (SIADH) in the postoperative period requiring replacement therapy [81].

40.9.3 Encephaloceles Repair

Encephaloceles occur due to failure of fusion of anterior neuropore during primary neurulation phase of embryogenesis, leading to protrusion of meninges and brain tissue mostly occurring in occipital and frontoethmoidal regions. Occipital encephaloceles are most common (70%) and usually contain meninges alone (meningocele) or with occipital lobes (meningoencephalocele). Ventricles may also be present along with brain tissue and meninges (meningoencephalocystocele). Occasionally, there may be other components of posterior fossa such as brainstem, cerebellum, intracranial vessels, and rarely torcula. The contents of the encephalocele along with the other associated congenital lesions determine the postoperative outcome [82].

Anaesthetic management poses several challenges to the anaesthesiologist. Apart from being associated with hydrocephalus, some of these can be of sizes even larger than the neonates' head and are called **giant occipital encephalocele**. The presence of a large occipital mass, restricted neck movements, short neck, co-existent hydrocephalus, and micrognathia imposes challenges in securing and maintaining the airway [83, 84]. Positioning the neonate for induction of anaesthesia needs care to prevent its rupture. Placing the encephalocele in a doughnut and raising the lower body to the same height can be done. Alternatively, neonate can be placed in lateral position [82, 85, 86], or the head of the neonate can be suspended beyond the head-end edge of the operating table and supported on the padded lap of the anaesthesiologist sitting at the head end, height adjusted to appropriate level, or supported by an assistant. Placing the head over a gel padded Mayfield horseshoe headrest allowing the encephalocele to hang freely beneath has also been reported. Despite the use of these manoeuvres, laryngoscopy and intubation can be difficult and difficult intubation aids including video laryngoscopes, flexible fibreoptic bronchoscope, and tracheostomy tube should always be ready. Administration of muscle relaxant must be preceded by confirmation of effective BMV. Some anaesthesiologists prefer endotracheal intubation while preserving spontaneous ventilation [86, 87]. If administered, succinylcholine is the preferred muscle relaxant due to anticipated airway difficulty. Alternatively, rocuronium can be used in institutions where sugammadex for rapid reversal is available. Movement of necks while airway management can cause brainstem compression and require careful watch on the vitals of the neonate. A co-existent ACM with symptoms of brainstem compression is associated with increased incidence of perioperative cardiorespiratory complications like arrhythmias, stridor, and postoperative apnea [88].

Surgery is conducted in the prone position that requires care of the eyes, ETT, and pressure points along with ensuring unrestricted respiratory movements. Injury of torcula, if it is present as a sac content, predisposes to cerebral deep vein thrombosis and consequent cerebral damage. There may be intracranial vessels that traverse through the encephalocele to further supply the normal brain parenchyma, and removal of such sac tissue can lead to brain infarction [82].

Cerebral malformation and lack of cerebral autonomic regulation predispose to development of hypothermia in the neonate with encephalocele who already has a large head size and large exposed surface area. Sudden loss of CSF can lead to hypotension, arrhythmias, and dyselectrolytemia. Sudden decompression can also lead to sudden traction of cerebral neurons and brainstem nuclei causing instantaneous cardiac arrest [89].

Presence of associated anomalies such as congenital heart disease can impact the perioperative anaesthetic management with its own set of problems. Anaesthetic considerations include all these concerns as discussed above along with the inherent concerns of neonatal age.

40.9.4 Meningomyeloceles Repair

Meningomyeloceles repair pose challenge in positioning the neonate for intubation. The sac can be placed in a doughnut and the remaining body can be lifted to prevent sac rupture. Presence of paraparesis below the level of the lesion warrants cautious use of succinylcholine. Bladder involvement necessitates repeated urinary catheterizations in future increasing the risk of latex allergy and hypersensitivity. Intraoperative neuromonitoring (IONM) has been deployed to minimize neurological damage during surgery and requires adjustments in doses of anaesthetic drugs and use of short-acting agents.

40.9.5 ACM Correction

ACM correction is present in almost all cases with MMC (>90%). The closure of NTD stops the outflow of CSF from the defect, leading to rise in ICP. The neonate must be followed up closely in the postoperative period for signs and symptoms of rising ICP as progressive hydrocephalus can occur which can worsen brainstem compression from ACM. This warrants an immediate VP shunt insertion. Posterior fossa decompression surgery is required if symptoms of brainstem decompression persist even after surgical treatment of hydrocephalus. Neonates with ACM leading to brainstem dysfunction have increased morbidity and mortality from cardiorespiratory events as mentioned above.

40.9.6 Craniosynostosis Surgery

Craniosynostosis is the premature intrauterine fusion of one or more cranial sutures, leading to abnormal skull growth. Multiple suture craniosynostosis may present with associated craniofacial abnormalities such as Apert's syndrome and Crouzen's syndrome. Surgical management includes strip craniectomy which should be carried out between 3 and 6 months of life to get the best result. Currently, endoscopic suturectomy for single suture involvement is the choice to prevent morbidities of open suturectomy such as blood loss and better wound healing [51]. The management of multiple suture craniosynostosis requires multidisciplinary approach for reconstruction of face with orbital advancements. Anaesthetic concerns include a difficult airway, sudden and massive blood loss, VAE, postoperative facial edema, and possible need for postoperative ventilation.

40.10 Neuroendoscopic Procedures

Neuroendoscopic procedures include ETV, placement of VAD, septostomy, shunt placement for multiloculated hydrocephalus, transaqueductal stenting for isolated fourth ventricle, and lavage for ventriculitis or IVH.

Schulz et al. stated that despite their fragility, neuroendoscopic procedures may play an important role in the treatment of disturbed CSF dynamics in preterm and term newborn infants and may be curative in few conditions like isolated lateral ventricle, isolated fourth ventricle, CSF diversion in multiloculated hydrocephalus, ventriculitis, and IVH [90, 91].

Preterm neonates have high incidence of IVH, post-haemorrhagic ventricular dilation (PHVD), and PHH (post-haemorrhagic hydrocephalus). Management options include placement of EVD (external ventricular drain), endoscopic ventricular lavage, VAD, and ventriculo-subgaleal shunts [35–38]. Early removal of blood degradation products and residual haematoma via endoscopic ventricular irrigation is feasible and safe for the treatment of PHH with the benefit of significantly lower shunt rates and fewer complications such as infection and development of multiloculated hydrocephalus compared to conventional CSF diversion techniques [92–94].

Currently, endoscopic procedures for single suture involvement craniosynostosis are being carried out to prevent morbidities of open suturectomy. Endoscopic strip craniectomy is minimally invasive technique that offers the advantages of decreased blood loss and improved wound healing. This procedure has been carried out successfully in infants with age as low as 4–5 weeks [50, 51].

ETV may not be feasible in neonates with small-sized ventricles. Although ETV carries low morbidity than open surgery, its use in treatment of hydrocephalus in neonates remains controversial [95, 96].

Endoscopic procedures are conventionally performed in the OT under GA; their duration may vary, but the anaesthetic technique employed should be such that it enables early awakening at the end of the surgery or procedure [97].

Anesthetic implications of neuroendoscopic procedures in neonates include:
- Wide variation in duration of the procedure.
- Hypothermia and bradycardia induced by administration of cold irrigation solution.
- Sudden dilation of ventricles by the irrigating fluid can raise the ICP stimulating Cushing reflex with refractory hypertension and bradycardia.

- Fenestration through a thickened floor can also cause bradycardia.
- Rarely, haemorrhagic complications can occur that might necessitate conversion to open craniotomy.
- Arrhythmias and neurogenic pulmonary edema following acute intracranial hypertension due to manipulation of the floor of the third ventricle and lack of egress of irrigation have been reported in children during ETV. However, efficacy of ETV in neonates remains controversial, and it may not be feasible with small size third ventricles [98–100].

40.11 Conclusion

Anesthetic-induced developmental neurotoxicity is known. Very low-birth-weight babies have poor and neurological and cognitive outcomes which can be worsened by cerebral injury due to cerebral hypoperfusion, metabolic derangements, co-existing disease, and surgery; aggressive management of intraoperative hypotension, hypo or hypercarbia, oxygenation, glycemia, and temperature control is warranted in neonates undergoing neurosurgery.

Technical advances in neurosurgery and sub-specialization in neonatal neurosurgery, anaesthesiology, and critical care have improved the outcome in pediatric patients with surgical lesions of the CNS; however, in neonates it is still evolving. Lack of literature and research results leaves the clinician to use ones' clinical knowledge and acquity to manage these highly vulnerable and risky patients, with equally risky surgical and anaesthetic management, for an optimum outcome.

Evidence-based management is still evolving in neonatal head and spine trauma. Fundamental knowledge of age-related differences in cerebrovascular anatomy and physiology is essential in the application of adult based head trauma protocols in neonates.

The advancement in minimally invasive surgical and monitoring techniques, IONM, anaesthesiology, and neurocritical care, in conjunction with multidisciplinary approach comprising neonatologist, pediatric neurosurgeon, and pediatric neuroanaesthesiologist, can pave way for correction of surgical lesions of the CNS in the neonatal period in the coming future. Further advances in techniques and experience will enable more surgeries to be safely performed in neonates with improved outcomes.

References

1. Pryds O. Control of cerebral circulation in the high-risk neonate. Ann Neurol. 1991;30(3):321–9. https://doi.org/10.1002/ana.410300302.
2. Furay C, Howell T. Paediatric neuroanesthesia. Cont Edu Anaesth Crit Care Pain. 2010;10(6):172–6. https://doi.org/10.1093/bjaceaccp/mkq036.
3. Rogers MC, Nugent SK, Traystman RJ. Control of cerebral circulation in the neonate and infant. Crit Care Med. 1980;8(10):570–4. https://doi.org/10.1097/00003246-198010000-00008.

4. Lassen NA, Christensen MS. Physiology of cerebral blood flow. Br J Anaesth. 1976;48(8):719–34. https://doi.org/10.1093/bja/48.8.719.

5. Vavilala MS, Lee LA, Lam AM. The lower limit of cerebral autoregulation in children during sevoflurane anesthesia. J Neurosurg Anesthesiol. 2003;15:307–12.

6. Doherty TM, Hu A, Salik I. Physiology, neonatal. Updated 2021 May 1. In: StatPearls [internet]. Treasure Island (FL): StatPearls Publishing. https://www.ncbi.nlm.nih.gov/books/NBK539840.

7. Wintermark M, Lepori D, Cotting J, et al. Brain perfusion in children: evolution with age assessed by quantitative perfusion computed tomography. Pediatrics. 2004;113:1642–52.

8. Lee JK. Cerebral perfusion pressure: how low can we go? Paediatr Anaesth. 2014;24:647–8.

9. Welch K. The intracranial pressure in infants. J Neurosurg. 1980;52(5):693–9. https://doi.org/10.3171/jns.1980.52.5.0693.

10. Parodi A, Rossi A, Severino M, et al. Accuracy of ultrasound in assessing cerebellar haemorrhages in very low birthweight babies. Arch Dis Child Fetal Neonatal Ed. 2015;100:F289–92.

11. McCann ME, Soriano SG. Perioperative central nervous system injury in neonates. Br J Anaesth. 2012;109(Suppl 1):i60–7.

12. Aquilina K. Neurosurgery of the newborn. In: MacDonald MG, Seshia MMK, editors. Avery's neonatology: pathophysiology and management of the newborn. 7th ed. Philadelphia, PA: Wolters Kluwer; 2015. p. 1017–33.

13. Juranek J, Salman MS. Anomalous development of brain structure and function in spina bifida myelomeningocele. Dev Disabil Res Rev. 2010;16(1):23.

14. Bhananker SM, Ramamoorthy C, Geiduschek JM, et al. Anesthesia related cardiac arrest in children: update from the pediatric Periop cardiac arrest registry. Anesth Analg. 2007;105:344–50.

15. Aisling M, Conran MD, Madelyn K. Anesthetic considerations in neonatal neurosurgical patients. Neurosurg Clin N Am. 1998;9(1):181–5.

16. Bodeliwala S, Kumar V, Singh D. Neonatal brain tumors: a review. J Neonatal Surg. 2017;6(2):30. https://doi.org/10.21699/jns.v6i2.579.

17. Qaddoumi I, et al. Characterization, treatment, and outcome of intracranial neoplasms in the first 120 days of life. J Child Neurol. 2011;26(8):988.

18. Crawford JR, Isaacs H Jr. Perinatal (fetal and neonatal) choroid plexus tumors: a review. Childs Nerv Syst. 2019;35(6):937–44. https://doi.org/10.1007/s00381-019-04135-x.

19. Aljared T, Farmer JP, Tampieri D. Feasibility and value of preoperative embolization of a congenital choroid plexus tumour in the premature infant: an illustrative case report with technical details. Interv Neuroradiol. 2016;22(6):732–5. https://doi.org/10.1177/1591019916665346.

20. Matschke J, Voss J, Obi N, et al. Nonaccidental head injury is the most common cause of subdural bleeding in infants <1 year of age. Pediatrics. 2009;124:1587–94.

21. Nicholas G, Copp A. Development of the vertebrate central nervous system: formation of the neural tube. Prenat Diagn. 2009;29:303–11. https://doi.org/10.1002/pd.2206.

22. Rehman B, Muzio MR. Embryology, week 2–3. In: StatPearls [internet]. Treasure Island (FL): StatPearls Publishing; 2021. https://www.ncbi.nlm.nih.gov/books/NBK546679/

23. Copp AJ, Adzick NS, Chitty LS, Fletcher JM, et al. Spina bifida. Nat Rev Dis Primers. 2015;1:15007. https://doi.org/10.1038/nrdp.2015.7.

24. Northrup H, Volcik KA. Spina bifida and other neural tube defects. Curr Probl Pediatr. 2000;30(10):313–32. https://doi.org/10.1067/mpp.2000.112052.

25. McComb JG. A practical clinical classification of spinal neural tube defects. Childs Nerv Syst. 2015;31(10):1641–57. https://doi.org/10.1007/s00381-015-2845-9.

26. Ocal E, Irwin B, Cochrane D, Singhal A, Steinbok P. Stridor at birth predicts poor outcome in neonates with myelomeningocele. Childs Nerv Syst. 2012;28(2):265–71. https://doi.org/10.1007/s00381-011-1585-8.

27. Shellhaas RA, Kenia PV, Hassan F, et al. Sleep-disordered breathing among newborns with Myelomeningocele. J Pediatr. 2018;194:244–247.e1. https://doi.org/10.1016/j.jpeds.2017.10.070.

28. McLone DG, Dias MS. The Chiari II malformation: cause and impact. Childs Nerv Syst. 2003;19(7–8):540–50. https://doi.org/10.1007/s00381-003-0792-3.
29. Gilbert JN, Jones KL, Rorke LB, et al. Central nervous system anomalies associated with meningomyelocele, hydrocephalus, and the Arnold-Chiari malformation: reappraisal of theories regarding the pathogenesis of posterior neural tube closure defects. Neurosurgery. 1986;18(5):559–64. https://doi.org/10.1227/00006123-198605000-00008.
30. McLone DG, Knepper PA. The cause of Chiari II malformation: a unified theory. Pediatr Neurosci. 1989;15(1):1–12. https://doi.org/10.1159/000120432.
31. Messing-Jünger M, Röhrig A. Primary and secondary management of the Chiari II malformation in children with myelomeningocele. Childs Nerv Syst. 2013;29:1553–62. https://doi.org/10.1007/s00381-013-2134-4.
32. Blount JP, Bowman R, Dias MS, Hopson B, et al. Neurosurgery guidelines for the care of people with spina bifida. J Pediatr Rehabil Med. 2020;13(4):467–77. https://doi.org/10.3233/PRM-200782.
33. Szabo EDZ, Luginbuehl I, Bissonnette B. Impact of anesthetic agents on cerebrovascular physiology in children. Pediatr Anesth. 2009;19:108–18. https://doi.org/10.1111/j.1460-9592.2008.02826.x.
34. Krovvidi H, Flint G, Williams AV. Perioperative management of hydrocephalus. BJA Edu. 2018;18(5):140–6. https://doi.org/10.1016/j.bjae.2018.01.007.
35. Thomale UW, Cinalli G, Kulkarni AV, et al. TROPHY registry study design: a prospective, international multicenter study for the surgical treatment of posthemorrhagic hydrocephalus in neonates. Childs Nerv Syst. 2019;35:613–9. https://doi.org/10.1007/s00381-019-04077-4.
36. Bock HC, Feldmann J, Ludwig HC. Early surgical management and long-term surgical outcome for intraventricular hemorrhage-related posthemorrhagic hydrocephalus in shunt-treated premature infants. J Neurosurg Pediatr. 2018;22(1):61–7. https://doi.org/10.3171/2018.1.PEDS17537.
37. Sartori L, Furlanis GM, Caliri SL, et al. Ultrasound-assisted neuroendoscopic lavage for intraventricular hemorrhage in a newborn: illustrative case. J Neurosurg. 2021; Case Lessons, 1(23), case 2196. https://thejns.org/caselessons/view/journals/j-neurosurg-case-lessons/1/23/article-CASE2196.xml
38. Tirado-Caballero J, Rivero-Garvia M, et al. Neuroendoscopic lavage for the management of posthemorrhagic hydrocephalus in preterm infants: safety, effectivity, and lessons learned. J Neurosurg Pediatr. 2020;26(3):237–46. https://thejns.org/pediatrics/view/journals/j-neurosurg-pediatr/26/3/article-p237.xml
39. van Lindert EJ, Liem KD, Geerlings M, et al. Bedside placement of ventricular access devices under local anaesthesia in neonates with posthemorrhagic hydrocephalus: preliminary experience. Childs Nerv Syst. 2019;35:2307–12. https://doi.org/10.1007/s00381-019-04361-3.
40. Jones S, Samanta D. Macrocephaly. In: StatPearls [internet]. Treasure Island (FL): StatPearls Publishing; 2021. https://www.ncbi.nlm.nih.gov/books/NBK560786/
41. McLone DG. Care of the neonate with a myelomeningocele. Neurosurg Clin N Am. 1998;9(1):111.
42. Thompson DN. Postnatal management and outcome for neural tube defects including spina bifida and encephalocoeles. Prenat Diagn. 2009;29(4):412.
43. Ntimbani J, Kelly A, Lekgwara P, et al. Myelomeningocele - a literature review. In: StatPearls [Internet] Treasure Island (FL): StatPearls Publishing; 2021. https://www.ncbi.nlm.nih.gov/books/NBK536959/
44. Cereda A, Carey JC. The trisomy 18 syndrome. Orphanet J Rare Dis. 2012;7:81. https://doi.org/10.1186/1750-1172-7-81.
45. Williams GM, Brady R. Patau syndrome. In: StatPearls. Treasure Island (FL): StatPearls Publishing; 2021. https://www.ncbi.nlm.nih.gov/books/NBK538347/
46. Chiriac DV, Hogea LM, Bredicean AC, et al. A rare case of Meckel-Gruber syndrome. Romanian J Morphol Embryol. 2017;58(3):1023–7.

47. Karnes PS, Day D, Berry SA, Pierpont ME. Jarcho-Levin syndrome: four new cases and classification of subtypes. Am J Med Genet. 1991;40(3):264–70. https://doi.org/10.1002/ajmg.1320400304.
48. Vernon MM, Powell D, Schultz AH, et al. Is routine preoperative transthoracic echocardiography necessary in newborns with myelomeningocele? J Perinatol. 2015;35(10):842–5. https://doi.org/10.1038/jp.2015.74.
49. Taylor GA, Madsen JR. Neonatal hydrocephalus: hemodynamic response to Fontanelle compression—correlation with intracranial pressure and need for shunt placement. Radiology. 1996;201(3):685.
50. Meier PM, Goobie SM, DiNardo JA, Proctor MR, et al. Endoscopic strip craniectomy in early infancy: the initial five years of anesthesia experience. Anesth Analg. 2011;112(2):407–14. https://doi.org/10.1213/ANE.0b013e31820471e4.
51. Goyal A, Lu VM, Yolcu YU, et al. Endoscopic versus open approach in craniosynostosis repair: a systematic review and meta-analysis of perioperative outcomes. Childs Nerv Syst. 2018;34(9):1627–37. https://doi.org/10.1007/s00381-018-3852-4.
52. Burrows PE, Robertson RL. Neonatal central nervous system vascular disorders. Neurosurg Clin N Am. 1998;9:155–80.
53. Zuccaro G, et al. Neurosurgical vascular malformations in children under 1 year of age. Childs Nerv Syst. 2010;26(10):1381.
54. Kothari R, Hodgson KA, Davis PG, et al. Time to desaturation in preterm infants undergoing endotracheal intubation. Arch Dis Child Fetal Neonatal Ed. 2021;106(6):603–7. https://doi.org/10.1136/archdischild-2020-319509.
55. Marshall TA, Deeder R, Pai S, Berkowitz GP, Austin TL. Physiologic changes associated with endotracheal intubation in preterm infants. Crit Care Med. 1984;12(6):501–3. https://doi.org/10.1097/00003246-198406000-00006.
56. Foglia EE, Ades A, Napolitano N, Leffelman J, et al. Factors associated with adverse events during tracheal intubation in the NICU. Neonatology. 2015;108(1):23–9. https://doi.org/10.1159/000381252.
57. Bang SR. Neonatal anesthesia: how we manage our most vulnerable patients. Korean J Anesthesiol. 2015;68(5):434–41. https://doi.org/10.4097/kjae.2015.68.5.434.
58. Kuan CC, Shaw SJ. Anesthesia for major surgery in the neonate. Anesthesiol Clin. 2020;38(1):1–18. https://doi.org/10.1016/j.anclin.2019.10.001.
59. Gevers M, van Genderingen HR, Lafeber HN, Hack WW. Accuracy of oscillometric blood pressure measurement in critically ill neonates with reference to the arterial pressure wave shape. Intensive Care Med. 1996;22:242–8.
60. Dannevig I, Dale HC, Liestol K, Lindemann R. Blood pressure in the neonate: three non-invasive oscillometric pressure monitors compared with invasively measured blood pressure. Acta Paediatr. 2005;94:191–6.
61. Dionne JM, Bremner SA, Baygani SK, Batton B, et al. Method of blood pressure measurement in neonates and infants: a systematic review and analysis. J Pediatr. 2020;221:23–31.
62. Kussman BD, Madril DR, Thiagarajan RR, et al. Anesthetic management of the neonate with congenital complete heart block: 16-year review. Paediatr Anaesth. 2005;15:1059–66.
63. Nafiu OO, Voepel-Lewis T, Morris M, et al. How do pediatric anesthesiologists define intraoperative hypotension? Paediatr Anaesth. 2009;19:1048–53.
64. Severinghaus JW, Lassen N. Step hypocapnia to separate arterial from tissue PCO_2 in the regulation of cerebral blood flow. Circ Res. 1967;20:272–8.
65. Oncel MY, Ozdemir R, Kahilogulları G, et al. The effect of surgery time on prognosis in newborns with meningomyelocele. J Korean Neurosurg Soc. 2012;51(6):359–62. https://doi.org/10.3340/jkns.2012.51.6.359.
66. Cherian J, Staggers KA, Pan IW, et al. Thirty-day outcomes after postnatal myelomeningocele repair: a National Surgical Quality Improvement Program Pediatric database analysis. J Neurosurg Pediatr. 2016;18(4):416–22. https://doi.org/10.3171/2016.1.PEDS15674.
67. Özdemir N, Özdemir SA, Özer EA. Kyphectomy in neonates with meningomyelocele. Childs Nerv Syst. 2019;35(4):673–81. https://doi.org/10.1007/s00381-018-4006-4.

68. Vanderhaegen J, Naulaers G, Van Huffel S, et al. Cerebral and systemic hemodynamic effects of intravenous bolus administration of propofol in neonates. Neonatology. 2010;98:57–63.

69. American Society of Anesthesiologists. Practice guidelines for preoperative fasting and the use of pharmacologic agents to reduce the risk of pulmonary aspiration: an updated report. Anesthesiology. 2011;114:495–511.

70. Newton R, Hack H. Place of rapid sequence induction in paediatric anaesthesia. BJA Edu. 2016;16(4):120–3. https://doi.org/10.1093/bjaceaccp/mkv024.

71. Flanders TM, Franco AJ, Hines SJ, et al. Neonatal intraoperative neuromonitoring in thoracic myelocystocele: a case report. Childs Nerv Syst. 2020;36:435–9. https://doi.org/10.1007/s00381-019-04380-0.

72. Gisi G, Boran OF. Anesthesia management during meningomyelocele repair alongside motor-evoked potentials in a newborn and a small infant. Childs Nerv Syst. 2020;36(11):3053–7. https://doi.org/10.1007/s00381-020-04579-6.

73. Aydinlar EI, Dikmen PY, Kocak M, et al. Intraoperative neuromonitoring of motor-evoked potentials in infants undergoing surgery of the spine and spinal cord. J Clin Neurophysiol. 2019;36(1):60–5. https://doi.org/10.1097/WNP.0000000000000523.

74. Fulkerson DH, Satyan KB, Wilder LM, et al. Intraoperative monitoring of motor evoked potentials in very young children. J Neurosurg Pediatr. 2011;7(4):331–7. https://thejns.org/pediatrics/view/journals/j-neurosurg-pediatr/7/4/article-p331.xml

75. Lalwani K, Aliason I. Cardiac arrest in the neonate during laparoscopic surgery. Anesth Analg. 2009;109(3):760–2. https://doi.org/10.1213/ane.0b013e3181adc6f9.

76. Slaughter LA, Patel AD, Slaughter JL. Pharmacological treatment of neonatal seizures: a systematic review. J Child Neurol. 2013;28(3):351–64. https://doi.org/10.1177/0883073812470734.

77. Hamid RKA, Newfield P. Pediatric neuroanesthesia: hydrocephalus. Anesthesiol Clin N Am. 2001;19(2):207–18. https://doi.org/10.1016/S0889-8537(05)70224-8.

78. Frim DM, Scott RM, Madsen JR. Surgical management of neonatal hydrocephalus. Neurosurg Clin N Am. 1998;9(1):105.

79. Morimoto K, et al. Two-step procedure for early neonatal surgery of fetal hydrocephalus. Neurol Med Chir (Tokyo). 1993;33(3):158.

80. Ventriculomegaly Trial Group. Randomised trial of early tapping in neonatal posthaemorrhagic ventricular dilatation: results at 30 months. Arch Dis Child Fetal Neonatal Ed. 1994;70(2):F129.

81. Müller-Scholden J, Lehrnbecher T, Müller HL, et al. Radical surgery in a neonate with Craniopharyngioma. Pediatr Neurosurg. 2000;33:265–9. https://doi.org/10.1159/000055967.

82. Singh N, Rao PB, Ambesh SP, Gupta D. Anaesthetic management of a giant encephalocele: size does matter. Pediatr Neurosurg. 2012;48(4):249–52. https://doi.org/10.1159/000346904.

83. Agrawal A, Lakhkar BB, Lakhkar B, Grover A. Giant occipital encephalocele associated with microcephaly and micrognathia. Pediatr Neurosurg. 2008;44(6):515–6. https://doi.org/10.1159/000187128.

84. Black SA, Galvez JA, Rehman MA, Schwartz AJ. Images in anesthesiology: airway management in an infant with a giant occipital encephalocele. Anesthesiology. 2014;120(6):1504. https://doi.org/10.1097/ALN.0b013e31829f028a.

85. Dey N, Gombar KK, Khanna AK, Khandelwal P. Airway management in neonates with occipital encephalocele - adjustments and modifications. Pediatr Anesth. 2007;17(11):1119–20. https://doi.org/10.1111/j.1460-9592.2007.02311.x.

86. Kokulu S, Karavelioğlu E. Anesthetic management in a newborn with a giant occipital encephalocele: a case report. J Anesth. 2013;27(5):793–4. https://doi.org/10.1007/s00540-013-1585-9.

87. Mayhew JF. Anesthsia in neonates with large encephaloceles. Pediatr Anesth. 2009;19(6):624. https://doi.org/10.1111/j.1460-9592.2009.03029.x.

88. Mahajan C, Rath GP, Dash HH, Bithal PK. Perioperative management of children with encephalocele: an institutional experience. J Neurosurg Anesthesiol. 2011;23(4):352–6. https://doi.org/10.1097/ANA.0b013e31821f93dc.

89. Mahajan C, Rath GP, Bithal PK, Mahapatra AK. Perioperative management of children with giant encephalocele. J Neurosurg Anesthesiol. 2017;29(3):322–9. https://doi.org/10.1097/ana.0000000000000282.

90. Schulz M, Bührer C, Spors B, Haberl H, Thomale UW. Endoscopic neurosurgery in preterm and term newborn infants--a feasibility report. Childs Nerv Syst 2013; 29(5):771–779. doi:https://doi.org/10.1007/s00381-012-2003-6.

91. Bowes AL, King-Robson J, Dawes W, et al. Neuroendoscopic surgery in children: does age at intervention influence safety and efficacy? A single-center experience. J Neurosurg Pediatr. 2017;20(4):324–8. https://doi.org/10.3171/2017.4.peds16488.

92. Etus V, Kahilogullari G, Karabagli H, et al. Early endoscopic ventricular irrigation for the treatment of neonatal Posthemorrhagic hydrocephalus: a feasible treatment option or not? A multicenter study. Turk Neurosurg. 2018;28(1):137–41. https://doi.org/10.5137/1019-5149.JTN.18677-16.0.

93. Cearns MD, Kommer M, Amato-Watkins A, et al. Opening and closure of intraventricular neuroendoscopic procedures in infants under 1 year of age: institutional technique, case series and review of the literature. Childs Nerv Syst. 2021;37(1):101–5. https://doi.org/10.1007/s00381-020-04895-x. Epub 2020 Sep 27.

94. Schulz M, Bührer C, Pohl-Schickinger A, et al. Neuroendoscopic lavage for the treatment of intraventricular hemorrhage and hydrocephalus in neonates. J Neurosurg Pediatr. 2014;13(6):706(1):101–105. https://doi.org/10.1007/s00381-020-04895-x.

95. Gorayeb RP, Cavalheiro S, Zymberg ST. Endoscopic third ventriculostomy in children younger than 1 year of age. J Neurosurg. 2004;100(5):427–9. https://doi.org/10.3171/ped.2004.100.5.0427.

96. Balthasar AJ, Kort H, Cornips EM, et al. Analysis of the success and failure of endoscopic third ventriculostomy in infants less than 1 year of age. Childs Nerv Syst. 2007;23(2):151–5. https://doi.org/10.1007/s00381-006-0219-z.

97. Meier PM, Guzma.n R, Erb TO. Endoscopic pediatric neurosurgery: implications for anesthesia. Pediatr Anesth. 2014;24(7):668–77. https://doi.org/10.1111/pan.12405.

98. Fritsch MJ, Kienke S, Ankermann T, et al. Endoscopic third ventriculostomy in infants. J Neurosurg. 2005;103(1 Suppl):50–3. https://doi.org/10.3171/ped.2005.103.1.0050.

99. Sufianov AA, Sufianova GZ, Iakimov IA. Endoscopic third ventriculostomy in patients younger than 2 years: outcome analysis of 41 hydrocephalus cases. J Neurosurg Pediatr. 2010;5(4):392–401. https://doi.org/10.3171/2009.11.PEDS09197.

100. Duru S, Peiro JL, Oria M, Aydin E, et al. Successful endoscopic third ventriculostomy in children depends on age and etiology of hydrocephalus: outcome analysis in 51 pediatric patients. Childs Nerv Syst. 2018;34(8):1521–8. https://doi.org/10.1007/s00381-018-3811-0.

Exstrophy Bladder or Ectopia Vesicae

41

Ranju Gandhi and Usha Saha

41.1 Introduction

The bladder exstrophy-epispadias-cloacal exstrophy complex is a constellation of ventral wall defects caused by a developmental abnormality 4–5 weeks after conception. Bladder exstrophy exists concomitantly with epispadias due to failure of lateral body wall folds to close in the midline, leaving the urethral meatus on the dorsum of the penis [1].

Bladder exstrophy /ectopia vesicae is a rare congenital malformation of the genitourinary system. The reported incidence is 1:10,000–50,000 live births, 2–3 times more common in male newborns. Basic anomaly is nonclosure of anterior bladder wall and anterior abdominal wall, exposing the bladder mucosa to the outside. This is associated with separation of pelvic bone, malrotation, so that the gap in the lower abdomen and pelvis is very wide. Urethra may not be closed properly with occurrence of epispadias. Management requires early closure of the bladder and abdominal wall along with pelvic osteotomy and approximation of pubic symphysis. Both intraoperative and postoperative management are very challenging both for the anesthesiologist and the surgeon. Postoperative pain management and pelvic and lower limb immobilization are imminent for several weeks until healing occurs. Babies have been operated in the neonatal period, but this is associated with high morbidity. This chapter will discuss the embryological abnormality responsible for the defect, various surgical components, and anesthetic management, and perioperative pain management [2].

R. Gandhi (✉)
Department of Anaesthesia, VMMC and Safdarjung Hospital, New Delhi, India

U. Saha
Department of Anesthesia, Critical Care, Pain and Palliative Care, LHMC, SSK and KSC Hospitals, New Delhi, India

41.2   Embryology

The bladder and ureterovesical junction are formed during 4–6 weeks of gestation and arise from the primitive urogenital sinus following subdivision of the cloaca. The bladder develops through mesenchymal-epithelial interactions between the endoderm of the urogenital sinus and mesodermal mesenchyme.

Various theories have been proposed for the genesis of **bladder exstrophy** or the **exstrophy-epispadias complex (EEC)** including obstruction or failure of mesenchymal migration [3], premature rupture of cloacal membrane [4] (prior to the fusion of the uro-rectal septum and the cloacal membrane), abnormal cell-cell interactions, and alteration in cell death. Another theory is persistence of pubic diastasis and open bony pelvis. The pelvic musculature rests behind the hindgut and urogenital sinus. Pubic diastasis is normal in early gestation, and by 8–10 weeks, the pubic bones rotate, with approximation and closure of the pubic symphysis. In pubic diastasis, because of malrotation of the pelvic bones, as the fetus grows and posterior musculature develops, it exerts anterior pressure, preventing normal rotation and approximation of the pubic bone and symphysis, disrupting closure of the bladder and abdominal walls, consequent exstrophy [5]. Three types of defects (EEC) may occur [6, 7]:

1. Cloacal exstrophy,
2. Classical bladder exstrophy, or
3. Epispadias. **OEIS complex** (Omphalocele, Exstrophy of the cloaca, Imperforate anus, and Spinal defects) is the most severe form of **EEC**. It is extremely rare with an incidence of 1:200,000–400,000 live births, sporadic in occurrence, with strong association with genetic defects, spina bifida, intersex, environmental exposures, twinning, and in vitro fertilization. Babies have specific facial features, developmental delays, and heart, skeletal, genitourinary, and neurological defects [8].

41.3   Pathophysiology

41.3.1 Bone Defect

They have a widened **pubic symphysis**, short pubic rami, retroverted acetabulum, wide sacroiliac joints, and larger sacrum [9]. **Spinal and Neurological** defects are present in nearly all babies including spina bifida occulta, scoliosis, hemivertebrae [10] neural tube defects (NTD), and tethered cord [11], and they add on to the severity of already present urinary and bowel incontinence. Other bony defects include clubfoot, tibial malformations, and congenital hip dislocation [8]. **Pelvic floor** musculature is abnormal, anus and bladder are more anterior [9], and these predispose female patients to uterine prolapse [12]. The **ventral abdominal wall** fascia is absent, umbilicus is more caudal position (at the upper limit), and with a small or large omphalocele depending on the degree of maldevelopment [8].

41.3.2 Anorectal Displacement

Anorectal displacement predisposes the baby to fecal incontinence. GI defects are very frequent in the form of imperforate anus, rectal stenosis, rectal prolapse [13], rudimentary hindgut, malrotation, and short bowel [8, 14].

41.3.3 Genitalia

Genitalia is profoundly abnormal, e.g., dorsal urethral meatus, epispadias, and short penis in males, and short stenotic vagina, bifid clitoris, and divergent labia in females [15]. **Bladder** is open anteriorly, undeveloped, small, and poorly compliant. Ureters enter the bladder at an abnormal angle with vesicoureteral reflux. Horseshoe kidney is very common in EEC [16].

41.4   Diagnosis and Postnatal Care

EEC can be diagnosed during prenatal sonography in the early second trimester and confirmed at 32 weeks of gestation [17]. Sonography findings are absent bladder filling, low set umbilicus, wide pubic rami, anterior anus, small genitalia, and lower abdominal mass [18], genitalia defects, and constant urine seepage. Male babies have epispadias, undescended testis, and/or inguinal hernia. Female babies may have epispadias, bifid clitoris, separated labia, absent vagina, and/or bifid uterus. Prenatal diagnosis allows for parental counselling, prognosis, and treatment approaches.

Postnatal diagnosis is by the evident defect. Babies must undergo renal, cardiac, pulmonary, and neurosurgical evaluation soon after birth. The exposed bladder and bowel segments should be covered with non-adherent dressing, kept clean using saline, and changed frequently. Evaluation under anesthesia (EUA) is done to ascertain the extent of defects and formulate management strategy. These babies should be managed at a tertiary neonatal center [19].

41.5   Surgical Management

Surgical repair of EEC is challenging because of the rarity and complexity of the defect. Basic repair is closure of the bladder, closure of anterior abdominal wall, approximation of the pubic rami, and epispadias and chordae correction. Bladder and abdominal wall closure should be done as early as possible, but pelvic osteotomy should be done only after 72 h age, when pelvis is still malleable.

41.5.1 Surgical Approaches Include

1. **CPRE- Complete Primary Repair of exstrophy**, preferred technique with low costless inflammation and fibrosis, improved bladder growth, and less need for urinary diversion [20– 24], and

2. **MSRE- Modern Staged Repair of Exstrophy** [25] that involves three surgeries: **The first stage** (within 2–3 days of life) includes bladder and abdominal wall closure, reconstruction of belly button, and osteotomy (>72 h age). **The second stage** (at 6–12 months of age) includes epispadias repair in boys, and urethral and labial repair in girls. **The third stage** (at 6–10 years age) for bladder neck reconstruction and bilateral ureteral reimplantation.

41.5.2 Other Surgical Approaches Described are

1. **Erlangen repair** - delayed complete one-stage repair at 8–10 weeks of age, allowing for stabilization and growth of the infant. Continence rates as similar to MSRE [26].
2. **Kelly repair** - an alternative staged repair, in which, instead of pelvic osteotomy, closure is accomplished through soft tissue mobilization from their attachment to the pelvic sidewall. Continence rates are similar to MSRE; however, the lower abdominal wall has an abnormal appearance [27].
3. **Warsaw approach** - is a two-stage approach, with early abdominal wall and bladder closure and lower extremity and pelvic immobilization, followed by additional surgeries at leisure [28].

41.5.3 Postoperatively

Postoperatively, these babies require immobilization of the pelvis and lower limbs for several weeks, especially if pelvic osteotomy has been done. This is extremely painful and continuous pain management for 4–6 weeks is essential. Immobilization can be achieved by:

(a) **External fixator-** Traction is adjusted according to the degree of pelvic diastasis as assessed on pelvic radiology, after 7–10 days of surgery and then at 4 weeks,
(b) **Spica cast application,** instead of painful external fixator, that creates problems with nursing care and feeding, immobilization can be achieved with similar results, or.
(c) **"Mummy wrapping"** the child's legs, though simple and less painful, is less secure and has poor results [29].

70% of these children can live without incontinence and with normal urethral voiding, and with minimal complication rate [30].

41.5.4 Preoperative Care

Preoperative care is directed towards less exposure of bladder and other viscera, and minimizing trauma and risk of infection. A non-adherent film dressing is applied, kept wet and cleaned with saline, and changed frequently as it becomes soaked with urine.

41.6 Preanesthetic Assessment

Components of PAE are:

1. A thorough assessment of the severity of the EEC defect,
2. Other organ systems, especially cardiac, pulmonary, and renal function assessment,
3. Discussion with the surgeon as to the plan of surgery, Primary or Staged, and.
4. Parental counselling and informed consent.

41.7 Anesthesia Concerns

(a) CPRE approach, though preferred, increases the risk of surgery and anesthesia because of prolonged duration (4–6 h), increased blood loss, hypothermia, and high complication rate (wound dehiscence, bladder prolapse, vesicocutaneous fistula, penile loss [31–33], and urinary incontinence [34, 35].
(b) MSRE approach has the disadvantage that it takes 10 years for full repair, but improves the safety in the neonate.

Preoperative investigations include Hb and complete blood counts, blood urea, serum creatinine and electrolytes, blood group and cross matching, and urinalysis (routine, microscopic examination, culture, and sensitivity).

41.8 Anesthesia Management

General principles of neonatal anesthesia need to be followed. Surgery requires general anesthesia, endotracheal intubation, and controlled ventilation. Two IV lines should be secured. Standard noninvasive monitoring is sufficient and includes ECG, NIBP, SpO_2, $EtCO_2$, and temperature. Central venous catheters are useful and can be considered as they can be utilized postoperatively for fluids, drug, TPN administration, as well as for blood sampling.

Caudal epidural catheter by ultrasound or landmark guided technique can be placed to facilitate intraoperative and postoperative analgesia. Catheter should be tunneled subcutaneously as it must be kept for 4–6 weeks, the entire postoperative period. Local anesthetic with additives (clonidine or dexmedetomidine) is preferred to fentanyl (short acting), and to morphine (respiratory depression). Measures should be taken to prevent hypothermia by use of fluid warmers and forced air blankets.

Care must be taken to prevent reopening of intracardiac shunts and PFC (persistent fetal circulation) and risk of ROP with high FiO_2.

41.9 Postoperative Management

- Pain management for 4–6 weeks,
- Antimicrobial prophylaxis (risk of infection due to stents, drains, pelvic fixator pins, osteotomy, and urine spillage). Other reasons are potential wound dehiscence and infection, pyelonephritis, vesicoureteral reflux, and additional surgical interventions,
- The wound should remain dry and free from tension,
- Pelvic and lower limb immobilization,
- Care to prevent accidental drag and removal of abdominal and bladder drains (suprapubic catheter), urethral catheter, and ureteral stents for the entire duration of immobilization,
- Early feeds or TPN,
- Care in a thermoneutral environment, and
- Adequate hydration and maintenance of volume status.

41.10 Conclusion

Management of bladder exstrophy has significantly changed over the last few decades. Surgery includes bladder and abdominal wall closure, pelvic osteotomy, postoperative traction and immobilization, pain and sedation management, nutritional management, and advanced pediatric nursing care. A team of pediatric urologists, orthopedic surgeons, anesthesiologists, pediatricians, pediatric nursing staff, and other hospital staff working together can provide the child with the best chance for a functional and cosmetic result. Most children can lead a dry life with normal urethral voidance and minimum complications.

References

1. El-Hattab AW, Skorupski JC, Hsieh MH, Breman AM, Petal. OEIS complex associated with chromosome 1p36 deletion: a case report and review. Am J Med Genet A. 2010;152A(2):504–11. https://doi.org/10.1002/ajmg.a.33226.
2. Massanyi EZ, Gearhart JP, Kost-Byerly S. Perioperative management of classic bladder exstrophy. Res Rep Urol. 2013;5:67–75. https://doi.org/10.2147/RRU.S29087. Published online 2013 Mar 12.
3. Vermeij-Keers C, Hartwig NG, van der Werff JF. Embryonic development of the ventral body wall and its congenital malformations. Semin Pediatr Surg. 1996;5(2):82–9.
4. Ambrose SS, O'Brien DP. 3rd surgical embryology of the exstrophy-epispadias complex. Surg Clin North Am. 1974;54(6):1379–90.
5. Beaudoin S, Barbet P, Bargy F. Pelvic development in the rabbit embryo: implications in the organogenesis of bladder exstrophy. Anat Embryol (Berl). 2004;208(6):425–30.
6. Muecke EC. The role of the cloacal membrane in exstrophy: the first successful experimental study. J Urol. 1964;92:659–67.

7. Martínez-Frías ML, Bermejo E, Rodríguez-Pinilla E, Frías JL. Exstrophy of the cloaca and exstrophy of the bladder: two different expressions of a primary developmental field defect. Am J Med Genet. 2001;99(4):261–9.
8. Diamond DA, Jeffs RD. Cloacal exstrophy: a 22-year experience. J Urol. 1985;133(5):779–82.
9. Stec AA, Pannu HK, Tadros YE, et al. Evaluation of the bony pelvis in classic bladder exstrophy by using 3D-CT: further insights. Urology. 2001;58(6):1030–5.
10. Cadeddu JA, Benson JE, Silver RI, Lakshmanan Y, et al. Spinal abnormalities in classic bladder exstrophy. Br J Urol. 1997;79(6):975–8.
11. McLaughlin KP, Rink RC, Kalsbeck JE, et al. Cloacal exstrophy: the neurological implications. J Urol. 1995;154(2 Pt 2):782–4.
12. Woodhouse CR, Hinsch R. The anatomy and reconstruction of the adult female genitalia in classical exstrophy. Br J Urol. 1997;79(4):618–22.
13. Stec AA, Baradaran N, Tran C, Gearhart JP. Colorectal anomalies in patients with classic bladder exstrophy. J Pediatr Surg. 2011;46(9):1790–3.
14. Hurwitz RS, Manzoni GA, Ransley PG, Stephens FD. Cloacal exstrophy: a report of 34 cases. J Urol. 1987;138(4 Pt 2):1060–4.
15. Ansari MS, Gearhart JP, Cervellione RM, Sponseller PD. The application of pelvic osteotomy in adult female patients with exstrophy: applications and outcomes. BJU Int. 2011;108(6):908–12.
16. Stec AA, Baradaran N, Gearhart JP. Congenital renal anomalies in patients with classic bladder exstrophy. Urology. 2012;79(1):207–9.
17. Ebert AK, Reutter H, Ludwig M, Rösch WH. The exstrophy-epispadias complex. Orphanet J Rare Dis. 2009;4:23.
18. Gearhart JP, Ben-Chaim J, Jeffs RD, Sanders RC. Criteria for the prenatal diagnosis of classic bladder exstrophy. Obstet Gynecol. 1995;85(6):961–4.
19. Nelson CP, Bloom DA, Dunn RL, Wei JT. Bladder exstrophy in the newborn: a snapshot of contemporary practice patterns. Urology. 2005;66(2):411–5.
20. Nelson CP, North AC, Ward MK, Gearhart JP. Economic impact of failed or delayed primary repair of bladder exstrophy: differences in cost of hospitalization. J Urol. 2008;179(2):680–3.
21. Dodson JL, Surer I, Baker LA, Jeffs RD, Gearhart JP. The newborn exstrophy bladder inadequate for primary closure: evaluation, management and outcome. J Urol. 2001;165(5):1656–9.
22. Baradaran N, Cervellione RM, Orosco R, Trock BJ, et al. Effect of failed initial closure on bladder growth in children with bladder exstrophy. J Urol. 2011;186(4):1450–4.
23. Oesterling JE, Jeffs RD. The importance of a successful initial bladder closure in the surgical management of classical bladder exstrophy: analysis of 144 patients treated at the Johns Hopkins Hospital between 1975 and 1985. J Urol. 1987;137(2):258–62.
24. McMahon DR, Cain MP, Husmann DA, Kramer SA. Vesical neck reconstruction in patients with the exstrophy-epispadias complex. J Urol. 1996;155(4):1411–3.
25. Jeffs RD. Functional closure of bladder exstrophy. Birth Defects Orig Artic Ser. 1977;13(5):171–3.
26. Ebert AK, Schott G, Bals-Pratsch M, Seifert B, Rösch WH. Long-term follow-up of male patients after reconstruction of the bladder-exstrophy-epispadias complex: psychosocial status, continence, renal and genital function. J Pediatr Urol. 2010;6(1):6–10.
27. Jarzebowski AC, McMullin ND, Grover SR, et al. The Kelly technique of bladder exstrophy repair: continence, cosmesis and pelvic organ prolapse outcomes. J Urol. 2009;182(Suppl 4):1802–6.
28. Baka-Jakubiak M. Combined bladder neck, urethral and penile reconstruction in boys with the exstrophy-epispadias complex. BJU Int. 2000;86(4):513–8.
29. Meldrum KK, Baird AD, Gearhart JP. Pelvic and extremity immobilization after bladder exstrophy closure: complications and impact on success. Urology. 2003;62(6):1109–13.
30. Baird AD, Nelson CP, Gearhart JP. Modern staged repair of bladder exstrophy: a contemporary series. J Pediatr Urol. 2007;3(4):311–5.

31. Schaeffer AJ, Stec AA, Purves JT, Cervellione RM, et al. Complete primary repair of bladder exstrophy: a single institution referral experience. J Urol. 2011;186(3):1041–6.
32. Husmann DA, Gearhart JP. Loss of the penile glans and/or corpora following primary repair of bladder exstrophy using the complete penile disassembly technique. J Urol. 2004;172(4 Pt 2):1696–700. discussion 1700–1701.
33. Alpert SA, Cheng EY, Kaplan WE, Snodgrass WT, et al. Bladder neck fistula after the complete primary repair of exstrophy: a multi-institutional experience. J Urol. 2005;174(4 Pt 2):1687–9. discussion 1689–1690.
34. Shnorhavorian M, Grady RW, Andersen A, Joyner BD, Mitchell ME. Long-term followup of complete primary repair of exstrophy: the Seattle experience. J Urol. 2008;180(Suppl 4):1615–9. discussion 1619–1620.
35. Hammouda HM, Kotb H. Complete primary repair of bladder exstrophy: initial experience with 33 cases. J Urol. 2004;172(4 Pt 1):1441–4. discussion 1444.

Biliary Atresia and Anesthetic Considerations

42

Sakshi Mahajan and Rakhee Goyal

42.1 Introduction

Extra hepatic biliary atresia is the commonest cause of neonatal cholestasis. It is characterized by progressive inflammation, fibrosis, and eventually obliteration of extra hepatic biliary tree, leading to obstruction of bile flow. If untreated, there will be death within 2 years of life due to liver failure, portal hypertension, and cirrhosis [1].

The incidence of biliary atresia is 1 in 5000–20,000 live births with greater prevalence in Asian population and in females (F:M::1.25:1) [2, 3].

Neonates have physiologic jaundice (serum bilirubin >5 mg/dL) up to 2 weeks of life, because of increased breakdown of erythrocytes and immature hepatic enzymes. It is mainly unconjugated hyperbilirubinemia. Jaundice persisting beyond 2 weeks of life in term neonates and 3 weeks of life in preterm neonates is pathological. Conjugated hyperbilirubinemia in neonates is always pathological and is defined as conjugated bilirubin >1 mg/dL or >20% of the total bilirubin [4, 5]. Biliary atresia is one of the most common causes of conjugated hyperbilirubinemia in neonates.

42.2 Classification

1. **Ohi Classification based on anatomical involvement, into three types** (Fig. 42.1) [6]:
   (a) Type I (5%)- affects the common bile duct.
   (b) Type II a- affects the common hepatic duct. The cystic and common bile duct are patent.

S. Mahajan (✉) · R. Goyal
Department of Anesthesia, Madhukar Rainbow Children's Hospital, New Delhi, India

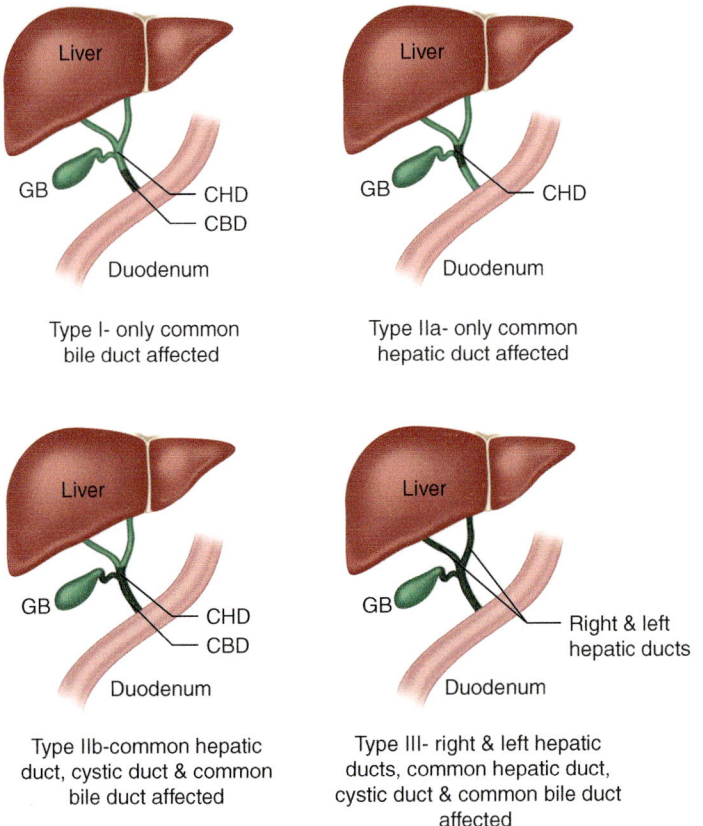

Fig. 42.1 Ohi classification of biliary atresia (CBD- Common Bile Duct, CHD- Common Hepatic Duct)

(c) Type II b- affects the common hepatic, common bile, and cystic ducts. The right and left hepatic ducts are patent.

(d) Type III (>90%)- is the commonest form and affects whole of the extra hepatic biliary system.

2. **Based on time of presentation, into two types:** [7]

(a) **Fetal form (syndromic form)** - is present in approximately 10% neonates and manifests within first 2 weeks of life. It is associated with other congenital anomalies and syndromes like **Biliary atresia splenic malformation syndrome**, and Polysplenia syndrome (**BASM Syndrome** - Polysplenia, situs inversus, intestinal malrotation, pre-duodenal portal vein, absent inferior vena cava (IVC), anomalous hepatic artery supply, cardiac defects) and is associated with poor outcome for both porto-enterostomy and hepatic transplant surgery.

(b) **Postnatal form (non-syndromic)** – is present in approximately 90% cases and manifests after 2 weeks, usually between 2–8 weeks. It is not associated with any other congenital anomalies and has a better prognosis as compared to the fetal form.

42.3 Pathogenesis

Various factors have been implicated in the pathogenesis of the disease [3, 8]:

1. **Defective embryogenesis** - extrahepatic biliary ducts are formed from ductal plate around 11–13 weeks of gestation. Ductal plate malformations may result in fetal biliary atresia.
2. **Genetic factors** involving inactivation or overexpression of certain genes.
3. **Viral infections** – most commonly associated viruses are reovirus3, rotavirus, and cytomegalovirus.
4. **Autoimmune causes** [9].

The postnatal form of biliary atresia may result from progressive inflammation of the biliary tree from exposure to virus, toxins, or autoimmune causes in the first few weeks of life [8].

42.4 Pathophysiology

42.4.1 Bilirubin Metabolism

80% of bilirubin comes from breakdown of hemoglobin and remaining from other heme containing proteins (myoglobin, cytochromes, etc.) [10]. Heme is taken up by reticuloendothelial cells and oxygenated to form biliverdin, which undergoes reduction by biliverdin reductase to form bilirubin. Bilirubin is water-insoluble and in the liver, it undergoes conjugation with glucuronic acid and becomes water-soluble which can be excreted in bile. In the gut, it undergoes hydrolysis to form stercobilinogen(urobilinogen) which then oxidizes to stercobilin. Stercobilin gives yellow color to stools. Some of the urobilinogen is reabsorbed from intestine into portal circulation (enterohepatic circulation), while some is excreted in the urine [11] (Fig. 42.2).

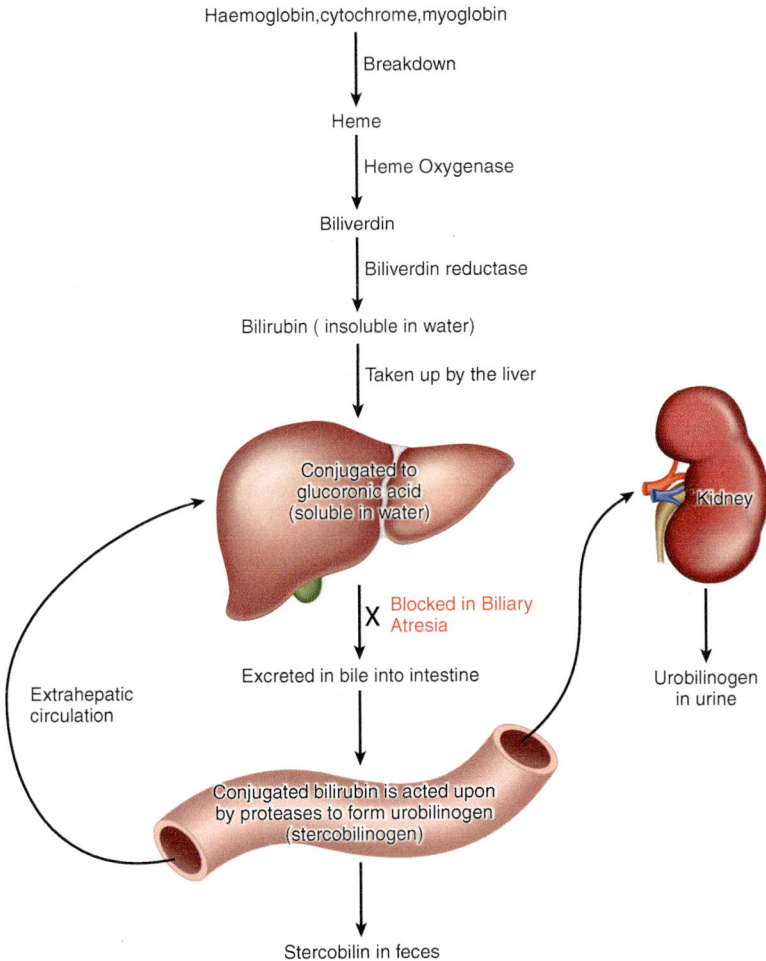

Fig. 42.2 Bilirubin metabolism and pathophysiology of biliary atresia

42.4.2 Pathophysiology

In biliary atresia, because of progressive inflammation of the biliary tract, there is obstruction to the excretion of bilirubin into bile duct, and this conjugated bilirubin starts accumulating in serum, leading to conjugated hyperbilirubinemia. No sterco-bilin is formed in the gut, thus acholic stools. Also, because of bile stasis there is activation of various cytokines like Tumor Necrosis Factor (TNF), Interleukin-6 (IL-6), TGF-Beta, Endothelin, Nitric Oxide(NO). These activated cytokines result in progressive fibrosis of the biliary tract and eventually cirrhosis of liver.

42.5   Signs and Symptoms

Most neonates are full term and have normal weight gain and appetite. Biliary atresia is characterized by a triad of jaundice, dark colored urine, and pale/acholic stools [1, 12].

In the fetal form, conjugated hyperbilirubinemia is present from the birth, whereas in postnatal form the physiological jaundice continues into conjugated hyperbilirubinemia. Any neonate having persistence of neonatal jaundice beyond 2 weeks of life should be worked up for biliary atresia [9].

Late presentation is associated with failure to thrive from liver failure, malabsorption of fat-soluble vitamins (vit A, D, E, K), vitamin K-dependent coagulopathy, and ascites. In late stages when the synthetic functions of liver are also affected, then coagulopathy becomes unresponsive to vitamin K supplementation [13].

42.6   Diagnosis

42.6.1 Laboratory Investigations [14]

1. **Serum bilirubin** - both total and direct bilirubin will be raised.
2. **Serum transaminases**- both ALT and AST levels are elevated.
3. **Alkaline phosphatase** - elevated levels are seen.
4. **Gamma glutamyl transpeptidase (GGT)** - is markedly increased and is used to differentiate biliary atresia from other forms of neonatal cholestasis.

42.6.2 Imaging Studies

1. **Ultrasonography**- enlarged liver and absent/contracted gall bladder is seen after 4 h of fasting [13].
2. **Doppler USG** - Hepatic artery resistance index is highly predictive of rapid deterioration in patients with biliary atresia. An index of more than 1 indicates very high mortality [15].
3. **Hepatobiliary scintigraphy (HIDA Scan)** – this use radioactive marker (Technetium Tc 99 m iminodiacetic acid). In biliary atresia uptake by the liver is normal, but there is no excretion of the isotope into the duodenum [16, 17].
4. **Percutaneous Liver biopsy** - shows fibrosis and inflammation in biliary ductules. It can help in differentiating between obstructive and hepatocellular causes of cholestasis, but it may be normal in initial stages, and serial biopsies are indicated [16].
5. **Intraoperative cholangiogram** - is the gold standard in diagnosis of biliary atresia [17].

42.7   Management

42.7.1 Medical Management Includes Supportive Treatment Like [14, 17]

- Oral antibiotics to prevent cholangitis.
- Urso-deoxy cholic acid to improve bile flow.
- Nutritional support in the form of oral fat-soluble vitamins.
- Role of corticosteroids is controversial.
- **Zinc sulfate** - in children with biliary atresia serum zinc levels are low and copper concentration is high [18]. High copper concentrations may aggravate hepatic fibrosis. Also, enzymes like DNA/RNA polymerases which help in liver regeneration contain zinc. Zinc sulphate has been used in neonatal unconjugated hyperbilirubinemia as it inhibits the enterohepatic cycle and decrease the bilirubin levels [19]. In a dose of 1 mg/kg 6 hourly, $ZnSO_4$ may have a protective effect on the liver and may also decrease bilirubin levels [20].

42.7.2 Surgery is the Definitive Treatment for Biliary Atresia

Early surgery (<6–8 weeks) has better results. **Kasai Porto Enterostomy** is done in three steps, via a large subcostal incision - [21]

1. Dissection at porta hepatis and removal of all atretic bile ducts. During this step, during exteriorization of liver and surgical retraction, there might be kinking of IVC, leading to decrease in venous return and severe hypotension,
2. Preparation of Roux-en-Y loop of jejunum, and.
3. Anastomosis of functional bile ducts to the jejunal loops which will allow bile drainage.

Prognosis depends on: [22]

1. Age at which surgery is done (< 8 weeks better prognosis),
2. Preoperative histology and remnant duct size,
3. Absence of portal hypertension,
4. Absence of congenital syndromes like BASM,
5. Post-op rapid clearing of bilirubin levels, and
6. Experience of surgical team.

Unfortunately, only 50–60% of Kasai Porto enterostomy are successful and most babies eventually need liver transplantation. Biliary atresia is in fact the most common indication for orthotopic liver transplant [6].

42.8   Anesthetic Management

A neonate with biliary atresia may require anesthesia for various procedures:

- Liver biopsy
- Intraoperative cholangiogram
- Upper GI endoscopy
- Kasai Porto enterostomy
- Revision surgeries

Anesthesia for these children is challenging not only because of their age, but also because of their pathology.

- **Airway**- these children should always be considered as full stomach because of abdominal distension due to ascites or hepatosplenomegaly. So, even for small procedures like endoscopy, airway should be secured with an endotracheal tube. Also, enlarged liver may cause splinting of diaphragm and decrease FRC, which makes them more prone to desaturation during periods of apnea as compared to normal infants [23].
- **Coagulopathy**- in early stages, coagulopathy is vitamin K-responsive as it is because of malabsorption of fat-soluble vitamins (vitamin K). In the later stages, when synthetic function of the liver also gets affected, then coagulopathy is because of decreased synthesis of clotting factors by the liver and is no longer responsive to vitamin K [24].
- **Drug metabolism**- hepatic metabolic function is affected in the late stages of the disease, so drug dosages may have to be altered [23].
- **Good postoperative pain relief** is required for early extubation. Doses of opioids and local anesthetics may have to be altered and post-op monitoring in NICU is essential.

42.9   Anesthetic Management of a Child Coming for Kasai Porto Enterostomy

42.9.1 Preoperative Preparation

1. **Medical management** is continued which includes:
   a. Injection vitamin K (1–2 mg/kg/day) IM for 3 days prior to surgery
   b. CBC, coagulation profile and LFT should be done
   c. Arrange for blood and FFP (10–15 ml/kg)
   d. NPO 4 hours for breast milk and 6 hours for formula feed
      Note - Written informed consent should be taken from the parents or guardians informing about the high risk of procedure, need for central venous access, need for postoperative ICU stay, and possible need for postoperative ventilation.

42.9.2 Intraoperative Management

Usually, the baby will have an IV canula in situ. In case not, then an inhalational induction can be done with sevoflurane in oxygen and nitrous oxide and then an IV can be placed. Obtaining a good IV line may be difficult in these neonates because of prolong hospital stay and multiple attempts at IV access. Venous access should preferably be achieved in upper limb veins which drain into SVC as IVC may get kinked or occluded intraoperatively when liver is exteriorized.

IV induction can be done using propofol since propofol metabolism is not much altered in liver disease as it is mainly metabolized via extra hepatic route [25, 26]. Barbiturates (Thiopentone), on the other hand, have a major hepatic metabolism and dose adjustment may be required [27]. Once induced, muscle relaxation can be achieved with atracurium or cisatracurium [28]. Cisatracurium has an advantage of less formation of laudanosine (a neurotoxic metabolite excreted by the liver). Trachea should be intubated with appropriate size endotracheal tube and a gastric tube (8–10 Fr) inserted.

A central line should be placed if coagulation profile is normal. In case of coagulopathy, a PICC line can be placed. Arterial cannulation is indicated in selected cases with cardiac anomalies.

Intraoperative monitoring includes ECG, pulse oximetry, NIBP, temperature, $EtCO_2$, and blood sugar. Central line may be used to measure CVP.

For maintenance of anesthesia, O_2 air mixture should be used. Nitrous oxide may cause distension of the gut and is better avoided [29]. Halothane should be avoided because of its potential hepatoxicity [27]. Desflurane, isoflurane, and sevoflurane can all be used for maintenance as all preserve hepatic blood flow and produce very little hepatotoxic metabolites [30]. Desflurane preserves hepatic flow better than sevoflurane. Also, it is metabolized to a lesser extent (0.02%) as compared to sevoflurane (5%). So, desflurane may be a better choice in these patients [31].

Opioids should be used intraoperatively for pain relief, preferably the short acting opioids like fentanyl or remifentanil. Morphine in a dose of 0.05–0.1 mg/kg has also been used [32].

42.9.3 Intraoperative Anesthetic Goals

Main intraoperative goals are to maintain euvolemia, euthermia, euglycemia, and hepatic blood flow.

i. **Euvolemia** - maintenance fluids are administered in the form of crystalloids, given at a rate of 10 mL/kg/h. 2% dextrose should be added in the first fluid as these babies are prone to hypoglycemia [33]. Blood sugars can be checked after 1–2 h, and dextrose added if sugars are low. Since it is a major open surgery, large volume fluid and blood losses are expected. Losses should be replaced with crystalloids. Blood loss exceeding 10% of total blood volume should be replaced by warm and fresh blood preferably not more than 5 days old [29].

ii. **Euthermia** should be always ensured by using warming blankets, in fluid warmers, warm irrigation fluids, warm blood, and blood products and covering the baby with cotton or plastic sheets.

iii. **Euglycemia** - Blood sugars are checked every 1–2 hours and dextrose added if sugar levels are low to maintain euglycemia.

EtCO$_2$ (End tidal carbon dioxide) should be maintained in normal range to prevent changes in hepatic and portal blood flow.

iv. **Hepatic Blood Flow** - Sudden drop in blood pressure is seen when liver is exteriorized. This is because of kinking of IVC (inferior vene cava) and consequent decrease in venous return to the heart. This is seen as decrease in amplitude of R wave on ECG [34], phenomenon known as **Brody's effect**. Fluid boluses of 10–20 mL/kg can be given to prevent hypotension [24], but avoid excessive fluids as this may lead to distension of liver capsule causing its rupture and hemorrhage. If hypotension is not corrected by 20 mL/kg fluid, then vasopressors should be started.

Sometimes, bradycardia may occur as a vagal response to liver traction. Releasing the traction usually is corrective in these cases. If it persists, atropine can be given.

v. **Extubation** - The neonate can be extubated at the end of surgery if respiratory efforts are adequate and no contraindication for extubation is present. The baby should be kept in NICU after surgery.

42.9.4 Postoperative Analgesia

Kasai Porto enterostomy is a major abdominal surgery and multimodal pain management is required for good recovery.

42.9.4.1 Epidural Block (Fig. 42.3)

Epidural block lowers the need for intra and postoperative opioids and also the need of postoperative ventilation [35]. An epidural catheter can be inserted from caudal, lumbar, or thoracic space. The tip of the catheter should be at T7–T8 thoracic level. It is important that care is taken while performing lumbar or thoracic epidural so as not to injure the spinal cord. The contraindications to epidural placement should be ruled out in every case (parental/ surgeon refusal, coagulopathy, spinal, or vertebral anomalies or any local or systemic infection) [36, 37].

Caudal block can also be given upto a volume of 1–1.5 mL/kg, using either bupivacaine or ropivacaine and additives (morphine) for extended pain relief but it is unlikely to cover all the required dermatomes [38].

42.9.4.2 Peripheral Nerve Blocks

Peripheral nerve blocks such as rectus sheath block, erector spinae block, and quadratus lumborum block can also be given, but under ultrasound guidance [39]. These are simple to perform and safer as there are no major vessels involved.

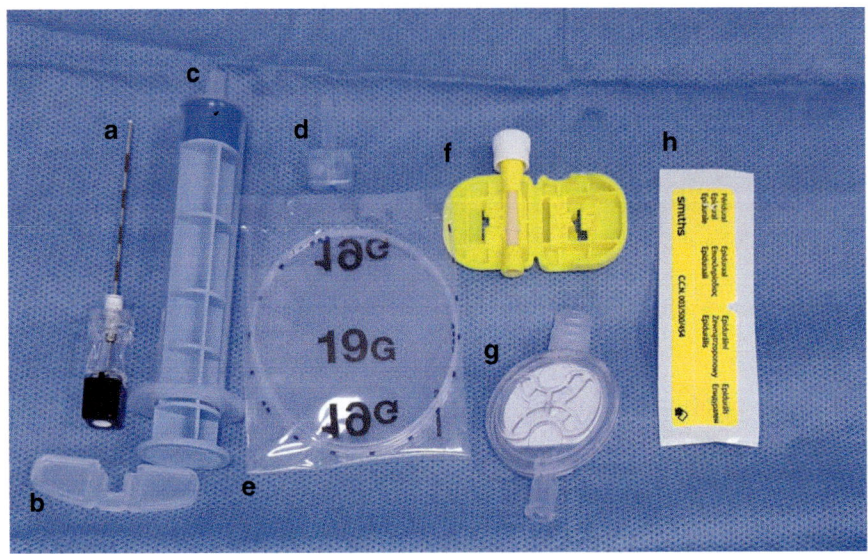

Fig. 42.3 Pediatric Epidural set (**a**) 19G Tuohy needle, 5 cm in length with transparent hub; (**b**) removable wings; (**c**) 10 mL loss of resistance syringe; (**d**) introducer; (**e**) 19G catheter; (**f**) luer-lock connector for the catheter; (**g**) bacterial filter; (**h**) label (yellow in color)

Continuous infusions can also be given, though the data are limited. Thoracic paravertebral block has also been used by some in these neonates [40].

Local anesthetics like bupivacaine or ropivacaine can be used with or without opioids. There are higher chances of cardiac toxicity with bupivacaine because of decreased hepatic clearance and increase in unbound fraction. But it has been seen that postsurgery there is an increase in level of alpha1 acid glycoprotein (AAG) and bupivacaine metabolism is similar in both infants with and without biliary atresia [41]. Recommended maximum dose of bupivacaine is 0.25 mg/kg/h in <4-month-old. Ropivacaine is less cardiotoxic and is a better option for epidural infusions in neonates. Recommended dose is 0.9–2 mL/kg bolus of 0.2% ropivacaine followed by infusion (0.2 mL/kg/h). The epidural infusions can be safely used for 48–72 h [42]. Postoperative removal of epidural catheter should be done only after getting a coagulation profile.

42.9.4.3 Intravenous Paracetamol
Intravenous paracetamol in a dose of 20 mg/kg bolus followed by 10 mg/kg 6 hourly is safe and provides a good pain relief [43, 44].

42.9.4.4 Systemic Opioids
Systemic opioids - synthetic and metabolic functions of liver are unimpaired at early stages. Also, because of the hepatic artery buffer response (HABR), the total hepatic blood flow is not altered in babies with biliary atresia. Thus, opioids usually

do not require dose modifications [32]. But postoperative monitoring to watch out for any respiratory depression is a must in patients receiving opioid infusion [45]. Naloxone should be readily available. Morphine can be used with a loading dose of 0.05 mg/kg followed by infusion with 10–40 mcg/kg/h up to a maximum of 1 mg/kg/day. Fentanyl can be used with a loading dose of 1mcg/kg followed by 1 mcg/kg/h. Tramadol has been also used in a dose of 1 mg/kg 12 hourly [24, 46]. Local infiltration at incision site also provides some pain relief.

42.10 Conclusion

Any neonate presenting with conjugated hyperbilirubinemia should be suspected of having biliary atresia. Most neonates are healthy, have good appetite and weight gain at presentation. Only presenting symptom of the disease may be jaundice persisting beyond 2 weeks of life. Early surgery has a better prognosis. Kasai Porto Enterostomy is challenging for the anesthetist. All precautions pertaining to normal surgical neonate must be kept in mind. In addition, these neonates may pose airway related challenges, may have coagulation abnormalities and altered drug metabolism. Good intraoperative and postoperative analgesia is also fundamental for expediting the recovery of the neonate after surgery. However, this procedure should be carried out in a center that has NICU and has provision for ventilation of these babies.

References

1. Hartley JL, Davenport M. Biliary atresia. Lancet. 2009;374:1704–13.
2. Davenport M. Biliary atresia: clinical aspects. Semin Pediatr Surg. 2012;21(3):175–84.
3. Asai A, Miethke A, Bezerra JA. Pathogenesis of biliary atresia: defining biology to understand clinical phenotypes. Nat Rev Gastroenterol Hepatol. 2015;12(6):342–52.
4. Ratnavel N, Ives NK. Investigation of prolonged neonatal jaundice. Curr Paediatr. 2005;15:85–91.
5. Feldman AG, Sokol RJ. Neonatal cholestasis: updates on diagnostics, therapeutics and prevention. Neoreviews. 2021;22(12): e819–36.
6. Ramachandran P, Safwan M, Reddy MS, Rella M. Recent trends in the diagnosis and management of biliary atresia in developing countries. Indian Pediatr. 2015;52(10):871–9.
7. Chardot C. Biliary Atresia Orphaned. J Rare Dis. 2006;1:28.
8. Zagory JA, Nguyen MV, Wang KS. Recent advances in the pathogenesis and Management of Biliary Atresia. Curr Opin Pediatr. 2015;27(3):389–94.
9. Sokol RJ, Mack C, Narkewicz MR, Karrer FM. Pathogenesis and outcome of biliary atresia: current concepts. J Pediatr Gastroenterol Nutr. 2003;37:4–21.
10. Kalakonda A, Jenkins BA, John S. Physiology, bilirubin. 2021. In: StatPearls [Internet]. Treasure Island (FL): StatPearls Publishing; 2022 Jan- PMID: 29261920.
11. Sticova E, Jirsa M. New insights in bilirubin metabolism and their clinical implications. World J Gastroenterol. 2013;19(38):6398–407.
12. Mogul D, Zhou M, Intihar P, Schwarz K, Frick K. Cost effective analysis of screening for biliary atresia with the stool card. J Pediatr Gastroenterol Nutr. 2015;60(1):91–8.
13. Bates MD, Bucuvalas JC, Alonso MH, Ryckman FC. Biliary atresia: pathogenesis and treatment. Semin Liver Dis. 1998;18(3):281–93.

14. Kelly DA, Davenport M. Current management of biliary atresia. Arch Dis Child. 2007;92:1132–5.
15. Green DW, Howard ER, Davenport M. Anaesthesia, perioperative management and outcome of correction of extrahepatic biliary atresia in the infant: a review of 50 cases in the King's college hospital series. Paediatr Anaesth. 2000;10:581–9.
16. Valle AS, Kassira N, Varela VC, Radu SC, Paidas C, Kirby RS. Biliary atresia epidemiology, genetics, clinical update, and public health perspective. Adv Paediatr. 2017;64(1):285–305.
17. Khalil BA, Perera MT, Mirza DF. Clinical practice: management of biliary atresia. Eur J Pediatr. 2010;169:395–402.
18. Sato C, Koyama H, Satoh H, Hayashi Y, Chiba T, Ohi R. Concentrations of copper and zinc in liver and serum samples in biliary atresia patients at different stages of traditional surgeries. Tohoku J Exp Med. 2005;207:271–7.
19. Mendez- Sanchez N, Martínez M, González V, Roldan- Valadez E, Flores MA, Uribe M. Zinc sulfate inhibits the enterohepatic cycling of unconjugated bilirubin in subjects with Gilbert's syndrome. Ann Hepatol. 2002;1(1):40–3.
20. Faal G, Masjedi HK, Sharifzadeh G, Kiani Z. Efficacy of zinc sulfate on indirect hyperbilirubinemia in premature infants admitted to neonatal intensive care unit: a double-blind, randomized clinical trial. BMC Pediatr. 2020;20:130.
21. Ramachandran P, Safwan M, Srinivas S, Shanmugam N, Vij M, Rela M. The extended Kasai portoenterostomy for biliary atresia: a preliminary report. J Indian Assoc Pediatr Surg. 2016;21(2):66–71.
22. Hanalioglu D, Ozen H, Karhan A, et al. Revisiting long term prognostic factors of biliary atresia: a 20 year experience with 81 patients from a single Centre. Turk J Gastroenterol. 2019;30(5):467–74.
23. Bromley P, Bennett J. Anaesthesia for children with liver disease. Cont Edu Anaesth Crit Care Pain. 2014;14:201–12.
24. Ganigara A, Ramavakoda CY, Bindu SB, Jadhav V, Aihole JS. Anesthetic management and perioperative outcome of infants with biliary atresia: a retrospective review of 40 cases from a tertiary care pediatric institute in India. Indian. J Clin Anesth. 2016;3(1):62–8.
25. Raoof AA, Van Obbergh LJ, Verbeeck RK. Propofol pharmacokinetics in children with biliary atresia. Br J Anaesth. 1995;74:46–9.
26. Smits A, Thewissen L, Caicedo A, Naulaers G, Allegaert K. Propofol dose-finding to reach optimal effect for (semi)- elective intubation in neonates. J Paediatr. 2016;179:54–60.
27. Rahimzadeh P, Safari S, Reza Faiz SH, Alavian SM. Anesthesia for patients with liver disease. Hepat Mon. 2014;14(7):e19881.
28. Simpson DA, Green DW. Use of atracurium during major abdominal surgery in infants with hepatic dysfunction from biliary atresia. Br J Anaesth. 1986;58:1214–7.
29. Jacob R. Anaesthesia for biliary atresia and hepatectomy in paediatrics. Indian J Anaesth. 2012;56:479–84.
30. Green DW, Ashley EM. The choice of inhalational anaesthetic for major abdominal surgery in children with liver disease. Paediatr Anaesth. 2002;12(8):665–73.
31. Soliman R, Yacoub A, Abdellatif M. Comparative effect of desflurane and sevoflurane on liver function tests of patients with impaired hepatic function undergoing cholecystectomy: a randomized clinical study. Indian J Anaesth. 2020;64:383–90.
32. Wang X, Qiao Z, Zhou ZJ, Zhuang PJ, Zheng S. Postoperative morphine concentration in infants with or without biliary atresia and its association with hepatic blood flow. Anaesthesia. 2014;69:583–90.
33. Bhardwaj N. Perioperative fluid therapy and intraoperative blood loss in children. Indian J Anaesth. 2019;63:729–36.
34. Ganigara A, Ramavakoda CY. Clinical evidence of Brody's effect in infants undergoing Kasai's portoenterostomy for biliary atresia. Paediatr Anaesth. 2014;24(11):1193–4.
35. Phelps HM, Robinson JR, Chen H, Luckett TR, Conroy PC, et al. Enhancing recovery after Kasai portoenterostomy with epidural analgesia. J Surg Res. 2019;243:354–62.

36. Seefelder C, Lillehei CW. Epidural analgesia for patients undergoing hepatic portoenteros-tomy (Kasai procedure). Paediatr Anaesth. 2002;12(2):193–5.
37. Bosenberg AT. Epidural analgesia for major neonatal surgery. Paediatr Anaesth. 1998;8:479–83.
38. Sato M, Lida T, Kikuchi C, Sasakawa T, Kunisawa T. Comparison of caudal ropivacaine-morphine and paravertebral catheter for major upper abdominal surgery in infants. Paediatr Anaesth. 2017;27(5):524–30.
39. Heydinger G, Tobias J, Veneziano G. Fundamentals and innovation in regional anaesthesia for infants and children. Anaesthesia. 2001;76(Suppl 1):74–88.
40. Kajikawa Y, Taguchi S, Kato T, Oshita K, Hamada H, Tsutsumi Y. Ultrasound- guided thoracic paravertebral block after surgery for biliary atresia in a neonate. J Japan Soc Clin Anesth. 2021;41(1):47–53.
41. Meunier JF, Goujard E, Dubousset AN, Samii K, Mazoit JX. Pharmacokinetics of bupivacaine after continuous epidural infusion in infants with or without biliary atresia. Anesthesiology. 2001;95:87–95.
42. Bosenberg AT, Thomas J, Cronje L, Lopez T, et al. Pharmacokinetics and efficacy of ropivacaine for continuous epidural infusion in neonates and infants. Paediatr Anaesth. 2005;15:739–49.
43. Pacifici GM, Allegaert K. Clinical pharmacology of paracetamol in neonates: a review. Curr Ther Res. 2015;77:24–30.
44. Allegaert K, Velde M, Anker J. Neonatal clinical pharmacology. Paediatr Anaesth. 2014;24(1):30–8.
45. Cravero JP, Agarwal R, Berde C, et al. The Society for Pediatric Anesthesia recommenda-tions for the use of opioids in children during the perioperative period. Pediatr Anesth. 2019;29:547–71.
46. Allegaert K, Anderson BJ, Verbesselt R, Debeer A, de Hoon J, Devlieger H, Van Den Anker JN, Tibboel D. Tramadol disposition in the very young: an attempt to assess in vivo cyto-chrome P-450 2D6 activity. Br J Anaesth. 2005;95(2):231–9.

Craniosynostosis: A Congenital Anomaly

43

Pratibha Jain Shah

43.1 Introduction

Anesthesia management in craniosynostosis surgery is complex and poses numerous challenges to the anesthesiologist. **Craniosynostosis** is a rare congenital developmental defect due to premature closure or fusion of one or more of the cranial sutures, before the brain is fully developed. Continued brain growth results in restricted growth of the skull perpendicular to the affected suture and compensatory cranium growth parallel to the affected suture in order to accommodate the growing brain, leading to distinct misshapen head as seen on 3D CT scan (at third day). Rarely, the meninges are pushed into the skull, giving the lattice appearance on CT scan. The overall prevalence of craniosynostosis is about 1 in 2000 to 1 in 2500 live births.

43.2 Classification of Craniosynostosis

1. Nonsyndromic or Isolated Craniosynostosis (IC):
   (a) It involves single suture and presents in 75–80% of the cases.
   (b) It is further classified depending on the suture affected into following (Fig. 43.1):
      i. Scaphocephaly or **sagittal synostosis or** dolichocephaly (55–60%): this is the most common type in which sagittal suture closes too early or prematurely. The head is long and narrow with frontal bossing and higher antero-posterior diameter.

P. J. Shah (✉)
Department of Anesthesiology, Pt JNMMC, Raipur, Chhattisgarh, India

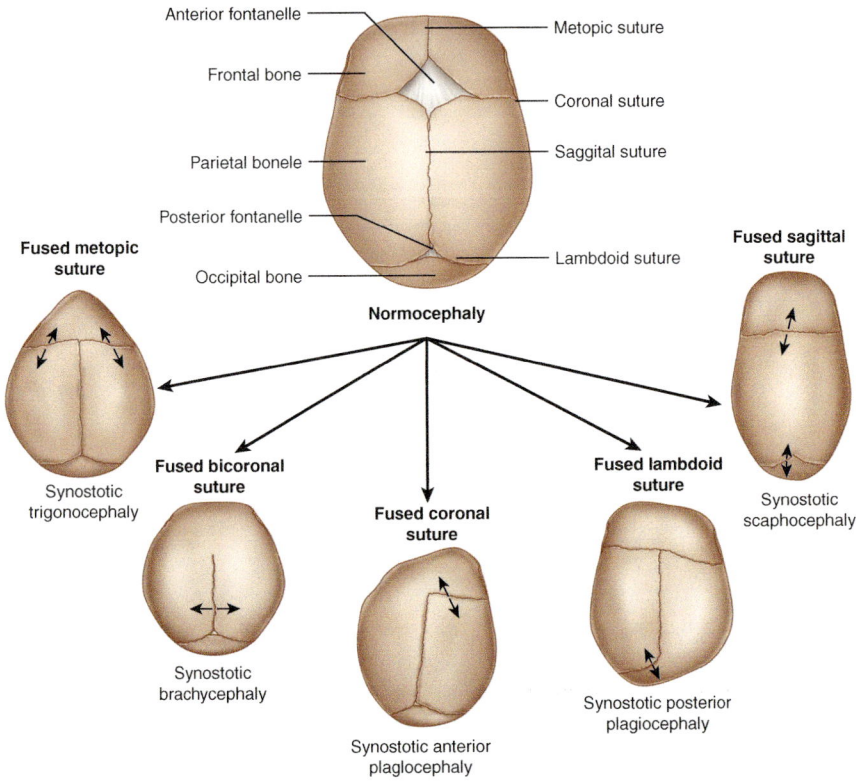

Fig. 43.1 Anatomical variation of craniosynostosis

    ii. Anterior plagiocephaly or **Coronal synostosis** (20–30%) - One of the coronal sutures closes too early or prematurely. Characteristic feature is flattened forehead on affected side, frontal bossing, and Harlequin sign (raised eye sockets - high supraorbital margins in radiographs, ipsilateral facial flushing, and nasal deviation).

    iii. Brachycephaly or **bi-Coronal synostosis** - Premature fusion of coronal sutures on both sides. Head is broad and short, flattened forehead and occiput, vertically long and prominent frontal bone, hypertelorism, and Harlequin type malformation.

    iv. Trigonocephaly or Metopic synostosis (10–15%) - Premature fusion of the metopic suture, characterized by narrow pointed forehead and broad occiput. Head looks triangular shaped when viewed from above.

    v. Posterior plagiocephaly or **Lambdoid synostosis** (3–5%) – this is the rarest type, from premature fusion of one lambdoid suture leading to flat occiput, tilting of skull to affected side, backward and downward displacement of ipsilateral ear, and contralateral frontal and occipital bossing.

    vi. Oxycephaly (turricephaly) – The fusion of all or most of the cranial sutures.

Table 43.1 Syndromes associated with craniosynostosis

Syndrome	Sutures involved	Presentation
Apert	Coronal suture	Midface hypoplasia, hypertelorism (bulging and wide-set eyes), beaked nose, underdeveloped jaw (that leads to crowded teeth), syndactyly of hands and feet, hearing loss, mild to moderate intellectual disabilities
Crouzon	Coronal, sagittal, and/or lambdoid sutures	Midface hypoplasia, beaked nose, exophthalmos, hypertelorism, cervical vertebral fusion, hearing loss, cleft lip/ palate, normal intelligence
Pfeiffer	Bi-coronal sutures	Hypertelorism, maxillary hypoplasia, broad thumbs, great toe, syndactyly, brachydactyly, hearing loss.
Muenke	Coronal suture (unilateral or bilateral)	Midface hypoplasia, hypertelorism, macrocephaly, hearing loss
Kleeblattschadel	Coronal and lambdoid sutures	"Beak-shaped" nose, maxillary hypoplasia with proptosis, ears displaced inferiorly, hydrocephalus

2. Syndromic or complex Craniosynostosis (SC):
   (a) Accounts for 20–25% of all cases of craniosynostosis.
   (b) It involves multiple sutures and is often associated with syndromes (cranial and extracranial anomalies like midface hypoplasia, skull base, and limb abnormalities).
   (c) The frequently associated syndromes with SC are Apert, Crouzon, Pfeiffer, Saethre–Chotzen, Carpenter, and Muenke syndromes (Table 43.1).
   (d) Most of these are autosomal-dominant, genetically inherited, involving mutations in genes encoding for fibroblast growth-factor (FGF) receptors.
   (e) These may be responsible for associated problems in 40–70% children with SC such as raised intracranial pressure (ICP), airway obstruction, feeding difficulties, behavioral issues, and psychological issues.

43.3 Etiology

- The cause of craniosynostosis is often unknown.
- The predisposing factors are either environmental (maternal smoking, in utero exposure to teratogens, intrauterine constraint, thyroid disease in mother, and fetal positioning), genetic (mutations), or maternal exposure to drugs (Clomiphene citrate).
- 20% craniosynostoses are autosomal dominant and due to genetic (FGF receptor) mutation.

43.4 Diagnosis

It is important to make a correct confirmatory diagnosis, as a misshapen head doesn't always indicate craniosynostosis. Deformational plagiocephaly also has flattened back of skull from spending a long time on one side of skull and can be treated with regular position changes, or with helmet therapy (cranial orthosis) to reshape the head.

- Clinical Features -.
  - The signs are usually noticeable at birth as abnormal-shaped skull and become more apparent during the first few months of life.
  - Signs and severity depend on number of fused sutures and the time of fusion.
  - Other signs are absence of soft spot on the skull, raised firm ridge along the affected sutures.
  - Slow or no growth of the head over time compared to body.
- Laboratory Investigations - Diagnosis should be confirmed by
  - Skull X-ray.
  - CT scan.
  - GRASE (gradient-and-spin-echo) MRI.
  - Genetic testing for FGF receptor genes.
  - USG cranium.

43.5 Complications

- Developmental Delay – depending on the type of craniosynostosis. Neonate with sagittal synostosis has a lower risk of learning disabilities compared to those with metopic, uni-coronal, or lambdoid synostosis.
- If left untreated- Permanent head and facial deformity, poor self-esteem, social isolation, raised ICP, and compression of the brain.
- Risk of raised ICP is more in syndromic type due to associated hydrocephalus, craniocephalic disproportion, airway obstruction, and abnormalities in venous drainage of brain.
- Unmanaged raised ICP - can result in developmental delays, cognitive impairment, lethargy, blindness, eye movement disorders, seizures, and rarely death.

43.6 Management

- Craniosynostosis presents with wide range of condition from otherwise well child with isolated single suture craniosynostosis to severe syndromic craniosynostosis.
- Mild cases don't need any treatment, if needed can be managed by specially molded helmet that assist in brain growth and correct the shape of the skull.
- Severe syndromic cases require surgery to relieve pressure on the brain, correct craniosynostosis, and allow normal brain growth and cognitive development.
- The **timing of the surgery** is contentious issues. It depends on the type of craniosynostosis and an underlying genetic syndrome.
  - Early surgery (3–6 months age) - has the advantage of softer bones where remodeling is easier. But the need for repeat surgeries along with physiologic

nadir of hemoglobin and blood volume at this age often coincides, leading to increase need for intra-operative blood transfusion.
- Late surgery (after 1 year of age) - usually discouraged due to risk of increased ICP and compression of the growing brain leading to seizures, developmental delay, and abnormal appearance. Bones of older children have loss of ossification properties with difficult remodeling necessitating bone grafting.
- Ideal timing - between the ages of 4 and 9 months.
- One reported case of craniosynostosis in which surgery was performed at 5 weeks because of evidence of impingement of brain growth in the image.
- Surgical approaches
  - Minimally invasive endoscopic surgery (Spring-assisted cranioplasty and suture release).
    Usually considered in babies up to 6 months of age.
    Advantage—smaller incision, less blood loss, and short (one-night) hospital stay.
  - Open surgery (Extended strip craniectomy, total vault reconstruction, fronto-orbital remodeling, posterior calvarial vault expansion) - Usually considered in older children after 6 months of age because of prolonged surgical time, more blood loss, need of massive transfusion, risk of venous air embolism, and longer hospital stay.

43.7 Anesthetic Management

The management of a surgical neonate with syndromic craniosynostosis is multidisciplinary, requiring coordinated and integrated approach among otorhinolaryngologist, ophthalmologist, plastic surgeon, neurosurgeon, and neuro-anesthesiologist.

Every patient is different in terms of associated syndromes, cosmetic appearance, and functional problems- therefore, a thorough preoperative assessment and the proposed surgical procedure should be individualized.

Challenges to the anesthesiologist:

1. Very young age.
2. Difficult airway (because of the abnormal head shape).
3. Prolonged duration of anesthesia.
4. Raised ICP.
5. Intraoperative Positioning – depending on the site and extent of surgery – supine, lateral, and prone.
6. Intraoperative Hypothermia.
7. High risk of perioperative complications - massive blood loss, venous air embolism.
8. Need of massive blood transfusion and coagulation therapy.
9. Need of postoperative ventilatory and intensive care support.
10. Syndrome-specific issues.
    (a) Baseline hematological, biochemical, and coagulation studies are essential.

(b) Optimize preoperative hemoglobin, with iron therapy or recombinant human erythropoietin.

(c) Counsel parents about specific anesthetic and surgical risks involved with the procedure (especially blood transfusion, venous air embolism).

(d) Expect difficult mask ventilation in case of midface hyperplasia.

(e) Access two intravenous lines.

(f) Invasive monitoring – intra-arterial pressure (IAP) monitoring when expecting rapid hemodynamic changes, massive blood loss, and need for repeated blood samples.

(g) Avoid factors that increase ICP (hypercapnia, hypoxia, acidosis, neck hyperextension, and raised central venous pressure).

(h) The reported incidence of VAE during craniosynostosis surgery is as high as 83%. It is usually asymptomatic and only 1–2% have significant hemodynamic compromise.

(i) Most of the patients are extubated at the completion of surgery.

(j) Delayed Recovery - Prolonged surgery, massive fluid shifts, large-volume and blood transfusions, effects of prolonged prone positioning, patient factors (preoperative airway obstruction or difficult breathing).

43.8   Conclusion

Craniosynostosis is a complex congenital anomaly due to premature closure of one of the skull sutures, which is characterized by mishappen skull and potential of complications such as raised ICP and venous air embolism specially in syndromic type. Small age of the patient, difficult airway, prolonged anesthesia, positioning, massive blood loss, hypothermia, and risks related to massive blood transfusion and venous air embolism, are main anesthetic concerns.

Pearls of Wisdom

- Craniosynostosis is a birth defect secondary to premature closure of one or more cranial sutures.
- Isolated, non-syndromic craniosynostosis is seen in 80% cases that doesn't require surgery.
- Scaphocephaly **(sagittal synostosis) is the most common and posterior plagiocephaly is the rarest type of isolated craniosynostosis.**
- Syndromic craniosynostosis is more complex involving multiple sutures, with associated cranial and extracranial anomalies. It usually requires surgical correction between 6 and 12 months of age.
- Anesthetic management in syndromic craniosynostosis is challenging due to young age, difficult airway, prolong anesthesia, massive blood transfusion, coagulation therapy, acid base and electrolyte changes, and hypothermia, which is further complicated by syndrome-specific issues.
- Positional plagiocephaly does not require surgical therapy.

Further Readings

Lin EE, Stricker PA. Anesthesia for craniofacial surgery. In: Soriano SG, McClain CD, editors. Essentials of pediatric neuroanesthesia. New York: Cambridge University Press; 2018. p. 86–91. https://doi.org/10.1017/9781316652947.011.

Pearson A, Matava CT. Anaesthetic management for craniosynostosis repair in children. BJA Edu. 2016;16(12):410–6.

Proctor MR, Meara JG. A review of the management of single-suture craniosynostosis, past, present, and future. J Neurosurg Pediatr. 2019;24:622–31.

Cystic Hygroma

44

Pratibha Jain Shah

44.1 Cystic Hygroma

A cyst is a fluid filled, thin walled, membranous, hollow cavity/sac (Oxford Dictionary). It is formed as a defence mechanism following repeated injury or mutation leading to uncontrolled cellular division. Hygroma is accumulation of watery fluid in a cyst.

Cystic hygroma (CH) was first described by Redenbacher in 1828. It is a cluster of cysts in the lymphatic system, due to a malformation in the embryonic stage of the fetus or an obstruction in the lymphatic system (like enlarged lymph nodes in lympho-reticulosis), restricting flow of lymph into the venous circulation. Lymph then accumulates in the lymphatic sacs in the vicinity. In a nuchal area, it collects in the jugular lymph sacs in the neck.

CH is the most common form of lymphangioma, but unlike others, it is benign, with no malignant potential. Histologically, it originates from the embryonic lymphatic vascular system.

CH is synonymous with cavernous lymphangioma, and lymphatic or chylous Cyst.

44.2 Lymphatic Circulation

CH being lymphatic in origin, it is relevant to know about lymphatic circulation in the body (Fig. 44.1).

P. J. Shah (✉)
Department of Anesthesiology, Pt JNM MC, Raipur, India

U. Saha (ed.), *Clinical Anesthesia for the Newborn and the Neonate*,
https://doi.org/10.1007/978-981-19-5458-0_44

837

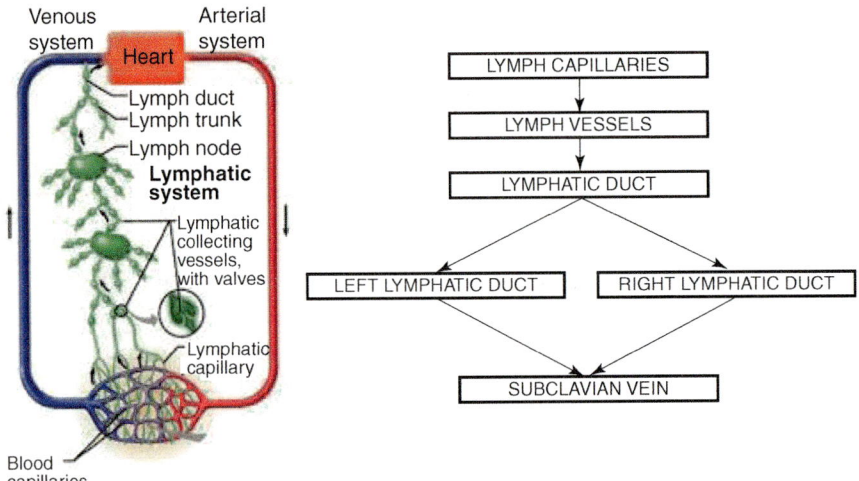

Fig. 44.1 The lymphatic system is made up of a network of thin lymphatic vessels with valves (allowing unidirectional flow) and lymph nodes. As blood flows, plasma leaks out from the blood vessels, mixes with the interstitial fluid, and is carried by lymphatics as Lymph, to the lymph nodes, where it is collected, filtered (removal of bacteria, abnormal cells) and drains into the venous system.

Lymph contains immune proteins, nutrients, and cell waste. It has an important role in immune response and disease resistance. Spleen, thymus, and tonsils are associated with the lymphatic system and immune response

44.3   Prevalence

CH can be detected in 1 in 100 fetus in the first trimester. The incidence is 1 in 800 pregnancies and 1 in 6000–8000 live births, with no gender preponderance. In 50% patients, it is present at birth, and most present in the childhood, by the age of 2 years. A very slow growing CH may present later in childhood or adults.

44.4   Location

CH being lymphatic in origin can occur anywhere within the body. Common sites are

- **Head and Neck** (face, mouth, cheek, and tongue) - 75%. About 70–80% are nuchal swellings, usually in the left posterior cervical triangle (Fig. 44.2). **Fleischmann's Hygroma** is a lymphatic cyst in the floor of the mouth. This is most challenging for the anesthesiologist.
- **Axilla** - 20%.

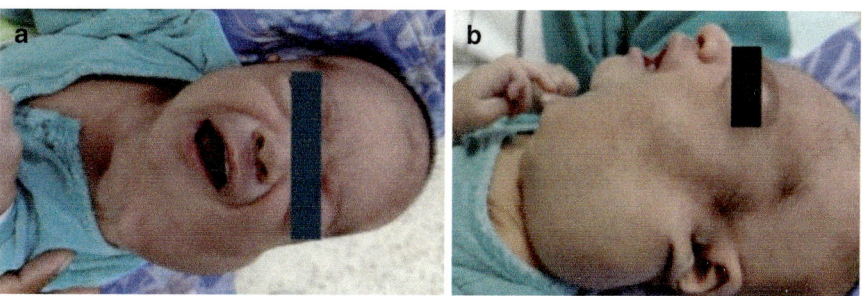

Fig. 44.2 Cystic hygroma left side of neck; (**a**) Front view (**b**) lateral view

– **Superior mediastinum and chest wall** - 5%.
– **Mesentery, retro-peritoneal, pelvis, and lower limbs** (leg, buttock, and groin).

44.5 Etiology (Table 44.1)

1. **Idiopathic** - The actual cause is **unknown.**
   Abnormal development of lymphatic vascular system, during embryonic stage, and abnormal endothelial differentiation may occur on its own or due to environmental and genetic factors.
2. **Environmental factors** include viral infections in the mother transmitted to the fetus, and maternal exposure to drugs or alcohol during pregnancy.
3. **Genetic factors** (in >50% cases). Common genetic syndromes are Turner syndrome (in 33% cases), Down syndrome, and Noonan syndrome. Other rare ones are Edward and Patau syndromes (details given below).

Lymphatic system may also be affected by **cardiac anomalies** with their consequent hemodynamic and tissue oxygenation disturbances, and anomalous lymphatic development.

Other causes such as **infections, malignancy, radiation, surgery, and trauma** may lead to occurrence of adulthood CH.

Table 44.1 Etiology of cystic hygroma

1.	Idiopathic	
2.	Environmental	Maternal viral infections and exposure to drugs and alcohol
3.	Genetic	Chromosomal anomalies and abnormal endothelial differentiation
(a)	Common syndromes	Turner syndrome Noonan syndrome Down syndrome
(b)	Uncommon syndromes	Edward syndrome, Patau syndrome
(3)	Congenital anomalies	Cardiac defects -hemodynamic and tissue oxygenation abnormalities
(4)	Other causes	Infection, malignancy, radiation, trauma, post-surgery

44.6 Various Syndromes (Table 44.1)

(a) **Turner syndrome** (45 X or 45 X0 = wholly or partially missing an X chromosome). This is not inherited disorder and occurs at random during cell division in early fetal life, in few or all cells of the body. In these females, there is abnormality in development of female features, changes in appearance, cardiac and fertility problems, and nuchal lymphogenesis.

(b) **Noonan syndrome** is an inherited autosomal dominant disorder of gene mutation that causes abnormal development of multiple body parts, with unusual facial features, short stature, cardiac defects, bleeding problems, skeletal abnormalities, and CH.

(c) **Down syndrome** (Trisomy 21 - extra chromosome 21) is not an inherited disorder. Composition of dermal collagen is altered which affects physical and mental development. These patients have typical facial features, intellect deficit, and learning disabilities.

(d) **Edward syndrome** (or Trisomy 18) - is not an inherited disorder but happens preconception, at random during egg or sperm formation by the process of disjunction. Many parts of the body are affected. Babies are born small, have cardiac defects, clenched fists, and overlapping fingers. Most babies die before or shortly after birth. They rarely survive 1 year of age.

(e) **Patau syndrome** (Trisomy 13) - is a rare serious genetic disorder in some or all cells of the body. Most babies die within 1 month of age or by 1 year of age. This is not an inherited disorder and occurs at random during cell division in early embryonic life. Babies have polydactyly, deformed feet (rocker bottom feet), holoprosencephaly (failure of brain to divide into two halves), microcephaly, mental deficiency, and microphthalmia.

44.7   Detection/Diagnosis

44.7.1 Prenatal Diagnosis

(a) **Ultrasound** – A routine **ultrasound** at 20 weeks of gestation may detect CH.
(b) **Genetic testing -** Karyotyping and α-fetoprotein levels by chorionic villus sampling and amniocentesis. **High alpha fetoprotein levels are suggestive of CH.**
(c) **Frequent ultrasounds** to watch for growth, changes in the cyst, and for complications.
(d) **Oligo/poly hydramnios** should alert the obstetrician for suspicion of CH.

Large cyst in the neck may cause death in Utero or at birth due to airway obstruction. Once detected, elective Caesarean section is planned at 38 weeks.

44.7.2 Postnatal investigations

Ultrasound, fluoroscopy, X ray neck, chest, CT scan, and MRI are done to confirm the antenatal diagnosis, and to see any changes in size and extension.

CT picture may show multiple fluid-filled loculi in the neck with tracheal compression and deviation.

Fast spin MRI provides better and more detailed image but is expensive.

To assess cardiopulmonary involvement, **angiography and ECHO** may be needed.

44.7.3 Presentation

Signs and symptoms depend on the size and anatomical location of the CH.

1. **Asymptomatic** – In a newborn, it may appear as a bulge under the skin, of slight bluish discoloration. It is a painless, non-tender, soft, cystic mass with facial disfiguration and neck extension and deviation.
2. **Symptomatic** - Lymphatic tumors progressively grow, enlarge, and become symptomatic. Depending on the rate of growth, patient may become symptomatic in the neonatal period or in childhood or later. Symptoms depend on its location.
   (a) **CH in the neck** – symptoms due to laryngo-pharyngeal compression and superior vena cava obstruction, deformity of face and neck, hyperextension and deviation of the neck, facial swelling, congestion, apnoeic attacks, breathing difficulty, stridor, feeding difficulty, and failure to thrive. Obstructive sleep apnea, difficulty in eating, and bone and teeth abnormalities occur with slow growing CH.
   (b) **Axillary or Groin CH** – difficulty in placing the limb in a normal neutral position, and risk of rupture of the cyst, infection and haemorrhage.
   (c) **CH on the chest** – chest wall deformity, breathing difficulty, infection, and bleeding.

(d) **Extension into the base of mouth** - cough, tachypnoea, breathing difficulty, chest retraction, stridor, and dysphagia (**Inspiratory stridor** = supraglottic obstruction, **Expiratory stridor** = subglottic/intrathoracic obstruction).

(e) **Mediastinal extension** may present with airway obstruction, compression and deviation of esophagus, trachea, laryngeal nerve, major vascular structures, and heart. Symptoms include severe hemodynamic compromise and respiratory obstruction, expiratory stridor, wheeze, gas exchange problems, dysphagia, and weight loss.

(f) **Complications** – If left untreated or ignored, patient may present with complications.
   - Significant cosmetic deformity.
   - Obstructive symptoms (stridor, wheeze, dyspnea, dysphagia, OSA, and nerve palsies).
   - Bleeding from injury to the skin over the cyst or its rupture.
   - Lymph discharging sinuses.
   - Recurrent infections and cellulitis.

44.7.4 Examination

- Soft cystic mass of variable size, facial deformity, head, neck, and tongue deviation.
- Signs of respiratory obstruction - laboured breathing, stridor, wheeze, and respiratory distress.
- Brilliant transillumination test.

44.8 Treatment OF CH

Outcome of a patient with CH is unpredictable because how and at what rate it grows or extends into the neighboring tissues is unpredictable. The list of treatment modalities for CH is as follows:

1. **No intervention** - Those detected early in pregnancy, often recede and disappear before birth.
2. **Observation, wait and watch** - Spontaneous regression with time occurs in some patients. In asymptomatic neonate, this is the best approach.
3. **Steroids** don't have much role.
4. **Sclerosing therapy** – intra lesion injection of sclerosing solution at weekly intervals to reduce its size and symptoms.
5. **Other modalities** - Chemotherapy, Radiotherapy, Radio-frequency ablation and Laser excision, have all been tried. They may reduce the cyst size temporarily, but it soon recurs.
6. **Surgical Excision** is the only definitive treatment. It can be done as a one stage or multistage procedure.

Remember

1. CH should never be drained or aspirated, because of risk of bleeding and infection.
2. Nonsurgical measures shrink the size of the CH and facilitate surgical dissection, but never cure completely.
3. They can be used to delay surgery in neonates till they become older.
4. Ideal age for surgery is 18 months to 2 years of age.
5. Often repetitive surgeries are needed due to its infiltrating nature.

44.9 Overall Role of Anesthesiologist

1. **Resuscitation and securing of the airway.**
2. **Diagnostic procedures – MRI, CT scan.**
3. **Sclerotherapy -** intralesional injection of sclerosing agent is a painful procedure and is done under general anesthesia.
4. **Non-surgical procedures** – Chemotherapy, Radiotherapy, Radio-frequency ablation, Laser excision.
5. **Surgical excision.**
6. **Postoperative airway management.**
7. **Anesthesia for postoperative problems and reoperation.**

Anesthetic considerations remain the same for all these procedures, except that these are usually short duration procedures, and are not corrective. So, the neonate is at a high risk of post-procedural airway obstruction and other post-surgical complications.

44.10 Indications for Surgery in Neonates

(a) Airway obstruction and respiratory distress.
(b) Feeding difficulty.
(c) Bleeding or leakage from the cyst.
(d) Multiple congenital anomalies.

44.11 Anesthetic Management

44.11.1 The Airway

As such airway management in neonates is challenging due to their **unique airway anatomy;** neck swelling further adds up because of the risk of sudden complete airway occlusion resulting in hypoventilation, apnea, and hypoxemia. A "Can't

Table 44.2 Anesthetic considerations

Preop	Induction and maintenance	Extubation and postoperative
Size/location Airway obstruction Intrathoracic extension Cong syndromes Heart defects	Premed – Atropine Avoid sedatives 100% O_2 by mask or hood NG tube and aspiration	Do not extubate ET and assisted vent – 24–48 H
Invest – CT, MRI, for extent Prophylactic steroids	CICV can occur Need to aspirate CH Maintenance of SR, gas induction, O_2 100%, Sevo/ H, attain plane of anesthesia for DL AI/ FOI Oral route No PEEP, low airway P	Complications Airway obstruction Hemorrhage Recurrent laryngeal & facial nerve injury, Cranial nerve injury -7th, 9th, 10th, 11th and 12th Infection, Injury to IJV, parotid duct, pharynx, muscles of neck Recurrence
Informed consent	Assistants	
IV line and IVF Monitoring equipment	ENT/Pead surg/cardiac surgeons	
Pead DA cart	OT prep for neonate	

Intubate, Can't Ventilate" (CICV) situation at induction is the most important complication at induction of anesthesia (Table 44.2).

The most important step in the anesthetic management is the securing of safe and reliable airway.

A detailed plan with different options for securing the airway should be sketched out prior to surgery and discussed with the assistants and surgeon.

44.11.2 Problems Frequently Encountered are Because of

a. Airway obstruction or potential for obstruction – care at intubation, anticipate CICV situation and avoid it.
b. Extension into the adjacent structures that create difficulty in securing the airway.
   - Laryngopharynx and pre-tracheal involvement.
   - Mediastinal compression or deviation of esophagus, trachea, laryngeal nerve, major vascular structures, and heart.
c. Concurrent medical diseases.
d. Concurrent congenital anomalies and associated syndromes.

e. Anemia, nutritional deficiencies, and metabolic disturbances.
f. Intraoperative invasive monitoring.
g. Airway problems intraoperatively - Accidental extubation (during neck extension), endobronchial migration of the tube (due to neck flexion and rotation).
h. Intraoperative hemorrhage and hemodynamic changes.
i. Post-operative respiratory obstruction (immediate or delayed).
j. Nerve injuries - Cranial nerves, facial, and recurrent laryngeal nerve.
k. Problems of newborn and neonate.
l. Long duration of surgery 4–6 h.

Note: Surgery for a giant CH should be undertaken in a tertiary care hospital where ENT, pediatric, and cardiothoracic surgical specialties are available along with NICU facilities.

44.11.3 Preoperative Preparation

- All neonates should undergo preoperative evaluation as thoroughly as possible, in view of the emergency nature of surgery, and asses for any invasion and its effects on the airway.
- **Informed written consent** explaining about possible difficult intubation, need for tracheostomy, and post-operative ventilation, should be obtained from the parents.
- Surgeons must explain about the risk of recurrence of the cys and other surgical complications.
- **Compression of esophagus** creates difficulty in swallowing and volume depletion. They should receive IV fluids preoperatively.
- **Compression or deviation of trachea** and difficulty in breathing necessitates intubation at birth or later.
- Newborns with huge CH may have difficulty in adapting to extrauterine environment and may have persistence of fetal circulation (PFC). The ET should be left in situ, connected to CPAP, so that adaptive changes can occur.
- Tracheal compression puts these neonates at risk of chest infection and congestion. Prophylactic antibiotics should be given.
- Feeding tube, placed orally, should be aspirated prior to induction.
- A difficult airway cart (*appendix*) with equipment appropriate for a neonate must be available (*ref Chapter on difficult airway*).
- An ENT surgeon should be at standby till the airway is secured in case of failed intubation. A surgeon must be standby to aspirate the cyst if CICV situation arises (aspiration is not routinely done as it makes surgical dissection more difficult). A cardiothoracic surgeon may also be made available.

44.11.4 Premedication

- Atropine 20 µg/kg oral/IM or 0/1 mg IV, or Glycopyrrolate, to dry airway secretions and as prophylaxis for possible bradycardia during induction and airway handling intraoperatively.
- Sedatives (midazolam 0.1 mg)/ketamine (0.5 mg/kg) may be given provided airway is secure. They are best avoided because of risk of exacerbating airway obstruction.
- Continuous O_2 by face mask.

44.11.5 Intraoperative Monitoring

Since CH lies closely to major vascular structures in the neck and thoracic outlet, massive bleeding during surgical dissection is a great risk. Blood grouping and crossmatching must be done and one unit of packed cells kept ready. This necessitates intense monitoring.

1. Noninvasive – Heart rate, NIBP, ECG, respiration, saturation, and $EtCO_2$.
2. Invasive - CVC (femoral or cubital vein) for fluid administration and packed cell transfusion, and intra-arterial line (femoral artery) for BP monitoring.
3. Temperature (rectal temperature) - Care to prevent hypothermia, due to extensive dissection, long duration, and possible blood loss must be taken (*ref chapter on thermoregulation*).
4. Urine output - Bladder catheterization.

Note – $EtCO_2$ monitoring is important as it will help detect ET problems early.

44.11.6 Induction and Intubation

Several options are available for induction and intubation, keeping the risk of occurrence of CICV situation in mind. Principles of safe induction in the neonate are as follows:

- Preoxygenation with 100% O_2 and avoidance of hypoxemia.
- Maintenance of spontaneous respiration till airway is secured.
- Avoidance of muscle relaxants.
- Inhalational induction with either Sevoflurane or Halothane is preferred over IV induction, as this allows better control of airway.
- IV ketamine (0.5 mg/kg IV) to aid induction and maintain bronchodilatation.
- Laryngoscopy and intubation in deeper plane of inhalational anesthesia.

- No blind intubation procedures or nasal route.
- If airway becomes obstructed following loss of consciousness, try to improve it by turning the patient lateral or semi-prone.
- Use oropharyngeal airway size 0. Avoid nasopharyngeal airway.
- Should the patient become apnoeic during induction, avoid IPPV. Instead use low pressure CPAP until return of spontaneous respiration. Then, try alternative methods of intubation.
- With an obstructed airway, it is difficult to achieve and maintain depth of anesthesia with inhalational agents and baby becomes hypoxic (Positive pressure ventilation via face mask does not ease obstruction).
- Needle aspiration of the cyst can help in airway maintenance, but being multilocular, one point aspiration may not be enough.
- Endotracheal tube size of 3–3.5 in a term neonate and 2.5–3.0 in a preterm neonate. A blunt ended curved stylet can help tube introduction in a partially visible glottis. Uncuffed ET to be used.
- Confirmation of intubation is done by 5-point auscultation and $EtCO_2$ monitoring to detect esophageal intubation.

44.11.6.1 Awake Intubation (AI)

- This requires great skill in a neonate, but if expertise and appropriate equipment and tubes are available, this is the best and safe option for securing the airway in a neonate with giant CH in the neck with respiratory symptoms.
- Due to reduced FRC and risk of hypoxemia, intubation time should not exceed 20 s (the apnea time).
- Neonatal fiberscopes with a O_2 port can circumvent the risk of hypoxemia while allowing time for intubation in case of difficulty.
- Ultra-thin bronchoscope over which 2.5–3 mm tracheal tube can be railroaded, can be used through LMA or directly while providing anesthetic gas mixture through another tube just inside the oral cavity.
- Rigid intubating bronchoscope aide intubation may be successful in case difficulty is encountered during fiberoptic intubation. A bougie is threaded through bronchoscope into the trachea, scope is removed, and appropriate size ET is railroaded over it.

Awake intubation may be associated with following risk:

(a) Trauma to gums, tongue, pharyngeal mucosa, and vocal cords, esp. when anatomy is not visible, and blind intubation is attempted.

(b) Stress-induced physiological changes - increase in blood pressure, heart rate, O_2 consumption, anterior fontanelle pressure, and intra cranial hemorrhage esp. in premature neonate.

44.11.6.2 Surgical Airway

Tracheostomy is the last option and should be performed by trained surgeon.

It is exceedingly difficult to reach the trachea especially if the CH is crossing over the midline. It is associated with a high risk of rupture of CH, bleeding, tracheal injury, hypoxemia, and aspiration.

44.11.6.3 Fixing of the ETT

- Sticking tapes or ribbon gauze usually used may get wet and loose from the cleaning solutions or blood under the drapes during surgery. They will also lie in the surgical field. ET should be **sutured** to the angle of the mouth to prevent inadvertent dislodgement or accidental extubation intraoperatively.
- Once ET placement is confirmed, **laryngeal packing** using wet ribbon gauze should be done around the tube to seal air leak and prevent aspiration of secretions and blood.
- Muscle relaxants and narcotic analgesics are given ONLY after securing the ET.

44.11.7 Maintenance of Anesthesia

- Balanced anesthesia with 2–4% Sevoflurane or 0.5–1% Halothane, muscle relaxants (Rocuronium 0.5 mg (repeated as and when required), analgesics (1–2 µg/kg Fentanyl) and controlled ventilation, using 40% O_2 in air or N_2O, via pediatric circuit or modified Ayre's T piece is the safest option.
- Give Prednisolone 5 mg IV as prophylaxis for airway edema.
- Ventilation should be controlled and with normal parameters (tidal volume of 5–6 mL/kg, airway pressure 12–15 cm H_2O, I:E::1:2).
- Low PEEP (3–5 cm H_2O) can be added if there is difficulty in maintaining saturation of 90–92% with an FiO_2 of 0.5–0.6.
- Excessively high intrathoracic pressure and PEEP further obstruct thoracic duct flow both by direct pressure on the duct and venous hypertension, and further increase the size of the cyst which makes surgical dissection more difficult.
- Do not ventilate using 100% O_2 for long due to risk of BPD and ROP.

Intraoperatively, anesthesiologist must be vigilant to detect ET dislodgment, endobronchial migration, obstruction or extubation.

44.11.8 Fluids and Blood Transfusion (Ref Chapter on IV Fluid Therapy)

Surgery is associated with high third space fluid losses (lymph in the cyst) and blood loss. Meticulous calculation of maintenance and replacement fluids must be done.

Blood loss must be carefully assessed. It is prudent to use a small bottle (100 mL size) as a trap in the suction line for accurate blood loss measurement.

These neonates may be anemic. Blood transfusion trigger is reached early as their allowable blood loss is zero. In a non-anemic neonate, allowable blood loss is 10% of total blood volume. Lost blood should be replaced with packed cells in 1:1 ratio, along with calcium supplement (1 mg/mL of blood) from a separate IV line (baby weighing 2.5 kg, total BV = 225 mL, 10% = 22–27 mL).

44.11.9 Extubation

After resection of the huge CH, even if the neonate meets the criteria for extubation (awake, good respiratory efforts and muscle power, hemodynamic stability), it is better to leave the ET in situ for 24–48 h and provide elective ventilation in the postoperative period, as they are at risk of delayed airway obstruction from laryngeal edema or secondary hemorrhage. On return of spontaneous respiration, ventilation can be changed to CPAP mode.

The effect of neuromuscular blockade will wear off on its own after 30–45 min. There is no need of using neostigmine and glycopyrrolate for reversal of residual neuromuscular block.

In case of injury to larynx or recurrent laryngeal nerve, babies may require intubation for a longer period with respiratory support.

44.12 Postoperative Complications

Surgical excision is associated with complications which increase the duration of hospital stay, need for NICU and ventilatory care, and re-exploration. These include the following:

1. Respiratory obstruction.
2. Hemorrhage.
3. Recurrent laryngeal and Facial nerve injury.
4. Cranial nerve damage - Injury to 7th, 9th, 10th, 11th and 12th nerves.
5. Wound infection.
6. Damage to neighboring structures – Internal jugular vein, parotid duct, pharynx, and muscles of the neck.
7. Recurrence (because of incomplete surgical excision).

44.12.1 Respiratory Obstruction

Respiratory obstruction is the most increased morbidity and even death. Causes may be:

- Secondary to reactionary edema of the airway and supraglottic edema, in initial 6–8 h of surgery.
- Airway collapse from possible tracheomalacia.
- Tongue edema.
- Rapid expansion of residual cyst due to hemorrhage.
- Edema of inflammation or cyst infection.
- Recurrent laryngeal and Hypoglossal nerve injuries.

Management

- **Reactionary edema** is a treatable cause if managed timely.
  - **Drugs** - IV dexamethasone and nebulization with racemic epinephrine.
  - **Humidified O$_2$.**
  - **Re-intubation** - In a neonate who has been extubated immediately after surgery, reintubation may be difficult and impossible. The usual ET size for this age is 3–3.5 id. Once laryngeal or airway edema occurs, airway becomes narrow and obstructed, and accommodate a smaller ET (size 2, 2.5).
  - **Tracheostomy** – is done if airway maintenance is required for a longer time (more than 4–5 days) but is more difficult. In an emergency, drainage of the local area may be lifesaving.
- Drains must be left in situ to prevent hematoma formation and respiratory obstruction.
- In the event of injury to hypoglossal nerve injury, tongue gets deviated, causing upper airway obstruction. The tongue must be stabilized by applying stitches at the dorsum and then traction.
- Cranial nerve injury takes a long time to heal or heal with residual deficit.
- Rapid expansion of the residual cyst (due to inflammation) requires urgent antimicrobial coverage.
- Dysphagia due to surgical interference with neural innervation to the muscles and tissues of hypopharynx and upper cervical esophagus is managed by providing feeds via the orogastric tube, parenteral nutrition, or both, until healing occurs or definitive treatment is undertaken.

44.13 Conclusion

- Though uncommon, neonates with a near fatal Giant CH can undergo successful anesthetic management for surgery, with proper evaluation, planning regarding airway management, coexisting anomalies, and postoperative complications.
- Good communication among the pediatric surgeon, anesthesiologist, ENT, and cardiac surgeons (in case of thoracic extension) is essential for efficient management.
- The key to a successful management includes identification of the potential problems, detailed preoperative evaluation with emphasis on airway assessment, and considering different options with a selection of an appropriate plan of anesthesia. Extubation should never be done in a hurry. Postoperative endotracheal tube and respiratory support can prevent airway related morbidity and mortality.
- Need for adequate fluid therapy, nutrition, and analgesia cannot be undermined.
- Recognition of potential adverse events in the postoperative period and prompt management can save life.

Contents of Difficult Pediatric Airway cart – airways (oropharyngeal and LMA), laryngoscopes (straight, curved, McCoy, and video laryngoscope), fibreoptic and rigid intubating bronchoscopes, ET tubes (sizes 2.0–4.0), stylets and bougies, Magill forceps, suction catheters, mini tracheostomy and cricothyrotomy kits, connectors of different sizes.

Further Readings

Abbas A, Mallhi AI, Alam SS, Mughal HMA. Cystic hygroma; difficult airway and the anesthetic considerations. Anaesth Pain Intensive Care. 2017;21(4):472–4.

Esmaeili MRH, Razavi SSB, Harofteh HRA, et al. Cystic hygroma: anesthetic considerations and review. JRMS. 2009;14(3):191–5.

Fleischmann's hygroma. Miller-Keane encyclopedia and dictionary of medicine, nursing, and allied health. 7th ed. © 2003 by Saunders, an imprint of Elsevier, Inc.

Kim H, Kim HS, Oh JT, Lee JR. Anesthetic management for neonate with giant cystic hygroma involved upper airway: a case report. Korean J Anesthesiol. 2011;60:209–13.

Rao KS, Shenoy T. Anesthetic management of a large cystic hygroma in a newborn. Anesth Essays Res. 2015;9:270–2.

Silay E, Coskuner I, Yildiz H, Bakan V, et al. Anaesthetic management of a neonate with giant cystic hygroma. Turk J Anaesthesiol Reanim. 2013;41(5):185–7. https://doi.org/10.5152/TJAR.2013.24.

Nesidioblastoma (Congenital Hyperinsulinism - CHI)

45

Pratibha Jain Shah

45.1 Introduction

Nesidioblastoma or persistent hyper insulinemic hypoglycemia of infancy (PHHI) or congenital hyperinsulinism (CHI) is a very uncommon yet life-threatening neuroendocrine cause of hypoglycemia. Its characteristic feature is recurrent episodes of severe, sustained, or persistent hypoglycemia due to elevated insulin levels, along with elevated C-peptide and proinsulin, beyond few hours of life. If not recognized promptly and managed, it may result in long-term neurological damage in the form of seizures, mental and psychological retardation, neurological deficits and even death from undiagnosed severe hypoglycemia. It is heterogenous clinically, genetically, and histopathologically.

George F Laidlaw in 1938 coined the term **"islet cell adenoma"** for neo-differentiation of islets of Langerhans from pancreatic duct epithelium. The term **Nesidioblastoma** was derived from the Greek words nesidion (islet) and blastos (germ). In 1989, Glaser proposed the term (PHHI), that replaced all other terms used previously.

45.2 Incidence

Incidence of symptomatic hypoglycemia is 4/1000 term and 6/1000 preterm newborns. Only 1% of these have nesidioblastoma (PHHI). It affects 1:50,000 live birth in random population and 1:2500 live birth in communities with significant consanguinities. There is slight male preponderance (M:F::1.2:1 in diffuse form and 1.8:1 for focal form). The most common age for presentation is in the neonates and infants and is rare after the age of 2 years.

P. J. Shah (✉)
Department of Anesthesiology, Pt JNM MC, Raipur, India

© The Author(s), under exclusive license to Springer Nature Singapore Pte Ltd. 2023
U. Saha (ed.), *Clinical Anesthesia for the Newborn and the Neonate*,
https://doi.org/10.1007/978-981-19-5458-0_45

45.3 Etiopathogenesis

PHHI is recessively inherited hyperinsulinism due to mutation of Sulfonylurea (SUR) genes and of genes regulating the function of ATP-dependent potassium channels on the β cell membrane. In some cases, it may be dominant and involves glucokinase and glutamate dehydrogenase genes.

There is overpopulation, maldistribution, and malfunctioning of β-cells which arise from the exocrine pancreatic ductal epithelium. Histologically, there is ducto-endocrine proliferation, supernumerary small endocrine groups, and large endocrine areas. It is analogous to non-insulinoma pancreatogenous hypoglycemic syndrome (NIPHS) in adults.

There are two types of PHHI: (a) focal and (b) diffuse.

(a) **Focal form (40%):** Presence of abnormal β cells in one or more focal areas inside the pancreatic tissue, each lesion 2.5–7.5 mm in diameter.
(b) **Diffuse form (60%):** Abnormal β cells present in all sections of the pancreas.

Antibodies to islets antigens are demonstrated in the serum of these patients but their role in pathogenesis is unclear. Elevated pituitary protein 7B2 is a diagnostic marker.

45.4 Clinical Presentation

- At birth - Macrosomia, mild to moderate hepatomegaly. Symptoms of hypoglycemia appear within 72 h of birth and can be adrenergic (anxiety, tremor, nausea, hunger, hypotonia, sweating, and palpitations) or neuroglycopenic (headache, lethargy, dizziness, diplopia, blurred vision, amnesia, seizures, confusion, and coma).
- Hypoglycemia -Normal blood sugar level in neonates is 40–60 mg/dL and <30 mg/dL in preterm and <40 mg/dL in term newborns is considered as hypoglycemia.
- Typical facies of hyperinsulinism - high forehead, large bullous nose, short columella, smooth philtrum, and thin upper lip.

45.5 Diagnosis (Box 45.1)

- Elevated insulin to glucose ratio to 0.4–2.7 (normal <0.4).
- Low ketone bodies, free fatty acids, and branched chain amino acids after 4–6 h of fasting.

> **Box 45.1 Diagnostic Criteria for PHHI and Differential Diagnosis**
>
> 1. Nonketotic hypoglycemia (blood sugar <36 mg/dL) both fasting/postprandial.
> 2. Hyperinsulinemia (>3 mU/L).
> 3. Need for high rate of glucose infusion (>10 mg/kg/min) to maintain blood sugar >54 mg/dL.
> 4. Rise in blood sugar following SC or IM glucagon (0.5 mg dose increases blood sugar by 18–36 mg/dL).
>
> **Differential Diagnosis** – Endocrine disorders (multiple endocrine neoplasia, hypopituitarism, hypothyroidism, adrenal insufficiency (maternal diabetes), IUGR (inborn error of metabolism), SGA (Patau and Beckwith-Wiedemann syndromes).

45.6 Management

Nesidioblastoma requires prompt management, otherwise may lead to irreversible brain damage and death.

45.6.1 Correction of Symptomatic Hypoglycemia

- High rate of 10% dextrose infusion (10–15 mg/kg/min). Up to 12.5% dextrose can be infused through a peripheral vein, but central vein is preferred because of high risk of peripheral venous thrombosis.
- Continuous feeding with glucose polymer orally or via nasogastric tube even during sleep to maintain blood glucose levels.

45.6.2 Drug Management

Three categories of drugs are used in management of PHHI (Table 45.1).

(a) **Drugs which inhibit insulin secretion-** Diazoxide, Somatostatin, Diphenylhydantoin, and Calcium channel blockers (Nifedipine) – these are the

Table 45.1 Drugs, their mechanism of action, and adverse effects

Drug	Mechanism of action	Adverse effects
Diazoxide	Inhibits pancreatic insulin release	Hypotension, salt and water retention, ↑BS, HR
Nifedipine	Calcium channel blocker	Hypotension, edema, dizziness, flushing
Octreotide	↓Growth hormone secretion	Dysglycemia, hypothyroidism, ECG changes
Hydrochlorothiazide	Inhibits Na reabsorption in duct	Hyperglycemia, hypotension, hyperuricemia
Glucagon	Insulin antagonism, glycogenolysis	Nausea, vomiting

primary drugs for long-term medical treatment of PHHI. **Diazoxide** is the first-line drug in management of PHHI. It can be administered orally in a dose of 8 mg/kg at 8 h intervals. It increases blood sugar by inhibiting release of insulin, stimulating release of catecholamines, and mobilizing glycogen. Hydrochlorothiazide (25 mg/alternate day) has similar action.

(b) **Drugs which antagonize the effect of insulin on tissues and increase hepatic glycogenolysis** - Epinephrine, Glucagon, and growth hormone. **Octreotide** (somatostatin analogue) is useful in diazoxide unresponsive babies and is given IV once a day in a dose of 2 mcg/kg. In higher doses, it may worsen hypoglycemia by inhibiting secretion of glucagon and growth hormone.

(c) **Drugs which destroy islet cells** – Streptozotocin or streptozocin, a naturally occurring alkylating antineoplastic agent, particularly toxic to the insulin-producing beta cells of the pancreas in mammals.

45.6.3 Surgical Resection

Surgery is indicated in babies not responding to medical management and for focal lesions amenable to surgical resection.

(a) **Resection of focal lesions.**
(b) **Sub-total pancreatectomy in case of diffuse lesion.**

45.7 Anaesthetic Management

45.7.1 Main Goal

1. To maintain adequate glycemic control (blood sugar 100–150 mg/dL) perioperatively to prevent hypoglycemia secondary to prolonged fasting, surgical manipulation of pancreas, and withheld dextrose infusion.
2. Frequent perioperative RBS monitoring every 15–30 min till discharge from recovery room because under GA mask all signs of hypoglycemia.
3. Thorough preoperative assessment and documentation of existing neurologic damage from previous hypoglycemic episodes.
4. Discontinue drugs which inhibit insulin release to attenuate exaggerated postoperative hyperglycemic effects.
5. Avoid prolonged fasting.

45.7.2 Anesthesia Technique

1. **Premedication** – Syrup Phenergan (0.5 mg/kg) for its anticonvulsant and anxiolytic effect.
2. **Difficult airway** in case of macrosomia.
3. **General anesthesia** with controlled ventilation and continuous epidural analgesia. The chosen anesthetic agent should not increase cerebral metabolic rate for

O_2 or cause further hypoglycemia. Thiopentone is suitable for induction. Among inhalation agents, Halothane and Isoflurane (inhibit pancreatic insulin release) are suitable. Avoid Sevoflurane as it may provoke convulsions.

4. **Muscle relaxants** – Atracurium or Rocuronium can be used for intubation and controlling ventilation. At the end of surgery, neostigmine and glycopyrrolate are used for reversal of residual neuromuscular blockade.
5. **Analgesia** – IV Fentanyl (1–2 μ/kg) supplemented with epidural Bupivacaine (0.25% 1 ml/kg) for intraoperative analgesia and continued postoperatively.
6. **IV fluids** - Surgery usually does not entail much fluid loss or blood loss. Use two IV lines – one for D 10 @ 10 mL/kg/min, and other for RL @ 1–2 mL/kg/min.
7. **Monitoring** – ECG, NIBP, SpO_2, $EtCO_2$, CVP, and temperature.

45.7.3 Postoperative Care

1. Post-surgery anticipate rise in blood sugar levels, as there is acute transition from hyperinsulinemic state to diabetic state.
2. Postoperatively, check blood sugar levels, reduce the rate of dextrose infusion, and start insulin drip according to blood sugar level to maintain euglycemia.
3. Start oral feeds as early as possible.

45.8   Conclusion

Nesidioblastoma is a neuroendocrine tumor characterized by severe, persistent hypoglycemia secondary to hyperinsulinemia, and if untreated may lead to irreversible brain damage and life-threatening complications. Surgical correction depends on the diffuse or focal form of disease. Anaesthetic management should focus on maintaining euglycemia through regular blood glucose monitoring and avoid excessive fasting. The chosen anesthetic drugs should not increase cerebral metabolic rate while maintaining glucose and insulin homeostasis.

Further Readings

Dardano A, Daniele G, Lupi R, Napoli N, et al. Nesidioblastosis and Insulinoma: a rare coexistence and a therapeutic challenge. Front Endocrinol. 2020;11:10. https://doi.org/10.3389/fendo.2020.00010.

Goel P, Choudhury SR. Persistent hyperinsulinemic hypoglycemia of infancy: an overview of current concepts. J Indian Assoc Pediatr Surg. 2012;17(3):99–103.

Mohamed HA. Nesidioblastosis: a review of anaesthetic implications: case report. Sudan Med J. 2016;52(3):140–5.

Patel K, Shikare M, Chavan D, Sawant P. Anesthetists approach in a neonate with Nesidioblastoma undergoing pancreatectomy. J Anaesthesiol Clin Pharmacol. 2013;29(3):384–6. https://doi.org/10.4103/09709185.117108.

Rahier J, Guiot Y, Sempoux C. Persistent hyperinsulinaemic hypoglycaemia of infancy: a heterogeneous syndrome unrelated to nesidioblastosis. Arch Dis Child Fetal Neonatal Ed. 2000;82(2):F108–12.

Soares AA, Karapurkar SA, Suresh SS. Anaesthetic management of nesidioblastosis in a newborn. J Postgrad Med. 1996;42:23.

Congenital Broncho-Biliary Fistula (CBBF)

46

Sakshi Mahajan and Rakhee Goyal

46.1 Introduction

Congenital broncho biliary fistula (**CBBF**) is a rare developmental abnormality with a fistulous communication between the respiratory and biliary tract. Clinical presentation, severity of symptoms, and prognosis depend on the size of the fistula and associated biliary tract malformations. We aim to make the reader aware of this rare yet life-threatening congenital abnormality, its clinical presentation, diagnostic and surgical modalities, and risks involved in a neonate undergoing corrective surgery. Under anesthesia management, points of specific concern in CBBF are discussed as other concerns remain the same as for any neonate coming for surgery.

46.2 Congenital BBF (CBBF)

Broncho-biliary fistula (BBF) is an uncommon clinical entity in which there is an abnormal connection between the biliary tract and the bronchus or elsewhere in the bronchial tree. There may be a connection with the trachea in some cases (trachea biliary fistula). BBF may be congenital or acquired. Acquired BBF may occur in older children and adults with obstruction in the biliary tract, and or abscess or hydatid cysts in the liver [1].

CBBF is of rare occurrence and was first reported by Neuhauser etal in 1952 [2]. Abnormal embryonic development of the foregut or abnormal fusion of the bronchial bud with the bile duct during the development in the early gestation period may create a connection between the biliary and respiratory tracts, giving rise to CBBF in the newborn. Its occurrence must be kept in mind in neonates with biliary tract anomalies, especially biliary atresia or congenital diaphragmatic hernia.

S. Mahajan (✉) · R. Goyal
Department of Anesthesia, Madhukar Rainbow Children's Hospital, New Delhi, India

U. Saha (ed.), *Clinical Anesthesia for the Newborn and the Neonate*, https://doi.org/10.1007/978-981-19-5458-0_46

46.3   Clinical Presentation

Time of presentation and severity of symptoms depends upon the size of fistula and associated biliary tract malformation. Symptoms can occur anytime from birth into the neonatal period and adulthood. Earlier the presentation, more severe is the disease, requiring early intervention. It is more common in females, and more involving the right main bronchus. However, connections at the level of carina or the left main bronchus have also been reported. [3, 4]

46.4   Pathophysiology

A neonate with biliary atresia may present with intermittent cyanosis, apnea, biliptysis (bile in saliva and its yellow discoloration), choking, and jaundice within a few days of birth. Bile in the bronchi and lungs can lead to chemical pneumonitis and respiratory distress. If diagnosis is not made, baby may continue to be treated for RDS, with grave outcome.

46.5   Diagnosis

Yellow green discoloration of the saliva or tracheal secretions should make one suspicious of the presence of a BBF. It can be confused with trachea-esophageal fistula (TEF), gastro-esophageal reflux disease (GERD), aspiration pneumonitis, or cardiac disease [1].

   Diagnostic modalities, besides clinical presentation, include bronchoscopy, CT chest, 3D-CT, Ultrasonography Contrast studies (bronchography, fistulogram, PTC, ERCP), MRCP, contrast-enhanced MRCP, and HIDA scan.

   Bronchoscopy is the first choice, in which abnormal opening can be seen in the trachea or bronchus.

   Chest CT and **3D- CT scans** may show abnormal branches of trachea, gas bubbles in the biliary tree, and a cone-shaped fissure-like protrusion on chest 3D-CT reconstruction [4].

   On **Ultrasonography,** accumulated gas in the bile duct and gall bladder, moving with baby's respiratory excursions, can be seen.

   Contrast studies like **bronchography** and **fistulogram** (using bronchial blocker) help delineate the defect before surgery [3, 4].

   PTC (Percutaneous transhepatic cholangiography) and ERCP (**Endoscopic retrograde cholangiopancreatography**) can show the origin and course of the fistula, bile duct anatomy, but are restricted for acquired BBF (ABBF) in adults, because of the complexity and trauma involved.

   MRCP and Contrast-enhanced MRCP outline the anatomy of the biliary tract and provide information on bile flow.

HIDA (Hepatobiliary iminodiacetic acid) scan (also known as cholescintigraphy or hepatobiliary scintigraphy) uses radioactive tracer and can be used for diagnosis and postoperative surveillance in neonates [5].

46.6   Treatment

The only definite treatment is Surgery. There are two major steps such as:

1. Identification, isolation, and closure or plugging of the BBF.
2. Establishing the connection between the biliary and gastrointestinal tract for bile drainage [6].

For good surgical results, the baby should be optimized in relation to the pulmonary function, oxygenation and gas exchange, and stabilization of the hemodynamics in the intervening preoperative period. These babies may require admission to NICU.

46.7   Surgery

Resection of the BBF can be done by Thoracoscopic route [4] or by Thoracotomy using extra pleural approach [5]. Open thoracotomy is preferred because of difficulty in maintaining ventilation during thoracoscopic approach in neonates. In severe cases, lobectomy may need to be undertaken.

Bronchoscopy guided Plugging of the fistula is less traumatic and with quick recovery but is limited for adult ABBF.

VATS (Video assisted thoracoscopic surgery) **is** less traumatic and quicker recovery after surgery for CBBF in a neonate, than thoracotomy.

Gunlemenz etal (2009) reported a newborn with CBBF of left main bronchus (respiratory distress and bilious tracheal discharge) and biliary atresia. Surgery included excision of fistula and re-establishing the biliary drainage system (Roux-en-Y cholecysto-jejunostomy). Creation of bile drainage route is important to avoid recurrence [6].

46.8   Preoperative Care

- Baby should not be kept supine. A propped-up position allows postural drainage of bile and prevents or reduces bile reflux [1].
- Quantity of each feed should be reduced.
- Adequate NPO period to reduce further risk of aspiration.
- During the fasting period, neonate must receive glucose containing IV fluids to maintain blood sugar >40 mg%.

- GI decompression (removal of collected air in the biliary tract) by placing a gastric tube, preferably by the oral route, left open for continuous drainage. This will also reduce bile reflux into the lung.
- IV antibiotics to be started.
- Loss of excessive bile can create fluid and electrolyte disturbances. Hence, hydration and electrolytes status must be checked and maintained.
- Somatostatin inhibits gastro-intestinal secretions and may be of some help [1].
- If the neonate is on mechanical ventilatory support, this must be continued till baby is transferred to the operation theater.
- Frequent endotracheal suctioning will be necessary to prevent soiling of other ipsilateral lobes and contralateral lung.

46.9 Ventilation Specifics in CBBF

Selection of proper mode of ventilation is important in BBF.

(a) Large volume and high pressure controlled ventilation may cause loss of air into the biliary tract through the fistula depending on its size. This may even open an otherwise collapsed, partially closed tract, while also reducing effective ventilation.
(b) Assisted−/controlled ventilation with low tidal volume and high respiratory rate must be adopted.
(c) High-frequency ventilation (HFV) is the preferred mode.
(d) Low pressure CPAP (enough to maintain SpO_2 (88–92%) is a safe option.

46.10 Anesthetic Management

Anesthesia management is extremely challenging in a neonate with BBF because of the following reasons:

- **Patient factors** – gestational age and body weight at birth, age (days or weeks) at the time of surgery, degree of lung soiling or damage, clinical condition (need for assisted ventilation or vasoactive drugs for hemodynamic control), and organ functions (Renal, Hepatic, and CVS).
- **Surgical factors** – type of surgery (open vs endoscopic), size and location of the fistula, surgical expertise, use of contrast media, and intraoperative cholecystography. [5] Depending on the extent of surgery, the surgical risk, duration of surgery, intraoperative bleeding, fluid shifts, and hypothermia will increase.
- **Anesthesia factors** – the usual care, precautions, and monitoring must be taken in the baby. Major anesthetic goal is to maintain good ventilation and prevent hypoxemia. Specific to BBF surgery, lung isolation is an essential requirement but is a problem in neonate. Airway is secured with the single lumen endotracheal tube. Bronchial blocker may be used to plug the fistula but is difficult in

neonates. Ventilation is controlled using low pressure high-frequency ventilation. Intraoperative lateral position and surgical retraction can exacerbate atelectasis and ventilation perfusion mismatch. Some air will always leak through the fistula and may cause inadequate ventilation. The contrast media is injected through the bile duct to delineate the fistulous tract and can spill into the lungs via the bronchial connection. Anesthetist must be ready to do tube suction immediately on injection of the dye [7].

- **Analgesia** – Intra- and post-operative pain relief can be provided by systemic opioids and paracetamol. Local infiltration at the incision site should always be done. Neuraxial block and thoracic epidural are good options along with general anesthesia.
- **Postoperative care** – baby is electively ventilated for few days and transferred to NICU, for care. Extubation is done once the lungs are fully expanded.

46.11 Conclusion

One should be alert to the occurrence of CBBF in a neonate presenting with recurrent pneumonia, respiratory distress, and yellow coloured saliva. Once suspected, appropriate investigations can confirm the diagnosis with timely corrective surgery. Preoperative stabilization is important. Surgery may be prolonged and there is risk of bile regurgitation during positioning and gut handling; hence, definitive airway with an endotracheal tube is advocated. There is no place for supraglottic devices. Since lung is involved, ventilation should always be controlled. Gentle ventilation can assist the surgeon in retracting the lung to identify the fistulous connection. Importance of intraoperative and postoperative analgesia is paramount. Besides specific care regarding the CBBF, all other care for a surgical neonate, including thermoregulation, must be always taken. Baby must be electively ventilated postoperatively, especially if surgery is extensive, prolonged and involves tracheal reconstruction. Anesthesiologist plays an important role in the outcome of the baby after surgery.

References

1. Liao GQ, Wang H, Zhu GY, Zhu KB, Lv FX, Tai S. Management of acquired bronchobiliary fistula: a systematic literature review of 68 cases published in 30 years. World J Gastroenterol. 2011;17(33):3842–9.
2. Neuhauser EB, Elkin M, Landing B. Congenital direct communication between the biliary system and respiratory tract. AMA Am J Dis Child. 1952;83:654–9. https://doi.org/10.1001/archpedi.1952.02040090100012.
3. Li TY, Zhang ZB. Congenital bronchobiliary fistula: a case report and review of the literature. Case Rep World J Clin Cases. 2019;7(7):881–90. https://doi.org/10.12998/wicc.v7.i7.881.
4. Bing Z, Chen R, Xing P, et al. Congenital bronchobiliary fistula: a case report and literature review. FrontPediatr. 2021;9:686827. https://doi.org/10.3389/fped.2021.686827.

5. Egrari S, Krishnamoorthy M, Yee CA, et al. Congenital bronchobiliary fistula: diagnosis and postoperative surveillance with HIDA scan. J Pediatr Surg. 1996;31(6):785–6. https://doi.org/10.1016/s0022-3468(96)90133-5. PMID: 8783103.
6. Gunlemez A, Tugay M, Elemen L, et al. Surgical experience in a baby with congenital bronchobiliary fistula. Ann Thorac Surg. 2009;87(1):318–20. https://doi.org/10.1016/j.athoracsur.2008.06.028.
7. Yin H, Zhao G, Du Y, et al. Anesthesia management in neonatal congenital bronchobiliary fistula: case report and literature review. BMC Anesthesiol. 2020;20:135.

Neonatal Malignancy and Anaesthesia

47

Shikhar More and Seema Mishra

47.1 Introduction

Neoplasms in the neonatal period are relatively rare with an expected incidence of 1 in 12,500–27,500 live births and comprise 2% of all childhood tumours [1].

Neonatal neoplasms are distinct from those occurring later in childhood or in adults with respect to their anatomical location, histology, tumour behaviour and treatment options. Although a majority of neonatal tumours are benign, malignant neoplasms are associated with high mortality, either due to perinatal or surgical complications or due to progression of disease itself. Due to the natural high cellular turnover in the neonatal period, histological diagnosis of malignancy is difficult. However, with increased understanding of association with various syndromes and availability of fetal imaging, tumours are frequently being diagnosed in the prenatal period, thus allowing for safe delivery, perinatal care and early decision-making. Care of neonates with neoplasm requires a state-of-art multidisciplinary approach comprising experts in high-risk pregnancy and neonatal care with pediatric oncology experts. This chapter aims to highlight the anaesthetic management of neonates who undergo surgery for neoplasms.

S. More
Department of Onco-Anaesthesia and Pain, Tata Medical Center, Kolkata, India

S. Mishra (✉)
Department of Onco-Anaesthesia and Palliative Medicine, Dr BRA, IRCH, AIIMS, New Delhi, India

47.2   Epidemiology of Neonatal Neoplasms

The etiology of neonatal tumours is not completely understood. It is likely that multiple factors including genetic predisposition, prenatal exposure to toxins, radiation, chemotherapy, maternal cancers, and chromosomal abnormalities may all contribute to the development and progression of neonatal tumours.

An analysis of SEER (Surveillance, Epidemiology, and End Results) programme data in the United States (2017) of 615 cases of neonatal malignancies found that solid tumours (n = 454) comprised the vast majority followed by leukaemias (n = 93) and CNS tumours (n = 68). The most common solid tumour was found to be Neuroblastoma (n = 174) followed by Germ cell tumours (n = 168). Neonates with solid tumours had the highest five-year survival of 71.2%, followed by leukaemias (39.1%) and CNS tumours (15%) [2].

There are a few single centre reports from India pertaining to neonatal tumours. A recent retrospective review of neonates who underwent surgery for neoplasms at the Postgraduate Institute of Medical Education and Research (PGIMER), Chandigarh, India, reported a total of 32 cases over 12 years [3]. The most common malignant tumour encountered was soft tissue sarcoma followed by teratomas. The overwhelming majority of benign tumours was sacrococcygeal teratoma (SCT). Other rare benign tumours were hamartomas and hemangioendotheliomas. About 16 neonates underwent SCT excision, while 6 underwent laparotomy including one liver resection and one nephroureterectomy. Other surgeries included those of the limbs, neck and abdominal and thoracic wall.

Another single centre experience from Meenakshi Medical Mission, Madurai, India, which included both benign and malignant tumours and "tumour like lesions" revealed that haemangiomas and lymphangiomas were most common among the 51 such cases over 5 years. Among "true" neoplasms, ovarian cysts were most common, followed by fibrosarcomas, neuroblastoma and teratomas. Malignant tumours comprised only around 15% of all tumours among which neuroblastoma was the most common [4].

Table 47.1 summarises the various neoplasms encountered in the neonates, their treatment modalities and potential anaesthetic exposures.

Many neoplasms diagnosed in the perinatal period are often composed of undifferentiated embryonic or fetal cells and remnants, which suggests genetic changes affecting the cell ability to differentiate. Thus, every neonate diagnosed with a tumour should be genetically screened. The presence of genetic syndromes has special implications in the peri-operative and overall management (Table 47.2).

Table 47.1 Neonatal neoplasms, presentation and management

Tumour type	Presentation	Management options
Neuroblastoma [5]	Most common malignant tumour Adrenal, paravertebral, thoracic, neck mass Spinal cord compression, Horner's syndrome, myoclonus Catecholamine excess: hypertension, sweating, flushing tachycardia	Ultrasound, CT, MRI Biopsy Primary surgery for resectable, low-risk cases Platinum/doxorubicin-based chemotherapy, stem cell transplant, radiotherapy in intermediate and high risk
Teratomas [6] Sacrococcygeal (SCT) Intracranial Cervical Retroperitoneal	Most common in neonates SCT – 30–60% of all teratomas Large vascular tumours Cardiac failure, hydrops fetalis, congenital heart disease	Usually diagnosed prenatal (ultrasound) Complete surgical removal is the goal of treatment Abdominoperineal approach for tumours with large pelvic components Platinum based chemotherapy for unresectable disease/positive margins
Soft tissue sarcoma (STS) [7] Fibrosarcoma Vascular tumours Rhabdomyosarcoma (RMS) Other fibroblastic/rhabdoid tumours	8–10% of all neonatal tumours Benign vascular tumours, fibromatoses more common RMS is most common malignant tumour Usually present as deep-seated mass in extremities, May involve head/neck, Torsion about 20%	Biopsy, immunohistochemistry essential in diagnosis RMS is primarily treated with chemotherapy, radiation; prognosis remains poor Primary surgery only if complete resection is possible with non-mutilating surgery Multimodal management followed by conservative surgery is most common.
Renal tumours [8] Congenial mesoblastic nephroma (CMN) Wilms' tumour (WT) Rhabdoid tumour Clear cell sarcoma	Around 5% of all perinatal tumours Prenatal: polyhydramnios, hydrops, premature delivery Abdominal mass, haematuria, hypertension Often associated with congenital cancer syndromes Pre-natal ultrasound diagnosis in majority of cases	Radical nephrectomy treatment of choice CMN and WT have favourable prognosis with good overall survival Chemotherapy is indicated in CMN if surgical margins are positive WT is often treated with a combination of surgery, chemotherapy and radiation

(continued)

Table 47.1 (continued)

Tumour type	Presentation	Management options
Liver tumours [9] Benign: Hemangiomas, Mesenchymal hamartomas, endotheliomas Malignant: Hepatoblastoma (HB), rhabdoid tumours, choriocarcinomas	Most hepatic tumours in newborns are benign HB most common malignant tumour, comprise 15% of all neonatal liver tumours Usually detected as abdominal mass on pre-operative scanning AFP levels for screening/ diagnosis Large vascular tumours may cause cardio-respiratory compromise	Symptomatic vascular tumours are optimised medically before attempts at surgical resection Outcomes in HB is dependent on complete surgical resection Chemotherapy includes vincristine, 5-FU, doxorubicin and may be given preoperatively to allow for complete resection
CNS tumours [10] Teratomas (most common, supratentorial) Astrocytoma, Choroid plexus papilloma, Medulloblastoma, Glioblastoma.	Rare in neonatal period, 14–41 cases per million live births Antenatal USG: large head, polyhydramnios, hydrops, hydrocephalus, macrocephalus, altered intracranial echogenicity Postnatal: Symptoms of raised ICP, hydrocephalus, lethargy, irritability Cranial nerve palsies, focal neuro-deficits, seizures etc	MRI for diagnosis which may require general anaesthesia Surgical resection and chemotherapy remain mainstay of treatment Radiation is avoided until 3 years of age Prognosis is poor due to difficulties with adequate surgical resection/chemotherapy

Table 47.2 Genetic syndromes associated with neonatal neoplasms [1]

Genetic syndrome	Tumours seen in perinatal period	Developmental defects
WAGR Syndrome – Wilms' tumour, aniridia, genitourinary abnormality, retardation (mental)	Wilms' tumour	Aniridia (absence of iris, glaucoma, cataract) Genitourinary abnormalities – undescended testis, bicornuate uterus Mental retardation, depression, attention deficit hyperactive disorder (ADHD), obsessive compulsive disorder (OCD), autism spectrum disorder
Denys-Drash syndrome (DDS) - progressive glomerulo nephropathy causing renal failure, genital abnormalities, Wilms' tumour	Wilms' tumour (50%)	Diffuse mesangial sclerosis leading to renal disease (focal/diffuse), usually presents with proteinuria, nephrotic syndrome, hypertension, end stage renal disease by 3 years of age Disorder of sexual development (ambiguous genitalia or phenotypically normal female external genitalia, internal genitalia are frequently dysplastic or inappropriate)

Table 47.2 (continued)

Genetic syndrome	Tumours seen in perinatal period	Developmental defects
Beckwith-Wiedemann syndrome (BWS)	Hepatoblastoma, adrenocortical carcinoma, Wilms' tumour (20%)	Overgrowth syndrome, macroglossia, macrosomia, renal abnormalities, unusual ear creases or pits, omphalocele, hemihypertrophy, neonatal hypoglycaemia
Congenital central hypoventilation syndrome (CCHS)	Neuroblastoma (3%)	Respiratory insufficiency, sleep apnea, Hirschsprung's disease
Mosaic variegated aneuploidy (MVA) syndrome – Some cells have abnormal number of chromosomes	Wilms' tumour, rhabdomyosarcoma, leukaemia (40%)	Facial dysmorphism, growth retardation, cataract, microcephaly, short stature, Dandy–Walker complex, eye abnormalities, seizures, intellectual disability
Li–Fraumeni syndrome	Brain tumour, bone or soft-tissue sarcoma, adrenocortical carcinoma	Inherited familial, mutation in tumour suppression gene (TP53)
Rhabdoid tumours	Atypical teratoid rhabdoid tumour - renal /extrarenal	
Retinoblastoma	Retinoblastoma (90%), sarcoma, melanoma, glioma, carcinoma	
Familial adenomatous polyposis	Hepatoblastoma (1%) colorectal/thyroid cancer, medulloblastoma, desmoid tumour	
Familial neuroblastoma	Neuroblastoma (30–70%)	
Medulloblastoma	Medulloblastoma (20%)	

47.3 Clinical Implications of Neoplasia in the Newborn

The diagnosis and treatment of a neoplasm in the neonatal period is a tremendous clinical challenge due to the delicate transitional physiology of the newborn respiratory and circulatory systems. There is also immense emotional and psychosocial impact on the parents which mandates effective communication regarding the disease, treatment processes, prognosis and long-term sequelae. The diagnostic modalities and treatment approach are unique to each set of tumours and needs multidisciplinary planning and coordination. Larger tumours can often be diagnosed on antenatal ultrasound, whereas undiagnosed small tumours may become symptomatic after birth.

Primary surgical excision during the neonatal period may be performed for teratomas, renal tumours, small sarcomas, and certain brain tumours. Neuroblastomas, liver tumours and soft tissue sarcomas are usually treated with chemotherapy with the aim of reducing the extent of surgery needed for complete removal. Large tumours compressing a vital organ may need emergent surgery and is associated with significant morbidity and mortality. It is worth noting that initiation of treatment is often preceded by a variable period of diagnostic investigations like radiological imaging, biopsies and histopathological confirmation, bone marrow examination, among others. Many of these procedures require anaesthesia for safe and smooth conduct. Treatment planning and medical optimisation of the newborn may delay initiation of therapy.

Treatment of these neoplasms may need various combinations of chemotherapy, surgery, radiation therapy depending on the cancer type, size and location and other prognostic factors. Treatment modalities have a narrow therapeutic window in this vulnerable population and potential toxicities can complicate the treatment process.

Combination chemotherapy uses multiple drugs which target the malignant cells at different stages of their cell cycle. Toxicity from these agents also involves normal tissues with high cellular turnover like bone marrow, mucosa, epidermis, and liver. Immature hepatic and renal systems, along with higher total body water and lesser adipose tissue, contribute to the development of toxicity. Bone marrow suppression and resulting thrombocytopenia and neutropenia are probably the most common forms of toxicity. Other manifestations include mucositis, dermatitis, vomiting, liver dysfunction and alopecia. Drug specific complications like anthracycline induced cardiomyopathy, renal toxicity due to platinum agents and bleomycin induced pulmonary fibrosis are often irreversible. Anaesthesiologists may be involved during placement of central venous catheters, management of painful mucositis and peri-operative care of patients who have received chemotherapy.

Radiation therapy is not preferred in neonates as it is likely to have adverse effects both immediate and in the long term. Oro-pharyngeal and gastro-intestinal mucositis are frequently seen as early complications of radiation which can lead to devastating nutritional, fluid and electrolyte abnormalities. Skin discolouration, desquamation and marrow suppression are fairly common. Long-term adverse effects of ionising radiation to immature and rapidly proliferating body tissues in neonates and infants are distinct from that of adults [11]. Cranial irradiation for brain tumours can lead to severe learning, cognitive, neurological, and neuroendocrine deficits. Increased somnolence after cranial irradiation can have potential implications for the anaesthesiologist.

Radiation damage to the bone can cause arrested chondrogenesis, severe growth retardation and scoliosis, cardiorespiratory and endocrine insufficiency, abdominal strictures, and adhesions. It is also being increasingly recognized that exposure to radiation in early life can itself lead to development of various malignancies including leukaemias and cancer of thyroid, breast, brain and soft tissues. These long-term sequelae of radiation in neonates and younger children has led oncologists to delay radiation until the child is older or avoid it altogether by incorporating surgery and chemotherapy in the treatment regimen [12]. In the rare occasion that a neonate requires anaesthesia for radiation therapy, absolute immobility is essential but for a very short duration. The logistics of non-operating room anaesthesia delivery and safe transfer of neonates is a formidable challenge. The setup should include adequately trained personnel, drugs, equipment and facilities for remote monitoring.

General anaesthesia with secure airway provides better conditions, specifically immobility, than conscious sedation and is associated with fewer cardiorespiratory side effects, in children [13].

A few oncologic emergencies may arise secondary to the effects of malignant process or as complication of therapy, e.g., spinal cord compression, raised intracranial pressure, superior vena cava syndrome, airway obstruction, and tumour lysis syndrome. These conditions require immediate attention and interventions, often involving the anaesthesiologist.

47.4 Common Malignant Lesions Seen in Neonates

47.4.1 Neuroblastoma

These are the most common malignant neoplasm in neonates and infants. They arise from the neural crest cells which mature into the sympathetic ganglia and adrenal glands and may potentially secrete catecholamines. Most neonatal neuroblastomas arise from the adrenal medulla, but may also be seen in thoracic or cervical sympathetic nervous system.

Neuroblastomas may often present in the neonatal period as an asymptomatic palpable abdominal mass. However, depending on the location and size of the tumour, a wide spectrum of disease spectrum has been reported.

Large abdominal tumours and metastatic hepatic masses may compromise respiration.

Posterior mediastinal masses may present with symptoms of airway compromise, Horner syndrome, and superior vena cava syndrome.

Paraspinal masses may cause paraplegia due to spinal cord compression.

Neuroblastomas may be associated with Beckwith-Wiedemann syndrome and Congenital Central Hypoventilation (CCH). They are seen as suprarenal masses on prenatal ultrasound. After birth, ultrasound, CT or MRI scans are used to confirm the diagnosis. Urinary catecholamines and their metabolites like vanillylmandelic acid or homovanillic acid are raised in most cases. However, unlike patients with pheochromocytoma, manifestations of excess circulating catecholamine are relatively rare in neuroblastoma. Biopsy of primary or metastatic lesions and bone marrow aspirates are used for histopathological confirmation.

Treatment is based on the size and extent of tumour, postnatal age and biological features. Watchful observation for spontaneous regression of small, solitary lesions is all that may be needed. Metastatic and high-risk neuroblastoma need aggressive treatment with a combination of chemotherapy, autologous stem cell transplant, surgery, and radiation. Chemotherapeutic agents used include cyclophosphamide, cisplatin, vincristine, and etoposide. Surgery is usually not undertaken in the neonatal period, for tumours that fail to resolve spontaneously and are compressing a vital organ.

47.4.1.1 Anesthetic Implications of Neuroblastoma Resection in Neonates [14–16]

- These neonates will require anaesthesia for biopsy, port or line placement or for surgery.
- Thorough preoperative evaluation should include location and extent of tumour, presence of airway or respiratory compromise or compression, SVC obstruction, hypertension, hyperdynamic circulation and catecholamine excess. Preoperative hypertension mandates a paediatric cardiology and is usually managed with adrenergic blockers.
- Presence of cancer syndromes and associated abnormalities like facial dysmorphism, macroglossia, intestinal atresia and Hirschsprung's disease should be looked for.
- Extensive surgery in the neonatal period is relatively rare, but when performed is usually emergent and extensive. Large tumour resection is associated with massive blood loss and volume shifts.
- Meticulous haemodynamic, fluid and blood management are essential. Invasive vascular lines for access or monitoring are needed. Crystalloids and 4% albumin can be used to maintain intravascular volume. Blood counts, coagulation profile and arterial blood gas monitoring at frequent intervals help guide intraoperative haemodynamic and gas exchange management.
- Intraoperative hypertension during tumour manipulation is common. Drug management includes Labetalol (0.25–1 mg/kg/h), Esmolol (50–200 mcg/kg/min), Sodium Nitroprusside (0.5–10 mcg/kg/min), or Nitroglycerin (0.5–10 mcg/kg/min) [17].
- Intermittent clamping of renal and splenic vessels may lead to oliguria and metabolic acidosis which improves with IV fluids and normalisation of urine output.
- Equally important is aggressive maintenance of normothermia and prevention of hypothermia.
- Regional anaesthetic and analgesic techniques are frequently employed along with GA.
- Neonates are nursed in the NICU postoperatively.

47.4.2 Germ Cell Tumors or Teratomas (GCT)

GCTs are the most common neoplasm in neonates, comprising 35–40% of all neonatal tumours [18]. Most common histological subtypes are teratomas, followed by yolk sac tumours. Teratomas are usually extragonadal, most frequently sacrococcygeal teratoma, but may occur elsewhere too (mediastinal, cervical, head neck, oropharyngeal, orbital, intracranial) [6].

SCT are often large and complex needing surgical treatment in the neonatal period itself. It has a 4:1 female preponderance and is often associated with other congenital abnormalities like genitourinary, congenital hip dislocation, congenital heart disease and oesophageal atresia. These tumours are highly vascular and if large, may cause high output cardiac failure due to intra tumour arterio-venous shunting and anaemia.

Neonatal teratomas are usually benign. Incidence of malignancy increases with age. A third of these tumours are mature and cystic, and may contain differentiated tissue like hair, bone, cartilage, and teeth. According to the intrapelvic involvement, SCTs are classified as type 1–4. The goal of treatment is complete surgical resection after birth. Removal of coccyx is important to reduce recurrence rate. Intrapelvic tumours may need abdominoperineal surgical approach. Aggressive removal of gastrointestinal or genitourinary structures is not recommended as it is associated with high morbidity. Even in the face of microscopically positive margins, recurrence rate and mortality are low. Chemotherapy is indicated in metastatic tumours or if surgical resection was incomplete.

47.4.2.1 Anesthetic Implications of GCT

Preanaesthetic evaluation should look for presence of associated congenital abnormalities like hydrocephalous, spina bifida, cleft lip and palate, and congenital cardiac and genitourinary malformations. Prematurity, presence of neurological deficit and cardiac failure are all associated with poor postoperative outcomes.

47.4.2.2 Intraoperative Management [19, 20]

1. Difficult airway may be encountered due to sub-optimal intubation position due to the presence of a large tumour. Rolls may be placed under the torso to lift the body above the plane of the tumour.
2. Adequate intravenous access is a must, central venous access may be necessary.
3. Caudal analgesia is not feasible. Epidural at a higher level may be used with caution, and if disease does not involve neural structures.
4. Surgery requires baby to be placed in prone position.
5. Prone positioning may worsen an already compromised respiratory system. Lung protective ventilation strategies, judicious application of PEEP, permissive hypercapnia and pressure-controlled ventilation is beneficial in reducing lung injury.
6. Major blood loss, its reduction and prompt management are crucial in achieving desired outcome. Margin for error is very small in estimation of losses; point of care haemoglobin and blood gas analysis yield valuable information.
7. Complications associated with major blood loss and massive transfusion such as hypovolemic shock, hypocalcaemia, dilutional coagulopathy, thrombocytopenia, DIC and hyperkalaemia are potential risks in neonates. Handling of large tumours also causes potassium release.
8. Prevention and management of hypothermia is important to reduce worsening of coagulopathy and deleterious metabolic effects.

47.4.3 Renal Tumours

Renal tumours in neonates though relatively rare, carry a good prognosis, with 5-year survival more than 90% [18]. These include mesoblastic nephromas, Wilms' tumour, rhabdoid tumours and clear cell sarcoma, and may be associated with Beckwith-Wiedemann, Denys-Drash, and WAGR syndromes.

Mesoblastic nephroma is the most common renal tumour in neonates (70% of all neonatal renal tumours) [8]. It can be diagnosed in prenatal imaging or as a palpable abdominal mass postnatal. Radical nephrectomy with negative margins is the ideal treatment with excellent prognosis.

Wilms' tumour comprises around 20% of all neonatal renal tumours [8]. They are usually unilateral except in familial Wilms' tumour which has autosomal dominant inheritance. Unlike mesoblastic nephroma, tumour invasion or thrombus in renal vein or inferior vena cava is fairly common. Patients may present with hypertension, haematuria, anaemia and polycythemia. Radical nephrectomy followed by chemotherapy and radiation is the usual treatment.

Rhabdoid renal tumours and clear cell sarcoma are both rare but aggressive tumours which are often metastatic at diagnosis.

47.4.3.1 Perioperative Management of Radical Nephrectomy [19]

1. Preoperative evaluation includes evaluation of the cardiorespiratory and GI function. Large tumours may impair gastric emptying and adequate precautions for full stomach is necessary. Presence of IVC thrombus or vascular involvement should alert anaesthesia team regarding possibility of large amounts of intraoperative blood loss. Renal function is usually well preserved but electrolyte and metabolic derangements secondary to GI effects may be present.
2. Adequate venous access, above the diaphragm, should be ensured, if possible, as large vascular bleed may need IVC clamping. Invasive haemodynamic monitoring should be employed in high-risk cases.
3. Careful attention to patient positioning is required as the surgery may be prolonged.
4. Risk of hypothermia and massive haemorrhage needs necessary care.
5. Neuraxial analgesic techniques should be part of multimodal analgesia.

47.4.4 Liver Tumours in Neonates [9]

Liver tumours include benign hamartomas, vascular tumours and hepatoblastoma. Most neonatal liver tumours are benign hemangiomas, mesenchymal hamartomas or endotheliomas. Although benign, being highly vascular, their management is challenging. Patients may present with large abdominal masses with significant cardiorespiratory compromise, and high output cardiac failure (due to intra-tumour arteriovenous shunting). Treatment is primarily medical with steroids, beta-blockers, and chemotherapy. Surgical intervention is indicated for symptomatic tumours not medically manageable. Other possible non-surgical interventions include arterial embolisation, and hepatic artery ligation.

Hepatoblastoma is the most common malignant liver tumour in neonates. Congenital hepatoblastoma accounts for 15% of all neonatal liver tumours [1]. It is usually an asymptomatic abdominal mass, jaundice, and ascites but liver functions are usually well preserved. It may be associated with Beckwith-Wiedemann syndrome, hemihypertrophy and Wilms' tumour. Metastatic disease in lungs, brain and bones may be present at diagnosis. Outcomes are generally good if complete resection is feasible. Removal of up to 80% of the neonatal liver has been reported with good outcomes. Chemotherapy includes cisplatin, vincristine, doxorubicin or 5-flurouracil.

47.4.4.1 Perioperative Management [21, 22]

1. Liver surgery in the neonate is a highly complex and specialised, that should be carried out in dedicated high-volume centres only.
2. Preoperative evaluation should include complete hemogram, renal function, and liver synthetic functions (albumin, PT-INR), and cardiac evaluation with echocardiography to rule out high output cardiac failure. One should be aware of any major vessel involvement and patency of the IVC.
3. Invasive arterial and CVP monitoring plays a vital role in effective management of rapid haemodynamic changes and blood loss. A rapid transfusion system should be kept ready. CVP as a lone parameter to guide haemodynamic management is not recommended.
4. Surgery involves mobilisation of liver from its ligamentous attachments. The mobilised liver may be entirely displaced out of the neonatal abdomen, which may lead to sudden fall in CVP and cardiac output. Vascular occlusion techniques are employed to reduce blood loss. The Pringle manoeuvre (control of hepatic artery and portal vein within the hepatoduodenal ligament) is used. Total hepatic excision with portal vein, supra hepatic and infrahepatic IVC clamping causes significant reduction in venous return and cardiac output, accompanied with tachycardia, and raised peripheral vascular resistance. Maintaining a low CVP (<5 cm/H_2O) helps in reducing blood loss, however adequate intravascular volume should be maintained to avoid severe hypotension especially during vascular clamping.
5. Point of care coagulation tests like thromboelastogram (TEG) should be used to diagnose and treat intraoperative coagulopathy.
6. Neuraxial analgesic techniques can be used provided there is no coagulopathy.

47.4.5 CNS Tumours in Neonates

These are rare in the neonatal period. Estimated incidence is 14–40 per million live births [1]. Intracranial teratomas are the most common primary CNS tumours in neonates followed by astrocytoma, ependymoma and primitive neuroectodermal tumours. Features on antenatal imaging include hydrocephalus, cranial asymmetry, and distorted anatomical landmarks. Postnatal presentation includes features of raised ICP, and non-specific symptoms (vomiting, lethargy, irritability, increasing head circumference). Bulging fontanelles, focal deficits and seizures are common in supratentorial tumours. Brainstem lesions present with cranial nerve palsies, abnormal eye movements and motor deficits. These tumours carry an unfavourable prognosis due to rapid proliferation and challenges associated with complete excision and adequate chemotherapy. Neonates who survive also have severe long-term morbidities like seizures, neurologic, cognitive, and neuroendocrine deficiencies [10, 18].

47.4.5.1 Anaesthetic Implications [23]

- Neonates with CNS neoplasms may have to undergo anaesthesia for diagnostic imaging, shunt placement or surgical tumour removal.
- The neurophysiology of neonates is very different than that of older children. The cerebral blood flow (CBF) is lower in premature (12 mL/100 gm/min) and in term neonates (25–30 mL/100 gm/min) compared to older children. The autoregulation curve is strictly maintained between 20 and 60 mmHg and sudden changes in blood pressure can be detrimental.
- Pre-operative neurological evaluation should include features of raised ICP, altered sensorium and cranial nerve palsies. Frequent vomiting and feed intolerance may lead to dehydration and electrolyte disturbances. Macrocephaly if present can lead to a difficult intubation.
- Intravenous induction and muscle relaxation to prevent increases in ICP is ideal. However, gas induction may be needed in case of difficult IV access. Since all volatile anaesthetics increase ICP, MAC < 1 should be maintained. Alternatively, TIVA can be used to maintain anaesthesia.
- Positioning a small neonate for neurosurgical procedure can be a challenge. Supine position with head turned to one side is used for supratentorial tumours and VP shunt placement. Care should be taken to secure the tube at the nondependent angle of mouth to prevent pooling of secretions. Prone position is used for posterior fossa surgeries. Careful padding of pressure points, proper limb positioning, and avoidance of abdominal compression is vital. Even small degrees of neck flexion and extension are enough to either cause endobronchial intubation or extubation and loss of airway.

Other care for hemodynamic and temperature management, fluid and blood replacement and maintenance of acid-base status remains as described above.

47.4.6 Leukaemias

These are rare in neonates and include acute myeloid, and lymphoblastic leukaemias [1]. Downs' syndrome is often associated with "transient" leukaemia which is potentially life threatening. Leukemic neonates may present with large hepatosplenomegaly, hyperleukocytosis, CNS involvement, and respiratory compromise due to diffuse pulmonary infiltrates or mediastinal lymph nodes. They may need anaesthesia for diagnostic and treatment purposes. Administration of even a single dose of dexamethasone can potentially lead to tumour lysis syndrome. Avoidance of rectal thermometers and strict asepsis is essential in immunocompromised neonates [19].

47.5 Summary

1. Neonatal neoplasms are uncommon; however, they carry a significant risk of morbidity and mortality.
2. Neonates with neoplasms may undergo anaesthesia for diagnostic and treatment purposes like central line placement, imaging and surgical excision.
3. Neonatal tumours are often associated with genetic cancer syndromes, congenital and developmental abnormalities in addition to the effects of the tumour itself.
4. Neuroblastomas and teratomas are the most common tumours for which surgical resection is undertaken in the neonatal period.
5. Large, vascular tumours may lead to cardiorespiratory compromise and compression of vital organs, necessitating emergent surgery.
6. Management of extensive blood loss, large volume transfusion, maintenance of normothermia and the delicate neonatal physiology makes surgical removal of tumours an extremely challenging ordeal in neonates.

References

1. Orbach D, Sarnacki S, Brisse HJ, Gauthier-Villars M, et al. Neonatal cancer. Lancet Oncol. 2013;14:e609–20. https://doi.org/10.1016/S1470-2045(13)70236-5.
2. Alfaar AS, Hassan WM, Bakry MS, Qaddoumi I. Neonates with cancer and causes of death; lessons from 615 cases in the SEER databases. Cancer Med. 2017;6:1817–26. https://doi.org/10.1002/cam4.1122.
3. Solanki S, Menon P, Samujh R, Gupta K, Rao KN. Clinical presentation and surgical management of neonatal tumors: retrospective analysis. J Indian Assoc Pediatr Surg. 2020;25:85. https://doi.org/10.4103/jiaps.JIAPS_241_18.
4. Chandrasekaran A. Neonatal solid tumors. Pediatr Neonatol. 2018;59:65–70. https://doi.org/10.1016/j.pedneo.2016.12.007.
5. Fisher JPH, Tweddle DA. Neonatal neuroblastoma. Semin Fetal Neonatal Med. 2012;17:207–15. https://doi.org/10.1016/j.siny.2012.05.002.
6. Lakhoo K. Neonatal teratomas. Early Hum Dev. 2010;86:643–7. https://doi.org/10.1016/j.earlhumdev.2010.08.016.
7. Ferrari A, Orbach D, Sultan I, Casanova M, Bisogno G. Neonatal soft tissue sarcomas. Semin Fetal Neonatal Med. 2012;17:231–8. https://doi.org/10.1016/j.siny.2012.05.003.
8. Isaacs H. Fetal and neonatal renal tumors. J Pediatr Surg. 2008;43:1587–95. https://doi.org/10.1016/j.jpedsurg.2008.03.012.
9. Isaacs H. Fetal and neonatal hepatic tumors. J Pediatr Surg. 2007;42:1797–803. https://doi.org/10.1016/j.jpedsurg.2007.07.047.
10. Bodeliwala S, Kumar V, Singh D. Neonatal brain tumors: a review. J Neonat Surg. 2017;6:30. https://doi.org/10.21699/jns.v6i2.579.
11. Paulino AC, Constine LS, Rubin P, Williams JP. Normal tissue development, homeostasis, senescence, and the sensitivity to radiation injury across the age spectrum. Semin Radiat Oncol. 2010;20:12–20. https://doi.org/10.1016/j.semradonc.2009.08.003.

12. Paulino AC. Treatment strategies to reduce radiotherapy late effects in children. J Radiat Oncol. 2013;2:121–8. https://doi.org/10.1007/s13566-012-0075-2.
13. Verma V, Beethe AB, LeRiger M, Kulkarni RR, Zhang M, Lin C. Anesthesia complications of pediatric radiation therapy. Pract Radiat Oncol. 2016;6:143–54. https://doi.org/10.1016/j.prro.2015.10.018.
14. Creagh-Barry P, Sumner E. Neuroblastoma and anaesthesia. Pediatr Anesth. 1992;2:147–52. https://doi.org/10.1111/j.1460-9592.1992.tb00190.x.
15. Kain ZN, Shamberger RS, Holzman RS. Anesthetic management of children with neuroblastoma. J Clin Anesth. 1993;5:486–91. https://doi.org/10.1016/0952-8180(93)90066-N.
16. Williams ES, Olutoye OA, Seipel CP, Aina T, editors. Clinical pediatric anesthesia, vol. vol. 1. Oxford: Oxford University Press; 2018. https://doi.org/10.1093/med/9780190678333.001.0001.
17. Gómez-Ríos MÁ, Nuño FC, Barreto-Calvo P. Anesthetic management of an infant with giant abdominal neuroblastoma. Braz J Anesthesiol (English Edition). 2017;67:210–3. https://doi.org/10.1016/j.bjane.2014.07.012.
18. Fernández KS. Solid tumors in the neonatal period. NeoReviews. 2014;15:e56–68. https://doi.org/10.1542/neo.15-2-e56.
19. Leduc LH. Neonatal and infant tumors. In: McCann ME, Greco C, Matthes K, editors. Essentials of anesthesia for infants and neonates. 1st ed. Cambridge: Cambridge University Press; 2018. p. 321–31. https://doi.org/10.1017/9781107707016.031.
20. Choudhury S, Kaur M, Pandey M, Jain A. Anaesthestic management of sacrococcygeal teratoma in infants. Indian J Anaesth. 2016;60:374. https://doi.org/10.4103/0019-5049.181620.
21. Bennett J, Bromley P. Anaesthesia for hepatic surgery, including transplantation, in children. In: James I, Walker I, editors. Core topics in Paediatric Anaesthesia. Cambridge: Cambridge University Press; 2013. p. 344–54. https://doi.org/10.1017/CBO9780511978906.036.
22. Mogane P, Motshabi-Chakane P. Anaesthetic considerations for liver resections in paediatric patients. South Afr J Anaesth Analg. 2013;19:290–4. https://doi.org/10.1080/22201173.2013.10872943.
23. Rath G, Dash H. Anaesthesia for neurosurgical procedures in paediatric patients. Indian J Anaesth. 2012;56:502. https://doi.org/10.4103/0019-5049.103979.

Neonatal Palliative Care: A Paradigm of Care

Gayatri Palat

48.1 Preamble

India accounts for more than a quarter of global neonatal deaths with current Neonatal Mortality Rate of 28 per 1000 live births. Prematurity, intra-partum-related complications, sepsis, and congenital anomalies are the leading causes of neonatal deaths. Almost 98% deaths due to asphyxia, 75% deaths due to prematurity and malformations, and 50% deaths due to sepsis occur in the first week of life. A significant number of these newborns get admitted to the NICU due to critical conditions, face unfavorable prognosis, and eventually require redirection of care with withholding or withdrawal of life-sustaining treatment after failure of intensive care.

Neonatal palliative care is the holistic management of supportive and end of life care for a neonate and their family in the situation where a life limiting condition has been identified. It starts from the point of diagnosis or recognition (including antenatal), and continues throughout the baby's life, death, and bereavement. It embraces physical, emotional, social, and spiritual components of suffering and focuses on the enhancement of quality of life for the baby and support for the family.

G. Palat (✉)
Department of Pain and Palliative Medicine, MNJ Institute of Oncology and RCC, Hyderabad, India

PAX India, Two Worlds Cancer Collaboration, Vancouver, Canada

© The Author(s), under exclusive license to Springer Nature Singapore Pte Ltd. 2023
U. Saha (ed.), *Clinical Anesthesia for the Newborn and the Neonate*,
https://doi.org/10.1007/978-981-19-5458-0_48

48.2   When to Refer to Palliative Care?

Babies who may require palliative care can be considered in five broad categories or
Triggers for Palliative Care Referral (Table 48.1).

Table 48.1 Triggers for palliative care referral

Clinical condition	Example
Antenatal/postnatal diagnosis of a condition that is not compatible with long-term survival	Bilateral renal agenesis, anencephaly, chromosomal abnormality
Antenatal/postnatal diagnosis of a condition which carries a high risk of significant morbidity or death	Severe bilateral hydronephrosis, impaired renal function, severe spina bifida
Babies born at the margins of viability where intensive care has been deemed inappropriate	22–24 weeks gestation
Postnatal conditions with a high likelihood of severe impairment of quality of life either when receiving life support or that may at some point require life support	Severe hypoxic ischemic encephalopathy (HIE)
Postnatal conditions which result in the baby experiencing "unbearable suffering" where palliative care is in baby's best interest	Severe necrotizing enterocolitis, refractory seizures from intraventricular hemorrhage

> Mrs. Shetty at 30 weeks of her pregnancy is diagnosed to have a baby with skeletal dysplasia. It is uncertain if the baby would survive the pregnancy or the delivery, and, if so, what the baby's life expectancy would be. The family is in great distress. The family was referred to palliative care team.

> Learning Point: Early palliative care referral recommended when a baby is diagnosed to have a limiting condition.

48.3   Developing a Palliative Care Plan

Developing a palliative care should be considered as soon as it's clear that the baby is moving towards imminent end of life care or when it is recognized that the baby has a life-threatening condition but could be transferred home or to a hospice.

48.4   Key Components of a Neonatal Palliative Care Plan

48.4.1 Early Integration of Palliative Care and Offering a Flexible Care Plan

An early palliative care intervention results in better quality of life for the baby and support to the family. The care plan must be continuously reviewed in the best interest of the baby. There should be flexibility in transitioning into and out of active, supportive or end of life care. Any changes should be documented and communicated.

48.4.2 Communication with the Parents and Shared Decision-Making

Parents form an integral part of a neonatal palliative care plan because they are surrogate decision-makers, navigate the complex healthcare system, and are often physically and emotionally exhausted due to uncertainty of decision-making and outcome, dealing with often unfriendly medical system, lack of social support system being away from home, and/or other socio-economic stressors. They may also be grieving for the loss of experience and joy of a normal pregnancy and birth. Under these conditions, it may not be easy for the parents to understand and take a complex and distressing decision easily.

48.4.2.1   Communication and Shared Decision-Making
Shared decision-making is accomplished when a person or family and their healthcare provider make decisions in a partnership. To achieve that -
- Every family should receive the news of their baby's diagnosis and prognosis in a face-to-face discussion in privacy and in a respectful, honest, and sensitive way.
- Be given the option of inviting other family members or close friends to be with them during this discussion.
- Encourage parents to actively participate in decision-making so that they feel a regaining sense of control of their parental role.
- Information must be shared in a clear, simple language that they can understand.
- The beliefs, values and family needs should be respected.
- Single session may not be enough and may require repeated sessions with the help of a multidisciplinary team.
- Phrases such as 'withdrawal of care' should be avoided as it may hint as if "giving up on" or "abandoning the treatment," and the family may feel as if they are giving permission to terminate their baby's life.

- The focus of discussion should be "what will be' rather than 'what will not be provided.' Phrases such as "We cannot cure your baby, but we will keep your baby as comfortable and pain free as possible", or "the focus of our treatment will be to keep the baby comfortable for as long as he/she lives," and "providing dignity" will be more appropriate.

Mrs. Shetty's Perspective

- "My baby Sitara was diagnosed to have severe congenital problem at my 36th week of pregnancy. The doctors thought she would die within days. I desperately needed to know all the details especially how she would be like when she was born and what would happen after birth and if it will be possible to hold her in my arms.
- When I met the palliative care team, they listened and made efforts to understand our concerns. They asked us questions like, 'what are your hopes?', 'What are your fears', and 'what would you like to know? 'The doctor and other team members answered to our questions slowly and gently, answered in a simple language which I could understand, were honest with their information and empathetic. The team referred to our baby Sitara by name, showing us they knew how real she was to us. The conversation transformed from something dreadful to something potentially meaningful.
- My Sitara died minutes after she was born but I was braced for it. I held her and this meant the world to me."

48.4.2.2 Making an Advance Care Planning

Making an advance care planning should be encouraged early in the consultation. It can includes both short-term and long-term goals of care and treatments such as resuscitation plan, what to do in the event of acute or further deterioration, withholding or discontinuing certain aspects of care (such as intubation/mechanical ventilation). It must be documented and shared with concerned members of the clinical care team.

48.4.3 Ensuring Adequate Symptom Control and Comfort Care

48.4.3.1 Basic Care

Basic comfort must be ensured to minimize distress and provide comfort by measures like cuddling, swaddling, Kangaroo care, breast feeding (if appropriate), keeping baby clean and dry, and warm.

48.4.3.2 Nutrition and Feeding

The goal of feeding at end of life is comfort, not provision of nutrition. A decision to continue nutrition and hydration may cause more harm like fluid overload, pain, excessive secretion and prolong the dying process. Breast feeding may be comforting for the baby as well as mother (Table 48.2). Tube feeding should be considered only if the baby expresses distress from hunger. Parenteral fluids and nutrition are rarely indicated.

48.4.3.3 Pain and Symptom Management

Baby Sitara is likely to have distressing symptoms like pain, dyspnea, agitation, secretions. Once in NICU, there is a high probability that the baby would undergo numerous painful diagnostic and therapeutic procedures (Table 48.3).

- Ensure impeccable assessment of pain (including procedural pain) and other distressing symptoms using standardized tools used for babies such as PIPS, NIPS, Neonatal Pain, Agitation, and Sedation Scale (N-PASS).
- Encourage non-pharmacological and pharmacological measures to reduce pain and distress due to painful procedures (Tables 48.5 and 48.6).
- Distressing symptoms should be anticipated and managed without hesitation (Table 48.7). The goal is to provide comfort. Short seizures may not distress the baby whereas air hunger may be distressing. Use of opioid medications is recommended to alleviate distressing symptoms like pain and dyspnea, e.g., use of morphine by the route best tolerated by the baby: oral, buccal, intravenous, or subcutaneous.

Table 48.2 Feeding in end of life care

If the baby develops symptoms of not absorbing feeds,
- Decrease the feed volume down to 50–100 mL/kg/day for hydration and comfort.
- Consider hourly feeding to maintain smaller volumes.
- Stop feeding if the baby is clearly not absorbing feeds, after discussing with the family.
- Ensure adequate mouth hygiene (wetting lips and cleaning mouth for comfort).

Table 48.3 Common painful procedures performed in NICU

Diagnostic	Therapeutic	Surgical
Adhesive tape removal	Arterial puncture	Suture
Bladder catheterization	Eye examination	Vascular cut down
Central line insertion / removal	Heel lancing	
Chest tube insertion/ removal	Lumbar puncture	
Chest physiotherapy	Bladder catheterization	
Dressing change	Venipuncture	
Gavage tube insertion		
Intramuscular injection		
Mechanical ventilation		
Peripheral venous catheterization		
PICC line insertion		
Tracheal intubation/ Extubation		

48.4.4 End of Life Care and Withdraw or Withhold Life-Sustaining Treatment

The interdisciplinary team once makes the decision in partnership with the family that the baby will require end-of-life care or a compassionate extubation, then -

- Agree upon a time and location for withdrawal of life-sustaining measures with the parents. A quiet room by the side of NICU may serve the purpose.
- Ask if parents would like to be present at the actual time of compassionate extubation.
- Discontinue intensive monitoring and investigations.
- Monitor for physical signs that suggest discomfort: crying, whimpering, changes in breathing pattern, gasping, excessive secretions, dry mouth, and ensure comfort.
- It may be difficult to predict how long it will take for the baby to die. Describe to parents what changes to expect as baby's condition deteriorates, such as skin color, breathing pattern, and gasps for air.
- Give specific treatment for symptom relief: morphine 0.15 mg/kg sublingual, or 0.05 mg/kg IV/SC every 15 min as required (for pain and air hunger).
- Allow family to spend time with the baby and create or make memories (Table 48.4).

Table 48.4 Making memories

- Offer family to hold any rituals important to them - naming ceremony/baptism/saying prayers.
- Encouraging family to spend time holding, bathing, clothing, and feeding the baby.
- Create memories by encouraging them to take pictures/videos of the baby with the family. A special memory boxes can be created to store footprints, locks of hair, plaster imprints of hands and feet, nametags, clothes the baby has worn.

- Mrs. Shetty and her family received consultations from the neonatal and palliative care team. It was agreed that active resuscitation would not be in the baby's best interest given the lethal condition. Goal of care as comfort care was established with mutual consensus.
- The baby was born with a poor APGAR Score. The family was allowed to spend time in a separate room by the side of NICU. They held the baby, said prayers, took pictures and did a quick naming ceremony. The mother wished to suckle her baby and was supported to do so. Baby was monitored for pain and distress by using scale like NIPS. Baby was kept comfortable, warm. Buccal Morphine and glycopyrrolate were used for pain, secretions.
- Baby died within a few hours in mother's arm and surrounded by family members. Palliative care team directed the family to necessary ambulance and funeral services and planned for a follow up bereavement call and support.

> **Learning point**: Early palliative care involvement results in better prepara-
> tion and family involvement, shared decision making, advance care planning,
> good symptom management and end-of-life-care for babies born with life
> limiting conditions.

48.4.5 After Death Plan

Allow the family to spend some time alone with the baby (the body). They may
require practical help with death declaration, mortuary, ambulance, funeral services,
verbal and written information about the process of getting the death certification.

48.4.6 Team Support

Allocate time for a follow-up debriefing meeting with the team after the death of the
baby. Dealing with death and dying of children is stressful. Peer and professional
help should be made available to the members of the team.

48.4.7 Bereavement

Parents may start experiencing anticipatory grief from the time of diagnosis or from
the time of delivery of the baby born with a life limiting condition. There are reports
of higher prevalence of complicated grief among these families. A dedicated
bereavement support system is highly recommended while planning a neonatal palliative care service.

48.5   Conclusion

Neonatal palliative care is a comprehensive, interdisciplinary model of care with the
aim of offering personalized care to the newborns affected by life limiting conditions
or complex medical conditions with uncertain prognosis. Palliative care team provides
emotional, spiritual and physical support to babies and families and help family to
make memories, spend time together, navigate complex decisions, and establish goals
of care. It should be an integral part of every NICU/ neonatal care set up.

Pearls of Wisdom
- Neonate palliative care should be an integral part of any program dealing with
  care of babies born with life-limiting conditions and diseases with uncertain
  prognosis.
- An early integration is recommended to treat symptoms, minimize suffering, and
  improve quality of life.
- Shared decision-making and advanced care planning in the baby's best interest
  and respecting family's values and wishes is recommended.

- Babies should be routinely screened and actively managed for pain, including procedural pain, and other distressing symptoms.
- Once baby approaches end-of-life care, the focus of care should be on enabling families to spend time with their baby, bonding and building memories, and comfort.
- Any health workers including volunteers dealing with children with life limiting conditions should receive training in the principles of palliative care and sensitive communication.

Appendix

Table 48.5 Non-pharmacological approach to procedural pain management

Interventions	Indications	Note
Sucrose	• For minor/or moderately painful short procedures in combination with other analgesics • Give 24–50% solution orally 2 min before the procedure • Analgesic effect is improved with addition of allowing infant to suck (follow sucrose with pacifier)	Contraindications • Unconscious, heavily sedated, absent gag reflex • Encephalopathy • Significant CNS depression • NEC
Breast feeding	• Only effective if infant has effective latch and feeds x 5 min prior to procedure.	
Non-nutritive sucking		Reduces acute procedural pain
Positioning		Swaddling- effective in preterm, Limited evidence in term baby
Kangaroo care	Should be maintained for 10–15 min post procedure to ensure neonate is fully relaxed and settled	Diminishes pain responses for term and preterm neonates
Environment	Keep babies clean, dry, minimally handled, quiet	

Table 48.6 Pharmacological management of procedural pain

Drug	Dose	Route	Note
Paracetamol	10–15 mg/kg	Oral/PR	Suitable for mild pain. Must be given 15–20 min before the procedure
EMLA (eutectic mixture of Lidocaine and Prilocaine)	Apply as occlusive dressing 1 h prior to procedure	Topical anesthesia on intact skin	Safe, approved for use in newborns for procedures like lumbar puncture, circumcision, vascular line insertion
Proparacaine 0.5%/ Tetracaine drops	Repeated as needed	Topical	Eye examination for ROP
Morphine	Term neonates *Oral/buccal: 50–100 mcg/kg q6h* *IV/SC: 25–50 mcg/kg q4-6h* *IV/SC infusion: Start 5–10 mcg/kg/h, then titrate to effect*		Safe and effective for neonates, when dosed correctly
Fentanyl	If ventilated: 1–2 mcg/kg If not: 0.5–1 mcg/kg	IV	Rapid onset, short duration Useful for procedures like tracheal intubation, extubation, suction, and chest tube insertion, vascular line insertion
Ketamine	0.5–2 mg/kg	IV	For chest tube and tracheal tube insertion

Table 48.7 Management of common symptoms in neonatal palliative care

Symptoms	Drugs	Dose	Route
Pain	Paracetamol	28–32 weeks GA – 20 mg/kg as a single dose, 10–15 mg/kg every 8–12 h, as necessary	PO
		>32 weeks GA – 20 mg/kg as single dose, 10–15 mg/kg every 6–8 h, as necessary	
		Preterm neonate (>32 weeks GA) – 7.5 mg/kg every 8 h Term neonate: 10 mg/kg every 4–6 h	IV infusion
	Morphine	50–100 mcg/kg every 6 h	PO
		25–50 mcg/kg every 4–6 h as per response	IV/SC
		5–10 mcg/kg/h as per response	IV/SC infusion
		3 × 24 h total IV dose	IV to PO conversion
	For breakthrough pain - 10 – 15% of total daily dose every 1–4 h Commence laxative (lactulose)		
	Fentanyl	Non-ventilated: 0.5–1 mcg/kg/per dose Ventilated: 1–2 mcg/kg/dose (repeated every 60 min, as per response)	IV/SC bolus
		0.5–2 mcg/kg/h as per response	IV/SC infusion

(continued)

Table 48.7 (continued)

Symptoms	Drugs	Dose	Route
Seizures	Midazolam	Initial dose 1–3 mg/kg/24 h increasing up to 7 mg/kg/24 h	IV/SC infusion
		300 mcg/kg as single dose, repeat once if necessary.	Buccal injection
Agitation / irritability	Consider comfort measures, e.g., changing nappy, gentle rocking, warmth, feeding		
	If pain is cause of agitation, start with PCM/sucrose. If no effect, start morphine		
	Midazolam	50–100 mcg/kg/dose 4 h	Buccal
Respiratory distress	Morphine	30–50% of the dose used for pain	PO/IV/SC
	Midazolam	0.25 mg/kg 2–4 h	PO
		0.05–0.15 mg/kg 2–4 h	IV bolus
Secretions	Glycopyrrolate	40–100 mcg/kg 3–4 times daily	PO
	Atropine eye drops	1–2 drops	On buccal mucosa
	Atropine	Injection solution, 20–40 µg/kg/dose 2–3 times a day	Applied to buccal mucosa

IV Intravenous, *PO* Subcutaneous, *SC* Subcutaneous

Further Readings

Cruz MD, Fernandes AM, Oliveira CR. Epidemiology of painful procedures performed in neonates: a systematic review of observational studies. Eur J Pain. 2016;20(4):489–98.

Hummel P, Puchalski M, Creech SD, Weiss MG. Clinical reliability and validity of the N-PASS: neonatal pain, agitation and sedation scale with prolonged pain. J Perinatol. 2008;28(1):55–60.

Lawrence J, Alcock D, et al. The development of a tool to assess neonatal pain. Neonatal Netw. 1993;12:59–66.

Sankar MJ, Neogi SB, Sharma J, Chauhan M, Srivastava R, Prabhakar PK, Khera A, Kumar R, Zodpey S, Paul VK. State of newborn health in India. J Perinatol. 2016;36:S3–8. https://doi.org/10.1038/jp.2016.183.

Stevens B, Johnston C, Petryshen P, Taddio A. Premature infant pain profile: development and initial validation. Clin J Pain. 1996;12(1):13–22.

http://www.icpcn.org/wp-content/uploads/2018/06/Neonatal-Palliative-care-guideline.FINAL_.pdf

https://www.togetherforshortlives.org.uk/wp-content/uploads/2018/01/ProRes-Perinatal-Pathway-for-Babies-With-Palliative-Care-Needs.pdf

https://www.neonatalnetwork.co.uk/nwnodn/palliative-care/

https://www.chelwest.nhs.uk/services/childrens-services/neonatal-services/links/Practical-guidance-for-the-management-of-palliative-care-on-neonatal-units-Feb-2014.pdf

COVID-19 and The Surgical Neonate

49

Pankhuri and Usha Saha

49.1 Introduction

Worldwide, as on November 18, 2021, there have been 255,732,876 coronavirus cases, and 5,138,966, deaths, with 231,148,033 recovered [1]. In India, from January 3, 2020, to November 17, 2021, there have been 34,466,598 confirmed cases of COVID-19 with 464,153 deaths reported to WHO. As of November 8, 2021, a total of 1,095,926,470 vaccine doses have been administered [2].

Transmission of COVID-19 to neonates primarily is through respiratory droplets, postnatal, when neonates are exposed to mothers or other caregivers with COVID infection. There is not much information regarding intrauterine, intrapartum, and peripartum transmission from an infected mother [3] (CDC 2020). COVID-19 has made anesthesia in neonates even more challenging. Taking proper precautions and following COVID guidelines while managing the patient in OTs will lead to better outcome in terms of patient's recovery and will reduce the risk of transmission to others. RTPCR has very high specificity (95%) and 63% sensitivity for nasal swab compared to 32% for pharyngeal swab [4, 5]. TrueNAT (cartridge-based nucleic acid amplification test) has also emerged as a testing method especially in mobile units and in containment zones [6].

Pankhuri
Department of Anesthesia, Critical Care, Pain and Palliative Care, Lady Hardinge Medical College, SSK and Kalawati Saran Childrens Hospitals, New Delhi, India

Department of Anesthesiology, Critical Care, and Palliative Care, Lady Hardinge Medical College, SSK and Kalawati Childrens Hospitals, New Delhi, India

U. Saha (✉)
Department of Anesthesia, Critical Care, Pain and Palliative Care, Lady Hardinge Medical College, SSK and Kalawati Saran Childrens Hospitals, New Delhi, India

In suspected or COVID-positive neonates, elective surgeries should not be undertaken, and full COVID guidelines should be followed when providing anesthesia for **emergency surgeries**. A simple measure, temperature check, is necessary for all patients before taking in OT. There should be designated operation theaters for COVID-positive/suspected cases. PAC should be done by the anesthetist in PPE. X-ray, ABG, and all routine investigations should be done. Evaluation for oxygen requirement, signs of shock, liver failure, and renal failure should be done. All care givers should practice infection prevention and control measures (mask, hand hygiene). Anesthesia induction and emergence should be smooth and equipment discarded or disinfected properly. Breathing circuit, mask, tracheal tube, and HME filters should be discarded after every patient.

49.2   COVID and Anesthesia for Neonates

COVID-19 pandemic, severe acute respiratory syndrome, caused by coronavirus 2 (SARS-CoV-2), is a major public health crisis threatening humanity in 2020 and 2021. It was declared a pandemic on March 11, 2020. Worldwide almost 25 crore 42 lakh people have suffered [1], and in India, 3.5 crore have tested positive, while 4.5 lakh have succumbed to COVID-19 (till November 15, 2021) [2, 7]. With exponential increase in the number of cases, worldwide, increasing trends in COVID-positive pediatric patients have also been observed.

Though less common in children (<18 years), and majority having mild symptoms or none at all, 10–20% of symptomatic children may need hospitalization, and 1–3% requiring intensive care.

As of November 2021, among 3.3 million COVID-19 deaths reported in the MPIDR COVerAGE database, 0.4% (over 11,700) occurred in under 20 years age, and out of these, 42% occurred in under 9 years age [8]. The second wave (April, 2021) witnessed drastic increase in COVID-related mortality in India, probably due to the following:

1. Less extensive and less effective lockdown in second wave than in first wave.
2. People were not taking the second wave seriously until it became full-blown, killing large number of people (as they had already witnessed and survived the first wave).
3. In second wave, entire households were becoming positive with new strains of mutated virus, with greater virulence than the previous strain.

The role of anesthetists became vital in this global health crisis because of their expertise in airway and ventilatory management, in providing anesthesia in COVID-positive patients for various surgeries, in critical and intensive care, and as fast response resuscitation team. This put the anesthetists at the highest risk of exposure to the virus, as they had to deal with the patient's airway, the route of transmission of virulent COVID-19. Here, we will be discussing COVID in neonates and challenges faced by the anesthesiologists during the anesthetic management in COVID-positive neonates undergoing surgery.

Transmission of COVID infection to neonates is by **respiratory droplets** during postnatal period from exposure to COVID-positive parents/caregivers, direct person to person, mainly through sneezing, coughing, and talking. These droplets may also land on surfaces, where the virus remains viable [3, 9, 10].

Symptoms and Signs: Median incubation period is 5.1 days (range 2–14 days). Period of infectivity starts 2 days prior to onset of symptoms, lasting up to 8 days. Most neonates remain asymptomatic or have mild symptoms such as fever, and rhinorrhea, features of upper respiratory tract infection. Depending on the viral load and innate immunity of the baby, symptoms may increase with tachypnea, regurgitation and vomiting, and loose motions. Respiratory symptoms are more common in neonates [10]. Few babies may develop severe symptoms in the form of pneumonia, cyanosis, labored breathing, lethargy, poor feeding, somnolence, and seizures. Other symptoms like sore throat, anosmia (**absence or impairment of the sense of smell),** and ageusia (**absence or impairment of the sense of taste**) cannot be elicited in neonates. Symptoms of COVID can be difficult to differentiate from other causes of respiratory difficulty in neonates like transient tachypnea of newborn (TTN), and respiratory distress syndrome (RDS). Risk of severe infection is more in premature neonates [3]. Therefore, prompt diagnosis and early treatment are required in such neonates.

Diagnosis: Early diagnosis is required in neonates born to COVID-positive mothers and neonates presenting with symptoms consistent with COVID for better prognosis and to prevent transmission to caretakers and hospital staff. COVID-19 testing is indicated in neonates who fall under the following categories [3]:

(i) Born to mothers with suspected COVID infection within 24 hrs of birth, and if testing is negative, it should be repeated at 48 h.
(ii) Born to mothers confirmed positive,
(iii) Asymptomatic neonate expected to be discharged within 48 h of birth,
(iv) Symptomatic babies,
(v) Neonates who require hospital admission for >48 h, and
(vi) Prior to elective surgery.

49.3   Tests Available for COVID Detection [3, 11]

1. **Reverse Transcription Polymerase Chain Reaction:** It amplifies a small, well-defined segment of DNA many folds, creating enough of it for analysis. Real-time PCR has the advantage of automation, higher-throughput and more reliable instrumentation, and high specificity (95%) and is the preferred method. The combined technique is described as **real-time PCR (RTPCR) or quantitative RTPCR (qRTPCR)** [4, 5]. Testing can be done by taking nasopharyngeal or throat swabs, saliva, deep airway material collected during suction, and feces. Its sensitivity is 63% for nasal swab, 32% for pharyngeal swab, 48% for feces, 72–75% for sputum, and 93–95% for bronchoalveolar lavage.
2. **Antigen Testing:**Antigen can be detected even before onset of COVID-19 symptoms. This gives rapid test results, but is less sensitive. Nasopharyngeal or ante-

rior nares swab or saliva is tested for the antigen, and has a specificity of 99.5%, and sensitivity of 56.8%.

3. **TrueNAT:** TrueNAT is a indigenously developed version of CB-NAAT (cartridge-based nucleic acid amplification test), also known as the GeneXpert test. This detects SARS-CoV-2 E-gene and the gene for the RNA-dependent RNA polymerase, in the nose or throat swab samples. It is quick, portable, and cheap and is used by mobile testing centers in containment zones. concordance with the reference standard assay and may be recommended for screening and confirmation of SARS-CoV-2 in the field settings [6].

4. **Antibody Tests:** SARS-CoV-2 antibody potency and protective period have not been established and do not imply immunity to a future infection.

Fallacious Results: Testing too early after birth can give higher false-positive results, because of nasal and throat contamination at birth or false negatives (RNA not detectable if exposure is soon after birth).

Prevention: All caregivers should practice infection prevention and control measures using mask and hand hygiene. The infected mother and the neonate should be isolated from others. Positive mothers should be allowed to breastfeed their babies if they have met the criteria for discontinuing isolation and as per CDC [3, 12] for the newborns:

(a) If 24 h have passed since last fever without antipyretics, and/or
(b) If 10 days have passed since first symptoms or 20 days since severe illness.

Neonate is kept under maternal care and with mother, but separation of mother and baby is required if

(a) Either mother or baby is very sick and needs to be treated under medicine.
(b) Higher risk for severe illness in baby. (e.g., preterm, low birth weight, underlying medical conditions)

49.4 Treatment in Pediatric Age Group [9, 13, 14]

(i) **Mild illness** (sore throat, rhinorrhea, cough, with normal respiration) can be managed by home isolation, supportive care, rest, adequate hydration and feeding, paracetamol (PCM) for fever (10–15 mg/kg/dose). If symptoms worsen, they must be reported. All admitted children are tested for CBC, LFT, RFT, coagulogram, CRP, D-dimer, fibrinogen, chest X-ray, blood culture. Admission of children with mild illness is indicated if there are associated comorbidities, such as chronic lung disease, symptomatic heart disease, chronic kidney disease, and neurological disorder. If inhaled medications are indicated, MDI should be used and nebulization is avoided.

(ii) **Moderate illness** (pneumonia, tachypnea >60/min in <2-month age, no signs of severe pneumonia/illness) is admitted to monitor progress, maintaining

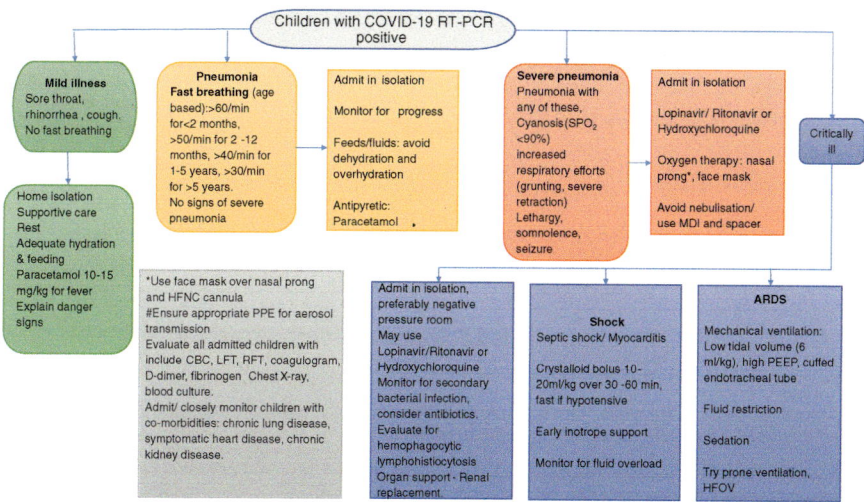

Chart 49.1 Management of COVID-19 in children (2 months–18 years) (Interim Protocol) [9]

hydration and feeding, avoiding over/dehydration, PCM for fever and amoxicillin if bacterial infection is suspected. O_2 therapy is started ($SpO_2 < 94\%$), and steroids given if rapid deterioration occurs.

(iii) **Severe illness** (severe pneumonia with cyanosis, desaturation, $SpO_2 < 90\%$, labored respiration, grunting, severe retraction, lethargy, somnolence, seizure, ARDS, sepsis, shock, MODS) requires admission to HDU/ICU, and evaluation for thrombosis, hemophagocytic lymphohistiocytosis, and organ failure. Steroids± remdesivir are started. E along with empiric antimicrobials. O_2 can be given via nasal prong, face mask, HFNC, or NIV to maintain target SpO_2 (>94%). Once stable, older children can be placed in awake prone positioning, with restrictive fluid therapy, and organ support. Dexamethasone (0.15 mg/kg per dose—max. 6 mg) twice a day for 5–14 days, depending on clinical response, is preferred over methylprednisolone/prednisolone. There are no pediatric trials on Remdesivir, and hence, its use is restricted to severe cases (presenting within 72 h of onset of symptoms) provided hepatorenal functions are normal. Dose in 3.5–40 kg is 5 mg/kg on first day and then 2.5 mg/kg once a day, for 5 days [9] (Chart 49.1).

49.5 Indications for ICU Admission in Neonates [13]

1. Need for mechanical ventilation,
2. Shock on vasopressor support,
3. Worsening mental status, and
4. Multiorgan dysfunction.

Intubation should be considered in case of RDS, desaturation (<90%) on noninvasive O_2 therapy, PaO_2/FiO_2 <200, PaO_2/FiO_2 <300 with hypotension on vasopressor support, or GCS < 8 with threatened airway [13]. During ventilatory support, **lung protective ventilation** is beneficial:

- Low tidal volume
- PEEP (positive end expiratory pressure)
- Ventilation in prone position.

49.6 COVID-19 Recommendations for Healthcare Workers (HCWs) (Minnesota 2021) [15]

- All HCW, regardless of vaccination status, should be tested for SARS-CoV-2 when symptomatic after a higher-risk exposure and when working in a facility experiencing an outbreak.
- Post-exposure testing should occur immediately upon identification of the case (but not earlier than 2 days after exposure) and at day 5–7 after exposure.
- Fully vaccinated HCWs (2 weeks after the last dose), if asymptomatic, do not need 14 days quarantine from work or community following exposure.
- Work restriction for 14 days should still be considered for HCW with underlying immune compromising conditions (e.g., organ transplantation, cancer treatment), or if signs or symptoms occur within 14 days of exposure.
- Unvaccinated HCWs should quarantine from work for 14 days following high-risk exposure.

49.7 COVID in Neonates and Anesthesia

49.7.1 Elective Surgery

  i. RTPCR is done within 72 h prior to surgery, and if COVID-positive, elective surgery is postponed until COVID negativity is achieved, as postoperative outcome of COVID-positive neonates is poor.
 ii. Optimization and prevention of worsening of infection. Patient should be categorized according to the symptoms and signs and early treatment started, and
iii. Prevention of transmission of infection to healthcare workers, OT and hospital staff, and other patients.
 iv. The suggested timing of elective surgery after recovery from COVID-19 is as follows [16]:
    1. 4 weeks for asymptomatic patient/recovery from mild nonrespiratory symptoms.
    2. 6 weeks for symptomatic patient (cough, dyspnea) who did not required hospitalization.
    3. 8–10 weeks for hospitalized patients.
    4. 12 weeks for patient who was admitted to ICU due to COVID-19 infection.

49.7.2 Emergency Surgery

(i) COVID-positive neonates and suspects should be taken up for **emergency surgery** with full precautions while following COVID guidelines when providing anesthesia.

(ii) Mandatory temperature check is necessary for all patients before taking in OT.

(iii) For **emergency surgery**, there should be designated OT for COVID-positive/suspected cases with sign board outside.

(iv) PAC should be done by the anesthetist in PPE.

(v) Severity of respiratory compromise should be determined.

(vi) X-ray, ABG, and all routine investigations should be done.

(vii) Evaluation for O_2 requirement, signs of shock, liver failure, and renal failure should be done.

49.8 Special OT Requirements for all COVID-Positive Patients

i. Adequate PPE should be available for all the staffs (Table 49.1, Figs. 49.1, 49.2, 49.3 and 49.4).

ii. Designated donning and doffing area should be present in or adjacent to the OT.

iii. HEPA (high-efficiency particulate air) filter should be attached to the expiratory end of corrugated breathing circuit before expired gas enters anesthesia machine. (In adult cases, an extra filter is also attached between Y piece of circuit and patient's mask/ETT/LMA. 2 filters in neonate circuit will increase Vd significantly, hence not advised).

iv. If gas analyzer is used, gases should be scavenged and not allowed to return to OT air.

Table 49.1 Personal protective equipment (PPE)

	Level 1	Level 2	Level 3	Level 4
Include	Surgical mask	Eye protection, surgical mask, disposable apron, gloves	Eye protection (goggles/ face shield/ visor), N- 95 mask, Long sleeve gown, Gloves, shoe covers	Eye protection, N-95 mask Overalls, Gloves, shoe covers
Use in	**Least risk areas** – offices, accounts, security, pharmacy	**Low risk areas** - OPD, non COVID ward, ABG/ ECG station	**In COVID areas** For short duration – < 4 hrs For brief interaction/ observation of patients (history taking, examination, blood sampling, taking swabs **In All Doffing areas**	**In COVID areas** • For longer duration - > 4 hrs • Close patient contact (NGT insertion, ET insertion/suction) **During CPR** **In OT during surgery** **In ER**

OPD – Outpatient department, ABG – Arterial blood gas, ECG -Electrocardiogram, NGT – Nasogastric tube, CPR- Cardiopulmonary resuscitation, OT – Operation theatre, ER – Emergency room

Fig. 49.1 Level 1 PPE

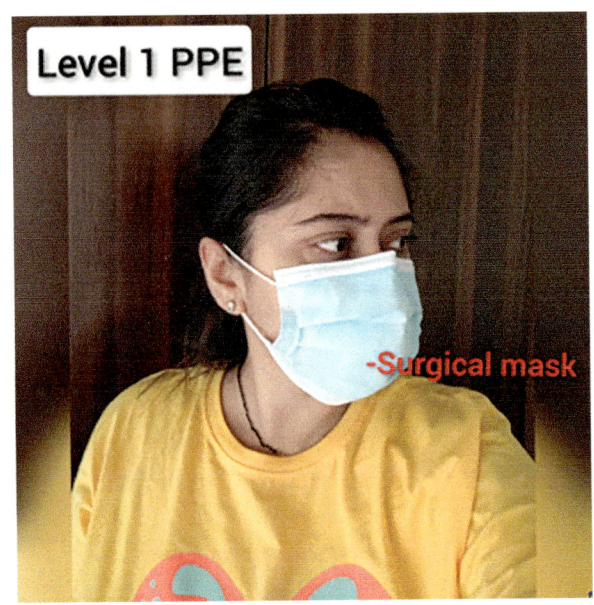

Fig. 49.2 Level 2 PPE

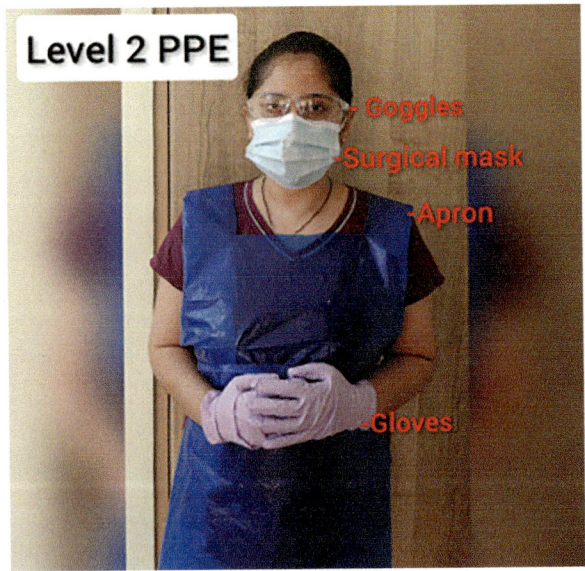

Fig. 49.3 Level 3 PPE

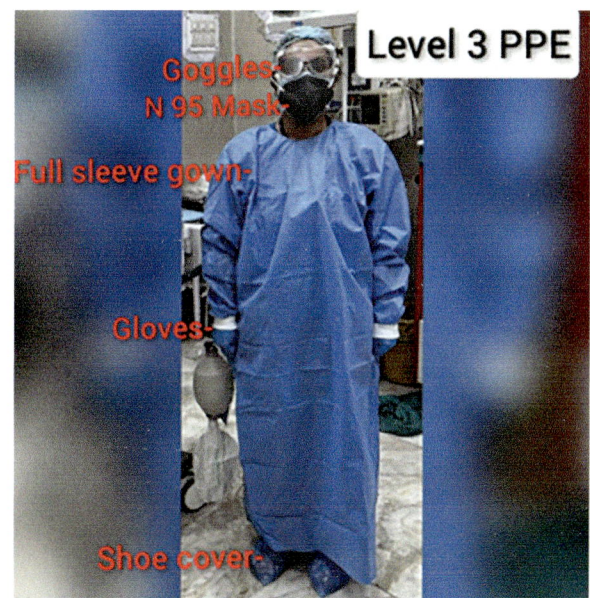

Fig. 49.4 Level 4 PPE

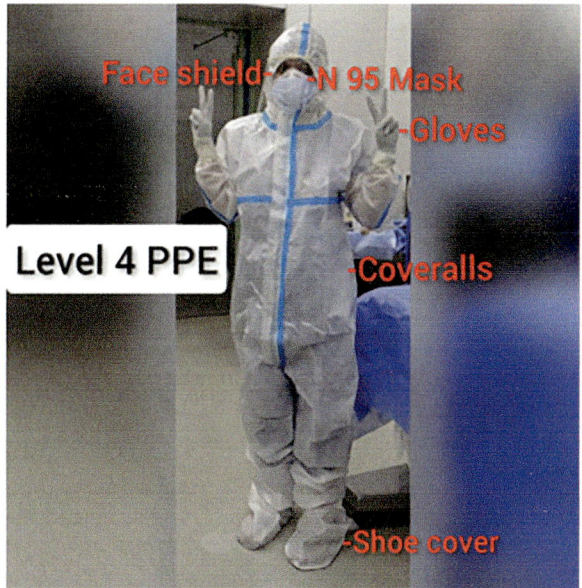

v. Preferably closed circuit should be used or kept available.

vi. Nondisposable equipment (monitors, keyboards) to be covered with transparent plastic.

49.9 Anesthetic Management

Anesthetic considerations and anesthesia management remain the same as discussed for neonates undergoing a particular surgery, with additional COVID care.

49.9.1 Choice of Anesthesia

General anesthesia is the choice in neonates. Regional anesthesia cannot be used as sole anesthetic technique, but can be utilized to reduce the requirements of anesthetic drugs, narcotics, and relaxants and improve postoperative recovery. Limited number of staff should be present in the OT, all wearing PPE, at any one time.

49.9.2 Monitoring

SPO_2, ECG, NIBP, PR, RR, temperature, urine output, and $EtCO_2$ should be monitored throughout. Additional monitoring depends on the baby's condition and surgical requirement.

49.9.3 Induction

Most experienced anesthetist should be the incharge of intubation as it decreases the number of attempts and exposure, as neonates are considered to have difficult airway. Person at the head end and technician should wear double gloves. Outer gloves are discarded after induction and intubation. mRSI (modified rapid sequence induction) avoids manual ventilation and potential aerosolization, while it is also preferred in sick neonates or those at risk of regurgitation and aspiration. If manual ventilation is indicated, small tidal volume at low pressure should be given.

i. Preoxygenation should be done with minimal gas flow and with tight seal.

ii. Video laryngoscopes (C-MAC, McGrath, TrueView) should be used with disposable blade. The blade should be resheathed immediately or kept in a separate tray after use. This helps reduce the exposure of the anesthetist who is intubating.

iii. ETT should be clamped before intubation and declamped only after connecting to the circuit.

iv. Ventilator should be kept on standby mode while intubating or when disconnection is required.

v. Positive pressure ventilation should be started only when cuff of ETT is inflated (not applicable if using uncuffed ETT in neonates).

vi. Auscultation is difficult with PPE, so position of ETT is confirmed visually while placing it, with chest rise on assisted ventilation, and $EtCO_2$ waveform.

49.9.4 Maintenance

- ETT and circuit disconnection should be minimized during surgery,
- Low gas flow technique should be used, preferably via closed circuit should be used (may not always be possible in neonates, hence extra care to be taken).
- Lung protective ventilation mode to be used, i.e., low tidal volume of 3–5 ml/kg, and low airway pressure (15–20 cm H_2O).

49.9.5 Emergence

- Should be smooth, avoid straining and coughing,
- High flow O_2, NIV (noninvasive ventilation), and nebulization should be avoided postoperatively.
- Neonates should be kept in designated postoperative room for COVID patients with monitors.

49.9.6 OT Equipment after Care

After patient has been shifted out of the OT, and all equipment must be cleaned and stored/kept before being used for the next patient:

- Airway equipment preferably uses disposable one-time use equipment especially that which is going to be in contact with the mucosa or secretions or expired gases. Breathing circuit, mask, ETT, LMA, oral airway, HME filter, gas sampling line, reservoir bag, soda lime, and forced air warming blanket should be bagged for disposal as contaminated waste, after every patient use.
- All used nondisposable airway equipment should be sealed in a double ziplocked plastic bag and then sent for decontamination and disinfection.
- The water trap and soda lime CO_2 absorber do not need to be replaced between COVID-19-positive patients if high-quality HMEF filters are used. Also, CO_2 absorber is alkaline and acts as virucidal. But, should water trap become contaminated, it should be discarded.
- The internal components of the anesthesia machine and breathing system do not need terminal cleaning if high-quality filters are used.

49.10 Conclusion

COVID-19, which started in December 2019 in China, was soon declared a pandemic after it started infecting and killing people around the globe. India has witnessed two waves affecting crores of people including children. Neonates born to suspected or COVID-positive mother can contract infection in postnatal period through droplet transmission.

Neonates presenting for surgeries during COVID pandemic should undergo detailed PAC and testing for COVID. Decision to proceed or delay surgery should be made after discussion with surgeon and weighing risk against benefits of surgery in COVID-positive neonates. If the surgery is planned, all the precautions should be taken by anesthetists, surgeons, and OT staffs to minimize the risk of transmission from the patients to healthcare workers.

Anesthetists should follow COVID guidelines during induction and intubation (most critical period when anesthetist is at risk of contracting COVID from a positive patient), during maintenance and emergence that can benefit the patient in terms of outcome and reduce the risk of spread of COVID. After surgery, proper sanitization and disposal of equipment and instruments should be done to prevent interpatient transmission in OT. In postoperative period, COVID-positive patients should be treated for the infection while monitoring for recovery.

Providing anesthesia to neonates is itself challenging, and COVID-19 has made it even more challenging, but it can be overcome by proper training, knowledge, following COVID protocols and taking required precautions.

References

1. Reported Cases and Deaths by Country or Territory. 18 Nov 2021. Worldometers.info/coronavirus/.
2. Coronavirus disease (COVID-19) pandemic. WHO Health Emergency Dashboard. https://www.who.int/emergencies/diseases/novel-coronavirus-2019.
3. Evaluation and Management Considerations for Neonates at Risk for COVID-19. Centers for Disease Control and Prevention (CDCP). Updated Dec. 8, 2020. https://www.cdc.gov/coronavirus/2019-ncov/hcp/caring-for-newborns.html
4. Bustin SA, Benes V, Garson JA, et al. The MIQE guidelines: minimum information for publication of quantitative real-time PCR experiments. Clin Chem. 2009;55(4):611–22. https://doi.org/10.1373/clinchem.2008.112797.
5. Logan J, Edwards K, Saunders N. Real-time PCR: current technology and applications. Caister Academic Press; 2009. ISBN 978-1-904455-39-4
6. Basawarajappa SG, Rangaiah A, Padukone S, et al. Performance evaluation of Truenat™ Beta CoV & Truenat™ SARS-CoV-2 point-of-care assays for coronavirus disease. Indian J Med Res. 2020; https://doi.org/10.4103/ijmr.IJMR2363_20.
7. COVID19 Statewise Status. MyGov.in. Covid19india.org 18 Nov 2021. https://www.mygov.in/corona-data/covid19-statewise-status.
8. Riffe T, Acosta E, Scholey J, et al. COVerAGE-DB: a database of COVID-19 cases and deaths by age. Identifier.: https://osf.io/mpwjq. 2021; https://doi.org/10.17605/OSF.IO/MPWJQ.
9. Guidelines for Management of COVID-19 in Children (below 18 years). Ministry of Health & Family Welfare. Government of India Protocol for Management of Covid-19 in

the Pediatric Age Group. MOHFW. GOI. 29.04.2021. https://www.mohfw.gov.in/pdf/GuidelinesforManagementofCOVID19inCHILDREN

10. COVID-19 (coronavirus) in babies and children—Mayo Clinic. 16 Nov 2021. https://www.mayoclinic.org/diseases-conditions/coronavirus/in-depth/

11. Covid -19 Testing- Part of a series on COVID-19 pandemic. https://en.wikipedia.org/wiki/COVID-19_testing.

12. Breastfeeding & Caring for Newborns. Centers for Disease Control and Prevention (CDCP). Updated Aug. 18, 2021. https://www.cdc.gov/index.htm

13. Sankar J, Dhochak N, Kabra SK, Lodha R. COVID-19 in children: clinical approach and management. Indian J Pediatr. 2020;87(6):433–42. https://doi.org/10.1007/s12098-020-03292-1.

14. COVID-19 in children: Clinical approach and management. https://nidm.gov.in/covid19/PDF/covid19/state/Meghalaya/107.pdf

15. Infection Prevention and Control: COVID-19. Minnesota Dept of Health. Updated 12 Nov 2021. https://www.health.state.mn.us/diseases/coronavirus/hcp/infectioncontrol.html.

16. ASA and APSF Joint Statement on Elective Surgery and Anesthesia for patients after COVID-19 infection. https://www.asahq.org/about-asa/newsroom/news-releases/2020/12/asa-and... December 8, 2020.

Ethics in Neonatal Anesthesia and Research

50

Anita Malik and Usha Saha

50.1 Introduction

It has always been felt that a medical person is above reproach and does all in good faith and is most competent. Physicians of the yore era put patient before self, family, money, and religion. Even in so far as testing and research were considered, patient had nothing to worry about, because the physicians were most reliable and trustworthy.

But somewhere in the modern-day practice, ethics took a back seat, where self-interest took the front seat, became more important than the patient. This led to some neglects and wrongs and led to errors of judgments that affected patient outcome adversely. Patients started doubting the trustworthiness of the physician and questioned their decisions.

This led to the necessity of stressing the importance of ethics to the physicians in their day-to-day clinical practice and in research. In this context, the International Covenant on Civil and Political Rights stated that "No one should be subjected to torture or to cruel inhumane or degrading treatment or punishment. In particular, no one will be subjected without his free consent to medical or scientific experimentation [1]." How this can be applicable to neonates remains to be seen.

In this chapter, we will go through how ethics developed in clinical medical practice and its role in research, especially in the newborns and neonates, and role and dilemmas of an anesthesiologist when faced with anesthetizing these preverbal babies undergoing surgery and how the anesthesiologist must safeguard self and

A. Malik (✉)
Department of Anesthesiology & Critical Care, King George's Medical University (KGMU), Lucknow, Uttar Pradesh, India

U. Saha
Department of Anesthesiology, Critical Care, Pain and Palliative Care, LHMC, SSK and KSC Hospitals, New Delhi, India

patient from any liabilities. Process of consent in its several forms is also discussed. This chapter is in two parts: first, role of ethics in Clinical practice and second, its role neonatal research.

Ethics is defined as moral code of conduct. They are the moral principles that govern a person's behavior or conducting of an activity.

It is the branch of philosophy that defines right and wrong, matters of value, and what is good for individuals and society.

Common value words used in ethical considerations are responsibility, integrity, honesty, respect, trust, openness, fairness, and transparency.

The four fundamental approaches to ethical discipline and decision-making framework, are [2]:

1. Utilitarian (outcome-based) ethics,
2. Deontological (duty-based) ethics,
3. Virtue (virtue-based) ethics and.
4. Communitarianism ethics—a person is a part of a community and that a person's social identity and personality are molded by community relationships.

50.2 Ethics in Clinical Practice and Neonatal Anesthesia

50.2.1 Clinical Ethics [2–5]

This is the application of moral code of conducts to the practice of medicine, biomedical science, education, and research. Clinical ethics assist physicians in identifying, analyzing, and resolving ethical issues that arise in day-to-day clinical practice. Ethical issues are of common occurrence, and it is important for the caretaker to identify them and resolve timely.

Ethical problems arise when the physician and patient face contradictions during the clinical management. **Contradictions give rise to ethical issues.**

Clinical ethics work on the principle that caretakers and patients (and families) and can work together to identify, analyze, and resolve any contradictions that may arise.

Hence, it is very important that every clinician be proficient in their knowledge of clinical ethics.

It is the responsibility of all personnel and staff involved in providing care to the patient that they maintain and follow the code of ethics and provide quality care.

Physicians and anesthesiologists must familiarize themselves with all aspects of ethics, including consent taking, principle of informed consent, and other forms of consent, be honest in their communication with the patient and family, maintain integrity and Confidentiality, be empathetic and are able to take care of issues such as end-of-life care, pain relief, patient rights, autonomy, and respect, and build trust in their relationship.

Clinical situations are not simple and attain complexities of varying degrees, involving a wide range of medical facts, varying circumstances, and patient's values, and at times, decisions must be reached quickly.

For example, when a patient refuses a particularly recommended treatment, essential for successful outcome, such as the Jehovah's Witness who refuses blood transfusion. Here, ethical issues arise because of patient's autonomy and right to make a choice (i.e., refuse blood transfusion), which may harm the patient (not getting necessary treatment), creating a moral dilemma for the treating physician.

Keeping the following key principles of medical ethics at the core of decision making process can help resolve many ethical issues:

(i) **Medical indications**—i.e., the treatment should benefit the patient (beneficence) and cause no harm (nonmaleficence).
(ii) **Patient preferences**—includes respect for patients right to decision making (autonomy), balancing with best possible treatment for a favorable outcome.
(iii) **Quality of life (QoL)**—the purpose of a medical management is improvement in the QoL, in balance with the above to factors.
(iv) **Contextual features**—like legalities, issues of justice and fairness, insurance claims, financial issues, and patient's paying ability, which can affect clinical decision making to a large extent.

50.2.2 Anesthesiologist's Dilemma

Role of anesthesiologist in the management of a surgical newborn and neonate is different from that of a neonatologist or a pediatrician. The anesthesiologist gets involved only when a baby requires surgery and often sees the neonate just prior to surgery in the holding area of the operation room. Dilemmas arise from the facts, that:

1. Diagnosis is already established, or in most cases, it is the most probable diagnosis.
2. Decision to operate is already made. Anesthesiologist is expected to administer anesthesia, irrespective of one's expert opinion regarding the criticality of surgery and the baby, especially in preterms, small for gestational age, low birth weight babies, and those with inborn medical and congenital problems.
3. In this age group, all surgeries are considered as critical and as an emergency, life or organ-saving procedures.
4. Investigations are ordered by the surgical team and are usually those that are necessary to establish the diagnosis.
5. Often most relevant investigations relevant from the anesthesia point of view are missing, and the surgical team is unwilling to wait for them or for the reports citing how imminent surgery is.
6. Many of these neonates have problems at transition, undiagnosed and untreated medical diseases, propensity for respiratory distress syndrome (RDS), intraventricular hypertrophy (IVH), bleeding diathesis, congenital heart disease (CHD), etc., that increase the risk of morbidity and mortality.

7. Most often or not, in case of adverse results, the blame is placed on the anesthesiologist.
8. Hence, the anesthesiologist must be highly experienced, be able to anticipate problems, prevent them, and manage in case they occur—often working in the blind.
9. The anesthesiologist must provide the best of care, make best choice regarding anesthesia techniques and drugs for induction, intubation and maintenance, use appropriate monitoring technique (invasive vs noninvasive), check OT appropriateness, adequately trained and efficient staff, anticipate and manage intraoperative fluid and blood loss, take a call on whether to extubate at the end of surgery or go for elective ventilation. These create ethical issues in the anesthetic management of the neonate, a patient who cannot communicate its problems.
10. Crying is the only symptom of any discomfort in these patients. More sick and critical a baby is, more is the chance that it will be listless, weak, with inability to even cry, either from the surgical disease or because of drugs administered (sedatives/analgesics) or from inability to move limbs (often splinted), or inadequate respiratory effort, and so on.
11. Since surgery must be undertaken, it is only ethical to provide good anesthesia, pain relief, maintain hemodynamic and volume status, maintain multiorgan function, cause no further harm, and reduce the suffering of the baby and parents.

Keeping the cardinal principles of ethics at the helm of decision making at any stage can go a long way in safeguarding the interests of both the neonate and the anesthesiologist.

50.2.3 Ethics in Neonatal Anesthesia

Providing anesthesia to a neonate requires a balance of clinical and ethical skills, as to what is best for neonates who cannot express their own interests. These principles must be adhered to in the clinical practice, during anesthesia, and throughout the perioperative care period.

Note:- As a rule of thumb, "magnitude of problems or risks is inversely proportional to the gestational age," and it is very important that all measures are taken to prevent further iatrogenic complications.

This can be easily achieved if the anesthesiologists follow the ethical principles:-

1. **Beneficence**—do good, do only that which will be beneficial, and promote the best interest of the neonate.
2. **Nonmaleficence**—primum non nocere (**do no harm**), such as pain, suffering, discomfort, disability, or death from treatment or disease.
3. **Autonomy**—right of competent patient in decision making. In neonates, this responsibility lies on the parents, and.

4. **Justice (social cooperation)**—judgment and decision that help to establish the anesthetist's primary duty toward the neonates, regarding them as individuals, even when they are clearly unable to express themselves, and also as to how the social benefits and the health care are distributed in the society. Broadly, it means to promote the greatest good for the greatest number for the distribution of resources **(macroallocation)**, while providing equal opportunity to each individual **(microallocation)**.

Ethical Concerns in neonatal anesthesia arise from the need to provide anesthesia, analgesia, monitoring, and intensive care, which the neonate should not be deprived of, in the face of knowing that these interventions may also have some adverse consequences. Some of these concerns are described below.

(i) **Decision making**—regarding the choice of anesthesia technique, choice of drugs, additional procedures, and need for invasive monitoring.

(ii) **Expert care and opinion**—if at any stage in the perioperative care, in the diagnosis and necessary investigations, and administration of anesthesia, there is need, expert opinion must be sought for, in the best interest of the neonate.

(iii) **Responsibility of care**—many different specialists and staff members are involved in the management of a neonate, and who has the responsibility of care must be decided beforehand. In a surgical neonate, the onus lies on the surgical specialist under whom the baby is admitted or on the operating physician. This may vary from institute to institute and country to country.

(iv) **Pain management**—all surgical neonates should receive good anesthesia and adequate pain relief, as there is proof that this improves neonatal outcome, as these newborns, neonates, and prematures do feel pain and exhibit stress responses that are adverse.

(v) **Blood transfusion and related issues**—transfusion of blood and blood products is not without any danger. Since the neonate cannot give consent, parental or surrogate decision makers prior consent must be obtained. In case of Jehovah's witness (those who refuse blood transfusion), appropriate adjustments in management must be made especially if surgery is associated with major blood loss.

(vi) **Consent taking**—this is an important aspect in the preoperative period and comes under various heads, such as consent, implied consent, informed consent, deferred consent, and continuing consent. All the requisites (provision of essential information to parents, responsibility of care, documentation) must be followed.

(vii) **Record keeping**—all consent documents and treatment records must be maintained including anesthesia records, drugs and dosages used, monitoring (invasive, noninvasive), vital parameters, IV fluids used, any intraoperative events, etc.

(viii) **Empathy** - This is the ability to understand what someone else is feeling or what it is like to be in their situation (putting yourself in their boots), to feel what others are feeling as if you are feeling it yourself, i.e., having feelings for the suffering baby and the parents. This can lead to several moral issues such as dilemma, distress, and uncertainty.

   (a) **Moral Dilemma**: It occurs when the physician feels the obligation to pursue one or more conflicting courses of action, e.g., when a conflict arises between action required by the principle of autonomy and by the principle of beneficence, such as CPR of the dying ex-premature neonate with a brain tumor or intracerebral bleed, or withdrawal of life support measures or treatment.

   (b) **Moral Distress**: It arises from the limits of viability—I do not agree with doing "everything," knowing or being aware of the probable outcome, breaking of bad news to the parents or relatives, end of life care, and.

   (c) **Moral Uncertainty**: It arises when the presenting issue is unclear, for example, in bronchopulmonary dysplasia or severe respiratory distress, where prognosis is poor, it is difficult to decide when or if to terminate and what to tell the parents in such a situation.

50.2.4 Communication with Parents

All information should be given to the parents with good communication. There is no scope for any miscommunication.

   (i) The way information is communicated influences parental understanding of the situation, their ability to discuss moral issues, and participate in decision making.

   (ii) Transparency and honesty in communication are crucial.

   (iii) Parents should be provided with accurate information from time to time.

   (iv) Information should be able to encourage and empower parents to make treatment choices.

   (v) There should be no miscommunication of facts.

   (vi) Information should be given in a manner and language understandable to the parents.

   (vii) This allows parental authority, physician to express his or her own clinical judgment, thus promote best interests of the newborn and the family.

50.2.5 Informed Consent

The principle of informed consent in the physician–patient (and family) relationship grew in early twentieth century. As patients (and families) became more aware of their rights and options, they became quick to allege negligence, when professionals failed to present all the options that a patient might choose to pursue, especially if the outcome is adverse. The rules for informed consent were first promulgated in the "Nuremberg Code (1947)" and later in the "Declaration of Helsinki (1964)" [6] and "Belmont Report," and codified in the "Code of Federal Regulations." A important points that emerged were as follow:

1. All interventions require consent to be taken, and more invasive an intervention is, greater is the need of consent.
2. A complication or an adverse outcome, and with inadequate or no consent, can make a physician (anesthesiologist) liable for "medical or clinical negligence" and legal action.
3. In newborns and neonates, this raises the question of "patient's capacity to consent **for surgery**" as [7]:
   - The neonates are largely regarded as an **extension of their parents.**
   - **Decision makers are parents.**
   - **Complete emphasis on parental autonomy** can, at times, compromise the right of the neonate to justice, beneficence, and nonmaleficence.
   - For **nonverbal children**, parents are supposed to act in the **best interest of their child.**
   - Before giving consent, parents should evaluate and ask themselves, especially when in doubt, **"if my child would be an adult, would he/she have given consent."**

50.2.6 Anesthetic Drug Use in Neonates [8–12]

A newborn baby is still in the process of adapting to the extrauterine life. The organs are all immature, not fully developed anatomically, physiologically, and functionally. This increases the anesthetists concern in the use of anesthetic drugs and their adverse effects on the developing brain and other body systems. Direct studies and research in this age group are scarce, and most literature is based on observational studies and experiences of the anesthesiologists when managing them for the surgery or in the ICU or during resuscitation. This issue is discussed later in the chapter (ethical issues in neonatal research). A few points of significance for a practicing anesthesiologist are enumerated here as follows:

   (i) **Urgent need for rigorous evaluation**.
  (ii) Studies indicate **anesthetic toxicity and neuronal apoptosis** in developing brain with long-term adverse outcomes (especially premature, multiple surgeries).
 (iii) Most anesthetic agents are **not adequately tested for safety or efficacy** in neonates.
 (iv) **Dosing** is often extrapolated from adult dosage experience.
  (v) **Many different drugs administered** concurrently.

(vi) Most drugs are approved by FDA for adult patients. Few drugs approved for use in neonates.

(vii) **Withholding anesthesia from neonates in need of surgery is unethical in itself.**

50.2.7 Legality and Neonatal Anesthesia

The possibility that anesthetics could harm the developing brain was identified in rodents, and since then, it has raised serious concerns in the anesthesia community, leading to U.S. FDA warning on the use of anesthetic agents in young children. Healthcare providers and policymakers are divided on the risks *versus* benefits of general anesthesia and surgery in pediatric populations. Concern was raised because of some studies where an association was found between early exposure to anesthesia and subsequent neurodevelopmental alterations. The prospective clinical trials addressing anesthetics in early age and long-term neurodevelopmental delay in children were carried out and published with good results. [8, 10, 12–15]

1. **In 1997, US legislation** encouraged more drug investigations in infants. This resulted in "more than 500 labeling changes to products regarding safety and efficacy in various pediatric ages." However, only 12 anesthetic agents were updated, and none in premature babies [16].

2. **EU (European Union) directive** proposed to prohibit all nontherapeutic research in children, but after heavy pressure from pediatricians, it was accepted, under the conditions that "clinical trials in minors may be undertaken only if some benefits for the group of patients is obtained from the trial and only where such research is essential to validate the data obtained on persons able to give informed consent. Additionally, such research should either relate directly to a clinical condition from which the minor concerned suffers or be of a nature that it can only be carried out on minors" [17].

3. **In 2003, USFDA approved** facilitated studies of anesthetic agents in children. Drugs which received approval for research included [16]:

    (i) **Intravenous agents**—propofol and ketamine,
    (ii) **Inhalational agents**—desflurane, sevoflurane, and isoflurane,
    (iii) **Opioids**—fentanyl, morphine, oxycodone, and remifentanil,
    (iv) **Benzodiazepine**—midazolam and lorazepam,
    (v) **Nondepolarizing muscle relaxants**—rocuronium,
    (vi) **Dexmedetomidine, and**
    (vii) **Lignocaine.**

    Results of These Studies emerged as:

    (a) **Sevoflurane** is safe and efficacious in neonates more than *9 days of age*, but there is a greater risk of **seizures.**
    (b) **Desflurane** is safe in children more than 2 *years of age.*

(c) **Propofol** is safe for *induction in children older than 3 years of age. It is safely used for maintenance as an infusion in infants more than 2 month of age. Safety of propofol in neonates has not been proven,* because studies are not done in this age group because of risk of high mortality.

(d) **Midazolam** can be used after modifying the dose schedule in neonates with congenital heart disease (CHD) and pulmonary hypertension. There is insufficient data to justify its routine use in neonates because of adverse neurologic outcome.

(e) **Fentanyl**—in 2005, it was established that fentanyl is safe in children above the age of 16 years. Its safety in children under 16 years of age is not established. The side effects that affect its safety profile in neonates and preterm are greater need for respiratory support and delay in starting enteral feeds, both when used as an infusion or as IV boluses.

(f) **Morphine** is frequently used in NICU setting for sedation and analgesia in sick neonates, especially on ventilatory support, and reported side effects include greater incidence of intraventricular hemorrhage (IVH) and EEG depression. Morphine is safe for use in older children (> 8–9 years age).

(g) **Xylocaine**—safety and efficacy of xylocaine are not proven in children under 12 years of age.

  Following this, only three anesthetic drugs received their approval for use **in neonates and preterms with proven safety profile.** They are as follows:

(I) **Dexmedetomidine.**
(II) **Remifentanil, and.**
(III) **Rocuronium.**

4. **SmartTots (strategies for mitigating anesthesia-related neurotoxicity in Tots) (2009)** [18].
   - A public–private partnership, launched by the U.S. Food and Drug administration (FDA) in collaboration with the International Anesthesia Research Society (IARS), in 2009.
   - The stakeholders include academic research institutions, medical professionals and societies, and government and nonprofit organizations.
   - There was insufficient evidence of a link between anesthesia use and damage to the developing brain in animals.
   - SmartTots aims to fund research to investigate various aspects of existing anesthetics, their administration, dosages, and exposure and to fill these gaps so as to make anesthesia and sedation safer for young children (under 5 years age), commonly undergoing surgeries for ear infections, tonsillectomy, hernia repair, and circumcision.
   - To establish new practice guidelines and new age-appropriate anesthetics.

5. **FDASIA (FDA Safety and Innovation Act) in USA and Europe (2012).**
   (i) FDA to obtain additional expertise in neonatal drug development and complex issues surrounding study design and outcome measures.
   (ii) Written requests to specifically include neonates so as to avoid unnecessary waivers. 25% of previous waivers were found to have been issued in error.
   (iii) Pediatric study plans for drugs to be submitted soon after completion of phase II trials in adults.
   (iv) Enhanced communication between different regulatory agencies.

6. **PANDA (2016)** Pediatric Anesthesia Neurodevelopment Assessment (PANDA) [12].

   This study was conducted in 105 children under the age of 3 years (critical time in brain development) undergoing inguinal hernia repair to examine whether single short exposure to GA (median of 80 min) had any effect on global cognitive function (IQ) later in life. IQ scores and secondary neurodevelopmental outcomes were assessed between the ages of 8 and 15, and outcome was compared for each child with a healthy, biologically related sibling of similar age, not exposed to anesthesia. There was no significant difference in outcome on comparison, although more children in the group exposed exhibited internalizing behavior (behaviors directed inward), needing evaluation.

7. **GAS study (2016)** (General Anesthesia Spinal) trial compared regional and general anesthesia for neurodevelopmental outcome and apnea in more than 700 children undergoing inguinal hernia repair during early life (under the age of 36 months), randomized to either sevoflurane-based GA or awake SAB. The study demonstrated no association between 1 h of GA and cognitive scores at the age of 2 years or IQ scores at the age of 5 years, compared to SAB [19].

8. **MASK (2018) study** (Mayo Anesthesia Safety in Kids) [10].

   This provided strong evidence that a short exposure to GA at a young age does not result in detectable alterations in neurodevelopmental outcome and that exposure to multiple anesthesia, before the age of 3 year, is associated with adverse neurodevelopmental outcomes. 997 children (411 unexposed, 380 singly exposed, and 206 multiply exposed) born between 1994 and 2007 were included. They underwent neuropsychological testing at ages 8–12 or 15–20 yr. The primary outcome was the full-scale intelligence quotient standard score of the Wechsler abbreviated scale of intelligence. Secondary outcomes included individual domains from a comprehensive neuropsychological assessment and parent reports.

   They concluded that anesthesia exposure before age 3 years was not associated with deficits in the primary outcome (IQ), although secondary outcomes (processing speed, fine motor abilities, executive function, behavior, and reading) were affected and that multiple, not single, exposures are associated with changes in neuropsychological domains associated with behavior and learning.

50.2.8 Pain Management

Until 1980s, almost half a century ago, pain and discomfort in the newborn were never considered a priority, and neonates, especially premature babies, were operated with little or no anesthesia and analgesia. In the NICU, babies rarely received sedation.

Advances in diagnosis, treatment, ongoing research, and advances brought about a change in the attitudes and practices in the neonatal anesthesia in early 80s, with the realization that:

(i) Newborn babies also do feel pain.
(ii) It is important to provide pain relief during surgery.
(iii) Anesthesia and analgesia are safe to use.
(iv) It is unethical not to provide adequate anesthesia and analgesia.

(v) Outcomes are better with good anesthesia and adequate analgesia.

(vi) May have "double effect" described by Partridge and Wall, (risk of mortality), and.

(vii) Groningen protocol [20] in Netherlands legalizes deliberate ending of life in newborns with extremely poor prognosis (downside of use of narcotics).

Today, providing anesthesia and pain relief is a standard norm and most physicians provide opioids with the intent to alleviate pain and promote comfort.

Authors Note: Whatever the result of these studies, anesthetists have been using drugs, according to their availability and their experience when faced with the dilemma of anesthetizing neonates, including ex premature, trying to keep in accordance with the ethical values and principles.

50.2.9 Anesthetic drugs that have been used in the past, in the surgical neonates, include the following

(a) **Inhalational agents**—halothane and even ether were routinely used for both induction and maintenance of anesthesia in the neonates, but with greatest of care because of the risk of myocardial depression and hypotension with halothane and delayed recovery with ether.

(b) **Intravenous anesthetic agents**—thiopentone was routinely used for induction and is even being used today, though in lower doses, despite theoretical recommendations of higher initial doses of anesthetic drugs because of greater proportion of body water to weight in this age group.

(c) **Sedatives**—diazepam in smaller doses was used but one tried to avoid using it because of its long half-life of 36 h in adults, which would further increase in a neonate due to the immature hepatic and renal function, and more severe effects on the immature brain, and delayed recovery.

(d) **Narcotics and analgesics**—pethidine and morphine have both been used to provide intraoperative analgesia and in NICU.

(e) **Local anesthetics**— xylocaine has been used for local infiltration, with the aim of reducing the requirement of inhalational agents and dose of narcotics.

50.3 Ethics in Neonatal Research

50.3.1 Development of Ethics in Human Research

For the progress in the field of medicine and development of better medical care, research is required. Consideration of appropriate study designs and ethical issues is important to investigate newer or currently available approaches for analgesia and anesthesia in neonates. Various conditions in neonates requiring treatment are pain/stress resulting from invasive procedures, surgical operations, and routine neonatal intensive care [21]. In general, children should not be at a disadvantage due to lack of knowledge and due to reduced research activity because of ethical issue constraints. However, the interpretation and implementation of ethical principles is not always straight forward [22]. While it is desirable that medical care of critically ill neonates should be based on best research evidence to ensure safe and efficacious treatment or procedures, in contemporary practice, this seldom happens [9, 23, 24].

For research on human subjects, three fundamental ethical principles as mentioned in the Belmont Report are respect for persons, beneficence, and justice. Respect for person acknowledges that each human being has value in himself (or herself) which must be preserved in all interaction between people. The principle of beneficence provides maximum possible benefits and minimum possible harms. The principle of justice implies that there should be no inequality in sharing the burden or risks with the benefits of research [25].

Privacy and confidentiality are also an integral part of ethics of research. Advancement in information technology and bioinformatics leading to the creation of larger, and more sophisticated, and increasingly interlinked databases will increase the issues of the ethics of confidentiality and data management [22].

50.3.2 Ethics in Human Research - Historical Facts

1. The Nuremberg Code of 1947 [26, 27].

   The judgment by the war crimes tribunal at Nuremberg laid down 10 standards to which physicians must conform when experimenting on humans which is now accepted worldwide. This established ethical guidelines for medical behavior (Table 50.1)

Table 50.1 Ethical guidelines—Nuremberg Code of 1947

(i)	Voluntary informed consent.
(ii)	The experiment should be such as to yield fruitful results for the good of society, unprocurable by other methods or means of study.
(iii)	The experiment should be designed and based on the results of animal studies and knowledge of natural history of the disease under study that the anticipated results justify the experiment.
(iv)	It should be conducted without unnecessary physical and mental suffering or injury.
(v)	No experiment should be conducted where there is a priori reason to believe that death or disabling injury will occur.
(vi)	The degree of risk should not exceed that determined by humanitarian importance of the problem.
(vii)	Conducted with proper preparations and adequate facilities to protect the subject against possible injury, disability, or death.
(viii)	Conducted by scientifically qualified persons, with highest degree of skill and care at all stages of the experiment.
(ix)	Subject should be at liberty to bring the experiment to an end at any time if he feels physically or mentally unable to continue.
(x)	The scientist in charge must be prepared to terminate the experiment at any stage, if there is cause to believe that continuation is likely to result in injury, disability, or death to the subject.

Table 50.2 Declaration of Helsinki (1964)

1. Physicians must consider the ethical, legal, and regulatory norms and standards for research in human subjects in their own country as well as international norms.
2. Research should be conducted in a manner that minimizes harm to environment.
3. Research involving humans must be conducted only by those with appropriate ethics and scientific education, training, and qualifications.
4. Appropriate compensation and treatment for subjects harmed during research must be ensured.
5. Measures to minimize the risks must be implemented.
6. Some vulnerable groups may have an increased likelihood of being wronged or incurring harm and should receive protection.
7. Research with a vulnerable group is justified if it is responsive to the health needs of that group and research cannot be carried out in another group.
8. Research must conform to scientific principles based on scientific literature, information, adequate laboratory, and animal data.
9. Design of research must be clearly described and justified in the protocol.
10. Informed voluntary consent is a must.
11. When the subject is incapable of giving consent, then the legally authorized representative (LAR) must give consent.
12. Every research study must be registered in a publicly accessible database before recruitment of the first subject.

2. Declaration of Helsinki 1964 (Amendment in 2013) [6, 28] (Table 50.2).

   The World Medical Association (WMA) developed the Declaration of Helsinki (DoH) as a statement of ethical principles for medical research involving human subjects. It addressed primarily the physicians and encouraged others involved in research to adopt these principles. In 2014, WMA celebrated 50 years of the adoption of DoH it states that -

   "It is the duty of the physician to promote and safeguard health, well-being, dignity, integrity, right to self-determination, privacy, and confidentiality of personal information of research subjects and patients. Medical progress is based on research that must include human subjects. Primary purpose of research involving humans is to understand the causes, development and effects of diseases, improve preventive, diagnostic, and therapeutic interventions (methods, procedures, treatments), but it can never take precedence over the rights and interests of the subject. Even the best proven interventions must be evaluated continually through research for their safety, effectiveness, efficiency, accessibility, and quality".

   General Principle is "The health of my patient will be my first consideration," and the International Code of Medical Ethics declares that "A physician shall act in the patient's best interest when providing medical care."

3. **Belmont Report** [25] was written in 1976, by the National Commission for the Protection of Human Subjects of Biomedical and Behavioral Research with the primary purpose to protect participants in clinical trials or studies, following the Tuskegee Syphilis Study, in which African Americans with syphilis were lied to and denied treatment for more than 40 years, and many died, infected others, and passed congenital syphilis onto their children. This study violated basic bioethical principles of autonomy, nonmaleficence, and justice.

4. **The National Commission for Protection of Human Subjects of Biomedical and Behavioral Research** (1979, in USA) enunciated 3 principles of ethics— **respect, beneficence, and justice.**
5. In 2005, **UNESCO** made **"Universal Declaration on Bioethics and Human Rights."**

50.3.3 Conduct of Biomedical Research in Children

Conduct of biomedical research in children raises several ethical issues. The lack of autonomy in children due to the cognitive and emotional level of maturity and the legal status to consent on their own behalf in research is an issue. To minimize research risks except in situations where the disease occurs only in children, it is required that animal studies and research on adults should precede studies with children. These concepts involve the basic ethical principles of beneficence and nonmaleficence. However, any system for protecting children involved in research should not unreasonably impede research on children that may potentially be beneficial to them in the future. A vulnerable set of patients should not be unduly exposed to research risks, which goes against the basic ethical principle of justice, just because they are available and their parents are not fully aware of their rights [29].

50.3.4 Guidelines for Research in Human

Research is essential for progress of science and development.

Inclusion of humans in research is essential for progress and development of science and medicine in adults.

Similarly, for progress in medicine in small children and neonates, research must include them as subjects of study.

But as stated above, all ethical principles must be adhered to in the planning and conduct of research in newborns, neonates, and premature babies, to safeguard their interest while looking for meaningful results:

1. **Enhancing knowledge** about human condition while maintaining sensitivity to Indian cultural, social, and natural environment.
2. Conducted under conditions that subject is not merely used for betterment of others, but is treated with **dignity and well-being, fairness, and transparency.**
3. Subjected to **evaluation and re-evaluation at all and any stage** of research— design, conduct, data analysis, and reporting of results.
4. **Negative results** are equally important as positive results and should form part of conclusion.
5. **Honesty toward the babies and parents at all levels.**
6. Four cardinal principles to be adhered to **beneficence, autonomy, nonmaleficence (primum non nocere), and justice/fairness** (Table 50.3).

Table 50.3 Principle for Research in Human—General Ethical Issues

1. Benefit-risk assessment and essentiality—maximum benefit, minimum risk
2. Informed voluntary consent (parent or LAR)
3. Nonexploitation, management, and compensation for research-related harm
4. Ensuring privacy and confidentiality
5. Professional competence
6. Distributive justice
7. Institutional arrangements and ancillary care during research and in case of a complication
8. Transparency, accountability, responsibility
9. Environmental and resource protection
10. There should be no conflict of interest, as these babies are unable to give their consent and are reliant on the medical care provider and parent or LAR
11. Selection of special/vulnerable groups
12. Post-research access and benefit sharing should be in the public domain

50.3.5 Consent

50.3.5.1 Informed consent

Informed consent guidelines which follow from the principle of respect for person provide information (including purpose, rationale, benefits, potential risks, and alternatives to participation), assessing comprehension of the information provided and ensuring the consent is voluntary and not influenced by the circumstances or persons involved [30]. Parental consent in neonatal research is influenced by the quality of the information delivered and the interaction between parents and investigators [30].

Detailed information is required in a way that makes it possible for parents to understand and make informed decisions. Parents must receive the relevant information, satisfactory information, information sheet, and opportunity to ask questions in order to give valid consent [31].

In emergency situations, like research in neonatal resuscitation and life-threatening emergencies when no surrogate consent can be taken, the parents/caregivers/legally acceptable representative (LAR) may not be in a situation to give consent. A deferred/delayed consent must be taken once the child has been stabilized. However, if the parents refuse the deferred consent, the patient should not be included in the research, and no further research-related procedures/data collection must be done from the patient. Also, the data previously collected prior to the consent process should not be used without the authorized adult's permission [29].

If one of the parents is a minor, then consent should not be taken from her/him. If both parents are minors, then enrolment of such a baby should be avoided as far as possible. To enroll such neonates for research, the investigators should provide adequate justification to the EC. A legally acceptable representative should provide an informed consent in such situations [29].

50.3.5.2 Validity of the Consent Process in Neonatal Research

Obtaining valid informed consent from parents at a really difficult time of their life in making a decision is quite challenging for the recruitment of preterm or sick neonates to clinical trials. Emotional influences upon decision making must be recognized and respected in clinical decisions about individual babies [31]. Based on a thematic analysis of interviews, only 59% of parents giving consent for neonatal trials had given valid consent, in terms of either voluntariness, competence, or informativeness (grasp of relevant information) according to self-reported problems with consent and a subgroup analysis showed that this problem was even greater when parents were giving consent for urgent or emergency research [32].

  (i) **Continuous Consent:** After initial agreement to participate, a continuing discussion with parents and further information after recruitment is provided. A concern of parents about receiving further information at a later stage when that might have affected their original decision sometimes affects continuous consent [33].

  (ii) **Enhanced Consent:** For some parents, additional material like a short summary of the trial and a set of frequently asked questions beside standard counseling was found to result in better understanding than conventional consent [34].

 (iii) **Deferred Consent:** In some emergency or critical care research settings like research on drugs used in resuscitation, it may not be possible to take formal consent. Deferred consent is suggested in such situations, where the process is split to give minimum information verbally, followed by full details and formal consent later [29].

Though the consent process might appear to play a very small role in protecting neonates from risk, the main responsibility lies with much better placed, research designers, and research ethical committees than most lay parents to make such judgments of risk [31].

50.3.6 Risks and Benefits

The efficacy and safety of drugs widely used in neonatal care require the scientific and ethical necessity of research on neonates but must be carefully designed to balance potential risks and benefits [12, 23, 24].

50.3.6.1   Classification of Risks [29]

Risks may be classified into four categories: **less than minimal, minimal, minor increase over minimal or low, and more than minimal or high risk.**

It is necessary to exercise individual judgment as these are just broad guidelines and the categorization of risk may vary from child to child even within the same research procedure, depending on the situation.

1. **Less Than Minimal Risk.**

    The probability of harm or discomfort is nil or not expected, like research on anonymous or nonidentified data/samples, data available in the public domain, and meta-analysis.

2. **Minimal Risk.**

The risk which may be anticipated as harm or discomfort not greater than those ordinarily encountered in daily life or during the performance of routine physical or psychological examinations or tests, provided it is carried out in a child-friendly way and after appropriate consent and is questioning, observing, and measuring the anthropometric parameters (such as height and weight). Procedures with minimal risk are history taking, physical examination, X-ray, and noninvasive bodily fluid collection (saliva or urine). The harm incurred is slight and temporary.

3. **Minor Increase Over Minimal Risk (Low Risk).**

There is a slight increase in the potential for harm or discomfort beyond minimal risk and include procedures that might cause transient pain or tenderness, small bruises or scars, or very slight, temporary distress, such as a blood test and oral sedation for diagnostic procedures.

4. **More Than Minimal Risk (High Risk).**

These are all the research procedures which have a risk over and above low risk with a potential to cause harm and include all interventional studies and invasive procedures such as lumbar or epidural puncture, nerve blocks, local infiltrations with LA drug, lung biopsy, liver biopsy, intravenous sedation for diagnostic procedures, surgeries, etc.

As the procedures included in a research projects do not occur in ordinary life and minimal risk is defined in terms of risks associated with everyday life for a child, the level of risk of the research needs to be considered against the level of risk a normal child would face in their everyday nonmedical life. The risk is applicable to everyday life of a healthy child in a stable society. If a standard procedure is replaced in a research where both have an element of risk, then the net increase in risk compared to risk of everyday life should be considered. EC differs in classifying minimal risk in practice in spite of guidelines [35]. The inherent riskiness of interventions should not be considered as risks of the research if the same procedures would necessarily be conducted as part of routine clinical care for eligible participant patients [36].

Framework of minimal risk, acceptable risk/benefit ratio and parental permission are the challenges for the researchers and policymakers to determine which study designs are morally acceptable [37].

There are varied views about the nature of the risks involved in research. The trial treatment or intervention should itself be viewed as a significant risk for the subject, if the outcome of the intervention is unknown and the context for the clinical trial is a potentially life-threatening condition for the subject [38]. A contradictory view is that it should not be viewed as a risk of the trial intervention but a risk of the disease and/or the situation, if the context for the trial is a potentially life-threatening condition [39]. Another view about risk in trials is that because the very information needed for fully informed consent is uncertain and under investigation, so fully informed consent is not possible for clinical trials [40].

50.3.6.2 Assessment of Risks and Benefits

The assessment of risks and benefits provides both an opportunity and a responsibility to gather systematic and comprehensive information about proposed research. It is a means to examine the properly designed proposed research for the researcher, a method for determining the justification of the risks presented to subjects for a review committee and assisting in the determination to participate in the research or not for prospective subjects.

50.3.6.3 Guidelines for Ethical Approval Based on Degree of Risk

For research procedures that are intended to provide potential direct diagnostic, therapeutic, or preventive benefit for the individual child participant, a risk category higher than minimal risk may be justified. For studies having interventions not intended to directly benefit the individual child participant, the risk levels should be minimum risk or low risk [29].

50.3.6.4 Vulnerability

Vulnerability and required safeguards are to be reconsidered by employing approaches that modify the research design, informed consent process, data collection procedures, study interventions, and research regulation to support the inclusion of vulnerable subjects while preserving their safety, welfare, and interests [41].

Unable to provide consent, and parents not able to understand the disclosed information, neonates are at risk of being provided with medications or practices of unproven safety and effectiveness, are the multiple vulnerabilities in a sick neonate, requiring emergency surgery [42].

The best way to conduct important research safely in a vulnerable patient population requires application of basic principles to the practicalities of the research projects, careful attention to the details of the study, flexibility in the application of the principles, and open deliberation [37].

In research involving vulnerable populations, the appropriateness of including them should itself be demonstrated.

Multiple variables affect judgment, like:

- Nature and degree of risk involved,
- Condition of the particular population, and,
- Nature and level of the anticipated benefits.

In the informed consent process, all relevant risks and benefits must be thoroughly documented.

50.3.7 Safeguard for All Studies in Humans

Not conducting research in neonates is detrimental and puts this age group at "**danger of being denied the right to benefit from research.**" This is unethical, but strict safeguards are needed for research to be carried out in these babies.

This raises an important question "**Why so few studies in neonates and pre-terms?" a few answers are as follows:**

1. This is a high-risk group and at risk of long-term disabilities.
2. There are significant liabilities in the form of high mortality and morbidity, especially in the surgical neonates.
3. Treatment is expensive both in the surgical and nonsurgical neonates. NICU stay is costly.
4. Lack of safety data to support drug safety and efficacy, especially anesthetic agents and drugs.
5. This group represents a small market.
6. All of the above are reasons for significant disincentives to conducting research in them.
7. Many Institutional Review Boards are adverse and believe it is unethical to conduct research in this group.
8. There is no standard anesthesia approach for management. Use of a drug or technique is based on anesthesiologists' expertise opinion and knowledge.

For each protocol submitted, the ethics committee must evaluate the study design, whether it answers the research question and the risks and burdens involved in the best possible way [31].

50.3.8 Guidelines for Research in Neonates [29]

Within the pediatric population, neonates represent the **most** vulnerable group.

1. Apart from this consideration study, protocols should also consider the potential long-term effects of interventions, including developmental effects.
2. Neonates should be researched when the findings of the study will have potential implications for neonatal healthcare.
3. When possible, older children should be studied before conducting studies in younger children and infants.
4. Ethical Committee (EC) should have an advisory member with expertise in neonatal research/care. It should scrutinize all research proposed in neonates for potential risks and carefully weigh against the possible benefits in this fragile population. EC should ensure a proper scientific review of the protocol by a competent person/s to remove any risks resulting from poor methodology. All measures to reduce risks should be undertaken.
5. Critically ill neonates should be considered for research even more carefully as the stress for parents or caretakers may interfere with their ability to an informed decision making, on behalf of their baby. Strategy of continuous consent can mitigate such problems.
6. The consent of one parent is required with research exposing the neonate to no or minimal risk or in studies that offer the prospect of direct benefit to the partici-

pant. However, for studies that do not offer the prospect of direct benefit or are high risk, consent from both parents is required. The exception being when only one parent has legal responsibility for the care and custody of the child, one parent is deceased, unknown, incompetent, or not reasonably available. The investigator has to provide adequate justification.

7. Approaches to modify research design, consent process, data collection procedure, study interventions, and research regulation to support and to preserve the safety, welfare, and interests of vulnerable subjects must be kept in mind [41].

In order to continue the ethical research in this area, potential solutions to the challenges to an ethically defensible consent process should be well identified. To build the evidence base for neonatal medicine, substantial advances in methodology and new ways of thinking to further refining the design and analysis of trials and studies in neonates continue [43].

Prospective RCTs involving neonates should be ethically permissible, with modifications in consent procedures, research design, and regulations for research oversight.

The quality of information and data available to professionals, families, and policymakers is frequently inadequate. Well-designed and appropriately powered clinical trials with effective recruitment and data collection can resolve uncertainty. If research cannot be conducted ethically, it will not serve its meaningful purpose to the society.

Table 50.4 summarizes why research is important in neonates, and safeguards to be adopted.

Table 50.4 Research in neonates

Why research in neonates?	– Is important and should be supported, encouraged, and conducted in an ethical manner. – They are not small adults. They have additional unique features. – Either the neonate itself or group of neonates should benefit from research. – In view of benefit for the neonates, the therapeutic burden is acceptable. – Always follow the norm of "minimal risk, minimal harm" as far as possible. – Undertaken only if comparable research in adults has no answers or cannot be done. – Research not directly of benefit to the neonate may not be unethical if it is likely to yield important information. – Not conducting research is also detrimental and unethical. – Strict safeguards are needed. – Legally valid consent should be obtained from a child, parent, LAR. – All proposals should be approved by institutional research EC involving experts.
Phase 1 studies	– For specific diseases for neonates. – Pharmacokinetics/dynamics are different from adults. – Are they acceptable—minimal risk/burden? – For RCTs—need to involve a group without treatment.
Phase 1 or 2 studies	– Can we give drugs to neonates who do not have an indication to receive that drug? – Should these studies only be done in neonates with a disease who ultimately might benefit from the drug?

50.3.9 Suggestions So That Neonates Can Benefit from Research

- Instead of adhering to the "**doctrine of informed consent**," one should use "**tailored approach**" to address issues of information, understanding, and consent.
- **Parental involvement strengthens them with** shared responsibility for safeguarding their baby's interests.
- Registering all clinical studies with a local and central body is mandatory.
- Publishing of the data irrespective of outcome is mandatory. Negative results are equally important as positive data.
- **Public attention—research results should be shared in public.** This helps dissipate information in the public and make them aware of the importance of research and about the need and nature of research in this venerable group.
- **Public awareness** enables parents to make rational decisions about participation in research.

50.3.10 Status in India [29]

The traditional Indian systems of medicine, homeopathy, ayurveda, unani, siddha, or indigenous system and allopathy, have followed the principal of "do not harm," even when there were no ethical guidelines or regulations.

Rapid advances in biomedical science and technology expanded the horizon of ethical dimensions. **ICMR** (Indian Council of Medical Research) and **CDSCO** (Central Drugs Standards Control Organization) are the two main bodies in India that regulate and maintain ethical standards into medical practice and research.

(i) In 1980, ICMR issued a policy on "ethical considerations involving human subjects" which were revised in 2000 and in 2006, taking into consideration the international standards.

(ii) In 2001, the "Indian Good Clinical Practice Guidelines for clinical drug trials in humans" was introduced under CDSCO. Several amendments were made in 2005, and Revised Guidelines were brought out in 2006.

(iii) Then in 2007, ICMR along with the Department of Biotechnology, introduced "Stem Cell Research and Therapy Guidelines."

(iv) Under the Drugs and Cosmetics Act, several amendments were made in 2013. In 2017, "National Guidelines for Stem Cell Research" were finalized.

(v) ICMR came out with the guidelines separately for biomedical research involving children in 2017 [29].

India is a country with unique challenges when applying the universal ethical principles whether in research or in clinical care. Some of the challenges arise from the following:

1. Sociocultural variability,
2. Varying standards of health care from place to place, village to village, city to city, and state to state,
3. Varying levels of education and level of understanding of information and legal and political will and understanding.

50.4 Key Points

1. All physicians and anesthesiologists must have competent knowledge of ethics and ethical guidelines.
2. Adoption of ethical principles can prevent many ethical problems and also help resolve ethical issues.
3. Four cardinal principles of ethics are beneficence, nonmaleficence, autonomy and respect, and justice (communitarism).
4. Easiest way to understand ethics is "by putting yourself in the same situation as the parent and think."
5. General anesthesia can be safely given. No definitive association of GA and adverse postoperative consequences.
6. Anesthesiologists must be aware of potential neurotoxicity of anesthetic drugs especially the inhalational anesthetic agents, on fine mental and intellect ability.
7. Long-term consequences become evident after five or six years or in teenage.
8. Regional anesthesia is **safer**, especially spinal anesthesia in premature neonates.
9. Regional techniques afford dual benefit—providing anesthesia and providing analgesia.
10. Prospective randomized trials involving neonates under certain conditions should be ethically permissible to allow inclusion of neonates in research [43].
11. Research in neonates should be carried out only if it is ethically acceptable.
12. Parents or LAR can give consent.
13. Extra safeguards are needed.
14. Consent procedures, modification of the research design, or regulations for research oversight may be required, especially if the studies are designed as pragmatic randomized clinical trials or as part of a learning healthcare system [43].
15. Results of research must be shared with the public.
16. Unrestricted sharing of results can aid parents and legal guardians of the neonates, in their decision making to participate in research and allow use in clinical management.

Authors' Note Whenever you are in doubt or dilemma in decision making, whether in clinical aspects or regarding research, especially when trying a new technique or drug or procedure, in neonates, try to place yourself in that situation, as a parent or a legal guardian of the baby, and ask whether I will use it on my patient or my baby or not?? If the answer is NO, then stop, and if the answer is YES, then go ahead.!!!

References

1. Universal Declaration of Human Rights (1948, art 5) and International Covenant on Civil and Political Rights ICCPR (1976, art 7).
2. Beauchamp TL, Childress JF. Principles of biomedical ethics. 7th ed. New York: Oxford University Press; 2010.
3. Waisel DB, Truog RD. An introduction to ethics. Anesthesiology. 1997;87:411–7.

4. Albert J, Siegler M, William W. Clinical ethics: a practical approach to ethical decisions in clinical medicine. 7th ed. McGraw Hill; 2010.

5. Post SG, editor. Encyclopedia of bioethics, vol. 5. 4th ed. New York: Simon & Schuster/ Macmillan; 2014.

6. World Medical Association. Declaration of Helsinki 1964–2014, 50 years of Evolution of Medical Research Ethics, 2014.

7. Wheeler R. Consent in surgery. Ann R Coll Surg Engl. 2006;88(3):261–4. https://doi.org/1 0.1308/003588406X106315.

8. Jevtovic-Todorovic V, Hartman RE, Izumi Y, Benshoff ND, et al. Early exposure to common anesthetic agents causes widespread neurodegeneration in the developing rat brain and persistent learning deficits. J Neurosci. 2003;23:876–82.

9. Davis JM, Connor EM, Wood AJ. The need for rigorous evidence on medication use in preterm infants: is it time for a neonatal rule. JAMA. 2012;308:1435–6.

10. Warner DO, Zaccariello MJ, Katusic SK, et al. Neuropsychological and behavioral outcomes after exposure of young children to procedures requiring general anesthesia: The Mayo Anesthesia Safety in Kids (MASK) Study. Anesthesiology. 2018;129:89–105. https://doi. org/10.1097/ALN.0000000000002232.

11. Davidson AJ, Sun LS. Clinical evidence for any effect of anesthesia on the developing brain. Anesthesiology. 2018;128:840–53.

12. Vutskits L, Culley DJ. GAS, PANDA, and MASK: no evidence of clinical anesthetic neurotoxicity! Anesthesiology. 2019;131:762–4. https://doi.org/10.1097/ALN.0000000000002863.

13. Sun LS, Li G, Miller TL, Salorio C, et al. Association between a single general anesthesia exposure before age 36 months and neurocognitive outcomes in later childhood. JAMA. 2016;315:2312–20.

14. McGowan FX, et al. Association between a single general anesthetic exposure before age 36 months and neurocognitive outcomes in later childhood. JAMA. 2016; https://doi.org/10.1001/ jama.2016.6967.

15. Davidson AJ, Disma N, de Graaff JC, Withington DE, et al. GAS consortium: Neurodevelopmental outcome at 2 years of age after general anaesthesia and awake-regional anaesthesia in infancy (GAS): an international multicentre, randomised controlled trial. Lancet. 2016;387:239–50.

16. FDA 2017: FDA Drug Safety Communication: FDA approves label changes for use of general anesthetic and sedation drugs in young children. 2017 Available at: https://www.fda.gov/ downloads/Drugs/DrugSafety/UCM554644.pdf.

17. European Union (EU) Clinical trials—Directive 2001/20/EC.

18. SmartTots (Strategies for Mitigating Anesthesia-Related Neuro-Toxicity in Tots) 2009.

19. McCann ME, de Graaff JC, Dorris L, Disma N, et al. GAS Consortium: Neurodevelopmental outcome at 5 years of age after general anaesthesia or awake-regional anaesthesia in infancy (GAS): an international, multicentre, randomised, controlled equivalence trial. Lancet. 2019;393:664–77.

20. Verhagen AAE. The Groningen Protocol for newborn euthanasia; which way did the slippery slope tilt? J Med Ethics. 2013;39(5):293–5. https://doi.org/10.1136/medethics-2013-101402.

21. Phil D, Anand JS, et al. Analgesia and anesthesia for neonates: study design and ethical issues. Clin Therapeutics. 2005;27(6):814–43.

22. Davidson AJ, O'Brien M. Ethics and medical research in children. Pediatr Anesth. 2009;19:994–1004.

23. Baer GR, Nelson RM. Ethics Group of the Newborn Drug Development Initiative Ethical challenges in neonatal research: summary report of the ethics group of the newborn drug development initiative. Clin Ther. 2006;28(9):1399–407.

24. Fleischman AR. Ethical issues in neonatal research involving human subjects. Semin Perinatol. 2016;40(4):247–53.

25. Ryan KJ. The Belmont Report: National Commission for the Protection of Human Subjects of Biomedical and Behavioral Research. The Belmont report. Ethical principles and guidelines for the protection of human subjects of research. J Am Coll Dent. 2014;81(3):4–13.

26. The Nuremberg Code (1947). BMJ. 1996;313(7070):1448.
27. Nuremberg Doctor's Trial. BMJ. 1996;313(7070):1445–75.
28. Declaration of Helsinki 1964 (Amendment in 2013).
29. National ethical guidelines for bio-medical research involving children, ICMR 2017.
30. Neyro V, Elie V, Thiele N, Jacqz-Aigrain E. Clinical trials in neonates: how to optimise informed consent and decision making? A European Delphi survey of parent representatives and clinicians. PLoS One. 2018;13(6):e0198097.
31. Wilman E, Megone C, Oliver S, Duley L, et al. The ethical issues regarding consent to clinical trials with pre-term or sick neonates: a systematic review (framework synthesis) of the empirical research. Trials. 2015;16:502.
32. Mason SA, Allmark PJ. Obtaining informed consent to neonatal randomized controlled trials: interviews with parents and clinicians in the Euricon study. Lancet. 2000;
33. Allmark P, Mason S. Improving the quality of consent to randomized controlled trials by using continuous consent and clinician training in the consent process. J Med Ethics. 2006;32(8):439–43.
34. Ballard HO, Shook LA, Iocono J, Bernard P, Hayes D Jr. Parents' understanding and recall of informed consent information for neonatal research. IRB. 2011;33(3):12–9.
35. Shah S, Whittle A, Wilfond B, et al. How do institutional review boards apply the federal risk and benefit standards for pediatric research? JAMA. 2004;291:476–82.
36. Lantos JD. U.S. research regulations: do they reflect the views of the people they claim to protect? Ann Intern Med. 2015;162:731–2.
37. Laventhal N, Tarini B, Lantos J. Ethical issues in neonatal and pediatric clinical trials. Pediatr Clin N Am. 2012;59(5):1205–20.
38. Cuttini M. Intrapartum prevention of meconium aspiration syndrome. Lancet. 2004;364(9434):560–1.
39. Vain N, Prudent L, Szyld E, Wiswell T. A difficult ethics issue. Lancet. 2004;364(9447):1751–2.
40. Tyson JE, Knudson PL. Views of neonatologists and parents on consent for clinical trials. Lancet. 2000;356(9247):2026–7.
41. Welch MJ, Lally R, Miller JE, Pittman S, Brodsky L, et al. The ethics and regulatory landscape of including vulnerable populations in pragmatic clinical trials. Clin Trials. 2015;12(5):503–10.
42. Kaye DK. The ethical justification for inclusion of neonates in pragmatic randomized clinical trials for emergency newborn care. BMC Pediatr. 2019;19:218.
43. Megone C, Wilman E, Oliver S, Duley L, et al. The ethical issues regarding consent to clinical trials with pre-term or sick neonates: a systematic review (framework synthesis) of the analytical (theoretical/philosophical) research. Trials. 2016;17:443.

Correction to: Effect of Anaesthesia on Developing Brain

Pratishtha Yadav and Nishkarsh Gupta

Correction to:
Chapter 8 in: U. Saha (ed.), *Clinical Anesthesia for the Newborn and the Neonate,* **https://doi.org/10.1007/978-981-19-5458-0_8**

The book was inadvertently published with an incorrect spelling of one of the author's names in Chapter 8 as Pratisa Yadav, whereas it should be Pratishtha Yadav.

The updated version of this chapter can be found at https://doi.org/10.1007/978-981-19-5458-0_8

Index

Printed by Printforce, United Kingdom